Dear Student,

As educators with over 40 years of experience teaching nursing students, we set out to write a book that will mentor students in the art and skills of health assessment and physical examination. We wrote this book with your needs in mind—you need to learn, practice, and apply health assessment skills in the classroom, in the laboratory, and in clinical setting. You need to be prepared to work in a variety of settings, with a diverse group of clients, with sensitivity to physical ability, heritage, beliefs and practices. Nurses are teachers, and part of your role is to promote the health and well-being of your clients. You will identify what they need to know based on your assessment techniques and the risk factors you find in their health histories.

We are thrilled to offer you our new textbook *Health & Physical Assessment in Nursing*. We hope you will find it an invaluable tool for success, with its true integration of text and media-based material. If you follow our suggestions, you will develop and refine your interviewing and assessment skills while you achieve your educational and professional goals.

Here are the three steps you can take using your textbook to succeed in this course:

1. Use the book to learn assessment techniques.

Read the *Overview* and *Anatomy and Physiology Review* at the beginning of each body system chapter. Learn and practice your interviewing techniques, follow the *Physical Assessment* process, and survey the *Abnormal Findings*. Use the *Health Promotion* feature to develop your own client education plans. The guide inside the front cover of your textbook will help you navigate through the sections of the chapters.

2. Demonstrate your skills.

Read the *Client Interaction* interview, then follow the story to the *Companion Website* to apply what you learned. Read the case study in *Application Through Critical Thinking* at the end of each chapter, and complete all the exercises and activities on the *Companion Website*. At **www.prenhall.com/damico** you can apply what you learned in the case, develop a teaching plan for the client, practice for the NCLEX-RN® exam—and much more.

3. Practice and test yourself.

Using the **Companion Website** and **Student CD-ROM,** test what you learned through a variety of activities and exercises tailored to your style of learning. For each chapter, you can experience animations, tutorials, review questions, and real-life cases. You will find numerous opportunities to practice NCLEX-RN® questions—especially alternative item format questions typically found in physical assessment. To access these rich resources, use the *Student CD-ROM* and the *Companion Website* at **www.prenhall.com/damico**.

Nursing is a dynamic and valuable profession, and we encourage and laud your choice to be a successful nurse. We wish you the best of luck as you embark on your education and your career!

Sincerely,

Donita D'Amico
Donita D'Amico

Colleen Barbarito
Colleen Barbarito

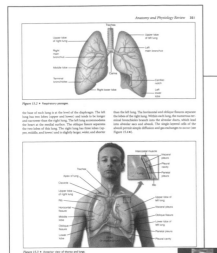

Start by reviewing A&P

Anatomy and Physiology Review gives you a refresher in an appealing visual format that brings A&P to life and provides a strong foundation for learning assessment techniques for that body system.

Learn interviewing techniques

Focused Interview Questions ask the client about general health, illness, symptoms, behaviors, pain, and lifespan.

Follow-up Questions help you gather more data from the interview.

Rationales help you understand why you need to ask these questions and how to apply the information you gather from the client's responses.

Learn step-by-step physical assessment techniques

Techniques and Normal Findings show you step-by-step the proper order of conducting a physical assessment.

The two-column format shows you side-by-side the expected and unexpected findings. The listing of common **Abnormal Findings** will help you learn the parameters of "normal." When applicable, we highlight *Special Considerations*, which alert you to variations you'll find in your client population and in the conditions discussed.

Each Physical Assessment section begins with a list of **Equipment** you will need to conduct the examination and a box of **Helpful Hints** that offers clinical pearls to prepare you for the examination and promote client comfort.

ALERT!

Be sensitive to the client's privacy, and limit exposure of body parts.

Alert! boxes advise you how to perfect physical assessment techniques and identify critical findings that the nurse should report immediately.

Recognize abnormal findings

The **Abnormal Findings** section shows you illustrations and photographs of abnormal findings, diseases, and conditions. This section helps you recognize these conditions and distinguish them from normal findings.

Provide health promotion and client education

The **Health Promotion** section links the *Healthy People 2010* objectives to **Client Education** goals for conditions affecting a specific body system—providing a complete picture of health promotion.

To help you prepare a teaching plan based on the assessment you performed, we link risk factors to important teaching points for clients—including lifespan, cultural, and environmental considerations.

1 Learn the techniques.

CLIENT INTERACTION

Ms. Tanish Thalia, age 32, reports to the Medi-Center with a chief complaint of pain, swelling, and redness at the nails of two fingers on her left hand. Following is an excerpt of the focused interview.

INTERVIEW

Nurse: Good morning. Ms. Thalia, I see from your information sheet that you have a problem with the fingernails of your left hand.

Ms. Thalia: Yes, I think it's my nails, but I'm not sure.

Nurse: The problem involves two digits of the left hand.

Ms. Thalia: Yes, the thumb and index finger are the only two. The other three seem to be okay.

Nurse: Looking at your nails, I see they are highly polished.

Ms. Thalia: Yes, I have them done professionally every 7 to 10 days. They were done 5 days ago.

Nurse: Are these your natural nails?

Ms. Thalia: Yes, I have silk wraps on all my nails to help make them stronger.

Nurse: Does the manicurist push and cut your cuticles?

Ms. Thalia: Yes, she does both. Do you think this is from having the manicure?

Nurse: It could be. I'm not sure. I need more information. When did you first notice the pain and swelling?

Ms. Thalia.: It started several days after I had my nails done, and now it seems to be getting worse. What is causing this?

Nurse: Is this the first time the manicurist did your nails?

Ms. Thalia: Oh no, Sally has been doing my nails for 3 years. This is the first time I have had anything like this.

Nurse: How much time are your hands and nails in water?

Ms. Thalia: Not much. I use gloves when I do the dishes.

ANALYSIS

The nurse uses open-ended statements to obtain the necessary information from Ms. Thalia. The nurse seeks clarification regarding the fingers involved and also confirms the condition of the nails, the frequency of care, and the type of care regarding cutting of the cuticles. When asked, Ms. Thalia is able to provide specific information regarding date of last manicure, symptoms involved, and the relationship between these two factors. The nurse does not make a judgment, and indicates more information is needed.

Please refer to the Companion Website at **www.prenhall.com/damico** and click on Chapter 11, the **Client Interaction** module, to answer questions about this case. In addition, see other resources for this chapter including NCLEX review questions and other interactive exercises and materials.

Interviewing skills

Found at the end of **Gathering the Data** sections, the **Client Interaction** case study brings interviewing skills alive by introducing you to rea clients. Read the interaction between the nurse and client, followed by the nurse's analysis of the situation. Then, go to *www.prenhall.com/damico* to pick up the rest of the story and complete the homework activities to practice your skills.

al Assessment in Nursing
■ BARBARITO

17 18 19 20 21 22 23 24 25 26 27   Site Search: Go

Chapter 16 > Client Interaction

Interaction

...ions are provided to challenge your thinking about this case. Answer each questions and compare your answers to the experts.
...he client presented in this case is 22 years old.

NCLEX-RN Review
Case Study
☐ Client Interaction
MediaLinks
MediaLink Applications
Audio Glossary
New York Times
Profile
Syllabus Manager

1. [Hint] **How might the approach change if the client is 82 years old?**

To create paragraphs in your essay response, type <p> at the beginning of the paragraph, and </p> at the end.

2. [Hint] **How might the approach change if the client is 14 years old?**

To create paragraphs in your essay response, type <p> at the beginning of the paragraph, and </p> at the end.

Assessment and documentation skills
Assessment Skills Laboratory Manual

The combination *Laboratory Manual* and *Study Guide* is intended to reinforce the content from the main text, as well as prepare the student for the skills laboratory and clinical experience. Each chapter begins with an overview, reading assignment, and list of key vocabulary terms to prepare the student for the review exercises. These exercises include study focus questions, anatomy and physiology labeling activities, multiple choice questions, and case studies. Finally, each chapter contains a documentation form and a clinical checklist to be used in the lab or clinical setting. These checklists will provide the student with the appropriate guidelines for a successful clinical experience.

Female Genitalia

Name: _____ Date: _____

Age: _____ LMP: _____

Gravida: _____ Parity: _____ AB: _____ Living Children: _____

History

Review of history related to female genitalia, gynecological, and sexual function:

YES|NO   IF YES, provide details:

Genitals and Gynecologic
☐ ☐ History of surgery
☐ ☐ Reproductive concerns
☐ ☐ Gynecologic problems
☐ ☐ Well woman exam
☐ ☐ Hormonal therapy
☐ ☐ Genital burning, itching
☐ ☐ Vaginal burning, itching
☐ ☐ Vaginal, genitalia lesions
☐ ☐ Vaginal discharge problems
☐ ☐ Vaginal dryness
☐ ☐ Previous infections, STDs
☐ ☐ Pain and/or cramping problems
☐ ☐ Menopause symptoms
☐ ☐ Cancer history

Last Pap test   Date: _____
                 Results: _____

Menstrual history   Date of menarche: _____
                     Date of last period: _____
                     Regularly: _____
                     Flow characteristics: _____
                     Premenstrual symptoms: _____
                     Dysmenorrhea: _____

Female Genitalia   Page 1 of 5
©2008 Pearson Education, Inc.

Critical thinking skills

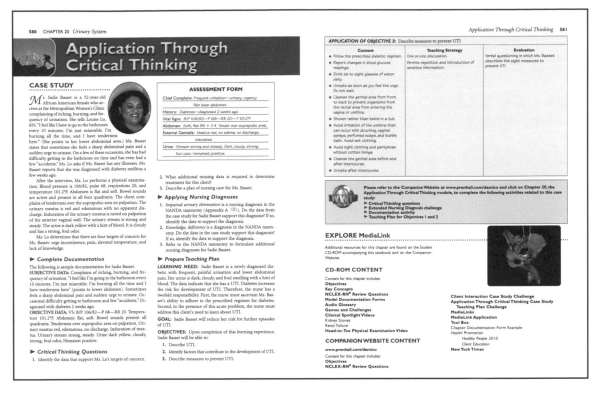

After reading through the chapter and practicing the techniques and steps of assessment, **Application Through Critical Thinking** gives you an opportunity to bring it all together and apply what you have learned.

The **Case Study** provides a real client scenario that details signs, symptoms, and interactions between the nurse and the client. Based on the information about this client, you can apply your knowledge through:

- **Critical Thinking Questions** that challenge you to think about your actions if you were the nurse in this scenario.

- **Applying Nursing Diagnoses** that ask you to identify NANDA Nursing Diagnoses that may apply to this client.

- **Complete Documentation** providing samples of documentation for the findings in this case study.

- **Prepare Teaching Plan** in which we identify the learning need and goals, and you prepare the client's teaching plan.

Go to *www.prenhall.com/damico* to complete these activities online and submit your responses as homework to your instructor.

EXPLORE MediaLink

Found at the end of each chapter, EXPLORE MediaLink encourages you to use the Student CD-ROM and Companion Website to apply what you learned from the textbook. You can preview the chapter-specific activities, animations, videos, and resources to help you demonstrate and test your new assessment skills.

2 Demonstrate your skills.

Watch, practice, and prepare for the NCLEX-RN® on the *Student CD-ROM.*

Your textbook is only part of the learning experience in health and physical assessment. We integrate the activities in the textbook with activities on the accompanying media resources. Chapter activities continue on the *Companion Website* and the *Student CD-ROM* to help you practice and apply your skills.

The bonus *Student CD-ROM* packaged with your textbook is an interactive study guide with numerous activities and resources for each chapter:

Key Concept Summaries—Quick access to key concepts from the textbook

NCLEX-RN® Review Questions—10 to 15 practice questions and rationales for all answers

Animations—Including heart and lung sounds to help you recognize normal and abnormal findings

Games and Challenges—Fun ways to test your knowledge and skills

Clinical Spotlight Videos—Learn more about diseases and abnormal findings

Audio Glossary—Pronunciations and definitions of key terms

Head-to-Toe Physical Examination Video—See how a nurse performs a complete assessment

Documentation Forms—For you to print and use in lab or in the clinical setting

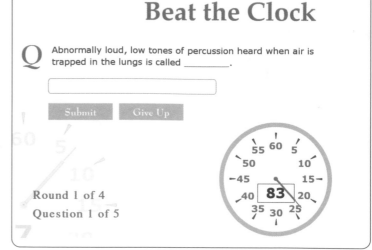

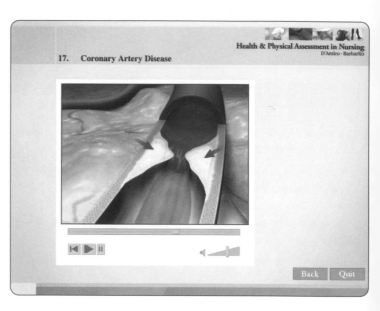

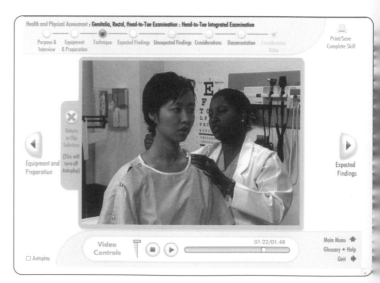

Apply your skills with homework, NCLEX-RN® reviews, and more on the *Companion Website*.

Health & Physical Assessment in Nursing
D'AMICO ■ BARBARITO

Home | Select Chapter: << prev 16 17 18 19 20 21 22 23 24 25 26 27 | Site Search: | Go | ?

**Chapter 16
Breasts and Axillae**

Home > Chapter 16 > Applying Nursing Diagnoses

Applying Nursing Diagnoses

Objectives
NCLEX-RN Review
Case Study
Applying Nursing Diagnoses
MediaLinks
MediaLink Applications
Audio Glossary
New York Times
Profile
Syllabus Manager

Review the case study again and answer the questions related to Nursing Diagnoses. When finished, compare your answers with the experts.

1. *Pain (chronic) is a diagnosis in the NANDA taxonomy. Do the data for Carol Jenkins support this diagnosis?*
[Hint]

To create paragraphs in your essay response, type <p> at the beginning of the paragraph, and </p> at the end.

2. *Identify additional nursing diagnoses from the NANDA taxonomy (see the appendix in the back of the textbook) for Carol Jenkins. Diagnosis _____*
[Hint]

To create paragraphs in your essay response, type <p> at the beginning of the paragraph, and </p> at the end.

Health & Physical Assessment in Nursing
D'AMICO ■ BARBARITO

Home | Select Chapter: << prev 16 17 18 19 20 21 22 23 24 25 26 27 | Site Search: | Go | ?

**Chapter 16
Breasts and Axillae**

Home > Chapter 16 > Documentation Challenge

Documentation Challenge

Objectives
NCLEX-RN Review
Case Study
Documentation Challenge
MediaLinks
MediaLink Applications
Audio Glossary
New York Times
Profile
Syllabus Manager

Consider this case with following information changed. Once you consider the information below, use the blank chart provided with this exercise to document your findings. New information about this case:

1. *Ms. Jenkins reports that she has a lump in her left breast. the lump was found 4 days ago while she was taking a shower. She has never had a lump before and is very frightened. Her best friend died last year from breast cancer. Ms. Jenkins's grandmother also died from breast cancer. She goes on to report that she has never had a mammogram. She is taking birth control pills.*
[Hint]

To create paragraphs in your essay response, type <p> at the beginning of the paragraph, and </p> at the end.

2. *The examination of Ms. Jenkins breasts reveals a hard irregular shaped lump about the size of a penny in the upper part of her breast near the axilla. It is difficult to move the lump. It wants to stay stationary. Ms. Jenkins reports that the lump is not tender to the touch.*
[Hint]

Health & Physical Assessment in Nursing
D'AMICO ■ BARBARITO

Home | Select Chapter: << prev 16 17 18 19 20 21 22 23 24 25 26 27 | Site Search: | Go | ?

**Chapter 16
Breasts and Axillae**

Home > Chapter 16 > Prepare the Teaching Plan

Prepare the Teaching Plan

Objectives
NCLEX-RN Review
Case Study
Prepare the Teaching Plan
MediaLinks
MediaLink Applications
Audio Glossary
New York Times
Profile
Syllabus Manager

Listed below is the Teaching Plan goal and objectives for this case. The textbook has shown how one of the objectives may be completed. Your challenge is to create the Teaching Plan for the remaining objectives.

1. *Goal Statement: the particpants in this learning program will have increased awareness of recommendations for screening for breast cancer.*
[Hint]

To create paragraphs in your essay response, type <p> at the beginning of the paragraph, and </p> at the end.

2. *Objectives:
1. Identify the recommended schedule for breast cancer screening.
2. Describe the methods for breast cancer screening.*
[Hint]

The *Companion Website* enhances and expands upon the textbook concepts by continuing the two case studies from the textbook. All activities provide you with response forms online that you can email to your instructor as homework or check your answers with immediate feedback. For each chapter, you will find:

NCLEX-RN® Review Questions—Over 300 new practice questions and rationales for all answers.

Client Interaction Case Study Challenge—Continuation of the textbook client interview and application questions

Application Through Critical Thinking Case Study Challenge—Provides a real client scenario that details signs, symptoms, and interaction between the nurse and the client. Based on the information about this client, you can apply your knowledge through:

- **Critical Thinking Questions**—Challenge you to think about your actions as if you were the nurse in this scenario.

- **Applying Nursing Diagnoses**—Asks you to identify NANDA Nursing Diagnoses that may apply to this client.

- **Complete Documentation**—Provides samples of documentation for the findings in this case study.

- **Prepare Teaching Plan**—Asks you to identify the learning need and prepare the client's teaching plan.

MediaLink Applications—Critical thinking activities and exercises direct you to a particular website to analyze data and information

MediaLinks—Websites and links to resources for physical assessment on the web

Tool Box—References and resources from the textbook

Practice and test yourself.

③

MyPhysicalAssessmentLab

Powered by Prentice Hall's **OneKey**, *MyPhysicalAssessment-Lab* offers Internet-based course management tools that accompany *Health & Physical Assessment in Nursing*. *MyPhysicalAssessmentLab* provides dependable and easy-to-use online homework, guided videos and animation tutorials, multimedia, and tests to help instructors reinforce and expand upon the concepts delivered in your class and skills lab. It provides instructors with a rich, flexible set of course materials, along with course management tools that make it easy to deliver all or a portion of your course online if you are using Blackboard or WebCT. Students can experience our virtual skills lab and perfect their physical assessment techniques. All of the interactive features of BlackBoard and WebCT are available to the class: discussion board, email, announcements, a calendar, chat rooms, and more.

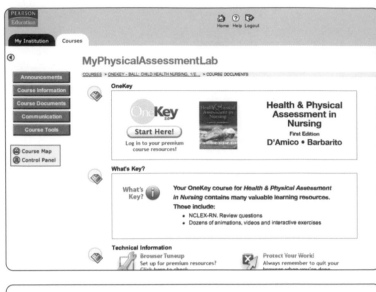

For Students

Clinical Checklists—Useful for both students and instructors, the checklists detail steps that the student should take in clinical.

Heart and Lung Sounds—For the cardiac and pulmonary chapters, students will have the opportunity to hear examples of normal and abnormal heart and ung sounds.

Case Studies—These scenarios detail a situation that the nurse might encounter and challenge the student to analyze the data and plan the nursing process and the client education activities.

Terminology Translator—Common medical terms are translated into Spanish.

Interactive Games and Challenges—From crossword puzzles to matching activities, students will have fun while drilling themselves on essential information.

Prentice Hall Real Nursing Skills—Complete Health Assessment videos with challenges and critical thinking questions

***Healthy People 2010* Activity**—*Healthy People 2010* standards for the select body system chapter are used in an application exercise.

NCLEX-RN® Review Questions—30-45 questions per chapter, including 10-15 new questions not found on the *Student CD-ROM* and *Companion Website*

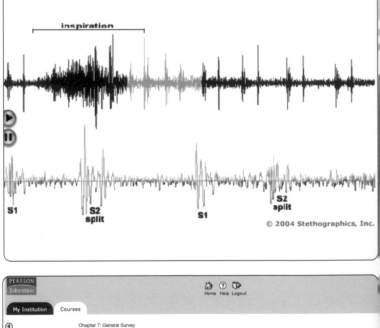

Powered by Prentice Hall's OneKey 2.0

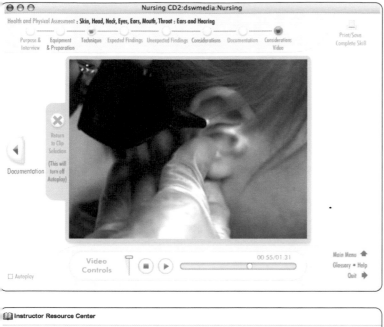

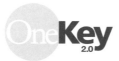

For Instructors

In addition to all the resources for the student course, instructors will have all their resources in one place:

Lecture Notes that correlate with each chapter.

PowerPoint® presentations that makes lectures easy, including:

- animations
- videos
- illustrations
- and text slides

Syllabus Manager offers features that facilitate students' use of *MyPhysicalAssessmentLab* and allow instructors to post their syllabi on the course.

Test Item File provides high-quality test bank of NCLEX-RN® items for each chapter, including alternative format items.

Research Navigator®—Provides the easiest way for students to start a research assignment or research paper. Complete with extensive help on the research process and two exclusive databases of credible and reliable source material, *Research Navigator* helps students quickly and efficiently make the most of their research time.

NOTE TO FACULTY—If you are using Blackboard or WebCT, ask your Prentice Hall Sales Representative for pricing information and how *MyPhysicalAssessmentLab* can help you make a difference for you and your students in the classroom, lab, and clinical setting. You can also go to *www.prenhall.com/nursing* for a demonstration.

Additional resources for student and instructor success.

We designed teaching and learning resources to expand and extend the textbook material and to bring it alive. The full complement of supplemental resources is available from your Prentice Hall sales representative.

Resources for student success

Clinical Handbook for Health & Physical Assessment in Nursing (ISBN 0-13-049478-X)
Provides essential information to you for clinical assignments, including details of physical assessment for each body system, and head-to-toe assessments for children, pregnant women, and older clients.

Assessment Skills Laboratory Manual
(ISBN 0-13-049477-1)
The combination Laboratory Manual and Study Guide is intended to reinforce the content from the main text, as well as prepare the student for the skills laboratory/ clinical experience. Each chapter begins with reading assignments, and list of key vocabulary terms to prepare the student for the review exercises. These exercises include study focus questions, anatomy and physiology labeling activities, multiple choice questions, and case studies. Documentation forms and clinical checklists can be used in the lab or clinical setting provide the student with appropriate guidelines for a successful clinical experience.

Prentice Hall's Real Nursing Skills: Health Assessment Nursing Skills
(ISBN 0-13-191525-8)
This three-CD resource offers students the complete foundation for competency in performing assessment skills. The CD-ROMs contain step-by-step techniques and rationales demonstrated in realistic video clips, animations, illustrations, and photographs. For each skill, students review: Purpose and Interview • Equipment • Preparation • Procedure • Expected Findings • Unexpected Findings • Considerations • Documentation • and Variations (if applicable).

Resources for instructor success

Instructor's Resource Manual (ISBN 0-13-049376-7)
This manual contains a wealth of material to help faculty plan and manage the health assessment course. It includes chapter overviews, detailed lecture suggestions and outlines, learning objectives, a complete test bank, teaching tips, and more for each chapter. The IRM also guides faculty on how to assign and use the text-specific *Companion Website*, *www.prenhall.com/ damico*, and the *Student CD-ROM*.

Instructor's Resource CD-ROM (ISBN 0-13-049378-3)
This valuable CD-ROM provides several tools to aid faculty in teaching physical assessment:

- Electronic version of Instructor's Resource Manual
- Complete PowerPoint® presentation featuring over 1,000 illustrations and over 350 text lecture slides
- Electronic test bank with over 300 questions in all NCLEX-RN® formats
- Over 130 animations and videos to project in the classroom
- Guidelines for using *MyPhysicalAssessmentLab* and other media resources that accompany this textbook

 Online Course Management
OneKey is all you need.
Convenience. Simplicity. Success.

Prentice Hall OneKey is an integrated online resource that brings a wide variety of supplemental resources together in one convenient place for both students and faculty. OneKey features everything you and your students need for out-of-class work, conveniently organized to match your syllabus:

- Interactive modules
- Text and image PowerPoint® presentations
- Animations and videos
- Case studies
- Course management tools
- Testing materials and gradebooks
- Customizable course content and online tests

OneKey content is available for download to locally hosted versions of BlackBoard and WebCT. For pricing information or a demonstration, please contact your Prentice Hall sales representative or go online to www.prenhall.com/nursing.

A note to instructors: Please use the following ISBN numbers to order the appropriate access code for your course.

Standard courses: ***MyPhysicalAssessmentLab***

 ISBN 0-13-227720-4   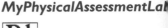 ISBN 0-13-228425-1

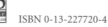 ISBN 0-13-219756-1   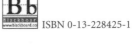 ISBN 0-13-238946-0

 * ISBN 0-13-173390-7   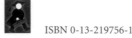 *Nationally hosted

Health & Physical Assessment in Nursing

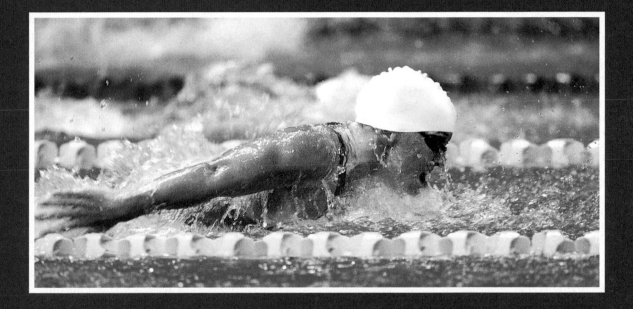

Donita D'Amico, MEd, RN
Associate Professor

William Paterson University
Wayne, New Jersey

Colleen Barbarito, EdD, RN
Assistant Professor

William Paterson University
Wayne, New Jersey

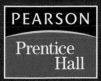

PEARSON

Prentice
Hall

Upper Saddle River, New Jersey 07458

Library of Congress Cataloging-in-Publication Data

D'Amico, Donita.
   Health and physical assessment in nursing / Donita D'Amico and Colleen Barbarito.
     p. cm.
   Includes bibliographical references and index.
   ISBN 0-13-049373-2
    1. Nursing assessment—Outlines, syllabi, etc. 2. Physical diagnosis—Outlines, syllabi,
etc. I. Barbarito, Colleen. II. Title.
   [DNLM: 1. Nursing assessment—methods—United States—Case Reports. 2. Physical
Examination—nursing—United States—Case Reports. 3. Healthy People Programs—United
States—Case Reports. 4. Holistic Nursing—methods—United States—Case Reports. WY
100.4 D158h 2007]
   RT48.D36 2007
   616.07'5—dc22

                        2005048928

Notice: Care has been taken to confirm the accuracy of information presented in this book. The authors, editors, and the publisher, however, cannot accept any responsibility for errors or omissions or for consequences from application of the information in this book and make no warranty, express or implied, with respect to its contents.

The authors and publisher have exerted every effort to ensure that drug selections and dosages set forth in this text are in accord with current recommendations and practice at the time of publication. However, in view of ongoing research, changes in government regulations, and the constant flow of information relating to drug therapy and drug reactions, the reader is urged to check the package inserts of all drugs for any change in indications of dosage and for added warnings and precautions. This is particularly important when the recommended agent is a new and/or infrequently employed drug.

Publisher: Julie Levin Alexander
Publisher's Assistant: Regina Bruno
Editor-in-Chief: Maura Connor
Acquisitions Editor: Pamela Fuller
Senior Managing Editor: Marilyn Meserve
Development Editor: Elisabeth Garofalo
Editorial Assistant: Melisa Baez, Gosia Jaros-White
Director of Manufacturing and Production: Bruce Johnson
Managing Production Editor: Patrick Walsh
Production Liaison: Cathy O'Connell
Production Editor: Amy Gehl, Carlisle Editorial Services
Manufacturing Manager: Ilene Sanford
Manufacturing Buyer: Pat Brown
Design Director and Cover Designer: Cheryl Asherman
Photography and Photo Research: Patrick Watson
Director of Marketing: Karen Allman
Senior Marketing Manager: Francisco Del Castillo
Marketing Coordinator: Michael Sirinides
Marketing Assistant: Patricia Linard
Associate Editor: Michael Giacobbe
Media Editor: John Jordan
Media Production Manager: Amy Peltier
Media Project Manager: Tina Rudowski
Composition: Carlisle Publishers Services, Inc.
Printer/Binder: Courier/Kendallville
Cover Printer: Phoenix Color
Cover Photo: Courtesy of Digital Vision/Getty Images, Inc.

Pearson Education Ltd.
Pearson Education Singapore, Pte. Ltd.
Pearson Education Canada, Ltd.
Pearson Education—Japan
Pearson Education Australia PTY, Limited

Pearson Education North Asia Ltd.
Pearson Educación de Mexico, S.A. de C.V.
Pearson Education Malaysia, Pte. Ltd.
Pearson Education, Upper Saddle River, New Jersey

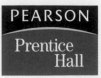

10 9 8 7
ISBN 0-13-049373-2

About the Authors

Donita D'Amico, MEd, RN

Donita D'Amico, a diploma nursing school graduate, earned her baccalaureate degree in nursing from William Paterson College. She earned a master's degree in Nursing Education at Teacher's College, Columbia University, with a specialization in Adult Health. Ms. D'Amico has been a faculty member at William Paterson University for more than 25 years. Her teaching responsibilities include physical assessment, medical-surgical nursing, nursing theory, and fundamentals in the classroom, skills laboratory, and clinical settings.

Ms. D'Amico coauthored several textbooks, including *Health Assessment in Nursing* and its companion clinical handbook by Sims, D'Amico, Stiesmeyer and Webster; as well as *Comprehensive Health Assessment: A Student Workbook* and *Modules for Medication Administration* with Dr. Colleen Barbarito.

Ms. D'Amico is active in the community. Within the university, she is a charter member of the Iota Alpha Chapter of Sigma Theta Tau International. She continues to serve at the chapter and state levels. She also serves as a consultant and contributor to local organizations.

Colleen Barbarito, EdD, RN

Colleen Barbarito received a nursing diploma from Orange Memorial Hospital School of Nursing, graduated with a baccalaureate degree from William Paterson College, and earned a master's degree from Seton Hall University, all in New Jersey. She received her Doctor of Education from Teacher's College, Columbia University. Prior to a position in education, Dr. Barbarito's clinical experiences included medical-surgical, critical care, and emergency nursing. Dr. Barbarito has been a faculty member at William Paterson University since 1984, where she has taught physical assessment and a variety of clinical laboratory courses for undergraduate nursing students and curriculum development at the graduate level.

Dr. Barbarito coauthored two books with Donita D'Amico—*Modules for Medication Administration* and *Comprehensive Health Assessment: A Student Workbook.* She published articles on anaphylaxis in *American Journal of Nursing* and *Coping with Allergies and Asthma.* Her research includes physical assessment and collaboration on revising a physical assessment project with results published as a brief in *Nurse Educator.* As a faculty member, Dr. Barbarito participated in committees to explore curricular change and to develop multimedia learning modules for critical thinking.

Dr. Barbarito is a member of Sigma Theta Tau International Honor Society of Nursing. She was an officer and serves as Faculty Advisor for the Iota Alpha Chapter at William Paterson University.

Contributors

A sincere and deep expression of thanks is extended to our chapter contributors. Their time, effort, and expertise so willingly given for the development and writing of each chapter helped foster the project's success.

Textbook Contributors

Lily Fountain, MS, RN
Clinical Instructor
University of Maryland
Baltimore, Maryland
Chapter 26, The Pregnant Female

Dawn Lee Garzon, PhD, APRN, BC, CPNP
Clinical Associate Professor
University of Missouri-St. Louis
Ladue, Missouri
Chapter 25, Assessment of Infants, Children, and Adolescents

Dorothy G. Herron, PhD, APRN, BC
Associate Professor
University of North Carolina
Greensboro, North Carolina
Chapter 27, Assessing the Older Adult

Sheila Tucker, MA, RD, LDN
Dietician and Part-time Faculty Member
Boston College
Chestnut Hills, Massachusetts
Chapter 9, Nutritional Assessment

Contributing Editor

June D. Thompson, DrPH, RN
Dr. Thompson is a research scientist for Florida Hospital in Orlando, Florida, and a writer and consultant for Prentice Hall Nursing. Dr. Thompson has been a writer and author for over the past 25 years and has had many published textbooks. In addition, she has a vast experience in developing and publishing multimedia educational products for nursing education.

Dr. Thompson has had a rich career in both education and practice. She considers herself a long-time emergency nurse and in her faculty position at the University of Texas Health Sciences Center, Houston, was responsible for developing the first emergency nursing master's program in the country. She has also served as the national president for the Emergency Nurses Association. In addition, Dr. Thompson has been an injury epidemiologist for the state of New Mexico, the director of Clinical Education and Research at the University of New Mexico Hospitals in Albuquerque, and faculty at the Ohio State University in Columbus, Ohio, and the University of Phoenix.

Student and Instructional Resources

Marianne Adam, MSN, RN, CRNP
Moravian College
Bethlehem, Pennsylvania
Distance Learning Course

Katrina Allen, MSN, RN, CCRN
Faulkner State Community College
Bay Minette, Alabama
Instructor's Resource CD-ROM
Distance Learning Course

Anita Althans, MSN, RNC
Our Lady of Holy Cross College
New Orleans, Louisiana
Instructor's Resource CD-ROM

Kimberly Attwood, MSN, BSN
Moravian College
Bethlehem, Pennsylvania
Distance Learning Course

Wanda Baker, RN, MN, FNP
Greenville Technical College
Greenville, South Carolina
Instructor's Resource Manual

Kristi Beam, RN, MSN
Jacksonville State University
Jacksonville, Alabama
Distance Learning Course

Kim Cooper, MSN, RN
Ivy Tech Community College
Terre Haute, Indiana
Instructor's Resource CD-ROM

Ann H. Crawford, PhD, RN, CNS
University of Mary Hardin-Baylor
Belton, Texas
Companion Website

Katherine H. Dimmock, EdD, MSN, RN, JD
Columbia College of Nursing
Milwaukee, Wisconsin
Student CD-ROM

Elizabeth Farren, PhD, MSN, BSN
Baylor University
Dallas, Texas
Laboratory Manual and Study Guide

Candace Gioia, RN, BSN, CNOR
Pinellas Technical Education Centers
St. Petersburg, Florida
Distance Learning Course

Janice Donaldson Hausauer, MS, RN, FNP
Montana State University
Bozeman, Montana
Student CD-ROM

Debra K. Hearington, MS, RN, CPNP
Virginia Commonwealth University
Richmond, Virginia
Instructor's Resource CD-ROM

Kelly Jones, MSN, RN, CNM
Cleveland Community College
Shelby, North Carolina
Distance Learning Course

Laurie Gasperi Kaudewitz, MSN, RNC, BSN
East Tennessee State University
Johnson City, Tennessee
Companion Website

Kathryn G. Magorian, MSN, RN
Mount Marty College
Yankton, South Dakota
Instructor's Resource CD-ROM

Dawna Martich, MSN, RN
American Healthways
Pittsburg Pennsylvania
Companion Website

Francine Parker, EdD, RN
Auburn University Montgomery
Montgomery Alabama
Distance Learning Course

Patricia Prechter, MSN, RN
Our Lady of Holy Cross College
New Orleans, Louisiana
Instructor's Resource CD-ROM

Betty Kehl Richardson, PhD, RN, BC, LMFT, LPC
Austin Community College
Austin, Texas
Instructor's Resource CD-ROM

Susan Scholtz, DNSc, RN
Moravian College
Bethlehem, Pennsylvania
Distance Learning Center

Lori Schumacher, MS, RN, CCRN
Medical College of Georgia
Augusta, Georgia
Distance Learning Course

Paula Dunn Tropello, EdD, RN, CNS, FNP
Troy University
Troy, Alabama
Companion Website

L. Diane Weed, PhD, RN, FNP
Troy University
Troy, Alabama
Distance Learning Course

Julie Will, MSN, RN
Ivy Tech Community College
Terre Haute, Indiana
Instructor's Resource CD-ROM

Thank You

We would like to extend our heartfelt thanks to more than 70 of our colleagues from schools of nursing across the country who have given their time generously over the past four years to help us create this learning program. These individuals helped us develop this textbook and media by reviewing chapters, art, and media, and by answering a myriad of questions right up until the time of publication. *Health & Physical Assessment in Nursing* has benefited immeasurably from their efforts, insights, suggestions, objections, encouragement and inspiration, as well as from their vast experience as teachers and nurses.

A special thank you to Janice Hausauer, MSN, RN, FNP, from Montana State University, who graciously shared her time and expertise with us from the very beginning of the book's development. Professor Hausauer helped us create a superior resource package by reviewing the entire book during its development, as well as every aspect of the supplement package. Her commitment to this project ensured a total teaching and learning package consistent with the textbook.

Martha Alkire, RN, MSN, CCRN, ACNP
Sacramento, California
Ella Anaya, RN, MSN, CNS
Kent State University
Cheryl A. Bean, DSN, APRN, BC, AOCN, ANP
Indiana University
Carla J. Beckham, MSN
Cumberland University
Sue Boyer, RN, MN
University of Illinois Chicago College of Nursing
Alice Brnicky, RN, MS
Texas Women's University
Jo Ann Bryan, RN, AND, NP-C, PA-C
Nurse Practitioner
Denise Burton, MS, RNC
Oklahoma City University
Randy Caine, EdD, RN, CS, CCRN, ANP-C
California State University-Los Angeles
Christina Calamaro, CRNP, CPNP, MSN, RN
University of Pennsylvania
Claudia Campbell, RN, BSN
Intermountain Health Care, Urban Central Regional Hospitals
Noreen Chikotas, MSN, CRNP, DEd, RN
Bloomsburg University
Pattie Clark, RN, MSN, ABD
Abraham Baldwin Agricultural College
Ann H. Crawford, PhD, RN, CNS
University of Mary Hardin-Baylor
Karen Cuvar, PhD, RN
Saint Louis University
Kelly Dempsey, MSN, RN, CCRN, ANP
Indiana University East
Nancy Dentlinger, RN, AS, MS, EdD, BS
Redlands Community College

Evelyn Duffy, MS, APRN, BC
Case Western Reserve University
Linda Dumas, RN, PhD
University of Massachusetts-Boston
Carrin L. Dvorak, RN, MSN
Cuyahoga Community College
Elizabeth Farren, PhD, RN
Baylor University
Arlinda Garner, MS, RN
College of the Mainland
Dawn Garzon, PhD, APRN, BC, CPNP
University of Missouri
Rebecca Gesler, RN, MSN
Saint Catharine College
Kristine Gill, RN, PhD
University of Akron
Winifred Guariglia, MSN, RN, CS, GNP
Bergen Community College
Karen Haghenbeck, PhD, FNP, RN, BC, CCRN, APRN
Pace University
Diana D. Hankes, PhD, APRN, BC
Carroll College
Janice Hausauer, MS, RN, FNP
Montana State University
Patricia Hawley, MAEd
Mecosta-Osceola Career Center and Ferris State University
Brenda Walters Holloway, MSN, CRNP
University of Alabama
Eva Humbach, MS, RN, FNP
Dominican College
Jacqueline Hutcherson, MSN, CNM
East Carolina University
Laurie Kaudewitz, RNC, MSN, BSN
East Tennessee State University

Deborah Kern, MSN, FNP
Montana State University
Joan King, MSN, PhD
Vanderbilt University
Maryanne F. Lachat, PhD, RNC
Georgetown University
Darlene Lacy
University of Mary Hardin-Baylor
Susan DeSanto-Madeya, DNSc, RN
University of Massachusetts-Boston
Gloria Kersey-Matusiak, PhD, RN
Holy Family University
Bonnie McCracken, RN
University of California Davis Health System
Karen Montalto, MSN, DNSc
Neumann College
Carol D. Morris, RN, MSN
Bellin College of Nursing
Terry Neal, MS, RN, FNPC
Indiana Wesleyan University
Gina Oliver, PhD, RN
University of Missouri
Carol Price, RN, MN
University of Texas at Tyler
Janet Purath, PhD, ARNP, BC
Washington State University
Barbara Resnick, PhD, CRNP, FAAN, FAANP
University of Maryland
Ted Rigney, RN, MS, CCRN, ACNP, NP
University of Arizona
Cheryl Robertson, MSN, CS, ANP, WHCNP-C
George Mason University
JoAnne Saxe, RN, MS, ANP
University of California San Francisco
Patricia Shaver, PhD, GNP, RNC, ANP
South Dakota State University
Mary H. Sizemore, RN, MSN, EdD, BSN
New Mexico State University
Elizabeth Sloand, MSN, RN, CPNP
Johns Hopkins University
Rachel Spector, PhD, RN
Culture Care Consultant

Carolyn Speros, DNSc, APRN, FNP
University of Memphis
Sheryl D. Stuck, RN, MSN, CS
Stark State College
Pat Tabloski, PhD, RNC
Boston College
Patricia Taylor, MSN
San Bernardino Valley College
Jean Taylor-Woodbury, BA, BS, MS
University of California-San Francisco
Alice Teall, MS, CRNP
Wright State University
Ellen Tim, RN, MSN, ANP-C
Duke University Medical Center
Paula Dunn Tropello, EdD, RN, CNS, FNP, MN
Wagner College
Douglas Turner, RN, PhD(c), MSN, CNS, CRNA
Forsyth Technical Community College
Shirley E. Van Zandt, MS, MPH, CRNP
Johns Hopkins University
Debra Walker, RN, DNSc, MSN
Samford University
L. Diane Weed, PhD, MSN, CRNP
University of Alabama at Huntsville
Lynne Weissman, RN, BSN, CPNP, MS
Dominican College
Virginia Weisz, MS, OGNP
Radford University School of Nursing
Rita Young, RN, MSN, CDE, CNS
University of Akron

Student Reviewers
Lynda Chesnes
Palm Beach Community College
Jennifer Long
Winona State University
Stacy McGarry
Winona State University
Elizabeth Menk
Winona State University
Sara Theobald
Winona State University

Preface

We wrote *Health & Physical Assessment in Nursing* and developed its rich media package to help instructors mentor students in the art and skills of health and physical assessment, as well as to help students develop and refine the assessment skills they need to care for a diverse population of clients in a variety of settings. The focus of this book is client assessment, recognizing that clients present a variety of physical, cultural, and spiritual experiences to nurses today. We approach assessment holistically, advocating the principles of health promotion and client education. We introduce concepts related to health, wellness, communication, culture, and education. As long-time teachers of assessment, we developed a system that surpasses the textbook alone—a way to help students learn the material effectively through true integration of the textbook and the media. For each chapter, the textbook concepts are extended onto the Student CD-ROM and the Companion Website through case studies and client education activities that make the material come alive.

Throughout development of our textbook, over 70 reviewers reacted positively to the accessibility and integration of *Health & Physical Assessment in Nursing:*

"The easy way of explaining health assessment and its components is the major strength of this textbook. I find it very easy to follow, with simple, yet appropriate terminology. It recognizes the early student as a novice and explains concepts in an easy-to-follow format."

—Laurie Kaudewitz
East Tennessee State University

"Integrating *Healthy People 2010* is up to date and not found in other textbooks our students use. I appreciate such integration of vital relevance to current issues in a text."

—Ella Anaya
Kent State University

About the Application Through Critical Thinking and Companion Website feature:

"The case study and critical thinking questions are done well. This is one of your best features. . . . I especially like the completeness of this content and how it flows from interview, physical assessment, care planning, and documentation. I would like this book for this feature alone. It makes things 'real' for the students and better prepares them for what they will be responsible for in the clinical setting."

—Ella Anaya
Kent State University

Organization of This Textbook

Health & Physical Assessment in Nursing is comprised of four units. Unit I, *Introduction to Health Assessment,* introduces health assessment concepts. The chapters within this unit establish a focus for comprehensive health assessment to promote health and well-being across the life span. Nursing assessment includes all of the factors that impact the client and health. Chapter 1 describes the knowledge, skills, and processes professional nurses use in holistic health assessment and health promotion. The professional nurse functions within the healthcare delivery system and has a responsibility to partner with other professionals and clients to maximize health. We introduce information about the *Healthy People 2010* initiatives that promote health, prevent illness, and that provide goals for healthcare services in the United States. We apply the *Healthy People 2010* initiatives in later chapters within the Health Promotion features. Chapter 2 explains the concepts of health and wellness, applying examples of several health promotion models. Chapter 3 discusses the importance of growth, development, and aging as factors that impact physical and psychosocial well-being. The client's heritage and spirituality have significant influences on the individual's health-related activities. Chapter 4 provides an overview of cultural concepts and describes methods to incorporate and address the client's culture, values, and beliefs in the assessment process. Chapter 5 describes psychological and social phenomena that the nurse must consider during a comprehensive assessment.

Unit II, *Introduction to Physical Assessment,* introduces physical assessment concepts. We describe techniques and equipment required for physical assessment in Chapter 6. Chapter 7 provides an in-depth explanation of the initial step of physical assessment—the general survey and measurement of vital signs. Chapters 8 and 9 discuss two important aspects of health assessment—pain and nutrition. Each chapter describes concepts related to these areas and includes measurements, methods, and tools to guide data gathering and interpretation of findings for clients across the life span. The client interview is the mechanism through which the nurse gathers subjective data. Subjective data refers to the client's own perceptions and recollections about health, illness, values, beliefs, and practices. Chapter 10 introduces an overview of how to conduct the client interview. The nurse's ability to communicate effectively is essential to the interview process. We include descriptions and examples of communication techniques in this chapter.

Unit III, *Physical Assessment,* introduces the methods and techniques that nurses use to obtain objective data. Objective data refers to measurable and observable behaviors. The chapters in Unit III are organized by body system, and each chapter begins with a review of anatomy and physiology. As we highlighted inside the front cover of the textbook, these highly structured chapters use a consistent format to walk students through the steps of assessment and build their skills step-by-step:

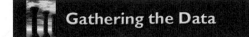
Gathering the Data

In **Gathering the Data,** students learn how to gather subjective data while conducting a client interview. We provide *Focused Interview Questions* that ask the client about general health, illness, symptoms, behaviors, pain, and lifespan. We also provide follow-up questions to help the student gather more data from the interview, as well as *Rationales* so the student understands why the nurse needs to ask these questions. We provide reminders about specific communication techniques to increase student confidence and competence while performing the health assessment.

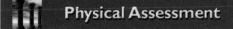
Physical Assessment

In **Physical Assessment,** we show the student how to collect objective data and conduct a physical assessment—from the preparation of the room and gathering of equipment, to greeting the client and the examination, to sharing findings with the client. The left column demonstrates step-by-step instruction for client preparation, position, details for each technique in assessment, and the expected findings. The right column includes corresponding abnormal findings and special considerations, such as an alternate method, technique or finding in relation to age, development, culture, or specific client condition. This format helps the student differentiate normal from abnormal findings while interpreting and analyzing data to plan nursing care. Hundreds of photos and illustrations help the student envision how to perform the techniques precisely and thoroughly. Documentation samples for each Physical Assessment section can be found on the *Companion Website,* with an example of narrative charting and a charting checklist. This allows the student to review and practice charting for each body system.

Abnormal Findings

In **Abnormal Findings,** we provide a vivid atlas of illustrations and photographs that feature examples of abnormal findings, diseases, and conditions. This section helps the student recognize these conditions and distinguish them from normal findings before they see them in the clinical setting.

Health Promotion

The **Health Promotion** section offers a detailed look at the *Healthy People 2010* goals for the particular body system, and follows with an overview of the related Client Education considerations.

Healthy People 2010—gives significance to the type of data a nurse must collect during health assessment and emphasizes the relevance of personal, family, and geographic history in relation to current and potential health problems. We highlight *Focus Areas, Prevalence, Objectives,* and *Actions* so the student will get an introduction to nationwide problems, but can quickly access information specific to the health needs and problems of a client.

Client Education—provides risk factors and client-oriented information designed to teach clients and family members strategies for managing symptoms of an illness, preventing illness, or maintaining optimal health. The content is based on behavioral, cultural, and environmental factors identified in *Healthy People 2010.*

Since health promotion is an important role for the nurse, this section shows the student how to link data collected from an assessment to risk factors and important teaching points for clients.

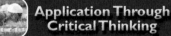
Application Through Critical Thinking

In **Application Through Critical Thinking,** we challenge students to apply critical thinking and diagnostic reasoning by working through a *Case Study.* After a detailed client scenario, students will answer critical thinking questions, identify possible nursing diagnoses, prepare documentation, and create a sample teaching plan. We provide examples to get the student started—and then we encourage students to use the *Companion Website* at www.prenhall.com/damico to submit their responses as homework to the instructor. Instructors will find answers to these activities in the *Instructor's Resource Manual,* along with guidelines for how to use the integrated textbook and website activities.

Unit IV, *Physical Assessment Across the Life Span,* contains three chapters that provide information about physical assessment of specialized client groups. These chapters describe how to conduct comprehensive head-to-toe assessments of infants and children, pregnant females, and older adults. While we focus on these special groups in Unit IV, we also integrate life span considerations throughout the book and especially in the interview questions and physical assessments for each body system in Unit III. This provides instructors with the flexibility of using this book in an integrated curriculum—where assessment techniques may be integrated into courses that cover maternity, pediatrics, and aging throughout the curriculum.

More Features That Help You Use This Book Successfully

On pages viii–ix earlier in this book, we showed you how to use the major sections and features of the textbook and media to be successful in this course. In addition, we offer the following features to further enhance the learning process and help you use this book successfully:

Key Terms at the beginning of the chapter identify the terminology the student encounters in conducting assessment and the pages where the student can find the definitions. We bold key terms and define them in the text, but the student may also refer to the comprehensive **Glossary** in the back of the textbook or the **Audio Glossary** on the Student CD-ROM and Companion Website.

Cultural Considerations

Cultural Considerations boxes are found in each chapter and highlight cultural differences that the nurse should consider while performing an assessment.

CLIENT INTERACTION

This feature teaches effective communication skills. It presents a brief clinical scenario and interaction between the client and nurse. The **Client Interaction** includes assessment cues to help the student develop strong communication skills by addressing body language, cultural sensitivity and values, language barriers, and noncompliant clients. These are common issues that present challenges to nurses, and the *Analysis* at the end of the interaction offers the student goals that the nurse needs to obtain with this specific client.

ALERT!

Individuals experiencing pain and dyspnea who are restless, anxious, and unable to follow your directions may need immediate medical assistance.

Alert! boxes remind students of specific nursing care tips or signs to be aware of when performing a physical assessment, and identify critical findings that the nurse should report immediately.

EQUIPMENT

examination gown and drape	skin marker
examination gloves	metric ruler
examination light	tissues
stethoscope	face mask

Equipment boxes help you prepare for the assessment by identifying the equipment you will need to conduct the examination.

HELPFUL HINTS

Providing an environment that is comfortable and private will reduce the client's anxiety. Each step in the procedure should be explained. It is important to tell the client when and if discomfort will accompany any examination.

At the beginning of the Physical Assessment section, the **Helpful Hints** provide suggestions and reminders about conducting the physical assessment. We offer clinical pearls to prepare the student for the examination and promote client comfort.

EXPLORE MediaLink

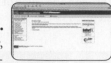

Found at the end of each chapter, **EXPLORE MediaLink** encourages the student to use the Student CD-ROM and Companion Website to apply textbook concepts. The student can preview the chapter-specific activities, animations, videos, and resources.

Additional Resources for Student and Instructor Success

We designed teaching and learning resources to expand and extend the textbook material and to mentor students in the art and skills of health assessment. For students, the text material is continued on the websites so they gain further understanding of what they've read and discussed by demonstrating what they have learned. For instructors, the full complement of supplemental resources is available from your Prentice Hall sales representative. Ask your Prentice Hall sales representative about the comprehensive teaching and learning package that accompanies *Health & Physical Assessment in Nursing*:

- ✔ *Clinical Handbook for Health Assessment*
- ✔ *Assessment Skills Laboratory Manual*
- ✔ Prentice Hall Real Nursing Skills: Health Assessment CD-ROMs
- ✔ Instructor's Resource Manual
- ✔ Instructor's Resource CD-ROM with TestGen and PowerPoint®
- ✔ Companion Website
- ✔ *MyPhysicalAssessmentLab* to accompany Blackboard or WebCT
- ✔ Online course management resources powered by OneKey

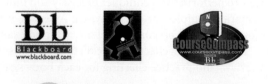

OneKey OneKey is all you need.
Convenience. Simplicity. Success.

Acknowledgments

This book would never have been completed were it not for the endless support, patience, and understanding of our families. We are especially grateful to Dianne and Jim for their immeasurable encouragement to bring this project to completion. Our special thanks to Minnie Lynch for her assistance with creating file after file, keeping us on schedule, and then getting the files to the right people. Thanks to our professional colleagues for their support, encouragement, and advice. A special thank you is extended to :

Barbara Kozier, Audrey Berman, and Shirley Snyder, authors of *Fundamentals of Nursing: Concepts, Process, and Practice,* for allowing us to adapt valuable words to enhance our chapter on pain assessment and images throughout our textbook.

Elisabeth Garofalo, Developmental Editor, our thanks for all that you have done. You have been our greatest cheerleader, and this we will always remember.

The staff at Prentice Hall—Maura Connor, Editor-in-Chief; Pam Fuller, Senior Acquisitions Editor; Mike Giacobbe, Associate Editor; and Pat Walsh, Cheryl Asherman, and Cathy O'Connell in production.

The staff at Carlisle Editorial Services, especially Amy Gehl, for keeping us on schedule and keeping track of the art program and paging schedules.

Pat Watson, for the wonderful photography.

Barbara Cousins, for the vivid illustrations.

Gosia Jaros-White, former editorial assistant, for those endless packages you sent to wherever we were, thank you.

June Thompson, thank you so much for your vision and your endless contributions to the textbook and the media.

Donita D'Amico
Colleen Barbarito

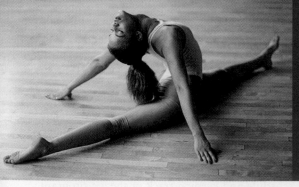

Dedication

We dedicate this book to our students.

You have provided us with the inspiration to write a book that

makes sense and can truly guide you in developing skills that you

will use throughout your professional lives.

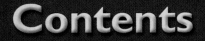

Contents

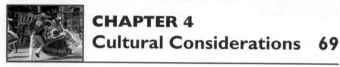

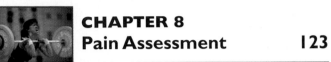

CHAPTER 8
Pain Assessment 123

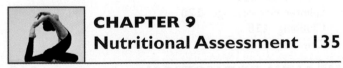

CHAPTER 9
Nutritional Assessment 135

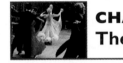

CHAPTER 10
The Health History 156

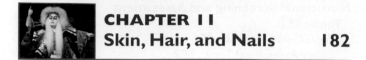

CHAPTER 12
Head, Neck, and Related Lymphatics 234

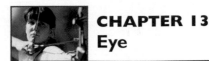

CHAPTER 13
Eye 263

CHAPTER 14
Ears, Nose, Mouth,
and Throat 304

CHAPTER 15
Respiratory System 348

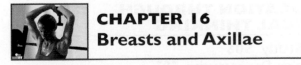

CHAPTER 16
Breasts and Axillae 397

CHAPTER 17
Cardiovascular System 425

CHAPTER 18
Peripheral Vascular
System   476

CHAPTER 19
Abdomen   510

CHAPTER 20
Urinary System   554

CHAPTER 23
Musculoskeletal System 666

CHAPTER 24
Neurologic System 730

UNIT IV
PHYSICAL ASSESSMENT ACROSS THE LIFE SPAN 782

CHAPTER 25
Assessment of Infants, Children, and Adolescents 782

CHAPTER 26
The Pregnant Female 821

**CHAPTER 27
Assessing the
Older Adult** 874

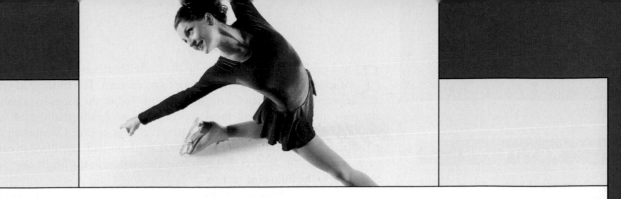

1

Health Assessment

MEDIALINK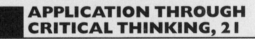

www.prenhall.com/damico

The CD-ROM in the back of this textbook and the Media-Link website contain NCLEX-RN® review questions, interactive exercises, case study challenges, animations, videos, documentation and checklist forms, and review materials. For a complete listing of the media content specific to Chapter 1, see the Explore MediaLink at the end of the chapter.

*T*he healthcare delivery system in the United States is changing. Historically, the focus of care has been illness and symptom centered. The individual entered the healthcare delivery system when illness was present. Today, the focus has changed. Emphasis of care now includes wellness, prevention of disease, health maintenance, and health promotion. The client is no longer the passive recipient of care. Clients take a more active role in the planning, decision making, and treatment modalities utilized in care. The role of the nurse is expanding. Factors that influence the change in the healthcare delivery system are described in the following sections.

Legislation, professional organizations, nurses, and consumers nationally and internationally have influenced reform of the healthcare delivery system. In 1978 the World Health Organization (WHO) prepared a primary healthcare report that emphasized health or well-being as a fundamental right and a social goal worldwide. Within the report is a stipulation that public institutions, governments, and consumers be involved in planning and delivering healthcare.

The American Nurses Association (ANA) outlined the profession's recommendations for reform of the healthcare system in *Nursing's Agenda for Health Care Reform (2004)*. The recommendations included restructuring the system to enhance access to primary care in community settings, fostering consumer responsibility in self-care and decision making about health, and facilitating the use of cost-effective providers. Further recommendations included development of standardized services to be provided to all residents and to be financed through private and public sources, planned change to reflect changes in demographics, reduction in healthcare costs, insurance reform, long-term care provision, and the institution of essential services.

Consumers are encouraging reform of the healthcare system to include wellness and quality of life, rather than simply treatment of disease. In addition, consumers value community health, health promotion, and disease prevention. These many changes in the delivery of healthcare impact the role of the professional nurse providing care. As a result, these aspects of nursing care are explained in this chapter and incorporated throughout this text. Nurses are taking on more responsibility. Health assessment has become an integral part of the expanded role of the nurse. Health assessment was always performed in a limited manner in the acute care setting. Today, nurses perform assessment in all settings and with clients of all ages and diversity. A description of the assessment process is included in a later section of this chapter. The subsequent chapters address specific areas of concern in assessment of the whole individual. The chapters in Unit III provide step-by-step guides for learning how to perform physical assessment of each of the systems. ∞ Nurses use the nursing process and critical thinking skills as the basis for the implementation of safe, competent client care.

The United States Department of Health and Human Services (USDHHS) joined the movement to reform healthcare in the *Healthy People* initiatives. These initiatives are based on the premise that individual health is closely related to the health of the community. Accordingly, the interactions of governments, professionals, communities, and individuals are required to improve access to healthcare and change the nation's health. The promotion of health of the individual and the community is an important focus of nursing practice. As such, nurses are an integral part of initiatives that address the health status of individuals and groups in the communities in which they live and work. One important initiative is *Healthy People 2010*.

HEALTHY PEOPLE 2010

Healthy People 2010: Understanding and Improving Health (USDHHS, 2000) presents a 10-year strategy intended to promote health and to prevent illness, disability, and premature death. Link to *Healthy People 2010* through the Companion Website. *Healthy People 2010* proposes 467 objectives to improve health. The objectives are organized into 28 focus areas (see Box 1.1). *Healthy People 2010* also identifies the following leading health indicators that reflect public health concerns in the United States:

- Physical Activity
- Overweight and Obesity

Box 1.1	Focus Areas in *Healthy People 2010*
Access to quality health services	Immunization and infectious diseases
Arthritis, osteoporosis, and chronic back problems	Injury and violence protection
Cancer	Maternal, infant, and child health
Chronic kidney disease	Medical product safety
Diabetes	Mental health and mental disorders
Disability and secondary conditions	Nutrition and overweight
Educational and community-based programs	Occupational safety and health
	Oral health
Environmental health	Physical activity and fitness
Family planning	Public health infrastructure
Food safety	Respiratory diseases
Health communication	Sexually transmitted diseases
Heart disease and stroke	Substance abuse
	Tobacco use
HIV	Vision and hearing

Data from: USDHHS (2000). *Healthy People 2010.* Washington, DC.

- Tobacco Use
- Substance Abuse
- Responsible Sexual Behavior
- Mental Health
- Injury and Violence
- Environmental Quality
- Immunization
- Access to Healthcare

Each of the leading health indicators is linked to the objectives to improve health. The indicators serve as a mechanism for the development of plans to improve health for both individuals and communities. Many of the plans to improve health incorporate promotion of screening for health problems, as well as preventive measures including immunization, increase in physical activity, and education regarding all aspects of health. The changing demographics in the United States as well as cultural, ethnic, geographic, linguistic, and socioeconomic differences are addressed in relation to health problems and plans to improve health in *Healthy People 2010*.

The *Healthy People 2010* initiative is so significant that it is incorporated throughout this text. Additionally, each chapter in Unit III addresses the assessment of systems of the body. ∞ The importance of gathering information about the systems and the actions that are suggested to promote health of the systems is linked with the related focus areas of *Healthy People 2010*. For example, the focus areas of tobacco use and respiratory diseases are linked with Chapter 15, "Respiratory System." ∞

This chapter provides an overview of the aspects of nursing practice and nursing skills required for the expanding role of the nurse. These include comprehensive assessment, nursing process, critical thinking, communication, documentation, and teaching. The skills and approaches required to meet the needs of diverse clients seeking advice and care in the changing healthcare system are illustrated throughout this text. Case studies provide opportunities to apply developing critical thinking skills. Simulated client interactions with analyses il-

lustrate communication techniques. Teaching plans, derived from case studies, provide examples of one of the most important interventions in health promotion and illness prevention. The process of health assessment is carefully explained in regard to the interview and hands-on physical assessment of the client in general and for each system of the body. Samples of documentation for each aspect of assessment provide guidelines and exemplify the requirements for documentation explained in this initial chapter.

Additionally, the succeeding chapters provide information about developmental, cultural, psychosocial, and environmental factors that impact health and influence approaches to assessment. Learning about assessment and all related factors is enhanced through the illustrations, photographs, tables, and figures in each chapter.

HEALTH

Traditionally, **health** has been thought of as the absence of disease. The terms *health* and *wellness* have been used interchangeably to describe the state when one is not sick. Today, these terms have clear distinctions in regard to definition and description of actions.

DEFINITIONS OF HEALTH

The World Health Organization presented a definition of health that remains active and relevant today. Health is defined as a state of complete physical, mental, and social well-being (WHO, 1947). Further, WHO describes health from a holistic approach in which the individual is viewed as a total person interacting with others. The individual functions within his or her physical, psychological, and social fields. These fields interact with each other and the external environment. The individual has the capability of maximizing the potential and fostering the most positive aspects of health. Models and mechanisms related to promotion of health are described in Chapter 2 of this text. ∞ Today, many definitions and models of health and wellness have been designed using these concepts. It is evident that health is far more than the absence of illness, disease, and symptoms.

The following definitions of health reflect the work of nursing theorists:

- A process and a state of being and becoming whole and integrated in a way that reflects person and environment mutuality (Roy & Andrews, 1999).
- The state of a person as characterized by soundness or wholeness of developed human structures and mental and bodily functioning that requires therapeutic self-care (Orem, 1971).
- A culturally defined, valued, and practiced state of well-being reflective of the ability to perform role activities (Leininger, 1991).
- A state of well-being and use of every power the person possesses to the fullest extent (Nightingale, 1860/1969).

MODELS OF HEALTH

The following are examples of models that explain the concept of health:

- The ecologic model developed by Leavell and Clark (1965) examines the interaction of agent, host, and environment. Health is present when these three variables are in harmony. When this harmony is disrupted, health is not maintained at its highest level and illness and disease occurs.

- In the clinical model, health is defined as the absence of disease or injury. The aim of the care by the health professional is to relieve signs and symptoms of disease, relieve pain, and eliminate malfunction of physiological symptoms.

- The eudaemonistic model views health as the actualization of a person's potential. Actualization refers to fulfillment and complete development. Illness would prevent self-actualization.

- According to Pender, Murdaugh, and Parsons (2002), the health promotion model defines health as the actualization of inherent and acquired human potential through goal-directed behavior, competent self-care, and satisfying relationships with others, while adjustments are made to maintain structural integrity and harmony with relevant environments.

Health is highly individualized and the definition one develops for self will be influenced by many factors. These factors will include but not be limited to age, gender, race, family, culture, religion, socioeconomic conditions, environment, previous experiences, and self-expectations.

Nurses must recognize that each client will have a personal definition for health, illness, and wellness. The behaviors one uses to maintain these changing states will be most individualized. Nurses must be aware of their own personal definition of health and at the same time accept and respect the client's definition of health, for this will influence practice. When health is defined in terms of physical change, the practice focus is on improvement of physical function. When health is considered to be reflective of physical, cultural, environmental, psychological, and social factors, the focus of nursing practice is more holistic and wide ranging. Any of the previously mentioned health models could be used by the professional nurse and other members of the health team as a paradigm for the design and delivery of healthcare.

HEALTH ASSESSMENT

Health assessment may be defined as a systematic method of collecting data about a client for the purpose of determining the client's current and ongoing health status, predicting risks to health, and identifying health-promoting activities. The data includes physical, social, cultural, environmental, and emotional factors that impact the overall well-being of the client. The health status will include wellness behaviors, illness signs and symptoms, client strengths and weaknesses, and risk factors. The scope of focus must be more than problems presented by the client. The nurse will use a variety of sources to gather the objective and subjective data. Knowledge of the natural and social sciences is a strong foundation for the nurse. Effective communication techniques and use of critical thinking skills are essential in helping the nurse to gather detailed, complete, relevant, objective, subjective, and measurable data needed to formulate a plan of care to meet the needs of the client. Health assessment includes the interview, physical assessment, docu-

mentation, and interpretation of findings. Each of these components is described in detail in Units II and III of this text. ∞ All planning for care is directed by interpretation of findings from objective and subjective data collected throughout the assessment process.

THE INTERVIEW

The **interview**, in which subjective data is gathered, includes the health history and focused interview. The data collected will come from primary and secondary sources. The primary source from which data is collected is the client, and the client is considered to be the direct source. An indirect or secondary source would include family members, caregivers, other members of the health team, and medical records.

Subjective data is information that the client experiences and communicates to the nurse. Perceptions of pain, nausea, dizziness, itching sensations, or feeling nervous are examples of subjective data. Only the client can describe these feelings. Subjective data is usually referred to as covert (hidden) data or as a symptom, when it is perceived by the client and cannot be observed by others. Family members or caregivers could report subjective data based on perceptions the client has shared with them. This information is most helpful when the client is very ill or unable to communicate, and is required when the client is an infant or child. However, to ensure accuracy, the nurse must validate subjective data obtained from other sources. The accuracy of subjective data depends on the nurse's ability to clarify the information gathered with follow-up questions and to obtain supporting data from other pertinent sources.

THE HEALTH HISTORY

The purpose of the **health history** is to obtain information about the client's health in his or her own words and based on the client's own perceptions. Biographical data, perceptions about health, past and present history of illness and injury, family history, a review of systems, and health patterns and practices are the types of information included in the health history. The health history provides cues regarding the client's health and guides further data collection. The health history is a most important aspect of the assessment process. Detailed information regarding the health history is presented in Chapter 10 of this text. ∞

THE FOCUSED INTERVIEW

The **focused interview** enables the nurse to clarify points, to obtain missing information, and to follow up on verbal and nonverbal cues identified in the health history. The nurse does not use a prepared set of questions for the focused interview. The nurse applies knowledge and critical thinking when asking specific and detailed questions or requesting descriptions of symptoms, feelings, or events. Therefore, the focused interview provides the means and opportunity to expand the subjective database regarding specific strengths, weaknesses, problems, or concerns expressed by the client or required by the nurse to begin to make reliable judgments about information and observations as part of planning care. In-depth information about the focused interview in health assessment is included in each chapter in Unit III of this text. ∞

PHYSICAL ASSESSMENT

Physical assessment is hands-on examination of the client. Components of physical assessment are the survey and examination of systems. Objective data gathered during physical assessment, when combined with all other reliable sources of information, provides a sound database from which care planning may proceed. **Objective data** is observed or measured by the professional nurse. This is also known as overt data or a sign since it is detected by the nurse. This data can be seen, felt, heard, or measured by the professional nurse. For example, skin color can be seen, a pulse can be felt, a cough can be heard, and a blood pressure can be measured. This objective data is needed to validate subjective data and to complete the database. The accuracy of objective data depends on the nurse's ability to avoid reaching conclusions without substantive evidence. The accuracy of objective data is also increased by attention to detail and verification. Unit II of this text provides information about the general survey and techniques for physical assessment. ⚭ Unit III includes detailed descriptions for physical assessment of systems. ⚭

In addition, data from all secondary sources including charts, reports from diagnostic and laboratory testing, family, and all healthcare professionals involved in client care are part of the database from which decisions about care are derived. Both subjective and objective data may further be categorized as constant or variable. *Constant data* is information that does not change over time such as race, sex, or blood type. *Variable data* may change within minutes, hours, or days. Blood pressure, pulse rate, blood counts, and age are examples of variable data.

DOCUMENTATION

Documentation of data from health assessment creates a client record or becomes an addition to an existing health record. The **client record** is a legal document used to plan care, to communicate information between and among healthcare providers, and to monitor quality of care. Further, the client record provides information used for reimbursement of services, is often a source of data for research, and is reviewed by accrediting agencies to determine adherence to standards.

Documentation is used to communicate information between and among the health professionals involved in the care of the client. In order for that communication to be effective, the nurse must adhere to the following guidelines for documentation. Documentation must be accurate, confidential, appropriate, complete, and detailed. When documenting, the nurse must use standard and accepted abbreviations, symbols, and terminology and must reflect professional and organizational standards (see Box 1.2).

Accuracy means that documentation is limited to facts or factual accounts of observations rather than opinions or interpretations of observations. When recording subjective data, it is important to use quotation marks and quote a client exactly rather than interpret the statement. In health assessment, accuracy also requires the use of accurate measurement and location of symptoms and physical findings. For example, rather than writing that the client had severe pain and swelling in the left lower extremity the nurse would document that a client had pain rated 8 on a scale of 1 to 10, and edema and redness on the dorsal surface of the foot over the first through third phalanges. Accuracy in documentation

Box 1.2	**Standard Abbreviations and Symbols**
abd	=	Abdomen
ADL	=	Activities of daily living
BP	=	Blood pressure
CBC	=	Complete blood count
CNS	=	Central nervous system
CVA	=	Costovertebral angle
Dx	=	Diagnosis
Ht	=	Height
Hx	=	History
LMP	=	Last menstrual period
mg	=	Milligram
P	=	Pulse
RR	=	Respirations rate
T	=	Temperature
VS	=	Vital signs
WBC	=	White blood cell
Wt	=	Weight
>	Means greater than
=	Means equal to
<	Means less than

requires the use of accepted terminology, symbols, and abbreviations. The use of accepted language in documentation provides for consistent interpretation of data as it is reviewed and used by healthcare professionals to monitor and oversee healthcare planning and delivery. Link to the Registered Nurses Association of British Columbia through the Companion Website. ⚭

Confidentiality means that information sharing is limited to those directly involved in client care. Information is considered appropriate for inclusion in a health record only if it has direct bearing on the client's health. Complete documentation means that all information required to develop a plan of care for the client has been included. In comprehensive health assessment, data from the health history, focused interview, and physical assessment are required for a complete record.

Protection of an individual's health information is regulated federally through the Health Insurance Portability and Accountability Act (HIPAA). Regulations under this law became effective in April 2003. The aim of the law was to create a national standard for privacy and to provide individuals with greater control over personal health information. Title II of the law, also known as Administrative Simplification, stipulates the requirements for maintaining the security and privacy of medical information. Healthcare providers, hospitals, and health insurance providers are required to follow policies to protect the privacy of health information. The HIPAA regulations protect medical records and other individually identifiable health information whether communicated in writing, orally, or electronically. Identifiable health information includes demographic information and any information that could identify an individual. For further information about HIPAA regulations, contact the USDHHS. Link to the U.S. Department of Health and Human Services through the Companion Website. ⚭

The types and amounts of documentation are determined by the purpose of the healthcare service and often by the setting. In emergency situations, data gathering and documentation focus on the immediate problem and factors that may influence or impact care decisions related to the emergency. For example, in an unconscious client, one would want to know if the altered level of consciousness was a result of a head injury in an otherwise healthy individual or associated with a previously diagnosed problem. In nonemergency situations in which a comprehensive health assessment will be conducted, documentation of all findings is required.

Data recorded during visits to healthcare providers or clinics for continued management of an existing condition is generally limited to findings indicating change, progress, or problems associated with the existing condition. Documentation for health screening and health promotion is often limited to the results of the screening process and referral information.

Documentation of data collected in health assessment should be completed as soon as possible. Recollection of details becomes difficult as time elapses. The nurse should record some details and notes during the data collection process, particularly direct client quotes and when precise information is required, such as the location of a lesion, wound, or abnormal finding. Immediacy of recording increases the accuracy of the information. It is important to explain the purpose of the documentation and inform the client at the outset that notes and forms will be used to record information.

Methods for documentation include narrative notes, problem-oriented charting, scales, flow sheets or check sheets, charting by exception, focus documentation, and computer documentation. Each of these will be described in the following paragraphs, and additional documentation exercises are provided throughout this text and on the Companion Website. Examples of each type of documentation appear in Figures 1.1 through 1.5 and are based on the following case study.

Janet Lewis, a 20-year-old female, came to the university health center. Ms. Lewis told the nurse, "I feel bloated and achy in my left side and it has increased over the past 3 or 4 days." In response to questions about appetite, Ms. Lewis responded, "I really don't feel like eating and I'm worried because I'm supposed to eat carefully. I recently had anemia and have been taking pills for it for a month." When asked about bowel elimination, she said, "My last BM was 4 days ago; it was hard pellets and dark colored." She responded to questions about gastrointestinal symptoms with the following: "I'm not nauseous and I haven't vomited." She further reported, "I had my last period 10 days ago." She told the nurse that her voiding was normal in amount and number of voids. Ms. Lewis brought the medication with her. The label read Fe gluconate 300 mg three times a day. Her physician instructed her to take the medication and have a follow-up visit in 1 month.

The physical examination revealed the presence of bowel sounds in all quadrants, dullness to percussion in the left upper and lower quadrants, firm distention, and tenderness in the left lower quadrant. There was no tenderness at the costovertebral angle (CVA). Hard, dry stool high in the rectum was identified on the rectal examination and a sample applied to a slide for occult blood testing. Blood was drawn for a complete blood count (CBC).

A rectal suppository was administered with a result, within 15 minutes, of a moderate amount of hard, dark stool. Ms. Lewis stated, "I feel a little better, but still achy." She was discharged to her dormitory with 30 ml of milk of magnesia (MOM) to take at bedtime. Ms. Lewis was advised to increase her fluid intake and continue to take the Fe gluconate as ordered. She was instructed to call the health center in the morning as a follow-up measure and to call her physician to schedule a visit and to discuss her laboratory results.

The nurse provided education as follows:

- Constipation and change in stool color are side effects of the Fe gluconate.
- Fe gluconate should be scheduled 2 hours after meals, with a full glass of water or juice.
- Increasing roughage by adding fresh fruits to the diet will help to reduce the constipation.

Narrative Notes

When implementing narrative notes, the nurse utilizes words, phrases, sentences, and paragraphs to record information. The information may be recorded in chronological order from initial contact through conclusion of the assessment, or in categories according to the type of data collected. The narrative record includes words, sentences, phrases, or lists to indicate judgments made about the data, plans to address concerns, and actions taken to meet the health needs of the client (see Figure 1.1 ●).

Narrative Note

A 20-year-old female seen because she "feels bloated" and has an "achiness" in her left side that has "increased over the past 3 or 4 days." She states she "really doesn't feel like eating" and that she is "worried" because she was "supposed to eat carefully" because she recently "had a problem with anemia" and has been "taking pills for it for a month." Brought medication with her. Label reads Fe gluconate 300 mg three times a day. She stated the doctor told her to take the pills until she has a return visit next month. She denies nausea and vomiting, last BM of dark hard pellets—4 days ago. LMP 10 days ago. Voiding "normal" amount and number of voids. On exam: VS-BP 110/66—P 88—RR 22. Color pale, skin warm and dry. Abdomen: distended, BS present x 4, dullness to percussion LUQ and LLQ, firm, tenderness to palpation LLQ. No CVA tenderness. Rectal exam: hard stool high in rectum, dark color. CBC drawn, stool for OB. Dulcolax suppository administered. Result—moderate hard, dark stool after 15 minutes—"feels a little better but still achy." Discharged to dorm with medication. Advised client to increase fluid intake, continue Fe gluconate as ordered. Education: 1. Side effects Fe—re: dark stool, constipation. 2. Schedule 2 hours after meals, take with full glass water or juice. 3. Increase roughage—fruits in diet. 4. Call in AM for follow-up. 5. Call PMD re: visit—lab results.

Figure 1.1 ● Narrative notes.

SOAP	
S	"I feel bloated and achy in my left side and it has increased over the past 3 or 4 days." "I really don't feel like eating." "I'm worried because I'm supposed to eat carefully." Because "I recently had anemia and have been taking pills for it for a month." "My last BM was 4 days ago; it was hard pellets and dark colored." "I'm not nauseous and I haven't vomited." "I had my last period 10 days ago."
O	Skin pale, warm, dry. VS-BP 110/66—P 88—RR 20 Abdomen: distended, BS+ × 4, dull percussion LUQ and LLQ, firm, tender LLQ Rectal: hard stool, dark
A	On Fe gluconate 300 mg three times a day—Anemia No history abdominal pain, discomfort, disease Constipation
P	Rectal suppository and laxative CBC, stool for occult blood Instruct: med, diet, fluid Follow up here and PMD

Figure 1.2 ● SOAP notes.

APIE	
A	"I feel bloated and achy in my left side and it has increased over the past 3 or 4 days." "I really don't feel like eating." "I'm worried because I'm supposed to eat carefully." "I recently had anemia and have been taking pills for it for a month." "My last BM was 4 days ago. It was hard pellets and dark colored." "I'm not nauseous and haven't vomited." "I had my last period 10 days ago." Skin pale, warm, dry. VS-BP 110/66—P 88—RR 20 Abdomen: distended, BS+ × 4, dull percussion LUQ and LLQ, firm, tender LLQ Rectal: hard stool, dark On Fe gluconate 300 mg three times a day—Anemia No history abdominal pain, discomfort, disease Constipation
P	Rectal suppository and laxative at bedtime CBC, stool for occult blood Instruct: diet, meds, fluids Follow up here and PMD
I	Dulcolax suppository administered Instruction
E	Moderate hard, dry dark stool "I feel a little better, but still achy."

Figure 1.3 ● APIE notes.

Problem-Oriented Charting

Problem-oriented records include the SOAP and APIE methods. The letters SOAP refer to recording **S**ubjective data, **O**bjective data, **A**ssessment, and **P**lanning. Subjective data is that reported by the client or reliable informant. Objective data is derived from the physical examination, client records, and reports. Assessment refers to conclusions drawn from the data. Planning indicates the actions to be taken to resolve problems or address client needs (see Figure 1.2 ●). The letters APIE refer to **A**ssessment, **P**roblem, **I**ntervention, and **E**valuation. When using this method, documentation of assessment includes combining the subjective and objective data. The nurse will draw conclusions from the data, identify and record the problem or problems, and plan to address these problems. Interventions are documented as they are carried out. Evaluation refers to documentation of the response to the plan (see Figure 1.3 ●).

Flow Sheets

Documentation of health assessment data can be accomplished through the use of scales, check sheets, or flowcharts. These forms are usually formatted for a specific purpose or need. They may use columns or categories for recording data and may include lists of expected findings with associated qualifiers for ranges of normal or abnormal findings. Charts and check sheets often provide space for narrative descriptions or comments (see Figure 1.4 ●).

Focus Documentation

Focus documentation is a method that does not limit documentation to problems, but can include client strengths. This type of documentation is intended to address a specific purpose or focus, that is, a symptom, strength, or need. A comprehensive health assessment may result in one or more foci for documentation. The format for focus documentation is a column to address subjective and objective data, nursing action, and client response (see Figure 1.5 ●).

Charting by Exception

Charting by exception is a system in which documentation is limited to exceptions from pre-established norms or significant findings. Flow sheets with appropriate information and parameters are completed. This type of documentation eliminates much of the repetition involved in narrative and other forms of documentation.

Computer Documentation

Computer-generated documentation may include all of the previously mentioned methods for recording data. The amount and types of information to be documented vary according to the computer program and the policies and standards of the agency in which computer documentation is utilized. The advantage in using most computer documentation is that it allows healthcare providers to use more time recording appropriate information and less time determining the correct terms, spelling, and descriptors.

Assessment of the Abdomen				
EXAM	**FINDINGS**			
Anterior				
INSPECTION				
Contour	_x_ Round	____ Flat	____ Protuberant	____ Scaphoid
Position of Umbilicus	midline			
Skin	Color pale, consistent with all other			
	Texture smooth			
	Lesions none			
Symmetry	Symmetrical			
Bulging	_x_ No ____ Yes			
Masses	_x_ No ____ Yes			
Movements	____ Waves _____			
	____ Pulsations _____			
AUSCULTATION				
Bowel Sounds	Present _x_ Yes ____ No			
	Quadrants _4_			
PERCUSSION	Tympany	Dull	Flat	Hyperresonant
LUQ	____	_x_	____	____
RUQ	____	____	____	____
RLQ	____	____	____	____
LLQ	____	_x_	____	____
PALPATION				
	Pain ____ Tenderness _x_ Location _LLQ_			
	Ascites ____ Yes _x_ No			
	Bladder ____ Palpable _x_ Nonpalpable			
Posterior				
PERCUSSION				
CVA	Pain _x_ No ____ Yes			

Figure 1.4 ● Check sheet.

Development of confidence and competence in documentation is an important part of nursing education. This text provides samples of recording for the client interview. Documentation of subjective and objective data collection for body systems is provided to guide and assist in the development of these skills.

INTERPRETATION OF FINDINGS

Interpretation of findings can be defined as making determinations about all of the data collected in the health assessment process. One must determine if the findings fall within normal and expected ranges in relation to the client's age, gender, and race and then the significance of the findings in relation to the client's health status and immediate and long-range, health-related needs. Interpretation of findings is influenced by a number of factors. These factors include the ability to obtain,

recall, and apply knowledge; to communicate effectively; and to use a holistic approach. Each of these factors is discussed in the following sections.

Knowledge

Nurses obtain, recall, and apply knowledge from physical and social sciences, nursing theory, and all areas of research that impact current nursing practice. For example, knowledge would include human anatomy and physiology and the differences that are associated with growth and development across the life span as well as characteristics specific to gender and race. Further, knowledge includes health-related and healthcare trends in groups and populations, such as the increased incidence of risk factors or actual illnesses in certain groups or populations. In the United States, for example, trends include increased longevity and increased in-

Date	Focus	Progress Note
01/20/09	Bowel Elimination	Data: "I feel bloated and achy in my left side and it has increased over the past 3 or 4 days." "I really don't feel like eating." "I'm worried because I'm supposed to eat carefully." "I recently had anemia and have been taking pills for it for a month." "My last BM was 4 days ago. It was hard pellets and dark colored." "I'm not nauseous and haven't vomited." "I had my last period 10 days ago."
		Skin pale, warm, dry. VS-BP 110/66—P 88—RR 20
		Abdomen: distended, BS+ × 4, dull percussion LUQ and LLQ, firm, tender LLQ
		Rectal: hard stool, dark
		On Fe gluconate 300 mg three times a day—Anemia, No history abdominal pain, discomfort, disease
		Constipation Action: Rectal supp administered
		Instruction Response: Moderate hard, dry dark stool
		"I feel a little better, but still achy."

Figure 1.5 • Focus notes.

cidence of obesity in children and adults particularly. The nurse must be able to access and use reliable resources in interpretation of findings. Resources include research, scientific literature, and charts, scales, and graphs to indicate ranges of norms and expectations about physical and psychological development. Examples include Denver Developmental scores, mental status examinations, weight and body composition charts, and growth charts prepared by centers for health statistics. Examples of charts and scales or links to information about measures are provided in each of the chapters in this text. Additionally, the nurse must be able to communicate effectively, to think critically, to recognize and act on client cues, to incorporate a holistic perspective, and to determine the significance of data in meeting immediate and long-term client needs.

Expectations about interpretation of findings change as one gains experience in nursing practice and with advanced practice preparation. The nurse must be able to recognize situations that require immediate attention and initiate care or seek appropriate assistance. (*If a client presented in an ambulatory care setting with dyspnea, the nurse would focus on providing measures to alleviate some symptoms, such as positioning and loosening constrictive clothing. The nurse would gather data that relates to the current problem and either arrange for transport to an acute care facility or seek assistance from an advanced nurse practitioner in the facility.*)

A nursing student is expected to recall and apply knowledge to discriminate between normal and abnormal findings and use resources to understand the findings in relation to wellness or illness for a particular client. Consider the findings from assessment of Julie Connor, a 12-year-old: asymmetrical shoulders and elevated right scapula on inspection of the posterior thorax, right lateral curvature of thoracic spine on palpation of vertebrae. The student would recall that scapulae should be symmetrical and the vertebrae should be aligned. The findings are interpreted as a deviation from the normal. The student would refer to available resources and learn that the findings are associated with scoliosis. More data would be required to confirm this and to determine the impact on Julie's current and future health.

Continued learning and actual experiences promote the ability to discriminate between normal and abnormal findings. In addition, one can recognize patterns that predispose individuals to illness or are indicative of specific illnesses, and implement and evaluate appropriate nursing care. Consider the following findings from assessment of James Long, a 46-year-old African American male: height 5′9″, weight 220 lb, BP 156/94, mother died at age 62 from cerebral vascular accident (stroke, brain attack), father died at age 42 from myocardial infarction (heart attack). Using knowledge of normal ranges of findings for vital signs, height, and weight, the BP and weight would be interpreted as abnormal findings. The findings indicate that this client has high blood pressure and is obese. The nurse applies knowledge of patterns associated with health problems to interpret the significance of the findings for this client. The nurse knows that hypertension occurs more frequently in African American males than in Caucasians and that family history of coronary artery disease, hypertension, and obesity increase the risk of both acquiring hypertension and the complications associated with it. Recommendations and plans for care for Mr. Long will be developed in collaboration with other healthcare professionals to address the immediate and long-term healthcare needs of reducing blood pressure and weight.

Communication

Effective communication is essential to the data-gathering process. **Communication** refers to the exchange of information, feelings, thoughts, and ideas. Communication occurs through nonverbal means such as facial expression, gestures, and body language. Verbal methods include spoken or written communication. A variety of verbal techniques, such as open-ended or closed questions, statements, clarification, and rephrasing, are used to gather information. The communication techniques must incorporate regard for the individual in relation to the purposes of the data gathering, the client's age, and the level of anxiety. In addition, the nurse must use techniques that accommodate language differences or difficulties, cultural influences, cognitive ability, affect, demeanor, and special needs. Communication in health assessment is further discussed in Chapter 10 of this text. ⨋ Sample client-nurse interactions appear in each chapter of Unit III. ⨋ For further information, link to Nursing Spectrum and to South Dakota State University through the Companion Website.

Holistic Approach

A holistic approach is an essential characteristic of nursing practice. **Holism** can best be defined as considering more than the physiological health status of a client. Holism includes all factors that impact the client's physical and emotional well-being. In a holistic approach, the nurse recognizes that developmental, psychological, emotional, family, cultural, and environmental factors will affect immediate and long-term actual and potential health goals, problems, and plans.

Developmental Factors

The developmental level of a client has an impact on health assessment. The source of information may vary depending on the age and developmental level of the client. Findings related to intellectual ability must be interpreted according to the assessed developmental level, not the stated age, in clients with developmental disabilities. Parents or guardians are the primary sources for information about children. The developmental level of the client also influences the approach to assessment, including the words and terminology. For example, assessment of a pregnant adolescent would be different from that of a 38-year-old woman pregnant for the third time.

Psychological and Emotional Factors

Psychological and emotional factors must be recognized as impacting physiological health and must be considered as predisposing or contributing factors when interpreting findings from a health assessment. One needs only to recall that anxiety triggers an autonomic response resulting in increased pulse and blood pressure to understand that relationship. Conversely, physical problems can impact emotional health. For example, childhood obesity can lead to problems with self-esteem and impact socialization and development. Psychological problems such as anxiety and depression may interfere with the ability to fully participate in health assessment. Grieving may limit one's ability to carry out required health practices or recognize health problems.

Family Factors

Family history of illness or health problems must be considered in health assessment and interpretation of findings. Individuals with a family history of some illnesses are considered at high risk for contracting that disease. For example, a female with a first-degree relative (mother, sister, daughter) with breast cancer has a risk almost three times higher than others of developing breast cancer herself. The nurse must recognize that family dynamics may influence one's approach to healthcare. In some families, health-related decisions are not made independently, but rather by the family leader or by group consensus. Circumstances within families can impact both physical and emotional health and must be considered as part of health assessment. For example, children of alcoholics are not only at risk for alcoholism, but also at risk for emotional issues not encountered by other children; therefore, one must view and interpret unexpected physical or emotional behaviors in relation to the alcoholic family situation.

Cultural Factors

Cultural factors must be considered when collecting data and interpreting findings. Culture impacts language, expression, emotional and physical well-being, and health practices. Findings regarding physical and emotional health must be interpreted in relation to the cultural norms for the client. For example, lack of eye contact during the interview would not be considered lack of ability to interact, depression, or a problem with attention in many Asian cultures. Care must be taken to provide clear explanations of abnormal findings, illnesses, and treatments because views of illness, causality, and treatment may have cultural influences. Refer to Chapter 4 of this text for further discussion of culture and cultural competence in nursing care. ⬤⬤

Environmental Factors

Internal and external environmental factors impact health assessment and interpretation of findings. The data must always be considered in relation to norms and expectation for age, race, and gender, and in relation to factors impacting the individual client. It is essential then to gather and use data from the health history, focused interview, and physical assessment when interpreting data.

INTERNAL ENVIRONMENTAL FACTORS. Data from the comprehensive health assessment provide cues about the client's internal environment, including emotional state, response to medication and treatment, and physiological or anatomical alterations that influence findings and interpretation. For example, the finding from assessment of Mrs. Bernice Hall, 49, is that she has dark, almost black, formed stools. This would be considered an abnormal finding since the normal finding would be brown-colored stools. However, Mrs. Hall stated during her health history that she has taken iron pills and eaten a lot of spinach and greens for years, and her stools have been that way ever since. Therefore, considering the internal environment of medication and diet, both of which darken the stool, the nurse interprets this as a normal finding for Mrs. Hall.

EXTERNAL ENVIRONMENTAL FACTORS. External environmental factors can also impact health, health assessment, and interpretation of findings. External factors include but are not limited to inhaled toxins such as smoke, chemicals, and fumes; irritants that can be inhaled, ingested, or contacted through the skin; noise, light, and motion; and any objects or substances one may encounter in the home, in schools, in workplaces, while shopping, or while traveling and carrying out normal activities. Consider assessment of Martha Whitman, a 22-year-old with back pain. The findings from the physical assessment are all within normal limits. Ms. Whitman stated that the pain started 2 weeks ago and has been getting worse with temporary relief from aspirin. Before referring this client for diagnostic studies, the nurse considered external environmental factors that may contribute to the back pain. The nurse asked about any activities or events associated with the onset of the pain. Ms. Whitman revealed that she had taken up quilting about 2 weeks ago, and has been sitting and working with an embroidery hoop almost every day for an hour or so. The additional information assists the nurse in interpretation of the back pain. The nurse recommends ways to sit and perform the quilting without straining the muscles of the back and will follow up to see if this relieves the pain. Consider the assessment of a toddler with nausea and vomiting. The nurse must consider gathering information about the circumstances surrounding the onset of the problem. For example, was the child in a new environment in which he could have ingested medications, cleaning fluids, or other toxic substances?

Health assessment includes the interview, physical assessment, documentation, and interpretation of findings. The preceding discussion with the accompanying examples illustrates the importance of knowledge, communication, and a holistic approach in health assessment. Collection of information and interpretation of findings are important components of nursing practice. Nursing practice is concerned with health promotion, wellness, illness prevention, health restoration, and care for the dying. The nursing process in which the nurse uses comprehensive assessment to identify a client's health status and actual or potential needs guides the practice of nursing. The nursing process then directs the nurse in the development of plans and the use of nursing interventions to meet those identified needs.

NURSING PROCESS

The **nursing process** is a systematic, rational, dynamic, and cyclic process used by the nurse for planning and providing care for the client. When first developed, the nursing process had four steps or phases: assessment, planning, implementing, and evaluation. Many nursing theorists have taken the original steps and expanded and clarified the meaning and action of each step. Most experts today accept a five-step process (see Figure 1.6 ●). These steps are assessment, diagnosis, planning, implementation, and evaluation. The nursing process can be used in any setting, with clients of all ages, and in all levels of health and illness.

Since the nursing process is client centered, the approach to nursing care becomes most specific to the client. The client can be the individual, family, community or population. The nurse uses critical thinking, therapeutic communication skills, and the knowledge of many arts and sciences when using the nursing process. Each step of the process will be defined here; however, greatest emphasis will be placed on assessment.

In the following sections, the steps of the nursing process are identified as discrete actions. However, in practice they are interrelated and overlap to some degree. The application and effective use of the nursing process is influenced by the ability of the nurse to obtain comprehensive, accurate data.

ASSESSMENT

Assessment, step 1 of the nursing process, is the collection, organization, and validation of subjective and objective data. The data collected forms the database used by the nurse. As the data change, the nurse must update the database. The database will describe the physical, emotional, and spiritual health status of the client. Strengths and weaknesses are identified as are responses to any treatment modalities.

Assessment begins at the moment the nurse meets the client and begins to gather information. Each piece of information collected about a client is a cue, because it hints at the total health status of the client. The baseline data acts as a marker during future assessment. This data becomes a guide for the nurse as to what questions to ask and what additional information is needed.

Consider the following situation. Mrs. Martha Jacobs is a 70-year-old female who tripped at home 2 weeks ago and suffered a sprain in her right ankle. Her initial treatment included an Ace bandage wrap, ice, and a nonsteroidal anti-inflammatory drug (NSAID) for discomfort. She was instructed to elevate the extremity for 3 days and to increase weight-bearing activity gradually. She is being seen in a follow-up visit and reports that her ankle is feeling much better, but she has abdominal discomfort.

When questioned about the problem, she stated, "My stomach has been kind of achy and it really started a couple of days ago." She replied to further questioning saying, "I've only had one or two little hard bowel movements in the last five days." She denied having a problem with bowel elimination in the past and stated, "I usually go once a day and it's soft." In response to further questions she stated that she has been "essentially, just sitting around, because I'm afraid to put too much weight on my ankle. I have been eating as usual, but I haven't been drinking so much because I hate to have to get up to use the bathroom."

A physical examination was conducted and the following were found: Bowel sounds were present in all quadrants, percussion revealed dullness in the left lower quadrant (LLQ), the abdomen was softly distended and nontender, and there were dry feces in the rectum.

Assessment refers to the collection of subjective and objective data in order to plan and provide care for the client. Recall that subjective data is information that the client experiences and reports to the nurse. Subjective data for Mrs. Jacobs include the following: achy stomach for a couple of days; one or two hard, little bowel movements in 5 days; fear of weight bearing; limited activity; eating solid foods; and decreased fluid intake.

Objective data is observed or measured by the nurse. The objective data for Mrs. Jacobs include the following: bowel sounds in all four quadrants of the abdomen, dullness to percussion in the LLQ, no tenderness, soft distention of the abdomen, and dry feces in the rectum.

DIAGNOSIS

Step 2 of the nursing process is diagnosis. The nurse uses critical thinking and applies knowledge from the sciences and other disciplines to analyze and synthesize the data. Client strengths, risks, and weaknesses are clearly identified. Data is compared to normative values and standards. Normative values and standards include but are not limited to charts for growth and development, laboratory values (hemoglobin, hematocrit, total cholesterol, blood glucose, etc.), the degree of flexion in the joints, the rate and characteristics of pulses, blood pressure, heart sounds, skin texture, core body temperature, language development, role performance, and interdependent functions.

Similar data is clustered or grouped together. The professional nurse makes a judgment after analysis and synthesis of collected data. This then becomes the **nursing diagnosis,** which is the basis for planning and implementing nursing care.

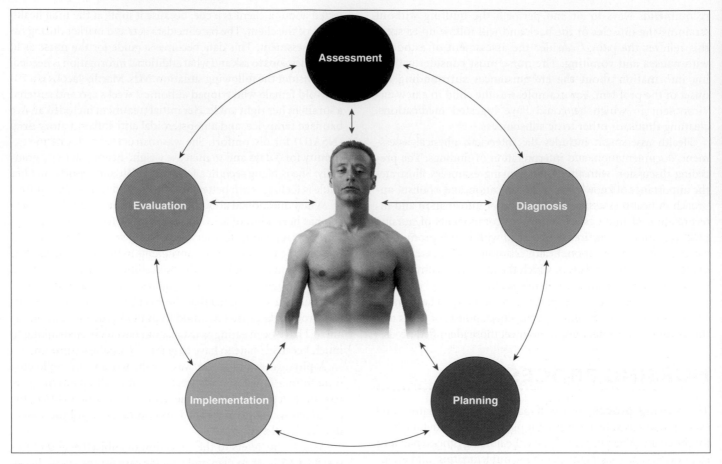

Figure 1.6 ● Nursing process.

The following is an analysis of the data from the previously cited assessment of Mrs. Jacobs. The analysis will describe the comparison to normative values and standards for the subjective and objective data, respectively. The achy abdomen is a deviation from normal because the abdomen is pain-free under normal conditions. One or two small, hard bowel movements in 5 days is considered an abnormal finding because stools are normally moist and because it is a deviation from the client's normal bowel pattern of soft stool, once daily. Fear of weight bearing is a normal finding. Most individuals experience anxiety after a painful injury. Older adults tend to feel anxious because they fear falling or further injury and potential loss of independence. However, "just sitting around" or immobility increases the risk, especially in older adults, for physical problems including elimination problems, weakness, and joint discomfort. Psychologically, the older adult may lose independence or become socially isolated. Eating as usual can be considered an abnormal finding in light of the fact that this client has decreased activity, change in elimination, and abdominal discomfort. Decreased fluid intake is an abnormal finding. The client understands the relationship between the amount of intake and the frequency and amount of urination; however, her actions increase her risk for other physical problems.

The findings from the physical examination include the presence of bowel sounds in all four abdominal quadrants. This is a normal finding. Bowel sounds are indicative of peristaltic activity. Dullness to percussion in the LLQ is an abnormal but not unexpected finding. The infrequency and characteristics of this client's

bowel movements indicate that feces are present in the rectum and descending colon. The abdomen is found to be nontender, which is a normal finding. Abdominal distention is an abnormal finding and indicative of stool and flatus accumulation in the bowel. Dry feces in the rectum are an abnormal but not unexpected finding because Mrs. Jacobs stated she had not been drinking much fluid. Moisture of the feces is related to fluid intake.

The analysis of assessment data includes clustering of information. The clusters consist of related pieces of information. The following clusters can be developed from the analysis of the objective and subjective data for Mrs. Jacobs.

● Achy, softly distended abdomen with dullness to percussion in the LLQ, infrequent hard stools with dry feces in rectum

● Eating regularly, decreased fluid intake

● Immobility, fear of weight bearing

After clustering the data, judgments are made and diagnoses are formulated. Diagnoses are generally two-part statements. The first part identifies the problem or strength demonstrated in the data and it is related to (R/T) the second part, that is, the likely cause of the problem. The following are several of many diagnostic statements that could be derived from the data for Mrs. Jacobs.

1. Constipation R/T lack of knowledge of the impact of fluid intake on bowel elimination

2. Immobility R/T fear of pain

3. Abdominal discomfort R/T constipation

A taxonomy, a conceptual framework for the formulation of nursing diagnoses, has been developed by the North American Nursing Diagnosis Association (NANDA). See Appendix A. ∞

Three types of nursing diagnoses are identified within the NANDA taxonomy: actual problems, risks for problems, and wellness issues. The following are examples of each type of diagnosis. *Ineffective breathing pattern* is a diagnostic statement, which exemplifies an actual problem. The statement *at risk for suicide* is representative of a diagnosis of a risk for a problem. An example of a diagnostic statement for wellness issues would be *readiness for enhanced family coping.*

Each NANDA diagnosis is composed of four components: a diagnostic label, a definition, defining characteristics, and risks or related factors. *Anxiety* is an example of a diagnostic label. Anxiety is defined as a state of mental uneasiness, apprehension, or dread in response to a perceived threat to oneself. Defining characteristics for anxiety include a verbal statement of anxiety (I feel anxious) or observed evidence including trembling, pallor, or a change in vital signs. Risks or related factors include physical or other factors that promote anxiety. For example, uncertainty about the outcome of a physical examination, uncertainty about the cause of a physical symptom such as a severe and prolonged headache, a job interview, or public speaking may promote anxiety.

NANDA diagnoses are formulated using a PES statement. The problem (P) is the diagnostic label, the etiology (E) includes the cause and contributing factors, and the signs and symptoms (S) are the defining characteristics. The PES statement of a diagnosis from the case study for Mrs. Jacobs would be written as follows: constipation (P) related to lack of knowledge (E) as evidenced by abdominal distention, achy abdomen, infrequent hard stool, and low fluid intake (S).

Each chapter in Unit III of this text includes a case study. ∞ The reader will be expected to analyze the data from the case studies in relation to critical thinking, the nursing process, and the development of nursing diagnoses.

PLANNING

Planning, step 3 of the nursing process, involves setting priorities, stating client goals or outcomes, and selecting nursing interventions, strategies, or orders to deal with the health status of the client. When possible, these activities need to include input from the client. Consultation or additional input may be needed from other healthcare professionals and family members. The developed nursing care plan acts as a guide for client care. This will help to enhance client strengths and help to negate, change, or prevent a weakness or problem for the client.

Planning, as previously stated, involves setting priorities, stating client goals, and selecting strategies to address the diagnoses. The priority for Mrs. Jacobs is to decrease her abdominal discomfort. This can be accomplished by addressing the factors that contribute to the problem. The nurse uses the diagnostic statements to develop goals and interventions. The goal is stated in terms of the expected client outcome, includes a time frame, and is derived from the first part of the diagnosis. The interventions are developed by determining the strategies to address the causes of the problem and are derived from the second part of the diagnostic statement.

The first diagnosis for Mrs. Jacobs, constipation R/T lack of knowledge of the impact of fluid intake on bowel elimination, will generate the following goal: The client will resume normal bowel elimination patterns within 72 hours.

The interventions are derived from the second part of the diagnosis. The intervention for Mrs. Jacobs will address her lack of knowledge about fluid intake in relation to bowel function. Therefore, the nursing intervention involves teaching Mrs. Jacobs.

IMPLEMENTATION

Implementation is step 4 of the nursing process. Now the care plan is put into action. Putting the nursing interventions into action, the professional nurse determines the client's need for assistance or the ability to function independently to achieve the stated goals. The professional nurse continues with the ongoing assessment of the client to update the database as behaviors change. The documentation of the implemented actions will include the client's response to nursing care. These actions will help meet the stated goals or outcomes, promote wellness, or convert illness to an improved state of health.

The intervention prescribed for Mrs. Jacobs, as previously stated, is teaching. Therefore, the nurse will teach Mrs. Jacobs by explaining the relationship of fluid intake to effective bowel function and include a discussion of the recommended amounts of fluid intake for adults. Providing information about the types of fluids that affect bowel elimination, such as fruit juices, would be part of the intervention.

EVALUATION

Step 5, the final step of the nursing process, is evaluation. The professional nurse compares the present client status to achievement of the stated goals or outcomes. At this time the nurse will need to modify the nursing care plan. This modification can be to continue, change, or terminate the nursing care plan based on goal achievement.

Evaluation refers to the determination that the goal has been achieved within the stated time frame. Recall that the goal for Mrs. Jacobs was to resume normal bowel elimination within 72 hours. The nurse must follow up with Mrs. Jacobs in 72 hours to determine if she has experienced a soft bowel movement on 2 consecutive days. This would indicate a return to normal bowel function for this client. If the goal has not been reached, the plan must be modified and further assessment or action may be required.

It is important to point out that several goals and interventions would be required to achieve the appropriate outcome for Mrs. Jacobs. Her bowel function is related to immobility and anxiety as well as decreased fluid intake. Goals would be derived for all diagnoses, and nursing interventions would be employed to address all of the causative factors.

CRITICAL THINKING

Critical thinking is a cognitive skill employed in all nursing activities and enhances the application of the nursing process. Alfaro-LeFevre (2003), defined and explained the critical thinking process. This work provided the foundation for the following discussion. **Critical thinking** is a process of purposeful and

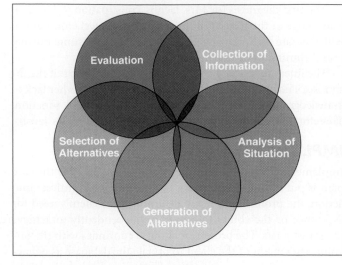

Figure 1.7 ● Elements of critical thinking.

creative thinking about resolutions of problems or the development of ways to manage situations. Critical thinking is more than problem solving; it is a way to apply logic and cognitive skills to the complexities of client care. It demands that nurses avoid bias and prejudice in their approach while using all of the knowledge and resources at their disposal to assist clients in achieving health goals or maintaining well-being.

When critically thinking about the client's health status, problems, or situations, one applies essential elements and skills. The five essential elements of critical thinking are collection of information, analysis of the situation, generation of alternatives, selection of alternatives, and evaluation. Figure 1.7 ● depicts the elements of critical thinking.

Each element has working skills to help the nurse be complete, thorough, and competent with the cognitive processes of critical thinking. Critical thinking skills are linked with each of the essential elements. The following discussion provides information and examples of the linkage of the elements and skills of critical thinking as they are applied in health assessment. Additionally, each chapter of Unit III includes a case study and questions to provide opportunities to apply critical thinking skills. ∞

COLLECTION OF INFORMATION

Collection of information, the first of the elements in critical thinking, involves the five skills of identifying assumptions, organizing data collection, determining the reliability of the data, identifying relevant versus irrelevant data, and identifying inconsistencies in the data (see Figure 1.8 ●). In use of this first skill, the nurse must be able to identify assumptions that can misguide or misdirect the assessment and intervention processes. For example, when interviewing a client, one must not assume that lack of eye contact indicates lack of attention, dishonesty, or apathy when it occurs in Asian, Native American, and other individuals.

The second skill of collection of information is organizing data collection. Collection of subjective and objective data must be carried out in an organized manner. In health assess-

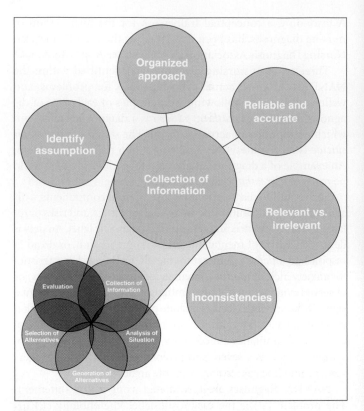

Figure 1.8 ● The five skills of the element Collection of Information.

ment the nurse first determines the client's current health status, level of distress, and ability to participate in the assessment process. The aim of data gathering in a client in acute distress is rapid identification of the problem and significant predisposing and contributory factors in order to select and initiate interventions to alleviate the distress. In nonacute situations, assessment follows an accepted and organized framework of survey, interview, and physical assessment.

The third skill of collection of information is determining the reliability of the data. One must recall that client information is valuable if it is reliable and accurate. The client is generally the best source of information, especially historical. However, physical and psychological factors may interfere with that capability. Information is then sought from a family member or caregiver who can provide reliable information. Other reliable sources of information include charts, medical records, and notes from other health professionals. One must also be certain that objective data is accurate. Measuring devices must be standardized, calibrated, and applied correctly.

A wealth of information is obtained when carrying out a comprehensive health assessment. One then applies the fourth critical thinking skill, which is to determine the relevance of the information in relation to the client's current, evolving, or potential condition or situation. Consider the relevance of nonimmunization or contraction of German measles in a male client seeking care for a fracture versus a 26-year-old sexually active female having an annual examination.

Identifying inconsistencies is the last of the skills associated with the element of collection of information. The nurse must be able to recognize discrepancies in the information. Further, one must determine if the inconsistency is a result of an oversight, misunderstanding, linguistic factor, or cultural factor. Indication of confusion, memory impairment, and subtle or overt communication indicating discomfort with a topic or area of questioning must also be considered. The following is an example of an inconsistency indicating misunderstanding. During the interview a client failed to identify a surgical repair of a fracture when asked about surgical procedures, but reported it when asked about the treatment for accidents or injuries. The inconsistency may not become apparent until the physical assessment takes place. A client may say that he or she has never used street drugs, but during the assessment the nurse may see track marks on the arms. The nurse must use care in communication while dealing with the inconsistency.

ANALYSIS OF THE SITUATION

The second element of critical thinking is analysis of the situation. The following five skills are linked to this element: distinguish data as normal or abnormal, cluster related data, identify patterns in the data, identify missing information, and draw valid conclusions (see Figure 1.9 ●).

The first of the skills is distinguishing normal from abnormal data. The nurse uses knowledge of human behavior as well as anatomy and physiology to compare findings with established norms in these areas. The nurse will use standards for laboratory results, diagnostic testing, charts, scales, and measures related to development and aging. The data must be analyzed in relation to expected ranges for age, gender, genetic background, and culture of the client. Consider the following situation: In a regularly scheduled checkup, John Morgan, age 31,

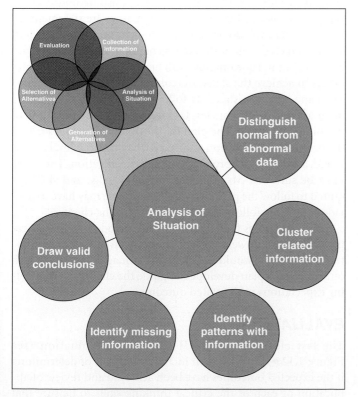

Figure 1.9 ● The five skills of the element Analysis of Situation.

undergoes a complete health assessment. He is found to have alopecia (hair loss) at the anterior hairline and thinning of the hair that has increased since his last visit. The nurse knows that alopecia occurs more frequently in men than in women, that in male pattern baldness the alopecia begins at the anterior hairline, and that alopecia is genetic and begins in early adulthood. When all other findings are within the normal limits for a 31-year-old male, the nurse considers the alopecia a normal finding in this client.

If the previously mentioned finding had occurred during an assessment of Margaret Lane, a 31-year-old female, the nurse would apply the same knowledge and consider alopecia an abnormal finding. Further, other findings would be carefully examined. In this situation, Ms. Lane stated in the health history, "I'm tired all the time. I must be anemic because I'm cold all the time and on top of all that I'm constipated." Additionally, she said, "I think I'm becoming irregular because I'm too tired to exercise and don't eat right and I guess that has messed up my periods too; it lasts much longer than it ever did." Findings during the physical assessment included pallor, weight gain, dry skin, and brittle nails. The nurse must now begin to apply the other skills associated with analysis of the situation.

When critically thinking, the nurse will cluster related information by sorting and categorizing information into groupings that may include but are not limited to cues, symptoms, body systems, or health practices. The following are clusters derived from the data about Ms. Lane:

- Skin dry, nails brittle, hair thinning and loss
- Constipation, irregularity, weight gain, "not eating right"
- Lack of exercise, tired, cold, pallor, "I must be anemic"
- Prolonged menstruation

Once the clustering has been completed, the nurse must apply the third skill of identifying patterns in the information. Use of this skill enables the nurse to get an idea about what is happening with the client and to determine if more information is required. The nurse must rely on knowledge and resources in identifying patterns. One might consider a pattern suggesting a nutritional or abdominal problem since information includes changes in eating, changes in bowel elimination, fatigue, and changes in the skin and hair. The data also suggest a metabolic or hormonal problem. However, the information is incomplete.

At this point the nurse would identify missing information, the fourth skill. Missing information would include but is not limited to onset of symptoms, medication history, family history of similar problems, and measures the client has taken to alleviate the problems. Additional information would include laboratory studies of hematologic, metabolic, or hormonal function.

The following is subjective data from the interview of Ms. Lane: *The symptoms had been going on for over a year, gradually getting worse. She didn't take any medications except Advil for a headache now and then. She knows of no one in her family with a problem like hers and she hasn't done anything except take laxatives sometimes, use hand cream, and try all kinds of hair care products that friends recommend.* The nurse explained the need for diagnostic studies. Ms. Lane obtained the requested laboratory and diagnostic testing and returned for a follow-up visit. The reports of several laboratory studies were as follows: Hgb 10 g/dl, Hct 30%, RBC 3.6, T_3 0.18, T_4 0.7 μg/dl, TSH 6.0 μU/ml, glucose 126.

The nurse has acquired information necessary to apply the last skill of drawing valid conclusions. This skill requires using all of one's knowledge and reasoning skills to draw logical conclusions about a problem or situation. The nurse concludes, based on history, objective findings in physical assessment, and diagnostic testing, that Ms. Lane has hypothyroidism. The critical thinking process continues as the nurse works with the client to develop a treatment plan for her problem.

Assessment is the focus of this text, and students will be applying the previously mentioned steps in the critical thinking process. To identify the importance of critical thinking to future practice, a discussion of the remaining elements and skills is included. These skills are essential to delivery of competent nursing care. The nurse gathers data, determines the meaning of the data, and decides what to do once information gathering is completed. The nursing actions often depend on the level of practice. For example, autonomous decisions such as diagnosis and treatment of disease by prescription of medication is within the role of the advanced practice nurse. For the generalist, data is shared with physicians who prescribe medical treatment. The generalist develops interventions such as education, support, and some modes for symptom relief as part of professional practice. Furthermore, the nurse brings a holistic approach to the client situation. Therefore, the nurse will collaborate with all healthcare professionals to be sure that plans are developed to meet individual physical and psychosocial needs.

GENERATION OF ALTERNATIVES

Articulating options and establishing priorities are the two skills associated with the critical thinking element of generation of alternatives (see Figure 1.10 ●). Articulation of options is simply stating possible paths to follow or actions to take to resolve a problem. There are several options for treatment of the client, Ms. Lane, cited previously: (1) Begin treatment with thyroid medication immediately as prescribed by the nurse practitioner, (2) delay the treatment with thyroid medication while continuing with diagnostic testing to establish the cause of the problem, (3) delay treatment with thyroid medication and seek a referral with an endocrinologist, or (4) initiate treatments to relieve symptoms.

Once the options have been enumerated, the nurse and client work together to establish priorities. This process must reflect the acuity of the problem and the client's ability to interpret the information required to weigh the advantages and disadvantages of each of the options in relation to health, lifestyle, cultural, and socioeconomic factors. The nurse knows the aim of therapy in hypothyroidism is to achieve and maintain normal thyroid functioning by administering thyroid replacement for the life of the client. Symptoms associated with hypothyroidism subside with thyroid replacement therapy. Immediate relief of discomfort can be achieved through dietary and activity modifications. The nurse shares this knowledge with Ms. Lane and priorities are established.

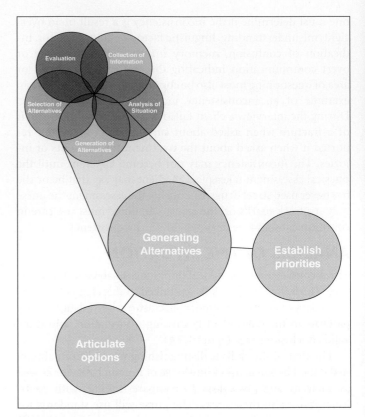

Figure 1.10 ● The two skills of the element Generating Alternatives.

SELECTION OF ALTERNATIVES

Selection of alternatives is the next element of critical thinking, and linked with it are the skills of developing outcomes and developing plans (see Figure 1.11 ●). Outcomes are statements of what the client will do or be able to do in a specific time period. The plan includes all of the actions required by the client independently or in coordination with healthcare professionals and others to achieve the stated outcomes. An overall outcome for Ms. Lane could be stated as follows: Ms. Lane will have and maintain normal thyroid levels within 5 weeks of initial dose of thyroid replacement. The plan for the outcome includes taking the prescribed medication as directed, having drug levels monitored, and reporting problems with the medication. The nurse must be sure that Ms. Lane has the knowledge and skills required to follow the plan. Therefore, the nurse may have to provide education, follow-up, and support for the client.

Some outcomes for Ms. Lane could include weight loss, return of normal bowel function, and improved nutritional status. A time frame would be determined for achievement of each outcome and a plan developed to guide the client toward meeting expectations in the stated outcomes.

EVALUATION

The last element in critical thinking is evaluation (see Figure 1.12 ●). This element includes the skills of determining if the expected outcomes have been achieved and review of application of each of the critical thinking skills to be sure that omissions and misinterpretations did not occur. In addition,

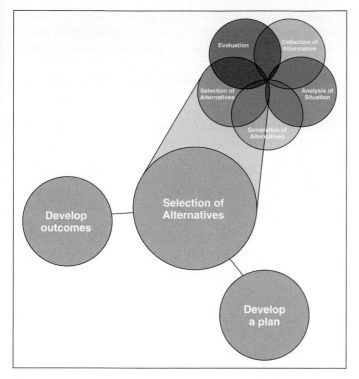

Figure 1.11 ● The two skills of the element Selection of Alternatives.

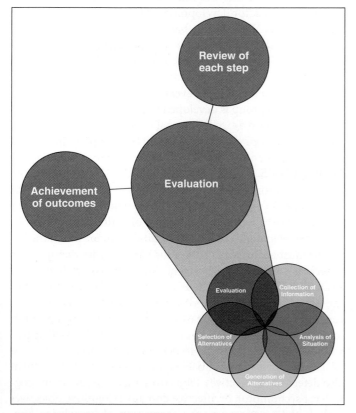

Figure 1.12 ● The two skills of the element Evaluation.

the nurse must evaluate thinking and judgment in the situation. One must be sure that decisions and actions were based on knowledge and the use of reliable resources and information. Furthermore, one must be sure that acts are based on moral and

ethical principles and that the effects of values and biases have been considered. The nurse would follow up with Ms. Lane to determine if each of the expected outcomes has been achieved in a timely manner.

ROLE OF THE PROFESSIONAL NURSE

The professional nurse provides care to the clients needing and seeking help. Nursing care is based on a strong knowledge base and the application of critical thinking. The knowledge base of the professional nurse is developed over time using information from the humanities and the biological, natural, and social sciences. Using research data, standards of care, and the nursing process, the professional nurse provides competent care. The client will be the individual, family, or community. The individual could be any age and at any developmental level. The actions of the professional nurse will be directed to promote health and wellness, treat and care for the ill, and care for the dying individual while being supportive to family members. To perform these actions, the nurse works in a variety of settings including hospitals, clinics, nursing homes, clients' homes, schools, and workplaces.

Regardless of the setting, the role of the professional nurse is multifaceted. Each situation requires the professional nurse to use critical thinking and the nursing process. To provide care and utilize the nursing process, the professional nurse must develop strong assessment skills. The gathering of complete, accurate, and relevant data is required. While gathering the subjective and objective data from the client, the nurse must be attuned to the signs, symptoms, behaviors, and cues offered by the client. The collected data varies as the status of the client changes. The professional nurse functions as a teacher, caregiver, client advocate, and manager of client care.

TEACHER

As a teacher, the nurse helps the client to acquire knowledge required for health maintenance or improvement, to prevent illness or injury, to manage therapies, and to make decisions about health and treatment. Teaching occurs in all settings and for a variety of reasons and may be informal or formal. Teaching is an important intervention to promote wellness and prevent illness. This intervention is enacted when collection and analysis of client data reveal a knowledge deficit, a need for education about an identified risk, or readiness to learn to enhance health. These three conditions represent the three types of diagnoses in the NANDA taxonomy: actual problems, risk for a problem, or a wellness issue. Teaching is such an important intervention that each chapter of Unit III of this text includes a section called Health Promotion in which common risk factors and intervention strategies are identified. ⏎ Further, each assessment chapter includes a teaching plan. The teaching plans included in this text and on the Companion Website are derived from case study information and are intended to illustrate this important nursing intervention.

Informal Teaching

Informal teaching generally occurs as a natural part of a client encounter. This type of teaching may be to provide instructions, to explain a question or procedure, or to reduce anxiety. For example, while asking about medications and the use of natural, herbal, or home remedies during the health history interview, the nurse may offer an explanation as follows: "This information is important because medications may interact with each other or with herbs and natural substances. The interaction can sometimes be harmful or change the effectiveness of one of your prescribed medications." The same information may be offered in response to a client statement or question such as, "What is so important that I have to go over my medications every time I come here?"

Explanations are offered to inform the client and often reduce anxiety. When performing a physical assessment, the nurse provides explanations. For example, "I would like you to take a deep breath in and out, through your mouth, each time I place the stethoscope on your chest. This will help me to clearly hear the air as it moves in and out of your lungs." The nurse may explain a technique during assessment of the musculoskeletal system as follows: "You will notice that I've asked you to push with both arms against my hands; that is so I can compare the strength of the left and right arms."

The following are additional examples of informal teaching. In response to parents' concerns about their infant's height and weight, the nurse explains how charts are used to assess growth and development and assists them to compare their child's data with that on the chart. A child with food allergies may approach the school nurse and ask, "I forgot my lunch today. Can I eat this packaged tuna thing from the machine?" The nurse will explain that the ingredients must be checked and may state, "I'll help you look at the container and we can determine if it is okay to eat."

Formal Teaching

Formal teaching occurs in response to an identified learning need of an individual, group, or community. Teaching plans are developed for formal teaching sessions. There are six components in teaching plans: the identified learning need, the goal, objectives, content, teaching strategies and rationales, and evaluation, as noted in Box 1.3. Teaching plans are developed to meet distinct needs of individual clients or common needs of individuals, groups, or communities. When developing or using previously developed teaching plans, the nurse must consider the age, gender, developmental level, culture, linguistic ability, dexterity, physical ability or limitations, and resources of the client or group. The selection of the content and methods for teaching and evaluation of learning should be influenced by the previously mentioned factors. For example, use of

Box 1.3	**Elements of a Teaching Plan**
• Learning Need	• Content
• Goal	• Teaching Strategy/Rationale
• Objectives	• Evaluation

printed materials would be inappropriate for a client with impaired vision or with limited literacy. The nurse would not include referral to Internet sites for clients without computer access. It would be best to suggest walking in a park or using a public facility for exercise rather than a health club for those with limited income. The following sections address each of the components of the teaching plan.

THE LEARNING NEED. Learning needs are identified as discrete knowledge deficits for an individual, or common needs of individuals and groups. Individual learning needs can be identified through the interview or in communication with a client throughout the assessment process. Consider the following situation. Janelle James, a 20-year-old female, states during the health history, "I do not perform self-breast examination. I don't know how to do it." Self-breast examination (SBE) is an important part of health promotion and disease prevention. Therefore, Janelle James has a need to learn about SBE.

The need for learning in individuals, families, and groups arises in response to lack of knowledge about common changes or risks that occur with aging, role change and development, illness, health promotion, and disease prevention. The following provides an example of a learning need for a group. A community center provides health promotion classes for senior citizens. The sessions are planned in collaboration with healthcare providers in the community. One session was developed to address the need for information about breast health because of the increased risk for development of breast cancer with aging.

THE GOAL. The goal is based on an identified learning need. The goal is written as a broad statement of the expected outcome of the learning. When considering the need for Janelle James, the goal would be broadly stated as follows: The client will accurately perform SBE every month.

A goal for a group is developed in response to identification of a learning need as well. The goal for the senior females with increased risk for breast cancer would be: The participants will follow recommended guidelines for breast cancer screening.

OBJECTIVES. In the teaching plan the objectives identify specific, measurable behaviors or activities expected of the client or group. Action verbs are used to denote the behavior or activity. Table 1.1 provides examples of action verbs. The objectives may include criteria or conditions under which the behavior must occur. An objective for Janelle James that includes criteria is written as follows: The client will correctly demonstrate SBE. Objectives include a time frame for completion of the objective. An example of a time frame for objectives for teaching a group about breast health would be written as follows: At the completion of the learning session, the participants will identify three measures to detect breast cancer.

The type of learning or behavior that is expected of the client also determines objectives. Objectives, therefore, are in the cognitive, psychomotor, or affective domains. Cognitive objectives include those concerning the acquisition of knowledge. Psychomotor objectives include the acquisition of skills. The affective domain refers to attitudes, feelings, values, and opinions. The expectation for Janelle James is that she will be able to perform a skill. The objective for performance of SBE is in the psychomotor domain. The example of an objective for the group

Table 1.1	Action Verbs for Development of Objectives	
DOMAIN	**ACTION VERBS**	
Cognitive	Appraises	Explains
	Changes	Generates
	Composes	Matches
	Concludes	Modifies
	Converts	Names
	Creates	Reorganizes
	Criticizes	Separates
	Defines	Solves
	Designs	States
	Diagrams	Subdivides
	Discriminates	Summarizes
Affective	Acts	Greets
	Adheres	Justifies
	Describes	Modifies
	Discusses	Presents
	Displays	Proposes
	Explains	
Psychomotor	Assembles	Fixes
	Calibrates	Makes
	Changes	Manipulates
	Demonstrates	Operates
	Dismantles	

learning about breast health is in the cognitive domain because it calls for the participants to identify three measures for breast cancer detection.

CONTENT. The content within a teaching plan refers to what will actually be taught. The objective for Janelle James states: The client will perform SBE. Therefore, the content must include the steps and actions required for SBE. The content to address the objective of identifying three measures for breast cancer detection would include information about SBE, annual examination by a healthcare provider, mammography, ultrasonic examination, and biopsy.

TEACHING METHODS. Teaching methods or strategies are the channels or avenues used to present the content. They must be suited to the needs of the learner and the type of learning that is expected. Psychomotor learning requires, for example in the case of Janelle James, demonstration as one teaching methodology. One-on-one discussion is a common strategy for individual client teaching. Group teaching strategies may include lecture, discussion, or role-play. Table 1.2 includes information about teaching methods.

EVALUATION. A plan for evaluation of learning is included in the teaching plan. In evaluation, one determines if the learning objectives have been achieved. The learning domain of the objective determines the methods for evaluation. Cognitive learning may be evaluated verbally through questions or in discussion with the client or by use of written measurements. Written evaluations include short answer, true-false,

fill-in, multiple-choice, and other types of tests. Members of the group learning about breast cancer detection, as described earlier, could be evaluated by a short answer quiz at the end of the session. Psychomotor learning is best evaluated by a demonstration of the skill expected in the objective. Janelle James would be evaluated through a return demonstration of SBE. Affective objectives are difficult to evaluate. Listening to the client and observing behavior that indicates feelings and values are effective methods. For example, one would determine if participants value prevention as part of health promotion and receive flu immunization. When evaluation reveals that learning has not taken place, the nurse may have to repeat all or part of the teaching.

CAREGIVER

The caregiver role has always been the traditional role of the nurse. Historically, physical care was the primary focus. Today, the nurse uses a holistic approach to nursing care. Using critical thinking and the nursing process, the professional nurse provides direct and indirect care to the client. Indirect care is accomplished with the delegation of activities to other members of the team. As client advocate the professional nurse acts as a protector. Clients are kept informed of their rights, given information to make informed decisions, and encouraged to speak for themselves. As a case manager, the professional nurse helps to coordinate care, manages the multidisciplinary team, and plans client outcomes within a specific time frame. Providing care, maintaining cost of care, and identifying the effectiveness of the plan are all responsibilities of the case manager.

ADVANCED PRACTICE ROLES

The advanced formal education and expanded roles of the nurse permit the professional nurse to function in advanced roles. These advanced roles include but are not limited to nurse researcher, practitioner, clinical specialist, administrator, and educator.

Nurse Researcher

The nurse researcher identifies problems regarding client care, designs plans of study, and develops tools. Findings are analyzed and knowledge is disseminated. The nurse performing the research adds to the body of knowledge of the profession, gives direction for future research, and improves client care.

Nurse Practitioner

The nurse practitioner, with advanced degrees and certified by the American Nurses Credentialing Center, practices independently in a variety of situations. At an agency or community-based setting, one could find a school nurse practitioner, family nurse practitioner, or gerontology nurse practitioner meeting the healthcare needs of clients seeking assistance.

Clinical Nurse Specialist

Clinical nurse specialists have advanced education and degrees in a specific aspect of practice. They provide direct client care, direct and teach other team members providing care, and conduct nursing research within the area of specialization.

Table 1.2	Teaching Methods		
TEACHING METHOD	**DOMAIN**	**ADVANTAGES**	**DISADVANTAGES**
Explanation	Cognitive	May be used for individual or group.	Passive learning.
One-on-One Discussion	Cognitive Affective	Learner participation. Clarification can be provided. Questions can be answered.	Requires time for discussion and to allow for questions.
Lecture	Cognitive	Useful for large groups. Facts presented in logical manner.	Passive learning.
Group Discussion	Cognitive Affective	Learners are more comfortable in groups. Allows participation of all members.	Can easily lose focus in a group discussion.
Case Study	Cognitive	Develops problem-solving skills. Allows learners to explore complex concepts.	Difficult to develop. Learners may have difficulty applying information to their own situation.
Role-Play	Cognitive Affective	Allows learners to appreciate different points of view. Learners actively participate.	Learners may be too anxious to participate. Effective in small groups only.
Demonstration	Psychomotor	Can be used with individuals and groups.	Passive learning.
Practice	Psychomotor	Learners actively involved. Hands-on experience.	Time consuming. Effective with small groups only to provide feedback.
Printed Material	Cognitive	Efficiently presents important information. Can supplement other teaching methods.	May not meet needs of low-literacy learners or those with language differences. Passive learning.
Media Audiovisual Presentation	Cognitive Affective Psychomotor	Can be used in all types of learning. Can supplement other teaching methods. Provides aural and visual stimulation.	Time consuming. Passive learning.
Computer-Assisted Instruction (CAI)	Cognitive Affective Psychomotor	Can be used with individuals and groups. Learning is active. Provides immediate feedback.	Requires equipment. Time consuming.

Nurse Administrator

Today, the role of the nurse administrator varies. Professional titles include vice president of nursing services, supervisor, or nurse manager of a specific unit. The responsibilities vary and could include staffing, budgets, client care, staff performance evaluations, consulting, and ensuring that goals of the agency are being accomplished. Advanced degrees are usually required for these positions. It is common to find nurse administrators with advanced degrees in several disciplines such as nursing and business administration.

Nurse Educator

The nurse educator, a nurse with advanced degrees, is employed to teach in a nursing program. This could be at a university, community college, or department of staff development in an agency providing nursing care. The educator is responsible for didactic and clinical teaching, curriculum development, clinical placement, and practice for students. The educator provides the student with the opportunity to practice assessment skills in a variety of settings with a diverse client population.

This chapter has presented an overview of concepts and processes important to health assessment. Aspects of nursing practice, knowledge, and skills required for the changing role of the nurse in today's healthcare arena have been introduced. These include health, comprehensive assessment, nursing process, critical thinking, communication, documentation, and teaching. An in-depth discussion of these important concepts is presented in succeeding chapters of this book. Development of knowledge, skills, and techniques is enhanced through the use of clinical examples and case studies. *Healthy People 2010*, the initiative to promote the health of individuals and communities, is developed as a feature in this text.

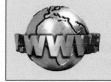

Application Through Critical Thinking

CASE STUDY

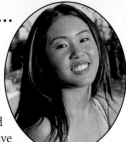

*M*ary Wong is a 19-year-old college freshman living in the dormitory. She has come to the University Health Center with the following complaints: Nausea, vomiting, abdominal pain increasing in severity, diarrhea, a fever, and dry mouth. She tells you, the nurse, "I have had abdominal pain for about 12 hours with nausea, vomiting, and diarrhea." These symptoms, she tells you, "all started after supper in the student cafeteria on campus."

You conduct an interview and follow it with a physical examination which reveals the following: symmetrical abdomen, bowel sounds in all quadrants, tender to palpation in the lower quadrants, guarding. Mary's skin is warm and moist, her lips and mucous membranes are dry.

► *Critical Thinking Questions*

1. Identify the findings as objective or subjective data.
2. Prepare a narrative nursing note from the data.
3. What factors must be considered in conducting the comprehensive health assessment of Mary Wong?
4. Prior to developing a nursing diagnosis, what must you do?

Please refer to the Companion Website at www.prenhall.com/damico and click on Chapter 1, the Application Through Critical Thinking module, to answer these and additional questions. In addition, complete NCLEX-RN® review questions and other interactive resources for this chapter.

EXPLORE MediaLink

Additional resources for this chapter are found on the Student CD-ROM accompanying this textbook and on the Companion Website.

CD-ROM CONTENT

Content for this chapter includes:
Objectives
Key Concepts
NCLEX-RN® Review Questions
Audio Glossary
Head-to-Toe Physical Examination Video

COMPANION WEBSITE CONTENT

www.prenhall.com/damico

Content for this chapter includes:
Objectives
NCLEX-RN® Review Questions

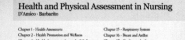
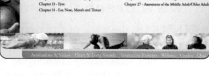

Application Through Critical Thinking
   Case Study Challenge
MediaLinks
MediaLink Application
Tool Box
   Focus Areas in *Healthy People 2010*
   Standard Abbreviations and Symbols
   Teaching Methods
New York Times

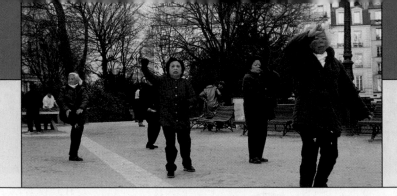

2

Wellness and Health Promotion

CHAPTER OBJECTIVES

Upon completion of this chapter, you will be able to:

1. Describe the concepts of wellness and health promotion.
2. Discuss theories of wellness.
3. Discuss perspectives of health promotion for the individual, family, and community.
4. Identify the leading health indicators in *Healthy People 2010.*
5. Discuss health promotion in relation to the nursing process.

MEDIALINK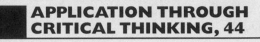

www.prenhall.com/damico

The CD-ROM in the back of this textbook and the Media-Link website contain NCLEX-RN® review questions, interactive exercises, case study challenges, animations, videos, documentation and checklist forms, and review materials. For a complete listing of the media content specific to Chapter 2, see the Explore MediaLink at the end of the chapter.

*I*n the modern world, wellness, health promotion, and health maintenance have become concerns to all. The client, the consumer of healthcare, is more active in the decision-making process related to healthcare issues. The client now has more control regarding the planning, implementation, and evaluation of strategies and outcomes of his or her health. As the healthcare delivery system has changed and become more complex, the roles of the healthcare providers, including the nurse, have expanded.

Individuals are currently more conscious of health and wellness. People have become more proactive regarding health and healthcare practices. This places a stronger emphasis on wellness, health promotion, and disease prevention. The *Healthy People 2010* initiative describes factors that influence individual and community health and wellness. The goals, leading health indicators, and focus areas of this important initiative are discussed in this chapter. Factors influencing health, identified in *Healthy People 2010*, are described in Unit I of this text. ⚭ Strategies that have been developed to promote wellness are then described and discussed in relation to health assessment in Unit III. ⚭

WELLNESS

Wellness describes a state of life that is balanced, personally satisfying, and characterized by the ability to adapt and to participate in activities that enhance quality of life. Concepts basic to wellness include self-responsibility and decision making regarding nutrition, physical fitness, stress management, emotional growth and well-being, personal safety, and healthcare.

WELLNESS THEORIES

Perceptions of wellness influence the nurse's approach to client care. When using a wellness perspective, the nurse focuses on the client's personal strengths and abilities to enhance health. The goals of nursing care are to assist the client to participate in health-promoting activities, prevent illness, and seek help for needs and problems. Additionally, the nurse focuses on the wellness concerns of the client and supports the client's spiritual and end-of-life needs. Theories regarding wellness have been developed and can assist nurses to clarify their perceptions of wellness. The theories of Dunn, Leavell and Clark, and Travis are presented in the following section.

Dunn

Dunn defined wellness for the individual as an integrated method of functioning that is oriented toward maximizing the potential of which the individual is capable. It requires the individual to maintain a continuum of balance and purposeful direction within the environment where he is functioning (Dunn, 1973). This theory is seen as a grid with two intersecting axes. Health intersects with environment, creating four quadrants (see Figure 2.1 ●). The health axis extends from peak wellness to death, creating various degrees of health and illness. The environmental axis moves from a most favorable environment to a most unfavorable environment. This model encourages the individual to maintain completeness and function at the greatest level of potential. It takes into consideration the uniqueness of the individual and the influence of family and community regarding healthcare practices.

Leavell and Clark

Leavell and Clark (1965) described primary, secondary, and tertiary levels of prevention in the healthcare system. In their model, actions are taken to maintain health, prevent illness, provide early detection of a disease, and restore the individual to the highest level of optimum functioning (see Figure 2.2 ●). The key word to emphasize the focus of primary prevention is *prepathogenic,* that is, before the development of disease or pathology. Actions are taken to prevent disease, illness, or injury. **Primary prevention** implies health and a high level of wellness for the individual. Immunizations, healthy diet, health teaching, genetic counseling, and correct use of safety equipment at work are examples of primary prevention strategies.

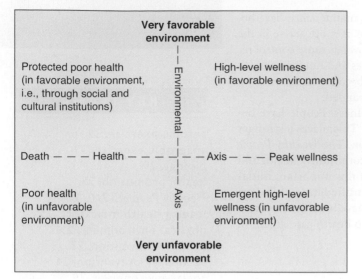

Figure 2.1 ● Dunn's model of wellness.

<table>
<tr><td>Wellness ——→ Illness ——→ Return to Wellness</td></tr>
</table>

Wellness ——→ Illness ——→ Return to Wellness

Prepathology ——→ Pathology ——→ Rehabilitation

| Primary | Secondary | Tertiary |
| Prevention | Prevention | Prevention |

Figure 2.2 ● Levels of prevention.

Table 2.1	**Levels of Prevention**	
LEVEL OF PREVENTION	**FOCUS**	**EXAMPLES**
Primary	Improving overall health Health promotion Prevention of illness, injury	Education about diet, exercise, environmental hazards, accident protection Immunization Assessment of risks for injury, illness
Secondary	Early identification of illness and treatment for existing health problems	Health screening and diagnostic procedures Regimens for treatment of illness Promotion of regular healthcare examinations across the life span
Tertiary	Return to optimum level of wellness after an illness or injury has occurred Prevention of recurrence of problems	Education to reduce or prevent complications of disease Referral to rehabilitation services

Early diagnosis of health problems, and prompt treatment with the restoration of health, is the focus of **secondary prevention.** Emphasis is on resolving health problems and preventing serious consequences. Screenings, blood tests, x-rays, surgery, and dental care are strategies utilized at this level of prevention.

Tertiary prevention is activity aimed to restore the individual to the highest possible level of health and functioning. Rehabilitation is the focus for tertiary prevention. Strategies include use of rehabilitation centers for orthopedic and neurologic problems. Teaching the client and family members

interventions to improve coping with a chronic illness and recognition of complications are examples of tertiary prevention strategies. Table 2.1 provides examples of nursing considerations in relation to the levels of prevention.

Travis

Travis and Ryan (1988) used a continuum to describe the state of health of the individual. At one end of the continuum is high-level wellness, and at the extreme other end is premature death. Between these two points are various degrees of health and illness. This model implies an ever changing state of health with the midpoint of the continuum being neutral (see Figure 2.3 ●)

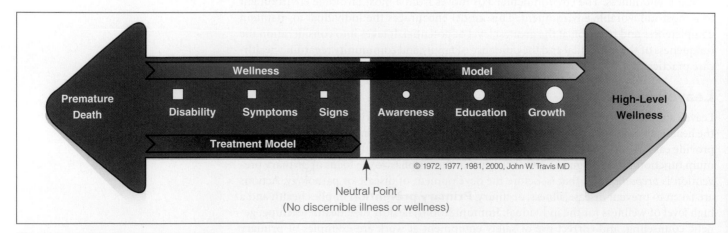

Figure 2.3 ● The illness/wellness continuum.

HEALTH PROMOTION

Health promotion refers to those actions used to increase health or well-being and the improvement of the health of individuals, families, and communities. Health promotion includes the prevention of disease and primary prevention measures, such as immunization.

DEFINITION

Pender, Murdaugh, and Parsons (2002) have defined **health promotion** as "behavior motivated by the desire to increase well-being and actualize human potential" (p. 7). Examples of health promotion activities include but are not limited to weight-control measures, exercise, management of stress, and coping with life experiences.

PERSPECTIVES ON HEALTH PROMOTION

An individual's health status or level of wellness is determined by risk factors, physical fitness, nutrition, health behaviors, and lifestyle. Certain risk factors cannot be controlled and these include age, genetic factors, biological characteristics, and family history. Individual health promotion includes the identification of lifestyle and environmental risks that influence the level of wellness and promoting efforts to reduce or eliminate the risks.

A variety of models have been developed to explain health promotion behaviors. These models assist in understanding individual behaviors in regard to health, are used in research related to health promotion, and guide interventions. These models include but are not limited to the health belief model, the theory of reasoned action/planned behavior, and the health promotion model.

Health Belief Model

The health belief model (Rosenstock, 1974) was developed to predict who would participate in health screenings or obtain vaccinations (see Figure 2.4 ●). According to the health belief model, the following individual perceptions influence the decision to act to prevent illness:

● One is vulnerable to an illness.
● The effects of the illness are serious.
● The behavior prevents the illness.
● The benefit of reducing a risk is greater than the cost of the preventive behavior.

Mediating variables influence individual perceptions. The first of the variables is perceived susceptibility, that is, the belief about the likelihood of developing an illness. Perceived severity is the second variable and refers to the individual's determination of how serious an illness would be. The severity includes physical, psychological, and social effects of illness. Another variable is the perceived cost of the health-promoting behavior. This refers to factors that interfere with the performance of a behavior. The individual must weigh physical and psychological cost versus the benefit.

The health belief model includes two constructs. These are cues to action and self-efficacy. Cues to action are internal and external stimuli that affect the individual's motivation to participate in health-promoting activities. For example, heart disease in a family member or the Great American Smokeout, a mass media campaign by the American Cancer Society, may motivate one to stop smoking. Self-efficacy refers to the level of confidence an individual has about the ability to perform the activity.

Last, mediating factors affect the health-promoting behaviors by influencing the perceptions of vulnerability, severity, effectiveness, and cost. Mediating factors include age, gender, ethnicity, education, and economic status.

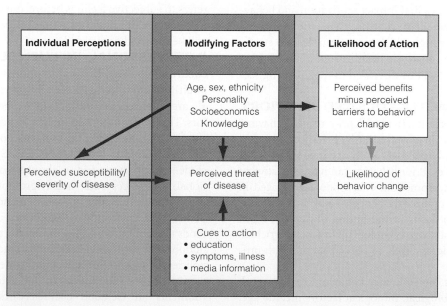

Figure 2.4 ● Health belief model.

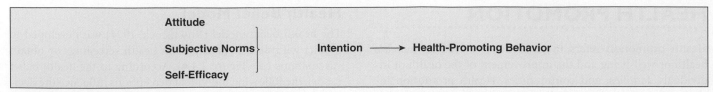

Figure 2.5 ● Theory of reasoned action/planned behavior.

Theory of Reasoned Action/Planned Behavior

The theory of reasoned action/planned behavior is a prediction theory representing a sociopsychological method for predicting health behavior (see Figure 2.5 ●). The theory of reasoned action/planned behavior is based on the assumptions that behavior is under volitional control and that people are rational beings. The theory holds that the intention to perform a behavior is a determinant in performance of the behavior.

Three variables affect the intention to perform a behavior: subjective norms, attitudes, and self-efficacy. *Subjective norms* refer to the individual's perception of what significant others believe or expect in relation to the individual's performance of a behavior. For example, whether one intends to begin a daily exercise program would be influenced by what one believes a spouse's opinion of the activity would be. *Attitudes* refer to value ascribed to a behavior. An attitude may be that eating a low-fat diet is a good way to prevent heart disease. *Self-efficacy* refers to the level of confidence in one's ability to perform a behavior (for example, feeling confident that a low-fat diet can be followed). According to the theory of reasoned action/planned behavior, an individual is likely to engage in health-promoting behavior when the individual believes that the benefit outweighs the cost.

Health Promotion Model

The health promotion model (Pender et al., 2002) is a competence model. Persons are depicted as "multidimensional and in interaction with interpersonal and physical environments as they pursue health." The model focuses on individual characteristics and behaviors, and variables that impact motivation and behavioral outcomes (see Figure 2.6 ●). The health promotion model provides a framework through which nurses can develop strategies to assist individuals to engage in health-promoting activities. Each aspect of the model will be discussed in the following sections of this chapter.

INDIVIDUAL CHARACTERISTICS AND BEHAVIORS. According to the health promotion model, prior related behaviors and personal factors have an effect on future behaviors. Prior related behaviors include knowledge, skill, and experience with health-promoting activities. Prior behavior can have a positive or negative effect on health promotion. When one has engaged in health promotion and recognized the benefit, it is likely that health-promoting behavior will occur in the future. Conversely, when health-promoting activities have been difficult or when barriers to participation arose, one is less likely to participate in health promotion in the future.

Personal factors that can influence behavior are biological, psychological, and sociological. Biological factors include age, gender, body mass index, strength, agility, and balance. Psycho-logical factors refer to self-esteem, motivation, and perceptions of one's health status. Socioeconomic status, education, race, and ethnicity are among the sociological factors considered within the health promotion model.

BEHAVIOR-SPECIFIC COGNITION AND AFFECT. Behavior-specific cognition and affect are variables that impact motivation to begin and continue activities to promote health. These variables include perceived benefit of action, perceived barriers to action, perceived self-efficacy, activity-related affect, interpersonal influences, and situational influences. Each of these variables is described in the following sections with appropriate examples.

PERCEIVED BENEFITS OF ACTION. Engagement in a particular behavior is determined by the belief that the behavior is beneficial or results in a positive outcome. Benefits may be intrinsic, such as stress reduction, or extrinsic, such as financial reward. Perceived benefits of actions motivate the individual to participate in health-promoting activities.

PERCEIVED BARRIERS TO ACTION. Barriers to participation in health-promoting activities may be real or imagined. The barriers include perceptions about the availability, expense, convenience, difficulty, and time required for an activity. Barriers are seen as hurdles and personal costs of participating in a behavior.

PERCEIVED SELF-EFFICACY. Perceived self-efficacy is a judgment of one's ability to successfully participate in a health-promoting activity to achieve a desired outcome. Individuals with high self-efficacy are more likely to overcome barriers and commit to health-promoting activity. Those with low self-efficacy have diminished efforts or cease participation in activities.

ACTIVITY-RELATED AFFECT. Activity-related affect refers to subjective feelings before, during, and after an activity. The positive or negative feelings influence whether a behavior will be repeated or avoided.

INTERPERSONAL INFLUENCES. Interpersonal influences are the individual's perceptions of the behaviors, beliefs, or attitudes of others. The family, peers, and health professionals are interpersonal influences on health-promoting behaviors. These influences also include expectations of others, social support, and modeling the behaviors of others.

SITUATIONAL INFLUENCES. Situational influences include perceptions and ideas about situations or contexts. Situational influences on health-promoting activities include perceptions of available options, demand characteristics, and aesthetics of an environment. Access to a cafeteria offering healthy foods at work or having a gym nearby are examples of available options that promote health. Demand characteristics include policies and procedures in employment and public environments. No-smoking policies in public buildings and work environments are demand characteristics that promote health. Aesthetics refers to physical and interpersonal characteristics of

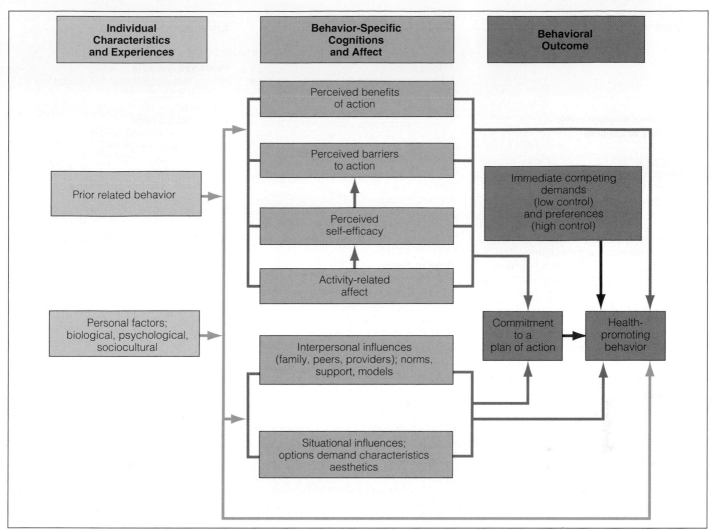

Figure 2.6 ● Health promotion model.

environments. Environments that are safe and interesting and that promote comfort and acceptance versus alienation are factors that facilitate health promotion.

Situational influences may be direct or indirect. For example, the requirement to wear protective eyewear and gloves in a microbiology laboratory creates a direct demand characteristic; that is, employees must comply with the regulation.

COMMITMENT TO A PLAN OF ACTION. Commitment to a plan of action includes two components. The first component is commitment to carry out a specific activity. The second component is identification of strategies for carrying out and reinforcing the activity. Commitment without strategies often leads to "good intentions" but results in failure to actually carry out the activity.

IMMEDIATE COMPETING DEMANDS AND PREFERENCES. Competing demands are alternative activities over which the individual has little control. These demands include family or work responsibilities. Neglect of competing demands may have a more negative impact on health than nonparticipation in a planned health-promoting activity. Competing preferences are alternative behaviors over which the individual has high control. The control is dependent upon the ability to self-regulate. Choosing to have lunch with a friend at

the health club rather than participating in the aerobics class is an example of choosing the competing preference over the health-promoting activity. Unless an individual can recognize, address, or overcome competing demands and preferences, a plan for health promotion may unravel.

BEHAVIORAL OUTCOMES. Health-promoting behavior is the expected outcome in the health promotion model. Health-promoting behaviors can lead to improved health, better functional ability, and improved quality of life across the age span.

An example of application of each of the models is presented in Figures 2.7 ● through 2.9 ●. The information is derived from the following case study.

Mr. Howard James is a 46-year-old African American. He is obese and has hypertension. There is a family history of heart disease. His father died at age 48 from a myocardial infarction (MI), an uncle is 54 years of age with congestive heart failure (CHF), and his brother, 52 years of age, was recently diagnosed with coronary artery disease (CAD). Mr. James is married and the father of two teenage children. He is an hourly employee at a local manufacturer. Mr. James was an athlete in the high school from which he graduated. He realizes that heart disease can create physical, emotional, family, and economic problems.

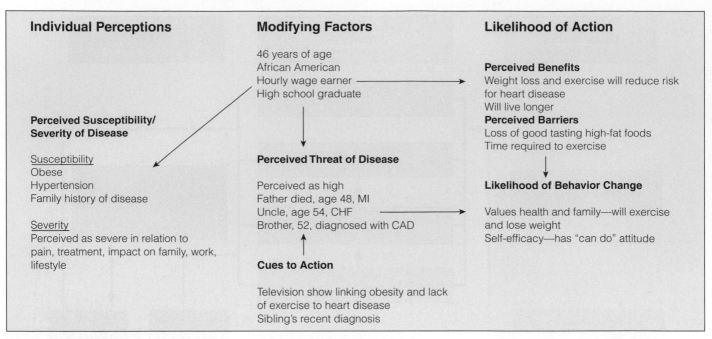

Individual Perceptions	Modifying Factors	Likelihood of Action

Figure 2.7 ● Application of the health belief model.

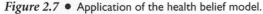

Attitude

"My weight is going to cause me to have a heart attack."

Subjective Norms

"My wife and kids would like me to lose this weight."

Self-Efficacy

"I know I can do this."

Intention

"I want to start a diet and exercise program."

Health-Promoting Behavior

"I am walking every day for 20 minutes and I have started a low-fat diet."

Figure 2.8 ● Application of the theory of reasoned actions/planned behavior model.

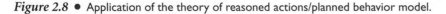

Mr. James has come to understand the risks his weight is causing through observation of family members with heart disease and after watching a television program about obesity and heart disease. He wants to begin activities to reduce his risk of heart disease. Mr. James will start an exercise and diet program with the support of his physician and family. After discussion of details and strategies, Mr. James will embark on a weight reduction program.

As stated earlier, the models for health promotion guide intervention. Nurses promote positive health-promoting behaviors by emphasizing the benefits of the behaviors, assisting the client to overcome barriers, and providing positive feedback for success. Personal factors influence health behaviors. Some of the factors such as age, gender, and family history cannot be changed. Nursing interventions will generally focus on factors that can be modified. However, it is also important to develop interventions to address factors that cannot be changed. For example, a client with a family history of colon cancer may avoid screening programs because of fear or a belief that the development of colon cancer is inevitable. Nurses can provide support for these clients and emphasize the importance of early detection in improved outcomes in colon cancer.

Health assessment and screening provides a rich database from which the nurse can assist the client, family, or community to identify the current health status, risks for illness or injury, strengths and weaknesses, and resources required to begin or continue appropriate health promotion activities. A variety of strategies including education, support, and modeling are used in health promotion. The nurse assists the individual to develop a plan of action and serves as a resource to guide the activity, monitor progress, and evaluate outcomes.

HEALTHY PEOPLE 2010

Health promotion of individuals, families, and communities is the focus of the agenda set forth in ***Healthy People 2010,*** a report by the United States Department of Health and Human Services (USDHHS) (2004). The *Healthy People 2010* report states that the health of individuals and the health of communities are closely

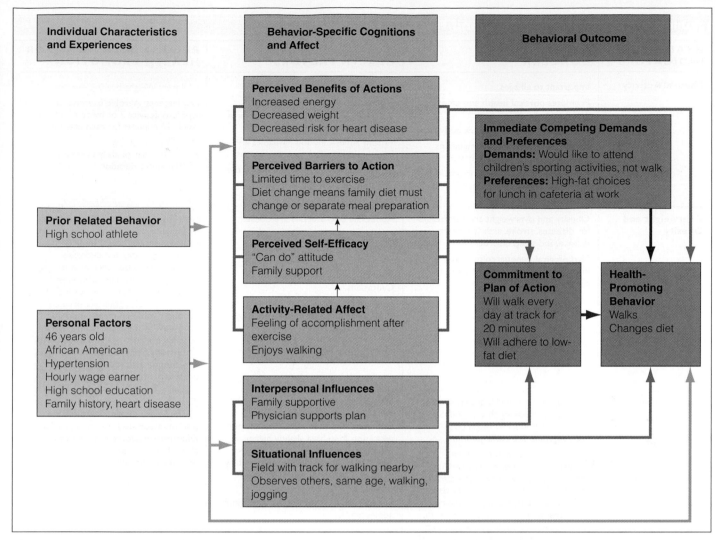

Figure 2.9 • Application of the health promotion model.

related. The goals of *Healthy People 2010* are to increase the length and quality of life and to eliminate health inequities. Ten leading health indicators related to significant public health concerns in the United States were identified in the report. The selection of the 10 indicators was based on the ability to motivate action, the ability to address the health concern, the availability of data to measure progress, and the relevance as public health issues. The 10 indicators are physical activity, overweight and obesity, tobacco use, substance abuse, responsible sexual behavior, mental health, injury and violence, environmental quality, immunization, and access to healthcare. Table 2.2 provides an overview of the concerns, factors, and recommendations for health promotion related to each of the health indicators. For more information about *Healthy People 2010,* contact the USDHHS. Link to *Healthy People 2010* through the Companion Website.

LEADING HEALTH INDICATORS

The discussion of **leading health indicators,** set forth in *Healthy People 2010,* provides a comprehensive view of factors that impact individual and community health and wellness. The factors affecting wellness in individuals, families, and communities as discussed in *Healthy People 2010* include biology,

behavior, social environment, physical environment, and policies and interventions. **Biology** includes genetic background, gender, race and ethnicity, family history, and problems occurring throughout life. Aging, diet, exercise, injury, infection, use of drugs and alcohol, and exposure to toxins change the individual's biology. Behaviors are the ways in which individuals respond to internal and external stimuli. **Social environment** refers to interactions between individuals and others as well as the institutions in an individual's community, including churches, schools, transportation systems, and protective services. The **physical environment** consists of all the things that are experienced through the individual's senses and some harmful elements such as radiation, ozone, and radon. Policies and interventions include a variety of services to promote health, prevent disease, and improve access to healthcare. Each of the 10 leading health indicators and the associated factors will be discussed in the following sections.

Physical Activity

Physical activity is important at all ages to maintain physical health, promote psychological well-being, and reduce the incidence of cardiovascular diseases, diabetes, and some forms

Table 2.2 Health Promotion and Health Indicators

HEALTH INDICATORS	CONCERN	HEALTH FACTORS	RECOMMENDATIONS FOR HEALTH PROMOTION
Physical Activity	Important to all ages. Promotes physical health and emotional well-being. Increases strength, decreases body fat. In children: Promotes and maintains skeletal development and mass. In older adults: Needed to maintain agility, reduce safety risks, and maintain independence in ADLs.	Men are more active than women. Higher income or education in individuals is related to higher levels of physical activity. African Americans and Hispanics are less physically active than Caucasians. Individuals over 75 years are less active than younger people.	Children: Weight-bearing exercise. Adolescents: Aerobic exercise or vigorous activity 3 or more times per week, 20 minutes for each activity session. Adults: Regular or daily physical activity of 30 minutes duration.
Overweight and Obesity	Obesity and overweight are risk factors for diabetes, stroke, arthritis, heart disease, and sleep disorders. Physiological, genetic, cultural, and environmental factors contribute to obesity.	About half of U.S. adults are obese. Obesity occurs more frequently in women. Obesity is higher in African American and Hispanic women than in Caucasians. Low-income adolescents are twice as likely to be obese as middle- and high-income adolescents.	Nutrition and exercise are important in maintaining or attaining healthy weight. Children should have 1 hour of exercise each day and decrease sedentary activities, such as watching TV. Dietary guidelines recommend consuming a variety of foods including vegetables, fruits, grains, fat-free dairy products, fish, lean meat, poultry, and foods low in sugar and saturated fat. Sensible portions are recommended. Counseling from healthcare providers is recommended for weight reduction programs.
Tobacco Use	More deaths in the U.S. are attributed to cigarette smoking than to AIDS, drug abuse, homicide, automobile accidents, and fire combined. Smoking is a risk factor for heart disease, breathing disorders, and lung cancer. Secondary smoke increases the incidence of asthma and bronchitis in children. Smoking during pregnancy increases the risk for premature birth, miscarriage, and SIDS. Use of chewing tobacco and cigars increases the risk of oral and GI cancers.	Individuals with low income and education are more likely to smoke than are those with higher income and education. Men have slightly higher rates of smoking than women. Native Americans, Alaska Natives, and military personnel have the highest smoking rates. Smoking habits most frequently begin in adolescence.	Cessation of smoking or never starting to smoke are the only methods to prevent associated risks and problems. Education of adolescents and children about hazards may decrease numbers who start smoking.
Substance Abuse	Alcohol and substance abuse are associated with health problems that include accidents, STDs, violence, and family problems. Alcohol use can increase the risk for heart and liver diseases. Alcohol use in pregnancy has been linked with low birth weight and fetal alcohol syndrome.	Drug and alcohol use in adolescents has been reported to fluctuate. Use of alcohol and/or drugs is reported to occur in around 20% of children between the ages of 12 and 17 years. Drug usage is higher in men in urban areas than in other groups.	Education about the risks associated with drugs and alcohol is warranted for children and adolescents. Counseling, therapy, and rehabilitation are among the options for drug users. Families may benefit from support groups.
Responsible Sexual Behavior	Unprotected sexual activity increases the risk for pregnancy, STDs, and HIV infection.	Unintended pregnancy rates are highest among teenagers, women over 40 years of age, and African American women. The majority of new cases of HIV occur in individuals under 25 years of age and are associated with sexual activity.	Education is essential about abstinence as the only sure method to reduce risks associated with sexual activity. Education about the use of condoms to reduce risks associated with sexual activity is also important.
Mental Health	Mental health enables individuals to perform productively in all aspects of their lives, to establish relationships with others, and to cope with life changes and problems. Depression contributes to disability and suicide.	Almost one fifth of the U.S. population is affected by mental illness annually. Depression accounts for the greatest number of cases of mental illness. Women are twice as likely as men to suffer from depression. Depression occurs more frequently in older adults.	Education about the signs of mental illness helps in getting diagnosis and treatment for mental illness. Medication and counseling are important components of treatment. Support groups are available for individuals and families coping with mental illness.

Table 2.2	Health Promotion and Health Indicators *(continued)*		
HEALTH INDICATORS	**CONCERN**	**HEALTH FACTORS**	**RECOMMENDATIONS FOR HEALTH PROMOTION**
Injury and Violence	Serious injuries can occur from motor vehicle accidents, falls, drownings, fires, poisons, and shootings.	Death associated with vehicular accidents occurs with the greatest frequency among those between 17 and 24 years of age. Alcohol use is associated with almost half of the vehicular fatalities in the U.S. Childhood homicides as a result of abuse increased in the 1990s. Almost half of gun-related deaths were homicides. Men are most frequently involved in homicide, and African Americans are five times more likely to be murdered than Caucasians.	Education about and the use of safety equipment can reduce injuries from accidents.
Environmental Quality	Environment includes the physical environment of air, water, and soil. The social environment includes housing, transportation, land use, development, and agriculture. Risks in the physical environment are related to exposure to chemical, biological, and physical agents that lead to respiratory and cardiovascular disease and cancer. The social environment exposes the individual to risks associated with the aforementioned agents as well as risks associated with stress, injury, or violence.	Data indicate that greater numbers of Hispanics, Asians, and Pacific Islanders live in areas that don't meet standards for air pollution than do Caucasians, African Americans, Native Americans, or Alaska Natives.	Education about risks is essential to health promotion. Stress the importance of waste treatment, food safety, and air quality. Reduction of smoking reduces hazards of secondhand smoke.
Immunization	Immunization can prevent disease, disability, and the spread of infection.	Caucasians have higher rates of immunization for pneumonia and influenza than do African Americans and Hispanics.	When recommendations in immunization schedules are followed, the incidence of many childhood illnesses is reduced. Immunization decreases the incidence of death or complications of infectious disease in older adults.
Access to Healthcare	Health insurance is the most significant factor in access to healthcare. When one is insured, regular healthcare and preventive practices are more likely to occur. Access to healthcare includes having a primary care provider or ongoing source of healthcare such as a clinic.	A significant number of Americans are without health insurance. Individuals between 18 and 24 years of age are most commonly lacking in ongoing healthcare. Higher levels of income and education influence access to healthcare. Longevity is increased in higher-income males. Lowest-income individuals have greater incidence of reduced activity related to chronic disease. Infant mortality is highest in mothers with less than 12 years of education. Those with higher education have greater understanding of information required to participate in practices beneficial to health.	Education is essential about the availability of services to those who are in low-income or noninsured populations.

of cancer. Physical activity increases skeletal and muscular strength, helps decrease body fat, is important in weight control, is indicated for reduction of depression, and improves emotional well-being. Regular physical activity is required in children to promote and maintain skeletal development and mass. In older adults, maintenance of agility through exercise reduces safety risks and enables individuals to continue independent activities of daily living (ADLs). Data indicate that in general men are more active than women, individuals of higher income and education are more physically active than those of low income and ed-

ucation, and African Americans and Hispanics are less physically active than Caucasians.

Regular physical activity reduces the risk for developing or dying from some of the leading causes of illness in the United States. Regular physical activity results in the following:

- Reduced risk of premature death
- Reduced risk of death from cardiovascular disease
- Reduced risk of development of diabetes
- Reduced risk of development of hypertension
- Reduced risk of development of colon cancer

- Reduction in depression and anxiety
- Weight reduction or control

Recommendations for physical activity developed through the Centers for Disease Control and Prevention (CDC) (2003) are as follows.

- Adults should:
  - Engage in moderate intensity physical activities for at least 30 minutes on 5 or more days of the week.
  - Engage in vigorous intensity activity for 20 minutes or more on 3 or more days of the week.
- Adolescents should:
  - Engage in moderate intensity activities for at least 30 minutes on 5 or more days of the week.
  - Engage in vigorous intensity exercise for 20 or more minutes on 3 or more days of the week.
- School-age children should:
  - Engage in 30 to 60 minutes of age and developmentally appropriate activity on all or most days of the week. Activity should occur in periods of 10 to 15 minutes and include moderate to vigorous intensity activities.

The level of intensity of exercise may be measured by use of the metabolic equivalent level (MET). The MET is used to estimate the amount of oxygen used during activity. One MET is the amount of energy required for a light intensity activity such as sitting quietly, reading a book, or talking on the phone. The average adult uses approximately 3.5 milliliters (ml) of oxygen per kilogram of body weight per minute for sitting quietly. The MET increases because the body has to work harder. Moderate intensity activities require 3 to 6 METs, and vigorous intensity activity requires more than 6 METs.

The intensity of an activity can be measured by determining if the heart rate is within a target zone. In moderate intensity exercise the heart rate should be 50% to 70% of the individual's maximum heart rate. In vigorous intensity activity the target heart rate is 70% to 85% of the maximum heart rate. Maximum heart rate is determined by subtracting the individual's age from 220. For example, the maximum heart rate for a 54-year-old would be calculated as 220 minus 54, which equals 166 beats per minute. In moderate intensity activity the target heart rate would be 83 at a 50% level and 116 at a 70% level. Table 2.3 provides examples of moderate and vigorous intensity activities.

Exercise may be categorized according to the type of muscle activity and source of energy. Muscle activities are classified as isotonic, isometric, or resistive. Isotonic exercise is also called dynamic exercise. In isotonic exercise the muscle shortens, producing contraction and active movement. Isotonic exercises increase the tone, strength, and mass of muscles; maintain joint flexibility; and improve circulation. Running, walking, cycling, and ADLs are examples of isotonic exercises.

Isometric exercises include those that affect muscle tension but do not result in muscle or joint movement. Isometric exercise is useful for strengthening abdominal, gluteal, and quadriceps muscles; for maintaining strength of immobilized muscles (for example, following a sprain or fracture); and for endurance training. Isometric exercise refers to exertion of pressure

Table 2.3	Physical Activities According to Level of Intensity
MODERATE INTENSITY	**VIGOROUS INTENSITY**
• Walking (3 to 4.5 mph) on a level surface • Walking the dog • Walking to class • Hiking • Roller-skating at a leisurely pace • Bicycling at 5 to 9 mph • Stationary cycling • Ballroom dancing • Tennis doubles • Golf • Softball • Gymnastics • Calisthenics • Recreational swimming • Playing on playground equipment • Skateboarding • Dodgeball • Gardening • Shoveling light snow • Moderate housework • Occupations that require periods of walking, pushing, pulling objects weighing less than 75 lb (maid service, waiting tables, patient care, farming, home building)	• Racewalking and aerobic walking at 5 mph or faster • Jogging • Running • Backpacking • Mountain climbing • Rollerblading at a brisk pace • Bicycling at 10 mph • High-impact aerobic dancing • Step aerobics • Boxing in the ring • Tennis singles • Karate, tae kwon do • Competitive sports • Tennis singles • Handball • Synchronized swimming • Swimming paced laps • Skipping • Jumping rope • Jumping jacks • Shoveling heavy snow • Heavy housework • Carrying heavy bags of groceries (25 lb or more) up stairs • Vigorous play with children • Occupations such as firefighting, masonry, mining, aerobics instructor, professional mover

against a solid object. Examples of isometric exercise would include tensing of thigh muscles and extending the arms and pushing against a wall.

Resistive exercise refers to muscle contraction against resistance. Resistive exercise can be isotonic, movement against resistance; or isometric, tension against resistance. An example of resistive exercise is lifting weights to increase the size and strength of pectoral muscles.

Exercises classified according to the source of energy include aerobic and anaerobic. **Aerobic exercise** refers to activity in which oxygen is metabolized to produce energy. Examples of aerobic activity include walking, jogging, swimming, and skating. Aerobic exercise can result in improved cardiovascular function and physical fitness. Guidelines for aerobic activity include exercise of 30 minutes or more on 3 to 5 days of the week and at an intensity that produces a heart rate of 220 beats per minute minus the age of the individual. **Anaerobic exercise** refers to activity in which the energy required is provided without using inspired oxygen. Anaerobic

6	no exertion
7	
	extremely light
8	
9	very light
10	
11	light
12	
13	somewhat hard
14	
15	hard (heavy)
16	
17	very hard
18	
19	extremely hard
20	

Figure 2.10 ● Borg rating of perceived exertion (Borg, 1998).

activity includes endurance training and is generally limited to short periods of vigorous activity.

Individuals may use two simple methods to assess the intensity of activity. The first method is the talk test. During light intensity activity a person should be able to sing. During moderate intensity activity, the individual should be able to carry on a conversation. The activity is considered vigorous if conversation is difficult due to being out of breath or winded.

The second measure of activity intensity is the perceived exertion rating. This rating is based on physical sensations experienced during activity. The sensations are rated subjectively and include increases in heart rate, respiratory rate, perspiration, and muscle fatigue. The individual is asked to assign a numerical rating to the activity performed. The scale ranges from 6 to 20, with 6 indicating no exertion and 20 indicating maximum exertion as presented in Figure 2.10 ●. Generally, a rating of 12 to 14 would be indicative of moderate intensity.

Overweight and Obesity

Overweight and obesity are risk factors for a number of diseases including heart disease, diabetes, stroke, arthritis, and sleep disorders. Additionally, obesity impacts emotional well-being as a result of discrimination or problems with body image or self-esteem. The number of obese individuals in the United States has risen dramatically since the 1980s. Physiological, genetic, cultural, environmental, and social factors contribute to obesity. Nutrition and exercise are important in attaining or maintaining a healthy weight. Dietary guidelines have been established for individuals ages 2 and older. Refer to

Chapter 9 for an in-depth discussion of nutrition. ⚭ The guidelines stress eating sensible portions of an assortment of foods such as vegetables and fruits, grains, fat-free dairy products, fish, lean meat, and poultry as well as foods low in sugar and saturated fat. Dietary guidelines also include the recommendation for exercise for adults and children when involved in maintaining or losing weight. Obesity occurs in approximately half of the adult population in the United States. Obesity is more prevalent among women than men and proportionately higher in African American and Mexican American women when compared to Caucasians. As stated in *Healthy People 2010*, low-income adolescents are twice as likely to be obese as compared to middle- and higher-income adolescents.

Tobacco Use

Cigarette smoking is responsible for more deaths in the United States than are HIV/AIDS, drug abuse, homicide, suicide, automobile crashes, and fire combined. Smoking is a risk factor for heart disease, breathing disorders, and lung cancer. Secondary smoke increases the incidence of asthma and bronchitis in children, and heart and lung diseases in adults. Smoking during pregnancy increases the risk for miscarriage, prematurity, and sudden infant death syndrome (SIDS). Smoking among adults has leveled off, but adolescent smoking has increased in the last decade. Use of chewing tobacco and cigar smoking also increase the risk for cancer of the mouth. Making a choice to never start smoking, or cessation of the use of tobacco products, are the only means to prevent the associated risks and problems. Individuals with low income and education are more likely to smoke than those with higher income and education. Men have slightly higher rates of smoking than women. In the United States, Native Americans, Alaska Natives, and military personnel have the highest smoking rates.

According to Fiore (2000), a desire to stop smoking has been expressed by more than 70% of smokers. Smoking cessation will result in immediate and long-term improvements in health. Assisting clients to stop smoking is a role of the healthcare professional to promote wellness.

Guidelines for clinicians have been developed and recommend assessment in relation to smoking and the desire to stop smoking. For smokers willing to stop, the guidelines include five As for use by healthcare providers: ask, advise, assess, assist, and arrange. These five As are implemented as follows:

1. Ask about smoking at every health visit.
2. Advise (that is, urge) all smokers to stop.
3. Assess the client's willingness to stop.
4. Assist or aid the client in quitting. Work with the client to develop a plan to quit while providing counseling, recommending pharmacotherapy, and providing resource materials.
5. Arrange for follow-up to determine progress or the need for further assistance.

Consumer information about nicotine addiction, difficulties involved with smoking cessation, benefits of smoking cessation, and steps for quitting are provided in a consumer guide through the USDHHS. The guidelines include the key steps of preparing, obtaining support, acquiring new skills and behaviors, obtaining and using medications correctly, and preparing for difficulties. Information about clinician and consumer guidelines for smoking cessation and about tobacco use is available through the USDHHS. Link to the USDHHS through the Companion Website.

Substance Abuse

The use of alcohol and illicit drugs has been linked with a variety of health problems including accidents, sexually transmitted diseases, violence, injury from accidents, and disruptions in families. Alcohol use can also increase the risk of heart and liver diseases. During pregnancy, alcohol use can result in fetal alcohol syndrome. Drug and alcohol use among adolescents has fluctuated over the past decade, although 10% to 20% of those between 12 and 17 years of age reported use of one or both substances. Drug use is higher among men and in urban areas.

There are indications that abuse of prescription drugs is rising in the United States. According to the National Institute on Drug Abuse (NIDA) (2002), almost 4 million people 12 years of age and older were using prescription drugs nonmedically. The drugs included pain relievers, sedatives, tranquilizers, and stimulants. Additionally, children between the ages of 12 and 17 and young adults between the ages of 18 and 25 were found to be the most frequent new users of prescription drugs for nonmedical purposes. In general, women and men are similar in rates of nonmedical use of prescription medications.

Prevention and identification of prescription drug abuse includes screening for abuse and symptoms associated with substance abuse. Ewing (1984) developed the CAGE questionnaire, which is a useful tool for assessment of alcohol and substance abuse. CAGE is a mnemonic for questions about **C**utting down on drinking, **A**nnoyance with criticism about drinking, **G**uilt about drinking, and using alcohol as an "**E**ye-opener".

Screening for prescription drug abuse is part of the health history in which one asks the client about prescription and over-the-counter medication use. Specific symptoms of prescription drug abuse can be identified during the health assessment. Healthcare providers must be alert to requests for increasing amounts of medication to relieve symptoms or for frequent refills of prescriptions.

Clients with chronic pain require the use of prescribed pain relievers. Healthcare providers often fear the risk of addiction and may underprescribe pain medication. Addiction to pain relievers is rare in individuals with chronic pain and long-term opioid use. Those who do become addicted have been found to have a history of psychological problems or prior drug abuse. Further information about pain is included in Chapter 8 of this text. ⚭ The NIDA is an excellent resource for information related to substance abuse. Information about commonly abused drugs, trends, research, prevention, and treatment can be found

at the Companion Website, which includes a link to the National Institute on Drug Abuse.

Responsible Sexual Behavior

Unprotected sexual activity increases the risk for pregnancy, sexually transmitted diseases (STDs), and infection with human immunodeficiency virus (HIV). Unintended pregnancy rates have been declining. They are highest among teenagers, women over 40, and African American women. STD occurs at a rate of almost 4 million new cases annually. Individuals below the age of 25 are reported to account for the majority of new cases of HIV, and the transmission of the disease is associated with sexual activity. Abstinence can ensure complete protection from infection and pregnancy. Correct use of condoms can reduce the incidence of risks associated with sexual activity.

In *Healthy People 2010,* one learns that prevention of STDs is dependent upon understanding the dynamics of the transmission of disease. The following factors impact the rate of infection in a population:

- The rate at which uninfected persons have sexual contact with infected persons
- The probability that exposure will lead to disease
- The time period during which an infected person remains able to spread the disease

Measures to act upon these factors include educational programs to increase the probability that changes in awareness, attitude, and behavior can occur. Measures include increased condom use, identification and treatment of persons with STDs, and active partner notification and treatment.

Primary healthcare providers have an active role in screening for behaviors that increase the risk for STDs. Examples of questions to be asked during a health assessment include the following:

- Are you sexually active?
- When was the last time you had sexual activity (oral, vaginal, anal)?
- When you had sexual activity, did you use a condom?
- Do you now have or have you had more than one sexual partner?
- Have you ever been treated for an STD?
- Have you had sexual activity with a partner who uses intravenous drugs?

Healthcare providers are expected to screen for symptoms of STDs during all aspects of health assessment, including the physical assessment. When risks or disease are identified, interventions are developed to treat the illness and to counsel individuals about methods to reduce the transmission of the disease. Additional information about problems related to sexual activity and illness is provided in Chapters 21 and 22 of this text. ⚭ For further information, contact the National Center for HIV, STD, and TB prevention (NCHSTP). Link to this center at the Companion Website.

Mental Health

Mental health enables an individual to perform productively, to establish relationships, and to adapt and cope with life changes and problems. According to the report in *Healthy People 2010*, one fifth of the population in the United States is affected by mental illness in one given year. Depression accounts for the greatest number of cases of mental illness. Depression contributes to disability and suicide. Mental illness has an impact on the individual, family, and community. Treatment includes medication and psychological counseling.

The impact of mental illness is economic and emotional. A mental illness may prevent an individual from obtaining or keeping a job. The employment difficulties can result in poverty for the individual and his or her family. Families may be further impoverished because health insurance reimbursement for mental health services is generally limited. Communities and societies face the economic burden of subsidizing diagnostic and treatment services and providing disability payments for those with mental illness while coping with lost productivity.

Mental illness is stressful for the individual and family. Family roles are often disrupted. Anxiety related to the mental illness and economic impacts often interferes with communication and interaction. Mental illness often results in the perception of social stigma (disgrace) for the individual and family. Stigmatization can result in reluctance to seek care. The stigmatized individual can experience decreased self-esteem, despair, and social isolation.

Perceptions about mental illness are affected by culture. For example, Asian Americans including those of Japanese, Chinese, Filipino, and Korean descent as well as Pacific Islanders, Vietnamese Americans, and Cambodian Americans perceive mental illness as a disgrace or taboo. As a result, the mentally ill are kept isolated, at home, as much as possible. However, Jewish Americans view attention to mental health to be as important as attention to physical health. For more information about culture and mental health, contact the Substance Abuse and Mental Health Service Administration (SAMHSA). A link to SAMHSA can be found at the Companion Website.

According to the National Institute of Mental Health (NIMH), depression may be present in more than 10% of clients seen by a primary healthcare provider. Depression may be difficult to diagnose because many illnesses present with symptoms such as fatigue, sleep disorders, pain, or other vague symptoms. In addition, clients may have other conditions that have similar symptoms. For example, depression may coexist with substance abuse, anxiety disorders, heart disease, and diabetes.

Screening for depression is accomplished through client interview and the use of screening tools. Screening questions in an interview include the following:

- Have you felt down, depressed, or hopeless in the past 2 weeks?
- Have you had little interest or pleasure in doing things?

When a client responds yes to the two questions, a diagnosis of depression necessitates the presence of at least four of the following symptoms. The symptoms must have persisted over 2 weeks and accompany impaired social and work functioning.

0	I do not feel sad.
1	I feel sad.
2	I am sad all the time.
3	I am so sad, I can't stand it.

Figure 2.11 ● Sample items from the Beck Depression Inventory.

- Significant weight loss or gain
- Disturbed sleep pattern
- Agitation or slowness
- Fatigue
- Loss of energy
- Feelings of guilt or worthlessness
- Inability to concentrate or make decisions
- Thoughts of death or suicide

Information about the following factors to consider can be obtained in the health history.

- Family history of depression
- Previous mental health disorder
- Two or more chronic illnesses
- Stress in the home or at work
- Multiple vague symptoms such as fatigue, loss of appetite, generalized aches, or pains
- Loss of interest in sexual activity

There are a variety of screening tools to detect depression. A frequently used tool is the Beck Depression Inventory. This 21-item instrument requires approximately 5 minutes to complete and can be used in clients from 18 to 80 years of age. Each of the items has four statements arranged in increasing severity. Figure 2.11 ● provides a sample item.

Mental disorders vary in their severity and impact on individuals, families, and communities. Mental disorders include depression, schizophrenia, bipolar disorder, obsessive compulsive disorder, and panic disorders. There is increasing progress in screening for and treatment of mental disorders. For more information about mental health disorders, trends, research, and treatment, contact the NIMH. Link to the NIMH through the Companion Website.

Injury and Violence

Serious injuries can occur from motor vehicle accidents, falls, drowning, fires, poison, and shootings. Table 2.4 describes application of the levels of prevention for specific aspects of this focus area. The greatest number of serious injuries result from motor vehicle accidents. Death as a result of motor vehicle accidents occurs with greatest frequency among those between 17 and 24 years of age. Alcohol has been associated with almost half of the traffic fatalities in the United States. Increased use of safety equipment and decreased driving after consumption of alcohol are considered the best way to reduce motor vehicle–related injuries and deaths. In the 1990s, childhood homicides increased as a result of child abuse, and almost half of firearm deaths were homicides. Men are most frequently involved in

Table 2.4	Levels of Prevention in Action		
	PRIMARY PREVENTION	**SECONDARY PREVENTION**	**TERTIARY PREVENTION**
Childhood	Educate parents about the use of bicycle safety helmets. Educate parents about recognition of the signs of head injury that require healthcare. Helmet use can reduce the risk of head injury by 85% (USDHHS, 2004).	Diagnostic procedures in head injury. X-ray, magnetic resonance imaging (MRI). Treatment of severe head injury. Head injuries are the most serious injury in pedacyclists in the U.S. (USDHHS, 2004).	Rehabilitation following head injuries. May require physical, cognitive, or emotional therapy. Emotional support for child and family dealing with disability.
Older Adulthood	Educate older adults regarding the following: Importance of exercise to increase strength and balance. Review of medications to determine side effects and interactions. Improving home safety including removal of throw rugs, improved lighting, installation of rails and grab bars. Vision examination. Importance of continued care for chronic conditions. These actions can reduce or modify risks for falls (National Center for Injury Prevention and Control, 2000).	Diagnostic procedures for hip fracture. Treatment of hip fracture. The majority of fractures in older adults are a result of falls (Bell, Talbot-Stern, & Hennessey, 2000). Hip fractures are among the most common fractures from falls in older adults (National Center for Injury Prevention and Control, 2000).	Rehabilitation following treatment for hip fracture. Education regarding measures to prevent further injury or disability.

homicide, and African Americans have five times the likelihood of being murdered when compared to Caucasians.

Workplace accidents and injuries and motor vehicle accidents are associated with fatigue. Fatigue, irritability, difficulty concentrating, and impatience can all occur when an individual experiences sleeping difficulties or lack of sleep. Requirements for sleep vary across the age span, but recommendations for sleep needs have been developed. These recommendations appear in Table 2.5.

Sleep is affected by aging, lifestyle changes, behavior, and illness. For example, middle-aged and older adults experience sleep disorders including sleep apnea, restless legs syndrome, and nocturia more than younger people. Illnesses such as arthritis, heart disease, respiratory disease, heartburn, and osteoporosis may interrupt or delay sleep. Medications may affect sleep, and mental disorders including depression and anxiety may result in sleep difficulties.

Nurses can use a variety of tools to assist clients to identify sleep problems. These include asking the client to record a sleep diary and using a list of questions to identify sleep difficulties. These questions include the following:

- Do you snore loudly?
- Have you observed that you stop breathing or gasp for breath during sleep?
- Do you feel drowsy or fall asleep while reading, when watching TV, while driving, or in other daily activities?
- Do you have unpleasant feelings in your legs when trying to sleep?
- Are there interruptions to your sleep (pain, dreams, light, temperature)?
- Do you have some trouble with sleep on 3 or more nights a week?

Recommendations for improving sleep include establishing a sleep routine with a regular bedtime and waking time. Other recommendations include the following:

- Avoid caffeine.
- Avoid alcohol.
- Get regular exercise.
- Establish a bedtime relaxation routine.
- Create a sleep conducive environment.

Table 2.5	Sleep Requirements Across the Age Span
AGE/STAGE	**HOURS OF SLEEP***
Infants/Babies	
0 to 2 months	10.5 to 18.5 hours
2 to 12 months	14 to 15 hours
Toddlers/Children	
12 to 18 months	13 to 15 hours
18 months to 3 years	12 to 14 hours
3 to 5 years	11 to 13 hours
5 to 12 years	9 to 11 hours
Adolescents	8.5 to 9.5 hours
Adults	7 to 9 hours
*Includes naps	

Environmental Quality

Environment includes the physical environment of air, water, and soil. The social environment includes housing, transportation, land use, development, and agriculture. Risks in the physical environment are related to exposure to chemical, biological, and physical agents that lead to respiratory and cardiovascular disease and cancer. The social environment exposes the individual to risks associated with the previously mentioned agents as well as risks associated with stress, injury, or violence. Policies have been enacted to reduce many physical and social environment threats including water treatment, food safety, waste management, and air quality programs. Data indicate that greater numbers of Hispanics, Asians, and Pacific Islanders reside in regions that do not meet standards for air pollution than do Caucasians, African Americans, Native Americans, or Alaska Natives. For information about environmental programs, methods to improve awareness, and increased knowledge about environmental issues, consult *Healthy People 2010*. Link to *Healthy People 2010* through the Companion Website.

Immunization

Immunizations can prevent disease, disability, and the spread of infection. Recommendations for childhood immunization have been developed and when followed reduce the incidence of many childhood illnesses. Recommendations for adults include pneumonia and influenza immunizations. Rates of immunization of adults have been reported as lower than those for children but are considered an effective way to decrease the incidence of death or complications of infectious disease in older adults. Caucasians have higher rates of immunization for pneumonia and influenza than do African Americans and Hispanics. Table 2.6 includes recommended schedules for childhood and adult immunization. For further information contact the National Immunization Program (NIP). A link to this program can be found at the Companion Website.

Access to Healthcare

Health insurance is the most significant factor in access to healthcare. When one is insured, regular healthcare and preventive practices are more likely to occur. Access to healthcare includes having a primary care provider or an ongoing source of healthcare, such as a clinic. A significant number of people under the age of 65 are without health insurance in the United States, and those between the ages of 18 and 24 are most commonly found to lack ongoing healthcare. Income and education are related to access to healthcare. Higher levels of education and income influence health and health promotion. For example, longevity is increased in higher-income males, while lowest-income individuals have greater incidence of reduced activity related to chronic disease. In addition, infant mortality is highest when mothers have had less than 12 years of education. Higher education is believed to influence health promotion because there is greater understanding of information required to participate in health beneficial practices.

Culture

Culture influences health promotion. Language barriers can prevent one from receiving or understanding information about all aspects of health and illness prevention. Culture influences social and physical behaviors that impact health. Individuals from some cultures often have difficulty understanding who to see or where to go to seek health services. These individuals often rely on family or cultural healers or practices and wait to seek treatment until the condition is serious. People from different cultures often have concerns about confidentiality, discrimination, and being treated inhumanely in the mainstream healthcare system. The nurse has a responsibility to advocate for clients, to assist them in navigating the healthcare system, and to provide care that incorporates the individual's health beliefs, practices, and cultural beliefs.

National standards for culturally and linguistically appropriate services (CLAS) have been issued by the USDHHS Office of Minority Health (OMH). These standards were developed to ensure that people entering the healthcare system will receive equitable and effective treatment in a culturally and linguistically appropriate manner. The standards are intended to be inclusive of all cultures; however, they are designed to address the needs of racial, ethnic, and linguistic population groups that experience unequal access to health services. For information about CLAS standards, contact the OMH through the link at the Companion Website.

HEALTH PROMOTION AND THE NURSING PROCESS

The nurse works with the client as the nursing process is applied in problem identification. The process continues through development and implementation of plans for care and is completed when the nurse and client evaluate the outcomes.

ASSESSMENT

Comprehensive assessment is essential to health promotion. Through the health history and physical assessment, the nurse gathers information about the client's current health status, risk factors, and predisposing factors associated with specific diseases. These risk factors are revealed through data about age, gender, race, and family history. The physical findings yield information including height, weight, and vital signs, and data about behaviors and practices. Additional assessments are conducted in relation to health promotion. These include physical fitness, nutritional status, a health risk appraisal, lifestyle inventories, assessment of current stressors, and stress management strategies. Social structure assessments include family and support systems, level of education, income, roles, and other activities. Areas included in most health risk appraisals are presented in Box 2.1. Information about health assessment tools is available through the National Center for Chronic Disease Prevention and Health Promotion (NCCDPHP). A link can be found at the Companion Website. Instruments for client self-assessment are available in written form, in English and Spanish, and online through organizations such as the American Diabetes Association and the American Heart Association. Link to these sites at the Companion Website. The CDC has established the Behavioral Risk Factor Surveillance System Survey. This comprehensive survey is available through the CDC link to the CDC through the Companion Website. Tools to assess risk, lifestyle, and stress include Lifescan, Health Risk Appraisal, Live Well, Wellness Appraisal, and Stress Assess. These tools are available at the Companion Website.

Table 2.6   Immunizations

Recommended Adult Immunization Schedule by Vaccine and Age Group
United States • October 2004–September 2005

AGE GROUP (yrs) ▶ VACCINE ▼	19–49	50–64	≥65
Tetanus, Diphtheria (Td)*	I dose booster every I0 years[1]		
Influenza	I dose annually[2]	I dose annually[2]	
Pneumococcal (polysaccharide)	I dose[3,4]		I dose[3,4]
Hepatitis B*	3 doses (0, I–2, 4–6 months)[5]		
Hepatitis A*	2 doses (0, 6–12 months)[6]		
Measles, Mumps, Rubella (MMR)*	I or 2 doses[7]		
Varicella*	2 doses (0, 4–8 weeks)[8]		
Meningococcal (polysaccharide)	I dose[9]		

*Covered by the Vaccine Injury Compensation Program.
See Footnotes for Recommended Adult Immunization Schedule on page 39.

| | For all persons in this group | | For persons lacking documentation of vaccination or evidence of disease | | For persons at risk (i.e., with medical/exposure indications) |

**The Recommended Adult Immunization Schedule is Approved by the Advisory Committee on Immunization Practices (ACIP),
the American College of Obstetricians and Gynecologists (ACOG) and the American Academy of Family Physicians (AAFP)**

This schedule indicates the recommended age groups for routine administration of currently licensed vaccines for persons aged ≥19 years. Licensed combination vaccines may be used whenever any components of the combination are indicated and when the vaccine's other components are not contraindicated. Providers should consult manufacturers' package inserts for detailed recommendations.

Report all clinically significant postvaccination reactions to the Vaccine Adverse Event Reporting System (VAERS). Reporting forms and instructions on filing a VAERS report are available by telephone, 800-822-7967, or from the VAERS website at *http://www.vaers.org*.

Information on how to file a Vaccine Injury Compensation Program claim is available at *http://www.hrsa.gov/osp.vicp* or by telephone, 800-338-2382. To file a claim for vaccine injury, contact the U.S. Court of Federal Claims, 717 Madison Place, N.W., Washington, DC 20005, telephone 202-219-9657.

Additional information about the vaccines listed above and contraindications for immunization is available at *http://www.cdc.gov/nip* or 800-CDC-INFO [800-232-4636] (English and Spanish).

(continued)

Table 2.6 **Immunizations** *(continued)*

Recommended Adult Immunization Schedule by Vaccine and Medical and Other Indications

United States • October 2004–September 2005

VACCINE ▼ INDICATION ►	Pregnancy	Diabetes, heart disease, chronic pulmonary disease, chronic liver disease (including chronic alcoholism)	Congenital immunodeficiency, cochlear implants, leukemia, lymphoma, generalized malignancy, therapy with alkylating agents, antimetabolites, CSF** leaks, radiation or large amounts of corticosteroids	Renal failure/end stage renal disease, recipients of hemodialysis or clotting factor concentrates	Asplenia (including elective splenectomy and terminal complement component deficiencies)	HIV*** infection	Health-care workers
Tetanus, Diphtheria (Td)*,1							
Influenza2		A, B			C		
Pneumococcal (polysaccharide)3,4		B	D	D, E, F	D, G		
Hepatitis B*,5				H			
Hepatitis A*,6		I					L
Measles, Mumps, Rubella (MMR)*,7						J	
Varicella*,8			K				

*Covered by the Vaccine Injury Compensation Program.
**Cerebrospinal fluid.
***Human immunodeficiency virus.
See Special Notes for Medical and Other Indications below. Also see Footnotes for Recommended Adult Immunization Schedule on page 40.

For all persons in this group	For persons lacking documentation of vaccination or evidence of disease	For persons at risk (i.e., with medical/exposure indications)	Contraindicated

Special Notes for Medical and Other Indications

A. Although chronic liver disease and alcoholism are not indications for influenza vaccination, administer 1 dose annually if the patient is aged ≥50 years, has other indications for influenza vaccine, or requests vaccination.

B. Asthma is an indication for influenza vaccination but not for pneumococcal vaccination.

C. No data exist specifically on the risk for severe or complicated influenza infections among persons with asplenia. However, influenza is a risk factor for secondary bacterial infections that can cause severe disease among persons with asplenia.

D. For persons aged <65 years, revaccinate once after ≥5 years have elapsed since initial vaccination.

E. Administer meningococcal vaccine and consider *Haemophilus influenzae* type b vaccine.

F. For persons undergoing elective splenectomy vaccinate ≥2 weeks before surgery.

G. Vaccinate as soon after diagnosis as possible.

H. For hemodialysis patients, use special formulation of vaccine (40 μg/mL) or two 20 μg/mL doses administered at one body site. Vaccinate early in the course of renal disease. Assess antibody titers to hepatitis B surface antigen (anti-HB) levels annually. Administer additional doses if anti-HB levels decline to <10 mIU/mL.

I. For all persons with chronic liver disease.

J. Withhold MMR or other measles-containing vaccines from HIV-infected persons with evidence of severe immunosuppression. (see *MMWR* 1998;47[No. RR-8]: 21–2 and *MMWR* 2002; 51[No. RR-2]:22–24).

K. Persons with impaired humoral immunity but intact cellular immunity may be vaccinated (see *MMWR* 1999;48[No. RR-06]).

L. No data to support a recommendation.

(continued)

Table 2.6   Immunizations *(continued)*

FOOTNOTES

Recommended Adult Immunization Schedule

United States • October 2004–September 2005

1. **Tetanus and diphtheria (Td).** Adults, including pregnant women with uncertain history of a complete primary vaccination series, should receive a primary series of Td. A primary series for adults is 3 doses; administer the first 2 doses at least 4 weeks apart and the 3rd dose 6–12 months after the second. Administer 1 dose if the person received the primary series and if the last vaccination was received ≥10 years previously. Consult recommendations for administering Td as prophylaxis in wound management (see *MMWR* 1991;40 [No. RR-10]). The American College of Physicians Task Force on Adult Immunization supports a second option for Td use in adults: a single Td booster at age 50 years for persons who have completed the full pediatric series, including the teenage/young adult booster.

2. **Influenza vaccination.** The Advisory Committee on Immunization Practices (ACIP) recommends inactivated influenza vaccination for the following indications, when vaccine is available. *Medical indications:* chronic disorders of the cardiovascular or pulmonary systems, including asthma; chronic metabolic diseases, including diabetes mellitus, renal dysfunction, hemoglobinopathies, or immunosuppression (including immunosuppression caused by medications or by human immunodeficiency virus [HIV]); and pregnancy during the influenza season. *Occupational indications:* health-care workers and employees of long-term–care and assisted living facilities. *Other indications:* residents of nursing homes and other long-term–care facilities; persons likely to transmit influenza to persons at high risk (i.e., in-home caregivers to persons with medical indications, household/close contacts and out-of-home caregivers of children aged 0–23 months, household members and caregivers of elderly persons and adults with high-risk conditions); and anyone who wishes to be vaccinated. For healthy persons aged 5–49 years without high-risk conditions who are not contacts of severely immunocompromised persons in special care units, either the inactivated vaccine or the intranasally administered influenza vaccine (FluMist®) may be administered (see *MMWR* 2004;53[No. RR-6]).
Note: Because of the influenza vaccine shortage in 2004, the Centers for Disease Control and Prevention (CDC) and the ACIP had modified the influenza vaccine recommendations (see *MMWR* 2004;53[39];923-924). These were further modified on December 17, 2004, and this schedule reflects those changes (i.e., routinely recommending influenza vaccination of persons 50-64 years of age) (see *MMWR* 2004;53[50]; 1183-1184).

3. **Pneumococcal polysaccharide vaccination.** *Medical indications:* chronic disorders of the pulmonary system (excluding asthma); cardiovascular diseases; diabetes mellitus; chronic liver diseases, including liver disease as a result of alcohol abuse (e.g., cirrhosis); chronic renal failure or nephrotic syndrome; functional or anatomic asplenia (e.g., sickle cell disease or splenectomy); immunosuppressive conditions (e.g., congenital immunodeficiency, HIV infection, leukemia, lymphoma, multiple myeloma, Hodgkins disease, generalized malignancy, or organ or bone marrow transplantation); chemotherapy with alkylating agents, antimetabolites, or long-term systemic corticosteroids; or cochlear implants. *Geographic/other indications:* Alaska Natives and certain American Indian populations. *Other indications:* residents of nursing homes and other long-term–care facilities (see *MMWR* 1997;46[No. RR-8] and *MMWR* 2003;52:739–40).

4. **Revaccination with pneumococcal polysaccharide vaccine.** One-time revaccination after 5 years for persons with chronic renal failure or nephrotic syndrome; functional or anatomic asplenia (e.g., sickle cell disease or splenectomy); immunosuppressive conditions (e.g., congenital immunodeficiency, HIV infection, leukemia, lymphoma, multiple myeloma, Hodgkins disease, generalized malignancy, or organ or bone marrow transplantation); or chemotherapy with alkylating agents, antimetabolites, or long-term systemic corticosteroids. For persons aged ≥65 years, one-time revaccination if they were vaccinated ≥5 years previously and were aged <65 years at the time of primary vaccination (see *MMWR* 1997;46[No. RR-8]).

5. **Hepatitis B vaccination.** *Medical indications:* hemodialysis patients or patients who receive clotting factor concentrates. *Occupational indications:* health-care workers and public-safety workers who have exposure to blood in the workplace; and persons in training in schools of medicine, dentistry, nursing, laboratory technology, and other allied health professions. *Behavioral indications:* injection-drug users; persons with more than one sex partner during the previous 6 months; persons with a recently acquired sexually transmitted disease (STD); all clients in STD clinics; and men who have sex with men. *Other indications:* household contacts and sex partners of persons with chronic hepatitis B virus (HBV) infection; clients and staff members of institutions for the developmentally disabled; inmates of correctional facilities; or international travelers who will be in countries with high or intermediate prevalence of chronic HBV infection for >6 months (http://www.cdc.gov/travel/diseases/hbv.htm) (see *MMWR* 1991;40[No. RR-13]).

6. **Hepatitis A vaccination.** *Medical indications:* persons with clotting factor disorders or chronic liver disease. *Behavioral indications:* men who have sex with men or users of illegal drugs. *Occupational indications:* persons working with hepatitis A virus (HAV)-infected primates or with HAV in a research laboratory setting. *Other indications:* persons traveling to or working in countries that have high or intermediate endemicity of hepatitis A. If the combined Hepatitis A and Hepatitis B vaccine is used, administer 3 doses at 0, 1, and 6 months (http://www.cdc.gov/travel/diseases/hav.htm) (see *MMWR* 1999;48[No. RR-12]).

7. **Measles, mumps, rubella (MMR) vaccination.** *Measles component:* adults born before 1957 can be considered immune to measles. Adults born during or after 1957 should receive ≥1 dose of MMR unless they have a medical contraindication, documentation of ≥1dose, or other acceptable evidence of immunity. A second dose of MMR is recommended for adults who 1) were recently exposed to measles or in an outbreak setting, 2) were previously vaccinated with killed measles vaccine, 3) were vaccinated with an unknown vaccine during 1963–1967, 4) are students in postsecondary educational institutions, 5) work in health-care facilities, or 6) plan to travel internationally. *Mumps component:* 1 dose of MMR vaccine should be adequate for protection. *Rubella component:* administer 1 dose of MMR vaccine to women whose rubella vaccination history is unreliable and counsel women to avoid becoming pregnant for 4 weeks after vaccination. For women of childbearing age, regardless of birth year, routinely determine rubella immunity and counsel women regarding congenital rubella syndrome. Do not vaccinate pregnant women or those planning to become pregnant during the next 4 weeks. For women who are pregnant and susceptible, vaccinate as early in the postpartum period as possible (see *MMWR* 1998;47[No. RR-8] and *MMWR* 2001;50:1117).

8. **Varicella vaccination.** Recommended for all persons lacking a reliable clinical history of varicella infection or serologic evidence of varicella zoster virus (VZV) infection who might be at high risk for exposure or transmission. This includes health-care workers and family contacts of immunocompromised persons; persons who live or work in environments where transmission is likely (e.g., teachers of young children, child care employees, and residents and staff members in institutional settings); persons who live or work in environments where VZV transmission can occur (e.g., college students, inmates, and staff members of correctional institutions, and military personnel); adolescents aged 11–18 years and adults living in households with children; women who are not pregnant but who might become pregnant; and international travelers who are not immune to infection. **Note:** Approximately 95% of U.S.-born adults are immune to VZV. Do not vaccinate pregnant women or those planning to become pregnant during the next 4 weeks. For women who are pregnant and susceptible, vaccinate as early in the postpartum period as possible (see *MMWR* 1999;48[No. RR-6]).

9. **Meningococcal vaccine (quadrivalent polysaccharide for serogroups A, C, Y, and W 135).** *Medical indications:* adults with terminal complement component deficiencies or those with anatomic or functional asplenia. *Other indications:* travelers to countries in which meningococcal disease is hyperendemic or epidemic (e.g., the "meningitis belt" of sub-Saharan Africa and Mecca, Saudi Arabia). Revaccination after 3–5 years might be indicated for persons at high risk for infection (e.g., persons residing in areas where disease is epidemic). Counsel college freshmen, especially those who live in dormitories, regarding meningococcal disease and availability of the vaccine to enable them to make an educated decision about receiving the vaccination (see *MMWR* 2000;49 [No. RR-7]). The American Academy of Family Physicians recommends that colleges should take the lead on providing education on meningococcal infection and availability of vaccination and offer it to students who are interested. Physicians need not initiate discussion of meningococcal quadrivalent polysaccharide vaccine as part of routine medical care.

(continued)

Table 2.6   Immunizations *(continued)*

Recommended Childhood and Adolescent Immunization Schedule

United States • 2005

AGE ▶ / VACCINE ▼	BIRTH	1 MO	2 MOS	4 MOS	6 MOS	12 MOS	15 MOS	18 MOS	24 MOS	4–6 YRS	11–12 YRS	13–18 YRS
Hepatitis B[1]	HepB #1	HepB #2 (→)			HepB #3				HepB Series			
Diphtheria, Tetanus, Pertussis[2]			DTaP	DTaP	DTaP		DTaP			DTaP	Td	Td
Haemophilus Influenzae type b[3]			Hib	Hib	Hib	Hib						
Inactivated Poliovirus			IPV	IPV		IPV				IPV		
Measles, Mumps, Rubella[4]						MMR #1				MMR #2	MMR #2	
Varicella[5]						Varicella				Varicella		
Pneumococcal Conjugate[6]			PCV	PCV	PCV	PCV				PCV / PPV		
Influenza[7]						Influenza (Yearly)				Influenza (Yearly)		
— Vaccines below this line are for selected populations —												
Hepatitis A[8]										Hepatitis A Series		

This schedule indicates the recommended ages for routine administration of currently licensed childhood vaccines, as of December 1, 2004, for children through age 18 years. Any dose not administered at the recommended age should be administered at any subsequent visit when indicated and feasible.

Indicates age groups that warrant special effort to administer those vaccines not previously administered. Additional vaccines may be licensed and recommended during the year. Licensed combination vaccines may be used whenever any components of the combination are indicated and other components of the vaccine are not contraindicated. Providers should consult the manufacturers' package inserts for detailed recommendations. Clinically significant adverse events that follow immunization should be reported to the Vaccine Adverse Event Reporting System (VAERS). Guidance about how to obtain and complete a VAERS form is available at **www.vaers.org** or by telephone, **800-822-7967**.

Range of recommended ages	Only if mother HBsAg(−)	Preadolescent assessment	Catch-up immunization

1. Hepatitis B (HepB) vaccine . All infants should receive the first dose of HepB vaccine soon after birth and before hospital discharge; the first dose may also be administered by age 2 months if the mother is hepatitis B surface antigen (HBsAg) negative. Only monovalent HepB may be used for the birth dose. Monovalent or combination vaccine containing HepB may be used to complete the series. Four doses of vaccine may be administered when a birth dose is given. The second dose should be administered at least 4 weeks after the first dose, except for combination vaccines which cannot be administered before age 6 weeks. The third dose should be given at least 16 weeks after the first dose and at least 8 weeks after the second dose. The last dose in the vaccination series (third or fourth dose) should not be administered before age 24 weeks.

Infants born to HBsAg-positive mothers should receive HepB and 0.5 mL of hepatitis B immune globulin (HBIG) at separate sites within 12 hours of birth The second dose is recommended at age 1–2 months. The final dose in the immunization series should not be administered before age 24 weeks. These infants should be tested for HBsAg and antibody to HBsAg (anti-HBs) at age 9–15 months.

Infants born to mothers whose HBsAg status is unknown should receive the first dose of the HepB series within 12 hours of birth. Maternal blood should be drawn as soon as possible to determine the mother's HBsAg status; if the HBsAg test is positive, the infant should receive HBIG as soon as possible (no later than age 1 week). The second dose is recommended at age 1–2 months. The last dose in the immunization series should not be administered before age 24 weeks.

2. Diphtheria and tetanus toxoids and acellular pertussis (DTaP) vaccine. The fourth dose of DTaP may be administered as early as age 12 months, provided 6 months have elapsed since the third dose and the child is unlikely to return at age 15–18 months. The final dose in the series should be given at age ≥4 years. **Tetanus and diphtheria toxoids (Td)** is recommended at age 11–12 years if at least 5 years have elapsed since the last dose of tetanus and diphtheria toxoid-containing vaccine. Subsequent routine Td boosters are recommended every 10 years.

3. *Haemophilus influenzae* type b (Hib) conjugate vaccine. Three Hib conjugate vaccines are licensed for infant use. If PRP-OMP (PedvaxHIB® or ComVax® [Merck]) is administered at ages 2 and 4 months, a dose at age 6 months is not required. DTaP/Hib combination products should not be used for primary immunization in infants at ages 2, 4, or 6 months but can be used as boosters after any Hib vaccine. The final dose in the series should be administered at age ≥12 months.

4. Measles, mumps, and rubella vaccine (MMR). The second dose of MMR is recommended routinely at age 4–6 years but may be administered during any visit, provided at least 4 weeks have elapsed since the first dose and both doses are administered beginning at or after age 12 months. Those who have not previously received the second dose should complete the schedule by age 11–12 years.

5. Varicella vaccine. Varicella vaccine is recommended at any visit at or after age 12 months for susceptible children, (i.e., those who lack a reliable history of chickenpox). Susceptible persons aged ≥13 years should receive 2 doses administered at least 4 weeks apart.

6. Pneumococcal vaccine. The heptavalent **pneumococcal conjugate vaccine (PCV)** is recommended for all children aged 2–23 months and for certain children aged 24–59 months. The final dose in the series should be given at age ≥12 months. **Pneumococcal polysaccharide vaccine (PPV)** is recommended in addition to PCV for certain high-risk groups. See *MMWR* 2000;49(RR-9):1–35.

7. Influenza vaccine. Influenza vaccine is recommended annually for children aged ≥6 months with certain risk factors (including, but not limited to, asthma, cardiac disease, sickle cell disease, human immunodeficiency virus [HIV], and diabetes) healthcare workers, and other persons (including household members) in close contact with persons in groups at high risk (see *MMWR* 2004;53[RR-6]:1–40). In addition, healthy children aged 6–23 months and close contacts of healthy children aged 0–23 months are recommended to receive influenza vaccine because children in this age group are at substantially increased risk for influenza-related hospitalizations. For healthy persons aged 5–49 years, the intranasally administered, live, attenuated influenza vaccine (LAIV) is an acceptable alternative to the intramuscular trivalent inactivated influenza vaccine (TIV). See *MMWR* 2004;53(RR-6):1–40. Children receiving TIV should be administered a dosage appropriate for their age (0.25 mL if aged 6–35 months or 0.5 mL if aged ≥3 years). Children aged ≤8 years who are receiving influenza vaccine for the first time should receive 2 doses (separated by at least 4 weeks for TIV and at least 6 weeks for LAIV).

8. Hepatitis A vaccine. Hepatitis A vaccine is recommended for children and adolescents in selected states and regions and for certain high-risk groups; consult your local public health authority. Children and adolescents in these states, regions, and high-risk groups who have not been immunized against hepatitis A can begin the hepatitis A immunization series during any visit. The 2 doses in the series should be administered at least 6 months apart. See *MMWR* 1999;48(RR-12):1–37.

(continued)

Table 2.6 Immunizations *(continued)*

Recommended Immunization Schedule for Children and Adolescents Who Start Late or Who Are More Than 1 Month Behind

United States • 2005

The tables below give catch-up schedules and minimum intervals between doses for children who have delayed immunizations. There is no need to restart a vaccine series regardless of the time that has elapsed between doses. Use the chart appropriate for the child's age.

CATCH-UP SCHEDULE FOR CHILDREN AGED 4 MONTHS THROUGH 6 YEARS

VACCINE	MINIMUM AGE FOR DOSE 1	MINIMUM INTERVAL BETWEEN DOSES			
		DOSE 1 TO DOSE 2	DOSE 2 TO DOSE 3	DOSE 3 TO DOSE 4	DOSE 4 TO DOSE 5
Diphtheria, Tetanus, Pertussis	6 wks	4 weeks	4 weeks	6 months	6 months[1]
Inactivated Poliovirus	6 wks	4 weeks	4 weeks	4 weeks[2]	
Hepatitis B[3]	Birth	4 weeks	8 weeks (and 16 weeks after first dose)		
Measles, Mumps, Rubella	12 mo	4 weeks[4]			
Varicella	12 mo				
Haemophilus influenzae type b[5]	6 wks	**4 weeks** if first dose given at age <12 months / **8 weeks (as final dose)** if first dose given at age 12–14 months / **No further doses needed** if first dose given at age ≥15 months	**4 weeks**[6] if current age <12 months / **8 weeks (as final dose)**[6] if current age ≥12 months and second dose given at age <15 months / **No further doses needed** if first dose given at age ≥15 months	**8 weeks (as final dose)** This dose only necessary for children aged 12 months–5 years who received 3 doses before age 12 months	
Pneumococcal Conjugate[7]	6 wks	**4 weeks** if first dose given at age <12 months and current age <24 months / **8 weeks (as final dose)** if first dose given at age ≥12 months or current age 24–59 months / **No further doses needed** for healthy children if first dose given at age ≥24 months	**4 weeks** if current age <12 months / **8 weeks (as final dose)** if current age ≥12 months / **No further doses needed** for healthy children if previous dose given at age ≥24 months	**8 weeks (as final dose)** This dose only necessary for children aged 12 months–5 years who received 3 doses before age 12 months	

(continued)

Table 2.6	Immunizations *(continued)*

Recommended Immunization Schedule for Children and Adolescents Who Start Late or Who Are More Than 1 Month Behind
United States • 2005

The tables below give catch-up schedules and minimum intervals between doses for children who have delayed immunizations. There is no need to restart a vaccine series regardless of the time that has elapsed between doses. Use the chart appropriate for the child's age.

CATCH-UP SCHEDULE FOR CHILDREN AGED 7 YEARS THROUGH 18 YEARS

	MINIMUM INTERVAL BETWEEN DOSES		
VACCINE	**DOSE 1 TO DOSE 2**	**DOSE 2 TO DOSE 3**	**DOSE 3 TO BOOSTER DOSE**
Tetanus, Diphtheria	4 weeks	6 months	**6 months**[8] if first dose given at age <12 months and current age <11 years **5 years**[8] if first dose given at age ≥12 months and third dose given at age <7 years and current age ≥11 years **10 years**[8] if third dose given at age ≥7 years
Inactivated Poliovirus[9]	4 weeks	4 weeks	**IPV**[2,9]
Hepatitis B	4 weeks	**8 weeks** (and 16 weeks after first dose)	
Measles, Mumps, Rubella	4 weeks		
Varicella[10]	4 weeks		

FOOTNOTES
Children and Adolescents Catch-up Schedules
United States • 2005

1. **DTaP.** The fifth dose is not necessary if the fourth dose was administered after the fourth birthday.

2. **IPV.** For children who received an all-IPV or all-oral poliovirus (OPV) series, a fourth dose is not necessary if third dose was administered at age ≥4 years. If both OPV and IPV were administered as part of a series, a total of 4 doses should be given, regardless of the child's current age.

3. **HepB.** All children and adolescents who have not been immunized against hepatitis B should begin the HepB immunization series during any visit. Providers should make special efforts to immunize children who were born in, or whose parents were born in, areas of the world where hepatitis B virus infection is moderately or highly endemic.

4. **MMR.** The second dose of MMR is recommended routinely at age 4–6 years but may be administered earlier if desired.

5. **Hib.** Vaccine is not generally recommended for children aged ≥5 years.

6. **Hib.** If current age <12 months and the first 2 doses were PRP-OMP (PedvaxHIB® or ComVax® [Merck]), the third (and final) dose should be administered at age 12–15 months and at least 8 weeks after the second dose.

7. **PCV.** Vaccine is not generally recommended for children aged ≥5 years.

8. **Td.** For children aged 7–10 years, the interval between the third and booster dose is determined by the age when the first dose was administered. For adolescents aged 11–18 years, the interval is determined by the age when the third dose was given.

9. **IPV.** Vaccine is not generally recommended for persons aged ≥18 years.

10. **Varicella.** Administer the 2-dose series to all susceptible adolescents aged ≥13 years.

Report adverse reactions to vaccines through the federal Vaccine Adverse Event Reporting System. For information on reporting reactions following immunization, please visit www.vaers.org or call the 24-hour national toll-free information line 800-822-7967. Report suspected cases of vaccine-preventable diseases to your state or local health department.

For additional information about vaccines, including precautions and contraindications for immunization and vaccine shortages, please visit the National Immunization Program Web site at www.cdc.gov/nip or call 800-CDC-INFO/800-232-4636 (English or Spanish)

PLAN DEVELOPMENT

Once data is gathered, the professional nurse works with the client to identify current, ongoing, or potential problems. Diagnoses are established and include problems and strengths. For example, problems may include obesity and smoking. A client's strength could be identified as physical fitness. Then goals and priorities are established to develop a plan to meet the needs of the client.

ROLES OF THE PROFESSIONAL NURSE

In implementing the plan, the nurse takes on the roles of educator, counselor, facilitator, nurturer, and role model. As educator, the nurse interprets and informs the client of the significance of findings from all of the completed assessments. Education then may consist of one-on-one sessions related to specific aspects of care or preventive measures as dictated by need. The nurse provides education about specific problems, risks, treatments, or behaviors and may have to provide education about resources available to meet the needs of the client and family.

As a counselor, the nurse creates and plans opportunities to discuss the implementation of specific activities and to review progress in behavior change or in goal attainment. The counseling role can occur in one-on-one sessions or with groups of clients involved in the same treatment, prevention, or promotion activity. In the facilitator role, the nurse may meet with the client's family to provide information, to encourage their participation with the client in health-related activities, or to promote family support for the client. As a facilitator, the nurse helps the client and family gain access to services and facilities required to meet the identified health needs.

The nurturing role of the nurse includes providing the types and amounts of support and encouragement that will assist clients to meet their health-related goals. The nurturing role is

Box 2.1	Areas of Assessment in Health Risk Appraisal

- Demographic information (age, gender, height, weight)
- Type and amount of exercise
- Occupation
- Smoking
- Twenty-four-hour dietary history
- Family history of heart disease, diabetes, cancer
- History of screening tests according to gender and age (mammography, prostatic specific antigen test PSA)
- Oral hygiene and dental care history
- Immunization history
- Personal history of illness
- Safety measures (seat belt, sunscreen, condom)
- Sexual activity and reproductive history
- Use of alcohol, illicit drugs, prescription drugs
- Emotional state or mood

particularly important when a client is attempting to change or modify a behavior. Lastly, the nurse models wellness and health-promoting behaviors and is willing to share experiences and difficulties in developing plans or meeting goals for healthy behaviors and lifestyles. Additionally, the nurse will identify individuals within the same culture or community who have experienced similar problems or have similar goals in relation to health promotion and wellness, with whom the client can interact and relate to as a model.

The nurse and client are involved in continual evaluation of progress in meeting goals. The evaluation process provides opportunities to address concerns. During evaluation, the client has the opportunity to modify, continue, or discontinue the plan. As a result of evaluation, priorities may be reordered or the methods and tactics may be changed.

Application Through Critical Thinking

CASE STUDY

You are participating in a health fair performing wellness screening. Gina Clark, a 22-year-old female, approaches your table. She states she is interested in seeing how healthy her habits are and wants to learn suggestions you have to help her feel better about her health. Your screening findings show a blood pressure of 132/83, pulse 88, respirations 18, temperature 98.2°F, height 5 ft. 4 in., and weight 190.

Gina reports that she drinks lots of soda and eats fast food several times each week. She does not like vegetables and tends to "snack" a lot rather than sitting down for prepared meals. She states she would like to eat better and to exercise, but she never seems to find the time. She had joined a gym with a friend about a month ago, but stopped going after 2 weeks when she became frustrated with sore muscles and lack of results. She would like to lose about 60 pounds and is interested in information on how to accomplish this goal. She tells you that because she is self-conscious about her weight, she does not socialize much or go out with friends. Her weight, she says, makes her feel uncomfortable. She slowly leans forward and quietly tells you that she is "repulsed" by her body and does not ever want to look in a mirror or have a picture taken. She indicates that whenever she is stressed about something, she tends to eat even more. "It is like a vicious cycle. I don't know what to do."

▶ Critical Thinking Questions

1. Describe the importance of wellness in comprehensive health assessment.

2. Where does the client see herself on the health-illness continuum?

3. What information is appropriate to share with Gina regarding healthy weight loss? (*Hint, review Healthy People 2010.*)

4. Construct at least three (3) nursing diagnoses that are appropriate for this client.

5. What data in the case study support these diagnoses?

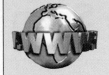

Please refer to the Companion Website at www.prenhall.com/damico and click on Chapter 2, the Application Through Critical Thinking module, to answer these and additional questions. In addition, complete NCLEX-RN® review questions and other interactive resources for this chapter.

EXPLORE MediaLink

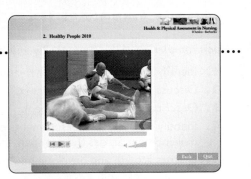

Additional resources for this chapter are found on the Student CD-ROM accompanying this textbook and on the Companion Website.

CD-ROM CONTENT

Content for this chapter includes:
Objectives
Key Concepts
NCLEX-RN® Review Questions
Audio Glossary
Clinical Spotlight Videos
   Healthy People 2010
Head-to-Toe Physical Examination Video

COMPANION WEBSITE CONTENT

www.prenhall.com/damico

Content for this chapter includes:
Objectives
NCLEX-RN® Review Questions

Application Through Critical Thinking
   Case Study Challenge
MediaLinks
MediaLink Application
Tool Box
   Levels of Prevention
   Health Belief Model
   Health Promotion Model
   Health Promotion and Health Indicators
   Immunizations
New York Times

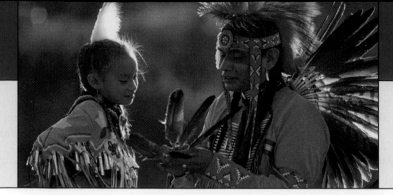

3

Health Assessment Across the Life Span

MEDIALINK

www.prenhall.com/damico

The CD-ROM in the back of this textbook and the Media-Link website contain NCLEX-RN® review questions, interactive exercises, case study challenges, animations, videos, documentation and checklist forms, and review materials. For a complete listing of the media content specific to Chapter 3, see the Explore MediaLink at the end of the chapter.

$\mathcal{K}$ nowledge of growth and development provides a framework for nursing assessment and planning effective nursing interventions. The focus of assessment is not a specific aspect of an individual's health. Rather, nursing assessment requires the ability to interpret how the complex interactions of heredity, environment, and physiological, cognitive, and psychological development affect an individual at a particular time. By developing an image of what is usual or expected of children and adults of various ages, the nurse has a basis for a comparison with the norm. This knowledge and an understanding of individual variations provide a foundation for assessment and appropriate nursing interventions that help individuals attain their maximum level of wellness.

The selected nursing interventions will support wellness and, at the same time, reflect the leading health indicators and goals of *Healthy People 2010*. The 10 leading health indicators that were presented in a table in Chapter 2 of this text apply to all age groups. ∞ The two broad goals of *Healthy People 2010* are to increase the quality of a healthy life and eliminate inequalities of health. Focus areas and objectives, derived from the two broad goals, have been formulated to assist the nurse to implement primary and secondary prevention strategies. Each of the assessment chapters in Unit III of this text provides information about specific focus areas and actions to promote health as outlined in *Healthy People 2010*. ∞

Growth and development are dynamic processes that describe how people change over time. The two processes are interdependent and interrelated. **Growth** involves measurable physical change and increase in size. Indicators of growth include height, weight, bone size, and dentition. Growth is rapid during the prenatal, neonatal, infancy, and adolescent stages of life; slows during childhood; and is minimal during adulthood. **Development** is an orderly, progressive increase in the complexity of the total person. It involves the continuous, irreversible, complex evolution of intelligence, personality, creativity, sociability, and morality. Development is continuous throughout the life cycle as the individual progresses through stages in physiological maturation, cognitive development, and personality development.

The pattern of growth and development is consistent in all individuals; however, the rate of growth and development varies as a result of heredity and environmental factors. Heredity is a determinant of physical characteristics such as stature, gender, and race. It may also play an important role in personality development as the determinant of temperament. Environmental factors affecting growth and development include nutrition, family, religion, climate, culture, school, community, and socioeconomic status.

PRINCIPLES OF GROWTH AND DEVELOPMENT

Four commonly accepted principles define the orderly, sequential progression of growth and development in all individuals:

1. Growth and development proceed in a **cephalocaudal**, or head to toe, direction. An infant's head grows and becomes functional before the trunk or limbs. A baby's hands are able to grasp before the legs and feet are used purposefully.

2. Growth and development occur in a proximal to distal direction, or from the center of the body outward. A child gains the ability to use the hand as a whole prior to being able to control individual fingers.

3. Development proceeds from simple to complex or from the general to specific. To accomplish an integrated act such as putting something in the mouth, the infant must first learn to reach out to the object, grasp it, move it to the open mouth, and insert it.

4. Differentiated development begins with a generalized response and progresses to a skilled specific response. An infant responds to stimuli with the entire body. An older child responds to specific stimuli with happiness, anger, or fear.

Although the classic theories of human development provide the foundation for nursing assessment, researchers are continuously evolving developmental theories that further define and explain human behavior. Additionally, interpretation of the classic theories

KEY TERMS

adolescence, 58
cephalocaudal, 47
cognitive theory, 48
development, 47
growth, 47
infant, 49
middle adulthood, 61
older adulthood, 63
preschooler, 54
psychoanalytic theory, 48
psychosocial theory, 49
school age, 56
toddler, 52
young adult, 61

broadens as societal changes and advances in technology redefine individuals' relationships, expectations, and goals. Behavior that is widely accepted or even the norm today was often considered unusual or abnormal a generation ago. For instance, the family unit is no longer assumed to be two parents with children but may now consist of a single parent, stepsiblings, halfsiblings, a surrogate mother, same-sex parents, or other configurations. What are the implications for development? Researchers also study innovations in technology. Children are bombarded with stimuli through television and videotapes, and they interact extensively with video games and computers. How do these affect the development of interpersonal skills? Advances in healthcare knowledge and technology have increased life expectancy, thus prolonging the span of productive years. This profoundly affects development, which continues until the individual dies.

THEORIES OF DEVELOPMENT

Three of the most influential classic theories of development are discussed here to provide a basic framework for nursing assessment. Although no one theory encompasses all aspects of human development, each is valuable as a framework for understanding, predicting, or guiding behavior.

COGNITIVE THEORY

Cognitive theory explores how people learn to think, reason, and use language. Jean Piaget theorized that cognitive development is an orderly, sequential process that occurs in four stages in the growing child. Each stage demonstrates a new way of thinking and behaving. Piaget believed that a child's thinking develops progressively from simple reflex behavior into complex, logical, and abstract thought. All children move through the same stages, in the same order, with each stage providing the foundation for the next. At each stage, the child views the world in increasingly complex terms. Piaget's stages of cognitive development are summarized below and discussed in more detail with each specific developmental stage later in this chapter.

Stage 1: Sensorimotor (Birth to 2 Years) The infant progresses from responding primarily through reflexes to purposeful movement and organized activity. *Object permanence* (the knowledge that objects continue to exist when not seen) and object recognition are attained.

Stage 2: Preoperational Skills (2 to 7 Years) Highly egocentric, the child is able to view the world only from an individual perspective. The new ability to use mental symbols develops. The child's thinking now incorporates past events and anticipations of the future.

Stage 3: Concrete Operations (7 to 11 Years) During this time period, the child develops symbolic functioning. Symbolic functioning is the ability to make one thing represent a different thing that is not present. The child is able to consider another point of view. Thinking is more logical and systematic.

Stage 4: Formal Operations (11 to Adulthood) The child uses rational thinking and deductive reasoning. Thinking

in abstract terms is possible. The child is able to deal with hypothetical situations and make logical conclusions after reviewing evidence.

PSYCHOANALYTIC THEORY

Sigmund Freud was an early theorist whose concepts of personality development provided the foundation for the development of many other theories. Freud believed that people are constantly adjusting to environmental changes, and that this adjustment creates conflict between outside forces (environment) and inner forces (instincts). The type of conflict varies with an individual's developmental stage, and personality develops through conflict resolution.

Psychoanalytic theory defines the structure of personality as consisting of three parts: the id, the ego, and the superego. The personality at birth consists primarily of the *id*, which is the source of instinctive and unconscious urges. The *ego* is the seat of consciousness and mediates between the inner instinctual desires of the id and the outer world. The ego, a minor nucleus at birth, expands and gains mastery over the id. In addition, it is the receiving center for the senses and forms the mechanisms of defense. The *superego* is the conscience of the personality, acting as a censor of thoughts, feelings, and behavior. The superego begins to form after age 3 or 4 years.

According to Freud's theory, children pass through five stages of psychosexual development, with each phase blending into the next without clear separation. Individuals may become fixated at a particular stage if their needs are not met or if they are overindulged. Fixation implies a neurotic attachment and interferes with normal development.

1. The *oral phase* occurs during the first year of life when the mouth is the center of pleasure. Sucking and swallowing give pleasure by relieving hunger and reducing tension.

2. The *anal phase* follows the oral phase and continues through about 3 years of age. The anus becomes the focus of gratification, and the functions of elimination take on new importance. Conflict occurs during the toilet-training process as the child is required to conform to societal expectations.

3. The *phallic phase* occurs during years 4 to 5 or 6, when the focus of pleasure shifts to the genital area. Conflict occurs as the child feels possessive toward the parent of the opposite sex and rivalry toward the parent of the same sex. These conflicts are referred to as the Oedipus and Electra complexes.

4. The *latency phase* occurs from 5 or 6 years of age to puberty. This is a time of relative quiet as previous conflicts are resolved and aggressiveness becomes latent. The child focuses energy on intellectual and physical pursuits and derives pleasure from peer and adult relationships and school.

5. The *genital stage* covers the period from puberty through adulthood. Sexual urges reawaken as hormonal influences stimulate sexual development. The individual focuses on finding mature love relationships outside the family.

PSYCHOSOCIAL THEORY

Erikson's psychosocial theory describes eight stages of ego development, but, unlike Freud, Erikson believed the ego is the conscious core of the personality. Erikson's **psychosocial theory** states that culture and society influence development across the entire life span. Erikson viewed life as a sequence of tasks that must be achieved with each stage presenting a crisis that must be resolved. Each crisis may have a positive or negative outcome depending on environmental influences and the choices that the individual makes. Crisis resolution may be positive, incomplete, or negative. Task achievement and positive conflict resolution are supportive to the person's ego. Negative resolution adversely influences the individual's ability to achieve the next task.

Stage 1: (Birth to 1 Year) presents the crisis of trust versus mistrust. The child who develops trust develops hope and drive. Mistrust results in fear, withdrawal, and estrangement.

Stage 2: (1 to 2 Years) is the crisis of autonomy versus shame and doubt. The child who achieves autonomy develops self-control and willpower. A negative resolution of the crisis results in self-doubt.

Stage 3: (2 to 6 Years) challenges the child to develop initiative versus guilt. Initiative leads to purpose and direction, whereas guilt results in lack of self-confidence, pessimism, and feelings of unworthiness.

Stage 4: (6 to 12 Years) is the crisis of industry versus inferiority. Industry results in the development of competency, creativity, and perseverance. Inferiority creates feelings of hopelessness and a sense of being mediocre or incompetent. Withdrawal from school and peers may result.

Stage 5: (12 to 18 Years) presents the challenge of identity versus role diffusion. Achieving ego identity results in the ability to make a career choice and plan for the future. Inferiority creates confusion, uncertainty, indecisiveness, and an inability to make a career choice.

Stage 6: (19 to 40 Years) is the time of intimacy versus isolation. Successful resolution allows the individual to form an intimate relationship with another person. Isolation results in the development of impersonal relationships and the avoidance of career and lifestyle commitments.

Stage 7: (40 to 65 Years) is the time of generativity versus stagnation. Positive crisis resolution results in creativity, productivity, and concern for others. Stagnation results in selfishness and lack of interests and commitments.

Stage 8: (65 Years to Death) is the time of integrity versus despair. Individuals conclude life, either appreciating the uniqueness of their lives and accepting death or feeling a sense of loss, despair, and contempt for others.

STAGES OF DEVELOPMENT

The most common and traditional approach used by developmental theorists to describe and classify human behavior is according to chronological age. Theorists attempt to identify meaningful relationships in complex behaviors by reducing them to core problems, tasks, or accomplishments that occur during a defined age range, or stage of life. Because theorists vary in their definitions of life stages, the following stages have been delineated to best illustrate the concepts of sequential development. It is important to remember that the ages are somewhat arbitrary. It is the sequence of growth, development, and observed behaviors that is meaningful during nursing assessment. For further information about infants and children, consult the National Center on Birth Defects and Developmental Disabilities (NCBDDD) and Bright Futures: Guidelines for Health Supervision of Infants, Children, and Adolescents. Link to their websites through the Companion Website.

INFANTS

An **infant** is a baby from 1 month of age to 1 year. During infancy, change is dramatic and occurs rapidly. The totally dependent newborn is transformed into an active child with a unique personality, all within the first year of life. The infant rapidly becomes mobile, often displaying a new skill each day. The developmental tasks of infancy are:

- Forming close relationships with primary caregivers
- Interacting with and relating to the environment

Physiological Growth and Development

Height, weight, and head circumference are the measurements used to monitor infant growth. At birth, most term infants weigh 2.7 to 3.8 kg (6.0 to 8.5 lb). During the first few days of life, many infants lose up to 10% of their birth weight but usually regain it by 14 days of age. Infants gain weight at a rate of 5 to 7 oz weekly during the first 6 months. Weight gain occurs in spurts rather than in a steady, predictable manner, with birth weight usually doubled in 4 to 6 months, and tripled by 1 year of age.

The average height of a normal term infant is 50 cm (20 in.) at birth. Height increases at a rate of about 2.5 cm a month during the first 6 months. An infant's height increases 50% during the first year of life.

Head circumference reflects growth of the skull and brain. At birth, the average term infant's head measures 35 cm (13.75 in.). Growth occurs at a monthly rate of 1.5 cm during the first 6 months, decreasing to 1 cm in the second 6 months. Ninety percent of head growth occurs during the first 2 years of life.

Dramatic changes occur within the organ systems of infants during the first year. The brain stem, which controls functions such as respiration, digestion, and heartbeat, is relatively well developed but lacks maturity at birth. As a result, these vital functions tend to be irregular during the early months of infancy, becoming regular with brain stem maturation by 1 year. The infant's nervous system is extremely immature at birth. Tremors of the extremities or chin are normal, reflecting immature myelinization. Much of the infant's physical behavior is reflexive (see Chapter 25 ⚭). These reflexes, or infant automatisms, disappear as myelinization of the efferent pathways matures. Myelinization of the efferent nerve fibers follows the cephalocaudal and proximodistal principles discussed earlier.

At birth, the infant's heart lies in an almost horizontal position and is large in relation to body size. With growth, the heart gradually shifts to a more vertical position. Although the ventricles are of equal size at birth, by 2 months of age the left ventricle develops better muscularity than the right. As the heart grows larger and the left ventricle becomes stronger, the low systolic blood pressure seen in the newborn rises, and the rapid heart rate of infants becomes slower.

At birth, the lungs are filled with fluid, which is quickly eliminated and absorbed as the lungs fill with air. The full complement of conducting airways is present, and the airway branching pattern is complete. The airways increase in size and length as the infant grows. Alveoli and respiratory bronchioles continue to grow after birth. The infant's thoracic cage is relatively soft, allowing it to pull in during labored breathing. Less tissue and cartilage in the trachea and bronchi also allow these structures to collapse more easily. Infants are obligatory nose breathers until 6 months of age. They gradually learn to breathe through their mouths by 3 or 4 months of age. Children use abdominal muscles more than thoracic muscles in respiration until 6 years of age.

Development of the eyes and visual acuity occurs rapidly during infancy. The inability of the infant to fixate consistently on an object, or not always being able to fixate the eyes together, is a result of immature eye muscles, which usually develop by 4 to 6 months of age. Infants see best at a distance of about 7.5 inches and have a visual acuity of about 20/150. Visual acuity rapidly develops to 20/40 by 2 years of age.

The ears and hearing are well developed at birth. The auditory (eustachian) tube, which connects the middle ear to the back of the throat in the nasopharynx, is shorter, wider, and more horizontal during infancy than during adult years. The size and position of the auditory tube gradually change with head growth.

Taste buds are present but immature at birth. Refined taste discrimination does not appear to develop until the infant is about 3 months old. Although the sense of smell is not refined in infancy, newborns are able to discriminate among distinctive odors and to recognize the smell of their mother's milk. The sense of touch is well developed at birth. Newborn infants show discriminating response to varied tactile stimuli.

Bone development, which begins before birth, continues during infancy. Ossification, the formation of bone, gradually occurs in the bony structures. Ossification is not complete until 14 years of age. While ossification is occurring, bones grow in length and width. Muscular growth occurs about twice as fast as that of bone from 5 months through 3 years. As muscle size increases, strength increases in response to appropriate stimulation.

Motor Development

Gross and fine motor skills develop in a predictable sequence, following the direction of maturation in the nervous system. Motor skill attainment in infancy provides milestones that mark normal development. Delay of early milestones may be an early indication of a developmental or neurologic abnormality. Table 3.1 shows how gross and fine motor skills develop during infancy. The age of skill attainment is an average, with some infants acquiring the skill somewhat earlier, some later. The Denver II is often used to assess the development of infants and children up to 6 years of age (see Chapter 25 ∞).

Table 3.1	Motor Skill Development in Infancy	
AGE	**GROSS MOTOR SKILLS**	**FINE MOTOR SKILLS**
1 month	Lifts head unsteadily when prone. Turns head from side to side. "Stepping" reflex when held upright. Symmetrical Moro reflex.	Hands held in fists. Tight hand grasp. Head and eyes move together. Positive Babinski reflex.
2 months	Holds head erect in midposition. Turns from side to back. Can raise head and chest when prone.	Holds a toy placed in hand. Follows objects with eyes. Smiles.
3 months	Holds head erect and steady. Holds head at 45- to 90-degree angle when prone. Stepping reflex absent. Sits with rounded back with support. May turn from front to back.	Plays with fingers and hands. Able to place objects in mouth.
4 months	When prone, uses arms to support self at a 90-degree angle. Can turn from back to side and abdomen to back. Sits with support.	Spreads fingers to grasp. Hands held predominantly open. Brings hands to midline.
5 months	Head does not lag and back is straight when pulled to sitting position. Reaches for objects. Moro reflex disappearing. Rolls from back to abdomen.	Grasps objects with whole hand. Transfers object from hand to hand.
6 months	Sits briefly without support. May crawl on abdomen.	Bangs object held in hand. Can release an object from hand. Reaches, grasps, and carries object to mouth. Uses all fingers in apposition to thumb for grasping.
7 months	Sits briefly with arms forward for support. Bears weight when held in a standing position.	Uses tips of all fingers against the thumb. May grasp feet and suck on toes.
8 months	Sits well alone.	Uses index and middle fingers against the thumb to grasp.
9 months	Creeps and crawls. Pulls to standing position.	Uses pincer grasp (thumb and forefinger). Sucks, chews, and bites objects. Holds bottle and places it in mouth.
10 months	Stands, cruises (walks sideways holding onto something).	Can clap, wave, and bring hands together to play "peek-a-boo."
11 months	Tries to walk alone.	Puts objects into container. Very precise pincer grasp.
12 months	Walks alone.	Positive Babinski reflex beginning to fade. Can hold a cup.

Language Development

Undifferentiated crying in early infancy communicates infants' needs. By 1 month of age, crying becomes differentiated as the pitch and intensity of the cry communicates various needs such as hunger, discomfort, anger, or pain. Infants are cooing with pleasure by about 6 weeks and babbling by 4 months. They begin to imitate the sounds of others by 9 to 10 months, although infants do not necessarily understand the meaning of their sounds. By 1 year, most infants say two to five words with meaning.

Cognitive Development

According to Piaget, infants are in the sensorimotor phase of cognitive development, during which the infant changes from a primarily reflexive response to being able to organize sensorimotor activities in relation to the environment. At birth, the infant responds to the environment with automatic reflexes. From 1 to 4 months, the infant perceives events as centered on the body and objects as an extension of self. By 4 to 8 months, infants gradually acknowledge the external environment (see Figure 3.1 •). They begin to develop the notion of *object permanence,* the concept that objects and people continue to exist even though they are no longer in sight. The infant first learns to search for a partially hidden object but does not search for one completely out of sight. By 9 to 10 months, the infant learns to search behind a screen for an object if it was seen to be placed there.

Psychosocial Development

According to Freud's psychoanalytic theory of personality, the id is present at birth. The unconscious source of motive and desires, the id operates on the "pleasure principle" and strives for immediate gratification. Infants are egocentric and do not differentiate themselves from the outside world. The id motivates infants, and infants view the world as existing solely for their gratification. When gratification is delayed, the ego develops as infants begin to differentiate themselves from the environment.

Infants are in what Freud called the oral stage of psychosexual development until 12 months of age. Most of their gratifi-

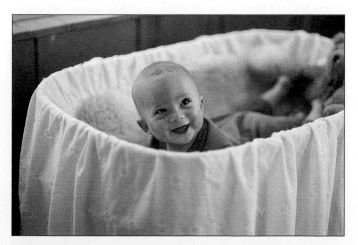

Figure 3.1 • An infant begins to notice the external environment by the age of 4 to 8 months.

cation is obtained from sucking nipples, hands, and objects, which satisfies the id's need for immediate gratification. Non-nutrient sucking on a pacifier, fingers, or thumb helps satisfy infants' need for oral gratification.

Erikson believed that the quality of care infants receive during the early months determines the degree to which they learn to trust themselves, other people, and the world in general. Erikson defined the primary task of infancy as developing a sense of trust or a sense of mistrust. Trust develops as the infant's basic needs are met through sucking, feeding, warmth, comfort, sensory stimulation, and other activities that convey the sense of love and security. Basic trust versus mistrust is not resolved only during infancy but is also a component of each successive stage of development. A basically trusting child may later develop a sense of mistrust when lied to by someone the child respects. However, the foundation for all later psychosocial development is laid in infancy because, according to Erikson, the consistency and quality of the parent-infant interaction directly affect the infant's development of ego identity, or self-concept.

All theorists of infant psychosocial development acknowledge the significance of the manner in which infants' needs are met. Although the concept of infant needs and the best way to meet them varies from theorist to theorist, it is clear that infants' needs extend beyond the physiological domain. Infants who lack sufficient social and cognitive stimulation exhibit signs of physical and affective imbalance. Children who receive adequate social and cognitive stimuli progress through sequentially more complex affective and social behaviors.

According to *attachment theory,* Brethertone (1992), a focused, enduring relationship between the infant and the primary caregiver is imperative for the healthy attainment of infant goals and is a precursor for relating appropriately to others in the future. Occurring over a period of months, attachment requires consistent, intimate interaction between the infant and primary caregiver. Many factors affect attachment. The infant and the primary caregiver each bring a unique temperament, personality, and style to the relationship. In addition, the primary caregiver's previous life experiences and preconceived expectations of the infant and parenting experience influence the attachment process.

The quality of attachment depends on what is often referred to as goodness of fit of the infant and primary caregiver. *Goodness of fit* refers to the concept that both the infant and primary caregiver must receive positive feedback and evoke a positive response in the relationship in order for attachment to develop. The crying infant who quiets in response to being held by the primary caregiver makes the primary caregiver feel successful. The infant who is difficult to console gives negative feedback with continued crying, making the primary caregiver feel unsuccessful and perhaps unloved. The primary caregiver transmits anxiety about parenting abilities to the infant, increasing the crying. By smiling and cooing in response to the primary caregiver's vocalizations, the infant encourages the caregiver to continue vocalizations, providing the infant with environmental stimulation.

By 3 months, the infant and primary caregiver achieve social synchrony, which is apparent in reciprocal vocal and affective exchanges. This mutually satisfying synchrony signals the end of the early adjustment period. The next step in attachment occurs at 3 to 5 months when the infant develops a clear preference for primary caregivers. As memory for absent objects emerges between 7 and 9 months, the infant's preference for primary caregivers creates the reaction of stranger anxiety.

Throughout the first year of life, the infant's crying serves as the signal of the need for comfort. Research has shown that infants whose mothers respond promptly to their cries in the first months of life cry less at 1 year. It is now well accepted that responding promptly to infants' cries helps establish a sense of internal security that fosters later independence. Concern over "spoiling" infants by promptly responding to their cries is no longer an accepted concept. Chronically inconsistent nurturing of infants may result in infants and toddlers uninterested in exploring, even in the presence of the caregiver. Some such children appear unusually clingy; others appear actively angry and distrustful, ignoring or resisting caregivers' efforts to comfort them.

Assessment of Infants

Frequent assessments during the first year provide opportunities to monitor the infant's rate of growth and development as well as to compare the infant with the norm for age. Height, weight, and head circumference measurements are plotted on an appropriate growth chart at each assessment. The three measurements should fall within two standard deviations of each other. More important, each measurement should follow the expected rate of growth, following the same percentile throughout infancy.

Accurate assessment combining information obtained by history, physical assessment, and knowledgeable observation allows early identification of common problems that may easily be resolved with early intervention. Often basic parent education and support remedy problems that, left untreated, could result in significant health problems or disturbed parent-child interactions later.

Overnutrition and undernutrition are identified by weight that crosses percentiles. In *overnutrition*, the rate of weight gain is accelerated and the rate of weight gain diminishes in *undernutrition*. Overnutrition may occur when caregivers do not learn to read infants' cues but instead assume that every cry signals hunger. Cultural beliefs that a fat baby is a healthy baby may also lead caregivers to overfeed infants.

Undernutrition may be caused by inadequate caloric intake resulting from lack of knowledge of normal infant feeding, a lack of financial resources to obtain formula, or inappropriate mixing of formula. Some quiet or passive infants do not demand feedings, and caregivers may misinterpret this passivity as lack of hunger.

Head growth that crosses percentiles requires evaluation as it may indicate *hydrocephalus* (enlargement of the head caused by inadequate drainage of cerebrospinal fluid). Early diagnosis and intervention for rapid head growth prevents or diminishes serious neurologic sequelae.

Parents and caregivers generally enjoy relaying infants' new developmental milestones and can accurately describe infants' abilities. An infant who seems to be lagging behind on milestones may not be receiving appropriate stimulation. Assessing caregivers' expectations and knowledge of infant development may reveal a knowledge deficit. Suggesting specific activities for caregivers to do with their infants may be the only intervention required. Infants who continue to lag further behind and are not achieving normal milestones require evaluation.

Healthy attachment is observed as a caregiver holds the infant closely in a manner that encourages eye contact. The caregiver looks at the infant, smiles, talks, and interacts with the infant. The infant responds by fixing on the caregiver's face, smiling, and cooing. The caregiver stays close to the infant, providing support and reassurance during examinations or procedures.

Failure to engage the infant through eye contact, to talk, or to smile limits available opportunities for the caregiver to receive positive feedback from the infant. The infant, in turn, finds efforts to engage the parent frustrating, resulting in decreased attempts to interact. A negative pattern is quickly established, requiring more extensive intervention the longer it persists. A thorough discussion of the assessment of infants is found in Chapter 25 of this text. ∞

TODDLERS

The **toddler** (1 to 3 years of age) is a busy, active explorer who recognizes no boundaries. Maturing muscles and developing language increase the toddler's ability to interact with the environment, allowing the child to gather information and learn with every experience. The major developmental tasks of being a toddler include the following:

- Differentiating self from others
- Tolerating separation from primary caregivers
- Controlling body functions
- Acquiring verbal communication

Physiological Growth and Development

The rate of growth decreases during the second year. The expected weight gain is about 2.5 kg (5.5 lb) between 1 and 2 years, and about 1 to 2 kg (2.2 to 4.5 lb) between 2 and 3 years. The average 3-year-old child weighs about 13.6 kg (30 lb).

Height growth is about 10 to 12 cm (4 to 5 in.) between 1 and 2 years, slowing to 6 to 8 cm (2.5 to 3.5 in.) between 2 and 3 years. Two-year-olds are approximately half of their adult size.

The head circumference of the toddler increases about 3 cm (1.25 in.) between the ages of 1 and 3 years. By 2 years the head is four fifths of the average adult size and the brain is 70% of the average adult size.

Alterations in the toddler's body proportions create striking changes in appearance as the child develops. Young toddlers appear chubby with relatively short legs and large heads. After the second year, the toddler's head becomes better proportioned, and the extremities grow faster than the trunk. Young toddlers have pronounced *lordosis* and protruding abdomens. With growth and walking, the abdominal muscles gradually develop, and the abdomen flattens.

Neurologic advances during the toddler years enable the toddler to progress developmentally. The increasing maturation of the brain contributes greatly to the child's emerging cognitive abilities. Myelinization in the spinal cord is almost complete by 2 years, corresponding to the increase in gross motor skills.

The toddler's cardiovascular system continues gradual growth. The gradual decrease in heart rate is related to the increasing size of the heart. The larger heart can pump blood more forcefully and efficiently. In addition, the toddler's capillaries constrict more efficiently to conserve body heat.

As the lungs grow in size, their volume and capacity for oxygenation also increase. This increased productivity of the lungs results in a decreased respiratory rate.

Visual acuity is close to 20/40 at 2 years and close to 20/30 by 3 years. Accommodation to near and far objects becomes fairly well developed in toddlers and continues with age. Taste and smell are well developed; taste and odor preferences and aversions are clearly communicated.

The toddler's changing body proportions are the direct result of musculoskeletal growth. Muscle grows faster than bone during the toddler years as muscle fibers increase in size and strength in response to increased use. Ossification slows after infancy but continues until maturation is complete. Long-shafted bones contain red marrow, which produces blood cells. The legs and feet of toddlers grow more rapidly than their trunks. The bowlegged appearance of young toddlers diminishes between 18 months and 2 years as the small-shafted bones rotate and gradually straighten the legs.

Motor Development

Gross and fine motor development continues at a rapid pace during the toddler years. The major accomplishments are listed below.

- *Fifteen months:* Walks independently, creeps upstairs, and is able to build a tower of two to three blocks.
- *Eighteen months:* Runs, climbs, pulls toys, and throws. Puts a block in large holes, scribbles, and builds a tower of four to five blocks.
- *Two years:* Tries to jump, and can walk up and down stairs. Can turn doorknobs, imitates a vertical stroke with crayon, uses a spoon without spilling, turns pages of a book, unbuttons a large button, and builds a tower of six to seven blocks.
- *Two and a half years:* Can stand on one foot for at least 1 second, can walk on tiptoe, jumps in place, goes up and down stairs using alternating feet, and catches a ball with arms and body. Is able to make a tower of nine large blocks, likes to fill containers with objects, will take things apart, can take off some clothing, buttons a large button, twists caps off bottles, and places simple shapes in correct holes.
- *Three years:* Pedals a tricycle, jumps from a low step, is toilet trained, can undress, puts own coat on, and catches an object with both arms. Begins to use blunt scissors, strings large beads, can copy a circle, can help with simple household tasks, can wash and dry hands, and can pull pants up and down for toileting.

Language Development

Language skills develop rapidly, progressing from a few single words at 1 year to hundreds of words used in sentences by 3 years. At 1 year, children express entire thoughts by one word, saying, for instance, "out" to express "I want to go out." Simple phrases are characteristic of the speech of 2-year-olds, such as "go car." Although their speech is simple, these children understand most of what is said to them. By 3 years, sentences are more complex and include more parts of speech.

Cognitive Development

The toddler continues in Piaget's sensorimotor stage until the age of 2 years, when the preoperational stage begins. Object permanence is fully developed by 18 to 24 months. The toddler is then able to conduct a search in many places for objects hidden from sight. As object permanence develops, toddlers develop the understanding that they are separate from the environment.

By age 2 the toddler acquires the ability to think of an external event without actually experiencing it. This is called mental representation. As a result, the toddler is now able to think through plans to reach a goal, rather than proceeding by trial and error.

With the preoperational stage, the child enters into the use of symbolic function. Instead of tying thoughts to the actual, the present, or the concrete, the child is able to think back to past events, think forward to anticipate the future, and think about what might be happening elsewhere in the present. Symbolic function enables the child to demonstrate delayed imitation: the child witnesses an event, forms a mental image of it, and later imitates it. In symbolic play, the child makes one object stand for something else, such as pretending that a laundry basket is a hat (see Figure 3.2 ●).

Psychosocial Development

According to Freud, the ego, which represents reason or common sense, continues to develop as the toddler experiences increased delays in gratification. The toddler years correspond to Freud's anal stage, during which the child takes great pleasure from expelling urine and, especially, feces. Toddlers may hold

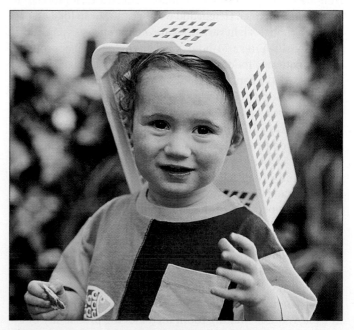

Figure 3.2 ● A toddler demonstrates symbolic play.

their stool, not wanting to give it up, or they may consider it a gift and object to its disposal. Toilet training takes on great significance as parents urge socially acceptable toileting while the child learns self-control and delayed gratification. Freud believed that the approach to toilet training and the child's reaction to it greatly influence the adult personality.

Toddlers' sense of trust developed during infancy leads them to a realization of their own sense of self. Realizing they have a will, they assert themselves in a quest for autonomy during Erikson's stage of autonomy versus shame and doubt. Parents are challenged to provide an environment in which toddlers may explore, while protecting them from danger and frustration above their level of tolerance. Parents provide a safe haven, with safe limits, from which the child can set out and discover the world, and keep coming back to them for support.

Erikson believed that toddlers who are not provided with safe limits by adults develop a sense of shame, or rage turned against themselves. Children who fail to develop a sense of autonomy, as a result of an overly controlling or permissive environment, may become compulsive about controlling themselves. Fear of losing self-control may inhibit their self-expression, make them doubt themselves, and make them feel ashamed.

Toddlers who have developed a firm attachment during infancy continue attachment behaviors during the toddler stage. Their repertoire of attachment behaviors becomes increasingly elaborate as they no longer seek prolonged body-to-body contact. Toddlers are sustained by only brief visual or physical contact with caregivers and can happily investigate new people and places. A secure attachment relationship in the first 2 years is characterized by the child's ability to seek and obtain comfort from familiar caregivers and by the child's willingness to explore and master the environment when supported by a caregiver's presence.

Assessment of Toddlers

Although the rate of growth of toddlers decreases, it proceeds in an expected manner. Height and weight continue to follow a percentile, although slight variations are often seen. Assessing caloric intake by obtaining a 24-hour recall gives clues to inappropriate feeding patterns. Toddlers generally feed themselves and begin to interact with the family at meals. A favorite food one week may be refused the next, causing frustration and confusion in caregivers. Concern for the toddler's health may precipitate a power struggle as parents try to force the toddler to eat. Poor weight gain may result as the toddler exerts a newfound independence by refusing to eat. Excessive weight gain occurs when caregivers use food to quiet or bribe their toddlers. Discussing appropriate eating expectations and weight gain helps parents resolve eating problems.

Since cooperation of the young toddler is unlikely, a health history is often the best way to assess development. Older toddlers are more willing to play with developmental testing materials or explore the environment while in proximity to a caregiver, enabling direct observations of development. Toddlers may not speak in a strange or threatening environment, making language assessment difficult. Listening to the child talk in a playroom or waiting room increases the probability of assessing the toddler's language.

The toddler wanders a short distance from a caregiver to explore, returning periodically to "touch base." After receiving reassurance and encouragement, the child is ready for further exploration. Exploration provides learning opportunities but also places the toddler at risk for accidental injury or poisoning.

Tantrums are a frequent occurrence. They are the result of unwanted limits or frustration. An attitude of calm understanding limits the duration of tantrums and keeps tantrums from becoming power struggles or attention-getting behavior.

Toddlers quickly turn to caregivers for comfort or when confronted with a stranger. Observing the adult-child interaction and listening to how the adult speaks to the child provides information on the quality of the relationship.

Continuous clinging of a toddler to a caregiver in a nonthreatening situation is unusual. Failure of the child to look to a caregiver for comfort and support may indicate that trust did not develop during infancy. Inappropriate caregiver expectations, such as expecting a toddler to sit quietly in a chair, may interfere with the normal progression of the toddler's development. Caregiver inattention to the activities of the child and failure to set limits result in the child's inability to develop self-control.

PRESCHOOL CHILDREN

The busy, curious **preschooler** (3 to 5 years of age) has an appearance and proportions closer to those of adults. The preschooler's world expands as relationships include other children and adults in settings outside the home. Developmental tasks during the preschool period include the following:

- Identifying sex role
- Developing a conscience
- Developing a sense of initiative
- Interacting with others in socially acceptable ways
- Learning to use language for social interaction

Physiological Growth and Development

Preschoolers tend to grow more in height than weight and appear taller and thinner than toddlers. Weight gain is generally slow at a rate of about 2 kg (4.5 lb) per year. The rate of height growth is about 7 cm (2.75 in.) per year.

The preschooler's brain reaches almost its adult size by 5 years. Myelinization of the central nervous system continues, resulting in refinement of movement. Most physiological systems continue to grow and are nearing maturity. Visual acuity remains approximately 20/30 throughout the preschool years. The musculoskeletal system continues to develop. Muscles are growing, and cartilage is changing to bone at a faster rate than previously. From 4 to 7 years, the active red bone marrow of earlier ages is gradually replaced by fatty tissue.

Motor Development

Gross and fine motor skills continue to be refined during the preschool years.

- *Three and a half years:* Skips on one foot, hops forward on both feet, kicks a large ball, and catches an object with hands. Cuts straight lines with scissors, manipulates large puzzle pieces into position, places small pegs in a pegboard, copies a circle, and unbuttons small buttons.

- *Four years:* Jumps well, hops forward on one foot, walks backward, and catches an object with one hand. Cuts around pictures with scissors, can copy a square, and can button small buttons.
- *Five years:* Can jump rope, and alternates feet to skip. May be able to print own name, copies a triangle, dresses without assistance, threads small beads on a string, and eats with a fork.

Language Development

Language becomes a tool for social interaction. As the preschooler's vocabulary increases, sentence structure becomes more complex, and the child becomes better able to understand another's point of view and share ideas. Speech should be 80% to 90% understandable by age 4. Sentences evolve from three or four words between 3 and 4 years, to six to eight words in grammatically correct sentences by 5 to 6 years.

Cognitive Development

Preschoolers are in the middle of Piaget's preoperational stage. Although symbolic thought is an immense milestone begun as a toddler, the preschooler's thinking continues to be rudimentary. Preschoolers continue to be egocentric and unable to see another's point of view. In addition, they feel no need to defend their point of view, because they assume that everyone else sees things as they do. Preschoolers demonstrate centration; they focus on one aspect of a situation and ignore others, leading to illogical reasoning. In addition, preschoolers believe that their wishes, thoughts, and gestures command the universe. The child believes that these "magical" powers of thought are the cause of all events.

Preschoolers enter Piaget's stage of intuitive thought at about 4 years. While egocentricity continues, older preschoolers are developing the ability to give reasons for their beliefs and actions and to form some concepts. They are limited by their inability to consider more than one idea at a time, making it impossible for them to make comparisons. Fantasy play begins to give way to play that imitates reality (see Figure 3.3 ●).

Psychosocial Development

The superego, or conscience, develops as the preschooler becomes more aware of other people's interests, needs, and values. The child learns right from wrong, developing an understanding of the consequences of actions. At this stage, the child's conscience is rigid and often unrealistic. With maturity, the conscience becomes more realistic and flexible.

As preschoolers become further aware of their separateness, gender awareness develops. They learn what makes girls different from boys during what Freud called the phallic phase. At this time, Freud believed that children have a romantic attraction to the parent of the opposite sex, making them rivals with their same-sex parent. The resulting fear and guilt are resolved as children identify with the same-sex parent, realizing they are unable to compete with the bigger, powerful parent. According to Freud, sexual urges are repressed, and the sex-related behaviors, attitudes, and beliefs of the same-sex parent are imitated.

Erikson believed that children's primary conflict at this stage is between initiative, which enables them to plan and carry out

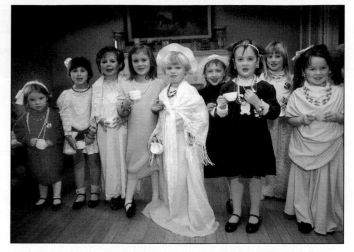

Figure 3.3 ● Preschoolers imitate reality in their play.

activities, and guilt over what they want to do. Their high level of energy, eagerness to try new things, and ability to work cooperatively characterize preschoolers. Children who are encouraged, reassured, and cheered on in their pursuits learn self-assertion, self-sufficiency, direction, and purpose. They develop initiative. Children who are ridiculed, punished, or prevented from accomplishing initiative develop guilt.

Preschoolers turn from a total attachment to their caregivers and begin to identify with them. A firm attachment during the early years allows preschoolers to detach from caregivers at this stage. This ability to detach enables children to explore new territory, learn new games, and form new relationships with peers.

Assessment of Preschool Children

Preschoolers' slowed rate of growth is often of concern to caregivers. The nurse can allay anxiety by showing the preschooler's growth chart and discussing eating expectations.

Preschoolers are generally pleasant, cooperative, and talkative. They continue to need the reassurance of a caregiver in view but do not need to return to the caregiver for comfort except in threatening situations. Talking with preschoolers about favorite activities allows the nurse to assess language ability, cognitive ability, and development. The nurse evaluates the child's use of language to express thoughts, sentence structure, and vocabulary. It may be possible to identify centration, magical thinking, and reality imitation as the child relays play activities. Lack of appropriate environmental stimulation may become evident, and the nurse may need to educate caregivers about age-appropriate activities for their children.

A clinging, frightened preschooler in a nonthreatening situation may be a child who lacks trust. Lack of communication between caregiver and child limits the child's ability to learn appropriate social interaction. In addition, the child does not have the opportunity to practice language skills or to obtain information by having questions answered. See Box 3.1 for a detailed listing of interventions, screenings, and counseling for ages birth to 10 years. A thorough discussion of the assessment of children is found in Chapter 25 of this text. ⚭

Box 3.1	Periodic Health Examination: Birth to 10 Years

Interventions Considered and Recommended for the Periodic Health Examination

Leading Causes of Death

Conditions originating in perinatal period
Congenital anomalies
Sudden infant death syndrome (SIDS)
Unintentional injuries (nonmotor vehicle)
Motor vehicle injuries

INTERVENTIONS FOR THE GENERAL POPULATION

Screening
Height and weight
Blood pressure
Vision screen (age 3–4 yr)
Hemoglobinopathy screen (birth)[1]
Phenylalanine level (birth)[2]
T_4 and/or TSH (birth)[3]

Counseling
Injury prevention
    Child safety car seats (age <5 yr)
    Lap-shoulder belts (age ≥5 yr)
    Bicycle helmet; avoid bicycling near traffic
    Smoke detector, flame retardant sleepwear
    Hot water heater temperature <120−130°F
    Window/stair guards, pool fence
    Safe storage of drugs, toxic substances, firearms, and matches
    Syrup of ipecac, poison control phone number
    CPR training for parents/caretakers
Diet and exercise
    Breastfeeding, iron-enriched formula and foods (infants and toddlers)

Diet and Exercise
    Limit fat and cholesterol; maintain caloric balance; emphasize grains, fruits, vegetables (age ≥2 yr)
    Regular physical activity
Substance use
    Effects of passive smoking
    Antitobacco message
Dental health
    Regular visits to dental care provider
    Floss, brush with fluoride toothpaste daily
    Advice about baby bottle tooth decay

Immunizations
Diphtheria-tetanus-pertussis (DTP)[4]
Oral poliovirus (OPV)[5]
Measles-mumps-rubella (MMR)[6]
H. influenzae type b (Hib) conjugate[7]
Hepatitis B[8]
Varicella[9]

Chemoprophylaxis
Ocular prophylaxis (birth)

INTERVENTIONS FOR HIGH-RISK POPULATIONS

Population	Potential Interventions
Preterm or low birth weight	Hemoglobin/hematocrit
Infants of mothers at risk for HIV	HIV testing
Low income; immigrants	Hemoglobin/hematocrit; PPD
TB contacts	PPD
Native American/Alaska Native	Hemoglobin/hematocrit; PPD; hepatitis A vaccine; pneumococcal vaccine
Travelers to developing countries	Hepatitis A vaccine
Residents of long-term care facilities	PPD; hepatitis A vaccine; influenza vaccine
Certain chronic medical conditions	PPD; pneumococcal vaccine; influenza vaccine
Increased individual or community lead exposure	Blood lead level
Inadequate water fluoridation	Daily fluoride supplement
Family h/o skin cancer; nevi; fair skin, eyes, hair	Avoid excess/midday sun, use protective clothing

[1]Whether screening should be universal or targeted to high-risk groups will depend on the proportion of high-risk individuals in the screening area, and other considerations. [2]If done during first 24 hr of life, repeat at age 2 wk. [3]Optimally between day 2 and 6, but in all cases before newborn nursery discharge. [4]2, 4, 6, and 12–18 mo, once between ages 4–6 yr (DTaP may be used at 15 mo and older). [5]2, 4, 6–18 mo, once between ages 4–6 yr. [6]12–15 mo and 4–6 yr. [7]2, 4, 6, and 12–15 mo, no dose needed at 6 mo if PRP-OMP vaccine is used for first 2 doses. [8]Birth, 1 mo, 6 mo; or, 0–2 mo, 1–2 mo, later, and 6–18 mo. If not done in infancy: current visit, and 1 and 6 mo later. [9]12–18 mo; or older child without hx of chickenpox or previous immunization. Include information on risk in adulthood, duration of immunity, and potential need for booster doses.

CRP, Cardiopulmonary resuscitation; *HIV,* human immunodeficiency virus; *TB,* tuberculosis; *PPD,* purified protein derviative; *STDs,* sexually transmitted diseases; *BCG,* bacille Calmette-Guérin.

Source: Adapted from U.S. Preventive Services Task Force: *Guide to clinical preventive services,* 2nd ed., Baltimore, 1996, Williams & Wilkins. For detailed high-risk definitions, see complete table at http://evolve.elsevier.com/Jarvis/.

SCHOOL-AGE CHILDREN

School age begins about the age of 6 years, when deciduous teeth are shed, and ends with the onset of puberty at about 12 years. Tasks of the school-age child include the following:

- Mastering physical skills
- Building self-esteem and a positive self-concept
- Fitting in to a peer group
- Developing logical reasoning

Physiological Growth and Development

Most children during the years from 6 to 10 reach a relative plateau, with growth occurring in a slow but steady manner. The average child gains about 3 kg (6.5 lb) and grows about 5.5 cm (2 in.) per year. Growth accelerates again at the onset of puberty, which occurs about age 10 for girls and age 12 for boys. During preadolescence (10 to 12 or 13 years), the growth of boys and girls differs. Growth in boys is generally slow and steady, and rapid in girls. Growth is variable, especially among girls at this age. Some girls of 11 years look like children, while others are starting to look like adolescents. By 12 years, some boys are beginning their growth spurt and demonstrating the onset of secondary sexual characteristics.

The body proportions of the school-age child are different from those of the preschooler. Children often appear gangly and awkward because of their proportionately longer legs, diminishing body fat, and a lower center of gravity. As increases in organ maturity and size occur, the child responds physiologically to illness in a more adult manner. The continuing maturation of the central nervous system (CNS) allows the child to perform increasingly complex gross and fine motor skills. Brain growth is slowed, with 95% of growth achieved by 9 years of age. Myelinization continues and is partly responsible for the transformation of the clumsy 6-year-old into the coordinated 12-year-old.

As cardiac growth continues, the diaphragm descends, allowing more room for cardiac action and respiratory expansion. The respiratory tissues achieve adult maturity, with lung capacity proportional to body size.

Most children achieve 20/20 vision by age 5 or 6 years. Visual maturity, including fully developed peripheral vision, is usually achieved by 6 or 7 years.

The most rapid growth during the school-age years occurs in the skeletal system. Ossification continues at a steady pace. Muscle mass gradually increases in size and strength, and the body appears leaner as "baby fat" decreases. As muscle tone increases, the loose movements, "knock-knees," and lordosis of early childhood disappear.

Motor Development

The gross motor skills of the 6- to 7-year-old are far better developed than fine motor coordination. Children of this age greatly enjoy gross motor activity such as hopping, roller-skating, bike riding, running, and climbing. The child seems to be in perpetual motion. Balance and eye-hand coordination gradually improve. The 6-year-old is able to hammer, paste, tie shoes, and fasten clothes. Right- or left-hand dominance is firmly established by age 6. By age 7, the child's hands become steadier. Printing becomes smaller, and reversal of letters during writing is less common. Many children have sufficient finger coordination to begin music lessons.

Less restlessness is seen in 7- and 8-year-old children, although they retain their high energy level. Increased attention span and cognitive skills enhance their enjoyment of board games. Improved reaction time increases sports ability.

Children between 8 and 10 years of age gradually develop greater rhythm, smoothness, and gracefulness of movements. They are able to participate in physical activities that require more concentrated attention and effort. They have sufficient coordination to write rather than print words, and they may begin sewing, building models, and playing musical instruments.

Energy levels remain high in children between 10 and 12 years of age, but activity is well directed and controlled. Physical skills are almost equal to those of the adult. Manipulative skills are also comparable to the precision exhibited by adults. Complex, intricate, and rapid movements are mastered with practice.

Language Development

The school-age child uses appropriate sentence structure and continues to develop the ability to express thoughts in words. Comprehension of language continues to exceed the school-age child's ability of expression. Vocabulary increases as the child is exposed to a wider range of reading materials and ideas in school and through association with peers.

Cognitive Development

Sometime around 6 or 7 years of age, children become what Piaget called operational. They are now able to use symbols to carry out operations, or mental activities, enabling them to perform activities such as reading and using numbers. The child becomes able to serialize, that is, order objects according to size or weight. In addition, the child begins to understand how to classify objects by something they have in common. Children commonly practice this new skill by collecting and frequently sorting collections of rocks, sports cards, shells, or dolls (see Figure 3.4 ●).

The school-age child develops an understanding of the principle of conservation, the ability to tell the difference between how things seem and how they really are. The child is able to see that transformation of shape or position does not change the mass or quantity of a substance. For instance, the child understands that two equal balls of clay remain equal when one ball is rolled into a "hot dog." In contrast, a younger child who has not mastered the principle of conservation believes the cylindrical shape is bigger because it is longer.

School-age children develop logical reasoning and understand cause-and-effect relationships. They can consider various sides of a situation and form a conclusion. Egocentrism decreases as the child becomes able to consider another's point of view. Although able to reason, the child is still somewhat limited by the inability to deal with abstract ideas.

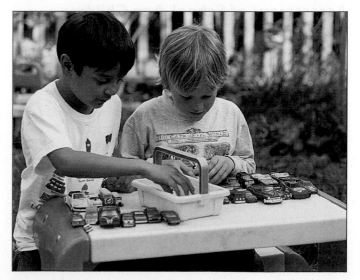

Figure 3.4 ● School-age children enjoy classifying objects.

Psychosocial Development

School-age children have accepted their sex roles and are now able to turn their energies to acquiring new facts, mastering skills, and learning cultural attitudes. Freud termed this the latency stage, considering it a time of relative sexual quiet. Curiosity about sex, and sexual and bathroom jokes demonstrate the ongoing sexual awareness of school-age children; however, the sexual turbulence of earlier and later stages is absent.

Erikson described the crises of this stage as industry versus inferiority. If children are motivated by activities that provide a sense of worth, they focus their attention on mastering skills in school, sports, the arts, and social interaction. Approval and recognition for their achievements result in feelings of confidence, competence, and industry. When children feel that they cannot meet the expectations of family or of society, they lose confidence, lack the drive to achieve, and develop feelings of inferiority and incompetence. The challenge of caregivers and teachers is to praise accomplishments and encourage skill development while avoiding criticism in areas in which children fail to excel. Providing successful experiences and positive reinforcement for children increases their opportunities to achieve.

Belonging to groups and being accepted by peers take on a new significance for school-age children. Children form clubs and gather in groups, often implementing strict rules or secret codes. They gradually become less self-centered and selfish as they learn to cooperate as part of a group. With this increased social exposure, children begin to question parental values and ideas. The family, however, remains the major influence on behavior and decisions.

As children enter the late school-age or preadolescent years (10 to 12 or 13 years), the caregiver-child relationship becomes strained as children begin to drift away from the family. Preadolescent children increasingly challenge parental authority and reject family standards as they discover that the family is "not perfect and does not know everything." Identification with a peer group increases, and children form a close relationship with a best friend. Some children begin to show an interest in others of the opposite sex. Preadolescents continue to want and need some restrictions, because their immaturity makes determining their own rules too frightening.

Assessment of School-Age Children

The slow, steady growth and changing body proportions of school-age children make them appear thin and gangly. Assessing children's intake of nutrients and calories and reviewing their growth charts reassures parents that their children are not too thin. The nurse can relieve family stress resulting from parents pushing their children to eat by educating parents to evaluate objectively their children's diets during the early school-age years. Older school-age children have an increase in appetite as they enter the prepubertal growth spurt. During the growth spurt, height and weight increase and may normally cross percentiles.

School-age children are eager to talk about their hobbies, friends, school, and accomplishments. Increasing neurologic maturity allows them to master activities requiring gross and fine motor control such as sports, dancing, playing a musical instrument, artistic pursuits, or building things. School-age children enjoy showing off newly acquired skills, and the family displays pride in their children's accomplishments.

School-age children frequently sort and classify collections of rocks, sports cards, dolls, coins, stamps, or almost anything. They are industrious in school, feeling pride in their accomplishments as they master difficult concepts and skills. The family provides positive feedback and encouragement to their children and speaks of their children's successes with pride.

Adult family members and school-age children communicate openly, with adults setting needed limits. Although peer relationships are becoming more important, the family remains the major influence during most of the school-age years. As children approach adolescence, the relationship with family may become strained as the children are drawn closer to peer groups and seek greater independence.

Children who lack hobbies or cannot think of any accomplishments may be environmentally deprived. Caregivers who are unable to think of anything positive to say about their children or who speak of them as a burden likely have a disturbed parent-child relationship. Children who lack encouragement and positive reinforcement at home for their achievements are at risk for gang recruitment. Gangs provide the "family" support children lack at home, increasing children's risk for violence, drug use, and illegal activity.

Problems in school may evolve at this time, with conflicts over grades and study time. The nurse can encourage the caregiver to help the child set a consistent place and time for homework. Caregivers should also be encouraged to communicate actively with the child's teacher. Teachers, adults, family members, and healthcare providers may identify learning disabilities at this time by careful observation.

ADOLESCENTS

Adolescence marks the transition from childhood to adulthood (12 to 19 or 20 years). Although all children undergo this transformation, passing through the stages of growth and development in a predictable sequence, the age and rate at which it occurs are highly variable. In a group of children of the same age, some look and act like children and some look and act like young adults. Adolescence is divided into three phases: early (10 to 13 years), middle (14 to 17 years), and late (17 to 21 years). The search for one's unique self or identity is the foundation of the tasks of this stage. Tasks of this period include the following:

- Searching for identity
- Increasing independence from parents
- Forming close relationships with peers
- Developing analytic thinking
- Forming a value system
- Developing a sexual identity
- Choosing a career

Physiological Growth and Development

An increase in physical size is a universal event during puberty, with maximum growth occurring prior to the onset of discernible sexual development. Pubertal weight gain accounts for about 50% of an individual's ideal adult body weight. While the percentage of body fat increases in females during puberty, it decreases in adolescent males. Pubertal height growth accounts for 20% to 25% of final adult height. The growth spurt generally begins between the ages of 12 and 14 in girls, and between 12 and 16 in boys, and lasts 24 to 30 months. Girls experience their fastest rate of growth at about 12 years, gaining 4.6 kg (10 lb) to 10.6 kg (23.5 lb) and growing 5.4 cm (2 in.) to 11.2 cm (4.5 in.). Boys experience their fastest rate of growth at about 14 years, gaining 5.7 kg (12.5 lb) to 13.2 kg (29 lb) and growing 5.8 cm (2.25 in.) to 13.1 cm (5.25 in.).

During puberty, the period of maturation of the reproductive system, primary and secondary sexual characteristics develop in response to endocrine changes. Primary sexual development includes the changes that occur in the organs directly related to reproduction, such as the ovaries, uterus, breasts, penis, and testes. Secondary sexual development includes the changes that occur in other parts of the body in response to hormonal changes, such as development of facial and pubic hair, voice changes, and fat deposits. Some changes such as increased activity in sebaceous and sweat glands occur as early as 9½ years of age in girls and at 10½ years of age in boys. Further information about changes in secondary sex characteristics is included in Chapters 21 and 22 of this text. ⬭ The Centers for Disease Control and Prevention (CDC) can be contacted at their website by linking through the Companion Website.

Brain tissue appears to reach maturity with puberty, and myelinization continues until the middle adult years. Because growth of the cerebrum, cerebellum, and brain stem is essentially complete by the end of the tenth year, the central nervous system (CNS) does not experience substantial growth during the pubertal period.

A cardiac growth spurt occurs during the prepubertal growth period, increasing cardiac strength, elevating the blood pressure, and stabilizing the pulse at a lower rate. Cardiac output becomes more dependent on stroke volume than heart rate.

During the growth spurt, rapid growth of the hands and feet occurs first, then growth of the long bones of the arms and legs, followed by trunk growth. Skull and facial bones change proportions as the forehead becomes more prominent and the jawbones develop. The growth rate slows after the onset of the external signs of puberty as ossification slows, and the epiphyseal maturation of the long bones occurs in response to hormonal influences. Since androgen influences bone density, the bones of males become more dense than those of females. Androgen also appears to be directly related to the significant increase in male muscle mass.

Cognitive Development

The period of adolescence corresponds to Piaget's stage of formal operations in which abstract thinking develops. Adolescents develop the ability to integrate past learning and present problems to plan for the future. They learn to use logic and solve problems by methodically analyzing each possibility. They use this new ability in scientific reasoning, and they create hypotheses and test them by setting up experiments. Analytic thinking extends to the adolescent's development of values. No longer content to accept what others say in an unquestioning manner, the adolescent can reason through inconsistencies and consider value options.

Psychosocial Development

According to Freud, sexual urges repressed during latency reawaken as adolescents enter the genital stage. Sexual gratification comes with finding a partner outside of the family.

Erikson described the conflict of adolescence as ego identity versus role diffusion. Homogeneous cliques support adolescents through the difficult search for their identity. They become very concerned with their bodies, their appearances, and their abilities, avoiding anything that would make them appear different. According to Erikson, the intolerance of others outside the clique displayed by adolescents is a temporary defense against identity confusion.

Adolescents' search for identity is stressful for adolescents and their families. The peer group becomes even more important than during the school-age years, providing a sense of belonging. Peer group participation allows adolescents to develop comfort in social participation (see Figure 3.5 ●). Peer group influence on clothing and hairstyles, beliefs, values, and actions may create tension between adolescents and their families. As personal identity evolves, adolescents begin to plan for a future career and prepare to enter adulthood.

Assessment of Adolescents

Caregivers rarely express concern that their adolescents are not eating. The pubertal growth spurt requires adolescents to increase their caloric intake dramatically, causing parents concern that they eat constantly but never seem full. Adolescents (particularly women) are at risk for developing eating disorders; feelings surrounding changes in the body should be explored.

Adolescents often communicate better with peers and adults outside of the family than with family members. Assessing adolescents with their parents and then one-on-one affords a more complete picture of their relationship and provides adolescents with an opportunity to freely express themselves and discuss concerns.

Adolescents are able to hold an adult conversation and are often happy to discuss school, friends, activities, and plans for the future. They tend to be anxious about their bodies and the rapid changes occurring. Often adolescents are unsure if what is happening to them is normal, and they frequently express somatic complaints.

As adolescents become more independent, adult family members become anxious over their evolving lack of control. Parents may be uncomfortable with adolescents' sexuality, rebellious dress and hairstyles, and developing values which may

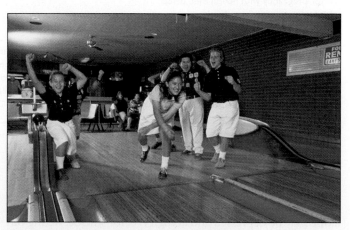

Figure 3.5 ● Peer group activity of adolescents.

Box 3.2	Periodic Health Examination: Ages 11–24 Years

Interventions Considered and Recommended for the Periodic Health Examination

Leading Causes of Death
Motor vehicle/other unintentional injuries
Homicide
Suicide
Malignant neoplasms
Heart diseases

INTERVENTIONS FOR THE GENERAL POPULATION

Screening
Height and weight
Blood pressure[1]
Papanicolaou (Pap) test[2] (females)
Chlamydia screen[3] (females <20 yr)
Rubella serology or vaccination hx[4] (females >12 yr)
Assess for problem drinking

Counseling
Injury prevention
  Lap/shoulder belts
  Bicycle/motorcycle/ATV helmets
  Smoke detector
  Safe storage/removal of firearms
Substance use
  Avoid tobacco use
  Avoid underage drinking and illicit drug use
  Avoid alcohol/drug use while driving, swimming, boating, etc.
Sexual behavior
  STD prevention: abstinence; avoid high-risk behavior; use condoms, female barrier with spermicide
  Unintended pregnancy: contraception

Diet and exercise
  Limit fat and cholesterol; maintain caloric balance; emphasize grains, fruits, vegetables
  Adequate calcium intake (females)
  Regular physical activity
Dental health
  Regular visits to dental care provider
  Floss, brush with fluoride toothpaste daily

Immunizations
Tetanus-diphtheria (Td) boosters (11–16 yr)
Hepatitis B[5]
MMR (11–12 yr)[6]
Varicella (11–12 yr)[7]
Rubella[4] (females >12 yr)

Chemoprophylaxis
Multivitamin with folic acid (females planning/capable of pregnancy)

INTERVENTIONS FOR HIGH-RISK POPULATIONS

Population	Potential Interventions
High-risk sexual behavior	RPR/VDRL; screen for gonorrhea (female), HIV, chlamydia (female); hepatitis A vaccine
Injection or street drug use	RPR/VDRL; HIV screen; hepatitis A vaccine; PPD; advice to reduce infection risk
TB contacts; immigrants; low income	PPD
Native Americans/Alaska Natives	Hepatitis A vaccine; PPD; pneumococcal vaccine
Travelers to developing countries	Hepatitis A vaccine
Certain chronic medical conditions	PPD; pneumococcal vaccine; influenza vaccine
Settings where adolescents and young adults congregate	Second MMR
Susceptible to varicella, measles, mumps	Varicella vaccine; MMR
Blood transfusion between 1978 and 1985	HIV screen
Institutionalized persons; healthcare/lab workers	Hepatitis A vaccine; PPD; influenza vaccine
Family h/o skin cancer; nevi; fair skin, eyes, hair	Avoid excess/midday sun, use protective clothing
Prior pregnancy with neural tube defect	Folic acid 4.0 mg
Inadequate water fluoridation	Daily fluoride supplement

[1]Periodic blood pressure for persons aged ≥21 yr. [2]If sexually active at present or in the past: q ≤3 yr. If sexual history is unreliable, begin Pap tests at age 18 yr. [3]If sexually active. [4]Serologic testing, documented vaccination history, and routine vaccination against rubella (preferably with MMR) are equally acceptable alternatives. [5]If not previously immunized: current visit, 1 and 6 mo later. [6]If no previous second dose of MMR. [7]If susceptible to chickenpox.
ATV, All-terrain vehicle; *STD*, sexually transmitted disease; *MMR*, measles-mumps-rubella; *TB*, tuberculosis; *HIV*, human immunodeficiency virus; *RPR*, rapid plasma reagin; *VDRL*, Venereal Disease Research Laboratories, *PPD*, purified protein derivative, *BCG*, bacille Calmette-Guérin.

differ from those of the parents. Communication between parents and adolescents is often challenging at this stage.

Severely restricting the activities and freedom of adolescents inhibits their ability to progress toward independence. Adolescents who lack social contacts and tend to spend much time alone may be depressed and at high risk for suicide. Acting out and risk-taking behaviors place adolescents at risk for serious injury from accidents or drug or alcohol use. Alliance with gangs places adolescents at risk for violence and participation in illegal activities.

See Box 3.2 for a detailed listing of interventions, screenings, and counseling for ages 11 to 24 years.

YOUNG ADULTS

The **young adult** (20 to 40 years) establishes a new life on a chosen career path and in a lifestyle independent of parents. Tasks of this period include the following:

- Leaving the family home
- Establishing a career or vocation
- Choosing a mate and forming an intimate relationship
- Managing one's own household
- Establishing a social group
- Beginning a parenting role
- Developing a meaningful philosophy of life

Physiological Development

During young adulthood, the body reaches its maximum potential for growth and development, and all systems function at peak efficiency. Skeletal system growth is completed around 25 years of age with the final fusion of the epiphyses of the long bones. The vertebral column continues to grow until about 30 years, adding perhaps 3 to 5 mm to an individual's height. Adult distribution of red bone marrow is achieved at about 25 years of age. Muscular efficiency reaches its peak performance between 20 and 30 years and declines at a variable rate thereafter.

Cognitive Development

According to Piaget, by young adulthood, cognitive structures have been completed. During the formal operations stage in adolescence, abstract thinking has been achieved. Formal operations characterize thinking throughout adulthood. Young adults continue to develop, however, as egocentrism diminishes and thinking evolves in a more realistic and objective manner.

Psychosocial Development

According to Erikson, the central task of young adults in their early 20s is intimacy versus isolation. During this stage, the young adult forms one or more intimate relationships. A secure self-identity must be established before a mutually satisfying and mature relationship can be formed with another person. The mature relationship requires the ability to establish mutual trust, cooperate with another, share feelings and goals, and completely accept the other person.

Other theorists believe that young adulthood consists of several stages. The 20s are generally accepted as the time of establishing oneself in adult society by choosing a mate, friends, an occupation, values, and a lifestyle. Around the age of 30, life is reassessed and the person either reaffirms past choices or deliberates changes. During the 30s, life again settles down, with the adult striving to build a better life in all aspects. It is a time of financial and emotional investment, and career advancement (see Figure 3.6 ●).

The decision whether to have children usually is made sometime during the young adult years. The addition of children requires major role adjustment and causes readjustment in a couple's relationship.

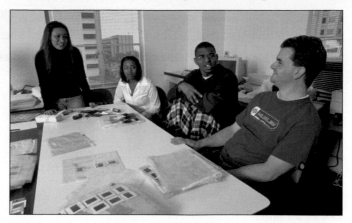

Figure 3.6 ● Young adults strive to advance their careers.

Assessment of Young Adults

Young adults are busy, productive, and healthy. At their maximum physical potential, young adults actively pursue sports and physical fitness activities. They refine their creative talents and enjoy activities with peers.

Young adults form an intimate partnership with another in a mature, cooperative relationship. Traditionally, this intimate relationship involved marriage. Increasingly, the relationship is formed and maintained without a formal marriage or between two people of the same sex. Developmentally, the important concept is the formation of the mature, intimate relationship.

People deciding to have children have many more choices than previously: surrogate motherhood, artificial insemination, in vitro fertilization, and other technological innovations. Deciding not to have children or delaying having children is increasingly accepted, as is the decision of single women to have children.

Young adults have chosen an occupation, established their values, and adopted a lifestyle. Career advancement, financial stability, and emotional investment characterize the young adult years.

The young adult without a steady job may lack direction and self-confidence. Marital discord may trigger feelings of failure and insecurity. Failing to achieve intimacy may place the young adult at risk for depression, alcoholism, or drug abuse.

See Box 3.3 for a detailed listing of interventions, screenings, and counseling for ages 25 to 64 years.

MIDDLE-AGED ADULTS

Middle adulthood (40 to 65 years) signals a halfway point, with as many years behind an individual as potentially ahead. This is a time of evaluation and adjustment, and its tasks include the following:

- Accepting and adjusting to physical changes
- Reviewing and redirecting career goals
- Developing hobbies and leisure activities
- Adjusting to aging parents
- Coping with children leaving home

Box 3.3	Periodic Health Examination: Ages 25–64 Years

Interventions Considered and Recommended for the Periodic Health Examination

Leading Causes of Death

Malignant neoplasms
Heart diseases
Motor vehicle and other unintentional injuries
Human immunodeficiency virus (HIV) infection
Suicide and homicide

INTERVENTIONS FOR THE GENERAL POPULATION

Screening

Blood pressure
Height and weight
Total blood cholesterol (men age 35–65, women age 45–65)
Papanicolaou (Pap) test (women)[1]
Fecal occult blood test[2] and/or sigmoidoscopy (≥50 yr)
Mammogram ± clinical breast exam[3] (women 50–69 yr)
Assess for problem drinking
Rubella serology or vaccination hx[4] (women of childbearing age)

Counseling

Substance use
  Tobacco cessation
  Avoid alcohol/drug use while driving, swimming, boating, etc.
Diet and exercise
  Limit fat and cholesterol; maintain caloric balance; emphasize grains, fruits, vegetables
  Adequate calcium intake (women)
  Regular physical activity

Injury prevention
  Lap/shoulder belts
  Motorcycle/bicycle/ATV helmets
  Smoke detector
  Safe storage/removal of firearms
Sexual behavior
  STD prevention: avoid high-risk behavior; use condoms/female barrier with spermicide
  Unintended pregnancy: contraception
Dental health
  Regular visits to dental care provider
  Floss, brush with fluoride toothpaste daily

Immunizations

Tetanus-diphtheria (Td) boosters
Rubella[4] (women of childbearing age)

Chemoprophylaxis

Multivitamin with folic acid (women planning or capable of pregnancy)
Discuss hormone prophylaxis (peri- and postmenopausal women)

INTERVENTIONS FOR HIGH-RISK POPULATIONS

Population	Potential Interventions
High-risk sexual behavior	RPR/VDRL; screen for gonorrhea (female), HIV, chlamydia (female); hepatitis B vaccine; hepatitis A vaccine
Injection or street drug use	RPR/VDRL; HIV screen; hepatitis B vaccine; hepatitis A vaccine; PPD; advice to reduce infection risk
Low income: TB contacts; immigrants; alcoholics	PPD
Native Americans/Alaska Natives	Hepatitis A vaccine; PPD; pneumococcal vaccine
Travelers to developing countries	Hepatitis B vaccine; hepatitis A vaccine
Certain chronic medical conditions	PPD; pneumococcal vaccine; influenza vaccine
Blood product recipients	HIV screen; hepatitis B vaccine
Susceptible to measles, mumps, or varicella	MMR; varicella vaccine
Institutionalized persons	Hepatitis A vaccine; PPD; pneumococcal vaccine; influenza vaccine
Healthcare/lab workers	Hepatitis B vaccine; hepatitis A vaccine; PPD; influenza vaccine
Family h/o skin cancer; fair skin, eyes, hair	Avoid excess/midday sun, use protective clothing
Previous pregnancy with neural tube defect	Folic acid 4.0 mg

[1]Women who are or have been sexually active and who have a cervix: q ≤3 yr. [2]Annually. [3]Mammogram q1–2 yr, or mammogram q1–2 yr with annual clinical breast examination. [4]Serologic testing, documented vaccination history, and routine vaccination (preferably with MMR) are equally acceptable alternatives.

ATV, All-terrain vehicles; *STD*, sexually transmitted disease; *TB*, tuberculosis; *RPR*, rapid plasma reagin; *VDRL*, Venereal Disease Research Laboratories; *HIV*, human immunodeficiency virus; *PPD*, purified protein derivative; *MMR*, measles-mumps-rubella.

Physiological Development

Functioning of the CNS during the early years of middle adulthood is normally maintained at the same high level achieved in young adulthood. Some individuals may experience a gradual decline in mental or reflex functioning as age advances past 50 because of changes in enzyme function, hormones, and motor and sensory functions. Decreased CNS integration may result in a slower, more prolonged, and more pronounced response to stressors.

Both men and women experience decreasing hormonal production during middle adulthood. During menopause, which usually occurs between ages 40 and 55, the ovaries decrease in size, and the uterus becomes smaller and firmer. Progesterone is not produced, and estrogen levels fall, resulting in the atrophy of the reproductive organs, vasomotor disturbances, and mood swings. Men experience a gradual decrease in testosterone, causing decreased sperm and semen production and less intense orgasms.

In individuals who become more sedentary over time, the heart begins to lose tone, and rate and rhythm changes become evident. Blood vessels lose elasticity and become thicker. Degeneration of cardiovascular tissues becomes a leading cause of death in individuals over age 45.

Lung tissues become thicker, stiffer, and less elastic with age, resulting in gradually decreased breathing capacity by age 55 or 60. Respiratory rates increase in response to decreasing pulmonary function.

Visual acuity declines, especially for near vision, and auditory acuity for high-frequency sounds decreases. Skin turgor, elasticity, and moisture decrease, resulting in wrinkles. Hair thins, and gray hair appears. Fatty tissue is redistributed in the abdominal area.

Bone mass decreases from age 40 until the end of middle adulthood. Calcium loss from bone tissues becomes pronounced in females. Muscle mass and strength are maintained in individuals who continue active muscle use. In those who lead a sedentary lifestyle, muscles decline in mass, structure, and strength. Muscle loss may also result from changes in collagen fiber, which becomes thicker and less elastic.

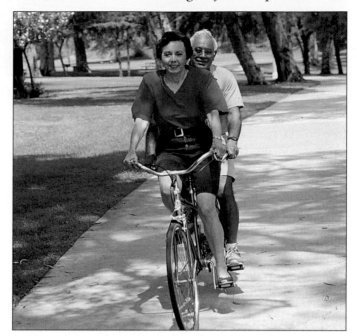

Figure 3.7 ● Middle adults usually have more time to focus attention on their relationships.

Cognitive Development

The middle adult's cognitive and intellectual abilities remain constant, continuing the abilities characteristic in Piaget's stage of formal operations. Memory and problem solving are maintained, and learning continues, often enhanced by increased motivation at this time of life. Life experiences tend to enhance cognitive abilities as the middle adult builds on past experiences.

Psychosocial Development

Erikson defined the developmental task of middle adulthood as generativity versus stagnation. He defined generativity as the concern for establishing and guiding the next generation. People turn from the self- and family-centered focus of young adulthood toward more altruistic activities such as community involvement, charitable work, and political, social, and cultural endeavors. Erikson believed that stagnation results if the need for sharing, giving, and contributing to the growth of others is not met. Stagnation refers to feelings of boredom and emptiness, which lead individuals to become inactive, self-absorbed, self-indulgent, and chronic complainers.

Some theorists believe the middle adult years begin with a transition during which a major reassessment of life accomplishments occurs. Typically the middle adult asks the question, "What have I done with my life?" People confront reality, accept that they cannot meet some goals, and emerge with redirected goals. Reassessment involves areas of career, personal identity, and family. The middle adult may reorder career goals or choose a new career path. Adjusting in a positive manner to children leaving home helps parents to focus attention on other relationships, find satisfying leisure activities, or pursue intellectual activities (see Figure 3.7 ●). Successful coping with the death of a parent helps people in middle adulthood come to terms with their own aging and death. Making financial plans and preparing for productive use of leisure time in retirement strengthen effective adaptation to retirement.

Assessment of Middle-Aged Adults

The adult in the middle years of life is satisfied with past accomplishments and involved in activities outside the family. Adjusting to the physical changes of aging, individuals develop appropriate leisure activities in preparation for an active retirement. Good financial planning during the middle adult years ensures financial security during retirement.

The middle adult years signal the end of childbearing and, most often, the end of child rearing. Individuals adjust to never having had children or to children leaving home. Couples renew their relationships or sometimes find they have little in common and separate. Some women choose to delay childbearing until their late 30s or early 40s, after establishing their careers. They begin their child-rearing years as many of their peers are completing this phase of life. Older mothers must make the transition from career women to mothers, even if they continue their careers.

The dissatisfied middle adult is unhappy with the past and expresses no hope for the future. Sedentary and isolated, the individual complains about life, avoids involvement, and fails to plan appropriately for retirement.

OLDER ADULTS

Individuals in **older adulthood** (65 years and older) vary greatly in their physical and psychosocial adaptation to aging. Developmental tasks of older adults include the following:

● Adjusting to declining physical strength and health
● Forming relationships within one's peer group
● Adjusting to retirement
● Developing postretirement activities that maintain self-worth and usefulness
● Adjusting to the death of spouse, family members, and friends
● Conducting a life review
● Preparing for death

Physiological Development

During the later years, there is an inevitable decline in body functions. The body becomes less efficient in receiving, processing, and responding to stimuli. The CNS experiences a decrease in electrical activity, resulting in slowed or altered sensory reception and decreases in reaction time and movement.

The cardiovascular system demonstrates degenerative effects in old age. Fatty plaques are deposited in the lining of blood vessels, decreasing their ability to supply blood to tissues. Systolic blood pressure increases as a result of the inelasticity of the arteries and an increase in peripheral resistance. Endocardial thickening and hardening throughout the heart decrease the efficiency of its pumping action. The valves become more rigid and less pliable, leading to reduced filling and emptying abilities. Cardiac output and reserve diminish, resulting in an inability to react to sudden stress efficiently.

Efficiency of the lungs decreases with age, increasing the respiratory effort required to obtain adequate oxygen. Vital capacity decreases, and residual air increases with age. The bronchopulmonary tree becomes more rigid, reducing bronchopulmonary movements. Ciliary activity decreases, allowing mucous secretions to collect more readily in the respiratory tree. As a result of diminished muscle tone and decreased sensitivity to stimuli, the ability to cough decreases.

Visual changes include loss of visual acuity, decreased adaptation to darkness and dim light, loss of peripheral vision, and difficulty in discriminating similar colors. Gradual loss of hearing is the result of changes in nerve tissues in the inner ear and a thickening of the eardrum. The senses of taste and smell decrease, and older adults are less stimulated by food than before. The gradual loss of skin receptors increases the threshold for sensations of pain and touch in the elderly.

Renal function is slowed by structural and functional changes associated with aging. Arteriosclerotic changes can reduce blood flow, impairing renal function. The kidney's filtering abilities become impaired as the number of functioning nephrons decreases with age. An enlarged prostate gland causes urinary urgency and frequency in men, and in women the same complaints are often due to weakened muscles supporting the bladder or weakness of the urethral sphincter. The capacity of the bladder and its ability to empty completely diminish with age in both men and women.

All bones are affected by a decrease in skeletal mass. Decreased density causes bones to become brittle and fracture more easily. Range of motion decreases as the tissues of the joints and bones stiffen.

Cognitive Development

Research continues into the effects of aging on cognitive abilities. Different kinds of cognitive functions seem to undergo different types, amounts, and rates of change in individual older adults. Functions dependent on perception rely on the acuity of the senses. When senses become impaired with aging, the ability to perceive the environment and react appropriately is diminished. Changes in the aging nervous system may also affect perceptual ability. Impaired perceptual ability diminishes the aging adult's cognitive capability.

Studies suggest that people who live in a varied environment that provides for continued use of intellectual function are often

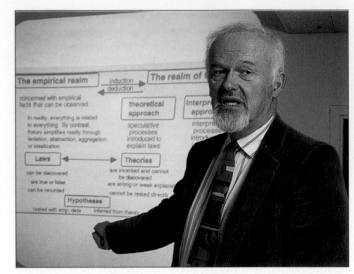

Figure 3.8 ● The ability to solve problems may be highly efficient in the older adult.

the ones who maintain or even strengthen these skills throughout life. Conversely, those who live in a static environment that lacks intellectual challenge may be the ones who most likely show some decline in intellectual ability with aging. Although learning and problem solving may not be as efficient in old age as in youth, both processes still occur to a greater extent than is often portrayed in stereotypes of older adults (see Figure 3.8 ●).

Psychosocial Development

The developmental task of late adulthood, according to Erikson, is ego integrity versus self-despair. When a review of life events, experiences, and relationships makes the adult content with life, the person attains ego integrity. Failure to resolve this last developmental crisis results in a sense of despair, resentment, futility, hopelessness, and fear of death.

Late adulthood requires lifestyle changes as well as review of one's past life. The adult adjusting to retirement must develop new activities to replace work and the role of worker. New friendships are established with peers of similar interests, abilities, and means. The person may pursue projects or recreational activities deferred during the working years, but activities are limited to those compatible with the physical limitations of old age. Lack of adequate income limits the activities and lifestyle of many older adults; financial resources enable them to be independent and look after themselves.

The lifestyle of later years is, to a large degree, formulated in youth. The person who was once gregarious and spent time with people continues to do so, and the person who avoided involvement with others continues toward isolation. Those who learned early in life to live well-balanced and fulfilling lives are generally more successful in retirement. The later years can foster a sense of integrity and continuity, or they can be years of despair.

Through the late adult years, the deaths of friends, siblings, and partner occur with increasing frequency. Reminded of the limited time left, the older adult comes to terms with the past and views death as an acceptable completion of life.

Box 3.4	Periodic Health Examination: Age 65 and Older

Interventions Considered and Recommended for the Periodic Health Examination

Leading Causes of Death

Heart diseases
Malignant neoplasms (lung, colorectal, breast)
Cerebrovascular disease
Chronic obstructive pulmonary disease
Pneumonia and influenza

INTERVENTIONS FOR THE GENERAL POPULATION

Screening
Blood pressure
Height and weight
Fecal occult blood test[1] and/or sigmoidoscopy
Mammogram ± clinical breast exam[2] (women ≤69 yr)
Papanicolaou (Pap) test (women)[3]
Vision screening
Assess for hearing Impairment
Assess for problem drinking

Counseling
Substance use
    Tobacco cessation
    Avoid alcohol/drug use while driving, swimming, boating, etc.
Diet and exercise
    Limit fat and cholesterol; maintain caloric balance; emphasize grains, fruits, vegetables
    Adequate calcium intake (women)
    Regular physical activity

Injury prevention
    Lap/shoulder belts
    Motorcycle and bicycle helmets
    Fall prevention
    Safe storage/removal of firearms
    Smoke detector
    Set hot water heater to <120–130°F
    CPR training for household members
Dental health
    Regular visits to dental care provider
    Floss, brush with fluoride toothpaste daily
Sexual behavior
    STD prevention; avoid high-risk sexual behavior; use condoms

Immunizations
Pneumococcal vaccine
Influenza[1]
Tetanus-dipththeria (Td) boosters

Chemoprophylaxis
Discuss hormone prophylaxis (women)

INTERVENTIONS FOR HIGH-RISK POPULATIONS

Population	Potential Interventions
Institutionalized persons	PPD; hepatitis A vaccine; amantadine/rimantadine
Chronic medical conditions; TB contacts; low income; immigrants; alcoholics	PPD
Persons ≥75 yr; or ≥70 yr with risk factors for falls	Fall prevention intervention
Cardiovascular disease risk factors	Consider cholesterol screening
Family h/o skin cancer; nevi; fair skin, eyes, hair	Avoid excess/midday sun, use protective clothing
Native Americans/Alaska Natives	PPD; hepatitis A vaccine
Travelers to developing countries	Hepatitis A vaccine; hepatitis B vaccine
Blood product recipients	HIV screen; hepatitis B vaccine
High-risk sexual behavior	Hepatitis A vaccine; HIV screen; hepatitis B vaccine; RPR/VDRL
Injection or street drug use	PPD; hepatitis A vaccine; HIV screen; hepatitis B vaccine; RPR/VDRL; advice to reduce infection risk
Healthcare/lab workers	PPD; hepatitis A vaccine; amantadine/rimantadine; hepatitis B vaccine
Persons susceptible to varicella	Varicella vaccine

[1]Annually. [2]Mammogram q1–2 yr, or mammogram q1–2 yr with annual clinical breast exam. [3]All women who are or have been sexually active and who have a cervix: q ≤3 yr. Consider discontinuation of testing after age 65 yr if previous regular screening with consistently normal results.

CPR, Cardiopulmonary resuscitation; *STD*, sexually transmitted disease; *TB*, tuberculosis; *PPD*, purified protein derivative; *HIV*, human immunodeficiency virus; *RPR*, rapid plasma reagin; *VDRL*, Venereal Disease Research Laboratories.

Assessment of Older Adults

Well-adjusted older adults maintain an active lifestyle and involvement with others and often do not appear their age. Lifestyle changes occur in response to declining physical abilities and retirement. Participation in activities that promote the elderly adult's sense of self-worth and usefulness also provides opportunities for developing new friendships with others of similar abilities and interests. Intellectual function is maintained through continued intellectual pursuits. Content with their life review, elderly adults enjoy their retirement years and accept death as the inevitable end of a productive life.

The older adult who has not successfully resolved developmental crises may feel that life has been unfair. Despair and hopelessness may be evident in the individual's lack of activity and bitter complaining. See Box 3.4 for a detailed listing of interventions, screenings, and counseling for ages 65 and older. A thorough discussion of the assessment of middle adults and older adults is found in Chapter 27 of this text. ∞

GROWTH AND DEVELOPMENT IN HEALTH ASSESSMENT

Health assessment includes gathering objective and subjective data, which is used to develop plans to maintain health or address health needs in clients of all ages. A comprehensive assessment includes data about physical, cognitive, and emotional growth and development. When conducting health assessments, the professional nurse must be able to obtain accurate data and interpret findings in relation to expectations and predicted norms and ranges for clients at various stages of physical and emotional development. Knowledge of anatomical and physiological changes as well as theoretical information about cognitive, psychoanalytic, and psychosocial events and expectations at each stage of human development are invaluable resources for the professional nurse.

Physical growth and development change across the age span. Stages from infancy through adolescence are marked by spurts of rapid growth and development. Health assessment includes the use of clinical growth charts to index individual client measurements of height and weight (and head circumference in infants) as expected normal values for age and gender (see Chapter 25 ∞). Additional indicators for normal growth and development throughout these stages are eating, sleeping, elimination, and activity patterns. Neurologic and sensory functions are assessed by monitoring development of speech and language, muscular growth, strength and coordination, and tactile sensibility.

Puberty is a period of rapid physiological growth and development. It occurs between the ages of 10 and 14 years in females and is marked by menarche, breast development, presence of pubic hair, and a spurt in height. In males, puberty occurs between the ages of 12 and 16 years and is characterized by a spurt in height, development of the penis and testicles, and presence of pubic hair. Young adulthood is the stage marked by completed growth in physical and mental structures. Physical development continues to be assessed by comparing individual findings to clinical growth charts and by assessing eating, sleeping, and activity patterns.

Middle age, occurring between the ages of 45 and 60 years, is another period in which dramatic changes in physical development occur. Primary changes are related to hormonal changes of the male and female climacteric. In addition, changes occur in all systems and include decreases in basal metabolic rate, muscle size, nerve conduction, lung capacity, glomerular filtration, and cardiac output. There is increased adipose tissue deposit, skeletal changes leading to decreases in height, as well as changes in tactile sensibility, vision, and hearing. The physical changes continue into the stage of older adulthood. The middle and older adult is at risk for obesity and health problems associated with it. Therefore, health assessment will include use of body mass index (BMI) to assess weight and risk for disease. Information about calculation of BMI is included in Chapter 9 of this text. ∞ In addition,

assessment will include checking the ability to carry out activities of daily living (ADL's), and regular testing of vision and hearing.

In addition to expectations about physical growth and development, there are also expectations about cognitive, psychosocial, and emotional development across the age span. For example, attachment is an essential element in infant development. Attachment refers to the tie between the infant and caregivers that promotes physical and psychosocial well-being. Assessment of attachment includes observation of interactions between the infant and caregivers for eye contact, apparent interest in the child, talking or cooing to the child, response to infant needs, and communication. Children are expected to develop language and cognitive abilities that enable them to learn and over time become independent beings. Young adults are expected to develop relationships with others and to become productive members of society. Maturity and aging lead individuals to contribute to the well-being of communities and their families and often to adapt to change and loss. Developmental milestones and crises occur in all stages of development and must be assessed. A variety of instruments and scales can be used to identify developmental delays, behavioral patterns, and responses that indicate potential or actual problems with emotional, cognitive, and psychosocial development and adaptation in children and adults of all ages. Table 3.2 includes a list and description of some of the instruments available to measure aspects of growth and development.

FACTORS THAT INFLUENCE GROWTH AND DEVELOPMENT

Factors that influence growth and development include nutrition, family, culture, race, and socioeconomic status. The following discussion provides examples of ways in which these factors impact growth and development.

NUTRITION

Nutrition is essential to physical and mental development. Growth patterns, in large part, are genetically determined. However, malnutrition can delay or prevent growth and development. Healthcare professionals routinely use measures of height and weight in comparison to clinical growth charts to identify slowed growth in children. Slowed growth is an early indicator of inadequate nutrition. The body is made up of water, fat, ash, and protein, and nutritional intake determines the amounts of each of these essential components. Alteration in one or more of the components affects development and health. Balanced nutrition promotes brain development in children and has been reported to prevent some forms of dementia in older adults. Further discussion of these concepts is included in Chapter 9 of this text. ∞

FAMILY

Family refers to a social system made up of two or more individuals living together, who are related by blood, marriage, or agreement. Families today may be identified as nuclear families, extended families, same-sex families, single-parent families,

Table 3.2	Instruments to Measure Growth and Development
Ages & Stages Questionnaire (ASQ)	This parent-completed questionnaire covers developmental areas of communication, gross motor, fine motor, problem solving, and personal-social.
Battelle Developmental Inventory	It tests developmental domains of cognition, motor, self-help, language, and social skills in children from birth through 8 years of age.
Brigance Screens	The screens assess speech-language, motor, readiness, and general knowledge at younger ages and also reading and math. Used from 21 to 90 months of age.
Eyberg Child Behavior Inventory (ECBI)	The ECBI is a parent report scale of conduct problem behaviors in children ages 2 to 16 years.
Family Psychosocial Screening	A clinic intake form identifies psychosocial risk factors associated with developmental problems including parental history of physical abuse as a child, parental substance abuse, and maternal depression.
Hassles and Uplifts Scale	This measures adult attitudes about daily situations defined as "hassles" and "uplifts." It focuses on evaluation of positive and negative events in daily life rather than on life events.
Life Experiences Survey	This self-administered questionnaire reviews life-changing events of a given year. Ratings are used to evaluate the level of stress one is experiencing.
McCarthy Scale of Children's Abilities	The McCarthy evaluates the general intelligence level of children ages 2½ to 8½. The scale identifies strengths and weaknesses in verbal, perceptual-performance, quantitative, memory, motor, and general cognitive skills.
Neonatal Behavioral Assessment Scale	The scale is used to assess newborns and infants up to 2 months of age. It measures 28 behavioral and 18 reflex items. It provides information about the baby's strengths, adaptive responses, and potential vulnerabilities.
Pediatric Symptom Checklist	This checklist of short statements identifies conduct behaviors and behaviors associated with depression, anxiety, and adjustment in children from 4 to 16 years of age. Item patterns determine the need for behavioral or mental health referrals.
Stanford-Binet Intelligence Scale: Fourth Edition	This test measures general intelligence. The areas of verbal reasoning, quantitative reasoning, abstract/visual reasoning, and short-term memory can be tested from age 2 to 23 years.
The Child Development Inventory	The scales measure social, self-help, gross motor, fine motor, expressive language, language comprehension, letters, numbers, and general development in children from 15 months to 6 years of age.
The Denver II	This test is administered to well children between birth and 6 years of age. The Denver II is designed to test 20 simple tasks and items in four sectors: personal-social, fine motor adaptive, language, gross motor.
The Mini-Mental Status Examination	This brief, quantitative measure of cognitive status in adults can be used to screen for cognitive impairment, to estimate the severity of cognitive impairment at a given point in time, to follow the course of cognitive changes in an individual over time, and to document an individual's response to treatment.
Wechsler Preschool and Primary Scale of Intelligence—Revised (WPPSI-R)	This is a standardized test of language and perception for children ages 4½ to 6.

stepfamilies, or single-state families. Families share bonds of affection or love, loyalty, commitment of an emotional or financial nature, continuity, and common shared values and rituals. Families help members to develop physically and emotionally by providing for the economic and safety needs of one another. Included in safety needs would be provision of appropriate nutrition to foster physical growth and development as well as objects, interactions, and activities that promote cognitive and emotional well-being. Family members provide support for each other during physical and emotional crises, and serve as models for social interaction, all of which impact individual members as they move through the stages of development from infancy to old age.

CULTURE

Growth and development is influenced by cultural factors. For example, perceptions of family roles, in particular those in child rearing, differ among cultures. Attachment is considered an essential element in psychosocial development. In Caucasian parents the trend is to have both paternal and maternal attachment occur early in the neonatal period. This differs among cultures. For example, in Cuban Americans, the mother is the primary caregiver and bonds with the child earlier and continually, while the father remains detached from infant care and only begins attachment behaviors when the child is able to walk and communicate. Culture influences the training and discipline of children, the value of developing cognitive skills, social interactions outside of the home that promote development, and attitudes to-

ward change, including illness and aging. In addition, for immigrants to the United States, language differences may impact the ability to communicate, to form social bonds outside of the cultural community, and to identify and utilize resources that foster development and provide support for individuals and families experiencing developmental and situational crises.

Differences in measures of growth and development have been noted between and among various ethnic groups. For example, newborn infants of African American, Indian, and Asian American populations have been reported to have lower birth weights than Caucasians. Females are generally smaller than males in all ethnic groups. Differences in weight, length, and head circumference have been noted in Mexican American and Caucasian children at 48 to 56 weeks of age. Mexican American children have shorter stature and greater weight than Caucasian children, while head circumference has been found to be greater in Caucasian children. In other reports, African American toddlers were found to have increased motor skills and earlier walking than did Caucasian toddlers.

SOCIOECONOMIC STATUS

Socioeconomic status is a major influence on growth and development. Overall, school-age children of low socioeconomic status have been found to have lower height and weight than those in other economic groups. Poverty impacts the ability to meet nutritional needs at all stages of development and increases exposure to environmental elements that influence health status and physical well-being. Socioeconomic status influences values and role expectations and behaviors regarding marriage, family, and gender responsibilities in parenting, education, and occupation. Income, values, and role expectations impact physical and psychosocial development across the age span. Further information about culture and psychosocial development is included in Chapters 4 and 5 of this text. ∞

Planning care for individuals is dependent upon comprehensive health assessment of health status and all of the factors that

impact health. Accurate interpretation of data requires one to use knowledge and resources in formulating judgments about findings. The previous discussion provided information about measures that assist in health assessment of physical and psychosocial growth and development across the life span. The U.S. Preventive Services Task Force has developed guidelines for health examination and recommendations for preventive strategies. These are available through the National Library of Medicine. Link to their website through the Companion Website.

Application Through Critical Thinking

CASE STUDY

*C*asey is a 2-year-old girl whose mother brought her in for a check-up. Her mother states that Casey does not have any problems that she has identified; she has no history of medical problems or diseases and her immunizations are up-to-date. The mother states she is very careful with what she feeds her family and that Casey has good eating habits. Casey's parents have some good friends whose youngest child is being carefully followed by his pediatrician because of what is thought to be "significant develop-

mental delays." Consequently, Casey's mother is very concerned about developmental milestones and wants her daughter "checked to make sure everything is all right." The mother states she has "read a lot of books" on child development, but asks many questions regarding care and needs of her child.

► *Critical Thinking Questions*

1. What are the expectations regarding physical development for a 2-year-old child such as Casey?
2. What level of language development is expected for a toddler?
3. Identify at least two standardized tools that are used to assess physical and psychosocial development across the age span.

Please refer to the Companion Website at www.prenhall.com/damico and click on Chapter 3, the Application Through Critical Thinking module, to answer these and additional questions. In addition, complete NCLEX-RN® review questions and other interactive resources for this chapter.

EXPLORE MediaLink

Additional resources for this chapter are found on the Student CD-ROM accompanying this textbook and on the Companion Website.

CD-ROM CONTENT

Content for this chapter includes:
Objectives
Key Concepts
NCLEX-RN® Review Questions
Audio Glossary
Animations
    Child Development
Head-to-Toe Physical Examination Video

COMPANION WEBSITE CONTENT

www.prenhall.com/damico

Content for this chapter includes:
Objectives
NCLEX-RN® Review Questions

Application Through Critical Thinking
    Case Study Challenge
MediaLinks
MediaLink Application
Tool Box
    Motor Skill Development in Infancy
    Periodic Health Examination: Birth to 10 Years
    Periodic Health Examination: Ages 11–24 Years
    Periodic Health Examination: Ages 25–64 Years
    Periodic Health Examination: Ages 65 and Older
New York Times

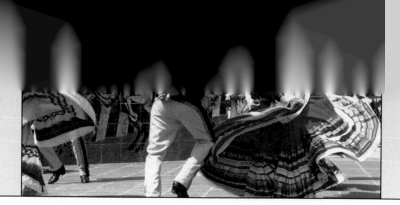

4

Cultural Considerations

MEDIALINK

www.prenhall.com/damico

The CD-ROM in the back of this textbook and the Media-Link website contain NCLEX-RN® review questions, interactive exercises, case study challenges, animations, videos, documentation and checklist forms, and review materials. For a complete listing of the media content specific to Chapter 4, see the Explore MediaLink at the end of the chapter.

*T*he United States is made up of people of many races, ethnicities, religions, and cultures. It is expected that the diversity in the United States will continue to expand throughout this century. It has been predicted that by 2050 the Asian population will have increased from 3% to 11%, African Americans from 12% to 16%, and the Hispanic groups from 9% to 21%. In addition, Arab, German, Brazilian, Greek, Egyptian, and Turkish groups are expected to increase. An individual's culture, race, and ethnicity impact beliefs about health, illness, and practices related to both. Although it is not possible to completely understand all cultures, the nurse must gain knowledge of several cultures. The nurse must continue to learn about other cultures and bring acknowledgment of personal cultural beliefs and values to each nurse-client encounter.

According to the American Nurses Association (ANA) (2003), knowledge of cultural diversity is vital in all areas of practice. This knowledge can strengthen the delivery of healthcare. Nurses need to understand how cultural groups perceive life processes, define health and illness, maintain health, determine the causes of illness, and provide care and cure. It is also important to understand the ways the cultural background of the nurse influences care. When nurses understand cultural diversity, apply cultural knowledge, and act in culturally competent ways, they can be more effective in assessing clients, developing culturally sensitive interventions, and influencing healthcare policy and practice.

CULTURAL COMPETENCE

Cultural competence refers to the capacity of nurses or health service delivery systems to effectively understand and plan for the needs of a culturally diverse client or group. Spector (2004) views cultural competence as a complex combination of knowledge, attitudes, and skills used by the healthcare provider to deliver services that attend to the total context of the client's situation across cultural boundaries. Incorporating the client's cultural values, beliefs, customs, and practices improves the nurse's ability to gather and interpret data and to plan care appropriate to meet the needs of diverse clients. The development of cultural competence is essential to nursing. Cultural competence develops over time through knowledge acquisition and experience. For access to case studies related to cultural care and information about cultural competence, link to Cultural Diversity in Nursing through the Companion Website.

A key goal in *Healthy People 2010* is to eliminate health disparities. One effort to eliminate disparities is the development of culturally and linguistically appropriate standards (CLAS). As described in Box 4.1, the CLAS standards are intended to correct current inequities and promote cultural competence in meeting the needs of racial, ethnic, and linguistic populations that experience unequal access to healthcare. For additional information, contact the National Center for Cultural Competence (NCCC) by linking through the Companion Website.

CULTURE

Spector (2004) defines **culture** as the nonphysical traits, such as values, beliefs, attitudes, and customs, that are shared by a group of people and passed from one generation to the next. Culture also defines how health is perceived, how healthcare information is received, how rights and protections are exercised, what is considered to be a health problem, how symptoms are perceived, and the type of treatment to be provided. Culture is learned generally within the family group, is shared by the majority within the culture, and changes in response to interactions with events in the external environment (see Figure 4.1 ●). Culture has also been identified as the way a population or group finds a shared meaning for information.

Culture may be divided into material and nonmaterial culture. Objects such as dress, art, utensils, and tools and the ways they are used are components of the *material culture*. *Nonmaterial culture* is composed of the verbal and nonverbal language, beliefs, customs, and social structures. Cultures may be further defined as macrocultures, that is, national,

---

Box 4.1   **National Standards for Culturally and Linguistically Appropriate Services in Healthcare**

1. Promote and support the attitudes, behaviors, knowledge, and skills necessary for staff to work respectfully and effectively with patients and each other in a culturally diverse work environment.

2. Have a comprehensive management strategy to address culturally and linguistically appropriate services, including strategic goals, plans, policies, procedures, and designated staff responsible for implementation.

3. Utilize formal mechanisms for community and consumer involvement in the design and execution of service delivery, including planning, policy making, operations, evaluation, training, and, as appropriate, treatment planning.

4. Develop and implement a strategy to recruit, retain, and promote qualified, diverse, and culturally competent administrative, clinical, and support staff that are trained and qualified to address the needs of the racial and ethnic communities being served.

5. Require and arrange for ongoing education and training for administrative, clinical, and support staff in culturally and linguistically competent service delivery.

6. Provide all clients with limited English proficiency (LEP) access to bilingual staff or interpretation services.

7. Provide oral and written notices, including translated signage at key points of contact, to clients in their primary language informing them of their right to receive interpreter services free of charge.

8. Translate and make available signage and commonly used written patient educational material and other materials for members of the predominant language groups in service areas.

9. Ensure that interpreters and bilingual staff can demonstrate bilingual proficiency and receive training that includes the skills and ethics of interpreting, and knowledge in both languages of the terms and concepts relevant to clinical or nonclinical encounters. Family or friends are not considered adequate substitutes because they usually lack these abilities.

10. Ensure that the clients' primary spoken language and self-identified race/ethnicity are included in the healthcare organization's management information system as well as any patient records used by provider staff.

11. Use a variety of methods to collect and utilize accurate demographic, cultural, epidemiological, and clinical outcome data for racial and ethnic groups in the service area, and become informed about the ethnic/cultural needs, resources, and assets of the surrounding community.

12. Undertake ongoing organizational self-assessments of cultural and linguistic competence, and integrate measures of access, satisfaction, quality, and outcomes for CLAS into other organizational internal audits and performance improvement programs.

13. Develop structures and procedures to address cross-cultural ethical and legal conflicts in healthcare delivery and complaints or grievances by patients and staff about unfair, culturally insensitive, or discriminatory treatment; difficulty in accessing services; or denial of services.

14. Prepare an annual progress report documenting the organizations' progress with implementing CLAS standards, including information on programs, staffing, and resources.

Source: U.S. Department of Health and Human Services. *National Standards for Culturally and Linguistically Appropriate Services in Health Care,* Final Report, March 2001, pp. 7–20.

---

racial, or ethnic groups within which microcultures exist based on age, gender, or religious affiliation. **Subcultures** exist within larger cultural groups. Subcultures are composed of individuals who have a distinct identity based on occupation, membership in a social group, or a specific ethnic heritage. For example, professional nurses are a subculture within the larger culture of healthcare professionals and further are part of the larger American culture (see Figure 4.2 •). Many individuals refer to themselves according to an ethnic heritage, such as Italian American, Greek American, or Arab American. These individuals form associations with others of the same ethnic origin to form a subculture within the larger American culture.

TERMS RELATED TO CULTURE

The terms *culture, race,* and *ethnicity* are often used synonymously. However, these terms refer to different aspects and characteristics

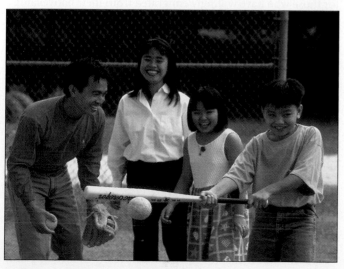

Figure 4.1 • Nuclear family interaction.

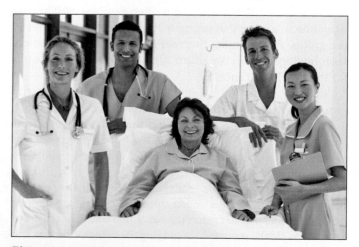

Figure 4.2 • Diversity within the subculture of nursing.

of populations and groups of people. These terms and others related to culture will be defined in the following sections.

RACE

Race refers to the identification of an individual or group by shared genetic heritage and biological or physical characteristics. Members of a given race have similarities in skin color, skeletal structure, texture of the hair, and facial features. Knowledge of the differences in racial characteristics is significant in health assessment since findings are interpreted according to norms for age, gender, and race. However, gene pools are becoming increasingly diverse. Skin color is not always a clear indication of racial identity. For example, dark-skinned individuals from Pakistan, Bangladesh, and parts of India are Caucasian by race. Additionally, racial blending is increasingly common in the United States. Many individuals identify themselves as biracial or multiracial. Definitions of racial and ethnic populations in the United States are provided by the Office of Minority Health (OMH). Link to their Website through the Companion Website.

ETHNICITY

The term *ethnic* refers to a group of people who share a common culture and who belong to a specific group. Ethnic groups are those with common social and cultural values over generations. **Ethnicity** is the awareness of belonging to a group in which certain characteristics or aspects such as culture and biology differentiate the members of one group from another. Ethnicity is defined by shared interest, ethnic heritage, religion, food, politics, or geography and nationality.

Ethnicity incorporates internal and external identification with a group. Internal identification means that one considers oneself a member of an ethnic group. For example, one may identify oneself as Arab, African, French, Irish, Italian, or Jamaican American. External identification means that those outside of the group perceive the person as a group member.

However, while "Asian American" is a recognized ethnic group, one must be aware that national origin is often a more important component of ethnicity. As a result, Asian Americans are likely to identify themselves, for example, as Japanese, Filipino, Vietnamese, Chinese, or Samoan.

In the United States, ethnicity is often demonstrated by participation in groups that promote the heritage or traditions of the group. For example, Emerald Societies exist to promote Irish heritage; Italian American social groups promote bonds for those of Italian ancestry.

Ethnicity refers to the degree of attachment with ancestral groups, heritage, or place of birth. Some ethnic identities such as Polish or Syrian are traced to locations in which ancestors were born outside of the United States. Ethnic groups such as Cajuns or Pennsylvania Dutch evolved from geographic regions within the United States.

Ethnocentrism is the tendency to believe that one's own beliefs, way of life, values, and customs are superior to those of others. Ethnocentrism creates the belief that one's own customs and values are the standard for judging the values, customs, and practices of others. Ethnocentrism can interfere with collection and interpretation of data as well as the development of plans of care to meet client needs. Awareness of one's own cultural beliefs, values, and biases can reduce ethnocentrism and foster culturally competent care.

DIVERSITY

Diversity is defined as the state of being different. Diversity occurs between and within cultural groups. Characteristics of diversity include nationality, race, color, gender, age, and religion. In addition, diversity is established by socioeconomic status, education, occupation, residence in urban versus suburban or rural areas, marital status, parental status, sexual orientation, and the time spent away from one's country of origin.

For example, Arab Americans are considered a cultural group in the United States. They share tradition as descendants of tribes of the Arabian Peninsula, and Arabic as a common language. However, diversity within this group is characterized by differences in religion, occupation, geography, and period of immigration to the United States. The early immigrants were Christians, seeking economic opportunity, and were from Libya and Syria. Later immigrants settled in urban areas of the northeastern United States and for the most part were self-employed or in managerial and professional occupations. In contrast, Arab immigrants after World War II were and continue to be predominantly refugees from nations undergoing political strife. These were mainly followers of the Islamic religion who settled in the midwestern and western United States and maintained strong ethnic ties to the nations from which they emigrated including Palestine, Iraq, Lebanon, and Egypt. Many Arab immigrants sought educational degrees or were professionals who remained in the United States.

ASSIMILATION

Assimilation refers to the adoption and incorporation of characteristics, customs, and values of the dominant culture by those new to that culture. For example, immigrants to the United States may assimilate over time and adopt the values of one culture over another. The assimilation process occurs more easily for those who have willingly emigrated from their native land.

Assimilation is affected by several factors including beliefs, language, age, and geography. Those who hold similar values and speak the language of the adopted country more easily assimilate. Assimilation occurs more easily in second-generation immigrants. For example, children born to Chinese parents in Western countries adopt Western culture easily, while parents tend to maintain the traditional culture. Chinese Americans living in "Chinatown" on the East and West Coasts of the United States are more likely to maintain much of their traditional Chinese cultural practices and beliefs.

Slow assimilation has occurred in the Cuban American population. Cuban Americans have established enclaves in Miami, Florida, and Union City, New Jersey. In these enclaves, Spanish remains the predominant language in the home and in many of the workplaces. The slow assimilation to English, as well as the isolation within Cuban communities, results in strong ethnic identity and some degree of insulation from the prevailing American culture.

CULTURAL PHENOMENA THAT IMPACT HEALTHCARE

Phenomena that impact the provision of healthcare to individuals of diverse cultures include communication, temporal relationships, family patterns, dietary patterns, health beliefs, and health practices. Understanding these phenomena is essential to comprehensive health assessment and to the delivery of safe and effective nursing care. Each of the phenomena will be discussed in the following sections. Table 4.1 provides an overview of characteristics considered as representative of beliefs and practices of a variety of cultural groups. It is important to note that differences in language, beliefs, values, and customs exist within cultural groups. Note that the table does not include all of the cultural groups one may encounter in practice.

Table 4.1	Cultural Phenomena Impacting Healthcare					
CULTURAL GROUP	**COMMUNICATION**	**TEMPORAL RELATIONS**	**DIETARY CONCERNS**	**FAMILY PATTERNS**	**HEALTH BELIEFS**	**HEALTH PRACTICES**
African Americans	Primary language is English. May use Black English, Pidgin, or Gullah. Highly verbal. Open communication about personal health and feelings with friends and family. Use touch readily with family and friends. Demonstrative facial expressions.	Relaxed about time. Present oriented.	High-fat, fried food diet. Early introduction of solids to infants. Muslims—no pork. Approximately 75% of African Americans are lactose intolerant.	Matriarchal. Value elders. Extended family closeness.	Sickness is a separation between God and humans. Health is harmony with nature. Illness is a disruption in harmony due to "bad spirits."	Religious and spiritual activities, especially prayer. Use home remedies, folk healers, and Western care. Often decreased access to healthcare.
Appalachians	English is the dominant language. May use Elizabethan or Chaucerian English. Pronunciation and word usage are generally local, not standard English. Concrete and direct in response to questions. Physical distancing in all settings during communication. Direct eye contact viewed as impolite.	In touch with rhythms of the body, not the clock. Present oriented.	Introduce foods including grease, coffee, and sugar to infants at early age. Snacks replace meals in adolescents. Limited knowledge of nutrition in health promotion and disease prevention.	Patriarchal. Older women preserve culture and impact healthcare decisions. Elders are respected. Obligation to family outweighs all other obligations.	Health includes body, mind, and spirit. Disease is not a problem unless it interferes with functioning. Fatalism—what happens is God's will.	Use folk remedies and self-medication. Seek help only when folk remedies fail and when condition becomes severe.
Arab Americans	Dominant language is Arabic. Colloquial language is used in everyday living. English is common second language. Use repetition, exaggeration, and gesturing. Outward display of emotion is demonstration of concern. Resist revelation of personal information. Sensitive to authority. Respond best to courtesy and initiating encounters with social conversation or "small talk." Touch between nonmarried individuals of the opposite sex is not acceptable.	Belief in predestination. Both good and evil are "God's will." Nonchalant about time.	Diet reflects USDA pyramid. Muslims eat no pork. Bread is served at every meal. Lamb and chicken are main meats. Muslims fast during month of Ramadan. No foods or fluids including water during daylight hours.	Patriarchal and hierarchical. The senior male member is the decision maker. Male role is to protect the women and family. Respect elders. Hijab—the covering of all but hands and face—provides protection for females.	Associate good health with good eating and fasting to cure disease. Good health means one has the ability to fulfill one's roles. Illness is attributed to diet, hot-cold shifts, exposure of the stomach during sleep, spiritual distress, envy, or the evil eye. Some belief in supernatural agents as the cause of disease.	Combine prayer with conventional medicine. Seek care for problems, not very involved in prevention. Not self-directive. The family oversees care. Disability and mental illness are social stigmas. Most respect is given to male physicians.

(continued)

COMMUNICATION

Communication refers to the verbal and nonverbal methods with which individuals and groups transmit information. Communication occurs between and among individuals for a variety of purposes. For example, cultural beliefs, customs, values, and morals are passed from generation to generation within a specific culture by communication. Communication provides information about a culture to those outside of the culture. Communication is the mechanism through which individuals establish relationships.

Table 4.1	**Cultural Phenomena Impacting Healthcare** *(continued)*					
CULTURAL GROUP	**COMMUNICATION**	**TEMPORAL RELATIONS**	**DIETARY CONCERNS**	**FAMILY PATTERNS**	**HEALTH BELIEFS**	**HEALTH PRACTICES**
Chinese Americans	Official language is Mandarin. Many dialects are spoken. Direct questions, instructions given in order, and simple sentences are best understood. May say they understand to avoid "loss of face." Share information when a trusting relationship is established. Dislike touch by strangers.	Time is cyclic as with the cycle of life. Two concepts regarding time: In "Chinese time," lateness is expected. In second view, punctuality is a sign of respect.	Regional differences exist. Rice is a staple in diet. Meat is included in diet but predominance is of vegetables and fruits. Genetic predisposition to lactose intolerance.	Male dominance. Children are highly valued, especially male children. Elders are venerated. Extended family is important, commonly with strong bonds and interdependence.	Two forces, yin and yang, are in balance to maintain health. Traditional concept of Qi as the vital force of life. Some is inherited; some is from the environment.	Traditional Chinese medicine, Western medicine, or both. Do not always provide information about all healthcare treatments and practices. Share medications with others. Herbal treatments are common. May distrust Western practitioners because of the pain and invasiveness of care.
Cuban Americans	Dominant language is Spanish. First generation prefers Spanish over English. Second generation uses English or Spanglish (mixing of the two languages). Value courtesy and respect. Speech is rapid and loud in volume.	Present oriented. Cuban time is followed in which there is a flexible period of 1 to 2 hours after a scheduled time for events to begin or for individuals to arrive at appointments.	High fat, starch, and calorie diet. Root crops (yams, yucca, malanga, plantains) are a large part of diet. Foods include rice, beans, beef, and pork. Meats are generally fried.	Patriarchal. Family is the most important social unit.	Health is associated with overweight. Fatalistic—believe they lack control over their lives. Santeria: folk practice with the use of herbs, rituals, and ceremonies to diagnose and cure illness.	Use of botanica to obtain traditional teas, potions, or poultices from plants. Family is the primary source of advice for healthcare. In the U.S.—accept Western medicine and seek primary provider and preventive services when accessible via insurance.
European Americans	Language: English. Insist on personal space. Tolerate embraces from close friends. In public, maintain neutral facial expression.	Future oriented.	Food types associated with holidays and social occasions (hot dogs at ball games, turkey at Thanksgiving). Influenced by ancestry. Rituals influence intake (coffee break).	Nuclear family is "professed" norm. Egalitarian power in family.	Health is individual responsibility. Believe in germ theory. Illness results from pathology or injury that can be prevented or dealt with.	Self-care practices. Use healthcare system for all aspects of healthcare. Use resources to learn about health and illness. Want to be involved in decision making regarding health and treatment.

Table 4.1	Cultural Phenomena Impacting Healthcare *(continued)*					
CULTURAL GROUP	**COMMUNICATION**	**TEMPORAL RELATIONS**	**DIETARY CONCERNS**	**FAMILY PATTERNS**	**HEALTH BELIEFS**	**HEALTH PRACTICES**
Filipino Americans	National language is Pilipino or Tagalog with 8 distinct dialects. English is second national language. Cadence and inflection are influenced by the ethnic language dialect. Contextual in communication. "Actions speak louder than words." Eye contact varies—some avoid with elders to show respect. Nodding is common during conversation but does not always indicate understanding—may mean simply listening.	Relaxed outlook on life. Filipino time means one can be 1 to 2 hours late for social appointments. In America, demand respect for punctuality.	Fish, chicken, and pork are primary sources for protein. Somewhat lactose intolerant. Salt and vinegar are used in food preparation and preservation. Rice, fruits, and vegetables are staples in the diet.	Egalitarian relationships. Respect is important and caring for aging parents is integral.	Fatalistic—accept events as up to God. Health is a result of balance. Illness is the result of imbalance, that is, personal irresponsibility or irregularity.	Share medications; take medications if they have been effective for others. Stoicism. Sick individual assumes dependent role and allows family to make decisions. Readily accept Western medicine but may also use folk healers.
Jewish Americans	English is the predominant language. First-generation immigrants may speak Yiddish. Hasidic males do not touch females other than their wife. Non-Hasidic—more informal.	Live for today but plan for the future and always have respect and honor for the past. Holidays and Sabbath begin at sunset.	Religious Jews follow Kosher rules—no pork, no dairy and meat at the same meal.	Family is the core unit of society. Genders share roles for work and child rearing. Respect and honor parents.	Each person has a duty to maintain physical and mental health. Preservation of life is paramount.	Health conscious. Respect for physicians. Follow instructions to maintain health and readily seek help for problems.
Mexican Americans	Dominant language is Spanish. There are many regional dialects. Speech is often high pitched, rapid, and loud. Eye contact is considered rude. Touch is acceptable. Reveal personal information when trust is established.	Present oriented. Relaxed concept of time. Schedules and appointment times are flexible.	Diet varies according to region. Rice, beans, and tortillas are staples. Species are used in preparation. Food is source for socialization.	Patriarchal. Machismo—men are wiser and stronger. Family takes precedence over work or any other obligation.	Fatalism—illness is God's will. Good health is equated with being free of pain. Belief in hot and cold theory of disease and evil eye.	Folk and Western medicine used—often dictated by economics. Stoicism. Physicians and nurses often seen as outsiders. Liberal use of OTC and antibiotic medications.
Native Americans	Dominant language varies with tribe. Many use English and native language. Some distrust of outsiders. Reveal personal information only when trust is established. Personal space requirement is greater than European Americans. Touch and eye contact vary with tribe.	Not future oriented. Time has little meaning or importance.	Corn is a staple in diet. Few fruits and vegetables. Lamb and fried chicken are frequent meat sources. Many are lactose intolerant.	Matrilineal. Grandmothers and mothers are most important. Elders are respected.	Wellness is equated with harmony with surroundings.	Medicine men are used to diagnose and treat disharmony. Variable acceptance of Western medicine.

(continued)

Table 4.1	Cultural Phenomena Impacting Healthcare *(continued)*					
CULTURAL GROUP	**COMMUNICATION**	**TEMPORAL RELATIONS**	**DIETARY CONCERNS**	**FAMILY PATTERNS**	**HEALTH BELIEFS**	**HEALTH PRACTICES**
Vietnamese Americans	Dominant language is Vietnamese. English is spoken by second generation. Personal feelings are not discussed openly with others. Eye contact is disrespectful. Touch is limited outside of the home. Silence is used to demonstrate negative emotions. Prefer more personal space than in other cultures.	Less concerned about the present and time schedules than are European Americans. Frequently late for appointments. Little attention to precise age.	Rice is a dietary staple. Fish, chicken, tofu, and green vegetables in abundance.	Patriarchal. Always includes an extended family structure. Immigrants are more egalitarian as women are increasingly employed and as they assimilate. Respect for elders.	Fatalism. Life is predetermined and illness is a punishment for wrongdoing. Good health is equated with harmony in hot and cold.	Family is the main provider of care. Prefer same-sex healthcare providers. Believe Western medicine is effective but not always accurate for them. As a result may over- or underuse prescribed drugs. Some use folk healers and prohibit female touching by healthcare providers—use a doll to explain and indicate problems.

Verbal Communication

Verbal communication includes spoken and written language. Diversity in language, word usage, and meaning has become an unavoidable part of life in the United States. According to the U.S. Census Bureau (2000) report, languages spoken at home by at least 14% of the population included Spanish, French, Creole, German, Italian, Asian, and/or Pacific Island languages. In addition, differences in word use and pronunciation exist in regions of the United States among English-speaking populations.

Verbal communication is essential to the provision of healthcare. The nurse must communicate with the client or family to:

- Obtain assessment data about physical and emotional health.
- Work with clients to identify strengths and weaknesses.
- Guide the pursuit of care to address problems and needs.
- Provide instruction regarding aspects of care.
- Evaluate progress toward health-related goals.

The tone of voice as well as the words spoken is of significance in many cultures. Loud tones of voice, for example, denote anger to Chinese Americans and are considered rude by Navajo Indians.

Linguistic differences can inhibit the communication that is essential to healthcare. Language differences can create barriers to initiating or maintaining contact with healthcare agencies or providers. Difficulties associated with language differences include the inability to make telephone contact and misunderstanding of dates, times, and locations for appointments. Language differences affect the amount and type of information that can be obtained during an interview and physical examination, and interfere with instruction regarding diagnostic testing and healthcare maintenance.

Nonverbal Communication

Nonverbal communication incorporates the gestures, facial expressions, and mannerisms that inform others of emotions, feelings, and responses that occur in interactions with others. Nonverbal behaviors include silence, touch, eye contact, lack of eye contact, distancing from others during communication, and posture (see Figure 4.3 ●). The nurse must recognize that each of these behaviors has personal and cultural significance and then interpret behaviors appropriately. In some cultures, silence is used to demonstrate respect for another person. In other cultures, silence indicates agreement. For example, in the Navajo culture, periods of silence are common. The silence indicates interest in what another is saying. The silence allows time for information processing. Not allowing this time can result in inaccurate responses or no response. Filipino Americans

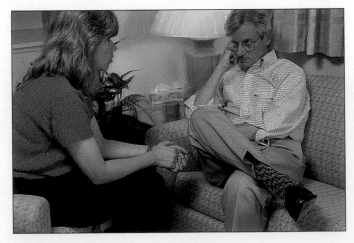

Figure 4.3 ● Nonverbal communication.

are comfortable with silence as well. They often use nodding of the head during communication, which may appear to indicate agreement or understanding but may simply mean "I hear you." In some cultures, casual touch is forbidden, and in many cultures the appropriate types of touch between members of the opposite sex are clearly delineated. Egyptian Americans are accustomed to close personal space, yet touch between individuals of different gender is limited to family members and in private. Personal space is greater for Navajos than for European Americans and so great in Appalachian American culture that members will stand at some distance from one another during social and healthcare situations.

TEMPORAL RELATIONSHIPS

Temporal relationships refer to an individual or group's orientation in terms of past, present, or future, as well as time orientation. There are cultural variations in temporal orientation. For example, the temporal orientation of the Cherokee is past oriented. Their actions are based on tradition and respect for ancestral practices. The European American culture is future oriented as demonstrated by the propensity to invest in the future and "save for tomorrow." Individuals from Hispanic or Chinese cultures are more likely to be "present," that is, concerned about the here and now. Another trait of European Americans is concern with time in terms of abiding by the clock, schedules, and punctuality. In other cultures and groups such as Cuban Americans, Mexican Americans, and Native Americans, time is not regarded to be as important.

FAMILY PATTERNS

Family patterns refer to the roles and relationships that exist within families. These roles and relationships include patterns for responsibilities, values, inclusion, and decision making. The roles and responsibilities of family members are often culturally specific in terms of age and gender. For example, patriarchal households, in which the male is responsible for all decisions including those related to healthcare, are common in Appalachian, Italian, and Filipino groups. African American groups are more likely to follow matriarchal patterns.

DIETARY PATTERNS

Nutritional intake has an impact on health from infancy through old age. The types and amounts of foods that individuals include in the diet are often culturally determined. In addition, certain foods and beverages as well as mealtimes are part of cultural rituals or accepted practices. For example, Americans are known for morning coffee or coffee break rituals, and those from Hispanic cultures are known to eat "dinner" late in the evening. Eating practices are also associated with culturally determined events or holidays. Muslims fast (no food or drink) from dawn to sunset during the month of Ramadan. Lent is a period during which Roman Catholics fast by eating just one full meal and two small meals on Ash Wednesday and Good Friday, and abstain from meat on Ash Wednesday and all Fridays until Easter. In the United States,

turkey is a traditional Thanksgiving meal. Certain foods are prohibited in some religious or cultural groups. For example, Muslims and Jews both prohibit the eating of pork. In most cultures, there are theories about nutrition and health. Different types of foods are selected, and food preparation practices vary according to needs in relation to health and illness. In Mexican, Iranian, Chinese, and Vietnamese cultures, a balance is sought between hot and cold foods to prevent illness as one of the aids for cure in certain illnesses. When a culture adheres to guidelines from the Western healthcare perspective, foods high in fat and salt are avoided as a way to prevent heart disease and some cancers.

HEALTH BELIEFS AND HEALTH PRACTICES

There are three general categories of health beliefs: the magico-religious, the biomedical, and the holistic health belief groups. In a magico-religious belief system, health and illness are believed to be controlled supernaturally or are seen as "God's will." This type of belief system is found in Hispanic and West Indian cultures in which illness may be attributed to "evil eye" or "voodoo."

Those who hold biomedical health beliefs consider illness to be caused by germs, viruses, or a breakdown in body processes and functions and believe that physiological human processes can be affected by human intervention. Individuals who follow traditional Western medical practice hold this belief.

In a holistic health belief system, one holds that human life must be in harmony with nature and that illness results from disharmony between the two. The holistic belief system is consistent with the concepts of yin and yang in the Chinese culture, the hot and cold theory of illness in some Hispanic cultures, and the dimensions of the medicine wheel as accepted by some Native Americans.

Health practices are influenced by one's health beliefs as well as economics, geography, knowledge, and culture. In some geographic regions and areas where there is limited access to Westernized healthcare, people often rely on folk healing or folk medicine. Folk healing is generally derived from cultural traditions and includes the use of teas, herbs, and other natural remedies to treat or cure illness. Seeking healthcare for illness and disease is one health practice that is influenced by culture. In many cultures, care is sought only when all other remedies have been exhausted or when the symptoms have become severe. This custom often results in complications and prolonged illness or hospitalization. This practice may be a result of stoicism exhibited in Appalachians and older European Americans, or as a result of lack of knowledge and understanding of the healthcare system or language barriers that can occur in other cultural groups who have immigrated to the United States.

Access to healthcare impacts one's health practices as well. Those in lower socioeconomic groups or without insurance are more likely to self-medicate, use folk or family remedies, and seek episodic acute care than those who have higher income levels and health insurance.

CULTURE IN COMPREHENSIVE HEALTH ASSESSMENT

Comprehensive health assessment refers to obtaining subjective and objective data that is used to identify client needs. The data is then used to develop and implement plans to meet those needs. Cultural data is essential to this process, because it informs the nurse about a variety of factors and practices that impact the current and future health status of the client. Cultural data in comprehensive assessment would include all of the cultural phenomena described in the previous section. Table 4.2 provides questions to guide the cultural assessment. This information enables the nurse to plan care according to specific needs and orientations of the client.

The nurse has an obligation to meet the needs of all clients. Therefore, knowledge of cultural and language differences is essential in current practice. The nurse must examine his or her own cultural values and beliefs, and reflect upon their significance to encounters and interactions with clients of diverse cultures. The nurse must continue to learn about a variety of cultures and languages. The NCCC provides a self-assessment checklist for healthcare personnel. The checklist provides examples of the beliefs, attitudes, and practices that promote cultural competence. For more information, link to the NCCC through the Companion Website.

When language differences exist, the nurse must use all resources possible to ensure that decisions are based on accurate information. These resources include the use of translators and written materials provided in the language of the client. Last, the nurse must seek information about community resources to meet the needs of the diverse cultural groups for whom care is provided.

Table 4.2	Guidelines for Cultural Assessment
Ethnicity	Does the client identify with a particular ethnic/racial/cultural group? Where was the client born? How long has the client lived in this country?
Communication	What language is spoken? Can the client communicate in English? If yes, both spoken and written? Does the client speak for self or defer to another? What nonverbal communication behaviors are observed (e.g., touching, eye contact)? What significance do these behaviors have for the nurse-client interaction?
Space	Observe the client's proximity to other people and objects within the environment. How does the client react to the nurse's movement toward the client? Assess the client's physical environment (especially important in home health nursing, community nursing, and long-term care nursing). What cultural objects within the environment have importance for health promotion/health maintenance?
Social Organization	What are the client's roles? Is the client the primary decision maker for healthcare behaviors? Must the client consult another to make health decisions? If yes, who? What other family members are important to the client's decision making? Are there cultural or religious leaders who are important in the client's health decision making? Is there a religious affiliation linked with cultural affiliation (e.g., Jewish, Latino Catholic)?
Time	What is the client's time orientation: past, present, or future? What is the significance of time for the client? Does the client talk about time in specifics, such as dates or times, or in generalities, such as "a long time" or "a short time"?
Environmental Control	How is health defined by the culture? What does the client believe to be the cause of the illness or health concern? Has the client used the services of cultural healers? What healing practices has the client used? Have folk healing behaviors been used? Is the client wearing or carrying any amulets or artifacts that are believed to have healing properties?
Biological Variations	Are there normal variations in anatomical characteristics (e.g., body structure or size, skin color, facial characteristics)? What are the dietary preferences of the client? Are the dietary preferences related to the client's ethnicity? Is the client at risk for nutritional deficiencies because of ethnicity (e.g., pernicious anemia, lactose intolerance)? Are there variations in physiological functioning related to the client's ethnicity or race (e.g., drug metabolism, alcohol metabolism)? Are there illnesses or diseases that the client is at risk for because of ethnicity or race (e.g., hypertension, diabetes mellitus, sickle-cell anemia)?

Source: Kozier, Barbara; Erb, Glenora; Blais, Kathleen; Wilkinson, Judith M., *Fundamentals of Nursing: Concepts, Process, and Practice,* 5th Edition, © 1998. Reprinted by permission of Pearson Education, Inc. Upper Saddle River, NJ.

This chapter provides an overview of some of the concepts related to culture. Approaches to cultural assessment are included in Chapter 3 and Chapter 10 of this text. ⬭ Unit III of this text provides information about the cultural considerations for assessment of specific body regions or systems. ⬭ In-depth discussions of heritage and cultural concepts can be found by linking to Cultural Diversity in Health and Illness through the Companion Website.

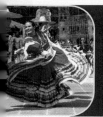

Application Through Critical Thinking

CASE STUDY

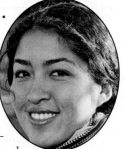

*S*ara Gulando is a 19-year-old nursing student performing a health screening of adults in an urban senior housing complex. The residents are from a variety of backgrounds including European, African, Native, Mexican, and Chinese Americans. Sara will work with these residents to screen for various health problems and determine their health habits and status. Sara comes from a small homogeneous town and has not had a great deal of exposure to individuals of different cultures and ethnic groups.

▶ Critical Thinking Questions

1. What expectations about health beliefs and practices should Sara bring to the experience?
2. What interview techniques should Sara use to determine the cultural identity of the residents?
3. What should Sara do to prepare for this experience?

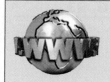

Please refer to the Companion Website at www.prenhall.com/damico and click on Chapter 4, the Application Through Critical Thinking module, to answer these and additional questions. In addition, complete NCLEX-RN® review questions and other interactive resources for this chapter.

EXPLORE MediaLink

Additional resources for this chapter are found on the Student CD-ROM accompanying this textbook and on the Companion Website.

CD-ROM CONTENT

Content for this chapter includes:
Objectives
Key Concepts
NCLEX-RN® Review Questions
Audio Glossary
Head-to-Toe Physical Examination Video

COMPANION WEBSITE CONTENT

www.prenhall.com/damico

Content for this chapter includes:
Objectives
NCLEX-RN® Review Questions

Application Through Critical Thinking
  Case Study Challenge
MediaLinks
MediaLink Application
Tool Box
  National Standards for Culturally and Linguistically
    Appropriate Services in Healthcare
New York Times

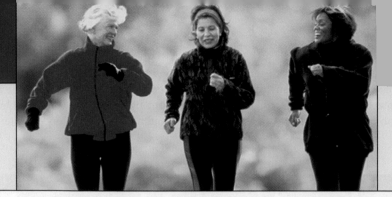

5

Psychosocial Assessment

MediaLink

www.prenhall.com/damico

The CD-ROM in the back of this textbook and the Media-Link website contain NCLEX-RN® review questions, interactive exercises, case study challenges, animations, videos, documentation and checklist forms, and review materials. For a complete listing of the media content specific to Chapter 5, see the Explore MediaLink at the end of the chapter.

$\mathcal{P}$sychosocial functioning includes the way a person thinks, feels, acts, and relates to self and others. It is the ability to cope and tolerate stress, and the capacity for developing a value and belief system. Psychosocial functioning is part of an intricate set of subsystems making up the human organism. These subsystems are interrelated components that make up an individual who is greater than a sum of parts. Assessment of the client must consider the interaction of body, mind, and spirit in their entirety rather than as separate body systems. When one part is missing or dysfunctional, all other parts of the individual are affected. Illness, developmental changes, or life crises may bring about changes in psychosocial functioning. The client may become stressed, may lose self-esteem, or may experience positive changes such as greater closeness with family. Changes in psychosocial functioning may, in turn, affect the client's physical health or response to treatment. For example, a client who is extremely stressed may not be able to understand or remember instructions for self-care, and a client who is socially isolated may not be able to get needed help at home. There is increasing evidence supporting the theory that mind-body interactions play a key role in both health and illness. No matter what the source of the client's concern, a psychosocial assessment can provide significant insights that help to individualize client care.

PSYCHOSOCIAL HEALTH

Psychosocial health can be defined as being mentally, emotionally, socially, and spiritually well (see Figure 5.1 ●). Psychosocial health includes mental, emotional, social, and spiritual dimensions. The mental dimension refers to an individual's ability to reason, to find meaning in and make judgments from information, to demonstrate rational thinking, and to perceive realistically. The emotional dimension is subjective and includes one's feelings. Social functioning refers to the individual's ability to form relationships with others. Included in the spiritual dimension are beliefs and values that give meaning to life.

FACTORS THAT INFLUENCE PSYCHOSOCIAL HEALTH

Psychosocial health is influenced by internal and external factors. Internal factors consist of one's genetic makeup, physical health, and physical fitness. External factors include the influence of those responsible for one's upbringing, and experiences in the social environment in which culture, geography, and economic status are contributory aspects. Additional factors to consider when addressing psychosocial health are self-concept, role development, interdependent relationships, and the abilities to manage stress, to cope with and adapt to change, and to develop a belief and values system.

INTERNAL FACTORS

Internal factors that influence psychosocial health include hereditary characteristics or those related to genetic makeup. In addition, the individual's physical health and level of fitness contribute to psychosocial health.

Genetics

As stated by the International Council of Nurses (2005), every health problem (with the exception of trauma) has a basis in genetics. With the completion of the Human Genome Project, gene-based testing and treatment are expected to dominate health care.

An individual's genetic makeup influences physical and psychosocial health throughout life. Research indicates that 60% to 65% of hypertension is inherited, children of manic-depressive parents have a slightly higher risk of experiencing that illness, and shyness is reportedly an inherited personality trait. Parents with attention deficit/hyperactivity disorder (ADHD) have an increased likelihood of having offspring with the disorder, and there appears to be a genetic link to conditions such as alcoholism and hypoglycemia.

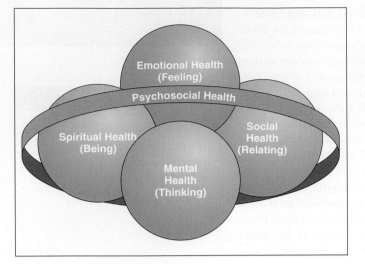

Figure 5.1 ● Psychosocial health.

Some studies of identical twins reveal that they often have the same habits, mannerisms, and perceptions of anxiety, even when raised separately.

Hereditary differences impact one's development in two ways. First, experiences impact hereditary predisposition for certain health problems. For example, an individual with a genetic predisposition to develop schizophrenia would likely develop the disease in a particular environment. Second, genetic characteristics result in reactions from others that can impact upon the developing personality. Consider the fact that body structure, appearance, and overall physical attractiveness are inherited. Most people respond more positively to children who are physically attractive than to those who are not. Repeated responses of a positive or negative nature can impact one's developing self-concept and self-esteem as well as overall behavior and interaction with others. Positive responses result in feelings of self-worth and confidence. Negative responses lead to low self-concept and may result in unmanageable levels of stress resulting in unacceptable behavior or mental illness. Furthermore, cognitive processes, including the abilities to think, perceive, remember, and make judgments, are dependent upon one's innate or inherited capacity and are enhanced or diminished in response to environmental and educational factors.

Physical Health

Physical health is associated with satisfaction of basic needs, quality of life, and psychosocial well-being. Research indicates that there is a mind-body-spirit connection. Physical health enables an individual to respond to stressors and, therefore, to adapt, cope with change, and grow as a functioning individual capable of personal and social interaction. Conversely, problems with health, particularly chronic illness, can negatively impact coping, adaptation, and personal and emotional fulfillment.

The mind-body-spirit connection is further explained as the body's response to thoughts and feelings. Positive and negative stress and anxiety may result in physical symptoms. Situations of positive and negative stress include marriage, childbirth, success in school or job performance, financial difficulties, the death of a friend or family member, or loss of a job. Physical symptoms that indicate a problem related to emotional stress or distress include the following:

- Back pain
- Chest pain
- Breathlessness
- Constipation
- Fatigue
- Hypertension
- Palpitations
- Dry mouth
- Nausea
- Weight loss or gain

Emotional **stress** affects health in several ways. First, stress affects the immune system resulting in increased susceptibility to infection. Second, during periods of stress or change, individuals are less likely to attend to habits that promote health such as eating nutritious meals or following an exercise routine. Last, some individuals use alcohol, tobacco, or drugs to "feel better."

Measures to deal with stress and reduce the negative impact on physical and emotional health include talking openly about feelings; thinking about positive aspects of life; using relaxation techniques such as meditation, yoga, prayer, or positive imagery; and following a regimen to promote health that includes healthy eating, exercise, and sleep.

Physical Fitness

Physical fitness is to the human body what fine-tuning is to an engine. It enables the body to perform up to its potential. Fitness can be described as a condition that helps individuals look, feel, and do their best. More specifically, physical fitness is:

> The ability to perform daily tasks vigorously and alertly, with energy left over for enjoying leisure-time activities and meeting emergency demands. It is the ability to endure, to bear up, to withstand stress, to carry on in circumstances where an unfit person could not continue, and is a major basis for good health and well-being. (President's Council on Physical Fitness and Sports, 2003, p. 2)

Physical fitness involves the performance of the heart and lungs, and the muscles of the body. Fitness, to some degree, influences qualities such as mental alertness and emotional stability, because what humans do with their bodies also affects what they can do with their minds. To maintain fitness, one must meet the needs for exercise, nutrition, rest, and relaxation, and follow practices to promote and preserve health. Recommendations related to physical activity were described in Chapter 2 of this text. ∞

EXTERNAL FACTORS

An individual's personality, sense of self, and role as a member of a larger society are influenced by a number of external factors. The manner and conditions in which a child is raised are an important influence. Additionally, the experiences during childhood and throughout life that are framed by culture, geography, and economic status contribute in great part to psychosocial well-being.

Family

Research indicates that children with consistent love, attention, and security grow into adults who are able to adapt to change and stress. Child rearing or caregiving generally occurs within a family unit. Families are considered social units of individuals who are related or live together over a period of time. Individual members in families have ongoing contact with each other; share goals, values, and concerns; and develop practices common to that specific group. Today, families involved in child rearing can be two-parent, single parent, heterosexual or homosexual domestic partnerships, blended or stepfamilies, adoptive families, or those in which grandparents, members of the extended family, or others provide childcare in the absence of parents.

Families influence psychosocial health because they are expected to provide for physical safety and economic needs; to help members develop physically, emotionally, and spiritually; and to help each individual develop an identity as self and member of the family. Families foster development of social skills, spiritual beliefs, and a value system. Families promote adaptive and coping skills and assist members to become part of the greater society. The ability to provide these basic needs is dependent upon the maturity of the caregivers and the support system available to them from family, community, and society.

Culture

Culture is a very complex system including knowledge, beliefs, morals, and customs that provide a pattern for living. Cultures may be composed of individuals from the same ethnic or racial group or background, in the same socioeconomic group, from the same geographic region, who practice a certain religion, and who share common values and beliefs. Culture influences the roles and relationships within families and groups that may be gender specific or determined by age. Culture dictates child rearing and health practices. Overall, behavior is defined by culture. The cultural norms affect physical, social, and mental well-being. An individual's experience and the ways in which one responds to stress, coping, and life situations are determined in great part by culture. Recall the details about the relationship of cultures and health described in Chapter 4. ∞

Geography

Geography refers to the country, region, section, community, or neighborhood in which one was born and raised, or in which one currently resides. The geography of an area affects family life and the development of individuals within families. Psychosocial health is influenced by the climate, terrain, resources, and aesthetics in varied locations. Community resources including schools, churches, healthcare facilities, transportation systems, support services, and safety systems affect the social development and emotional well-being of individuals within the community. Individuals in urban areas are subjected to stressors associated with crowded conditions, congestion, and crime rates higher than in other areas. Residents of rural areas may experience the stressors of limited resources and isolation.

In addition, in the United States one must consider the geographic impacts on psychosocial health that accompany regional characteristics, immigration, and the increased mobility of individuals and families. Some regions in the United States have a highly ethnic character. This character shapes the individual's self-concept and the ways one appraises, is appraised, and interacts with others from within and without the regional/ethnic norm. Immigrants face the stress of adapting to new geographical characteristics and cultural norms. Communities into which immigrants settle and the individuals within them must adapt to the differences in language, customs, morals, values, and roles of the immigrant population. Children of immigrants face the difficulty of being raised in a family with "old world" values and norms, while growing and developing as members of their adopted community and culture. Because of economic demand or opportunity, families tend to move more frequently today than in the past. Adults and children then must adjust to the culture of the new location, the loss of the familiar, and the stress of separation from family and friends.

Economic Status

Economic status affects the formation of values and attitudes. Values and role expectations related to marriage, gender roles, family roles, sex, parenting, education, housing, leisure activities, clothing, occupation, and religious practice are influenced by an individual or family's economic status. In the United States, the higher the income the more likely it is that individuals and families will have achieved higher levels of education, or provide for higher levels of education for their children. Better education leads to greater occupational opportunity, better housing, and the ability to participate in a variety of leisure activities. These advantages contribute to the development of high self-worth and self-esteem and result in individuals and families better equipped to manage and adapt to life changes. Those in lower economic groups or in poverty are focused on the present, that is, the immediate needs of self or family including the basic needs of food, clothing, and shelter. Self-esteem and self-image are often lower in poor individuals and families. Continual confrontation with the results of the disparities in income may result in anger, frustration, difficulty in coping, family disturbances, abnormal behaviors, and mental illness. Many times these individuals lack any form of health insurance and do not know how to access the healthcare delivery system.

ADDITIONAL FACTORS IN PSYCHOSOCIAL HEALTH

Additional factors to consider in psychosocial health are self-concept, role development, interdependent relationships, and the abilities to manage stress, to cope and adapt to change, and to develop a belief and value system.

Self-Concept

Self-concept refers to the beliefs and feelings one holds about oneself. A positive self-concept is essential to a person's mental and physical health. Individuals with a positive self-concept are better able to develop and maintain interpersonal relationships and resist psychological and physical illness.

Self-concept develops over time as a person reacts to and learns from interactions with others. As an individual develops across the life span, the interactions move from the immediacy of contact with caregivers as children to contact with individuals in the greater environment.

Body image and self-esteem are components of self-concept. Body image is the way one thinks about physical appearance, size, and body functioning. Self-esteem refers to the sense of worth or self-respect of an individual. All aspects of self-concept affect psychosocial health. Psychosocially healthy people have a realistic sense of self, adapt to change, develop ways to cope with problems, and form relationships that promote growth and development. In contrast, psychosocially unhealthy individuals often have problems with self-concept, which manifest as pessimism, social isolation, feelings of worthlessness, neglect of physical health, depression, anxiety, substance abuse, or suicidal thoughts (see Figure 5.2 ●).

Role Development

Role development refers to the individual's capacity to identify and fulfill the social expectations related to the variety of roles assumed in a lifetime. Roles are reciprocal relationships in which expectations exist for each participant. Examples of reciprocal roles are child-parent, student-teacher, employee-employer, as well as the reciprocal roles of spouse, sibling, friend, and neighbor. Roles are learned through socialization. The earliest learning generally occurs within the family when children observe and model adult behavior. When role development is healthy and occurs in a supportive environment, self-concept and psychosocial well-being are enhanced as the individual gains confidence in the ability to interact with others according to societal norms. However, nonsupportive, violent, or abusive family relationships are stressful and can lead to unsuccessful role relationships. Individuals who receive support and understand role expectations are able to meet the challenges of changing roles as they develop and mature. Individuals who have experienced family stress have conflicting views of role expectations, or are unclear of social norms. They often experience frustration or a sense of inadequacy associated with fear or negative judgment from others if their performance is not in accordance with expectations for new or changing roles.

Interdependent Relationships

Interdependent relationships are those in which the individual establishes bonds with others based on trust. Interdependent relationships are characterized by mutual reliance and

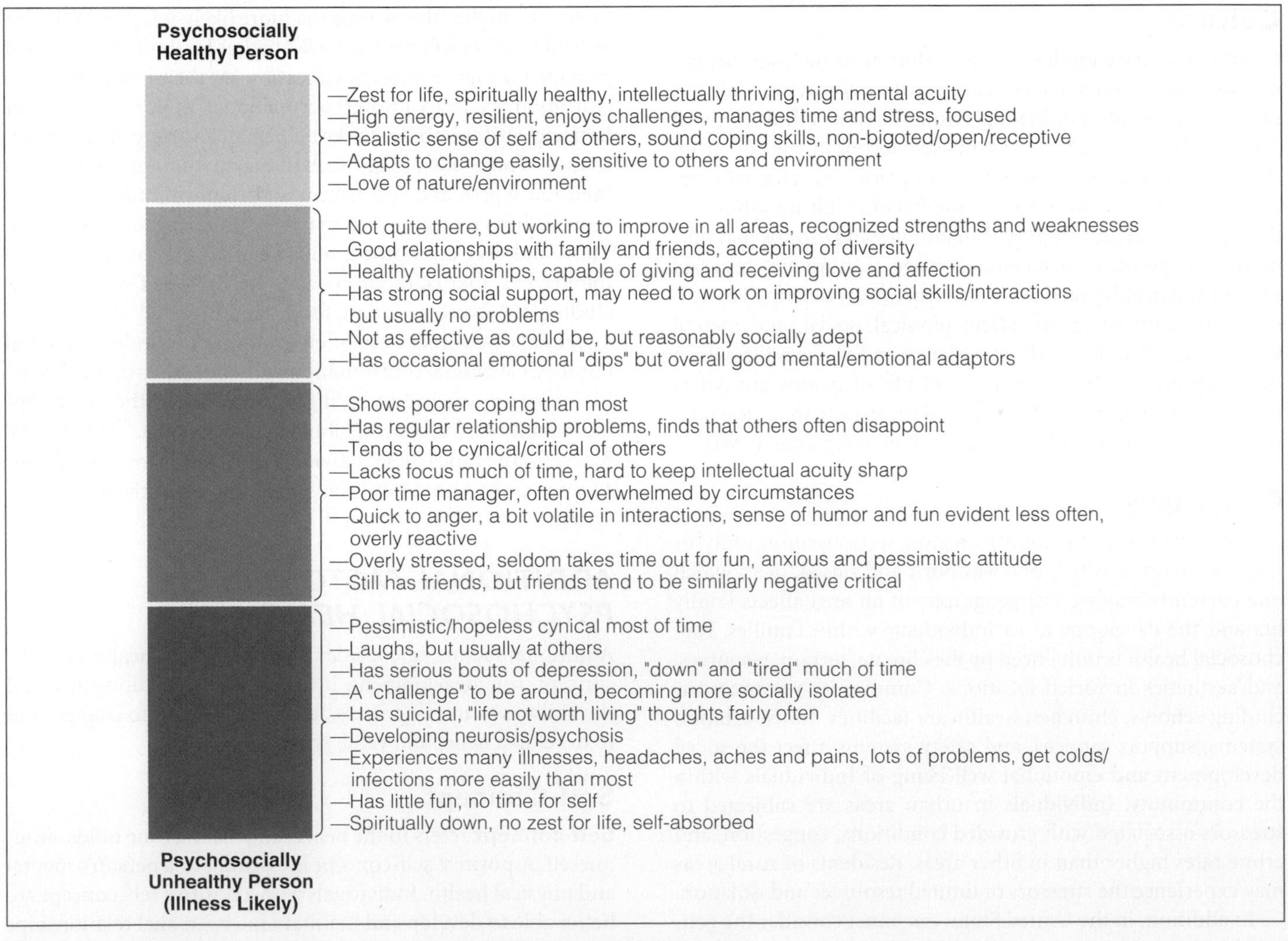

Psychosocially Healthy Person

—Zest for life, spiritually healthy, intellectually thriving, high mental acuity
—High energy, resilient, enjoys challenges, manages time and stress, focused
—Realistic sense of self and others, sound coping skills, non-bigoted/open/receptive
—Adapts to change easily, sensitive to others and environment
—Love of nature/environment

—Not quite there, but working to improve in all areas, recognized strengths and weaknesses
—Good relationships with family and friends, accepting of diversity
—Healthy relationships, capable of giving and receiving love and affection
—Has strong social support, may need to work on improving social skills/interactions but usually no problems
—Not as effective as could be, but reasonably socially adept
—Has occasional emotional "dips" but overall good mental/emotional adaptors

—Shows poorer coping than most
—Has regular relationship problems, finds that others often disappoint
—Tends to be cynical/critical of others
—Lacks focus much of time, hard to keep intellectual acuity sharp
—Poor time manager, often overwhelmed by circumstances
—Quick to anger, a bit volatile in interactions, sense of humor and fun evident less often, overly reactive
—Overly stressed, seldom takes time out for fun, anxious and pessimistic attitude
—Still has friends, but friends tend to be similarly negative critical

—Pessimistic/hopeless cynical most of time
—Laughs, but usually at others
—Has serious bouts of depression, "down" and "tired" much of time
—A "challenge" to be around, becoming more socially isolated
—Has suicidal, "life not worth living" thoughts fairly often
—Developing neurosis/psychosis
—Experiences many illnesses, headaches, aches and pains, lots of problems, get colds/infections more easily than most
—Has little fun, no time for self
—Spiritually down, no zest for life, self-absorbed

Psychosocially Unhealthy Person (Illness Likely)

Figure 5.2 ● Psychosocially healthy person versus psychosocially unhealthy person.

support. According to Roy and Andrews (1999), these relationships are based on the human needs of love, respect, and value for another. These important relationships include the individuals that one identifies as the significant other and one's support system. The ability to form, maintain, and adapt to changes in interdependent relationships is impacted by the individual's self-esteem. Individuals generally choose loving and close relationships with those who have similar levels of self-esteem. For example, when two people with high self-esteem form a loving and caring relationship, the high self-esteem is reinforced. Conversely, individuals with low self-esteem choose relationships with others with low self-esteem. As a result, feelings of negative self-worth are reinforced. Positive self-esteem enhances psychosocial health and enables the individual to grow and develop, adapt to change, solve problems, make decisions, maintain physical well-being, and seek help when needed for physical or emotional difficulties. Further, quality of life and length of life, which are measures of psychosocial health, have been linked to positive interdependent relationships.

Stress and Coping

Stress and coping are the individual's physical and emotional response to psychosocial or physical threats called stressors. An automobile accident, a failing grade, an illness, and loss of a job are examples of stressors. However, stress is not the event itself, but the individual's response to it. Events that are highly stressful for one individual may not be stressful for another. The stress response may include familiar physical symptoms such as sweaty palms or a pounding heart. The immediate physical reaction to stress is also referred to as the fight-or-flight response. Physical response to long-term stress may include symptoms such as habitually cold hands or suppression of immune function. The emotional reactions to stress may include difficulty sleeping, inability to concentrate, or anxiety. Positive as well as negative events may produce stress. The physical signs of stress include the following:

- Increased heart rate
- Decreased blood clotting time
- Increased rate and depth of respirations
- Dilated pupils
- Elevated glucose levels
- Dilated skeletal blood vessels
- Elevated blood pressure
- Dilated bronchi
- Increased blood volume
- Contraction of the spleen
- Increased blood supply to vital organs
- Release of T lymphocytes

Stress, in itself, is not bad. In fact, stress can sometimes motivate or enhance performance. Coping mechanisms are what an individual uses to deal with threats to physical and mental well-being. Like other patterns of behavior, patterns of coping with stress stem from early development when the child models the

ways significant people in his or her life have coped with and dealt with stress.

Spiritual and Belief Patterns

Spiritual and belief patterns reflect an individual's relationship with a higher power or with something, such as an ideal, a group, or humanity itself, that the person sees as larger than self and that gives meaning to life. The outward demonstration of spirituality may be reflected in religious practice, lifestyle, or relationships with others. A moral code is often included in one's belief patterns. A moral code is the internalized values, virtues, and rules one learns from significant others. It is developed by the individual to distinguish right from wrong. An individual's spiritual beliefs and moral code are affected by culture and ethnic background.

According to McSherry and Ross (2001), methods to assess spirituality and spiritual needs include direct questioning, indicator tools, and values clarification tools. Stoll (1979) introduced direct questioning as a method to assess spirituality. Stoll incorporated four basic areas for questioning: the client's concept of God, sources of hope and strength, religious practices, and the relationship between spiritual beliefs and health.

When using indicator tools, the nurse will observe verbal or nonverbal behaviors that indicate a spiritual need. Expressions of anger and crying are behaviors indicative of distress. Verbal cues would include statements such as, "Why do I deserve this?"

Additional measures for spiritual assessment include the spiritual well-being scale (SWBS). This scale is a 20-item instrument that examines religious and existential well-being. The SWBS is a paper-pencil instrument currently available in English and Spanish. The standard method is for the scale to be self-administered, and it takes 10 to 15 minutes to complete. The SWBS can be accessed at their Website through a link at the Companion Website.

Anadarajah and Hight (2000) developed the use of HOPE questions to use as a formal spiritual assessment in the client interview. The mnemonic HOPE is explained as follows. **H** refers to questions about the client's spiritual resources. These include sources of hope, meaning, love, and comfort. **O** refers to participation in or association with organized religion. **P** includes personal spiritual practices. **E** refers to the effects of healthcare and end-of-life issues. Table 5.1 includes questions for the HOPE approach to spiritual assessment.

Hodge (2001) described a narrative framework for spiritual assessment. This qualitative instrument incorporates a spiritual history and a framework to identify spiritual strengths as shown in Table 5.2.

The Joint Commission on Accreditation of Healthcare Organizations (JCAHO) also provides standards and recommendations regarding elements of spiritual assessment. JCAHO states, "Spiritual assessment should, at a minimum, determine the client's denomination, beliefs, and what spiritual practices are important to the client. This information would assist in determining the impact of spirituality, if any, on the care/services being provided and will identify if any further assessment is needed" (JCAHO, 2004).

Table 5.1	HOPE Approach to Spiritual Assessment
H Spiritual Resources	What are your sources of **hope** or comfort? What helps you during difficult times?
O Organized Religion	Are you a member of an **organized religion?** What religious practices are important to you?
P Personal Spirituality	Do you have **spiritual beliefs,** separate from organized religion? What **spiritual practices** are most helpful to you?
E Effects on Care	Is there any conflict between your beliefs and the **care** you will be receiving? Do you hold beliefs or follow practices that you believe may affect your **care?** Do you wish to consult with a religious or spiritual leader when you are ill or making decisions about your **healthcare?**

Source: Anadarajah, G., & Hight, E. (2000). *Spirituality and medical practice: Using the HOPE questions as a practical tool for spiritual assessment.* www.aafp.org/.

Table 5.2	Narrative Spiritual Assessment

Part I. Narrative Framework—Spiritual History

Sample Interview

1. Describe your personal and family religious traditions. (Include importance of religion and religious practices.)
2. What practices were important to you in youth? How have those experiences influenced your life?
3. How would you describe your religiosity or spirituality today? Do you believe your spirituality provides strength? How?

Part II. Interpretive Framework—Evokes Spiritual Strengths

1. Affect: How does spirituality affect joy, sorrow, coping? What part does spirituality play in providing hope?
2. Behavior: What rites or rituals do you use or follow? Do you have a relationship with a religious community or leader?
3. Cognition: Describe your current beliefs. Do your beliefs affect the ways you deal with difficulties or impact healthcare decisions?
4. Communion: What is your relationship with God? How do you communicate? Does your relationship help you in difficult times?
5. Conscience: Describe your values. How do you determine right and wrong?
6. Intuition: Have you experienced spiritual hunches, premonitions, or insights?

Source: Adapted from Hodge, D. R. (2001). Spiritual assessment: A review of major qualitative methods and a new framework for assessing spirituality. *Social Work, 46*(3), 8037–8046.

THE NURSING PROCESS IN PSYCHOSOCIAL ASSESSMENT

The professional nurse uses knowledge, effective communication skills, and critical thinking in application of the nursing process in psychosocial assessment. In conducting psychosocial assessment, the professional nurse uses a holistic approach in assessing the client's responses to life experiences and the environment. The information is used to formulate nursing diagnoses and to plan care for the client.

ASSESSMENT

When assessing psychosocial health the nurse gathers data related to several important areas. These include psychosocial concern, self-concept and beliefs, stress and coping mechanisms, and reasoning ability.

Psychosocial assessment begins before the initial interview when the nurse gathers information from the medical record relating to past emotional or psychiatric problems as well as physiological illnesses that may have affected the client's psychological or social functioning. For example, psychosocial problems may be related to brain tumors, multiple sclerosis, or bipolar disorder.

During the initial interview, the nurse gathers more information about the client's social history (e.g., marital status and occupation), history of growth and development, past emotional problems, response to crises and illnesses, and family history of emotional or psychiatric illness. If an area of heightened concern is discovered, the nurse may focus on that area during the initial interview and may also conduct a focused interview

at a later time during the course of the client's care. During the focused interview, the nurse uses information obtained from the medical history, the initial interview, and subsequent client interactions to help the client do a careful inventory of past and current psychosocial health status.

Psychosocial Well-Being

The nurse conducts an interview focused on psychosocial well-being when:

- The information collected during the health history indicates psychosocial dysfunction.
- The client's behavior during the initial interview is anxious, depressed, erratic, or bizarre.
- More information is needed to determine if any relationships exist between past disease processes and potential emotional or psychiatric concerns.

In some situations a psychosocial concern is not apparent at the time of the initial interview but becomes apparent at a later time, such as when a client learns of a negative prognosis or undergoes disfiguring surgical procedures. In these cases, the nurse should seek a focused psychosocial interview whenever the emotional problem becomes apparent. The case study (see Figure 5.3 ●) describes a situation where anxiety and fear impeded a client's recovery from a physical illness. Only after the nurse focused on the emotional impact of the illness was the client able to respond to therapy.

In some situations the client's primary health concern is psychosocial in nature. Clients with substance abuse, depression,

---

CASE STUDY

Mrs. Ada Sweeney, a 54-year-old grandmother, was admitted to intensive care with gastrointestinal bleeding. Over the next few days, Mrs. Sweeney was diagnosed with severe ulcerative colitis, anemia, and dehydration. Although the physician initiated an aggressive therapeutic medical regimen, Mrs. Sweeney failed to respond to therapy and continued to experience diarrhea accompanied by gastrointestinal bleeding, elevated temperatures, and severe abdominal pain. One evening the nurse on duty, Indira Singh, discovered Mrs. Sweeney crying in her room. Ms. Singh then used a focused interview to gather information regarding the behavior Mrs. Sweeney was demonstrating. "I'm worried about my grandson," Mrs. Sweeney told the nurse. "I'm raising him and his sisters until their mother is able to come back for them." Mrs. Sweeney went on to tell Ms. Singh that her daughter had been sent to prison on drug charges and there was no one else to care for her four children. "I do the best I can, but there's never enough money to go around, and I'm terrified the authorities will take the children away from me." Ms. Singh questioned Mrs. Sweeney about her immediate and extended family, income, job, and available support systems. After Ms. Singh reviewed the data she gathered during the focused interview, it became clear that Mrs. Sweeney's anxiety and fear over the future of her grandchildren was interfering with her recovery.

Within the next few days the social service department at the hospital found a state program that provided a homemaker for the children until their grandmother recovered, assisted the family in obtaining food stamps, and began a search for better housing. Mrs. Sweeney immediately began to show a response to her nursing and medical treatment and was able to leave the hospital within 2 weeks.

Figure 5.3 ● Case study.

neurosis, or psychosis fall into this category. In these situations, the nurse should integrate the questions outlined here as part of the focused interview into the initial interview during the first contact with the client, family, or friends.

The focused interview should be structured to obtain the most information with the fewest questions. Clients may feel uncomfortable answering questions about themselves, making it difficult for the nurse to gather accurate and detailed data regarding the psychosocial aspects of the client's life. The following sections include a variety of questions to use as a guide for collecting information about the client's past history of psychosocial and physiological problems as well as the five areas of psychosocial functioning.

History of Psychosocial Concerns

Some psychosocial concerns begin early in life and reappear whenever a client faces a major stressor or life crisis. The way the client coped with problems and treatment modalities in the past can be useful information for planning for the client's current problems. The following questions are helpful in eliciting this information:

1. Describe any emotions you find yourself frequently experiencing both currently and in the past.
   When the nurse assesses clients, a complete psychosocial history is helpful in determining whether the current health problem is related to previous psychosocial dysfunction.

2. If you have had an emotional problem in the past, were you treated for it? What kind of treatment did you have? Was the treatment successful? Who gave you the treatment? When? Do you still have the problem?
   This information is helpful in developing the current nursing care plan if previous methods of treatment were successful.

3. Do you use alcohol or drugs? If so, what do you use, how much, and how often? Have you had any treatment for substance abuse? What kind of treatment? Where?
   Substance abuse may be the underlying cause of physiological or psychosocial health problems or may be the result of some other underlying problem.

4. Have you had any eating problems such as anorexia, bulimia, or binge eating? Were you treated? How? By whom? When?
   A client who has an eating disorder may be in denial and unable to give accurate information on this question. If an eating disorder is suspected, the nurse should look for the diagnostic cues during the physical assessment.

History of Physiological Alterations or Diseases

When being treated for medical-surgical conditions, clients and their families may be unaware that the physical problems may be related to or caused by an underlying psychosocial problem. An understanding of the body-mind interaction, both positive and negative, can help nurses and clients realize when covert cognitive, perceptual, or affective problems are related to the overt signs and symptoms. Sometimes the underlying problem does not surface immediately but becomes apparent only after several days of nursing care.

The following questions are helpful for uncovering additional information:

1. Describe any chronic illnesses you have had.
   Clients with recent onset of chronic illnesses often have problems complying with treatment or adjusting to living with the condition.

2. How has your illness changed your mood or feelings? When you are nervous or anxious, how does your body feel?
   A physiological condition may be an underlying cause of anxiety, nervousness, or other abnormal behavior. Conversely, abnormal psychosocial behavior may aggravate or cause a physiological condition.

3. Have you had any of the following health problems: arthritis? asthma? bowel disorders? heart problems? glandular problems? headaches? stomach ulcer? skin disorders? If so, describe how the condition has affected your life.

These conditions sometimes have both a psychological and physiological component. The presence of the condition may signal an underlying psychosocial disturbance.

Self-Concept

It is difficult to gather significant data about self-concept, because most clients find it embarrassing to answer questions about themselves. Clients feel more comfortable divulging this information after a positive nurse-client relationship has been established and when the nurse integrates questions into general conversation.

The following questions are helpful in obtaining additional information about self-concept:

1. How would you describe yourself to others?
   Asking clients to describe themselves is an excellent technique for determining how they perceive themselves.

2. What are your best characteristics? What do you like about yourself?

3. What would you change about yourself if you could?
   This is a positive way of asking a client to talk about negative self-perceptions.

4. Would you describe yourself as shy or outgoing?

5. Do you consider yourself attractive? Sexually appealing? If no, why not?
   The client's self-perception of attractiveness and sex appeal may reveal problems with self-image.

6. Have your feelings about your appearance changed with this illness? If so, how?
   Self-image may change if the illness or treatment has caused a change in appearance.

7. Who comes first in your life: your spouse, children, friends, parents, or yourself?

8. Do you have difficulty saying no to others?
   Clients who are depressed, feel hopeless, or feel powerless have difficulty with assertiveness.

9. Do you like to be alone?
   Clients with positive self-concept enjoy spending time by themselves, but those who indicate that they'd rather be alone most of the time may be experiencing emotional problems.

10. Describe your social life. What do you do for fun?
    Clients who are unable to answer this question may be depressed or out of touch with reality.

11. What are your hobbies or interests? Do you spend much time pursuing them?

12. For heterosexuals only. Are you comfortable relating to the opposite sex? If no, why not?
    Persons with self-concept or self-image problems may experience difficulty relating to the opposite sex.

13. Are you comfortable with your sexual preference? If not, why not?
    Clients who are homosexual and have not learned to accept their sexuality may experience a self-image problem.

14. Do you have any concerns about your sexual function? If so, what?

Family History

The nurse should explore this area more fully if the health history indicates a family history of psychosocial dysfunction. Although no member of the family may have been diagnosed as being mentally ill, the nurse should explore individual as well as family dysfunction.

The nurse should ask the following questions in relation to the client's parents, siblings, and extended family in the case of a child, and also in relation to the client's current family if an adult.

1. Describe any problems your family may have had with mental disorders.
   Some mental disorders such as schizophrenia are familial, that is, the illness recurs in the same family over several generations.

2. What were your major responsibilities in your family?

3. Describe your relationships with your parents and extended family.
   The nurse should look for family dysfunction problems such as schisms (families in chronic controversy), disengagement (detached relationships), or enmeshment (family interactions that are intense and focus on power conflicts rather than affections) as the client describes his or her family life.

4. What is your birth order in your family? How many brothers and sisters do you have? Are your sisters and brothers older or younger?
   Age and gender birth order influence how an individual relates to other men and women throughout life.

5. Describe your relationship with your siblings growing up at home. Did you and your siblings have problems getting along? If so, how did you solve them?
   The way a client learned to handle stress and conflict with siblings as a child influences the way the client handles these issues throughout life.

6. What members of your extended family (grandparents, aunts, uncles, cousins) were important to you as you grew up? How did they influence you?
   Significant others shape an individual's self-concept and self-esteem. Descriptions of significant others help the nurse understand why clients feel and act as they do.

7. Did you have death or losses in your family as you grew up? How did your parents teach you to cope with the loss? How did they cope with the loss?
   Clients who are depressed may not have learned how to deal with loss as a child and may have difficulty dealing with the loss of a loved one or with their own or a significant other's declining health status.

8. Were your parents divorced or remarried during your childhood? If so, whom did you live with? Describe your life growing up with a single parent or stepparent.
   Children who are products of a divorce may carry emotional scars into adulthood, affecting their psychosocial health and indirectly affecting their physical health status.

9. Describe how your parents raised you. How did it affect you?
   Clients who were raised by parents who had serious emotional problems, or who were abused by their parents, are more likely to have emotional problems as adults.

10. How did your family deal with adversity and conflict?
    Clients learn to deal with problems from their family. Knowing how the client learned to deal with problems as a child helps the nurse understand how the client might deal with the present health problem.

11. When disagreement arose in your family, how was it solved? Who sided with whom?
    In dysfunctional families, schisms result causing family members to align themselves into coalitions against other family members, such as parents against children, father and sons against mother and daughters, and sisters against brothers.

Other Roles and Relationships

It is also important for the nurse to ask questions about other roles and relationships in the client's life.

1. Describe your relationships with your friends, neighbors, and coworkers.

2. Do you belong to any social groups? Community groups?

3. Who is your closest friend? How do you maintain your friendship?
   An individual's ability to form close relationships indicates a healthy self-concept. An individual who consistently fails to form close relationships may have a self-concept problem.

4. Is your closest friend the most important person in your life? If not, who is the most important person in your life? Explain why.

Stress and Coping

A person learns coping mechanisms from significant others during early childhood and throughout life. The ability to cope is also greatly affected by the number and severity of stressors that have occurred in a person's life. One method for assessing stress in a client's life is to administer the Holmes social adjustment rating scale (see Table 5.3). The items on this scale represent stressors that may occur in a person's life. Since stress is a response to events, not the events themselves, not all people are equally stressed by these events. However, on average, the higher the client's score, the more likely it is that the individual has responded with stress. As a result, the individual is more likely to experience stress-related disorders (e.g., headaches, asthma, skin rashes, back pain, frequent colds, anxiety). The scale demonstrates that positive life events should also be part of a psychosocial assessment, because these positive events can be just as stressful as negative events in a person's life.

The following questions are helpful to gather additional information about the client's stress and coping mechanisms.

1. What do you do for relaxation? For recreation?

2. What is your greatest source of comfort when you are feeling upset?
   This question identifies the client's coping mechanisms.

3. Who do you call when you need help?
   This question identifies important persons in the client's support system.

4. What is the greatest source of stress in your life at the present time? How have you coped with similar situations in the past?
   A person who has successfully coped with stress in the past may be able to call upon these coping skills to deal with current problems.

5. Describe how you are dealing with your illness. Have you had difficulty adjusting to: changes in your appearance? ability to carry out activities of daily living? relationships? If so, describe how you feel.
   Clients who have undergone severe, sudden changes that are apparent to others frequently have difficulty adjusting to these changes.

6. Do you take any drugs, medications, or alcohol to cope with your stress? If so, describe what you are taking.
   Clients who are experiencing stress are at risk for becoming addicted to these substances, especially if there is a family history of drug or alcohol abuse.

7. Are you experiencing any of the following: sadness? crying spells? insomnia? lack of appetite? weight loss? weight gain? loss of sex drive? constipation? fatigue? hopelessness? irritability? indecisiveness? confusion? pounding heart or pulse? trouble concentrating?
   These may indicate a high level of stress or major depression.

8. Have you ever considered taking your life? If so, describe what you would do.
   Clients who are suicidal often admit their intentions if questioned directly. Clients are at high risk for suicide if they can describe a method for committing the suicide and have the necessary means at their disposal. (See Box 5.1 for characteristics of the suicidal client.)

The Senses and Cognition

Clients who are out of contact with reality may display illusional, delusional, and hallucinatory speech and behaviors, such as talking to themselves (auditory hallucinations); reacting to objects, noises, or other people in strange ways (illusions); or discussing false beliefs (delusions). Direct questioning may increase the client's anxiety and escalate the abnormal behavior or cause confusion. The nurse should use direct questioning only when the client appears to be in control and in touch with reality.

The following questions are helpful to gather additional information. The nurse should preface these questions by first explaining to the client that some of the questions may seem silly or unimportant, but that they are helpful in assessing memory.

1. What is your name?

2. How old are you?

3. Where were you born?

4. Where are you right now?

5. What day of the week is it? What is the date?
   Questions 1 through 5 determine whether the client is oriented to person, place, and time.

6. What would you take with you if a fire broke out?
   The client's ability to make a judgment is tested here.

7. Count backward from 10 to 1.
   Tests cognitive function.

8. What did you have for breakfast?
   Tests recent memory.

9. Who were the last two presidents?
   Tests remote memory.

Table 5.3 Holmes Social Readjustment Scale

EVENT	EVENT VALUE
1. Death of a spouse	100
2. Divorce	73
3. Marital separation	65
4. Jail term	63
5. Death of a close family member	63
6. Personal injury or illness	53
7. Marriage	50
8. Fired at work	47
9. Marital reconciliation	45
10. Retirement	45
11. Change in health of family member	44
12. Pregnancy	40
13. Sex difficulties	39
14. Gain of a new family member	39
15. Business readjustment	39
16. Change in financial state	38
17. Death of a close friend	37
18. Change to different line of work	36
19. Change in number of arguments	35
20. Mortgage or loan over $10,000	31
21. Foreclosure of mortgage or loan	30
22. Change in responsibilities at work	29
23. Son or daughter leaving home	29
24. Trouble with in-laws	29
25. Outstanding personal achievement	28
26. Spouse begins or stops work	26
27. Begin or end school	26
28. Change in living conditions	25
29. Revision of personal habits	24
30. Trouble with boss	23
31. Change in work hours or conditions	20
32. Change in residence	20
33. Change in schools	20
34. Change in recreation	19
35. Change in church activities	19
36. Change in social activities	19
37. Change in sleeping habits	16
38. Change in number of family get-togethers	15
39. Vacation	13
40. Christmas	12
41. Minor violations of the law	11
Total Points	

Directions for completion: Add up the point values for each of the events that you have experienced during the past 12 months.

Scoring

Below 150 points:

The amount of stress you are experiencing as a result of changes in your life is normal and manageable. There is only a 1 in 3 chance that you might develop a serious illness over the next 2 years based on stress alone. Consider practicing a daily relaxation technique to reduce your chance of illness even more.

150 to 300 points:

The amount of stress you are experiencing as a result of changes in your life is moderate. Based on stress alone, you have a 50/50 chance of developing a serious illness over the next 2 years. You can reduce these odds by practicing stress management and relaxation techniques on a daily basis.

Over 300 points:

The amount of stress you are experiencing as a result of changes in your life is high. Based on stress alone, your chances of developing a serious illness during the next 2 years approaches 90%, unless you are already practicing good coping skills and regular relaxation techniques. You can reduce the chance of illness by practicing coping strategies and relaxation techniques daily.

Source: From Holmes, T., & Rahe, R. J. (1967). Social Readjusting Rating Scale. *Journal of Psychosomatic Research, 11,* 213–218. Elsevier Science Ltd., Pergamon Imprint, Oxford, England.

10. Describe what the following statement means: People who live in glass houses shouldn't throw stones.
Tests the client's ability to do abstract or symbolic thinking.

11. Are you having any problems thinking? If so, describe what happens.
The client may not be able to answer this question if a thought disorder is present. Clients with bipolar disorders and who are manic describe their thoughts as "racing."

12. Do you have trouble making decisions? Describe what happens when you have to make a decision.

The inability to make decisions may indicate depression or low self-esteem.

13. Do you ever hear voices, see objects, or experience other sensations that don't make sense? If so, describe your experiences.
The client who is out of touch with reality may experience auditory, visual, gustatory, somatic, and olfactory hallucinations (hearing, seeing, tasting, feeling, and smelling stimuli that are not real). Discussing hallucinatory experiences in detail may reinforce them for the client; therefore, it is important not to dwell on these symptoms with the client.

Box 5.1	Characteristics of the Client Who Is at the Highest Risk for Suicide

The following characteristics may indicate that a client is at increased risk for suicide. While one of the following items alone may not indicate a client is contemplating suicide, the more factors present, the more likely that the client is at increased risk.

- Single, divorced, or widowed
- Socially isolated, or little or no support system
- History of suicide attempts
- Family history of suicide
- Recent loss, i.e., divorce, threat of or loss of a loved one; loss of a job, money, or social status
- History of drug abuse or alcoholism
- History of mental illness
- Depressed or recovering from depression
- Severe anxiety or fear
- Serious or physical illness, with impaired lifestyle or altered body image
- Sleep dysfunction
- Expressing feelings of hopelessness, powerlessness, rejection, or punishment
- Arranging personal affairs, i.e., taking out an insurance policy, planning a funeral, canceling social engagements, preparing a will, or giving possessions away
- Verbalizing suicidal thoughts, i.e., "Sometimes I think I'd be better off dead" or "I give up"
- Sudden or unexplained behavior change
- Feelings of ineffective communication, or family members rejecting attempts at communication
- Feelings of increased life responsibilities
- Crying for no obvious reason
- Certain demographic variables such as gender (suicide rates are higher for men), race (suicide rates are higher for Caucasians and Native Americans), age (suicide rates are higher between 15 and 24 years), both ends of the socioeconomic scale

14. If you hear voices, do they tell you what you must do?
    The nurse asks this question to determine if the client is experiencing command hallucinations. These are dangerous hallucinations that may lead the client to self-destructive behavior or to harm others.

15. Do you ever misinterpret objects, sounds, or smells? If so, please describe.
    Clients who are very anxious or out of contact with reality may experience illusions (misinterpretation of environmental stimuli).

The content of a client's hallucinations and delusions is important to assess in order to provide for the client's safety and the safety of others. Command hallucinations tell clients to carry out acts against themselves or others that are usually harmful. The command hallucinations may be part of an elaborate delusional system in which clients feel persecuted or in danger. In some cases, clients are disturbed by these thoughts and share them with others. In other situations, however, clients keep their thoughts to themselves, and these thoughts do not become apparent until they commit some violent act. A client who demonstrates these symptoms should be referred to a psychiatric/mental health nurse or clinical specialist who has the skill and expertise needed to uncover hallucinatory and delusional thinking without exacerbating the symptoms.

Spiritual and Belief Systems

The questions in this section determine how clients' ethical, moral, and religious values affect their health status. Often the client's statements about values play an important role in how the nurse should implement care. It is important to be sensitive to the client's reaction to these questions when assessing this area, because the client's spiritual life and belief systems may be very personal.

The nurse should also be careful about querying a client who is hallucinating or is delusional, because the questions can exacerbate delusional or hallucinatory behavior.

The spiritual and belief systems of clients usually derive from their culture and ethnic background. A client may have beliefs about health and illness, God, or the supernatural that are culturally derived. The nurse needs to understand that these issues play an important role in the client's ability to cope with a psychosocial health concern or illness.

The following questions are used to assess the client's spiritual and belief systems and the cultural and ethnic considerations surrounding them. While collecting this information, the nurse should observe the client's verbal and nonverbal behavior, interpersonal relationships, and immediate environment.

1. Describe your ethnic and cultural background.
   Clients from some ethnic and cultural groups are more likely to have health-related beliefs and practices that have an impact on nursing care (see Chapter 4 ⬭).

2. To whom do you go for help regarding your health (doctor, nurse, practitioner, folk healer, medicine man, or other healer)?
   The nurse is more likely to gain the client's compliance if the client's folk healer is included in the planning stage.

3. What are your beliefs about life, health, illness, and death?
   The nurse needs this knowledge about the client's health-related beliefs to develop an individualized plan of care.

4. Does religion or God play a part in your life? If so, what is it?
   The nurse should incorporate the client's religion and faith in God in the plan of care if they are important to the client.

5. What part do hope and faith play in your life? Is your faith helpful to you during times of stress? If so, describe how.

6. Has your present health concern affected your spiritual life? If so, describe how.

7. Do your spiritual beliefs help you cope with illness or stress? If so, describe how.

8. Have you experienced any anger with God or a higher being or force because of things that have happened to you? If so, describe how you feel.
   Clients who feel anger toward God or a higher force may project this anger toward family, friends, and healthcare providers.

9. Do you believe your illness is a punishment for past sins or wrongdoing?
   Clients who feel they are being punished may feel guilty and lose the ability to cope with the illness.

10. If you use prayer, describe how you use it to cope with life or stress.
    The nurse should incorporate the client's use of prayer in the plan of care if it is meaningful to the client.

11. Are you affiliated with any religion?

12. Describe any religion-related nutrition or health practices that you must follow.

13. Are you concerned about the morality or ethical implications of any of the treatments planned for you?

Physical Observation

During the initial or focused interview, the nurse should also observe the client's general appearance, posture, gait, body language, and speech patterns. The client's general appearance includes the manner of dress, personal hygiene, and grooming.

- The client should be clean and well groomed. The clothes should be clean, worn properly, and appropriate for the client's age and the time and place. The nurse must be careful not to impose his or her own standards when judging the dress of another.

- Abnormal speech patterns may indicate anxiety, fear, or altered thought processes (see Box 5.2). The nurse should observe the coherence and organization of the client's speech. The client's speech should be logical and sequential.

- Clients may demonstrate the following: talking to themselves (auditory hallucinations); reacting to objects, noises, or other people in strange ways (illusions); or manifesting erratic beliefs (delusions). The client may appear to be aphasic or incoherent. These clients may be experiencing altered communication, altered thought processes, and ineffective coping.

- The client who is dirty, disheveled, or unshaven or who has a body odor may have an altered body image caused by a low self-esteem. The nurse should further assess the client for changes in skin integrity due to unclean conditions and look for signs of ringworm, pediculosis, or other skin problems (see Chapter 11 ⚭).

The nurse should next observe the client's posture, gait, and general body language.

- The client's posture should be erect and relaxed. The body language should be open with direct eye contact unless inappropriate for the client's ethnic group. Movements should be fluid, relaxed, and spontaneous. A closed, guarded posture with poor eye contact may indicate fear, anxiety, or defense mechanisms. The client who paces, wrings hands,

appears restless, or exhibits tics (involuntary movements) may also be experiencing anxiety. A slow, shuffling gait may indicate depression or poor contact with reality.

The nurse must also observe the facial expression and affect. The expression and affect should be appropriate for the conversation and circumstances.

- An unusually sad (depressed) or extremely happy (euphoric) demeanor that is inappropriate for the circumstances, labile (rapid) mood swings, or flat affect (absence of emotional expression) may indicate difficulty coping.

Finally, the nurse should notice the content and manner of speech. The content, tone, pace, and volume of the speech should be appropriate for the situation.

Measures, scales, and instruments are available to assess particular aspects of psychosocial health including quality of life, social support, stress, and psychosocial well-being. For example, the Centers for Disease Control and Prevention (CDC) uses "healthy day measures" to assess quality of life in populations. Box 5.3 includes questions used in healthy day measures. For further information, contact the CDC through the link at the Companion Website.

Other measures to assess particular aspects of psychosocial health include the Multidimensional Health Profile–Psychosocial (MHP–P). An instrument designed to screen for psychosocial problems, the MHP–P assesses life stress, coping, social supports, and mental health. For a sample score report, contact their Website through the link at the Companion Website.

One may also use the Duke Social Support and Stress Scale (DUSOCS). This is a 24-item self- and interviewer-administered instrument to measure family and nonfamily support and stress. Psychological well-being may be assessed with a variety of scales including the delighted-terrible scale, the faces scale, the ladder scale, and the life satisfaction index. Each of these provides a system to rank the client's perceptions of well-being. For more information, go to DUSOCS through the link at the Companion Website.

Box 5.2	**Abnormal Speech Patterns Associated with Altered Thought Processes**

- Loud, rapid, pressured, and high-pitched
- Circumlocution (inability to communicate an idea due to numerous digressions)
- Flight of ideas (jumping from one subject to another)
- Word salad (a conglomeration of multiple words without apparent meaning)
- Neologisms (coining new words that have symbolic meaning to the client)
- Clanging (rhyming conversation)
- Echolalia (constant repetition of words or phrases that the client hears others say)

Box 5.3	**Healthy Days Measures**

The CDC uses a set of questions called the "Healthy Days Measures." These questions include the following:

1. Would you say that in general your health is
   a. Excellent
   b. Very good
   c. Good
   d. Fair
   e. Poor
2. Now thinking about your physical health, which includes physical illness and injury, for how many days during the past 30 days was your physical health not good?
3. Now thinking about your mental health, which includes stress, depression, and problems with emotions, for how many days during the past 30 days was your mental health not good?
4. During the past 30 days, for about how many days did poor physical or mental health keep you from doing your usual activities, such as self-care, work, or recreation?

Source: United States Department of Health and Human Services, Centers for Disease Control and Prevention, National Center for Chronic Disease Prevention and Health Promotion.

ORGANIZING THE DATA

Once the nurse has collected the data from all of the various sources, the information is sorted, grouped, and categorized. Each diagnostic cue falls under one of the psychosocial functioning groups mentioned earlier in this chapter: self-concept, roles and relationships, stress and coping, the senses and cognition, and spiritual and belief systems. After the diagnostic cues have been grouped and clustered under one of the psychosocial groups, the nurse determines the final nursing diagnoses.

The following case study demonstrates how diagnostic cues obtained during the assessment lead to nursing diagnoses related to psychosocial well-being and function.

Mr. Abe Johnson, a transient passing through town, was admitted to the local hospital emergency room after being arrested for disturbing the peace and possession of heroin. The guards at the jail had brought him to the hospital after they were unable to control his violent behavior. When approached by the admitting nurse, Ms. Quan, Mr. Johnson shouted, "Don't come near me with that gas machine! The High Lord has told me that I control the secret of life and death, and if you touch me you must die!" The nurse recognized that Mr. Johnson had seen the stethoscope she carried as a "gas machine." After observing Mr. Johnson's manner and tone for a few minutes, she also noted that he was hearing voices. Ms. Quan knew that Mr. Johnson's behavior could become violent if he continued to experience command hallucinations. She removed the stethoscope from around her neck and showed it to Mr. Johnson. She said, speaking in a quiet calm voice, "This is the stethoscope that I use to listen to a client's heart. Sometimes I use it to take blood pressures. Would you like to look at it?" As Mr. Johnson doubtfully held the stethoscope and rapidly and repeatedly turned it over, she said, "Most stethoscopes are black and silver but mine is white and gold. I think it's a pretty color, don't you?" Mr. Johnson threw the stethoscope back at Ms. Quan, mumbling "OK." After a few minutes she said, "You've been brought to the hospital, Mr. Johnson. I'm Ms. Quan, your nurse, and I'm here to take care of you. Have you noticed that even though I've been helping you remove your clothes, nothing has happened to me?"

In this clinical situation, the nurse showed Mr. Johnson respect and concern for his feelings and well-being. She did not, however, validate his perceptions about the stethoscope or acknowledge the voices he heard. Instead, she reinforced reality for him by describing the white and gold stethoscope and pointing out that he had no special power to harm her.

The nurse then clustered the information gained from the assessment and identified the significant cues demonstrated by Mr. Johnson:

- Hallucinations
- Delusions
- Illusions
- Fearful thoughts
- Irritability
- Inaccurate interpretation of environment

Ms. Quan reviewed all the data and saw the following factors as contributing to Mr. Johnson's problems:

- Substance abuse
- Transient lifestyle

Then, after reviewing the assessment data, identifying contributing factors, and clustering the information, Ms. Quan formulated diagnoses and a plan of care.

The holistic approach to nursing holds that the individual must be viewed as a total being, by which body, mind, and spirit continuously interact with self and with the environment. The psychosocial assessment is a key component that must be integrated into the nurse's holistic approach to data collection. This assessment guides the nurse toward a true and accurate picture of the client as a total human being.

Application Through Critical Thinking

CASE STUDY

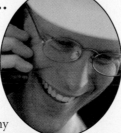

Luke Van Hoff, a 44-year-old engineer, has recently been transferred from a suburban town office to a larger firm in an urban area. His wife and three school-aged children will join him at the completion of the school year.

Luke is currently residing in company housing while house hunting on the weekends.

He was eager to take the new position because it meant a significant increase in income.

You are the nurse in the corporate health office who will conduct a comprehensive health assessment of this new employee.

▶ Critical Thinking Questions

1. What psychosocial issues will be addressed in the interview?
2. Analyze the data in the case study and describe how the psychosocial health of Mr. Van Hoff will be impacted.
3. Select the tools that would be appropriate for psychosocial assessment of Mr. Van Hoff.

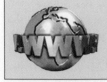

Please refer to the Companion Website at www.prenhall.com/damico and click on Chapter 5, the Application Through Critical Thinking module, to answer these and additional questions. In addition, complete NCLEX-RN® review questions and other interactive resources for this chapter.

EXPLORE MediaLink

Additional resources for this chapter are found on the Student CD-ROM accompanying this textbook and on the Companion Website.

CD-ROM CONTENT

Content for this chapter includes:
Objectives
Key Concepts
NCLEX-RN® Review Questions
Model Documentation Forms
Audio Glossary
Head-to-Toe Physical Examination Video

COMPANION WEBSITE CONTENT

www.prenhall.com/damico

Content for this chapter includes:
Objectives
NCLEX-RN® Review Questions
Application Through Critical Thinking
  Case Study Challenge

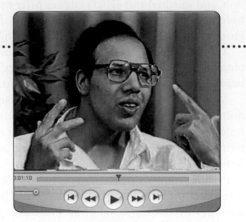

MediaLinks
MediaLink Application
Tool Box
  HOPE Approach to Spiritual Assessment
  Characteristics of the Client Who Is at the Highest Risk for
  Suicide
New York Times

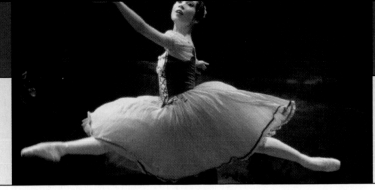

6

Techniques and Equipment

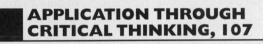

MEDIALINK

www.prenhall.com/damico

The CD-ROM in the back of this textbook and the Media-Link website contain NCLEX-RN® review questions, interactive exercises, case study challenges, animations, videos, documentation and checklist forms, and review materials. For a complete listing of the media content specific to Chapter 6, see the Explore MediaLink at the end of the chapter.

*U*nit I of this book identified and discussed many concepts to be considered when assessing the overall health status of the client. ∞ These concepts include but are not limited to health, wellness, growth and development, culture, and psychosocial considerations. Much of the data gathered in relation to these concepts is subjective and is obtained through client interviews during the health history and focused interview sessions. For example, when a client reports feeling "pins and needles" in his left foot, or feelings of "nausea" after drinking cold water, subjective data is being reported and collected.

Objective data must be gathered as part of the **database.** This is accomplished through the physical assessment of the client. The objective data is obtained by using the four basic or cardinal techniques of physical assessment: inspection, palpation, percussion, and auscultation. Special equipment and the senses of the nurse are used to measure, observe, touch, and listen to sounds of the body. A safe, comfortable environment conducive to client comfort, dignity, and privacy is essential. Individual clients will react differently to each situation. The nurse must obtain client permission to proceed, make the client feel comfortable, and communicate with the client throughout the physical assessment.

BASIC TECHNIQUES OF PHYSICAL ASSESSMENT

When performing physical assessment, the nurse will utilize four basic techniques to obtain objective and measurable data. These techniques are inspection, palpation, percussion, and auscultation and are performed in an organized manner. This pattern of organization varies when assessing the abdomen. The sequence for abdominal assessment is inspection, auscultation, percussion, and palpation. Percussion and palpation could alter the natural sounds of the abdomen; therefore, it is important to auscultate and listen to the unaltered sounds. This sequence is further discussed in Chapter 19 of this text. ∞

INSPECTION

Inspection is the skill of observing the client in a deliberate, systematic manner. It begins the moment the nurse meets the client and continues until the end of the client-nurse interaction (see Figure 6.1 ●). Inspection always precedes the other assessment skills and is never rushed. Most novice nurses feel uncomfortable staring at the client; nevertheless, careful scrutiny provides critical assessment data. The nurse should talk to the client, help the client relax before proceeding with inspection, and avoid the temptation to touch the client. It is important to complete inspection of the client before using any of the other techniques. However, if the client is a child, the nurse may need to vary the approach to secure the child's attention and cooperation.

Inspection begins with a survey of the client's appearance and a comparison of the right and left sides of the client's body, which should be nearly symmetrical. As the nurse assesses each body system or region, he or she inspects for color, size, shape, contour, symmetry, movement, or drainage. When inspecting a large body region, the nurse should proceed from general overview to specific detail. For example, when inspecting the leg, the nurse surveys the entire leg and then focuses on each part, including the thigh, knee, calf, ankle, foot, and toes in succession. One should remember to look at the client, listen for natural sounds, and use the sense of smell to detect odors. Use of each of the senses enhances the findings.

Throughout inspection, the nurse applies the skills of critical thinking to analyze the observations and determine the significance of the findings to the general health of the client. The nurse must know the anticipated findings regarding inspection of a body part. The nurse asks: Are the findings considered to be within normal parameters or unexpected findings? Are the findings consistent with other diagnostic cues? What other information is needed to support this finding?

Although the nurse will perform most of the inspection without the help of instruments, some special tools for visualizing certain body organs or regions are important. For example, the ophthalmoscope is used to inspect the inner aspect of the eye. This and other instruments used to enhance inspection are discussed later in this chapter.

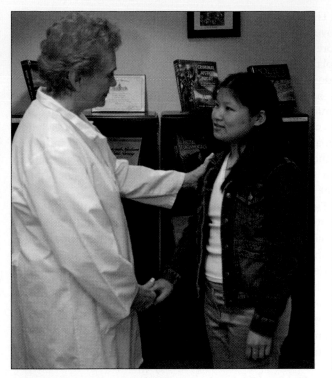

Figure 6.1 ● Inspection of client.

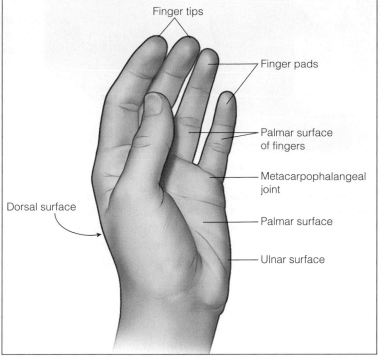

Figure 6.2 ● Sensitive areas of the hand.

Finger tips

Finger pads

Palmar surface
of fingers

Metacarpophalangeal
joint

Palmar surface

Ulnar surface

Dorsal surface

PALPATION

Palpation is the skill of assessing the client through the sense of touch to determine specific characteristics of the body. These characteristics include size, shape, location, mobility of a part, position, vibrations, temperature, texture, moisture, tenderness, and edema. The approach used by the professional nurse to obtain this data is important. The nurse must be gentle and obtain the confidence of the client. The hand of the nurse must be moved slowly and intentionally. The nurse must learn how much pressure to use during palpation with the examination hand. Too much pressure may produce pain for the client. Too little pressure may not permit the nurse to perceive the data accurately. This is a skill that requires practice and is developed over time.

The hand has several sensitive areas; therefore, it is important to use the part of the hand most responsive to body structures and functions. The nurse will use the fingertips, finger pads, base of the fingers, palmar surface of the fingers, and the dorsal and ulnar surfaces of the hand (see Figure 6.2 ●).

The finger pads are used for discrimination of underlying structures and functions such as pulses, superficial lymph nodes, or crepitus. Vibratory tremors felt through the chest wall are known as **fremitus.** Fremitus can be vocal, when the client speaks, or tussive, during coughing. Vibrations are best perceived by the examiner when using the base of the fingers (metacarpophalangeal joints). The palmar aspect of the fingers is used to determine position, consistency, texture, size of structures, pain, and tenderness. The dorsal surface of the fingers is most sensitive to temperature. The ulnar surface of the hand including the finger is most sensitive to vibrations such as fremitus. Remember, the dominant hand is always more sensitive than the nondominant hand.

The fingertips are used in percussion and will be discussed later in this chapter.

Light Palpation

During palpation, the nurse should use light, moderate, or deep pressure depending on the depth of the structure being assessed and the thickness of the layers of tissue overlying the structure. One must always begin with light palpation. This is the safest, least uncomfortable method and allows the client to become accustomed to the nurse's touch. Light palpation is used to assess surface characteristics, such as skin texture, pulse, or a tender, inflamed area near the surface of the skin. For light palpation, the finger pads of the dominant hand are placed upon the surface of area to be examined. The hand is moved slowly and the finger pads, at a depth of 1 cm (0.39 in.), form circles on the skin during assessment as demonstrated in Figure 6.3 ●.

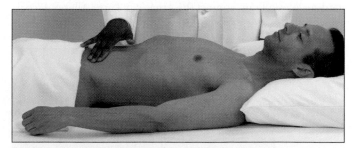

Figure 6.3 ● Light palpation.

Moderate Palpation

Moderate palpation is used to assess most of the other structures of the body. For moderate palpation, the nurse uses moderate pressure, places the palmar surface of the fingers of the dominant

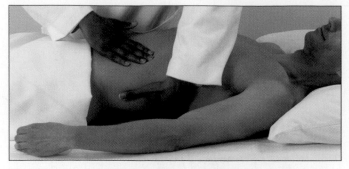

Figure 6.4 ● Moderate palpation.

hand over the structure to be assessed, and presses downward approximately 1 to 2 cm (0.25 to 0.5 in.), rotating the fingers in a circular motion. Now the nurse can determine the depth, size, shape, consistency, and mobility of organs, as well as any pain, tenderness, or pulsations that might be present (see Figure 6.4 ●).

Deep Palpation

Deep palpation is used to palpate an organ that lies deep within a body cavity such as the kidney or spleen, or when overlying musculature is thick, tense, or rigid such as in obesity or with abdominal guarding. The nurse should use more than moderate pressure by placing the palmar surface of the fingers of the dominant hand on the skin surface. The extended fingers of the nondominant hand are placed over the fingers of the dominant hand, pressing and guiding the fingers downward. This technique provides extra support and pressure and allows the nurse to palpate at a deeper level, from 2 to 4 cm (0.75 to 1.5 in.). All palpation must be used with caution; however, greatest caution must be used with deep palpation. Deep palpation can cause pain and disrupt underlying pathology (see Figure 6.5 ●).

Before beginning the technique of palpation, the nurse should explain to the client what is about to happen. It is difficult to feel underlying structures if the client is tense or frightened. Therefore, it is important to help the client relax and become comfortable before proceeding. To help prevent discomfort, the nurse should warm the hands; keep fingernails short, smooth, and trimmed; and not wear jewelry. Nonsterile gloves should be used if open skin areas or drainage were noted during inspection. Gloves may be latex or nonlatex materials. The nurse should ask clients if a known latex allergy exists. For more information regarding latex allergy, contact the American Latex Allergy Association at their Website through the Companion Website.

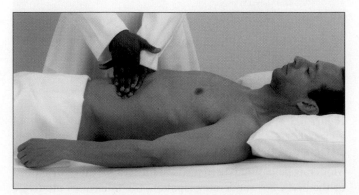

Figure 6.5 ● Deep palpation.

The nurse should proceed slowly, using smooth, deliberate movements, and avoid abrupt changes. Most clients will be more relaxed if the nurse talks to them during the examination, explaining each movement in advance. For example, during an abdominal assessment, the nurse might say, "I'm going to place my hand on your abdomen next. Tell me if you feel any discomfort and I will stop right away. How does it feel when I press down in this area?" It is a good idea to touch each area before palpating it. This touch informs the client that the examination of the area is about to begin and may prevent a startled reaction. Known painful areas of the body are usually the last area to be palpated.

Through palpation the nurse perceives data from the assessment and applies critical thinking. The nurse must be able to anticipate the findings regarding palpation of a body structure. Examples of critical thinking questions include: Should light, moderate, or deep pressure be used? If so, why? Are the findings consistent with normative parameters or are they unexpected findings? Does the client report any discomfort or pain during the process of palpation? Are the findings consistent with other diagnostic cues? What other information is needed to support this finding?

PERCUSSION

Percussion is the third technique used by the nurse to obtain data when performing physical assessment. **Percussion** comes from the Latin word *percutire*, meaning to strike through. Therefore, the nurse strikes through a body part with an object, fingers, or reflex hammer, ultimately producing a measurable sound. The striking or tapping of the body produces sound waves. As these waves travel toward underlying structures, they are heard as characteristic tones. The procedure is similar to a musician striking a drum, creating a vibration heard as a musical tone. Percussion is used to determine the size and shape of organs and masses, and whether underlying tissue is solid or filled with fluid or air.

Three methods of percussion can be used: direct percussion, blunt percussion, and indirect percussion. The part of the body to be percussed indicates the method to be used.

Direct Percussion

Direct percussion is the technique of tapping the body with the fingertips of the dominant hand. It is used to examine the thorax of an infant and to assess the sinuses of an adult as illustrated in Figure 6.6 ●.

Blunt Percussion

Blunt percussion involves placing the palm of the nondominant hand flat against the body surface and striking the nondominant hand with the dominant hand. A closed fist of the dominant hand is used to deliver the blow. This method is used for assessing pain and tenderness in the gallbladder, liver, and kidneys as shown in Figure 6.7 ●.

Indirect Percussion

Indirect percussion is the technique most commonly used because it produces sounds that are clearer and more easily interpreted. A hammer or tapping finger used to strike an

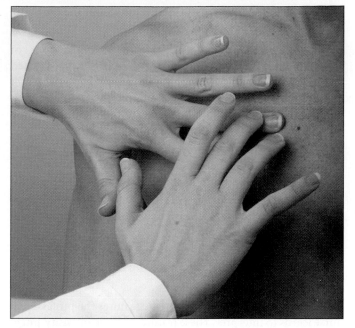

Figure 6.8 ● Indirect percussion.

object is called a **plexor,** derived from the Greek word *plexis.* **Pleximeter,** from the Greek word *metron,* meaning measure, refers to the device that accepts the tap or blow from a hammer (see Figure 6.8 ●).

To perform indirect percussion, the hyperextended middle finger of the nondominant hand is placed firmly over the area being examined. This finger is the pleximeter. It is important to keep the other fingers and the palm of this hand raised in order to avoid contact with the body surface. Pressure from the other fingers and palm on the adjacent surface muffles tones being produced. Using only wrist action of the dominant hand to generate motion, the nurse delivers two sharp blows with the plexor. The plexor is the fingertip of a flexed middle finger of the dominant hand. The plexor makes contact with the distal phalanx of the pleximeter and is immediately removed. When the plexor maintains contact with the distal phalanx, the sound waves are muffled. Enough force should be used to generate vibrations and ultimately a sound without causing injury to the client or self. Some helpful percussion hints are:

- Ensure that motion is from the wrist, not the forearm or plexor finger.
- Release the plexor finger immediately after the delivery of two sharp strikes.
- Ensure that only the pleximeter makes contact with the body.
- Use the tip of the plexor finger, **NOT** the finger pad, to deliver the blow.
- Use two strikes and then reposition the pleximeter. Delivery of more than two rapid consecutive strikes creates the "woodpecker syndrome" and sounds are muffled.

Sounds

Interpreting a percussion tone is an art that takes time and experience to develop. The amount of air in the underlying structure being percussed is responsible for the tone being produced. The more dense the tissue is, the softer and shorter the tone.

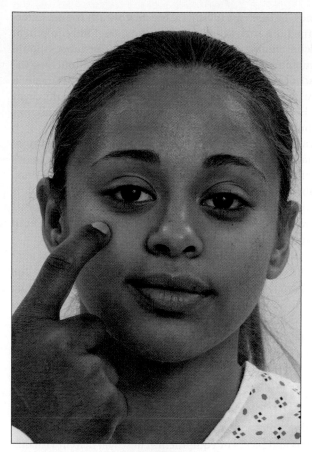

Figure 6.6 ● Direct percussion.

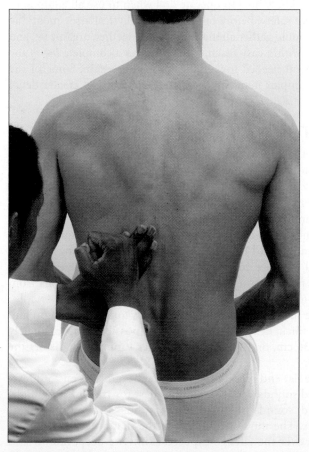

Figure 6.7 ● Blunt percussion.

The less dense the tissue is, the louder and longer the tone. The five percussion sounds are classified as follows:

1. **Tympany** is a loud, high-pitched, drumlike tone of medium duration characteristic of an organ that is filled with air. It is heard commonly over the gastric bubble in the stomach or over air-filled intestines.

2. **Resonance** is a loud, low-pitched, hollow tone of long duration. It is the normal finding over the lungs.

3. **Hyperresonance** is an abnormally loud, low tone of longer duration than resonance. It is heard when air is trapped in the lungs.

4. **Dullness** is a high-pitched tone that is soft and of short duration. It is usually heard over solid body organs such as the liver.

5. **Flatness** is a high-pitched tone, very soft, and of very short duration. It occurs over solid tissue such as muscle or bone.

Percussion sounds have characteristic features the professional nurse learns to interpret. These features include intensity, pitch, duration, and quality.

Intensity or *amplitude* of a sound refers to the softness or loudness of the sound. The louder the sound is, the greater the intensity or amplitude of the sound. This is influenced by the amount of air in the structure and the ability of the structure to vibrate.

Pitch or *frequency* of the sound refers to the number of vibrations of sound per second. Slow vibrations produce a low-pitched sound while a high-pitched sound comes from more rapid vibrations.

Duration refers to the length of time of the produced sound. This time frame ranges from very short to very long with variation in between.

Quality refers to the recognizable overtones produced by the vibration. This will be described as clear, hollow, muffled, or dull.

Like other assessment skills, the nurse perceives data from the assessment of the client and applies critical thinking. The nurse must be able to anticipate and identify the produced sound. Is this sound the expected sound? Is this sound considered to be within the normative range for this body part? Does the client report any discomfort or pain during percussion? Are the findings consistent with other diagnostic cues? What other information is needed to support this finding?

AUSCULTATION

Auscultation is the skill of listening to the sounds produced by the body. When auscultating, one uses both the unassisted sense of hearing and special instruments such as a stethoscope. Body sounds that can be heard with the ears alone include speech, coughing, respirations, and percussion tones. Many body sounds are extremely soft, and a stethoscope is needed to hear them. Stethoscopes work not by amplifying sounds but by blocking out other noises in the environment. Use of the stethoscope is described later in this chapter.

Auscultating body sounds requires a quiet environment in which the nurse can listen not just for the presence or absence of sounds, but also for the characteristics of each sound. External distractions such as radios, televisions, and loud equipment should be eliminated whenever possible. The nurse should avoid rubbing against client's clothes or drapes, or touching the stethoscope tubing since these actions produce sounds that will obscure the sounds of the body. It is important to keep the client warm, because shivering is uncomfortable and also obscures body sounds.

Sounds are described in terms of intensity, pitch, duration, and quality. For example, the nurse might note that a client's respirations are loud, high-pitched, long, and raspy. Many times the nurse will hear more than one sound at a time. It is important to focus on each sound and identify the characteristics of each sound. Closing the eyes and concentrating on each sound might help the nurse focus on the sound.

The nurse uses critical thinking with the technique of auscultation. The nurse must know the expected sound in the body region being auscultated. Is this sound considered to be within the normative range for this body region? Are unusual sounds heard? Are these findings consistent with other diagnostic cues? What other information is needed to support this finding?

EQUIPMENT

Throughout physical assessment the nurse will use various instruments and pieces of equipment. These will help in visualizing, hearing, and measuring data. It is the responsibility of the nurse to know how to operate and when to use all equipment for client safety. Before beginning the physical assessment, the nurse should gather all the equipment together, organize it, and place it within easy reach. Table 6.1 gives a complete list of the equipment needed for a typical screening exam. Some of the more complex items on the list are discussed in greater detail below or in later chapters.

STETHOSCOPE

The stethoscope is used to auscultate body sounds such as blood pressure, heart sounds, respirations, and bowel sounds. The stethoscope has three parts: the binaurals (earpieces), the flexible tubing, and the end piece. The end piece contains the diaphragm and the bell (see Figure 6.9 ●). To be effective in blocking out environmental noise, the stethoscope must fit. The binaurals should fit snugly but comfortably, sloping forward, toward the nose, to match the natural slope of the ear canals. (Most manufacturers supply several different binaurals from which to choose.)

The tubing that joins the binaurals to the diaphragm and bell is thick, flexible, and as short as possible (approximately 30 to 36 cm, or 12 to 18 in.). Longer tubing may distort the sound.

The flat end piece, called the diaphragm, screens out low-pitched sounds and, therefore, is best for transmitting high-pitched sounds such as lung sounds and normal heart sounds. The nurse should place the diaphragm evenly and firmly over the client's exposed skin. The deep, hollow end

| Table 6.1 | Equipment Used During the Physical Assessment |

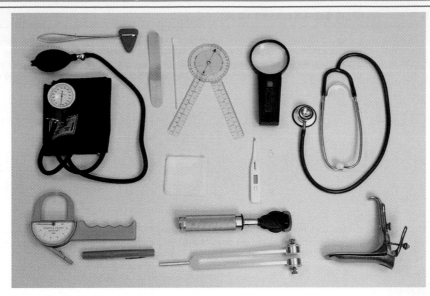

EQUIPMENT	USE
Cotton balls or wisps	Test the sense of touch
Cotton-tipped applicators	Obtain specimens
Culture media	Obtain cultures of body fluids and drainage
Dental mirror	Visualize mouth and throat structures
Doppler ultrasonic stethoscope	Obtain readings of blood pressure, pulse, and fetal heart rate
Flashlight	Provide a direct source of light to view parts of the body
Gauze squares	Obtain specimens; collect drainage
Gloves	Protect the nurse and client from contamination
Goggles	Protect the nurse's eyes from contamination by body fluids
Lubricant	Provide lubrication for vaginal or rectal examinations
Nasal speculum	Dilate nares for inspection of the nose
Ophthalmoscope	Inspect the interior structures of the eye
Otoscope	Inspect the tympanic membrane and external ear canal
Penlight	Provide a direct light source and test pupillary reaction
Reflex hammer	Test deep tendon reflexes
Ruler, marked in centimeters	Measure organs, masses, growths, and lesions
Skin-marking pen	Outline masses or enlarged organs
Slides	Make smears of body fluids or drainage
Specimen containers	Collect specimens of body fluids, drainage, or tissue
Sphygmomanometer	Measure systolic and diastolic blood pressure
Sterile safety pin	Test for sensory stimulation
Stethoscope	Auscultate body sounds
Tape measure, flexible, marked in centimeters	Measure the circumference of the head, abdomen, and extremities
Test tubes	Collect specimens
Thermometer	Measure body temperature
Tongue blade	Depress tongue during assessment of the mouth and throat
Tuning fork	Test auditory function and vibratory sensation
Vaginal speculum	Dilate the vaginal canal for inspection of the cervix
Vision chart	Test near and far vision
Watch with second hand	Time heart rates, fetal pulse, or bowel sounds when counting

(continued)

Table 6.1   Equipment Used During the Physical Assessment *(continued)*

SPECIAL EQUIPMENT	USE/DESCRIPTION
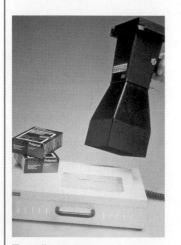 Goniometer	Measures the degree of joint flexion and extension. Consists of two straight arms of clear plastic usually marked in both inches and centimeters. The arms intersect and can be angled and rotated around a protractor marked with degrees. The nurse places the center of the protractor over a joint and aligns the straight arms with the extremity. The degree of flexion or extension is indicated on the protractor.
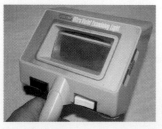 Skinfold calipers	Measures the thickness of subcutaneous tissue. The nurse grasps a fold of skin, usually on the upper arm, waist, or thigh, keeping the sides of the skin parallel. The edges of the caliper are placed at the base of the fold and the calipers tightened until they grasp the fold without compressing it.
Transilluminator	Detects blood, fluid, or masses in body cavities. Instruments manufactured for transillumination are available, or a flashlight with a rubber adapter may be used. In either case, the light beam produced is strong but narrow. When directed through a body cavity, the beam produces a red glow that reveals the presence of air or fluid.
Wood's lamp	Detects fungal infections of the skin. The Wood's lamp produces a black light, which the nurse shines on the skin in a darkened room. If a fungal infection is present, a characteristic yellow-green fluorescence appears on the skin surface.

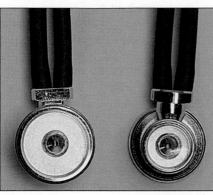

A

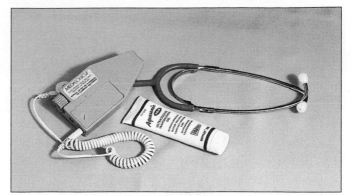

Figure 6.11 ● Doppler ultrasonic stethoscope.

Figure 6.9 ● A, stethoscope with both a bell-shaped and flat-disc amplifier. B. Close-up of a flat-disc amplifier (left) and a bell amplifier (right).

clude an assortment of interchangeable diaphragms and bells in different sizes for different purposes; for example, smaller diaphragm pieces are used for examining children.

DOPPLER ULTRASONIC STETHOSCOPE

A Doppler ultrasonic stethoscope uses ultrasonic waves to detect sounds that are difficult to hear with a regular stethoscope, such as fetal heart sounds and peripheral pulses (see Figure 6.11 ●). It operates on a principle discovered in the 19th century by Johannes Doppler, the Austrian physicist who found that the pitch of a sound varies in relation to the distance between the source and the listener. To the listener, the pitch sounds higher when the distance from the source is small, and lower when the distance from the source is great.

The way to eliminate interference is to apply a small amount of gel to the end of the Doppler probe (the transducer), which may resemble a wand or a disk. When using the Doppler ultrasonic stethoscope to assess the pulse, the nurse turns it on and places the probe gently against the client's skin over the artery to be auscultated. It is important to avoid heavy pressure, because it may impede blood flow. The probe sends a low-energy, high-pitched sound wave toward the underlying blood vessel. As the blood ebbs and flows, the probe picks up and amplifies the subtle changes in pitch, and the nurse will hear a pulsing beat.

piece, called the bell, detects low-frequency sounds such as heart murmurs. It is placed lightly against the client's skin so that it forms a seal but does not flatten to a diaphragm. Either end piece may be held against the client's skin between the index and middle fingers of the examiner (see Figure 6.10 ●). Friction on the diaphragm or bell from coarse body hair may cause a crackling sound easily confused with abnormal breath sounds. This problem can be avoided by wetting the hair before auscultating the area. Stethoscopes usually in-

OPHTHALMOSCOPE

An ophthalmoscope is used to inspect internal eye structures. Its main components are the handle, which holds the battery, and the head, which houses the aperture selector, viewing aperture, lens selector disk, lens indicator, lenses of varying powers of magnification, and mirrors (see Figure 6.12 ●).

The light source shines light through the viewing aperture, which is adjusted to select one of five apertures (see Figure 6.13 ●).

1. The large aperture is used most often. It emits a large, full spot for viewing dilated pupils.
2. The small aperture is used for undilated pupils.

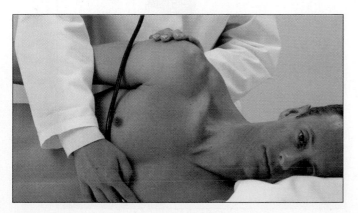

Figure 6.10 ● Nurse using a stethoscope.

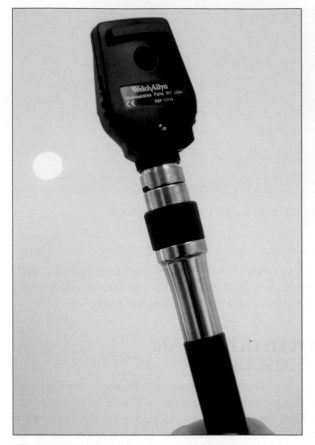

Figure 6.12 ● Ophthalmoscope demonstrating aperture.

3. The red-free filter shines a green beam used to examine the optic disc for pallor or hemorrhaging, which appears black with this filter.
4. The grid allows the examiner to assess the size, location, and pattern of any lesions.
5. The slit allows for examination of the anterior eye and aids in assessing the elevation or depression of lesions.

The lens selector dial must be rotated to bring the inner eye structures into focus. While looking through the viewing aperture, one rotates the lens selection dial to adjust the convergence or divergence of the light. At the zero setting, the lens

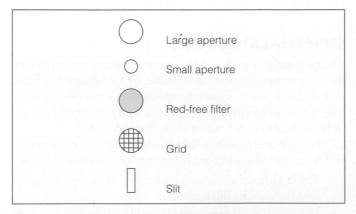

Large aperture

Small aperture

Red-free filter

Grid

Slit

Figure 6.13 ● Apertures of ophthalmoscope.

neither converges nor diverges the light. The lens dial is moved clockwise to access the numbers in black, which range from +1 to +40. These lenses improve visualization in a client who is farsighted. The lens dial is moved counterclockwise to access the red numbers, which range from −1 to −20. These lenses improve visualization if the client is nearsighted. See Chapter 13 for a more detailed discussion of assessment of the eye. ○○

OTOSCOPE

The otoscope is used to inspect external ear structures. The main components of the otoscope are the handle, which is similar to that of the ophthalmoscope, the light, the lens, and specula of various sizes (see Figure 6.14 ●). The specula are used to narrow the beam of light. The nurse should select the largest one that will fit into the client's ear canal. If a nasal speculum is not available, the otoscope can be used to inspect the nose. In this case, the nurse should use the shortest, broadest speculum and insert it gently into the client's naris. See Chapter 14 for a more detailed discussion of assessment of the ears and nose. ○○

Special equipment is required for assessment of several body systems. For example, the reflex hammer is used in the neurologic assessment and the vaginal speculum in assessment of the female reproductive system. Each chapter in Unit III of this text provides a discussion of specialized equipment and uses in physical assessment of a particular system. ○○

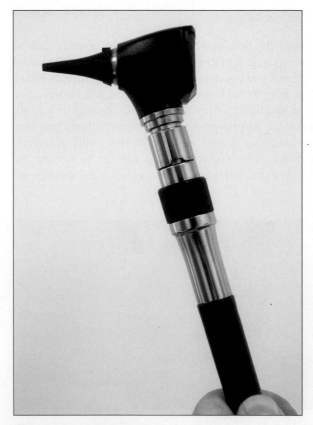

Figure 6.14 ● Otoscope.

PROFESSIONAL RESPONSIBILITIES

Throughout all aspects of the assessment process, the nurse must apply critical thinking while providing a safe and comfortable environment for the client. The nurse must identify cues presented by the client and apply critical thinking to determine the relevance of this data. The safe external environment created by the nurse includes comfort, warmth, privacy, and the use of Standard Precautions.

CUES

In addition to developing the skills of inspection, palpation, percussion, and auscultation, the nurse must be able to recognize the relative significance of the many visual, palpable, or auditory cues that may be present during an assessment. **Cues** are bits of information that hint at the possibility of a health problem. In other words, the nurse needs to know what to look for. To become skilled at cue recognition, nurses should cultivate their senses until they readily perceive even slight cues. For example, some things that are noticed during an initial survey or inspection of the client may hint at an underlying health problem. Swelling (edema) of the legs provides a cue to assess for heart problems. Bruising (ecchymosis) of the skin is a cue to ask the client about recent falls, trauma, injury, anticoagulant medication, or a bleeding problem. Grimacing, guarding (protective posture), or wincing when a client moves or a body part is moved during assessment are cues to examine for underlying joint and muscle problems or masses. Cues that suggest hearing loss include not following directions, looking at the examiner's lips during conversation, or speaking in a loud voice. Asymmetry of facial expression is a cue to assess function of the cranial nerves. Odors are cues to suggest a problem with hygiene or drainage from an orifice or wound. Cue recognition develops with practice, but beginners can acquire the skill by observing an experienced nurse, by practicing on partners, by studying the visual aids in this text, and by using the many videos, animations, skills, and clinical simulations available on the Companion Website of this book.

CRITICAL THINKING

Throughout the assessment process, the nurse gathers subjective and objective data. Recall that subjective data is reported by the client during the interviews, and the objective data comes from the physical assessment and the application of the four techniques of inspection, palpation, percussion, and auscultation. These data form the database reflecting the health status of the client. During this process the presented cues must be interpreted.

The interpretation of cues and other collected data utilizes the process of critical thinking. Being organized when collecting data, the nurse looks for inconsistencies and checks to be sure the data is accurate. The data is compared to normative values and ranges. Data is clustered and patterns are identified. Missing information is identified and, after the database is completed, valid conclusions are drawn. At this time priorities are established, outcomes and a plan are developed, and evaluation then follows.

Once cues are recognized and data is collected, the nurse must be able to interpret the findings. Is a particular finding normal, or does it indicate an alteration in the client's health? Normal data are assessment findings that fall within an accepted standard range for a specific type of data. For example, the normal range for the adult pulse rate is 60 to 100 beats per minute. A pulse of 76 is therefore considered normal. Some healthy individuals exhibit characteristics that are outside the standard range for a specific type of data. Such findings are considered variations from the norm. For example, a long-distance runner with a pulse of 48 resulting from regular cardiovascular conditioning exhibits a variation from the norm for pulse rate. Findings that are outside the range for a specific type of data and that may indicate a threat to the client's health are considered unexpected findings or deviations from the norm. For example, an irregular, thready pulse rate of 120 is an unexpected finding that could indicate the presence of a harmful condition. It is important to note that not all unexpected findings indicate the presence of a disease or disorder. For example, fatigue in a 20-year-old student may indicate anemia or infection, or it may be caused simply by a lack of sleep.

PROVIDING A SAFE AND COMFORTABLE ENVIRONMENT

The physical assessment may be performed in a variety of settings, including a clinic, a hospital room, a school nurse's office, a corporate health services office, or a client's home. No matter where the location, the nurse is responsible for preparing a setting that is conducive to the client's comfort and privacy. The examination room should be warm, private, and free from distractions and interruptions. Overhead lighting must ensure good visibility and be free of distortion. A portable lamp to highlight body surfaces and contours may be needed.

The client should be positioned on a sturdy examination table with a firm surface that is covered with a clean sheet or paper cover. Though not as efficient, a firm bed will suffice if an examination table is not available. The table must be placed to allow the nurse easy access to both sides of the client's body. The table's height should allow the nurse to perform the examination without stooping. The nurse should also have a stool to sit on during certain parts of the examination and a small table or stand to hold the examination equipment.

The examination should be individualized according to the client's personal values and beliefs. Some clients, for example, may request that a family member be present during the examination. Some may ask for a nurse of the same sex. Some female clients may object to breast and vaginal examinations, regardless of the gender of the examiner, and some male clients may refuse penile, scrotal, and rectal examinations. A thorough assessment of the client's culture, religious beliefs, and environment, as described in previous chapters, may help the nurse to anticipate these needs. Although explaining the reason for a certain procedure may help the client understand its benefit, a nurse must never attempt to influence or coerce the client to agree to any procedure. In all cases, the nurse must document which procedures took place and any that were refused.

Many clients experience anxiety before and during a physical examination. These feelings may stem from fear of pain, embarrassment at being looked at and touched by a stranger, or worry about the outcome of the examination. The nurse can alleviate the client's anxiety by approaching the examination gradually, first by communicating with the client, then by performing simple measurements such as height, weight, temperature, and pulse, which most clients find familiar and nonthreatening. As these measurements are taken, the client will have the opportunity to ask additional questions and to become accustomed to the nurse's presence.

In most cases, clients should urinate before the examination. Voiding helps clients feel more comfortable and relaxed and facilitates palpation of the abdomen and pubic area. If urinalysis is to be done, the client should be instructed in obtaining a clean-catch specimen and given a container for the urine sample.

After ensuring that the examination room is warm, the nurse shows the client how to put on the examination gown and leaves the client to undress in privacy. It may be helpful to assure the client that it is all right to leave underpants on until just before the genital examination. Before reentering the examination room, the nurse should knock to alert the client.

Drapes are used to preserve the client's privacy and to provide warmth. When invasive procedures such as vaginal or rectal examinations are performed, drapes provide an aseptic field. When used properly, a drape exposes only the part of the body being examined and covers the surrounding area. Drapes are available in a variety of shapes and materials from simple rectangular sheets made of linen, to disposable drapes made of paper lined with waterproof plastic (see Chapter 22 ⚭).

The physical examination may be an exhausting experience for a client who is elderly, debilitated, frail, or suffering from a chronic illness, since the nurse must examine every part of the body, and the client must make frequent changes in position. Consequently, the nurse should consider the client's age, health status, level of functioning, and severity of illness at all times and adapt the examination accordingly. In addition, the nurse can conserve the client's energy by moving around the client during the examination, rather than asking the client to move, and by carrying out the examination as quickly and efficiently as possible. The techniques and approaches for physical assessment vary for children, pregnant females, and older adults. Special considerations for assessment of these groups are included in each assessment chapter in Unit III. ⚭ Further, Chapters 25 through 27 provide in-depth information about assessment of infants, children, adolescents, pregnant females, and older adults. ⚭

Before beginning the physical examination, the nurse should wash his or her hands in the presence of the client. Hand washing not only protects the nurse and the client, but also signals that the nurse is providing for the client's safety. Nonsterile exam gloves should be available and used appropriately during the examination. The bell and diaphragm of the stethoscope should be cleaned after the assessment of each client to prevent the spread of infection.

Some situations that arise during a physical examination pose a potential hazard for the client. For example, a client might become light-headed and dizzy from taking deep breaths during a respiratory assessment, or fall when asked to touch the toes during a musculoskeletal assessment. A client who is frail, weak, debilitated, or suffering from a chronic illness is at greatest risk. Throughout the procedure, it is necessary to anticipate potential hazards and modify the examination to prevent them. In addition, some examination techniques may injure the client if used indiscriminately. For example, vigorous, deep palpation of a throbbing mass might lead to a ruptured abdominal aneurysm.

Before beginning the examination, the nurse should thoroughly explain to the client what is to follow and encourage the client to ask questions. If the client does not speak the nurse's language, it is important to secure the assistance of a translator. If the client's hearing is impaired, the nurse must find someone who knows sign language.

During the examination, the nurse should explain each step in advance so that the client can anticipate the nurse's movements. Clients are more relaxed and cooperative during the procedure when they understand what is about to happen. This is also an opportunity to provide client teaching. For example, while inspecting the client's skin, the nurse may want to discuss the long-term effects of sun exposure. Sharing information with clients during the examination may alleviate their anxiety, enhance their understanding, and give them a sense of partnership in their healthcare.

At times, the nurse may note an unexpected finding and want to call in another examiner to check the finding. In such instances, it is best simply to inform the client that another examiner is being asked to check the assessment. Because the finding may be normal, it is best to avoid alarming the client.

In many healthcare institutions, the client is asked to sign a consent form for the physical examination, especially if invasive procedures such as a vaginal or rectal examination or blood studies are to be performed. It is the nurse's responsibility to ensure that the client understands the procedures to be performed and that all necessary consent forms are signed.

STANDARD PRECAUTIONS

Throughout the physical assessment, the professional nurse is required to apply the principles of asepsis. The Centers for Disease Control and Prevention (CDC) and the Occupational Safety and Health Administration (OSHA) have provided guidelines to protect the client and healthcare workers. Hand washing, use of gloves, use of protective barriers, disposal of sharps, handling of specimens, and proper disposal of body wastes are included in the guidelines. Each healthcare agency has created agency policies based on these guidelines. A nurse working at an agency is responsible for knowing the policies and following the guidelines. Refer to Appendix B to review Standard Precautions or link to the CDC through the Companion Website.

Application Through Critical Thinking

CASE STUDY

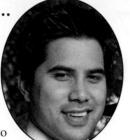

*A*s part of a comprehensive health assessment course, Jose Espero, a student nurse, must conduct a physical assessment of a child between the ages of 2 and 5 years and an adult over the age of 65. Jose contacts the parents of a 3-year-old African American female for consent to carry out the assessment. The parents have asked Jose to meet with them and explain in detail what he will be doing prior to giving consent.

In addition a 73-year-old Asian male residing in an assisted living facility has consented to the physical assessment.

► *Critical Thinking Questions*

1. What should be included in the explanation of the assessment procedures to the parents and the older adult?
2. What factors will influence application of physical assessment techniques for each of the clients?
3. Identify the equipment Jose must prepare for the physical assessment.
4. What safety and comfort issues must be addressed when conducting the assessment for the child and the adult?

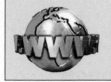

Please refer to the Companion Website at www.prenhall.com/damico and click on Chapter 6, the Application Through Critical Thinking module, to answer these and additional questions. In addition, complete NCLEX-RN® review questions and other interactive resources for this chapter.

EXPLORE MediaLink

Additional resources for this chapter are found on the Student CD-ROM accompanying this textbook and on the Companion Website.

CD-ROM CONTENT

Content for this chapter includes:
Objectives
Key Concepts
NCLEX-RN® Review Questions
Model Documentation Forms
Audio Glossary
Games and Challenges
Head-to-Toe Physical Examination Video

COMPANION WEBSITE CONTENT

www.prenhall.com/damico

Content for this chapter includes:
Objectives
NCLEX-RN® Review Questions

Application Through Critical Thinking
   Case Study Challenge
MediaLinks
MediaLink Application
Tool Box
   Equipment Used During the Physical Assessment
New York Times

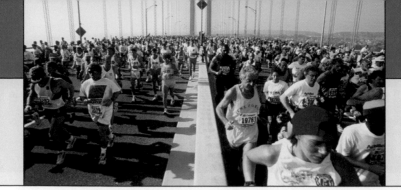

7
General Survey

CHAPTER OBJECTIVES

Upon completion of this chapter, you will be able to:

1. Describe the general survey as part of a comprehensive health assessment.
2. Identify the components of the general survey.
3. Measure vital signs.
4. Discuss the factors that affect vital signs.
5. Apply critical thinking during the initial nurse-client encounter.

MEDIALINK

www.prenhall.com/damico

The CD-ROM in the back of this textbook and the Media-Link website contain NCLEX-RN® review questions, interactive exercises, case study challenges, animations, videos, documentation and checklist forms, and review materials. For a complete listing of the media content specific to Chapter 7, see the Explore MediaLink at the end of the chapter.

CHAPTER OUTLINE

APPLICATION THROUGH CRITICAL THINKING,

$\mathcal{T}$ he **general survey** begins during the interview phase of a comprehensive health assessment (see Figure 7.1 ●). While collecting subjective data, the nurse observes the client while developing initial impressions about the individual's health and formulating strategies for the physical assessment. The observation includes what is seen, heard, or smelled during the initial phase of assessment. Clues that are uncovered during the general survey will guide the nurse during later assessment of body regions and systems. These clues will help to determine the client's ability to participate in all aspects of the assessment process. For example, the client having pain will need to have pain relief. The client having trouble breathing, dyspnea, will need assistance before proceeding. Remember, pain and dyspnea are two of the many factors that will influence the client's ability to participate in the assessment. These concepts are discussed in detail in Chapters 8 and 15 of this text. ⚭ Upon completion of the general survey, the professional nurse will assess height, weight, and vital signs. Information about each of these important phases of comprehensive health assessment is discussed in the sections to follow. The data obtained in the general survey forms a guide for all physical assessment.

KEY TERMS

diastolic pressure, 116
functional assessment, 120
general survey, 109
hyperthermia, 113
hypothermia, 113
oxygen saturation, 116
pain, 119
pain rating scales, 119
pulse, 114
respiratory rate, 116
sphygmomanometer, 117
systolic pressure, 116
temperature, 113
vital signs, 113

COMPONENTS OF THE GENERAL SURVEY

The general survey is composed of four major categories of observation: physical appearance, mental status, mobility, and behavior of the client. Specific observations are required in the general survey. The following sections identify these required observations. During the general survey the professional nurse will determine if the observed behaviors fall within an expected range for the gender, age, genetic background, and culture of the client. The nurse must also determine the ability of the client to participate in all aspects of the process before proceeding.

PHYSICAL APPEARANCE

The client's physical appearance provides immediate and important cues to the level of individual wellness. Thus, beginning with the initial meeting, the nurse notes any factors about the client's physical appearance that are in any way unexpected. For example, the nurse might note that a client appears undernourished, seems older than his or her stated age, has a frown, is smiling, or has skin color that is pale, flushed, ruddy, or cyanotic.

Body shape and build may indicate the client's general level of wellness. The body should be symmetrical and the proportions regular: The client's arm span should approximate the height, and the distance from the pubis to the crown of the head should roughly equal the distance from the pubis to the sole of the foot. The client's height and weight should be within normal ranges for age and body build. Extreme thinness or obesity may indicate an eating disorder. The nurse must consider the client's lifestyle, socioeconomic level, and environment.

MENTAL STATUS

The nurse assesses the client's mental status while the client is responding to questions and giving information about health history. The nurse notes the client's affect and mood, level of anxiety, orientation, and speech. Findings in these areas may be evaluated further during the assessment of the client's psychosocial status and neurologic system.

The nurse assesses clients for orientation to person, place, and time. Clients should typically be able to state their name, location, the date, month, season, and time of day. In most cases, the nurse will be able to sense a client's orientation during the initial interview. If the client appears confused, the nurse should ask him or her to respond to the following: "Tell me your name." "Where you are now?" "What is today's date?" and "What time is it?" If the client cannot respond or responds incorrectly, a more detailed assessment of mental status must be performed. See Chapter 25 for details on how to perform this assessment in children. ⚭

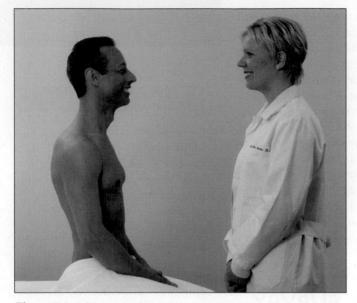

Figure 7.1 • The nurse begins the general survey.

MOBILITY

The nurse observes the client's gait, posture, and range of motion (the complete movement possible for a joint). Normally, the client walks in a rhythmic, straight, upright position with arms swinging at each side of the body. The shoulders are level and straight. Difficulty with gait and posture, such as stumbling, shuffling, limping, or the inability to stand erect, calls for further evaluation. Range of motion should be fluid and appropriate to the age of the client. The nurse will observe deviations from the normal that include weakness, stiffness, or involuntary motor activity. See Chapter 23 for information on assessing the musculoskeletal system and range of motion. ∞

BEHAVIOR OF THE CLIENT

An assessment of the client's behavior includes information about the following factors: dress and grooming, body odors, facial expression, mood and affect, ability to make eye contact, and level of anxiety. The way in which clients dress may provide clues to their sense of self-esteem and body image. However, the nurse must consider many factors before drawing conclusions based on a client's appearance. For example, a client who wears clothing that is inappropriate for the situation or weather may be blind, mentally ill, experiencing situational grief or anxiety, or mentally fit but unable to buy other clothes due to financial constraints.

The nurse observes the client for cleanliness and personal hygiene. The client who is dirty or has a strong body odor or poor dental hygiene may be depressed, have poor self-concept, or lack knowledge about personal hygiene practices. However, one must consider the client's environment before drawing conclusions. For example, a client who is dirty may have just come from working on a construction site.

The nurse assesses the client's emotional state by noting what the client says, the client's body language, facial expression, and the appropriateness of the client's behavior in relation to the situation and circumstances. The client should exhibit comfort in talking with the examiner. Giggling when answering questions about bowel movements may simply indicate embarrassment, whereas giggling when describing the death of a loved one may be an example of inappropriate affect.

The nurse also assesses the client for apprehension, fear, and nervousness. Like affect and mood, the client's level of anxiety is revealed through speech, body language, and facial expression. During the health assessment, the client may exhibit anxiety due to embarrassment, fear of pain, or worry about the outcome of the examination. If the client's anxiety seems to have no cause, the client must be evaluated further. To obtain a relative impression of the level of anxiety, clients may be asked to rate their feelings of anxiety on a scale of 0 to 10. The nurse uses the client's response as an indicator of the need for further assessment and as a baseline for future assessment of anxiety levels.

The nurse assesses the client's speech for quantity, volume, content, articulation, and rhythm. The client should speak easily and fluently to the nurse or to an interpreter. Disorganized speech patterns, silence, or constant talking may indicate normal nervousness or shyness, or may signal a speech defect, neurologic deficit, depression, or another disorder.

AGE-RELATED CONSIDERATIONS

It is important to consider the developmental stage of the child or adolescent when assessing for each of the previous factors. The appearance of the younger child reveals a great deal of information about the child's parents or caretakers, and the appearance of an older child gives clues about self-care. For instance, a child 3 years of age whose skin and clothes are dirty may be a victim of neglect, while a 13-year-old in the same condition may lack knowledge about proper hygiene.

The nurse should note the child's interaction with the parents or caretakers. Their relationship should exhibit mutual warmth and caring. Signs of child abuse include clinging to a parent or strong attachment to a parent because of fear of parental anger; absence of separation anxiety in a child who, because of developmental stage, would ordinarily demonstrate it; avoidance of eye contact between caretaker and child; a caretaker's demonstration of disgust with a child's behavior, illness, odor, or stool; flinching when people move toward the child; and regression to infantile behavior.

The dress, grooming, and personal hygiene of an older adult may be affected by limitations in mobility from arthritis, cardiovascular disease, and other disorders, or by a lack of funds.

The gait of an older adult is often slower and the steps shorter. To maintain balance, older adults may hold their arms away from the body or use a cane. The posture of an older adult may look slightly stooped because of a generalized flexion, which also causes the older adult to appear shorter. A loss in height may also be due to thinning or compression of the intervertebral disks.

The behavior of the older adult may be affected by various disorders common to this age group, such as vascular insufficiency and diabetes. In addition, medications may affect the client's behavior. Some medications may cause the client to feel anxious, and others may affect the client's alertness, orientation, or speech. Older adults are likely to have one or more chronic conditions associated with age, such as arthritis, hypertension, or diabetes. As a result, older adults must consume several prescription medications. Overmedication may occur because older adults seek care from multiple healthcare providers without collaboration regarding treatment. Multiple medications may combine to produce dangerous side effects. Additionally, the schedules for multiple medications may be confusing and result in overmedication, forgotten doses, negative side effects, or ineffectiveness of medication. Therefore, the nurse must conduct a thorough assessment of the client's medication schedule and history.

MEASURING HEIGHT AND WEIGHT

The nurse measures the client's height and weight to establish baseline data and to help determine health status. The client should be asked about height and weight before taking any measurements. Large discrepancies between the stated height and weight and the actual measurements may provide clues to the client's self-image. Alternatively, discrepancies in weight may indicate the client's lack of awareness of a sudden loss or gain in weight that may be due to illness.

HEIGHT

The nurse uses a measuring stick attached to a platform scale or to a wall to measure height. The client should look straight ahead while standing as straight as possible with heels together and shoulders back. When using a platform scale, the nurse raises the height attachment rod above the client's head, then extends and lowers the right-angled arm until it rests on the crown of the head. The measurement is read from the height attachment rod (see Figure 7.2 ●). When using a measuring stick, the nurse should place an L-shaped level on the crown of the client's head at a right angle to the measuring stick (see Figure 7.3 ●).

WEIGHT

A standard platform scale (see Figure 7.4 ●) is used to measure the weight of older children and adults. It is best to use the same scale at each visit and weigh the client at the same time of day in the same kind of clothing (e.g., the examination gown) and without shoes. If using a digital scale, the nurse simply reads the weight from the lighted display panel. Otherwise, the scale is calibrated by moving both weights to 0 and turning the knob until the balance beam is level. The nurse moves the large and small weights to the right and takes the reading when the balance beam returns to level. Special bed and chair scales are available for clients who cannot stand.

Average height and weight for adult men and women are available in charts prepared by governmental agencies and insurers. Table 7.1 illustrates average acceptable weights for adults. The body mass index (BMI) is considered a more reliable indicator of healthy weight. The BMI and other measures in relation to weight are discussed in Chapter 9 of this text. ∞

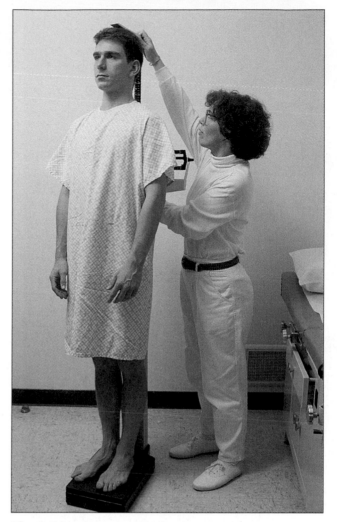

Figure 7.2 ● Measuring the client's height with a platform scale.

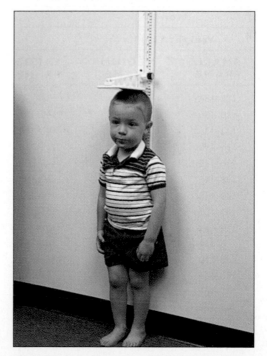

Figure 7.3 ● Measuring a child's height with a measuring stick.

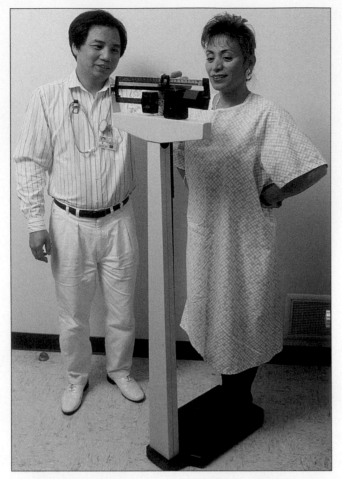

Figure 7.4 • Measuring the client's weight with a standard platform scale.

AGE-RELATED CONSIDERATIONS

To measure an infant's length, the nurse places the child in a supine position on an examining table that is equipped with a ruler, headboard, and adjustable footboard. The nurse positions the head against the headboard, extends the infant's leg nearest the ruler, and adjusts the footboard until it touches the infant's foot. The space between the headboard and footboard represents the length of the infant. Alternatively, the nurse places the infant on a standard examination table, extends the infant's leg, marks the paper covering at the infant's head and foot, and measures the distance between the markings (see Figure 7.5 •).

Infants are weighed on a modified platform scale with curved sides to prevent injury. The scale measures weight in grams and in ounces. The nurse places the unclothed baby on the scale on a paper drape and watches the baby to prevent a fall (see Figure 7.6 •). Measurements are taken to the nearest 10 g (0.5 oz).

Children over the age of 2 or 3 years may be weighed on the upright scale or seated on the infant scale. The child's underpants should be left on. To measure height, the nurse uses the platform scale or a measuring stick attached to the wall, as for an adult. By the age of 4, most children enjoy being weighed and measured and finding out how much they have grown. Growth and development are discussed in Chapter 3 of this text. ⚭

The height of older adults may decline somewhat as a result of thinning or compression of the intervertebral disks and a general flexion of the hips and knees. Body weight may decrease because of muscle shrinkage. The older client may appear thinner, even when properly nourished, because of loss of subcutaneous fat deposits from the face, forearms, and lower legs. At the same time, fat deposits on the abdomen and hips may increase.

| Table **7.1** | 1999 Metropolitan Height and Weight Tables, Men and Women, Ages 25 to 59 |

Men				Women			
	Weight (lb)*				Weight (lb)*		
HEIGHT	SMALL FRAME	MEDIUM FRAME	LARGE FRAME	HEIGHT	SMALL FRAME	MEDIUM FRAME	LARGE FRAME
5'2"	128–134	131–141	138–150	4'10"	102–111	109–121	118–131
5'3"	130–136	133–143	140–153	4'11"	103–113	111–123	120–134
5'4"	132–138	135–145	142–156	5'0"	104–115	113–126	122–137
5'5"	134–140	137–148	144–160	5'1"	106–118	115–129	125–140
5'6"	136–142	139–151	146–164	5'2"	108–121	118–132	128–143
5'7"	138–145	142–154	149–168	5'3"	111–124	121–135	131–147
5'8"	140–148	145–157	152–172	5'4"	114–127	124–138	134–151
5'9"	142–151	148–160	155–176	5'5"	117–130	127–141	137–155
5'10"	144–154	151–163	158–180	5'6"	120–133	130–144	140–159
5'11"	146–157	154–166	161–184	5'7"	123–136	133–147	143–163
6'0"	149–160	157–170	164–188	5'8"	126–139	136–150	146–167
6'1"	152–164	160–174	168–192	5'9"	129–142	139–153	149–170
6'2"	155–168	164–178	172–197	5'10"	132–145	142–156	152–173
6'3"	158–172	167–182	176–202	5'11"	135–148	145–159	155–176
6'4"	162–176	171–187	181–207	6'0"	138–151	148–162	158–179

*Weight in pounds. Men; allow 5 lb of clothing. Women: allow 3 lb of clothing.

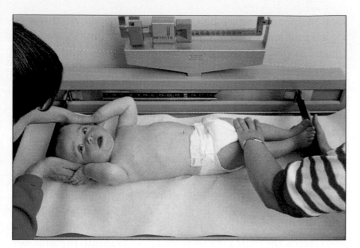

Figure 7.5 ● Measuring an infant's length.

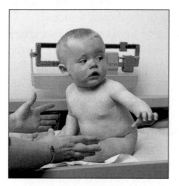

Figure 7.6 ● Weighing an infant.

MEASURING VITAL SIGNS

Vital signs include body **temperature, pulse, respiratory rate, blood pressure,** and **pain.** Measurement of oxygen saturation may be included when taking vital signs. The nurse measures vital signs to obtain baseline data, to detect or monitor a change in the client's health status, and to monitor clients at risk for alterations in health.

MEASURING BODY TEMPERATURE

The body's surface temperature—the temperature of the skin, subcutaneous tissues, and fat—fluctuates in response to environmental factors and is therefore unreliable for monitoring a client's health status. Instead, the nurse should measure the client's core temperature, or the **temperature** of the deep tissues of the body (e.g., the thorax and abdominal cavity). This temperature remains relatively constant at about 37°C, or 98.6°F.

Sensors in the hypothalamus regulate the body's core temperature. When these hypothalamic sensors detect heat, they signal the body to decrease heat production and increase heat loss (e.g., by vasodilation and sweating). When sensors in the hypothalamus detect cold, they signal the body to increase heat production and decrease heat loss (e.g., by shivering, vasoconstriction, and inhibition of sweating).

Factors That Influence Body Temperature

A variety of factors may influence normal core body temperature. These include:

- **Age.** The core temperature of infants is highly responsive to changes in the external environment; therefore, infants need extra protection from even mild variations in temperature. The core body temperature of children is more stable than that of infants but less so than that of adolescents or adults. However, older adults are more sensitive than middle adults to variations in external environmental temperature. This increased sensitivity may be due to the decreased thermoregulatory control and loss of subcutaneous fat common in older adults, or it may be due to environmental factors such as lack of activity, inadequate diet, or lack of central heating.

- **Diurnal variations.** Core body temperature is usually highest between 8:00 p.m. and midnight, and lowest between 4:00 and 6:00 a.m. Normal body temperature may vary by as much as 1.0°C or 1.8°F between these times. Some individuals have more than one complete cycle in a day.

- **Exercise.** Strenuous exercise can increase core body temperature by as much as 2°C or 5°F.

- **Hormones.** A variety of hormones affect core body temperature. For example, in women, progesterone secretion at the time of ovulation raises core body temperature by about 0.35°C or 0.5°F.

- **Stress.** The temperature of a highly stressed client may be elevated as a result of increased production of epinephrine and norepinephrine, which increase metabolic activity and heat production.

- **Illness.** Illness or a central nervous system disorder may impair the thermostatic function of the hypothalamus. **Hyperthermia,** also called fever, may occur in response to viral or bacterial infections, or from tissue breakdown following myocardial infarction, malignancy, surgery, or trauma. **Hypothermia** is usually a response to prolonged exposure to cold.

Routes for Measuring Body Temperature

Core body temperature was once typically measured with a mercury-in-glass thermometer. Mercury, a toxic liquid metal, can pose a health threat to the individual and community. Although the amount of mercury in each thermometer is small, the adverse effects are high and multidimensional when the instrument breaks and the liquid escapes from the container. Agencies are banning the sale and use of mercury-filled glass thermometers. Alcohol and galinstan are two products replacing mercury in glass thermometers. For more information, link to the U.S. Environmental Protection Agency through the Companion Website. Today, nurses are more likely to use an electronic thermometer (see Figure 7.7 ●), which gives a highly accurate reading in only 2 to 60 seconds. These portable, battery-operated devices consist of an electronic display unit, a probe, and disposable probe sheaths. The nurse attaches the appropriate probe to the unit, covers it with a sterile sheath, and

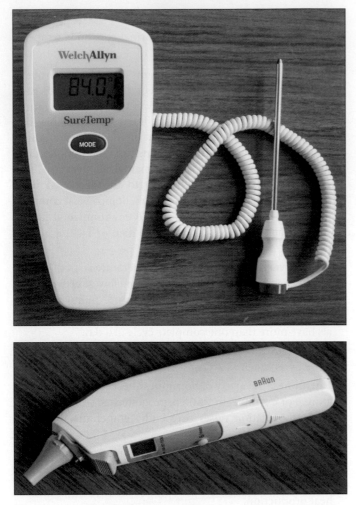

Figure 7.7 • Electronic thermometers.

inserts it into the body orifice. The probe is left in place until the temperature appears on the liquid crystal display (LCD) screen. There are four routes for measuring core body temperature: oral, rectal, axillary, or tympanic.

ORAL. The oral temperature is the most accessible, accurate, and convenient method. While glass thermometers may be used in the home setting, because of the possiblity of breaking and mercury exposure, they are no longer used in the clinical setting.

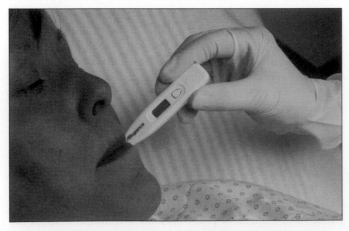

Figure 7.8 • Placement of the thermometer for an oral temperature.

Oral temperatures may be evaluated by using an electronic or digital probe device. Place the covered probe at the base of the tongue in either of the sublingual pockets to the right or left of the frenulum (see Figure 7.8 •), and instruct the client to keep the lips tightly closed around the thermometer. The thermometer is left in place until the device beeps or shows indication that the measurement is completed. After removing the thermometer, the nurse either discards the disposable sheath or cleans the device. The temperature reading will be in the display window.

RECTAL. A rectal temperature is taken if the client is comatose, confused, having seizures, or unable to close the mouth. It is important to use prelubricated thermometer covers and put on disposable examination gloves. The client should be in a side-lying position. The nurse asks the client to take a deep breath and then inserts the thermometer from 1.5 to 4 cm into the anus, being careful not to force insertion of the thermometer. The probe is left in place until there is a beep or the device indicates that the reading is completed. Remove the probe, dispose of the disposable sheath, and obtain the reading in the display window.

AXILLARY. Occasionally, the nurse needs to take an axillary temperature. This is the safest method and is less invasive than the oral or rectal routes, especially for infants and young children. Because of the variability of probe positioning, many authorities, consider the axillary route to be least accurate. For an axillary temperature, the nurse places the thermometer in the client's axilla and assists the client in placing the arm tightly across the chest to keep the thermometer in place.

TYMPANIC. The tympanic temperature can be taken only with an electronic thermometer. Using infrared technology, it measures a client's core body temperature quickly and accurately. This method is the most comfortable and least invasive for the client. The measuring probe resembles an otoscope. The nurse gently places the covered tip of the probe at the opening of the ear canal, being careful not to force the probe into the ear canal or occlude the canal opening. After about 2 seconds, the client's temperature reading will appear on the LCD screen.

MEASURING THE PULSE RATE

The heart is a muscular pump. The left ventricle of the heart contracts with every beat, forcing blood from the heart into the systemic arteries. The amount of blood pumped from the heart with each heartbeat is called the *stroke volume*. The force of the blood against the walls of the arteries generates a wave of pressure that is felt at various points in the body as a **pulse**. The ability of the arteries to contract and expand is called *compliance*. When compliance is reduced, the heart must exert more pressure to pump blood throughout the body.

Location of Pulse Points

The apical pulse is felt at the apex of the heart. Figure 7.9 • illustrates the location of the apical pulse for a child under 4 years, a child 4 to 6 years, and an adult. The peripheral pulse is the pulse as felt in the body's periphery, for example, in the neck, wrist, or foot. Figure 7.10 • shows eight sites where the peripheral pulse is most easily palpated. In a healthy client, the peripheral pulse rate is equivalent to the heartbeat. Alterations in the client's health can weaken the peripheral pulse, making it difficult to detect. Thus,

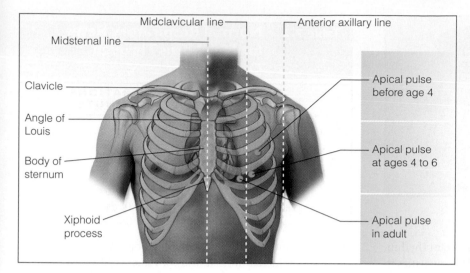

Figure 7.9 ● Location of the apical pulse in a child under age 4, a child ages 4 to 6, and an adult.

assessment of the peripheral pulse is an important component of a thorough health assessment.

Factors That Influence Pulse Rate

A variety of factors may influence the normal pulse rate. These include:

- **Age.** The average pulse rate of infants and children is higher than that of teens and adults. After age 16, the pulse stabilizes to an average of about 70 beats per minute (bpm) in males and 75 bpm in females.
- **Gender.** As previously noted, the average pulse rate of the adult male is slightly lower than that of the adult female.
- **Exercise.** The pulse rate normally increases with exercise.
- **Stress.** In response to stress, fear, and anxiety, the heart rate and the force of the heartbeat increase.
- **Fever.** The peripheral vasodilation that accompanies an elevated body temperature lowers systemic blood pressure, in turn causing an increase in pulse rate.
- **Hemorrhage.** Pulse rate increases in response to significant loss of blood from the vascular system.
- **Medications.** A variety of medications may either increase or decrease the heart rate.
- **Position changes.** When clients sit or stand for long periods, blood may pool in the veins, resulting in a temporary decrease in venous blood return to the heart and, consequently, reduced blood pressure and lowered pulse rate.

Palpation of the Radial Pulse

The peripheral pulse site most commonly used is the radial pulse. The radial pulse is palpated by placing the pads of the first two or three fingers on the anterior wrist along the radius bone (see Figure 7.11 ●). If the pulse is regular, the nurse counts the beats for 30 seconds and multiplies by 2 to obtain the total bpm. If the pulse is irregular, the nurse counts the beats for a full minute.

Four factors are considered when assessing the pulse: rate, rhythm, force, and elasticity. A pulse rate of less than 60 bpm, called *bradycardia*, may be found in a healthy, well-trained athlete. A pulse rate over 100 bpm, called *tachycardia*, may also be found in the healthy client who is anxious or has just finished exercising.

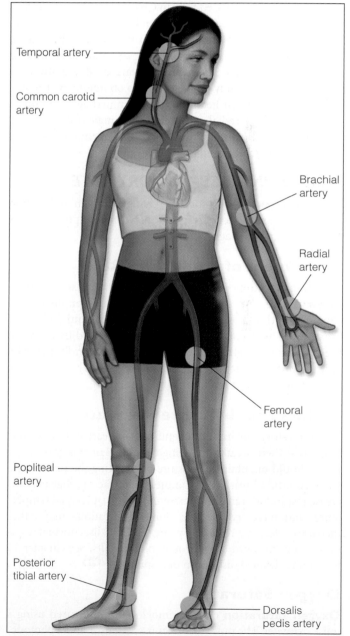

Figure 7.10 ● Body sites where the peripheral pulse is most easily palpated.

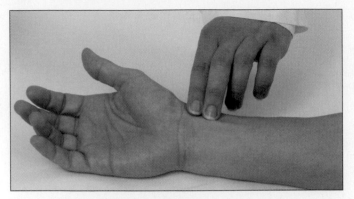

Figure 7.11 • Palpating the radial pulse.

Table 7.2	Normal Respiratory Rates for Newborns Through Older Adults	
AGE		**RESPIRATIONS PER MINUTE**
Newborn		30–80
3–9 years		20–30
10–15 years		16–22
16–adult		15–20
Adult		12–20
Older adult		15–25

The pulse of a healthy adult has a relatively constant rhythm; that is, the intervals between beats are regular. Irregularities in heart rhythm are discussed fully in Chapter 17 of this text. ∞

The nurse assesses the force of a pulse, or its stroke volume, by noting the pressure that must be exerted before the pulse is felt. A "full, bounding" pulse is difficult to obliterate. It may be caused by fear, anxiety, exercise, or a variety of alterations in health. A "weak, thready pulse" is easy to obliterate. It also may indicate alterations in health such as hemorrhage. The nurse palpates along the radial artery in a proximal-to-distal direction to assess the elasticity of the artery. A normal artery feels smooth, straight, and resilient.

MEASURING RESPIRATORY RATE

The human body continuously exchanges oxygen and carbon dioxide through the act of respiration. Normal respiratory rates are dependent upon age.

Assessment of Respiratory Rate

Counting the number of respirations per minute assesses **respiratory rate.** The nurse observes the full respiratory cycle (one inspiration and one expiration) for rate and pattern of breathing. The client's respiratory rate is assessed by counting the number of breaths for 30 seconds and then multiplying by 2. If the nurse detects irregularities or difficulty breathing, the respirations are counted for one full minute.

Factors That Influence Respiratory Rate

The respiratory rate in some clients may increase if they become aware that their breaths are being counted. For this reason, the nurse should maintain the posture of counting the radial pulse while counting breaths per minute. Other factors that may increase respiratory rate include exercise, stress, increased temperature, and increased altitude. Some medications may either increase or decrease respiratory rate. Table 7.2 lists normal respiratory rates for newborns through older adults. See Chapter 15 for a more detailed discussion of respiration. ∞

Oxygen Saturation

Oxygen saturation of the hemoglobin is measured using a pulse oximeter. The pulse oximeter uses a sensor and a photodetector to determine the light sent sand absorbed by the hemoglobin. The reported percentage represents the light absorbed by oxygenated and deoxygenated hemoglobin. A value of 95% to 100% is considered normal, while a value of 70% is considered to be life threatening. This noninvasive procedure allows oxygen saturation values to be easily obtained and rapidly updated. Pulse oximetry can detect hypoxemia before symptoms such as cyanosis (blue color) of the skin appear.

MEASURING BLOOD PRESSURE

Blood ebbs and flows within the systemic arteries in waves, causing two types of pressure. The **systolic pressure** is the pressure of the blood at the height of the wave, when the left ventricle contracts. This is the first number recorded in a blood pressure measurement. The **diastolic pressure** is the pressure between the ventricular contractions, when the heart is at rest. This is the second number recorded in a blood pressure measurement.

Circulatory Factors That Influence Blood Pressure

Factors that influence blood pressure include but are not limited to the following:

- Cardiac output is the amount of blood ejected from the heart. Cardiac output is equal to the stroke volume, or amount of blood ejected in one heartbeat (measured in milliliters per beat), multiplied by the heart rate (measured in bpm). Cardiac output averages about 5.5 L/min (liters per minute).

- Blood volume is the total amount of blood circulating within the entire vascular system. Blood volume averages about 5 L in adults. A sudden drop in blood pressure may signal sudden blood loss, as with internal bleeding.

- Peripheral vascular resistance is the resistance the blood encounters as it flows within the vessels. Peripheral resistance is in turn influenced by various factors, such as vessel length and diameter. Two of the most important factors influencing peripheral resistance are blood viscosity and vessel compliance.

- Blood viscosity is the ratio between the blood cells (the formed elements) and the blood plasma. When the total amount of formed elements is high, the blood is thicker, or more viscous. The molecules pass one another with greater difficulty, and more pressure is required to move the blood.

- Vessel compliance describes the elasticity of the smooth muscle in the arterial walls. Highly elastic arteries respond readily and fully to each heartbeat. Rigid, hardened arteries, as are found with arteriosclerosis, are less responsive, and greater force is required to move the blood along.

Note that blood in the systemic circulation flows along a pressure gradient from central to peripheral; in other words, pressure is higher in the arterioles than in the capillaries, and higher still in the aorta. The average blood pressure of a healthy adult is 120/80 mm Hg.

Additional Factors Affecting Blood Pressure

Additional factors that influence blood pressure include but are not limited to the following:

- **Age.** Systolic blood pressure in newborns averages about 78 mm Hg. Blood pressure rates tend to rise with increasing age through age 18 and then tend to stabilize. In older adults, blood pressure rates tend to rise again as elasticity of the arteries decreases.
- **Gender.** After puberty, females tend to have lower blood pressure than males of the same age. Reproductive hormones may influence this difference because blood pressure in women usually increases after menopause.
- **Race.** American males of African ancestry over the age of 35 tend to have higher blood pressures than American males of European descent.
- **Obesity.** Blood pressure tends to be higher in people who are overweight and obese than in people of normal weight of the same age.
- **Physical activity.** Physical activity (including crying in infants and children) increases cardiac output and therefore increases blood pressure.
- **Stress.** Stress increases cardiac output and arterial vasoconstriction, resulting in increased blood pressure.
- **Diurnal variations.** Blood pressure is usually lowest in the early morning and rises steadily throughout the day, peaking in the late afternoon or early evening.
- **Medications.** A variety of medications may increase or decrease blood pressure.

Blood pressure is also affected by alterations in health. Any condition that affects the cardiac output, peripheral vascular resistance, blood volume, blood viscosity, or vessel compliance can affect blood pressure.

Assessment of Blood Pressure

An accurate measurement of blood pressure is an essential part of any complete health assessment.

CLIENT PREPARATION. It is important to reassure the client that the procedure for taking blood pressure is generally quick and painless. The client should be at rest for at least 5 minutes before taking a blood pressure measurement and up to 20 minutes if the client has been engaging in heavy physical activity. Client anxiety may also cause a temporary elevation of blood pressure.

EQUIPMENT. The nurse measures blood pressure with a blood pressure cuff, a **sphygmomanometer,** and a stethoscope. There are various cuff sizes as shown in Figure 7.12 ●. The cuff consists of an inflatable bladder, which is covered by cloth and has two tubes attached to it. One of these tubes ends in a

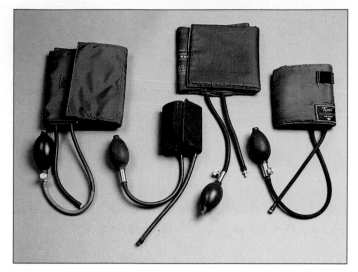

Figure 7.12 ● A variety of cuff sizes: a small cuff for an infant, small child, or frail adult; a normal adult-size cuff; and a large cuff for measuring the blood pressure on the leg or on the arm of an obese adult.

rubber bulb with which to inflate the bladder. A small valve on the side of the bulb regulates air in the bladder. When the valve is loosened, air in the bladder is released. After the valve is tightened, pumped air remains in the bladder. The second tube attached to the bladder ends in a sphygmomanometer, a device that measures the air pressure in the bladder. There are two types of sphygmomanometers: aneroid and mercury. The aneroid sphygmomanometer has a small, calibrated dial with a needle. It is more portable but less reliable than the mercury type. The mercury sphygmomanometer has a calibrated cylinder filled with mercury. To determine the blood pressure, the nurse reads the measurement corresponding to the crescent-shaped top of the column of mercury. (*Note:* The use of mercury sphygmomanometers is being discontinued in healthcare settings.) The bladder of the blood pressure cuff must fit the length and width of the client's limb. If the bladder is too narrow, the blood pressure reading will be falsely high. The width of the bladder should equal 40% of the circumference of the limb. The length of the bladder should equal 80% of the circumference of the limb. Note that the circumference of the client's limb, and not the age of the client, determines the cuff used. Automatic monitors can be used to measure blood pressure. These devices include a cuff attached to an electronic monitor. Application of the cuff is the same as in the manual method. The monitor provides a reading on an LCD screen of the systolic, diastolic, and mean blood pressures.

THE PROCEDURE. Blood pressure measurements are usually taken by placing the cuff on the client's arm and auscultating the pulse in the brachial artery. The nurse must use common sense when choosing which arm to use for the measurement. For example, blood pressure should not be measured in an arm on the same side as a mastectomy or an arm with a shunt. If blood pressure cannot be measured in either arm because of disease or trauma, a thigh blood pressure may be taken, using the popliteal artery, or a leg blood pressure may be taken, using the posterior tibial or dorsalis pedis arteries.

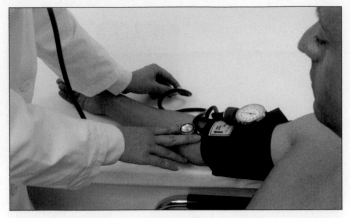

Figure 7.13 ● Measuring the client's blood pressure.

To measure the blood pressure in the client's arm, the nurse follows these steps:

1. Place the client in a comfortable position in a quiet room.
2. Confirm that the blood pressure cuff is the appropriate size for the client's arm.
3. Remove any clothing from the client's arm.
4. Slightly flex the arm and hold it at the level of the heart with the palm upward.
5. Palpate the brachial pulse.
6. Place the cuff on the arm with the lower border 1 inch above the antecubital area making sure that the cuff is smooth and snug. One finger should fit between the cuff and the client's arm. Be sure that the center of the bladder is over the brachial artery. Many cuffs have an arrow to indicate the center of the bladder, thus the part of the cuff to be over the artery.
7. Palpate the radial pulse.
8. Close the release valve on the pump.
9. Inflate the cuff until the radial pulse is no longer palpable and note the reading on the sphygmomanometer. This is the palpatory systolic blood pressure.
10. Place the diaphragm of the stethoscope over the brachial pulse (see Figure 7.13 ●).
11. Pump up the cuff until the sphygmomanometer registers 30 mm Hg above the palpatory systolic blood pressure (the point at which the radial pulse disappeared).
12. Release the valve on the cuff carefully so that the pressure decreases at the rate of 2 to 3 mm Hg per second.
13. Note the manometer reading at each of the five Korotkoff phases (see Box 7.1). The first sound is recorded as the systolic blood pressure and the last sound is recorded as the diastolic blood pressure.
14. Deflate the cuff rapidly and completely.
15. Remove the cuff from the client's arm.

AGE-RELATED CONSIDERATIONS

The client's age can impact the methods and equipment used to assess vital signs. The following sections address age-related considerations.

Box 7.1	**Korotkoff's Sounds**

When measuring blood pressure, auscultate to identify five phases in a series of sounds called Korotkoff's sounds, named after the Russian surgeon who first described them. These five phases are:

Phase 1: The period initiated by the first faint, clear, tapping sounds. These sounds gradually become more intense. To ensure that they are not extraneous sounds, identify at least two consecutive tapping sounds. *Rationale:* The tapping sounds occur when the cuff pressure has decreased enough to allow the first spurts of blood into the artery.

Phase 2: The period during which the sounds have a swishing quality. *Rationale:* The swooshing sounds occur as the blood flows turbulently through the partially occluded artery and the vessel walls vibrate from the impact.

Phase 3: The period during which the sounds are tapping sounds similar to Phase 1 sounds, but they are crisper, higher-pitched, and more intense. *Rationale:* During Phase 3, blood flows through the artery during systole, but the pressure in the cuff is still high enough to cause the artery to collapse during diastole.

Phase 4: The period during which the sounds become muffled and have a soft, blowing quality. *Rationale:* The pressure in the cuff is now low enough so that the artery no longer collapses completely during any part of the cardiac cycle.

Phase 5: The point at which the sounds disappear. *Rationale:* The absence of sound reflects the absence of pressure in the cuff. Normal blood flow is inaudible.

Document the blood pressure measurements as follows:

- The systolic pressure is the point at which the first tapping sound is heard (Phase 1).
- In adults, the diastolic pressure is the point at which the sounds become inaudible (Phase 5).
- In children, the diastolic pressure is the point at which the sounds become muffled (Phase 4).
- Some institutions may require you to record readings at both Phase 4 and Phase 5 for all clients, regardless of age. In such cases, document the three readings as systolic pressure, first diastolic pressure, and second diastolic pressure. Note that the second diastolic pressure may be zero; that is, muffled sounds may be audible even when the cuff is completely deflated. Finally, in cases when muffled sounds (Phase 4) are never heard, record a dash for the Phase 4 reading.

Source: American Heart Association. "Recommendations for Human Blood Pressure Determination by Sphygmomanometers." Publication number 7001005 (1987), pp. 3–5.

Temperature

Respirations and pulse rate are assessed before measuring rectal temperature in infants because taking a rectal temperature may cause an infant to cry. Holding the infant in a lateral position with the knees flexed onto the abdomen, or prone on the nurse's lap, the nurse separates the infant's buttocks with the nondominant hand and inserts the thermometer with the dominant gloved hand. The nurse should use a blunt-tipped thermometer, insert it no more than 2.5 cm or 1 in., and hold on to the exposed end. To avoid the risk of rectal perforation, an axillary temperature may be taken rather than a rectal temperature in newborns. The nurse should take the axillary temperature also in toddlers and older children whenever possible to eliminate their anxiety over the invasive rectal procedure. An oral route may be used as early as age 5 if the child is able to keep his or her mouth closed and does not bite on the glass thermometer. Electronic thermometers, which are unbreakable and register quickly, are particularly useful with children.

Body temperature in the older adult may be reduced because of decreased thermoregulatory control and loss of subcutaneous fat. Older adults are more sensitive to environmental changes in temperature, possibly because of lack of physical activity, inadequate diet, or inability to afford adequate heating.

Pulse

The apical site is used for children younger than age 2. In preschool children, the nurse uses the brachial site and counts the pulse for a full minute. It is important to pay attention to any irregularities in rhythm, such as sinus arrhythmia, which is not uncommon in children. The pulse rate of the healthy older adult is in a range from 60 to 100 bpm. The radial artery may feel rigid if there is loss of elasticity in the arterial walls.

Respirations

The nurse should count respirations for one full minute in infants, because the breathing pattern may show considerable variation from a series of rapid breaths to brief episodes of apnea. The respiratory rate in older adults may be increased to accommodate a decrease in vital capacity and inspiratory reserve volume.

Blood Pressure

A Doppler stethoscope is used when measuring blood pressure in infants and in children under the age of 2. In children over the age of 2, it is imperative that the nurse use the correct size cuff and a small diaphragm for the stethoscope. The American Heart Association recommends that, in children, diastolic pressure be read at the beginning of Korotkoff phase 4, when the sounds become muffled. The heart pumps against increased resistance, and systolic blood pressure increases as the systemic arteries lose elasticity with increasing age.

PAIN—THE FIFTH VITAL SIGN

Assessment of **pain** is essential in comprehensive health assessment. Pain is an entirely subjective and personal experience. When pain is present, it impacts every aspect of an individual's health and well-being. Pain can be acute and chronic, severe or mild, but overall it is an experience unique to the individual. The perception of pain and the ways in which the individual responds to pain vary according to age, gender, culture, and developmental level. When conducting a pain assessment, the nurse must consider all factors influencing the individual's experience with pain. Refer to Chapter 8 of this text for a thorough discussion of pain. ⚭

PAIN ASSESSMENT

The nurse typically initiates pain assessment because many individuals do not discuss their pain until asked about it. Pain assessment consists of two phases. The first phase is a pain history, and the second phase is observation of behaviors and responses to pain.

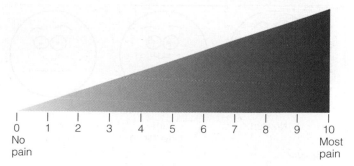

Figure 7.14 ● Pain rating intensity scale.

Pain History

A pain history includes collection of data about the location, intensity, quality, pattern, precipitating factors, actions aimed at relief of pain, impact on activities of daily living (ADLs), coping strategies, and emotional responses.

LOCATION. The nurse should ask the client to point to the specific location of pain. Charts in which body outlines are depicted are a useful method for children and adults to accurately identify the site of pain. When recording the location, the body outline charts may be used. The nurse is also expected to record locations, using appropriate terminology in relation to the proximity or distance from known landmarks (e.g., pain in substernal area 3 cm below the xiphoid process).

INTENSITY. The intensity of pain is most accurately assessed through the use of **pain rating scales** (see Figure 7.14 ●). Most scales use a numerical rating of 0 to 5 or 0 to 10, with 0 indicating the absence of pain. Descriptors accompany the number ratings in many scales. The descriptors assist the client to "quantify" the intensity of the pain. For children and adults who cannot read or are unable to numerically rate their pain, faces rating scales are available (see Figure 7.15 ●). Numbers accompany each facial expression so that pain intensity can be identified.

QUALITY. Quality of pain is assessed by asking the client to apply an adjective to the pain. For example, pain may be experienced as burning, stabbing, piercing, or throbbing. Children may have difficulty describing pain; therefore, it is important to use familiar terminology, such as "boo-boo," "feel funny," or "hurt." The nurse must use quotation marks to record the description of the pain in the exact words spoken by the client.

PATTERN. The pattern of pain refers to the onset and duration of the pain experience. In addition, the nurse assesses whether the pain is constant or intermittent. If the pain is intermittent, the nurse must assess the length of time without pain or between episodes of pain.

PRECIPITATING FACTORS. A variety of factors can precipitate pain. These precipitating factors include activity, exercise, and temperature, or other climactic changes. Fear, anxiety, and stress can also precipitate pain.

ACTIONS TO ACHIEVE PAIN RELIEF. Assessment of pain includes gathering data about the measures taken by the client to relieve or alleviate the pain. The nurse will inquire about the use of medications, home and folk remedies, and alternative or complementary therapies, such as acupuncture, massage, and imagery. The nurse must also gather data about the effectiveness of the measures.

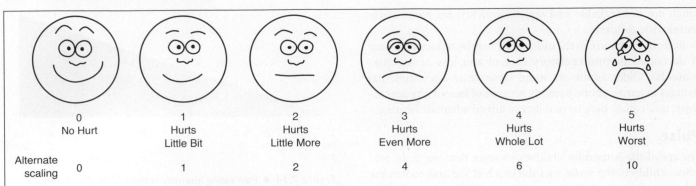

Brief word instructions: Point to each face using the words to describe the pain intensity. Ask the child to choose face that best describes own pain and record the appropriate number.

Original instructions: Explain to the person that each face is for a person who feels happy because he has no pain (hurt) or sad because he has some or a lot of pain. Face 0 is very happy because he doesn't hurt at all. Face 1 hurts just a little bit. Face 2 hurts a little more. Face 3 hurts even more. Face 4 hurts a whole lot. Face 5 hurts as much as you can imagine, although you don't have to be crying to feel this bad. Ask the person to choose the face that best describes how he is feeling.

Rating scale is recommended for persons age 3 years and older.

Figure 7.15 ● The Wong-Baker "FACES" pain rating scale.
Source: From Hockenberry, MJ, Wilson D., Winkelstein ML: *Wong's Essentials of Pediatric Nursing*, ed. 7, St. Louis, 2005, p. 1259. Used with permission. Copyright Mosby.

IMPACT ON ACTIVITIES OF DAILY LIVING. Assessment of the impact of pain on ADLs enables the nurse to understand the severity of the pain and the impact of the pain on the client's quality of life. ADLs include work, school, household and family management, mobility and transportation, leisure activities, and marital and family relationships. The nurse may ask the client to rate the impact of the pain on each of the ADLs.

COPING STRATEGIES. There are a variety of ways in which individuals cope with pain. Various coping strategies include but are not limited to prayer, yoga, tai chi, chi quong, support groups, distraction, relaxation techniques, or withdrawal. The strategies are often unique to the individual or reflect cultural values and beliefs. The nurse attempts to identify coping strategies employed by the client and to determine if they are effective in pain management.

EMOTIONAL RESPONSES. An assessment of the client's emotional response to pain is important. Pain, especially chronic or debilitating pain, can result in depression, anxiety, and physical and emotional exhaustion. The emotional response to pain is often related to the type, intensity, and duration of pain.

Observation

The observation phase of the pain assessment includes the direct observation of the client's behavior and physiological responses.

BEHAVIOR. A variety of behaviors indicate the presence of pain. Many of these behaviors are nonverbal or consist of vocalizations. Behaviors indicative of pain include facial grimacing, moaning, crying or screaming, guarding or immobilization of a body part, tossing and turning, and rhythmic movements.

PHYSIOLOGICAL RESPONSES. The site of the pain and the duration of the pain influence physiological responses to pain. The sympathetic nervous system is stimulated in the early stage of acute pain. The response is demonstrated in elevation of blood pressure, pulse and respiratory rates, pallor, and diaphoresis. Parasympathetic stimulation often accompanies visceral pain. This results in lowered blood pressure and pulse rate, and warm dry skin.

THE FUNCTIONAL ASSESSMENT AS PART OF THE GENERAL SURVEY

Nurses use their observational skills in many situations. When making observations, nurses are continually thinking about the data and using their knowledge of the physical, behavioral, and social sciences to interpret the findings. The findings are interpreted according to the expected norms for clients in relation to age, gender, race, development, and culture.

FUNCTIONAL ASSESSMENT DEFINED

The **functional assessment** is an observation to gather data while the client is performing common or routine activities.

FUNCTIONAL ASSESSMENT DURING THE GENERAL SURVEY

During the general survey of a healthy client, the nurse will observe the client while performing the following common activities: walking into the examination room, taking a seat for the interview, and moving the arms and hands to arrange clothing or to shake hands as an introduction. The nurse will also observe the facial expression while these acts occur. From this brief encounter, the nurse applies knowledge to begin to gather and interpret data about the client's mobility and strength, and the symmetry of the face and parts of the body.

CRITICAL THINKING

When applying the critical thinking process, the professional nurse uses a variety of skills that culminate in assisting clients to make healthcare decisions.

The following case study and analysis is presented to demonstrate the application of critical thinking in the functional assessment of a client as part of the general survey.

The nurse conducted a comprehensive health assessment of a 70-year-old African American female who was new to the clinic. The interaction began when the nurse went to the waiting area to bring the client to the interview area. The following occurred: As the nurse entered the waiting area, all of the clients looked up. The nurse called out "Jane Carter" and looked about the room. An African American female with gray hair seen under a brightly colored scarf said, "Here I am. I'll be right there." The woman rose slowly, pushing herself up with her hands placed on the arms of the chair. The nurse heard a soft "mmm, oh my." The client gathered her purse and reached for a cane resting next to the chair. As the client approached, the nurse noted that she had smooth skin on her face and hands. She was approximately 5′4″ and obese. She walked slowly toward the nurse, with the cane in her right hand. She moved her left leg stiffly. As she moved through the door, she asked, "Will I have to sit down again now? I'm mighty stiff."

As stated early in this chapter, the general survey begins with the initial encounter with the client and provides cues about the client. The observations from the brief case study include the following:

- All of the clients looked up when the nurse entered the waiting area.
- When a name was called, an African American female with graying hair responded.
- The woman rose slowly.
- The woman used her arms to push herself out of the chair.
- The woman uttered "oh my" while rising.
- The woman gathered her purse and reached for a cane.
- The woman had smooth skin on her face and hands.
- The woman was approximately 5′4″ tall and was obese.
- She walked slowly.
- She held the cane in her right hand.
- The movement of the left leg was stiff.
- As she entered the exam area, she asked, "Will I have to sit down again now? I'm mighty stiff."

In applying critical thinking the nurse will begin to sort information and determine an approach to continue data gathering. The nurse considers each of the observations in terms of normal and abnormal findings in relation to the age, gender, race, and culture of the client. Interpretations of the nurse's observations in the preceding case study are as follows:

- All the clients looked up when the nurse entered the room.
  The client was aware that someone entered the room; this indicates that her vision and hearing are intact. This is considered a normal finding.
- The client responded when her name was called.
  This is further indication that hearing is intact. This is a normal finding.
- The client had graying hair.
  This is an expected finding in a 70-year-old female.
- The client rose slowly.
  This is an expected finding in an older adult because of decreased muscle tone and strength.
- The client used her arms to push herself out of the chair.

This is an indication of diminished strength in the lower extremities. This is an expected finding in an older adult because of decreased muscle tone and strength. This requires follow-up to determine the actual muscle strength of the client.

- The client uttered "oh my" while rising.
  This indicates discomfort or surprise. This is initially interpreted as an abnormal finding. Discomfort is indicative of an underlying problem. In this case, the problem may be musculoskeletal.
- The client gathered her purse and reached for a cane.
  This indicates that the client is alert and cognizant of her surroundings and the need to gather her personal items. This is a normal finding. The reaching for the cane suggests she has a musculoskeletal problem requiring its use. This is an abnormal finding and requires follow-up to ascertain the underlying problem.
- The client had smooth skin on her face and hands.
  This finding suggests that the client is in a state of fluid and nutritional balance and that she follows hygiene practices. This has the suggestion of being a normal finding. However, the nurse will consider other factors during the assessment.
- The client was approximately 5′4″ tall and was obese.
  Obesity is an abnormal finding. However, the nurse knows that obesity occurs with more frequency in African American females than in Caucasians and that weight gain occurs with aging.
- She walked slowly.
  This is expected in older adults who have lost muscle and skeletal mass and strength. This requires further evaluation in relation to the client's need to push herself up from the chair while uttering "oh my."
- She held the cane in her right hand.
  The ability to hold the cane indicates coordination in the right extremity. The nurse must follow up to determine the reason for the use of the cane and whether the client has been using the cane appropriately in relation to the underlying problem.
- The movement of the left leg was stiff.
  This is an abnormal finding. The nurse must determine the underlying cause. This is suggestive of a musculoskeletal problem. However, there may be a neurologic problem.
- As she entered the exam area, she asked, "Will I have to sit down again now? I'm mighty stiff."
  This response indicates the client's concern with movement. The statements are not unexpected in relation to observations about the movements and gait of the client. This statement forces the nurse to make a rapid decision about the process of the health assessment. The nurse must quickly gather more data to determine the client's ability to participate in all aspects of the assessment.

The preceding analyses demonstrate that a great deal of information can be obtained through observation. In this situation much information is missing. As this information is gathered, the nurse will determine the relevance of each piece of data to the overall situation. The nurse applies critical thinking throughout the comprehensive health assessment while working with the client to meet health-related needs.

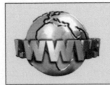

Application Through Critical Thinking

CASE STUDY

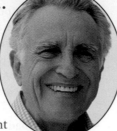

*I*t was a Friday morning. You were the nurse who conducted a physical examination of Joseph Miller, a 73-year-old, Caucasian male. You began with a client interview during which the following occurred.

The client entered the room, looked right at you, smiled, and stated "How do you do?" in a clear voice. When you introduced yourself, he gave a firm handshake, then held both of your hands in his and commented, "Boy, you sure have cold hands." He walked steadily to the chair you indicated, but held onto the desk while getting seated. You informed the client of the purpose of the interview. He stated "no" when asked if he had any specific complaints or problems. He then shrugged his shoulders and commented, "I don't think I have anything special going on, I'm here for my three-month check and I expect to get a clean bill of health." You asked him to sign an admission form. He put on reading glasses, perused the form, and signed.

When asked about current medications, the client stated "I have them with me, let me show you." He then took out three medicine bottles. He read each label and commented as follows about each. "This is Pardivil, it's for my blood pressure; this one is ferrous sulfate, that's iron, I have some anemia; this last one is Digit, I take it every other day for my heart." He frowned and said, "This bottle is nearly empty." After opening the bottle and looking at the contents he said, "Yup, just as I thought, I only have three pills left so I'll have to fill it. I'll be out of pills by Thursday and the drug store is always packed just before the weekend."

You continued the interview and concluded it by telling the patient you were going to check his blood pressure, pulse, temperature, and weight before escorting him to the examination room.

▶ *Critical Thinking Questions*

1. What are the findings from the case study for Mr. Miller?
2. How would you interpret the findings in relation to the categories for observation in the general survey?
3. Which findings indicate the need for follow up in interview or physical assessment?
4. What factors must be considered when evaluating the vital signs assessment for Mr. Miller?

Please refer to the Companion Website at www.prenhall.com/damico and click on **Chapter 7,** the **Application Through Critical Thinking** module, to answer these and additional questions. In addition, complete **NCLEX-RN®** review questions and other interactive resources for this chapter.

EXPLORE MediaLink

Additional resources for this chapter are found on the Student CD-ROM accompanying this textbook and on the Companion Website.

CD-ROM CONTENT

Content for this chapter includes:
Objectives
Key Concepts
NCLEX-RN® Review Questions
Model Documentation Forms
Audio Glossary
Animations
    Anatomical Landmarks
Head-to-Toe Physical Examination Video

COMPANION WEBSITE CONTENT

www.prenhall.com/damico
Content for this chapter includes:
Objectives

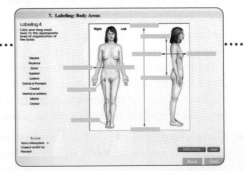

NCLEX-RN® Review Questions
Application Through Critical Thinking
    Case Study Teaching Plan Challenge
MediaLinks
MediaLink Application
Tool Box
    Normal Respiratory Rates for Newborns Through Older Adults
New York Times

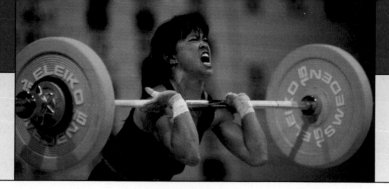

8

Pain Assessment

MEDIALINK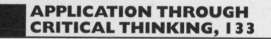

www.prenhall.com/damico

The CD-ROM in the back of this textbook and the Media-Link website contain NCLEX-RN® review questions, interactive exercises, case study challenges, animations, videos, documentation and checklist forms, and review materials. For a complete listing of the media content specific to Chapter 8, see the Explore MediaLink at the end of the chapter.

*P*ain is a highly unpleasant sensation that affects a person's physical health, emotional health, and well-being. Healthcare professionals include pain as a component of vital signs assessment. Pain assessment is identified as the fifth vital sign.

Assessment of pain requires a strong knowledge base regarding the concept of pain and methods to collect information about the pain experience. Accurate assessment of pain is essential to develop, monitor, and evaluate the effectiveness of pain relief interventions.

Pain assessment, treatment, and relief present one of the greatest challenges to the nurse and other members of the healthcare team. The nurse has a primary role regarding the collection and analysis of data, the implementation of treatment modalities, and the evaluation of the client regarding pain experiences.

DEFINITION OF PAIN

Pain comes from the Greek word *poinē* meaning penalty, implying the person is paying for something. An individual's perception of pain is influenced by age, gender, culture, and previous experience with pain.

Pain has been defined as "whatever the experiencing person says it is, existing whenever he or she says it does" (McCaffery & Pasero, 1999, p. 5). Pain is a universal experience. Everyone experiences pain at some time and to some degree. It is a highly subjective, unpleasant, and personal sensation that cannot be shared with others. This sensation can be associated with actual or potential tissue damage. Pain can be the primary problem or associated with a specific diagnosis, treatment, or procedure.

No two people experience pain in the same manner. It can occupy all of a person's thinking, force changes in the ability to function on a daily basis, and produce changes in the individual's life. For the client, it is a difficult concept to describe, thus making pain treatment and relief most difficult.

The nurse cannot see or feel the pain being experienced by the client; however, the effects produced by the pain will be assessed. These changes can be physiological, psychological, and behavioral in nature.

PHYSIOLOGY OF PAIN

Pain is a complex, subjective, multidimensional phenomenon that is not clearly understood. Theories that have been developed to explain the conceptual and physiological aspects of pain include specific theory, pattern theory, and gate control theory.

THEORIES OF PAIN

The concept of specific theory explains the complexity of pain. This theory demonstrates that pain neurons are as specific and unique as other specific neurons (taste, smell) in the body. The special pain neurons transport the sensation to the brain for interpretation. The transport occurs in a straight line to the brain, making the pain equal to the injury. This theory does not include a consideration of any psychological component to pain.

The pattern theory indicates that individuals will respond in a different manner to a similar stimulus. This theory implies the pattern of the stimulus is more important than the specific stimulus. It does not take into consideration the psychosocial component to pain.

According to Melzack and Wall's gate control theory (1965), peripheral nerve fibers carrying pain impulses to the spinal cord can have their input modified at the spinal cord level before transmission to the brain. Synapses in the dorsal horns act as gates that close to keep impulses from reaching the brain, or open to permit impulses to ascend to the brain.

Small-diameter nerve fibers carry pain stimuli through a gate, but large-diameter nerve fibers going through the same gate can inhibit the transmission of those pain impulses—that is, close the gate (see Figure 8.1 ●). The gate mechanism is thought to be

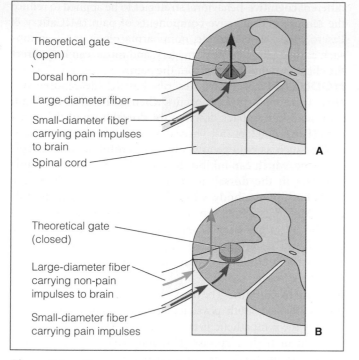

Figure 8.1 ● Gate control theory. A. open gate, B. closed gate.

situated in the substantia gelatinosa cells in the dorsal horn of the spinal cord. Because a limited amount of sensory information can reach the brain at any given time, certain cells can interrupt the pain impulses. The brain also appears to influence whether the gate is open or closed. For example, previous experiences with pain affect the way an individual responds to pain. The involvement of the brain helps explain why painful stimuli are interpreted differently by different people. Although the gate control theory is not unanimously accepted, it does help explain why electrical and mechanical interventions as well as heat and pressure can relieve pain. For example, a back massage may stimulate impulses in large nerves, which in turn close the gate to back pain.

NERVOUS SYSTEM

The nervous system must receive and interpret a stimulus to allow the individual to recognize the pain process. How pain is transmitted and perceived is not completely understood. Whether pain is perceived and to what degree depends on the interaction between the body's analgesia system and the nervous system's transmission and interpretation of stimuli.

Nociception

The peripheral nervous system includes primary sensory neurons specialized to detect tissue damage and to evoke the sensations of touch, heat, cold, pain, and pressure. The receptors that transmit pain sensation are called **nociceptors.** These pain receptors or nociceptors can be excited by mechanical, thermal, or chemical stimuli (see Table 8.1). The physiological processes related to pain perception are described as **nociception.** Four processes are involved in nociception: transduction, transmission, perception, and modulation (Paice, 2002).

TRANSDUCTION. During the transduction phase, noxious stimuli (tissue injury) trigger the release of biochemical mediators (e.g., prostaglandins, bradykinin, serotonin, histamine, substance P) that sensitize nociceptors. Noxious or painful stimulation also causes movement of ions across cell membranes, which excites nociceptors. Pain medications can work during this phase by blocking the production of prostaglandin (e.g., ibuprofen) or by decreasing the movement of ions across the cell membrane (e.g., local anesthetic).

TRANSMISSION. The second process of nociception, transmission of pain, includes three segments (McCaffery & Pasero, 1999). During the first segment, the pain impulse travels from the peripheral nerve fibers to the spinal cord. Substance P serves as a neurotransmitter, enhancing the movement of impulses across the nerve synapse from the primary afferent neuron to the second-order neuron in the dorsal horn of the spinal cord (see Figure 8.2 ●). Two types of nociceptor fibers cause this transmission to the dorsal horn of the spinal cord: C fibers, which transmit dull, aching pain; and A-delta fibers, which transmit sharp, localized pain. The second segment is

Table 8.1	Types of Pain Stimuli
STIMULUS TYPE	**PHYSIOLOGICAL BASIS OF PAIN**
Mechanical	
1. Trauma to body tissues (e.g., surgery)	Tissue damage; direct irritation of the pain receptors; inflammation
2. Alterations in body tissues (e.g., edema)	Pressure on pain receptors
3. Blockage of a body duct	Distention of the lumen of the duct
4. Tumor	Pressure on pain receptors; irritation of nerve endings
5. Muscle spasm	Stimulation of pain receptors (also see chemical stimuli)
Thermal	
Extreme heat or cold (e.g., burns)	Tissue destruction; stimulation of thermosensitive pain receptors
Chemical	
1. Tissue ischemia (e.g., blocked coronary artery)	Stimulation of pain receptors because of accumulated lactic acid (and other chemicals, such as bradykinin and enzymes) in tissues
2. Muscle spasm	Tissue ischemia secondary to mechanical stimulation (see above)

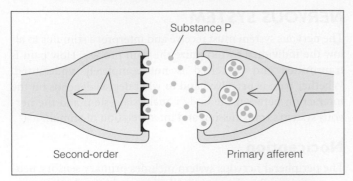

Figure 8.2 ● Substance P assists the transmission of impulses across the synapse from the primary afferent neuron to a second-order neuron in the spinothalamic tract.

transmission from the spinal cord, and ascension, via spinothalamic tracts, to the brain stem and thalamus (see Figure 8.3 ●). The third segment involves transmission of signals between the thalamus and the somatic sensory cortex where pain perception occurs.

Pain control can take place during this second process of transmission. For example, opioids (narcotics) block the release of neurotransmitters, particularly substance P, which stops the pain at the spinal level.

PERCEPTION. The third process, perception, occurs when the client becomes conscious of the pain. It is believed that pain perception occurs in the cortical structures, which allows for

different cognitive-behavioral strategies to be applied to reduce the sensory and affective components of pain (McCaffery & Pasero, 1999). For example, nonpharmacologic interventions such as distraction, guided imagery, and music can help direct the client's attention away from the pain.

MODULATION. Often described as the "descending system," this fourth process occurs when neurons in the brain stem send signals back down to the dorsal horn of the spinal cord (Paice, 2002, p. 75). These descending fibers release substances such as endogenous opioids, serotonin, and norepinephrine, which can inhibit the ascending noxious (painful) impulses in the dorsal horn. These neurotransmitters are taken back by the body, which limits their analgesic usefulness (McCaffery & Pasero, 1999). Clients with chronic pain may be prescribed tricyclic antidepressants, which inhibit the reuptake of norepinephrine and serotonin. This action increases the modulation phase that helps inhibit painful ascending stimuli.

Responses to Pain. The body's response to pain is a complex process that has both physiological and psychosocial aspects. Initially the sympathetic nervous system responds, resulting in the fight-or-flight response. The body adapts to the pain as the parasympathetic nervous system takes over, reversing many of the initial physiological responses. This adaptation to pain occurs after several hours or days of pain. The actual pain receptors adapt very little and continue to transmit the pain message. The person may learn to cope through cognitive and

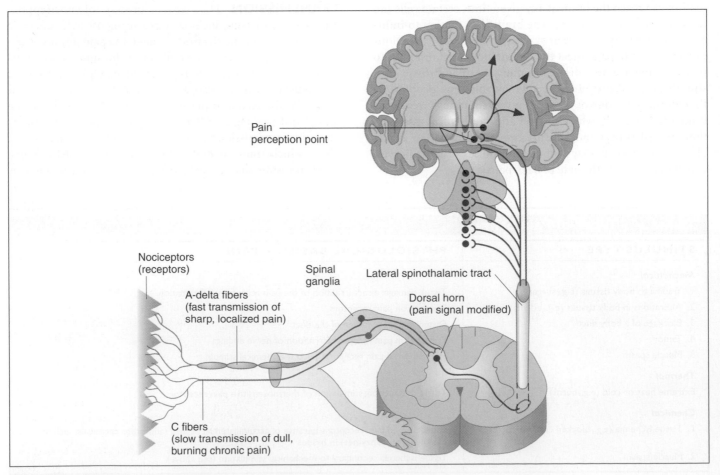

Figure 8.3 ● Physiology of pain perception.

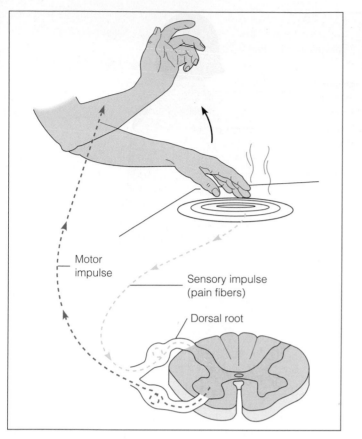

Figure 8.4 ● Proprioceptive reflex to a pain stimulus.

Table 8.2	Comparison of Acute and Chronic Pain

ACUTE PAIN	CHRONIC PAIN
Mild to severe	Mild to severe
Sympathetic nervous system responses:	Parasympathetic nervous system responses:
Increased pulse rate	Vital signs normal
Increased respiratory rate	
Elevated blood pressure	
Diaphoresis	Dry, warm skin
Dilated pupils	Pupils normal or dilated
Related to tissue injury; resolves with healing	Continues beyond healing
Client appears restless and anxious	Client appears depressed and withdrawn
Client reports pain	Client often does not mention pain unless asked
Client exhibits behavior indicative of pain: crying, rubbing area, holding area	Pain behavior often absent

behavioral activities, such as diversions, imagery, and excessive sleeping. The individual may seek out physical interventions to manage the pain, such as analgesics, massage, and exercise.

A proprioceptive reflex also occurs with the stimulation of pain receptors. Impulses travel along sensory pain fibers to the spinal cord. There they synapse with motor neurons, and the impulses travel back via motor fibers to a muscle near the site of the pain (Figure 8.4 ●). The muscle then contracts in a protective action. For example, when a person touches a hot stove, the hand reflexively draws back from the heat even before the person is aware of the pain.

NATURE OF PAIN

Pain, a subjective and personal experience, can be described in many ways. The type of pain, the point of origin, and the duration of pain are several ways that the nurse and other members of the healthcare team may describe pain.

TYPES OF PAIN

Pain may be described in terms of duration, location, or etiology. When pain lasts only through the expected recovery period from illness, injury, or surgery, it is described as **acute pain,** whether it has a sudden or slow onset and regardless of the intensity. **Chronic pain** is prolonged, usually recurring or persisting over 6 months or longer, and interferes with functioning. Chronic pain can be further classified as chronic malignant pain when associated with cancer or other life-threatening condi-

tions, or as chronic nonmalignant pain when the etiology is a nonprogressive disorder. Such disorders include cluster headaches, low back pain, and myofascial pain dysfunction. Acute pain and chronic pain result in different physiological and behavioral responses, as shown in Table 8.2.

Pain may be categorized according to its origin as cutaneous, deep somatic, or visceral. **Cutaneous pain** originates in the skin or subcutaneous tissue. A paper cut causing a sharp pain with some burning is an example of cutaneous pain. **Deep somatic pain** arises from ligaments, tendons, bones, blood vessels, and nerves. It is diffuse and tends to last longer than cutaneous pain. An ankle sprain is an example of deep somatic pain. **Visceral pain** results from stimulation of pain receptors in the abdominal cavity, cranium, and thorax. It tends to appear diffuse and often feels like deep somatic pain, that is, burning, aching, or a feeling of pressure. Visceral pain is frequently caused by stretching of the tissues, ischemia, or muscle spasms. For example, an obstructed bowel will result in visceral pain.

Pain may also be described according to where it is experienced in the body. **Radiating pain** is perceived at the source of the pain and extends to nearby tissues. For example, cardiac pain may be felt not only in the chest but also along the left shoulder and down the arm. **Referred pain** is felt in a part of the body that is considerably removed from the tissues causing the pain. For example, pain from one part of the abdominal viscera may be perceived in an area of the skin remote from the organ causing the pain (see Figure 8.5 ●).

Intractable pain is highly resistant to relief. One example is the pain from an advanced malignancy. When caring for a client experiencing intractable pain, nurses are challenged to use a number of methods, pharmacologic and nonpharmacologic, to provide pain relief.

Neuropathic pain is the result of current or past damage to the peripheral or central nervous system and may not have a stimulus, such as tissue or nerve damage, for the pain. Neuropathic

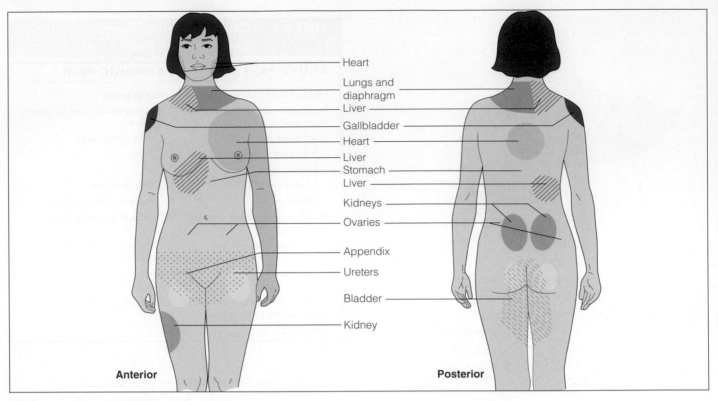

Figure 8.5 ● Sites of referred pain.

pain is long lasting, is unpleasant, and can be described as burning, dull, and aching. Episodes of sharp, shooting pain can also be experienced (Hawthorn & Redmond, 1998). Examples of this pain include trigeminal neuralgia and peripheral neuropathy.

Phantom pain, which is perceived in a body part that is missing (e.g., an amputated leg) or paralyzed by a spinal cord injury, is an example of neuropathic pain. This can be distinguished from *phantom sensation,* that is, the feeling that the missing body part is still present. The incidence of phantom pain can be reduced when analgesics are administered via epidural catheter prior to the amputation.

CONCEPTS ASSOCIATED WITH PAIN

When a person perceives pain from injured tissue, the pain threshold is reached. An individual's **pain threshold** is the amount of pain stimulation the person requires to feel pain. A person's pain threshold is fairly uniform; however, it can change. For example, the same stimuli that once produced mild pain can at another time produce intense pain. Excessive sensitivity to pain is called **hyperalgesia.**

Two additional terms used in the context of pain are pain sensation and pain reaction. **Pain sensation** can be considered the same as pain threshold; **pain reaction** includes the autonomic nervous system and behavioral responses to pain. The autonomic nervous system response is the automatic reaction that often protects the individual from further harm, for example, the automatic withdrawal of the hand from a hot stove. The behavioral response is a learned response used as a method of coping with pain.

Pain tolerance is the maximum amount and duration of pain that an individual is willing to endure. Some clients are unable to tolerate even the slightest pain, whereas others are willing to endure severe pain rather than be treated for it. Pain tolerance is widely influenced by psychological and sociocultural factors.

FACTORS INFLUENCING PAIN

Factors that influence the individual's perception of and reaction to pain include developmental stage, psychosocial development, and the environment.

DEVELOPMENTAL CONSIDERATIONS

The age and developmental stage of a client will influence both the reaction to and the expression of pain. Age variations and related nursing interventions are presented in Table 8.3.

The field of pain management for infants and children has grown significantly. It is now accepted that anatomical, physiological, and biochemical elements necessary for pain transmission are present in newborns, regardless of their gestational age. The American Academy of Pediatrics and the Canadian Paediatric Society (2000) have recommended that environmental, nonpharmacologic, and pharmacologic interventions be used to prevent, reduce, or eliminate pain in neonates. Physiological indicators may vary in infants, so behavioral observation is recommended for pain assessment (Ball & Bindler, 2003). Children may be less able than an adult to articulate their experience or needs related to pain, which may result in their pain being undertreated.

Older adults constitute a major portion of the individuals within the healthcare system. The prevalence of pain in the older population is generally higher due to both acute and chronic disease conditions. Pain threshold does not appear to

Table 8.3	Age Variations in the Pain Experience	
AGE GROUP	**PAIN PERCEPTION AND BEHAVIOR**	**SELECTED NURSING INTERVENTIONS**
Infant	Perceives pain.	Give a glucose pacifier.
	Responds to pain with increased sensitivity.	Use tactile stimulation. Play music or tapes of a heartbeat.
	Older infant tries to avoid pain; for example, turns away and physically resists.	
Toddler and Preschooler	Develops the ability to describe pain and its intensity and location.	Distract the child with toys, books, pictures. Involve the child in blowing bubbles as a way of "blowing away the pain."
	Often responds with crying and anger because child perceives pain as a threat to security.	Appeal to the child's belief in magic by using a "magic" blanket or glove to take away pain.
	Reasoning with child at this stage is not always successful.	Hold the child to provide comfort.
	May consider pain a punishment.	Explore misconceptions about pain.
	Feels sad.	
	May learn there are gender differences in pain expression.	
	Tends to hold someone accountable for the pain.	
School-age Child	Tries to be brave when facing pain.	Use imagery to turn off "pain switches."
	Rationalizes in an attempt to explain the pain.	Provide a behavioral rehearsal of what to expect and how it will look and feel.
	Responsive to explanations.	
	Can usually identify the location and describe the pain.	Provide support and nurturing.
	With persistent pain, may regress to an earlier stage of development.	
Adolescent	May be slow to acknowledge pain.	Provide opportunities to discuss pain.
	Recognizing pain or "giving in" may be considered weakness.	Provide privacy.
	Wants to appear brave in front of peers and not report pain.	Present choices for dealing with pain. Encourage music or TV for distraction.
Adult	Behaviors exhibited when experiencing pain may be gender-based behaviors learned as a child.	Deal with any misconceptions about pain.
	May ignore pain because to admit it is perceived as a sign of weakness or failure.	Focus on the client's control in dealing with the pain.
	Fear of what pain means may prevent some adults from taking action.	Allay fears and anxiety when possible.
Older Adult	May have multiple conditions presenting with vague symptoms.	Thorough history and assessment is essential.
	May perceive pain as part of the aging process.	
	May have decreased sensations or perceptions of the pain.	Spend time with the client and listen carefully.
	Lethargy, anorexia, and fatigue may be indicators of pain.	
	May withhold complaints of pain because of fear of the treatment, of any lifestyle changes that may be involved, or of becoming dependent.	Clarify misconceptions.
	May describe pain differently, that is, as "ache," "hurt," or "discomfort."	Encourage independence whenever possible.
	May consider it unacceptable to admit or show pain.	

change with aging, although the effect of analgesics may increase due to physiological changes related to drug metabolism and excretion (Eliopoulos, 2005).

PSYCHOSOCIAL CONSIDERATIONS

Family, culture, religion, and other factors influence the individual's ability to express and accept treatment modalities regarding pain.

Ethnic background and cultural heritage have long been recognized as influencing both a person's reaction to pain and the expression of that pain. Behavior related to pain is part of the socialization process. For example, individuals in one culture may learn to be expressive about pain, whereas individuals from another culture may learn to keep those feelings to themselves and not bother others. Chinese Americans are usually

stoic and therefore may request little or no pain medication. Arab Americans believe pain is punishment, and suffering is viewed as atonement. Arab American women express pain verbally to family members, whereas the men are stoic. Expression of pain by the man is viewed as an indication of weakness.

Cultural background can affect the level of pain that a person is willing to tolerate. In some Middle Eastern and African cultures, self-infliction of pain is a sign of mourning or grief. In other groups, pain may be anticipated as part of the ritualistic practices, and tolerance of pain may signify strength and endurance. There are significant variations in the expression of pain. Studies have shown that individuals of northern European descent tend to be more stoic and less expressive of their pain than individuals from southern European backgrounds.

Nurses have their own attitudes and expectations about pain. Andrews and Boyle (2003) pointed out that healthcare has been dominated by white Anglo-Saxon Protestants, and most nurses have been influenced by these values and beliefs. For example, nurses may place a higher value on silent suffering or self-control in response to pain. They may expect clients to be objective about pain and to be able to provide a detailed description of the pain. Nurses may deny or downplay the pain they observe in others (Andrews & Boyle, 2003, p. 410). Therefore, nurses must identify their own personal attitudes about pain in order to provide culturally competent care for clients in pain.

ENVIRONMENTAL CONSIDERATIONS

Environmental factors will influence a person's ability to identify and seek relief for pain. The external environment includes a variety of stimuli for pain. Objects that may contribute to pain include restrictive clothing, ill-fitting shoes, or furniture and other objects in the work and home environments that cause pressure, strain, discomfort, or pain in healthy or already painful areas of the body. The ability to move freely influences the person's ability to avoid or control painful stimuli.

Family members and support systems, including members of the health team, are factors in the external environment that must be considered. A strange environment such as a hospital, with its noises, lights, and activity, can compound pain. The lonely person who is without a support network may perceive pain as severe, whereas the person who has supportive people around may perceive less pain. Some people prefer to withdraw when they are in pain; others prefer the distraction of people and activity around them. Family caregivers can be a significant support for a person in pain. With the increase in outpatient and home care, families are assuming an increased responsibility for pain management. Education related to the assessment and management of pain can positively affect the perceived quality of life for both clients and their caregivers (McCaffery & Pasero, 1999).

Expectations of significant others can affect a person's perceptions of and responses to pain. In some situations, girls may be permitted to express pain more openly than boys. Family role can also affect how a person perceives or responds to pain. For instance, a single mother supporting three children may ignore pain because of her need to stay on the job. The presence of support people often changes a client's reaction to pain. For example, toddlers often tolerate pain more readily when supportive parents or nurses are nearby.

The internal environment includes individual perceptions and experiences related to pain. Previous pain experiences alter a client's sensitivity to pain. People who have experienced pain or who have been exposed to the suffering of someone close are often more threatened by anticipated pain than people without a pain experience. The success or lack of success of pain relief measures influences a person's expectations for relief. For example, a person who has tried several pain relief measures without success may have little hope about the helpfulness of nursing interventions.

Some clients may accept pain more readily than others, depending on the circumstances. A client who associates the pain with a positive outcome may withstand the pain amazingly well. For example, a woman giving birth to a child or an athlete undergoing knee surgery to prolong his career may tolerate pain better because of the benefit associated with it. These clients may view the pain as a temporary inconvenience rather than a potential threat or disruption to daily life.

By contrast, clients with unrelenting chronic pain may suffer more intensely. They may respond with despair, anxiety, and depression because they cannot attach a positive significance or purpose to the pain. In this situation, the pain may be looked upon as a threat to body image or lifestyle and as a sign of possible impending death.

Anxiety often accompanies pain. The threat of the unknown and the inability to control the pain or the events surrounding it often augment the pain perception. Fatigue also reduces a person's ability to cope, thereby increasing pain perception. When pain interferes with sleep, fatigue and muscle tension often result and increase the pain; thus a cycle of pain–fatigue–pain develops. People who believe that they have control of their pain have decreased fear and anxiety, which decreases their pain perception. A perception of lacking control or a sense of helplessness tends to increase pain perception. Clients who are able to express pain to an attentive listener and participate in pain management decisions can increase a sense of control and decrease pain perception.

ASSESSMENT

Accurate and timely client assessment is imperative for effective pain management. Poorly managed or untreated pain will influence every aspect of an individual's health and well-being. Pain assessment is considered the fifth vital sign. The strategy of linking pain assessment to routine vital sign assessment and documentation ensures pain assessment for all clients. Because pain is subjective and experienced uniquely by each person, nurses need to assess all factors affecting the pain experience—physiological, psychological, behavioral, emotional, and sociocultural.

The extent and frequency of the pain assessment varies according to the situation. For clients experiencing acute or severe pain, the nurse may focus only on location, quality, severity, and early intervention. Clients with less severe or chronic pain can usually provide a more detailed description of the experience. Frequency of pain assessment usually depends on the pain control measures being used and the clinical circumstances. For example, in the initial postoperative period, pain is often assessed whenever vital signs are taken, which may be as often as every 15 minutes and then extended to every 2 to 4 hours. Following pain management interventions, pain intensity should be reassessed at an interval appropriate for the intervention. For example, following the intravenous administration of morphine, the severity of pain should be reassessed in 20 to 30 minutes.

Because many people will not voice their pain unless asked about it, pain assessments must be initiated by the nurse. It is also essential that nurses listen to and rely on the client's perceptions of pain. Believing the person experiencing and conveying the perceptions is crucial in establishing a sense of trust.

Pain assessments consist of two major components: (a) a pain history to obtain facts from the client and (b) direct observation of behavioral and physiological responses of the client. The goal of assessment is to gain an objective understanding of a subjective experience.

PAIN HISTORY

A detailed history to obtain subjective data from the client is essential for successful treatment and relief from pain. During the history taking and focused interview, the nurse provides clients an opportunity to express in their own words how they view pain. It also gives the nurse an opportunity to observe the body language or nonverbal communication of the client. The responses made by the client will help the nurse understand the meaning of pain to the client and the coping strategies being used. Each person's pain experience is unique, and the client is the best interpreter of the pain experience.

FOCUSED INTERVIEW

During the focused interview, qualitative and quantitative information regarding pain will be collected. The qualitative data will include location, duration, and characteristics of the pain. The quantitative data will provide information regarding the intensity of the pain. This subjective data will be obtained using closed and open-ended questions. Follow-up questions may be needed for greater clarification regarding the pain experience. Sample questions are provided for the nurse to use to obtain the subjective data. This list of questions is not all-inclusive but represents the types of questions required in a comprehensive focused interview. Additional questions specific to a body system will be found in the assessment chapters in Unit III of this text. ∞

Questions Regarding Location

1. Where is your pain?
2. Does the pain move or is it just in one place?
3. Are you able to point to or put your finger on the painful area?
   Questions 1 to 3 give the client the opportunity to specifically locate the pain and identify the body parts involved. An alternative method would be to give the client a picture of the body and ask him or her to color the areas of the body affected by the pain.

Questions Regarding Intensity

1. How bad is the pain now?
2. Using a scale of 0 to 10, with 0 being no pain and 10 being the worst possible pain, how would you rate your present pain level?
   Questions 1 and 2 give the client the opportunity to describe the present level or intensity of the pain being experienced at the present time.
3. An alternative method would be to give the client a pain intensity scale (see Figure 7.14 on p. 119 ∞) and ask the client to place a mark to correspond to the pain being experienced. The nurse should be sure to use an appropriate tool for the client. Rating scales include use of numbers and pictures, and they are language specific.

Questions Regarding Quality

1. What does the pain feel like?
2. Describe your pain.
   Questions 1 and 2 give clients the opportunity to describe the pain using their own words.
3. An alternative method would be to list the possible descriptive terms and ask the client to respond yes or no to each descriptor. The terms include *deep, superficial, burning, aching, pressure like, dull, sharp, shooting, stabbing, piercing, crushing,* or *tingling.*
   This is a comprehensive and easy way to elicit information regarding the quality of the pain.

Questions Regarding Pain Pattern

1. Do you have pain now?
2. When did the pain begin?
3. Is the pain constant or intermittent?
4. How long does the pain last?
   These questions give the client the opportunity to explain a pattern associated with pain.

Questions Regarding Precipitating Factors

1. What do you think started the pain?
   This question elicits client perceptions about the cause of pain.
2. What were you doing just before the pain started?
   This question is intended to identify triggers or factors related to the onset of pain.
3. Have you been under a great deal of stress lately?
   This is an attempt to determine a link to psychosocial factors or psychogenic sources of pain.

Questions Regarding Pain Relief

1. What have you done to relieve the pain?
2. Did it work?
3. Have you used this before? When?
4. Why do you think it worked (or didn't work) this time?
   Questions 1 to 4 provide the client the opportunity to discuss what actions have been taken to help decrease or eliminate the pain.
5. An alternative method to questions 1 to 4 would be to list the possible strategies and ask the client to respond yes or no to each strategy. These include:
   Do you take a prescribed pain pill?
   Do you take an over-the-counter medicine for the pain?
   Do you change your diet in any way when you have pain?
   Do you use an ice pack or heating pad on the pain?
   Do you use prayer?
   Do you or a family member perform some ritual?
   Do you rest when you have the pain?
   Do you do anything that has not been mentioned?

   When the client responds yes, the nurse must then determine the effectiveness of the strategy.

Questions Regarding Impact on Activities of Daily Living

1. Describe your daily activities.
2. How well are you able to perform these activities?
3. Does the pain in any way hinder your ability to function?
   Questions 1 to 3 encourage the client to describe the ability to function independently on a daily basis.
4. An alternative method would be to list possible daily activities and ask the client to respond with a yes or no if the pain hinders the ability to perform the actions.

   Examples include:

   Do you have difficulty sleeping?

   Has your appetite changed?

   Are you able to get out of bed without help?

   Do you have difficulty walking, standing, sitting, or climbing stairs?

   Are you able to perform your work activities?

   Are you able to concentrate at school, work, or home?

   Are you able to drive? To ride in a car?

   Do you have mood swings?

   Do you find yourself being short with family members and friends?

Questions Related to Coping Strategies

1. Describe how you deal or cope with the pain.
2. Are you in a support group for pain?
3. What do you do to decrease the pain so you can function and feel better?
   Questions 1 to 3 enable the client to share his or her coping strategies. These may be unique to the individual and may reflect family values and cultural beliefs.

Questions Related to Emotional Responses

1. Emotionally, how does the pain make you feel?
2. Does your pain make you feel depressed?
3. Does your pain ever make you feel anxious, tired, or exhausted?
   Questions 1 to 3 give the nurse the opportunity to explore with the client emotional feelings. These feelings are often related to the type, intensity, and duration of pain.

PHYSIOLOGICAL RESPONSES

Assessment of client behaviors will include the collection of objective data. There are wide variations in nonverbal responses to pain. For clients who are very young, aphasic, confused, or disoriented, nonverbal expressions may be the only means of communicating pain. Facial expression is often the first indication of pain, and it may be the only one. Clenched teeth, tightly shut eyes, open somber eyes, biting of the lower lip, and other facial grimaces may be indicative of pain. Vocalizations like moaning and groaning or crying and screaming are sometimes associated with pain.

Immobilization of the body or a part of the body may also indicate pain. The client with chest pain often holds the left arm across the chest. A person with abdominal pain may assume the position of greatest comfort, often with the knees and hips flexed, and move reluctantly.

Purposeless body movements can also indicate pain—for example, tossing and turning in bed or flinging the arms about. Involuntary movements such as a reflexive jerking away from a needle inserted through the skin indicate pain. An adult may be able to control this reflex; however, a child may be unable or unwilling to do so.

Rhythmic body movements or rubbing may indicate pain. An adult or child may assume a fetal position and rock back and forth when experiencing abdominal pain. During labor a woman may massage her abdomen rhythmically with her hands. Because behavioral responses can be controlled, they may not be very revealing. When pain is chronic there are rarely overt behavioral responses because the individual develops personal coping styles for dealing with pain, discomfort, or suffering.

Physiological responses vary with the origin and duration of the pain. Early in the onset of acute pain the sympathetic nervous system is stimulated, resulting in increased blood pressure, pulse rate, respiratory rate, pallor, diaphoresis, and pupil dilation. The body does not sustain the increased sympathetic function over a prolonged period. Therefore, the sympathetic nervous system adapts, making the physiological responses less evident or even absent. Physiological responses are most likely to be absent in people with chronic pain because of central nervous system adaptation. Thus, it is important that the nurse assess more than the physiological responses, because they may be poor indicators of pain.

ASSESSMENT TOOLS

Assessment tools have been developed to help the client use measurable terms to describe the pain being experienced. The same tool will help the nurse obtain precise data needed to implement treatment modalities and evaluate pain relief.

The tool should be easy to use, tabulate, and score. It should be in the language of the client, and it should be used consistently. The nurse must teach the client, family members, and other members of the healthcare team correct use of the tool. All tools have advantages and disadvantages. It is the responsibility of the nurse to identify these factors before implementation of the appropriate tool.

Tools used for pain assessment are designed and classified as unidimensional or multidimensional tools. A unidimensional tool will seek data regarding one aspect of pain. Many times this single element relates to the intensity of pain. Numeric rating scales, visual analogue scales, the Oucher Scale, and the Poker Chip Scale are examples of unidimensional tools.

A multidimensional tool will seek data regarding more than one factor of pain. These tools look at intensity and other elements, including affective and sensory elements. The McGill Pain Questionnaire, short and long form, is an example of a multidimensional tool.

UNIDIMENSIONAL TOOLS

Assessment tools employed by the nurse help clients describe their pain. Unidimensional tools are used to help determine the client's level of acute pain. The tool is called unidimensional since it assesses one aspect of pain. These tools can be used in any clinical setting across the age span. It is important for the nurse to use the tool consistently throughout the assessment, treatment, and reassessment of the client. Because they measure just one element of the pain experience, unidimensional tools can lead to inadequate use of treatment modalities.

The Numeric Rating Scale asks the client to describe pain intensity with a number. The selected number then equates to pain severity. The Simple Verbal Descriptive Scale is another unidimensional tool. The individual is presented with six descriptive words and is asked to select one that corresponds to the present level of intensity.

The Body Diagram tool presents an outline of the body. The individual is asked to mark the picture showing the location of the pain. Shading of the body parts by the client will describe the intensity of the pain. The Oucher Scale has been designed for children. Pictures of faces ranging from neutral to distressed are presented, and the child selects the one representing his or her level of pain.

MULTIDIMENSIONAL TOOLS

The multidimensional assessment tools assess two or more elements of pain. These tools go beyond pain intensity. They assess the nature, location, mood, and impact of pain regarding activities of daily living. The McGill Pain Questionnaire is available in a long and short form, and is used when pain is prolonged. The long form measures intensity, location, pattern, sensory dimensions, and affective dimensions of pain. The short form measures intensity, sensory dimensions, and affective dimensions of pain.

The Brief Pain Inventory is another multidimensional scale used for assessment of pain. This tool provides information on pain and how pain interferes with the person's ability to function. Questions on this tool address medications, relief, individual beliefs, and quality of life.

Many tools are available to assist the client and nurse to assess, treat, and evaluate pain, and to measure the effectiveness of the treatment modalities. Tools must be appropriate for the age, culture, language, and cognitive abilities of the individual.

This chapter emphasizes pain as both physiological and emotional. Pain perception may be increased when a client also experiences anxiety, fatigue, or depression. The psychological aspect of pain is a subjective and personal experience influenced by age, culture, religion, and past experience with pain.

Pain assessment requires respect for the client's beliefs and attitudes about pain. Establishing a caring relationship, listening to the client, and using comprehensive interview techniques are essential in the assessment of pain. Numeric scales and surveys assist the nurse in quantifying pain.

Successful management of pain is dependent upon an accurate assessment of the type and degree of pain the client is experiencing as well as the identification of underlying causes.

The assessment data is used by the nurse in interaction with the client and other health professionals to develop a plan for pain management. The holistic approach to nursing assessment of pain permits the plan to reflect the individual beliefs, needs, and wishes of the client.

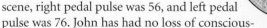

Application Through Critical Thinking

CASE STUDY

John Taylor, age 12, was hit by a car while riding his bicycle. He has several injuries and is brought to the emergency department at the local community hospital. The emergency technician informs the staff his right leg was splinted at the scene, right pedal pulse was 56, and left pedal pulse was 76. John has had no loss of consciousness; however, his respirations are 32 and shallow. He is crying and tells the nurse he has a lot of pain in his right leg and cannot seem to catch his breath.

The emergency department physician asks for a chest x-ray immediately, starts supportive oxygen therapy, and gives direction for administration of pain medication.

► Critical Thinking Questions

1. How and when should the nurse assess the pain in this patient?
2. What pain scale tool, if any, would be appropriate to use?
3. What additional information regarding pain is needed?
4. What role will the parents have at this time?

► Applying Nursing Diagnoses

1. What diagnostic statement from NANDA is appropriate for the client experiencing pain?
2. Identify the subjective and objective data for John Taylor that support the NANDA nursing diagnosis of *pain, acute*.

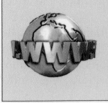

Please refer to the Companion Website at www.prenhall.com/damico and click on Chapter 8, the Application Through Critical Thinking module, to answer these and additional questions. In addition, complete NCLEX-RN® review questions and other interactive resources for this chapter.
► Critical Thinking questions
► Extended Nursing Diagnosis challenge
► Documentation activity

EXPLORE MediaLink

Additional resources for this chapter are found on the Student CD-ROM accompanying this textbook and on the Companion Website.

CD-ROM CONTENT

Content for this chapter includes:
Objectives
Key Concepts
NCLEX-RN® Review Questions
Model Documentation Forms
Audio Glossary
Games and Challenges
Head-to-Toe Physical Examination Video

COMPANION WEBSITE CONTENT

www.prenhall.com/damico

Content for this chapter includes:
Objectives
NCLEX-RN® Review Questions

Application Through Critical Thinking
   Case Study Teaching Plan Challenge
MediaLinks
MediaLink Application
Tool Box
   Types of Pain Stimuli
   Comparison of Acute and Chronic Pain
   Age Variations in the Pain Experience
New York Times

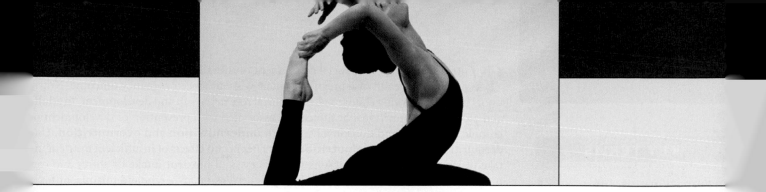

9

Nutritional Assessment

MEDIALINK

www.prenhall.com/damico

The CD-ROM in the back of this textbook and the Media-Link website contain NCLEX-RN® review questions, interactive exercises, case study challenges, animations, videos, documentation and checklist forms, and review materials. For a complete listing of the media content specific to Chapter 9, see the Explore MediaLink at the end of the chapter.

*N*utritional health is a crucial component of overall health across the life span. The nutritional health of a pregnant female will influence pregnancy outcome. Nutritional health in growing children plays a central role in growth and development. In adults and older adults, nutritional health can be associated with prevention or development of chronic disease in conditions involving both **undernutrition** and **overnutrition.** Undernutrition, also called **malnutrition,** describes health effects of insufficient nutrient intake or stores. Overnutrition results from excesses in nutrient intake or stores and can manifest itself in conditions such as obesity, hypertension, hypercholesterolemia, or toxic levels of stored vitamins or minerals.

The determination of an individual's nutritional status is based upon the foundation of a thorough nutritional assessment. The assessment portion of the nursing care process incorporates the gathering and interpretation of data often used as part of a nutritional assessment. This data then creates the base for later development of appropriate nursing and nutritional interventions aimed at preserving or improving nutritional health.

DEFINING NUTRITIONAL HEALTH

Nutritional health can be defined as the physical result of the balance between nutrient intake and nutritional requirements. For example, an individual who consumes excess saturated fat may be at risk for elevated blood cholesterol and cardiovascular disease. This person may therefore be considered to have poor nutritional health due to overnutrition. A pregnant female who consumes less than required amounts of folic acid may place her unborn child at risk for certain birth defects, such as neural tube defects, and could be considered in poor nutritional health due to undernutrition. A client who consumes adequate nutrition to meet individual needs and avoids habitual excesses and insufficiencies would be considered in good nutritional health.

Many factors can influence nutritional health. When gathering data for a nutritional assessment, it is important to realize common risk factors for a poor nutritional status. Overnutrition in the form of excess dietary intake of fat, especially saturated fat, has been associated with an increased risk of atherosclerosis. Overweight and obesity are linked with increased risk of hypertension, cardiovascular disease, type 2 diabetes, some cancers, degenerative joint disease, and other conditions. Additionally, excess body weight has been shown to increase the risk of all-cause mortality in adults 30 to 74 years of age. In the United States, 63% of males and 55% of females 20 to 74 years of age are considered overweight or obese, a statistic that has increased by 25% over the past 30 years. The prevalence of obesity and overweight has doubled in children and adolescents in the last 30 years to 13% and 14%, respectively. Excess alcohol intake is associated with chronic liver disease and cirrhosis, the 12th leading cause of death in the United States according to the National Center for Health Statistics at the Centers for Disease Control and Prevention (CDC).

Undernutrition is less common than overnutrition in the United States, but can have devastating physical health consequences when **protein-calorie malnutrition** or other nutrient deficiencies develop. Undernutrition can lead to growth faltering, compromised immune status, poor wound healing, muscle loss, physical and functional decline, and lack of proper development. Generally, individuals at risk for undernutrition include those who have a chronic illness or are poor, elderly, hospitalized, restrictive eaters (from chronic dieting or disordered eating), or alcoholics. An individual can have both overnutrition and undernutrition, such as an overweight child who consumes no fruit or vegetables. Box 9.1 outlines additional risk factors for overnutrition and undernutrition to consider when conducting a nutrition assessment.

The U.S. Department of Health and Human Services, Office of Disease Prevention and Health Promotion, has established a collaborative public health initiative called *Healthy People* aimed at increasing the quality and years of healthy life in the U.S. population and

Box 9.1	**Risk Factors for Poor Nutritional Health**

Undernutrition

- Chronic disease, acute illness, or injury
- Multiple medications
- Food insecurity—lack of free access to adequate and safe food
- Restrictive eating due to chronic dieting, disordered eating, faddism, or food beliefs
- Alcohol abuse
- Depression, bereavement, loneliness, social isolation
- Poor dental health
- Decreased knowledge or skills about food preparation and recommendations
- Extreme age—premature infants or adults over 80 years of age

Overnutrition

- Excess intake of fat, sugar, calories, or nutrients
- Alcohol abuse
- Sedentary lifestyle
- Decreased knowledge or skills about food preparation and recommendations

Box 9.2	**Cultural and Socioeconomic Influences on Nutritional Health**

Overweight and Obesity

- Over 60% of adults age 20 to 74 years are overweight, with 27% classified as obese.
- Up to 15% of children age 6 to19 years are overweight.
- Prevalence of obesity has increased in the three major racial and ethnic groups.
- Prevalence of overweight is highest among Mexican American males.
- Prevalence of obesity is highest among Mexican American females.
- Hypertension, a comorbidity of overweight and obesity, affects 23% of adults in the United States.
- Prevalence of hypertension is highest among the Black population.
- Adults of low socioeconomic status have twice the rate of overweight or obesity compared to those of medium and high socioeconomic status.

Undernutrition

- Undernutrition can contribute to growth retardation. By definition, 5% of children would be expected to be at the 5th percentile for height. However, up to 15% of Black children have growth retardation in the first year of life, and 11% of Asian and Pacific Islander children have growth retardation during the second year.
- Up to 60% of older adults in dependent care or hospitals are malnourished.
- Adequate folic acid and iron status are important for healthy outcomes during pregnancy. Pregnant Mexican American females are more likely than other ethnic groups to have iron deficiency and low folic acid levels. Females of lower economic status and those with less education are also more likely to have inadequate folic acid or iron status.
- Black women and adolescents under age 15 years are more likely to have insufficient gestational weight gain and deliver low birth weight babies than other populations.

Poverty and Food Insecurity

- Among Americans, the prevalence of poverty was 12.1% in 2002.
- Children under age 18 experience a 16.7% poverty rate.
- Prevalence of poverty is highest among Black (24.1%) and Hispanics (21.8%).

Source: Healthy People 2010. 19 Nutrition and Overweight. www.healthypeople.gov/Document/HTML/VOLUME2/19 Nutrition.htm; retrieved 06/24/2005.

reducing health disparities. The *Healthy People 2010* objectives targeting overweight, obesity, and issues of undernutrition are important reminders to the clinician of the central role nutrition plays in overall health across the life span. The increasing prevalence of overweight and obesity in the United States, as well as the statistics on nutritional health disparities, illustrate the importance of nutritional screening and assessment as the first step toward reaching these important goals. The *Healthy People 2010* feature on page 153 lists objectives that influence nutritional health. Box 9.2 outlines the cultural and socioeconomic influences that may affect nutritional health.

NUTRITIONAL ASSESSMENT

A nutritional assessment is the foundation upon which nursing diagnoses are developed and later the implementation of goals and objectives in the nursing care process are created. The prevention or treatment of malnutrition and overnutrition first requires a nutritional assessment. Determination of an individual's nutritional status should be accomplished while gathering data for a nursing assessment.

Nutritional assessment techniques and tools vary in their level of sophistication and depth. No one piece of data can give a complete nutritional assessment. Many parameters used to assess nutritional status can be affected by nonnutritional influences such as disease, medication, or environment. This illustrates the need to gather data from varying resources. Generally, an assessment done using multiple variables will be more valuable than an assessment made with limited data. In some healthcare situations, not all parameters or data are available. The nurse must rely upon available information and sharp clinical judgment when making an assessment.

Varying medical diagnoses or issues specific to the life span will also influence pertinent parameters and techniques used in assessing a client's nutritional status. For example, measuring waist circumference may be of use when assessing potential overnutrition in adults, but would be of little nutritional use when assessing either a client with ascites or a pregnant female.

A registered dietitian (RD) is generally responsible for completing a comprehensive nutritional assessment in most acute or long-term care settings; a nurse may do this as well and is most often the frontline clinician to obtain the data needed for a nutritional assessment. A nurse is ideally situated to identify nutritionally at-risk clients needing further intervention targeting nutritional health.

The components used in a nutritional assessment include nutritional history, the physical assessment, anthropometric measurements, and laboratory values. Several validated assessment tools exist to streamline the nutritional assessment process for use in a variety of healthcare settings or with specific populations. Other tools exist that simply screen for risk factors for poor nutritional health and facilitate necessary referrals to appropriate clinicians.

NUTRITIONAL HISTORY

A careful nutritional history is part of a comprehensive nutritional assessment and is best accomplished using more than one tool. A diet recall, a food frequency questionnaire, and a food record are components of a nutritional history that can be complemented with a focused interview for more specific information.

Diet Recall

A **diet recall,** also called a 24-hour recall, can be done quickly in most settings to obtain a snapshot assessment of dietary intake. A client is asked to verbally recall all food, beverages, and nutritional supplements or products consumed in a set 24-hour period. Obtaining a recall for both a weekday and one weekend day will strengthen the data obtained. The nurse should ask primarily open-ended questions to appear nonjudgmental and not hint at "correct" answers to questions. The nurse should begin the diet recall by asking, "Tell me what you ate yesterday (or on a specific day). When was the first time you had something to eat or drink in the day?" This type of questioning avoids asking the assuming "What did you have for breakfast?" Clients may feel judged if they admit they skip breakfast or too embarrassed to admit missing a meal. The result may be an inaccurate recall where clients contrive answers they feel the nurse is seeking. Gentle prompting to obtain complete information is often needed. The nurse should ask about all food from meals and snacks, all liquids, including alcohol, and any use of nutritional supplements such as herbs, vitamins and minerals, or diet and sports nutritional products. One must determine whether fortified versions of common foods are consumed in order to assess nutrient intake accurately. Many foods are now fortified and should not be overlooked as significant sources of vitamins and minerals. Cereals and juices are examples of fortified foods to which nutrients not normally found in the product, such as calcium, have been added. A family member may participate in the interview with the permission of the client or if the client is unable to give a recall. Accuracy of a secondhand recall, even from a family member, has been found to be variable.

A best estimate of portion sizes will improve the accuracy of a recall. It is easy to over- and underestimate portion sizes of foods and liquids without a visual comparison. Life-size culturally appropriate food models are available. Digital photographs are less cumbersome and easily available as well. It is not always convenient to carry facsimiles to different settings where the nurse may be interviewing a client. In such cases, use of the food analogies in Figure 9.1 • can be helpful.

There are drawbacks to exclusive use of a diet recall for a nutritional history. A 24-hour recall is simply a 1-day example of intake and may not be indicative of normal habits. Other types and amounts of intake may occur on different days that were not assessed. Clients may have significant food habits that occur occasionally but not on the day recalled. The use of dietary supplements or alcohol often does not occur in the same fashion each day, yet it is crucial information to assess. Many other important data related to diet could be overlooked by relying on the recall alone. The accuracy of the recall relies heavily on the

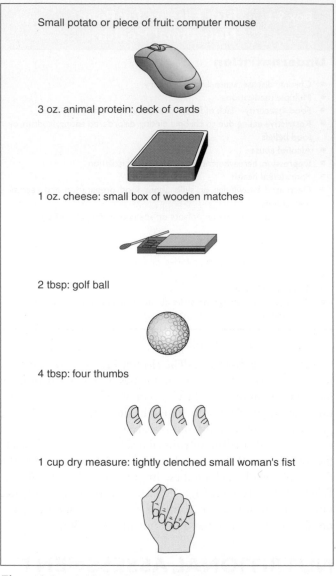

Small potato or piece of fruit: computer mouse

3 oz. animal protein: deck of cards

1 oz. cheese: small box of wooden matches

2 tbsp: golf ball

4 tbsp: four thumbs

1 cup dry measure: tightly clenched small woman's fist

Figure 9.1 • Analogies for estimating portion size.

memory of the client and good interviewing skills of the nurse. Repeated diet recalls taken during subsequent healthcare visits can be used for comparison purposes and validation of intake.

Underreporting bias can occur with all parts of a nutritional history and may become apparent during the recall. Clients seeking the social approval of the nurse or wanting to avoid disapproval for their habits may underreport. Underreporting occurs for all ages and is seen more often in smokers, the obese, and individuals with lower educational and socioeconomic levels. Additionally, alcohol and drug use are frequently underreported. A nonjudgmental approach during the nutritional history will provide an environment conducive to full answers by the client. Combining the recall with a food frequency assessment and a focused interview will yield the best information upon which to base an assessment.

Food Frequency Questionnaire

A **food frequency questionnaire** assesses intake of a variety of food groups on a daily, weekly, or longer basis. This questionnaire helps to fill in some of the missing data not captured by a 24-hour

Table 9.1	Food Frequency Questionnaire					
FOOD	**VARIETY**	**TYPE**	**AMOUNT PER DAY**	**AMOUNT PER WEEK**	**LESS THAN ONCE PER WEEK (LIST)**
Fruit	Juice	apple	12 oz		
	Fresh	melon		1 cup	
	Canned/frozen	none			
Vegetables	Green	varied		1–2 x	
	Other	squash		1x	
Dairy	Milk	low fat	2 cups		
	Cheese				1x month
	Yogurt	never			
Protein	Animal	poultry or fish	each night		
	Plant	soyburger or tofu		1–2x	
Fats	Saturated	butter	1–2 pats		
	Unsaturated	olive oil		tbsp	
Fluids	General	water	4 oz 4x with meds		
	Caffeine	tea	each a.m.		
	Alcohol	wine		3x	
Sweets and Sugars		cookies	2x		
Supplements	Vitamin/mineral	multivitamin	one		
	Herbal	echinacea			4–5x year for cold
	Other: Over-the-counter weight loss product	cannot recall ingredients			tried once and stopped, complains of feeling dizzy

recall to provide a more balanced assessment of intake. For example, a 24-hour recall may indicate no fruit intake while a food frequency assessment finds two servings of fruit and one serving of juice daily. Food frequency questionnaires can be formal instruments composed of a checklist of food groups and foods or shorter questionnaires aimed at gathering general information. All food, beverage, and supplement groups should be included. Clients can fill out longer checklists before or after an interview but may find such tools cumbersome. Shorter questionnaires can be administered verbally and are more practical. Table 9.1 is an example of a basic food frequency questionnaire.

Food Record

Keeping a food record or diary for up to 3 days can provide supplemental information for a nutritional history. Recording two sequential weekdays and a weekend day works well. Food diaries longer than 3 days in length tend to be recorded retrospectively with a loss of accuracy. Underreporting bias should also be considered when evaluating a food diary.

Focused Nutritional History Interview

A diet recall, food frequency questionnaire, or food diary can be used alone or in combination as parameters in a quick nutritional assessment. Conducting a more focused interview along with these tools, either as part of a nursing assessment or just concerning nutrition, will give the clearest picture of nutritional status.

A nutrition-focused interview can easily dovetail with a diet recall. As the recall is conducted, pertinent ancillary questions can be asked. For example, a client may report drinking cranberry juice at breakfast because of intolerance to citrus fruits. The nurse could then use that cue to ask if there are other intolerances or food allergies, before getting back on track to the recall. The remainder of the needed nutrition history data can be gathered from the client and the medical chart after the recall portion of the interview. This more extensive form of a nutritional history assesses current habits but also can assess former habits. Past chronic dieting, supplement use, and therapeutic diets are examples of important historical data to gather. Box 9.3 outlines data topics to gather during the focused interview in addition to diet recall data. Table 9.2 is an example of a nutritional history form combining diet recall, food frequency, and focused interview data.

PHYSICAL ASSESSMENT

The physical assessment portion of a nutritional assessment consists of two parts: **anthropometric** measurements and a head-to-toe physical assessment of a client. Anthropometric measurements include any scientific measurement of the body. Pertinent data from the medical history and examination should be considered during this portion of a nutritional assessment. The healthcare setting and the client's needs dictate the depth of data gathered. Height, weight, and measurements of body fat and muscle composition are anthropometric measurements. At times, estimated measurements and alternative techniques for obtaining anthropometric data may be necessary due to specific circumstances that make standard measurement difficult or impossible.

Height

Measurement of height is needed in adults to make an accurate assessment of weight status. In children, height is monitored on a continuum to assess growth and, indirectly, nutritional status. See Chapter 7 for accurate height assessment methods. ⌘

Box 9.3	Nutritional History Data

Food

- All meals and snacks
- All liquids, including water, alcohol, and caffeinated beverages
- Use of fortified foods
- Preparation methods
- Portion sizes
- Grocery habits

Beliefs and Practices

- Adherence to a therapeutic diet for medical reasons or due to food allergy or food intolerance
- Cultural or religious influences on food choices and practices
- Faddism—trendy food and nutrition beliefs
- Lifestyle diet choices—vegetarianism, vegan diet, avoidance of certain foods or food groups
- **Pica**—if present: types of substances eaten, source, and amounts
- Meal patterns—number and frequency of meals and snacks, missed meals, location of meals

Supplement and Medication Use

- Vitamin and mineral use—dose, frequency, and constituents
- Herbal use—dose, frequency, and constituents
- Over-the-counter weight loss or sports supplements—dose, frequency, and ingredients
- Over-the-counter and prescription medications to assess for drug-nutrient interactions or drug-herb interactions

Socioeconomic and Educational Influences

- Education and literacy level
- Knowledge and skills related to food and nutrition
- Social environment—assess for isolation and social support system
- General economic status and access to adequate food (food security)
- Functional capacity related to Activities of Daily Living (ADL) and Independent Activities of Daily Living (IADL) (such as shopping, meal preparation, self-feeding)
- Activity level
- Presence of substance abuse—drugs, alcohol, which can interfere with adequate diet

Box 9.4	Calculating Weight Loss Percentage

A community health nurse is visiting the senior center for a seasonal flu shot clinic. Miss M., an 80-year-old female, complains that she needs to sew new elastic into her skirt as the old elastic is not working to keep the skirt on her waistline. The nurse wonders if she has lost some weight since the last visit and weighs her. She weighs 108 lb, down from 120 lb 6 months ago.

(120 lb prior weight − 108 lb current weight)/120 lb prior weight =
12 lb weight loss / 120 lb prior weight = 0.10
0.10 × 100 = 10% weight loss in 6 months

lowed in children and pregnant females to monitor growth and development. Weight guidelines for children and pregnant females are outlined in the Nutritional Assessment Across the Life Span section on pages 149 and 150. When obtaining a weight history, the nurse should look for prior documentation of actual weight if available. Otherwise, open-ended questions can be asked such as, "When was the last time you were weighed?" followed by, "What did you weigh then?" The nurse may also ask for weights at specific points in time as a cross-check: "What did you weigh this past summer before coming to college?" The nurse should not simply ask, "Has your weight changed recently?" as the client may not have an accurate answer or not want to divulge any known gain or loss. The nurse can discern whether weight change has occurred by asking for specific weight information and calculating any noted differences.

Unintentional weight loss of 5% of body weight or more over a month or 10% or more over 6 months is considered clinically significant and warrants attention. Weight change is calculated using the following formula.

$$[(\text{prior weight} - \text{current weight}) / \text{prior weight}] \times 100 = \% \text{ weight change}$$

Box 9.4 outlines an example of calculations used to determine percent weight change.

Body Mass Index

Body mass index (BMI) is widely used to assess appropriate weight for height using the following formula: BMI = weight (kg)/ height^2 (meters). Parameters have been established to delineate underweight, healthy weight, and overweight standards in adults based on current scientific findings of morbidity and mortality prevalence associated with various BMI values. The National Heart, Lung, and Blood Institute (NHLBI), along with WHO, have established internationally used classifications for BMI, which are outlined in Table 9.3. Many charts, tables, and nomograms exist to make BMI calculations quick and easy for clinical application.

Exclusive use of BMI as an indicator of weight status makes the assumption that all individuals have equal body composition at each given weight. Also, it assumes that every person of the same weight has the same amount of muscle mass, body fat, and bone mineral content. This generalization has not been found to be true and therefore represents a clinical limitation to the use of BMI

When no means of obtaining measured height is feasible, self-reported height may be used. Every effort should be made to obtain a current measured height, but this is not always possible. The accuracy of self-reported heights can be questionable. Men, women, and adolescents have been reported to overstate self-reported height by up to 2 cm. Adults over the age of 60 years have been reported to overstate height by approximately 2.5 cm. When self-reported heights are used, documentation should note this.

Weight

Current body weight and weight history are essential components of a nutritional assessment. Every effort should be made to obtain actual weight since self-reported weights are often underreported in men and women. In the individual with undetected weight loss, self-reported weight could delay proper nutritional intervention by masking the clinical change. See Chapter 7 for accurate methods to determine the client's weight. ⊂⊃

Weight history is crucial to determine the presence of any intentional or unplanned weight losses. Weight history is also fol-

Table 9.2   Nutrition Assessment Form

NUTRITION EVALUATION

Name: ....   Date: ....

Home Address: ....   Referred By: ....

....

Phone: ....

Age: ....   Signed Consent/Date: ....

Height (Ht).................	Weight (Wt).............	Recent wt change	Max/Min wts.................	Client goal ....
Body fat %.................	Wt Hx	Exercise	Ex. freq/duration	Other activities ....
Medical Hx/Dx	Rx and OTC meds.........	Vits/minerals................	Supplements.................	Herbs ....
Previous Diets	Food allergies/ intolerances..................	Food prep/refrig	Restrictive? .... Binge?........................ Purge?........................ Laxatives?................... Other?........................	Living with ....

Diet Hx: ....   Diet Hx: ....

M-F ....   Weekends ....

FOOD FREQUENCY

Fruit (indicate day/week/other)

vit C ....

other ....

....

Vegetables

green ....

other ....

Grains/starch

whole grain...

other ....

Dairy (indicate day/week/other)

milk/yogurt ....

cheese..

other ....

Animal protein

....

....

Plant protein

....

....

Fats (indicate day/week/other)

saturated..

polyunsaturated ....

monounsaturated ....

Sugars/sweets

....

....

Fluids-water

other ....

caffeinated ....

alcohol...

Source: Provided courtesy of Sheila Tucker, MA, RD, LDN.

---

alone when assessing weight. Athletic people with little body fat and ample muscle mass can be classified as overweight using BMI despite a visual assessment that reveals a high level of fitness. Likewise, an individual's BMI may fall within the classification of healthy, yet the person may have little muscle mass and excess body fat.

BMI classifications exist as generic standards of height-weight comparisons for the general population. Racial differences have been observed in body composition that may warrant more specific BMI classifications for various population groups. Asian adults have been reported to have a higher proportion of body fat mass at a given BMI than Caucasians. African American adults have greater muscle mass and bone mineral density at a given BMI than Caucasians. Additionally, ethnic differences within race categories have been observed. For example, Chinese adults have been observed to have proportionately higher body fat mass at a given BMI than Polynesians. Further study is warranted to establish valid BMI health classifications for various population groups. These drawbacks

Table 9.3   Classification of Body Mass Index (BMI) in Adults

BMI	CLASSIFICATION
<16	Severe malnutrition
16–16.99	Moderate malnutrition
17–18.49	Mild malnutrition
18.5–24.9	Normal
25–29.9	Overweight
30–34.9	Obese class 1
35–39.9	Obese class 2
≥40	Obese class 3

Source: Department of Health and Human Services. National Heart, Lung, and Blood Institute. from www.nhLbi.nih.gov/health/public/heart/obesity; retrieved 06/24/2005

indicate the problem of using BMI as a sole indicator of weight status or nutritional health and are an excellent example of the need to use multiple parameters when conducting an assessment.

Height-Weight Tables

Height-weight tables have been used in the past to assess body weight in adults, but are no longer a standard. Such tables outlined reference weights for given heights for both males and females or were gender specific. Table 9.4 is an example of a current height-weight table based on BMI calculations presented in an easy-to-use form.

Use of such height-weight tables has the same limitations as does use of BMI as a sole indicator of weight status. Differences in body composition go largely unaccounted for and the clinician must remember to assess each person for these individual differences.

Waist Circumference

Excess, centrally located abdominal fat deposition is considered to be an independent risk factor for cardiovascular disease in adults. Measurement of waist circumference can be included in a comprehensive nutritional assessment, especially when risk factors for cardiovascular disease exist. The NHLBI considers waist circumference greater than 102 cm in males and greater than 88 cm in females indicative of risk.

Waist circumference should be measured with a spring-loaded measuring tape to ensure reliable tension is applied with each measurement. Use of the bony landmark on the lateral border of the ilium is recommended when marking a site guide for the measurement. Figure 9.2 ● depicts the location of this landmark. Standing behind the client and palpating the right hip can locate the lateral ilium. A line should be drawn at the uppermost lateral line of the ilium at the midaxillary point.

Table 9.4 Height–Weight Table with BMI Calculation

Locate the height of interest in the left-most column and read across the row for that height to the weight of interest. Follow the column of the weight up to the top row that lists the BMI. BMI of 19–24 is the healthy weight range, BMI of 25–29 is the overweight range, and BMI of 30 and above is in the obese range.

BMI	19	20	21	22	23	24	25	26	27	28	29	30	31	32	33	34	35
HEIGHT							WEIGHT IN POUNDS										
4'10"	91	96	100	105	110	115	119	124	129	134	138	143	148	153	158	162	167
4'11"	94	99	104	109	114	119	124	128	133	138	143	148	153	158	163	168	173
5'	97	102	107	112	118	123	128	133	138	143	148	153	158	163	158	174	179
5'1"	100	106	111	116	122	127	132	137	143	148	153	158	164	169	174	180	185
5'2"	104	109	115	120	126	131	136	142	147	153	158	164	169	175	180	186	191
5'3"	107	113	118	124	130	135	141	146	152	158	163	169	175	180	186	191	197
5'4"	110	116	122	128	134	140	145	151	157	163	169	174	180	186	192	197	204
5'5"	114	120	126	132	138	144	150	156	162	168	174	180	186	192	198	204	210
5'6"	118	124	130	136	142	148	155	161	167	173	179	186	192	198	204	210	216
5'7"	121	127	134	140	146	153	159	166	172	178	185	191	198	204	211	217	223
5'8"	125	131	138	144	151	158	164	171	177	184	190	197	203	210	216	223	230
5'9"	128	135	142	149	155	162	169	176	182	189	196	203	209	216	223	230	236
5'10"	132	139	146	153	160	167	174	181	188	195	202	209	216	222	229	236	243
5'11"	136	143	150	157	165	172	179	186	193	200	208	215	222	229	236	243	250
6'	140	147	154	162	169	177	184	191	199	206	213	221	228	235	242	250	258
6'1"	144	151	159	166	174	182	189	197	204	212	219	227	235	242	250	257	265
6'2"	148	155	163	171	179	186	194	202	210	218	225	233	241	249	256	264	272
6'3"	152	160	168	176	184	192	200	208	216	224	232	240	248	256	264	272	279
	HEALTHY WEIGHT						OVERWEIGHT					OBESE					

Source: Evidence Report of Clinical Guidelines on the Identification, Evaluation, and Treatment of Overweight and Obesity in Adults, 1998. NIH/National Heart, Lung and Blood Institute (NHLBI).

Reported in Dietary Guidelines for Americans, 2005 U.S. Department of Health and Human Services. www.heathiers.gov/dietaryguidelines. Retrieved June 26, 2005.

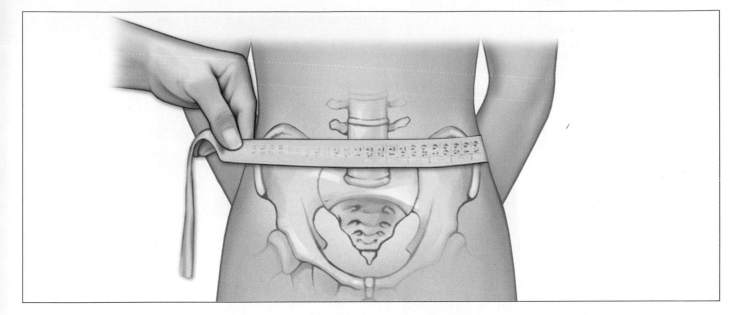

Figure 9.2 • Landmarks for waist circumference.

Other references suggest measuring waist circumference just below the umbilicus, but this can be unreliable since an obese state can change the position of the umbilicus. Waist circumference should be measured at the marked midaxillary line while keeping the measuring tape parallel to the floor. Measurement should be done directly on the surface of the skin and not over clothing. It has been suggested that taking measurements with the client in front of a mirror is helpful to ensure a true horizontal extension of the measuring tape, especially in those who are obese or have wider hips than waist. The spring-loaded measuring tape should be pulled taut but should not compress the skin. Uneven tension on the measure between sequential measurements will alter reliability of waist circumference measurements.

Waist circumference validity can be limited by obesity when increases in abdominal fat mass become pendulous due to the effects of gravity and no longer are situated along the waistline. Increases in abdominal subcutaneous fat and increases in body weight may not always be reflected by increases in waist circumference. Additionally, waist circumference is not a valid nutritional tool for use in adults with ascites, for pregnant females, or for those with other medical conditions associated with increases in fat-free abdominal girth, such as polycystic kidney disease.

Body Composition Measurement

More specific assessment of body fat and muscle mass than weight alone can be made using skinfold measurements or technological instruments. Muscle mass is also referred to as **somatic protein** stores or skeletal muscle. This second tier of anthropometric measurements can assess body composition of just two components, fat and fat-free mass, or in multicomponents, which can include more precise analysis of fat-free mass for muscle, bone, and fluid components. Increasing levels of technology and updating of older reference values to include

multicomponent analysis will allow more valid assessment of body composition in the future.

SKINFOLD MEASUREMENTS. Skinfold thickness measurements can estimate subcutaneous body fat stores. Measurements taken at up to eight sites on the body are believed to be predictive of overall body fat composition. Skinfold measurements are made using professional grade calipers and a flexible measuring tape. Plastic calipers should not be used. The technique for properly grasping the skinfold layers and subcutaneous fat takes practice before reliable measurements can be made. Both skinfold layers and subcutaneous fat are pinched and then held gently between the thumb and forefinger with care taken not to grasp underlying muscle. The fold is then measured between the calipers for each marked site on the body. If a distinct separation of subcutaneous fat and muscle cannot be accomplished when grasping the skinfold, body composition results will not be representative. The caliper jaws should be placed perpendicular to the fold and left in place for several seconds after tension is released to allow for even compression before the reading is taken. Three measurements should be taken at each site and then averaged. The right side of the body is used for taking skinfold measurements.

The tricep skinfold (TSF) is the site most often used to estimate subcutaneous fat because of easy access to this measurement in most situations. Tricep measurements are done at the midpoint of the arm equidistant from the uppermost posterior edge of the acromion process of the scapula and the olecranon process of the elbow. A measuring tape should be used to determine this midpoint on the back of the upper arm, and the site should be marked for reference. It is helpful to have the client flex the arm at a 90-degree angle while locating the bony landmarks and measuring the midpoint. However, the arm should hang freely during the skinfold measurement itself. Figure 9.3 • illustrates the location of the TSF measurement.

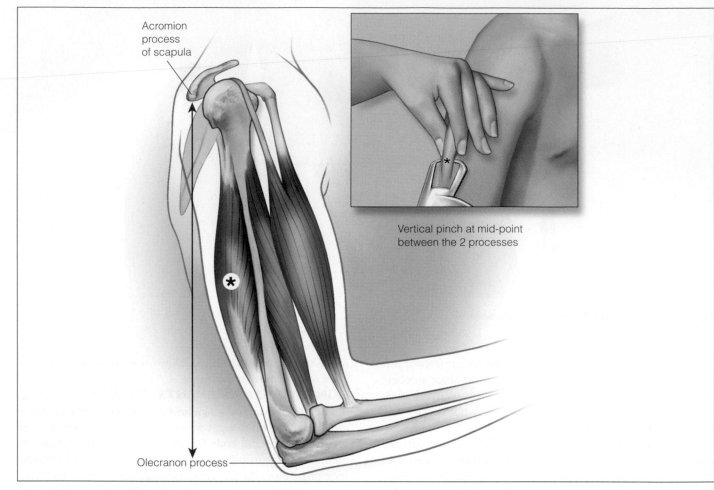

Acromion
process
of scapula

Vertical pinch at mid-point
between the 2 processes

Olecranon process

Figure 9.3 • Landmarks for tricep skinfold measurement.

Other sites that can be used for skinfold measurements include the chest, subscapular, midaxillary, suprailiac, abdomen, and upper thigh.

Measurement values for each skinfold site can be evaluated in two ways. First, they may be compared to reference values that are specific for gender, age, race, and fitness level. Reference values are simply descriptions of body composition compiled from subjects in population studies and should not be considered the same as a standard. References values allow the clinician to assess an individual's measurements compared to others in a similar, well-defined population group. Standards, however, are values that are known to be desirable targets for health regardless of population norms.

Commonly used reference values to assess skinfold measurements in some populations are over 20 years old. Older references were not obtained from diverse population groups, making them difficult to apply to the wider population that exists today. Newer reference standards are constantly being published and are becoming more population specific, but no widely used single reference exists. Therefore, the nature of human diversity requires even more research to be done in this area to appreciate the variety of reference values needed for racial, ethnic, age, fitness, and gender categories. Age-related differences in body fat distribution necessitate specific skinfold references for older adults as the relationship between

specific site subcutaneous fat measurements and total body fat is different than in younger adults. Changes in skin elasticity and connective tissue also affect skinfold accuracy with age.

MIDARM MUSCLE CIRCUMFERENCE AND CALF CIRCUMFERENCE. Circumference measurements of limbs can be used alone or in conjunction with skinfold measurements to provide additional or confirmational body composition information. Midarm muscle circumference (MAMC) is obtained by measuring midarm circumference (MAC) at the same site as the tricep skinfold. A spring-loaded flexible measure is used to provide tension without compressing the skin. Calf circumference is measured at the site of maximum calf width, which can be determined by placing the measure around the calf and sliding it along the calf until a maximum value is noted. Limb circumferences are measured in centimeters in adults.

BIOELECTRICAL IMPEDANCE ANALYSIS. Bioelectrical impedance analysis (BIA) is a noninvasive tool for assessing body composition employing principles of electroconduction through water, muscle, and fat. In traditional BIA, electrodes are placed on the dorsal surfaces of the right foot and hand with the client in the supine position on a nonconductive surface. Calculations are based on the knowledge that muscle and fluids have a higher electrolyte and water content than does fat and thus conduct electrical current differently. Altered hydration and altered skin temperature will cause measurement error by altering

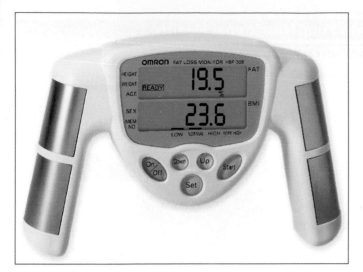

Figure 9.4 ● Handheld BIA device.

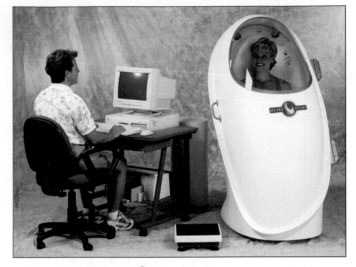

Figure 9.5 ● BOD POD® Body Composition Tracking System.

electrical current flow. Clients should be well hydrated when employing BIA technology, or dehydration will slow conductivity and give a falsely high body fat measurement. Equations used to predict body fat composition with BIA need to be population specific. Standard error for BIA measurements approximates skinfold measurements at 3% to 4%, provided correct equations are used and the client is hydrated. In comparison to the difficult and sometimes unreliable measuring of skinfold thicknesses in clients who are elderly or obese, BIA technology may provide more accurate results in these two groups. Newer BIA devices are being manufactured for easier clinical use (see Figure 9.4 ●). Handheld body fat analyzer devices measure segmental electrical impedance from arm to arm rather than the traditional whole-body method.

NEAR-INFRARED INTERACTANCE. Infrared interactance devices measure body fat at specific sites by passing infrared light through tissue and measuring reflected light. Predictive equations estimate body fat composition at the site. Gender, body weight, height, frame size, and fitness level are included in the calculation to determine total body fat percentage. Generally this measurement is performed on the bicep. Small, handheld near-infrared devices are available for clinical use. Standard error for near-infrared measurement exceeds 3.5% and can be as high as 5.5%; error is greater with increased body fat.

LABORATORY BODY COMPOSITION. Several other more sophisticated and expensive tools exist for measuring body composition. These are primarily used in laboratory research and not in clinical situations. Underwater weighing, dual x-ray absorptiometry (DEXA), and body plethysmography are examples of research tools. Underwater weighing requires the client to be completely submersed underwater to measure water displacement by the body. Regression equations calculate body fat based on known density of fat-free and fat tissue. Underwater weighing has long been called the gold standard for body composition although it utilizes only a two-component model and does not measure bone mineral content or total body water. DEXA takes advantage of x-ray technology to measure a multicomponent model of body composition and is quickly becoming the research tool of

choice. *Plethysmography* measures air volume displacement by the body using similar methodology to underwater weighing. Clients are measured in a small chamber called a BOD POD® Body Composition Tracking System (see Figure 9.5 ●).

Body Fat References or Standards

Standards of body fat percentage that are associated with health or morbidity and mortality have not been established. Many sources agree that a minimum essential body fat percentage exists. A minimum of 3% body fat in men and 12% in women is considered essential. These minimums are the lowest value compatible with health, but optimal body fat is higher and should be determined on an individual basis. It is recommended that a range of body fat be given rather than a specific target due to the errors associated with predicting specific values. A range of 12% to 20% body fat in men and 20% to 30% in women has been suggested for health, but more research is necessary to develop population-specific recommendations. Research aimed at development of future standards and references for body fat percentage will address the relationship between BMI and body fat percentage and allow the nurse a clearer assessment of body composition traits associated with health risks. Age-specific recommendations are also needed.

Physical Assessment

A visual head-to-toe physical assessment can yield findings that may be indicative of normal or abnormal nutritional status. Like all other components of a nutritional assessment, the physical assessment is most useful when used in conjunction with other nutritional assessment parameters. Table 9.5 outlines physical findings associated with poor nutritional health.

Data that is gathered as part of the physical assessment is also pertinent to the nutritional assessment. Existing medical diagnoses and treatment such as medication or surgical plans are important when evaluating nutritional status. Physical findings such as poor dental health, problems with chewing or swallowing, gastrointestinal complaints, functional decline in physical or mental status, and declining vision, taste, or smell all have negative effects on nutritional health.

Table 9.5	Clinical Findings Associated with Poor Nutritional Health		
BODY PART	**FINDING**	**POTENTIAL DEFICIENT NUTRIENT**	**EXAMPLE**
Hair	Dull, sparse, brittle hair Dyspigmentation (**flag sign**) Alopecia	Protein Protein, biotin, or zinc	Alopecia
Face	Moon face Pallor	Protein Iron	
Eyes	Dry mucosa (**xerophthalmia**), blindness and night blindness, Bitot's spot Pale conjunctiva Yellow subdermal fat deposits around lids (**xanthelasma**)	Vitamin A Iron High cholesterol	Night blindness Bitot's spot
Mouth Lips	Cracks at corners (**angular stomatitis**), inflammation (**cheilosis**)	Riboflavin	Angular stomatitis

Table 9.5	Clinical Findings Associated with Poor Nutritional Health *(continued)*

BODY PART	FINDING	POTENTIAL DEFICIENT NUTRIENT	EXAMPLE
Tongue	Smooth, beefy red or magenta (**glossitis**)	Niacin, pyridoxine (B₆), riboflavin	
	Atrophic papillae	Iron	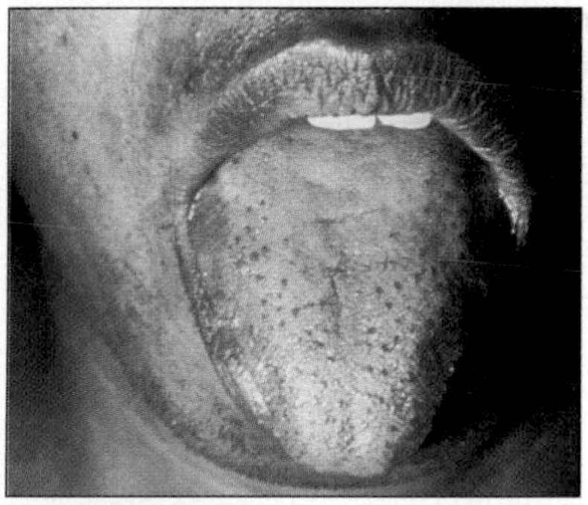
	Diminished taste (hypogeusia)	Zinc	
Teeth	Delayed eruption	Vitamin D	
	Caries in baby	May indicate baby-bottle tooth decay	
	Mottled enamel	Excess fluoride	

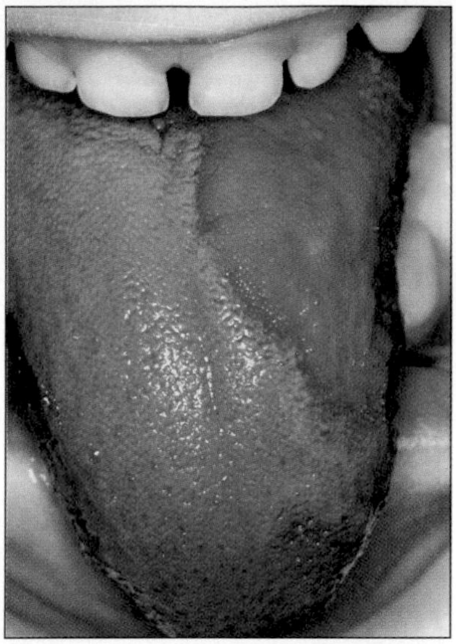

Glossitis

Atrophic papillae

BODY PART	FINDING	POTENTIAL DEFICIENT NUTRIENT	EXAMPLE
Gums	Spongy, bleeding	Vitamin C	

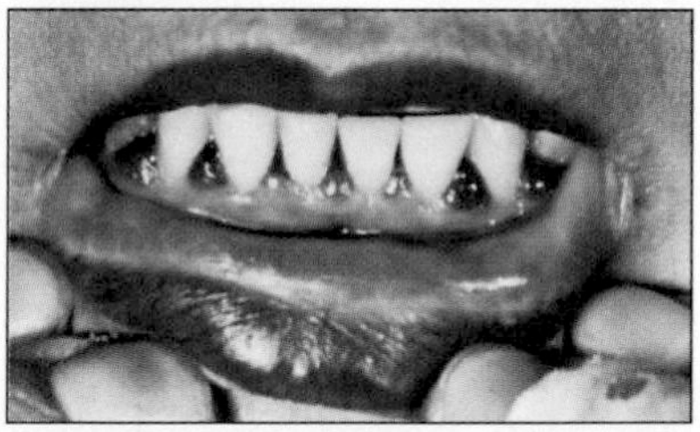

Spongy, bleeding

BODY PART	FINDING	POTENTIAL DEFICIENT NUTRIENT	EXAMPLE
Glands	Increased thyroid (goiter)	Iodine	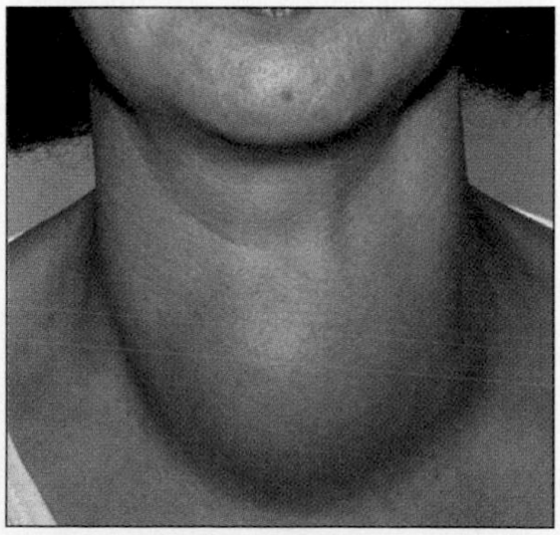
	Increased parotid size	Protein-calorie or bulimia	

Goiter

(continued)

Table 9.5   Clinical Findings Associated with Poor Nutritional Health *(continued)*

BODY PART	FINDING	POTENTIAL DEFICIENT NUTRIENT	EXAMPLE
Skin	Poor wound healing/decubitus ulcer	Protein, calories, vitamin C, zinc	Pellagra
	Follicular hyperkeratosis (goosebump flesh)	Vitamin A	
	Dry, scaly	Vitamin A, essential fatty acids, zinc	
	Photosensitive symmetrical rash (pellagra)	Niacin	
	Bruising (purpura)	Vitamins C and K	
	Pinpoint hemorrhages (petechiae)	Vitamin C	
Skeleton/ Trunk	Stunted growth	Protein-calorie, zinc	Rickets
	Ascites	Protein	
	Beading on ribs (rachitic rosary), bowed legs (**rickets**), widened epiphysis, narrow chest (pigeon breast)	Vitamin D	
	Loss of fat, muscle wasting	Protein, calories	
Genitalia	Hypogonadism	Zinc	

Table 9.5	Clinical Findings Associated with Poor Nutritional Health *(continued)*		
BODY PART	**FINDING**	**POTENTIAL DEFICIENT NUTRIENT**	**EXAMPLE**
Limbs	Pitting edema Loss of fat, muscle wasting	Protein Protein, calories	Depressions of pitting edema lower leg
Nails	Spoon-shaped (**koilonychia**) ridges	Iron	
Nervous System	Hyporeflexia, confabulation Dementia, confusion, ataxia, neuropathy Neuropathy Tetany	Thiamine Vitamin B$_{12}$ Excess vitamin B$_6$ Calcium, magnesium	
Cardiac	Arrhythmia	Potassium, magnesium	

BIOCHEMICAL ASSESSMENT— LABORATORY MEASUREMENTS

Several biochemical parameters are commonly used in a nutritional assessment. No one laboratory value is unique in its sensitivity to predict nutritional status as each has confounding reasons for abnormal values. As in the case of physical findings of malnutrition, laboratory values may not reflect current known nutrition status as half-lives and body pools of plasma components vary.

The biochemical assessment and laboratory measurements along with their significance, values, and findings are summarized in Table 9.6.

CULTURAL CONSIDERATIONS FOR THE NUTRITIONAL ASSESSMENT

Religious and cultural influences on health, nutrition beliefs, and food habits vary among and within ethnic groups. It is important to ask specific questions about these influences to understand how they affect or are interpreted by the individual client. Assumptions and generalizations based on the client's association with a cultural or ethnic population will not provide the nurse with accurate personal information about the client.

During the physical assessment and anthropometric portion of the assessment, careful and sensitive questioning of the client

or a translator is needed to determine whether issues exist that may interfere with the gathering of data. Removal of certain garments may be prohibited; this can interfere with obtaining accurate weight, determining body measurements, or assessing clinical signs and symptoms. Examination or touching by a member of the opposite sex may be taboo. The nurse should engage in decision making with the client on how best to proceed when such issues are present. Box 9.5 outlines cultural nutritional considerations.

NUTRITIONAL ASSESSMENT ACROSS THE LIFE SPAN

From infancy to older adulthood, specific consideration needs to be given to each population's unique, nutritional health parameters. Normal growth and development during childhood, the nutritional needs for a healthy pregnancy, and health maintenance and disease prevention in adulthood all provide additional parameters to consider when conducting a nutritional assessment.

The Pregnant Female

Nutritional health plays a primary role in a successful pregnancy. A mother's preconception nutritional status, appropriate weight gain, and adequate nutrition during pregnancy are important contributing factors to the health of a newborn. A

Table 9.6	Biochemical Assessment Laboratory Measurements	
LABORATORY MEASUREMENT	**SIGNIFICANCE**	**VALUES AND FINDINGS**
Albumin	Low albumin levels can be indicative of depleted visceral protein status and malnutrition. Dehydration or overhydration will lead to false levels due to hemoconcentration or dilution.	Expected 3.5 to 5 g/L Half-life in days 14 to 20 Mild malnutrition 2.8 to 3.4 g/L Moderate malnutrition 2.1 to 3.4 g/L Severe malnutrition < 2.1 g/L
Prealbumin	Also called thyroxine-binding prealbumin, has a long half-life and is therefore felt to provide a more current picture of protein status than does albumin. Prealbumin is an acute-phase reactant protein and is affected by inflammation and infection. Hemoconcentration or dilution will cause false values.	Expected 150 to 350 mg/L Half-life in days 2 to 3 Mild nutrition 110 to 150 mg/L Moderate malnutrition 50 to 109 mg/L Severe malnutrition < 50 mg/L
Transferrin	Responsible for iron binding and transport.	Expected > 200 mg/dL Half-life in days 8 to 10 Mild nutrition 180 to 200 mg/L Moderate nutrition 160 to 180 mg/L Severe nutrition < 160 mg/L
Total Lymphocyte Count	Evaluates nutrition when confounding medical conditions such as cancer or immunosuppressive drugs interfere with nutritional assessment.	Expected TLC is 2,000 to 3,500 cells/mm^3. Plasma level below 1,500 cells/mm^3 may indicate malnutrition and poor immunocompetence.
Delayed Skin Hypersensitivity Testing	A delayed response to intradermal injection of foreign substances such as *Streptococcus* or *Candida*.	Delayed or no response may indicate malnutrition, poor immune system, or no previous exposure.
Cholesterol	High cholesterol may indicate overnutrition or undernutrition.	≥200 mg/dL is associated with cardiovascular disease. ≤160 mg/dL may indicate malnutrition.
Nutritional Anemia Assessment	Poor nutrition may be evidenced by low stores of iron, folic acid, vitamin B_{12}.	*Macrocytic anemia* as evidenced by deficient folic acid or vitamin B_{12} level. *Microcytic anemia* as evidenced by decreased red blood cell volume. *Iron deficiency anemia* as evidenced by low plasma hemoglobin and hematocrit.
Nitrogen Balance	Measured to estimate adequacy of dietary intake.	*Nitrogen balance* as evidenced by nitrogen intake equals nitrogen loss. *Catabolism* occurs when there is a negative nitrogen balance. *Anabolism* occurs when the intake of protein and calories exceeds the nitrogen loss.
Plasma Proteins	Albumin, prealbumin, and transferrin are each used to assess visceral protein status.	
Immunocompetence	A depressed immune status can result from malnutrition, disease, medication, or other disease treatments.	

comprehensive nutritional assessment of a pregnant female includes all the parameters of a general assessment with some additional pregnancy-specific data assessed. See Chapter 26, The Pregnant Female for further details. ⚭

Infants, Children, and Adolescents

Nutrition plays a crucial role in the growth, physical development, and cognitive development of infants and children. Undernutrition can lead to growth faltering and developmental delays or stunting, the effects of which can be permanent. Overnutrition can set the stage for chronic disease. Overweight and obese children, especially those with one or more overweight or obese parents, are more likely to become overweight adults. Accurate assessment of nutritional health can help ensure positive outcomes or serve as the necessary foundation for needed nutritional interventions. It is essential for a nurse to have the knowledge and skills to identify nutritionally at-risk children. In many commu-

nity settings, such as schools, early intervention clinics, or well-child clinics, the nurse is often the only healthcare professional conducting an assessment that includes nutritional parameters. See Chapter 25, for a discussion of nutritional assessment of infants, children and adolescents. ⚭

Adults

Nutritional assessment of the adult focuses on evaluating the issues of both overnutrition and undernutrition. Overnutrition and undernutrition are not mutually exclusive conditions. For example, an obese individual can have nutrient deficiencies from poor quality intake that contains excess calories. Food habits developed early in life and maintained may help to promote good health well into adulthood and older adulthood.

The general components of a nutritional assessment are all pertinent when assessing an adult. The presence of a chronic disease or condition may become a significant factor affecting

Box 9.5	Cultural Diet Influences

- Cultural and religious beliefs and traditions can affect food choices, beliefs, and practices in many ways from the number of meals eaten in a day to choices of foods, preparation methods, and overall food beliefs.
- Diversity exists within cultural and religious groups. It is important to avoid applying general knowledge about cultural and religious food practices to all people within a group; instead explore individual interpretation and influences.
- Assess common dietary staples as well as foods believed to be associated with health or symbolic benefits. Some food is thought to promote health or cure conditions. Other beliefs may be related to life span issues, such as the proper diet during pregnancy for easy delivery or to make the "hot" condition "colder."
- Many religious groups have dietary laws that are observed differently by subgroups within the population. Consumption of kosher meats, fasting, and avoidance of certain foods such as pork, crustaceans, birds of prey, beef, or other animal products are examples.
- Ask about food practices and special meals for special occasions and holidays. Some religious groups fast during parts of some religious holy days.
- Discuss food preparation methods. A variety of cultures make similar type dishes but prepare them differently—for example, using different fats like bacon drippings, lard, oils, or ghee clarified butter.
- Ask about medicinal herb use as this varies among cultures and is often an important aspect of health beliefs.
- Explore to what extent any acculturation has taken place and traditional practices changed once living in a new dominant culture. Ask whether new foods have been added along with traditional foods, whether foods have been substituted for different newer versions, and whether any traditional foods have been omitted. In some cases, traditional diets are healthier than the diet in the new culture, and encouragement to maintain healthy traditions may be helpful.

nutritional health. Medications can have nutritional health implications. Lifestyle choices, socioeconomic status, education, and cultural influences can affect nutrition status in addition to dietary habits. Box 9.3 outlines pertinent nutritional history data to obtain when assessing the adult.

The Older Adult

Regular nutritional assessment of the older adult is essential. Good nutritional health is an important component of ensuring autonomy into older adulthood. Undernutrition can affect quality of life, morbidity, and mortality. Protein-energy malnutrition is considered an independent risk factor for mortality in older adults recently discharged from the hospital. Skeletal muscle loss, functional decline, altered pharmacokinetics, depressed immune status, and increased risk of institutionalization all can result from malnutrition in the older adult. The prevalence of malnutrition in the elderly population is unfortunately significant, affecting up to 60% of institutionalized or hospitalized older adults and up to 13% of those in the community.

Quality of life issues related to overnutrition are also important in the older population. Overweight and obesity are risk factors for degenerative joint disease and potential functional and mobility problems. Comorbid conditions associated with overweight, such as diabetes and cardiovascular disease, may require treatment intervention, therapeutic diets, and medications that impact nutritional health.

Poor nutrition occurs along a continuum. In the older adult, changes in nutrition health can go undetected if only strict cut-off values are observed to diagnose nutrition issues. Most general nutritional assessment parameters are applicable to the elderly population, but the nurse should be mindful of *any* change in nutrition status in the older adult, even when measured values and parameters remain within normal limits. See Chapter 27, for a discussion of nutritional assessment in the older adult. ⚭

NUTRITIONAL SCREENING AND ASSESSMENT TOOLS

Nutritional assessment data can be gathered and evaluated in a comprehensive fashion, or a more formal validated tool can be used to streamline the process. Numerous nutritional screening and assessment tools exist, but none is considered the gold standard for use in most populations. Until a consensus is reached defining malnutrition, a variety of nutritional screening and assessment tools will continue to be published.

Nutritional screening tools are used for quick assessment of risk factors for poor nutritional health. Screening tools are not meant for diagnostic purposes and are instead used to triage clients who may require further assessment or intervention. Screening tools give a rough estimate of nutrition risk or status. Nutritional assessment tools are generally more comprehensive than screening tools for the goal of identifying or diagnosing malnutrition. Not all assessment or screening tools are validated for use in the populations where they are being used. Lack of validation may lead to frequent missed diagnoses or incorrect diagnoses of poor nutritional health. Sharp clinical judgment by the nurse is a necessary adjunct to any tool.

FOOD GUIDE PYRAMID

Dietary Guidelines for Americans is published jointly every 5 years by the Department of Health and Human Services (HHS) and the Department of Agriculture (USDA). The *Guidelines* provide authoritative advice for people 2 years and older about how good dietary habits can promote health and reduce risk for major chronic diseases. The most recent guidelines, released January 2005, provide a *new* comprehensive Food Guide Pyramid and an interactive website that may be used for individual food guide planning and diet analysis (see Figure 9.6 ●). This site is located at *www.mypyramid.gov*. The nurse can compare the diet recall or nutrition history data to the distribution of food groups recommended and make a general assessment of diet adequacy. The number and size of food servings included in the Food Guide Pyramid are generic and should be adjusted for more active or less active individuals. The interactive website at *www.mypyramid.gov* permits the user to factor in age, gender, activity, and food preferences. The benefit of the new pyramid is that it is flexible and molds to the individual. Instead of needing special food pyramids for various age or culture groups, the new website has the richness of choice to meet all needs.

Anatomy of MyPyramid

One size doesn't fit all
USDA's new MyPyramid symbolizes a personalized approach to healthy eating and physical activity. The symbol has been designed to be simple. It has been developed to remind consumers to make healthy food choices and to be active every day. The different parts of the symbol are described below.

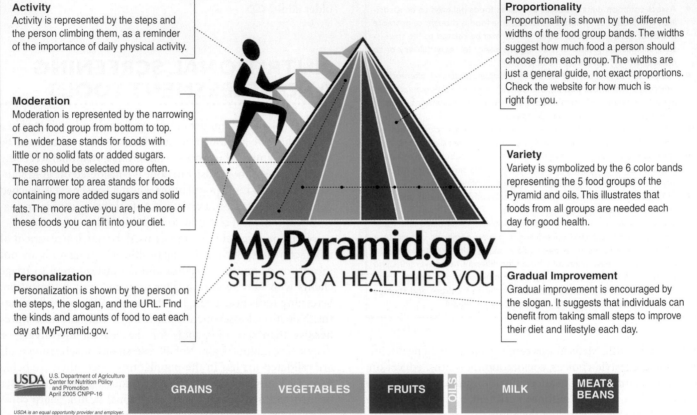

Activity
Activity is represented by the steps and the person climbing them, as a reminder of the importance of daily physical activity.

Moderation
Moderation is represented by the narrowing of each food group from bottom to top. The wider base stands for foods with little or no solid fats or added sugars. These should be selected more often. The narrower top area stands for foods containing more added sugars and solid fats. The more active you are, the more of these foods you can fit into your diet.

Personalization
Personalization is shown by the person on the steps, the slogan, and the URL. Find the kinds and amounts of food to eat each day at MyPyramid.gov.

Proportionality
Proportionality is shown by the different widths of the food group bands. The widths suggest how much food a person should choose from each group. The widths are just a general guide, not exact proportions. Check the website for how much is right for you.

Variety
Variety is symbolized by the 6 color bands representing the 5 food groups of the Pyramid and oils. This illustrates that foods from all groups are needed each day for good health.

Gradual Improvement
Gradual improvement is encouraged by the slogan. It suggests that individuals can benefit from taking small steps to improve their diet and lifestyle each day.

MyPyramid.gov
STEPS TO A HEALTHIER YOU

USDA
U.S. Department of Agriculture
Center for Nutrition Policy and Promotion
April 2005 CNPP-16

USDA is an equal opportunity provider and employer.

GRAINS | VEGETABLES | FRUITS | OILS | MILK | MEAT& BEANS

Figure 9.6 ● Food pyramid.

OTHER ASSESSMENT TOOLS

In addition to global and comprehensive resources such as *www.mypyramid.gov,* there are specialized screening tools that many clinicians have found helpful. Samples and details of the tools may be found on the Companion Website that accompanies this textbook. See *www.prenhall.com/damico,* Chapter 9.

The REAP Tool

The REAP (The Rapid Eating and Activity of Client) tool is a food and eating questionnaire for clients to complete before a clinic or office visit. The questions, which range from diet and food choices to activity and exercise, are intended to provide a focused interview during a comprehensive assessment.

The WAVE Tool

WAVE is an acronym standing for **W**eight, **A**ctivity, **V**ariety in diet, and **E**xcess related to overnutrition, calories, foods, and alcohol. This handy pocket card reminds the health care professional of the important components to assess during the examination.

The DETERMINE Checklist

DETERMINE is an acronym standing for **D**isease, **E**ating Poorly, **T**oothloss/mouth pain, **E**conomic Hardship, **R**educed social contact, **M**ultiple medicines, **I**nvoluntary weightloss/gain, **N**eeds assistance in selfcare, **E**lder years above 80 years.

The DETERMINE checklist may be used to assess the nutritional status of the older adult. The mnemonic scores the nine warning signs of poor nutrition in the older adult. The scoring of the tool provides a stratified nutritional risk score. This tool has been validated for use with community-based elderly.

The Minimum Data Set

The Minimum Data Set (MDS) is a component of the Residential Assessment Instrument mandated for all clients in Medicare certified healthcare facilities. The MDS nutritional components are to be included in admission assessments for all residents as well as quarterly and annual updates. Any changes in client status that involve a nutritional component of the MDS require a complete reassessment of nutritional status.

Mini Nutritional Assessment and Subjective Global Assessment

The Mini Nutritional Assessment (MNA) and Subjective Global Assessment (SGA) have both been validated for use in the nutritional assessment of older adults. The SGA has also been used in assessment of other populations since its development over 20 years ago. The MNA is a newer tool with extensive data validating its use with older adults. The MNA can be included as a routine component of a physical examination or as a quick bedside tool.

View all of these specialized tools on the Companion Website at www.prenhall.com/damico. Click on Chapter 9 and look for the Nutrition Assessment Tools. ⦾ The Mini Nutritional Assessment Tool is also located in Appendix G. ⦾

 Refer to the Companion Website at **www.prenhall.com/damico** and click on the **Documentation** module for documentation samples and documentation practice exercises.

Health Promotion

HEALTHY PEOPLE 2010
NUTRITIONAL OBJECTIVES

Overarching goals of *Healthy People 2010* are to increase the quality and years of healthy life and to eliminate health disparities. Issues related to overweight and obesity are considered among the leading health indicators monitored to track progress toward achievement of overall goals. Objectives include the following:

- Increase the proportion of adults who are at a healthy weight.
- Reduce the proportion of adults who are obese.
- Reduce the proportion of children and adolescents who are overweight or obese.
- Reduce growth retardation among low-income children under age 5 years.
- Increase the proportion of persons age 2 years and older who meet the dietary recommendations for calcium and consume at least:

- two daily servings of fruit
- three daily servings of vegetables, with at least one green or dark orange vegetable
- six daily servings of grain products, with at least three whole grain choices
- Increase the proportion of people age 2 years and older who consume less than:
  - 10% of calories from saturated fat
  - 30% of calories from total fat
  - 2,400 mg of sodium
- Reduce iron deficiency among young children and females of childbearing age.
- Reduce low birth weight and very low birth weight.
- Increase the proportion of pregnancies begun with an optimum folic acid level.

CLIENT EDUCATION
UNDERNUTRITION

RISK FACTORS

- Insufficient gestational weight gain

- Iron deficiency in pregnant female, infant, or child

- Insufficient folic acid intake during pregnancy

- Inadequate calcium and vitamin D intake

- Inadequate dietary intake in older adults

CLIENT EDUCATION

- Provide clients with information on need for weight gain during pregnancy. Outline nutrient-dense food choices to support gain.
- Teach clients or caregivers about role of iron and important food sources. Reinforce use of iron supplement in pregnant female.
- Provide clients with list of good sources of folic acid. Emphasize role of folic acid in avoidance of birth defects.
- Teach clients about importance of calcium and vitamin D in bone health. Outline good sources of these nutrients.
- Teach clients about healthy eating and importance of maintaining nutritional health with aging process.

OVERNUTRITION

RISK FACTORS

- Obesity/overweight

- Excessive intake of cholesterol/saturated fat

- Excessive intake of dietary supplements

CLIENT EDUCATION

- Advise clients of risks associated with excess body weight. Educate clients about healthful ways to lose weight.

- Discuss relationship between diet and heart disease with clients. Educate clients on steps to take toward lowering intake of foods that increase blood cholesterol.

- Educate clients on dangers of oversupplementation with herbs, sports nutrition products, vitamins, and minerals. Emphasize a healthy balanced diet in place of the need for supplements.

Source: Healthy People, 2010. 19. Nutrition and Overweight. Retrieved June 24, 2005, from www.healthypeople.gov/Document/HTML/VOLUME2/19Nutrition.htm.

Application Through Critical Thinking

CASE STUDY

*H*arry Chien is an 89-year-old widower brought to the clinic by his niece who is concerned about his diminished dietary intake. His past medical history is significant for mild hypertension, which is treated with a diuretic and a 2-g sodium therapeutic diet. Physical examination reveals blood pressure of 110/75 and pulse of 72. Height is 5′8″, and weight is 156 lb. Weight 6 months prior was 175 lb. Significant laboratory measures: albumin 3.0 mg/dl. Urinalysis sent: sample dark and scant volume. His skin appears dry with dry axillae and petechiae on trunk and arms. His eyes are sunken. Temporal wasting is noted as well as diminished subcutaneous fat stores on limbs. The exam of the oral cavity reveals poorly fitting dentures, spongy gums, and deep tongue furrows.

Upon talking to Mr. Chien, the nurse learns that food does not taste the same to him anymore. He blames this on his low-sodium diet. His niece reports that she takes her uncle grocery shopping each week and has noticed that his pantry at home has many of the items still there from the prior week. She tells the nurse that her uncle is a retired professional chef and used to love to cook until the last few months. He has resorted to heating food in the microwave and often overcooks it. Mr. Chien states he overheats the food because the microwave is unpredictable. His niece is reading her concerns from a list she has made and passes the list to her uncle for further comment. The nurse notices he squints at the list and then says he has nothing to add.

The nurse conducts a diet recall that reveals:

Breakfast:	Large mug black coffee
	Either cold cereal (flake type, not fortified) and whole milk or 2 pieces of toast or 1 English muffin with butter and jelly
	6 oz apple juice or cider, unfortified
Midday meal:	Sandwich on white bread—either tuna salad, peanut butter and jelly, or sliced turkey with mayonnaise and iceberg lettuce. Used to add tomato to sandwich but "can't be bothered cutting up one."
	Occasionally heats leftovers from restaurant meal with niece; usually has enough for two or three reheated meals during week. Pasta or meat and potato or rice type meals. No vegetables. Overheats and discards often.
	Cookie
	Cup of tea with whole milk and 2 tsp sugar
Evening:	6 oz ready-to-eat pudding
	4 oz milk with comment "no liquids after 7 p.m. or I have to get up all night"

Mr. Chien takes no nutritional supplements of any kind. The nurse asks further questions about the lack of fruit and vegetables and learns that it has been almost 6 months since Mr. Chien had fruit other than applesauce or apple juice. He also has stopped eating vegetables in the same time frame. He states that he cannot be bothered preparing either type of food, but on further questioning admits that he is having difficulty chewing some foods and some vision problems that make food preparation difficult or unsafe.

► Complete Documentation

The following is a sample documentation from the nutrition assessment of Harry Chien.

SUBJECTIVE DATA: Brought by niece who notes diminished intake. c/o low Na1 rx causing hypogeusia with secondary anorexia. Also c/o difficulty chewing, vision changes. Diet recall 5 2 meal/day pattern with no liquids after 7 p.m. Liquid intake, 32 oz/day (only 10 oz noncaffeine). No fruit/vegetable 3 6 mos.

OBJECTIVE DATA: VS: BP 110/75—Pulse 72. Height 5'8", weight 156 lb. BMI 23.5. Weight 6 months ago 175 lb. Albumin 3.0 mg/dl, UA pdg: sample dark and scant. Skin and axillae dry/petechiae present. Temp/limb wasting noted. Eyes sunken. Oral cavity: spongy gums, poorly fitting dentures, tongue furrows. Medications: HCTZ.

► Critical Thinking Questions

1. How would the data from the case study be clustered to identify the problem areas?

2. How should the nurse interpret the data related to Mr. Chien's fruit and vegetable intake?

3. What additional data would the nurse require to develop a plan of care for Mr. Chien?

► Applying Nursing Diagnoses

The NANDA taxonomy (see Appendix A 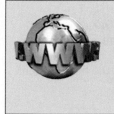) includes the following nursing diagnoses: *dentition, impaired; skin integrity, impaired;* and *oral mucous membrane, impaired.*

1. Do the data from the case study support these nursing diagnoses? If so, identify the data.

2. Identify nursing diagnoses from the NANDA taxonomy that address the self-care and dependency issues for Mr. Chien and identify the data that support your conclusions.

3. Develop additional nursing diagnoses for Mr. Chien and provide PES (problem, etiology, signs or symptoms) statements.

Please refer to the Companion Website at www.prenhall.com/damico and click on Chapter 9, the Application Through Critical Thinking module, to complete the following activities related to this case study:
► **Critical Thinking questions**
► **Extended Nursing Diagnosis challenge**
► **Documentation activity**

EXPLORE MediaLink

Additional resources for this chapter are found on the Student CD-ROM accompanying this textbook and on the Companion Website.

CD-ROM CONTENT

Content for this chapter includes:
Objectives
Key Concepts
NCLEX-RN® Review Questions
Model Documentation Forms
Audio Glossary
Games and Challenges
Clinical Spotlight Videos
    Bulimia
    Anorexia
    Eating Disorders
    Overweight Children
Head-to-Toe Physical Examination Video

COMPANION WEBSITE CONTENT

www.prenhall.com/damico

Content for this chapter includes:
Objectives
NCLEX-RN® Review Questions

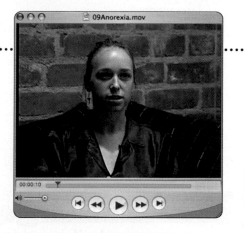

Application Through Critical Thinking
    Case Study Teaching Plan Challenge
MediaLinks
MediaLink Application
Tool Box
    Risk Factors for Poor Nutritional Health
    Calculating Weight Loss Percentage
    Classification of Body Mass Index (BMI) in Adults
    Biochemical Assessment Laboratory Measures
    Health Promotion
        Healthy People 2010
        Client Education
New York Times

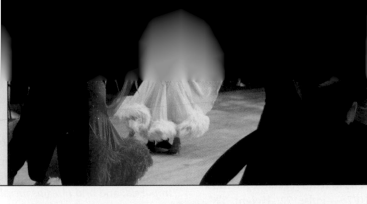

10

The Health History

CHAPTER OBJECTIVES

Upon completion of this chapter, you will be able to:

1. Discuss the purpose of the nursing health history.
2. Describe communication skills used by the professional nurse when conducting a health history.
3. Identify barriers to effective nurse-client communication.
4. Describe the influence of culture on nurse-client interactions.
5. Discuss the professional characteristics used in establishing a nurse-client relationship.
6. Discuss the phases of the client interview.
7. Describe the components of the nursing health history.
8. Obtain a health history.
9. Develop a genogram.

MEDIALINK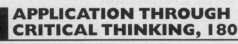

www.prenhall.com/damico

The CD-ROM in the back of this textbook and the Media-Link website contain NCLEX-RN® review questions, interactive exercises, case study challenges, animations, videos, documentation and checklist forms, and review materials. For a complete listing of the media content specific to Chapter 10, see the Explore MediaLink at the end of the chapter.

The health assessment interview provides an opportunity to gather detailed information about events and experiences that have contributed to a client's current state of health. The **health history** is a comprehensive record of the client's past and current health. The health history is gathered during the initial health assessment interview, which usually occurs at the client's first visit to a healthcare facility. This database is updated with each visit. The purpose of the health history is to document the responses of the client to actual and potential health concerns. Thus, the health history includes a wellness assessment covering questions on how the client optimizes health and well-being in such areas as nutrition, stress management, and social interaction.

The health history performed by the nurse has a different focus from the medical history performed by the physician. Although both consist of subjective data, the focus of the medical history is to gather data about the cause and course of disease. Thus, the medical history focuses on the disease rather than on the client and the client's lifestyle practices. For example, the physician may ask a client to relate the details of the range of motion in the left hip to determine the cause of abnormal movement and to prescribe a specific treatment. The nurse obtains the same information, but uses it to determine the extent to which the client will need support and teaching regarding ambulation and performance of activities of daily living (ADLs), such as getting dressed independently at home. The nurse and the physician gather the same information for different purposes. The nursing health history may produce information about a medical diagnosis, but the focus is on the client's response to the health concern as a whole person, not just on one or two body parts or systems.

COMMUNICATION SKILLS

Effective communication skills play an important role in developing a nurse-client relationship, conducting the health assessment interview, and collecting data for the health history. Communication is also important in educating, guiding, facilitating, directing, and counseling the client. The nurse cannot develop trust, establish rapport, or carry out nursing interventions for clients without knowledge of communication techniques. For example, nurses may need to modify their communication skills when dealing with younger or older clients. The younger nurse teaching the elderly client about ways to add fiber to the diet may need to use a serious and respectful communication technique. Conversely, an older nurse counseling a teenage client regarding safe and responsible sexual practices may need to make special efforts to create an informal atmosphere that allows the teenager to open up and speak freely.

Communication is the exchange of information between individuals. During the communication process an individual, sometimes called the sender, develops an idea and transmits it in the form of a message to another person, or receiver. The receiver perceives the message (the sender's transmitted idea) and interprets it. Once the receiver interprets the meaning, the receiver formulates a response and transmits it back to the sender as feedback. **Encoding** is the process of formulating a message for transmission to another person. To encode an idea, the sender has to choose the words, body language, signs, or symbols that will be used to convey the message. Decoding is the process of searching through one's memory, experience, and knowledge base to determine the meaning of the intended message (see Figure 10.1 ●).

To communicate successfully, the client must be able to accurately decode the messages the nurse sends. For example, communication may break down if the nurse uses words the client does not understand or behaves in a manner that is frightening to the client. Communication may also break down if the nurse fails to decode the client's messages accurately by not listening actively and attentively.

INTERACTIONAL SKILLS

Interactional skills are actions that are used during the encoding/decoding process to obtain and disseminate information, develop relationships, and promote understanding of self and others. Nurses use a variety of interactional skills during the communication

KEY TERMS

attending, 158
communication, 157
concreteness, 163
empathy, 163
encoding, 157
false reassurance, 160
focused interview, 166
genogram, 173
genuineness, 163
health history, 157
health pattern, 171
interactional skills, 157
listening, 158
paraphrasing, 158
positive regard, 162
preinteraction, 164
primary source, 170
reflecting, 159
secondary source, 164
summarizing, 160

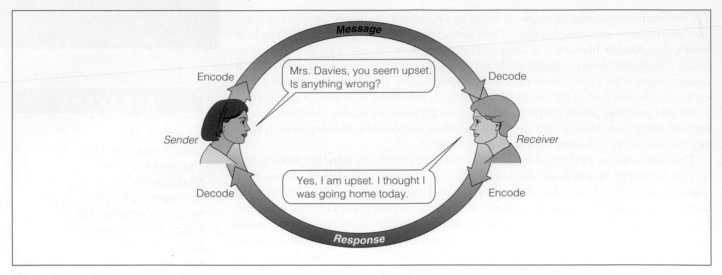

Figure 10.1 ● The communication process.

process to gather assessment data from the client, family, significant others, and healthcare personnel. The interactional skills that are helpful during an interview include listening, attending, paraphrasing, leading, questioning, reflecting, and summarizing (see Table 10.1). The nurse uses these interactional techniques to help the client communicate information thoroughly and also to confirm that the nurse has understood the client's communication correctly.

Listening

Listening is paying undivided attention to what the client says and does. It involves interpretation of what has been said. Listening is a basic part of the communication process and is the most important interactional skill. People who have not developed listening skills have problems relating to others and difficulty attaining their goals. Successful listening involves taking in the client's whole message by hearing the words as well as interpreting body language. Successful listening is an active process requiring effort and attention on the part of the nurse (see Figure 10.2 ●). It is important to push thoughts about the day's schedule or the next client from one's mind while listening to a client and to give full attention to the client, so as not to miss some of the message. The nurse should note not only the words the client speaks, but also the tone of voice and even what the client does not say. The woman who states, "My mother died last week" and immediately moves on to another topic of discussion has told the nurse a lot about how she is dealing with a death in her family.

Attending

Giving full attention to verbal and nonverbal messages is called **attending**. Body language may be as much as 93% of the message a client sends. Body language, or nonverbal messages, also provides significant information that the nurse might otherwise overlook and signals information that the client may have omitted intentionally or unintentionally. For example, a male client who feels expressing pain is a weakness may deny that he

is in pain. However, his facial expression, guarded reaction to abdominal palpation, and drawn position in bed send a message of severe pain. Because body language can send messages such as hostility, defensiveness, or confusion, the nurse must tune in to the client's nonverbal as well as verbal messages. Nonverbal cues such as posture, eye contact, makeup, dress, accessories, and items in the client's environment (books, a rosary, or photographs) tell a significant story and add more depth to the intended message. Attentive listening skills also include encouraging the client to speak by making comments such as "I see" and "Go on."

Paraphrasing

Communication skills include checking to make sure that the nurse has understood the client accurately by paraphrasing. **Paraphrasing** means that the nurse restates the client's basic message. For example, the client may say, "I don't really know if I should have this test." The nurse would paraphrase by saying, "You haven't received enough information yet to make a decision."

Leading

Nurses use leading skills to encourage open communication. These skills are most effective when starting an interaction or when trying to get the client to discuss specific health concerns. Leading skills are especially helpful in getting clients to explore their feelings and to elaborate on areas already introduced in the discussion. The leading techniques nurses commonly use when interviewing a client include direct leading, focusing, and questioning.

Questioning

Questioning is a very direct way of speaking with clients to obtain subjective data for decision making and planning care. Questioning techniques include closed and open-ended questions. *Closed questions* limit the client's response to yes, no, or one-word answers ("Were you feeling angry when your mother

Table 10.1 Interactional Skills

SKILL/DEFINITION	TECHNIQUE	EXAMPLES
Attending Giving the client undivided attention.	• Use direct eye contact if appropriate for culture. Look at the client during the conversation. • Lean toward the client slightly. • Select quiet area with no distractions for interview. • Convey unhurried manner; avoid fidgeting and looking at watch.	Nurse arranges with peers for no interruptions during interview. Nurse sits facing client, remains alert, and focuses on what client is saying.
Paraphrasing/Clarification Restating the client's basic message to test whether it was understood.	• Listen for the client's basic message. • Restate the client's message in your own words. • Ask the client if your words are an accurate restatement of the message.	*Client:* "I toss and turn all right. Sometimes I can't get to sleep at all. I don't know why this is happening. I've always been a deep sleeper." *Nurse:* "It sounds like you're not getting enough sleep. Is that right?"
Direct Leading Directing the client to obtain specific information or to begin an interaction.	• Decide what area you want to explore. • Tell the client what you want to discuss. • Encourage the client to follow your lead.	"Let's discuss the pain in your back." "When did your symptoms begin?"
Focusing Helping the client zero in on a subject or get in touch with feelings.	• Use focusing when the client strays from the topic or uses tangential speech. • Listen for themes, issues, or feelings in the client's rambling conversation. • Ask the client to give more information about a specific theme, issue, or feeling. • Encourage the client to emphasize feelings when giving this information.	"Describe how you feel when you can't sleep." "Did you say you were angry and frustrated before you went to bed? Go over that again."
Questioning Gathering specific information on a topic through the process of inquiry.	• Use open-ended questions whenever possible. Avoid using questions that can be answered with "yes," "no," "maybe," or "sometimes." • Ask the client to express feelings about what is being discussed. • Ask questions that help the client gain insight.	"What did you mean when you said your back was breaking?" "How did you feel after you talked to your boss?"
Reflecting Letting the client know that the nurse empathizes with the thoughts, feelings, or experiences expressed.	• Take in the client's feelings from verbal and nonverbal body language. • Determine which combination of "cues" you should reflect back to the client. • Reflect the "cues" back to the client. • Observe the client's response to the reflected feelings, experience, or content.	*Feelings:* "It sounds like you're feeling lonely." "It must really be frustrating not to be able to get enough sleep." *Experience:* "You're yawning. You must be tired." "You act as if you're in pain." *Content:* "You think you're going to die." "You believe the medication is helping."
Summarizing Tying together the various messages that the client has communicated throughout the interview.	• Listen to verbal and nonverbal content during the interview. • Summarize feelings, issues, and themes in broad statements. • Repeat them to the client, or ask the client to repeat them to you.	"Let's review the health problems you've identified today."

said that?"). *Open-ended questions* are purposely general and encourage the client to provide additional information. Examples of open-ended questions include "Tell me what brought you here today" or "You said that your ankle hurts. Tell me more about that."

Reflecting

Reflecting is repeating the client's verbal or nonverbal message for the client's benefit. It is a way of showing the client that the nurse empathizes or is in tune with the client's thoughts, feelings, and experiences. For example, Mr. Bates, a 60-year-old with diabetes, is admitted to an outpatient clinic to be evaluated for a possible amputation of his right lower leg because of gangrene. During the clinic visit, Mr. Bates sits in a chair in the examination room with his head in his hands. When the nurse begins to question him, he looks up and says, "Leave me alone. Nothing you can do will help. I might as well be dead." The nurse's response might be, "Mr. Bates, may I sit here for awhile? I can see that you are upset" (reflecting feeling). "You must feel angry that this is happening to you" (reflecting content). This example demonstrates that thoughts, feelings, and experiences are reflected at the same time.

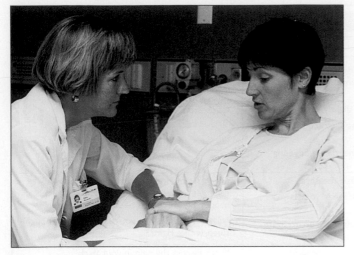

Figure 10.2 ● The nurse conveys attentive listening through a posture of involvement.

Summarizing

Summarizing is the process of gathering the ideas, feelings, and themes that clients have discussed throughout the interview and restating them in several general statements. Summarizing is a useful tool because it shows clients that the nurse has listened and understood their concerns. It also allows clients to know that progress is being made in resolving their health concerns and signals closure of the interview. One strategy is to read back to the client what has been documented and then ask, "Is that correct?"

BARRIERS TO EFFECTIVE CLIENT INTERACTION

In some situations the nurse may unknowingly hinder the flow of information by using nontherapeutic interactions (interactions that are harmful rather than helpful). Nontherapeutic interactions interfere with the communication process by making the client uncomfortable, anxious, or insecure. Some interactions that can be most harmful if used during the health assessment interview are false reassurance, interrupting or changing the subject, passing judgment, cross-examination, use of technical terms, and insensitivity.

FALSE REASSURANCE

False reassurance occurs when the nurse assures the client of a positive outcome with no basis for believing in it. False reassurance deprives clients of the right to communicate their feelings. Examples include "Everything will be all right" or "Don't worry about not being able to sleep at night. You'll be fine." False reassurance can be implied by the tone of voice used by the nurse in the communication process.

INTERRUPTING OR CHANGING THE SUBJECT

Interrupting the client or changing the subject shows insensitivity to the client's thoughts and feelings. In most cases this happens when the nurse is ill at ease with the client's comments and is unable to deal with their content. Clients who show extreme emotion (e.g., anger, weeping) during the interview, who ask intimate questions about the nurse's personal life, or who are sexually aggressive in the presence of the nurse may make the nurse uncomfortable during the interview. In these instances, the nurse must recognize what it is about the client's behavior that is making him or her uncomfortable and deal with the situation at hand in a professional manner rather than changing the subject. For example, "Your questions about my personal life are making me feel uncomfortable. We need to talk about what is concerning you today instead."

PASSING JUDGMENT

Judgmental statements convey a strong message that the client must live up to the nurse's value system to be accepted. These statements imply nonacceptance and discourage further interaction. Examples include "Abortion is the same as murder" or "You're not following your diet."

CROSS-EXAMINATION

Asking question after question during an assessment interview may cause the client to feel threatened, and the client may seek refuge by revealing less information. Because all interviews include many questions, the nurse should be careful not to make clients feel that they are being cross-examined with an endless barrage of questions. It is helpful to pause between questions and ask how the client is tolerating the interview to this point. Encouraging clients to express their feelings about the pace and nature of the interview makes them feel more at ease.

TECHNICAL TERMS

Whenever possible, the nurse should use lay rather than technical terms and avoid jargon, slang, or clichés. Terms such as *anterior* and *posterior* are useful for nursing and medical personnel but are more confusing to the client than the terms *front* and *back*. It is best to avoid the use of initials and acronyms unless they are commonly accepted as everyday language. For instance, most clients will understand the term AIDS but not prn (as necessary).

SENSITIVE ISSUES

Nurses often need to ask clients questions that are sensitive and personal. The client may feel uncomfortable providing information about such concerns as abuse, homelessness, emotional and psychological problems, use of drugs and alcohol, self-image, sexuality, or religion. Discomfort with these issues may cause the client to lapse into silence. It is important to be sensitive to the client's need for silence. The client may need to reflect on what was said or to come to grips with emotions the question has evoked before proceeding. The nurse also watches for nonverbal signs, such as tear-filled eyes or wringing of hands, which indicate the client's need to pause for a moment. After a period of silence, if the client does not resume the conversation, the nurse may need to prompt the client by saying, "After that, what happened?" or "You were saying . . . " Certain questions may cause a client to cry. The nurse should offer tissues, let the client cry, and wait until the client is ready to proceed before asking additional questions. Some clients may feel that they need permission to cry. A nurse who sees that the client is holding back tears can give the client permission to cry by saying, "I know that you are upset. It is all right to cry." If the client reacts to questions about sensitive issues with anger, the nurse should acknowledge what the client is feeling: "I can see that you are angry. Please tell me why." If the client becomes angry, the nurse should acknowledge the anger, apologize, and wait to resume the interview until the client's anger dissipates. Asking the client sensitive questions may make the nurse uncomfortable. A nurse who anticipates being uncomfortable with certain questions should take time to reflect upon and come to terms with these feelings before beginning the interview. Role-playing the situation with another nurse as the client or mentally visualizing how to react in the anticipated situation will help avoid uncomfortable feelings during the interview. When asking sensitive questions, it is best to be direct and honest with the client: "I feel uncomfortable asking you such personal questions, but I need the information to complete your plan of care." Communication strategies like these will help the nurse conduct a thorough and effective interview in these sensitive situations.

THE INFLUENCE OF CULTURE ON NURSE-CLIENT INTERACTIONS

Differences in culture and the ways in which they are demonstrated have a significant impact on the interactions that occur in the nurse-client relationship. The professional nurse must be prepared to recognize and adapt the interactional processes to cultural differences. Further, nurses must not allow their own cultural values and practices to bias the impressions of the client, nor to impair the interaction.

DIVERSITY

How a sender encodes a message and a receiver decodes it depends on a combination of factors such as culture, ethnicity, religion, nationality, education, health status, and level of intelligence. When two people differ in any of these ways, each must be more open to the other person's way of thinking and foster mutual understanding.

The nurse is careful not to bring cultural stereotypes to the communication process. Each individual, whether client or nurse, has some degree of ethnocentrism; that is, the individual sees a culturally specific way of life as being the "normal" way. Nurses must not impose their own culturally specific values on clients. Avoiding cultural bias requires effort because these values may be so ingrained that they may surface unconsciously during communication. All people have a right to have their cultural heritage recognized as valuable. No one culture is better than another. The nurse who works in a community with clients from many cultures and nationalities should learn as much as possible about the culture, values, and belief systems of the clients who present for healthcare. The best way to learn is by asking and observing the "cultural experts," clients, and clients' families.

In the United States, many individuals are often uncomfortable with silence and speak constantly to avoid any lag in the conversation. In Vietnam, a talkative individual could be perceived as impatient, inconsiderate, and superficial. The nurse who makes a lot of small talk while interviewing a client of Vietnamese descent may find it difficult to obtain information from the client. A Cantonese client using English as a second language may misplace stress on syllables and use short vowels. A nurse from a different cultural background may think this client is angry, curt, impatient, or rude, resulting in miscommunication.

Consider the following situation: Mrs. Pearl Robinson, a 76-year-old African American who has lived most of her life in the rural South, had her blood pressure checked at the local senior citizen center while visiting her daughter in Detroit. The nurse who checked Mrs. Robinson told her that her blood pressure was high and suggested that she see her family physician as soon as possible. Mrs. Robinson interpreted the nurse's statement to mean that she had "high blood," a simple condition the "old folks talked about." Mrs. Robinson believed she could treat "high blood" by drinking vinegar and water and eating salty foods. In this situation, the difference in cultural and regional background between Mrs. Robinson and the nurse contributed to the difference in the way each one encoded and decoded the term *high blood pressure* (see Figure 10.3 ●).

BODY LANGUAGE

Body language is extremely important when developing the nurse-client relationship. If the nurse and the client are from different cultures, body language is an even more critical part of the communication process. Simple body movements such as eye contact, handshakes, or posture may carry different messages in different cultures. For example, some Native American communities consider direct eye contact an invasion of privacy and a firm handshake aggressive. The nurse of Northern European descent might believe that a client who avoids direct eye contact is suspicious and cannot be trusted and that a weak handshake translates into a weak personality. The nurse of Asian descent might believe that the outgoing and talkative client of Italian descent is being rude.

Although nurses should attempt to individualize communication styles to ethnic groups, they must not make assumptions about the ethnicity of clients. The differences among individuals in a group are often greater than the differences between the groups themselves. For example, a client or nurse of Japanese descent who is a fourth-generation American differs little in communication style from an American of European descent. As another example, consider the reverse of the earlier situation with Mrs. Robinson. The client, Mrs. Robinson, is a well-educated, urban woman, but the nurse assumes that, simply because Mrs. Robinson is of African American descent, she must believe in the concept of "high blood." The potential for miscommunication in this situation is even greater than in the first example. Nurses must never stereotype clients

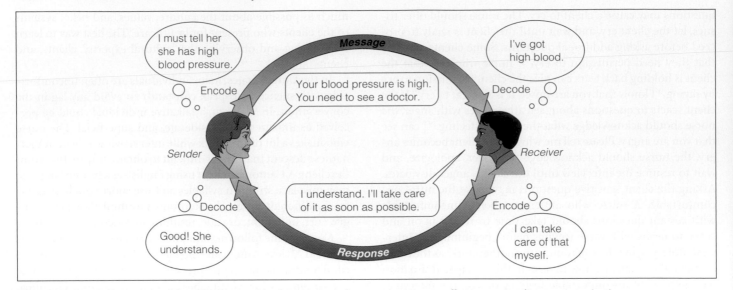

Figure 10.3 ● Differences in cultural or regional background may become barriers to effective nurse-client communication.

because they are of a different culture, are from a different country, or practice a different religion. Rather, it is the nurse's responsibility to learn about a client's culture and use this knowledge as a basis for developing a meaningful nurse-client relationship.

COMMUNICATING WITH LANGUAGE DIFFERENCES

Communication is challenged if the client does not speak the same language as the nurse or uses the language of the dominant culture, such as English, as a second language. If the client does not speak the same language, the nurse should bring in a translator to assist with the interview. It is helpful to meet with the translator before approaching the client to discuss the purpose of the interview, the terms the nurse needs to use, the kinds of information the nurse needs to collect, and the confidentiality of the subject matter. Learning a few key health-related terms in the client's language contributes to developing trust and establishing an effective nurse-client relationship.

During the interview, the seating should be arranged so that the client can see the nurse and the translator at the same time without turning the head from side to side. The nurse looks at the client, not the translator, as the interview progresses. It is important to avoid discussing the client with the translator, leaving the client out of the conversation. Throughout the interview, the nurse asks questions one at a time using clear, concise terms. Even clients who are not bilingual may understand some of the words that are used. Although some clients speak English extremely well as a second language, they may have some difficulty communicating their thoughts when overcome by extreme stress. It is not uncommon for clients who speak fluent English to revert back to their native language during times of stress. If this is the case, the nurse should follow the recommendations for clients who do not speak English. A translator is usually not needed unless the client is extremely stressed or in severe pain. Some clients communicate better in writing or understand the written word better than the spoken word, so it

is a good idea to have a pencil and paper readily available. Box 10.1 provides guidelines for interviewing clients who do not speak English.

PROFESSIONAL CHARACTERISTICS TO ENHANCE THE NURSE-CLIENT INTERACTION

Clients are more willing to discuss their health issues if they perceive that they are in a trusting, helping relationship and have developed a sense of rapport or mutual trust and understanding with the interviewing nurse. Carl Rogers, founder of the humanities psychology movement, developed client-centered therapy. Rogers defined the helping relationship as one "in which at least one of the parties has the intent of promoting the growth, development, maturity, improved functioning, and improved coping with life of the other" (1957, pp. 27–32). Nurses who establish helping relationships with their clients believe that the positive aspects of the helping relationship are shared by the nurse as well as the client.

The nurse interviewer's attitude plays an important role in the success of the interview. The client is more likely to cooperate if the nurse conveys a willingness to help and assist the client. According to Rogers (1951), Brammer, Abrego, and Shostrum (1993), Carkhuff (2000), and other social psychologists, a helping person possesses the characteristics of positive regard, empathy, genuineness, and concreteness.

POSITIVE REGARD

Positive regard is the ability to appreciate and respect another person's worth and dignity with a nonjudgmental attitude. Nurses who respect their clients value their individuality and accept them regardless of race, religion, culture, ethnic background, or country of origin. Clients sense positive regard

Box 10.1 — Guidelines for Interviewing Clients Who Do Not Speak English

- Be open to ways you can communicate effectively. Imagine yourself entering a care setting where few people speak your language. Your sensitivity to this fear and unease will be your greatest strength in providing quality care for your client.
- Determine what language your client speaks. Your first assumption may not be correct. For example, South American immigrants may speak one of a variety of Native American dialects, Portuguese, or Spanish.
- Make sure the client can read and write, as well as speak, in the native language. Be alert for any confusion.
- Learn key foreign phrases that will help you communicate with the client.
- Find friends, relatives, neighbors, or other nurses who can help you translate. Try to obtain a phone number for this person. You may need immediate help with a question or emergency.
- Find out if your healthcare facility has access to translators. It is best to have an official translator when you give instructions or obtain consent.
- Look at your *client* while telling the translator what to say. This helps your client feel connected to you and conveys meaning through body language and facial expression.
- Use clear simple language. For example, don't tell the translator to ask for a clean-catch specimen, instead explain what you mean step by step.
- Pause frequently for the translator.
- Ask the translator to provide the proper context for any colloquial expressions your client may use.

If You Can't Find a Translator

- Develop cards with phrases or illustrations to aid communication. Have several translators review the cards before using them.
- Use written handouts for client teaching. These can be developed or purchased. Look for handouts with plenty of diagrams.

in nurses by their demeanor, attitudes, and verbal and nonverbal communication.

EMPATHY

Empathy is "the capacity to respond to another's feelings and experiences as if they were your own" (Cormier, Cormier, & Weiser, 1984, p. 22). Nurses demonstrate empathy by showing their understanding and support of the client's experience or feelings through actions and words. Empathy allows the nurse to see the issues through the client's eyes, fostering understanding of the client's health concerns.

GENUINENESS

Genuineness is the ability to present oneself honestly and spontaneously. People who are genuine present themselves as down-to-earth and real. To be genuine, nurses must convey interest in, and focus on, the situation at hand, giving the client their full attention. They use direct eye contact, facial expressions appropriate to the situation, and open body language. Facing the client, leaning forward during conversation, and sitting with arms and legs uncrossed are examples of open body language. A genuine person communicates in a congruent manner, making sure that verbal and nonverbal messages are consistent. The nurse who tells a client to "take your time" during the interview, but constantly looks at the clock, gives a

mixed or incongruent message. Genuineness and congruent communication promote rapport and trust with the client.

CONCRETENESS

For the nurse, **concreteness** means speaking to the client in specific terms rather than in vague generalities. For instance, saying "I need this information to help you to plan a diet to lower your cholesterol level" is more specific than "I need this information to plan your nursing care." The more specific statement promotes understanding and a sense of security in the client. Speaking to the client in concrete terms implies that the nurse respects the client's ability to understand and recognizes the client's right to know the details of the plan of care.

THE HEALTH HISTORY INTERVIEW

The health history interview is the exchange of information between the nurse and the client. This information, along with the data from the physical assessment, is used to develop nursing diagnoses and design the nursing care plan. Unlike other types of interviews nurses conduct, the health history interview is a formal, planned interaction to inquire about the client's health patterns, ADLs, past health history, current health issues, self-care activities, wellness concerns, and other aspects of the client's health status. In most situations, nurses use a special health history tool to collect assessment data. The health history is a critical component of the comprehensive health interview.

SOURCES OF INFORMATION

A variety of sources of information are included in a comprehensive health assessment. In the health history portion, subjective data is gathered. Therefore, the professional nurse will seek to obtain information from the most reliable source.

The Primary Source

The primary and best source of information for the health assessment interview is the client. The client is the only one who can describe personal symptoms, experiences, and factors leading to the current health concern. In some situations, the client may be unable or unwilling to provide information. For example, a client who has had a cerebral vascular accident (brain attack) may not be able to understand what is being said or verbalize a response. The nurse carefully evaluates the client who is unable to give accurate and reliable information and uses another source of information if indicated. The following clients may be unable to provide accurate and reliable information:

- Infants or children
- Clients who are seriously ill, comatose, sedated, or in substantial pain
- Clients who are developmentally disabled
- Clients disoriented to person, place, or time
- Clients with psychosocial concerns
- Clients who cannot speak the common language
- Aphasic clients

In some situations an adult client is able but unwilling to provide certain types of information because of fear, anxiety, embarrassment, or distrust. Some reasons why clients may be hesitant to share information include:

- *Fear of a terminal diagnosis.* A client may not be ready to cope with the stress of a terminal illness and deny its possibility.
- *Fear of undergoing further physical examination.* A claustrophobic client may deny problems because of fear of a magnetic resonance imaging (MRI) scan.
- *Embarrassment.* A male client may refuse to discuss urinary problems because he fears catheterization or rectal examination.
- *Fear of legal implications.* An alcoholic client involved in a car accident may fear revealing the addiction to alcohol.
- *Fear of losing a job.* An airline pilot may be reluctant to admit visual problems or hearing loss.
- *Lack of trust.* A client with AIDS who wishes the diagnosis to remain private may fear a breach in confidentiality.

Secondary Sources

A **secondary source** is a person or record that provides additional information about the client. The nurse uses secondary sources when the client is unable or unwilling to communicate. For example, the parent or caregiver is the source of information for a child who cannot communicate. Secondary sources are used to augment and validate previously obtained data. The most commonly used secondary sources are significant others to whom the client has expressed thoughts and feelings about lifestyle or health status, and medical and other records containing descriptions of the client's subjective experience. The interviewing nurse should not overlook the attending physician and other healthcare personnel who have cared for the client as excellent secondary sources of information.

Clients often share their personal experiences, feelings, and emotions with significant others. A significant other is a person who has won the client's respect and who holds a position of importance in the client's life. A significant other may be a family member, lover, cohabitant, legal guardian (if the client is a minor or legally incompetent), close friend, coworker, pastor, teacher, or health professional. These individuals often provide a different viewpoint or perspective about the client's stresses and thoughts, attitudes, and concerns about daily life and illness. The significant other who has the closest relationship with the client is usually the most accurate source of information when the client is unable or unwilling to speak.

Whenever possible, the nurse should obtain the client's permission before requesting information from another person. This simple act of courtesy demonstrates respect for the client's privacy and goes a long way in establishing a mutual sense of trust. Obtaining the client's verbal and written permission also prevents potential accusations concerning invasion of privacy.

The nurse must be cautious when collecting client data from another person. This information may be prejudiced by that person's own bias, life experience, and values, and may not be a true reflection of the client's own thinking. Every attempt must be made to validate secondary information by verifying it with the client, by observation, or by confirming the information with at least one other source. The nurse does not seek secondary information if the client is competent but unwilling to provide personal information and has not granted the nurse permission to explore information with secondary sources. The nurse should respect the wishes and confidentiality of the client and attempt to obtain the information at a later time.

The medical record is an excellent source of accurate subjective and objective data about the client. The subjective statements made by the client and recorded in the nursing progress notes provide insight about the client's symptoms and feelings. Nursing progress notes, descriptions of client responses to treatment, physicians' progress notes, treatment plans, medical histories, laboratory results, and vital signs are examples of excellent secondary resources the nurse can use to develop the nursing care plan. The nurse also investigates medical records from previous hospitalizations or clinic visits. If the medical record is available, it should be reviewed before the health assessment interview because it provides cues to actual and potential health problems to explore. During the interview, one should always validate any information from a secondary source, especially if it conflicts with the client's statements during the interview.

PHASES OF THE HEALTH ASSESSMENT INTERVIEW

The health assessment interview is divided into three phases: preinteraction, the initial or formal interview, and the focused interview. The first two phases provide information the nurse uses along with information from the physical assessment to develop the total client database, formulate nursing diagnoses, and initiate the nursing care plan. The third phase, the focused interview, occurs throughout all stages of the nursing process. Its purpose is to gather, clarify, and update additional client data as it becomes available.

The focused interview is used to validate probable or hypothetical nursing or collaborative diagnoses. After the initial interview, the nurse develops several hypothetical nursing diagnoses. Before making a final diagnosis, the nurse conducts a focused interview along with a physical assessment to gather additional data. This additional data is then compared with defining characteristics of the probable diagnoses to determine the most appropriate nursing diagnosis for the client. The chapters in Unit III contain focused interview questions for each body region or system. ∞

Phase I: Preinteraction

The **preinteraction** phase is the period before first meeting with the client. During this time, the nurse collects data from the medical record, previous health risk appraisals, health screenings, therapists, dietitians, and other healthcare professionals who have cared for, taught, or counseled the client, and family members or friends. The nurse reviews the client's name, age, sex, nationality, medical and social history, and current health concern. If necessary, the nurse also reviews literature describing recent research, new treatments, medication, prevention strategies, and self-care interventions that might have a bearing on the client's care.

The nurse uses information obtained during the preinteraction phase to plan and guide the direction of the initial interview.

Nurses are more likely to conduct a successful interview if they know in advance, for example, that the client has an emotional problem, is deaf, speaks a foreign language, or is a triathlete.

Information about the client is not the nurse's only consideration during the preinteraction stage. During this phase, the nurse reflects upon his or her own strengths and limitations. For example, a nurse opposed to abortion may have difficulty interviewing a client who is considering an abortion. In this situation, the nurse's anxiety could interfere with the collection of data and the provision of nursing care. Nurses should be aware of their own feelings and prejudices and plan how to interact with the client. For instance, a nurse who has had an experience similar to the client's would decide whether to reveal that to the client.

The nurse chooses the setting and time before the initial interview takes place. A quiet, private place where few distractions or interruptions will occur is most conducive to a successful interview. The client will feel more relaxed and comfortable if the area has subdued lighting, moderate temperature, and comfortable seating. More chairs should be provided if family members or an interpreter will be present. A glass of water and tissues should be available for the client's use. The most ideal setting is one that is private because the presence of another person might hinder the client's ability to be free and open. If the client is hospitalized, the nurse should hold the interview in a private conference room if one is available. The nurse can also hold the interview in the client's room, preferably with no roommates present. If this is not possible, the nurse should select a quiet time of day for the interview, draw bedside curtains or place a screen for privacy, and use a subdued level of speech. In the home setting, a quiet room or even the backyard may be used as long as the client is comfortable and no distractions are present.

The nurse should sit facing the client at a comfortable distance without using a table, a desk, or any other barrier that might make communication difficult. When possible, the nurse and the client should be on the same level. If the nurse sits in a chair that is higher than the client's or stands at the bedside, it places the client in an inferior position that might make the client uncomfortable. A distance of approximately 1.5 to 4 ft between the nurse and the client is most likely to make the client feel at ease. Moving closer than 1.5 ft may invade the client's intimate space, and clients from some cultures may consider this impingement on private space aggressive or seductive. Although 1.5 to 4 ft is the average distance, each person's personal space differs slightly. If the client moves back in the chair, suddenly crosses arms and legs, or seems anxious, the nurse may be invading the client's intimate space. If so, the nurse should move back until the client seems more relaxed. A translator or family member who is present to assist with the interview should sit on one side of the client so that conversation flows easily (see Figure 10.4 ●).

The interview should be scheduled at a time that is convenient for the nurse and the client. The interview should not interfere with cooking dinner, picking up the children after school, or work. If the client is hospitalized, the nurse takes care not to schedule the interview at the same time diagnostic tests or treatments are scheduled, during mealtimes, or during visiting hours. The interview should be postponed if the client is in pain, has been sedated recently, is upset, or is confused.

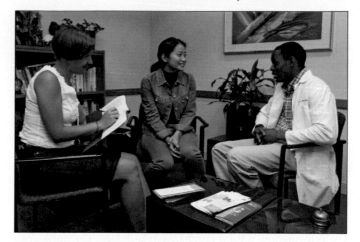

Figure 10.4 ● A translator may help facilitate interaction with a client who does not speak English.

Phase II: The Initial Interview

The initial interview is a planned meeting in which the nurse interviewer gathers information from the client. In most cases, the nurse uses a health history form to collect the data to avoid overlooking any area of information. The nurse gathers information about every facet of the client's health status and state of wellness at this time. This data will be used to develop tentative nursing diagnoses. In addition to providing data, the initial interview also helps establish a nurse-client relationship based on mutual trust and communication, and gives the nurse insight into the client's lifestyle, values, and feelings about wellness, health, and illness. The health assessment interview is an anxiety-producing situation for most clients. In few other situations is a person required to tell a stranger such intimate details about personal history, health habits, or physical and emotional problems. The nurse has a great responsibility to allay these fears and anxieties so that the client can communicate as effectively as possible. One way to make clients feel at ease is to address them by their title (Dr., Mrs., Mr., Ms.) and family name (last name) rather than given name (first name). It is important to ask permission to use the client's given name, since some clients may feel the nurse is being overly familiar or inappropriate. In this case, the client will be reluctant to divulge personal information.

The nurse begins by describing the interviewing process, explaining its importance, and telling the client what to expect. The nurse might say something like this: "Good morning, Mr. Bradley. I'm Janet Goebel, the nurse responsible for your care today. To plan the care, I need some additional information. For about the next 45 minutes I would like to find out as much as possible about you and why you are here. Since we will be talking about a variety of things, I'll be jotting down some notes as we speak. Please stop me at any time if you don't understand a question or need more information about something. Some questions have to do with personal and private areas such as your beliefs, family, income, emotions, and sexual activity. Everything we discuss will be held in strict confidence. However, you may choose not to disclose some information."

Notice several things about these introductory remarks. First, the nurse introduced herself and described the purpose of the interview in a friendly, caring tone intended to make the client feel at ease. Second, the nurse gave the client a time frame and said notes would be taken during the interview. This advance notice is important, because some clients become threatened or anxious when the nurse writes down information. Third, the nurse encouraged the client to interrupt or ask questions at any point during the interview. Finally, the nurse reinforced the privacy and confidentiality of the interview.

After making the introductory comments, the nurse will begin to seek information about the client's health status. The opening questions are purposely broad and vague to let the client adjust to the questioning nature of the interview. For instance, "What led up to your seeking assistance with your health?" If the nurse begins the interview with a series of very specific personal questions, the client may begin to "shut down," giving less and less information, until no exchange takes place. The nurse continuously assesses the client's anxiety level as the interview continues. Restlessness, distraction, and anger are signs that the client perceives the interview as threatening. The nurse will elicit the best information from clients by asking carefully thought-out and clearly stated, open-ended questions throughout the interview.

After gathering sufficient information, the nurse proceeds with closure of the interview. The nurse indicates that the interview is almost at an end and gives the client an opportunity to express any final questions or concerns. For example, "Is there anything else you would like to discuss or ask about, since our time is just about at an end?" It is important to take a few minutes to summarize the information gathered in the interview and to identify key health strengths as well as concerns. The nurse should review what the client can expect next with regard to nursing care. A final step is to thank the client: "I've appreciated your time and cooperation during the interview."

Phase III: The Focused Interview

The nurse uses the **focused interview** throughout the physical assessment, during treatment, and while caring for the client. The purpose of the focused interview is to clarify previously obtained assessment data, gather missing information about a specific health concern, update and identify new diagnostic cues as they occur, guide the direction of a physical assessment as it is being conducted, and identify or validate probable nursing diagnoses.

Consider the following situation: Mr. Joseph Bradley is a 36-year-old stockbroker who is a new client at the outpatient clinic. He told the nurse during the initial interview that he experiences severe abdominal pain, nausea, and bloating after eating spicy foods and that this is why he has decided to seek help. Later that day when Mr. Bradley was admitted to the hospital, the same nurse used a focused interview to elicit the following information from the client: He drinks at least 10 cups of coffee and smokes two packages of cigarettes a day, tends to forget to eat when feeling stressed, uses over-the-counter medication to treat his heartburn, and recently lost a large amount of money in the stock market. When questioned further, Mr. Bradley confirmed that his pain sometimes occurs at times when he has not eaten spicy food. By using a focused interview, the nurse clarified information that had been previously obtained (the client's abdominal pain is not associated with spicy food), included ad-

ditional needed information, and identified several new cues not observed before (caffeine and nicotine intake, stress, and anxiety). It is not unusual for clients like Mr. Bradley to fail to give complete information during the initial interview because of anxiety, distrust, discomfort, or confusion.

Nurses use the focused interview continuously to update diagnostic cues because signs, symptoms, and client health concerns often change from moment to moment or day to day. Nurses perform most focused interviews during routine nursing care. For example, while bathing a man who recently had surgery, the nurse focuses on the client's discomfort by asking pertinent questions about his pain. Examples of focusing questions or statements a nurse might use in this situation to update information include: "Is the pain as severe as it was yesterday?" "Describe the pain you are experiencing now."

In some cases, the information that the nurse learns during the focused interview plays an important part in how physical assessment is performed. For example, if the client states that he is experiencing severe pain in the upper right quadrant of the abdomen, the nurse would examine this area last. Beginning the assessment with the nontender areas permits the nurse to establish the borders of the affected area. Examination of a painful area can exacerbate symptoms, increase the pain, and force termination of the assessment process.

In Mr. Bradley's situation, the nurse's initial hypothetical nursing diagnosis was pain related to consumption of spicy foods, as evidenced by abdominal discomfort, nausea, and abdominal distention. However, with the additional information obtained during the focused interview, the nurse changed the nursing diagnosis to *Pain related to nicotine and caffeine intake, stress, and missed meals, as evidenced by abdominal discomfort, nausea, and abdominal distention.* In view of the new information, the nurse added the following nursing diagnosis: *Anxiety related to financial losses, as evidenced by chain smoking, forgetting meals, increased intake of coffee, and agitation.*

THE HEALTH HISTORY

The goal of the interview process is to obtain a health history containing information about the client's health status. In many healthcare settings, both inpatient and outpatient settings, the nurse and physician complete separate health histories regarding the client. The nursing health history focuses on the client's physical status, patterns of daily living, wellness practices, and self-care activities as well as psychosocial, cultural, environmental, and other factors that influence health status. As nurses gather information during the nursing history, they allow clients an opportunity to express their expectations of the healthcare staff as well as the agency or institution. The information in a nursing health history is used along with the subsequent data from the physical assessment to develop a set of nursing diagnoses that reflect the client's health concerns.

A medical history, by contrast, focuses on the client's past and present illnesses, medical problems, hospitalizations, and family history. The major aim of the medical history is to determine a medical diagnosis that accounts for the client's physiological alteration.

Although nursing and medical histories tend to overlap in some areas, neither format alone presents a true picture of the client's total health status and health needs. Combining the nursing and medical history into one format, the complete health history, provides the most comprehensive source of information for assessing the client's total health needs. Integrating the salient features from the nursing and medical history has distinct advantages for both the client and the caregivers. The information in the health history directs coordinated or collaborative medical and nursing treatment plans that complement one another. The health history saves both the staff and the client time and energy, because the client has to provide significant information only once. Using a health history fosters communication among members of the healthcare team, because they all share its contents. The health history, therefore, fosters effective communication and collaboration between and among the nurse, physician, and other healthcare providers.

COMPONENTS OF THE HEALTH HISTORY

Most healthcare settings have developed nursing and medical health history forms for collecting the data, organizing it, and ensuring that the interviewer does not omit any information. The nursing health history form is organized in a variety of ways in different institutions, agencies, or facilities. That organization often reflects a conceptual framework or nursing model used by that facility. The required information remains constant regardless of which framework or nursing model is used, how the information is labeled, or how the data is categorized. For instance, Orem's model is organized according to self-care deficits (Orem, 1991); Gordon's, according to 11 functional health patterns (Gordon, 1990); and Doenges's, according to 13 diagnostic divisions (Doenges & Moorhouse, 1990). Nonethe-

less, all models focus on the current health concerns along with an additional broad focus on all aspects of the client's lifestyle and response to the environment.

In general, health histories include the following groups of information (see Table 10.2):

- Biographical Data
- Present Health or Illness
- Past History
- Family History
- Psychosocial History
- Review of Body Systems

The information gathered for each of the components of the health history serves a purpose in health assessment and in application of the nursing process for each client. Responses to the questions asked in the health history provide specific information about the individual. The nurse will use professional judgment in determining the significance of the responses, the need for follow-up questioning, and the relevance of information to meeting the health needs of the client.

Biographical Data

The biographical data include the client's name and address, age and date of birth, birthplace, gender, marital status, race, religion, occupation, information about health insurance, and the reliability of the source of information. When possible, the client completes a form that elicits this data. Otherwise, the interviewing nurse documents it.

Gathering biographical data is an important initial step in understanding the client. The biographical data provides a data set from which the nurse can begin to make judgments. The biographical data will be used to relate and compare individual

---

Table 10.2 Health History Format

I. Biographical Data	III. Past History	Family
Name	Medical	Social Structure/Emotional Concerns
Address	Surgical	Self-Concept
Age	Hospitalization	
Date of Birth	Outpatient Care	VI. Review of Body Systems
Birthplace	Childhood Illnesses	Skin, Hair, and Nails
Gender	Immunizations	Head, Neck, and Lymphatics
Marital Status	Mental and Emotional Health	Eyes
Race	Allergies	Ears, Nose, Mouth, and Throat
Ethnic Identity/Culture	Substance Use	Respiratory
Religion and Spirituality		Breasts and Axillae
Occupation	IV. Family History	Cardiovascular
Health Insurance	Immediate Family	Peripheral Vascular
Source of Information/Reliability	Extended Family	Abdomen
	Genogram	Urinary
II. Present Health or Illness		Male Reproductive
Reason for Seeking Care	V. Psychosocial History	Female Reproductive
Health Beliefs and Practices	Occupational History	Musculoskeletal
Health Patterns	Education	Neurologic
Medications, Prescription and Over the Counter	Financial Background	
	Roles and Relationships	

characteristics to established expectations and norms for physical and emotional health. Furthermore, the biographical data provides information about social and environmental characteristics that impact physical and emotional health.

A thorough discussion of each of the pieces of information in the biographical data section of the health history is presented in the following sections. This information is presented to assist the reader in developing and refining the skills required in meeting the healthcare needs of clients.

NAME AND ADDRESS. The client's name and address are generally the first pieces of biographical data to be collected. Listening to the client state his or her name and address provides the first opportunity to assess the client's ability to hear and speak. The client's address reveals information about the client's environment. The nurse will associate the environment with known health benefits and risks. For example, individuals living in crowded urban environments are at risk for problems associated with heavy vehicular traffic including respiratory problems from exhaust. Conversely, access to a variety of healthcare facilities and services is usually greater in urban areas than in rural areas.

AGE AND DATE OF BIRTH. The client's age and date of birth are requested in the biographical data. Establishing the age of the client permits the nurse to begin evaluation of individual characteristics in relation to norms and expectations of physical and social characteristics across the age span. For example, the skin of a 20-year-old is expected to be smooth and elastic, while the skin of a 70-year-old would be expected to have wrinkles and decreased elasticity. The client's age also influences behavior, communication, and dress. For example, one would expect that the vocabulary of an 18-year-old would be greater than that of a 6-year-old. It is expected that adolescent clothing and appearance will be influenced by trends more frequently than will that of older adults.

GENDER. The client's gender is an element of the biographical data. There are differences according to gender in terms of physical development, secondary sex characteristics, and reproduction. For example, males have greater muscle mass than do females. Fat distribution in the thighs, hips, and buttocks is seen in females in greater amounts than in males. Males develop coarse facial hair as a beard while females do not. Moreover, there are health risks associated with sexual differences. For example, although breast cancer can occur in males it occurs more frequently in females. Osteoporosis occurs in both sexes; however, postmenopausal females are at greater risk. Adolescent males are at greater risk for injury from motor vehicle accidents than are females; however, adolescent females have a higher incidence of eating disorders than do boys.

BIRTHPLACE. The biographical data includes identification of the client's birthplace. Identification of the birthplace allows the nurse to determine the environmental and cultural factors that impacted or contributed to the client's current state of health and well-being. For example, in the United States, individuals who are born and live in areas where coal mining accounts for much of the industry are at greater risk for respiratory diseases such as black lung, emphysema, and tuberculosis than are individuals who are born in coastal or mountain areas of the western United States. Further, individuals born in tropical areas outside of the United States are more likely to have been exposed to parasitic diseases than are those born within the United States.

It is important to determine the length of time the client spent in and near the place of birth, and the places in which the client lived before locating to the current residence. Cultural, environmental, and geographic characteristics of regions and nations influence the health and well-being of the inhabitants. For example, there is an increase in the number of Chinese women who smoke, particularly among those who emigrate to the United States. Further, geographic moves force the individuals to adapt and adjust to new cultural norms. Problems in development may result when frequent moves prohibit individuals from forming and maintaining attachments to family and friends. It is important to understand the characteristics of the areas in which clients were born and where they resided throughout their lives. Knowledge of the characteristics of cities, communities, and regions beyond one's own experience is difficult. For example, a nurse who was born and lived in or near New York City can describe an urban and suburban environment that encompasses a highly developed area in terms of industry, business, and entertainment with a transportation and highway system that permits rapid travel and access to business and leisure activities, schools, and a variety of healthcare facilities. That nurse will understand that there are communities within New York City that reflect ethnic, cultural, economic, and social differences. Yet, that same nurse may not be able to describe the characteristics of locations beyond New York City. Persons who emigrated to the United States may have knowledge about their location of origin and the region in which they now reside. However, they may not be able to describe the physical environment of regions beyond their experience. All nurses encounter clients who were born or lived in cities, regions, or countries with which they have little specific knowledge. Therefore, nurses must ask clients to describe the locations in which they were born or resided over time, using questions or statements such as the following:

- Is the place you were born in a city?
- Is the region in which you lived close to a large city?
- Tell me about the place where you were born.

To find out about the physical and environmental characteristics of each location, the nurse will include questions such as these:

- Was the area you grew up in an industrial area?
- Was the place where you were born a farming area?
- How far did you have to travel to shop or go to school or get to a healthcare facility?
- How many people reside in that city?

MARITAL STATUS. Marital status is another element of the biographical data. Marital status indicates if the client is single, married, widowed, or divorced. The above-mentioned designations refer to heterosexual relationships. To ensure that individuals who are from differing sexual orientations have an opportunity to identify a significant relationship, the nurse should ask the client if he or she is now or has ever been in a long-term or committed relationship with another person. It is helpful to determine the length of marriage, relationship, widowhood, and divorced status.

The client's marital or relationship status provides initial information about the presence of significant others who may provide physical or emotional support for the client. In addition, when a client relates the loss of a significant other through death or divorce, the nurse begins to evaluate emotional responses and coping ability expected in relation to the event and length of time from the event. The nurse also considers the information in relation to expectations for development. Developmental theorists such as Erikson, discussed in Chapter 3 of this text, have described stages across the life span, which include the establishment of intimate relationships. ∞ Marriage and establishing intimate relationships is known as a hallmark of young adulthood. Intimacy and sharing in relationships outside of marriage is an essential developmental process when one is single and during middle and older adulthood when one is widowed.

RACE. Race refers to classification of people according to shared biological and genetic characteristics. The nurse can begin to identify characteristics of the client in relation to expectations, norms, and risk factors associated with race. For example, skin coloration is an important health indicator in relation to oxygenation and in identification of jaundice. Assessment of African Americans, Asians, and Caucasians differs because of the levels of melanin, which alters the coloration of the skin across racial lines. Low levels of hemoglobin, as in anemia, can be assessed as pallor in Caucasians and Asians, but in African Americans is best assessed by examining the oral mucosa and assessing capillary refill. Jaundice is best assessed by examination of the sclera of the eye in Asians, who ordinarily have a yellowish skin color or tone. Further, the bone density of African Americans is higher than that of Caucasians or Asians. The following are some health problems associated with racial differences.

- African Americans have a higher incidence of hypertension and hypertension-related kidney failure than Caucasians.
- African Americans have a lower incidence of osteoporosis than Asians or Caucasians.
- Caucasians are at greater risk for peripheral arterial disease than are African Americans.

It is important to note that there has been and continues to be a racial blurring in the United States. Many individuals identify themselves as biracial or as having mixed racial origins. Therefore, expectations, norms, and risks are not as clearly delineated as they have been in the past. Assessment requires careful history taking.

RELIGION. Religion generally refers to an organizing framework for beliefs and practices and is associated with rites, rituals, and ceremonies that mark specific life passages such as birth, adulthood, marriage, and death. Religious beliefs often influence perceptions about health and illness. Religions can impose certain restrictions that impact health, such as not eating pork in the Jewish and Muslim religions.

The nurse will ask the client the following questions or use the following statements to elicit information.

- What is your religion or religious preference?
- Have you ever belonged to a religious group?
- How long have you followed the religion?
- Do you adhere to all of the rules of the religion?
- Tell me how your religion influences your health.

- Are there beliefs that govern your life?
- Tell me how your beliefs affect your relationships with others.

Additional information about the role of religion in the client's life is obtained when asking about health practices, when asking about family history, and when obtaining psychosocial information (see the complete cultural assessment in Box 10.2).

Box 10.2	**Cultural Assessment**

1. What racial group do you identify with?
2. What is your ethnic group?
3. How closely do you identify with that ethnic group?
4. What cultural group does your family identify with?
5. What language do you speak?
6. What language is spoken in your home?
7. Do you need an interpreter to participate in this interview?
8. Would you like an interpreter to be with you when health issues are discussed?
9. Are there customs in your culture about talking and listening, such as the amount of distance one should maintain between individuals, or making eye contact?
10. How much touching is allowed during communication between members of your culture and between you and members of other cultures?
11. How do members of your culture demonstrate respect for another?
12. What are the most important beliefs in your culture?
13. What does your culture believe about health?
14. What does your culture believe about illness or the causes of illness?
15. What are the attitudes about healthcare in your culture?
16. How do members of your culture relate to healthcare professionals?
17. What are the rules about the sex of the person who conducts a health examination in your culture?
18. What are the rules about exposure of body parts in your culture?
19. What are the restrictions about discussing sexual relationships or family relationships in your culture?
20. Do you have a preference for your healthcare provider to be a member of your culture?
21. What do members of your culture believe about mental illness?
22. Does your culture prefer certain ways to discuss topics such as birth, illness, dying, and death?
23. Are there topics that members of your culture would not discuss with a nurse or doctor?
24. Are there rituals or practices that are performed by members of your culture when someone is ill or dying, or when they die?
25. Who is the head of the family in your culture?
26. Who makes decisions about healthcare?
27. Do you or members of your culture use cultural healers or remedies?
28. What are the common remedies used in your culture?
29. What religion do you belong to?
30. Do most members of your culture belong to that religion?
31. Does that religion provide rules or guides related to healthcare?
32. Does your culture or religion influence your diet?
33. Does your culture or religion influence the ways children are brought up?
34. Are there common spiritual beliefs in your culture?
35. How do those spiritual beliefs influence your health?
36. Are there cultural groups in your community that provide support for you and your family?
37. What supports do those groups provide?
38. What do you expect from the healthcare providers in this agency?

OCCUPATION. The client's occupation is part of the biographical data. Information about the client's occupation is important in determining if physical, psychological, or environmental factors associated with work impact the client's health. For example, coal mining is associated with black lung disease. Those employed in law enforcement and safety are at risk for physical injury and experience psychological stresses associated with ensuring one's own safety and that of the community.

HEALTH INSURANCE. Health prevention, health seeking, and health maintenance behaviors are influenced by the ability to pay for services. Therefore, the nurse will ask the client questions regarding health insurance, the type of insurance, and the services that are covered within the insurance plan. For example, the nurse will ask 65-year-old clients if they are enrolled in Medicare A and B and if they have a supplemental insurance. Health insurance alone does not indicate the client's inclination to participate in healthcare. For example, uninsured individuals seek and receive healthcare in clinics and through other low- or no-cost means, and others are private payers for health services. Prior to the nursing interview, clerical staff may obtain information about health insurance.

SOURCE OF INFORMATION. The biographical data must identify the source of the information for the health history. The usual source of information is the client, who is the **primary source**. Secondary sources of information include family members, friends, healthcare professionals, and others who can provide information about the client's health status. The use of translators or interpreters must be indicated when recording the source of information.

RELIABILITY OF THE SOURCE. Reliability of the source means that the person providing information for the health history is able to provide a clear and accurate account of present health, past health, family history, psychosocial information, and information related to each of the body systems. The client is considered to be the most reliable source. Determining reliability of the client includes assessing the ability to hear and speak and the ability to accurately recall health-related past events. However, parents or guardians must serve as the source of information for children. Secondary sources are used when the client cannot participate in the interview because of physical or emotional problems. Secondary sources are selected when their knowledge of the client is sufficient to provide thorough and accurate information. A complete health history may be impossible, for example, when a person has no living relatives or friends who can provide information, when the client is unable to provide information because of a language barrier and no translator is available, and in an emergency when the client is unable to respond and sources of information cannot be identified.

Present Health-Illness

The history of present health or illness includes information about all of the client's current health-related issues, concerns, and problems. The history includes determination of the reason for seeking care, as well as identification of health beliefs and practices, health patterns, health goals, and information about medication and therapies.

REASON FOR SEEKING CARE. The client usually gives the reason for seeking care when the nurse asks, "Why are you seeking help today?" or "What is bothering you?" The reason for seeking care, sometimes written as the chief complaint, is an important part of the health history picture. The nurse explores the reason for seeking care because it provides the first indicators for possible nursing diagnoses and sets the direction of the rest of the health history interview. It is not appropriate, however, to attempt to develop nursing diagnoses at this point. The client has given minimal information, and no physical assessment or diagnostic testing has been performed. Instead, the nurse develops a list of statements that reflect the client's major reasons for seeking care. Each statement is a brief, concise, and time-oriented description of the client's concern. Here are some examples of statements describing reason for seeking care:

- Substernal chest pain since 9:00 a.m.
- Swelling in lower legs and feet for the past 2 weeks
- Physical examination needed for football team by next Tuesday
- Weight gain of 10 lb since discontinuing daily walking regimen

The client's own words should be used to document the reason for contact whenever possible: "I've lost 15 pounds in the last 3 weeks" or "I've lost the feeling in my right arm and hand." The nurse explores the onset and progression of each behavior, symptom, or concern the client relates. Also, the nurse asks clients how their concern has affected their lives and what expectations they have for recovery and subsequent self-care. The answers to these questions provide valuable information about clients' ability to tolerate and cope with the stress brought on by their health concern and healthcare.

HEALTH BELIEFS AND PRACTICES. A person's beliefs about health and illness are influenced by heritage, exposure to information, and experiences. Culture and heritage influence an individual's perceptions about internal and external factors that contribute to health and cause illness and the practices the individual follows to prevent and treat health problems. For example, Mexicans believe that health is largely God's will and is maintained by practices that keep the body in balance. Mexicans also believe that many diseases are caused by disturbance in the hot and cold balance of the body. Navajo Indians believe that health is related to achieving harmony with nature. Illness is explained as disruption in harmony, which is caused by some acts on the part of the ill person or by having a curse placed upon the person. Navajos seek the care of a healer or "medicine man" to determine what the individual has done to disrupt harmony and to restore harmony through a healing ceremony. Mexicans will eat foods that oppose the diseases associated with hot and cold imbalances. Cold foods such as fruit, barley, fish, and vegetables are eaten to combat hot diseases that include infections and kidney diseases.

In the United States and in many Westernized countries, beliefs about health and illness are derived from a scientific approach. The scientific approach includes "germ theory" as applied in infectious diseases; knowledge of changes in body structures and functions associated with aging including arthritis, menopause, and vision changes; as well as the understanding that diet and lifestyle choices influence health and illness. Health practices include seeking healthcare from healthcare providers who use scientific methods to diagnose and treat illness. Healthcare practices include following recommendations for disease prevention including screening for risks, screening for early detection of problems, and immunization.

Two factors have influenced perceptions of health and healthcare practices in the United States. The first factor is that people of all nations have emigrated and continue to emigrate to the United States. As a result, the beliefs and practices of these individuals, families, and groups influence the ways in which individual healthcare is managed. Many of the immigrant populations have adapted to and use the healthcare system in the United States but retain cultural practices. For example, clients with an Irish heritage believe that eating a healthy diet, getting proper sleep, and not going outdoors with wet hair promote health. These clients are likely to use home remedies for colds and headaches. These remedies include the use of tea and honey for a sore throat and applying a wet rag to the head for headaches. Cuban Americans are accustomed to Westernized approaches to all aspects of healthcare, yet many consult an elder or use a *botanica* for herbal treatments before seeking care and continue the use of herbs while receiving prescribed treatments. The adoption of Westernized or scientific beliefs and practices is influenced by the length of time from immigration and often by the age of the client. Conversely, the exposure to and knowledge of a variety of cultural beliefs and healthcare practices has promoted the adoption of many treatments, remedies, and therapies from those cultures by healthcare practitioners in the United States. For example, acupuncture, which is part of traditional Chinese medicine, has become a widely accepted therapy.

Culture influences the client's perceptions of healthcare providers as well. For example, African Americans recognize the doctor as the head of the healthcare team. Arab Americans, Jewish Americans, and Chinese Americans hold physicians in high regard. Mexican Americans respect healthcare professionals but fear seeking care because of concerns about confidentiality. The view of nurses is often dependent upon the cultural view of women's roles in society and a lack of respect for those viewed as subservient to the physician. In many cultures, the assistance of a family member or cultural healer is sought before that of a healthcare professional. Furthermore, health-seeking behaviors are influenced by the type of illness, language barriers, and concerns that family and cultural rituals surrounding care of the sick and dying will not be respected or permitted.

The second factor to influence health beliefs and practices is the availability of information. Healthcare information is widely available in all forms of media, through educational programs, and in literature provided by healthcare and community organizations. The Internet is responsible for dissemination of healthcare information to a growing number of computer owners and users. Increased information about preventive and treatment services has promoted a different approach to healthcare. Clients who use a variety of information sources are more likely to be informed about recommendations for screening and preventive measures for themselves or family members according to age. Informed clients are more likely to seek therapies they have read or heard about, to question recommended therapies, or to seek many opinions about therapy. There are risks associated with the use of the Internet for healthcare information. Clients may not be able to judge the reliability of the source. In addition, healthcare products are available for purchase through the Internet. Clients may purchase and use products that interfere with current therapies or are harmful.

The following are questions or statements used to obtain information about the client's health beliefs and practices:

- What do you think it means to be healthy?
- What are the reasons people become sick?
- Do the members of your family think about health and illness the same way that you do?
- Tell me about your own health.
- What do you do to take care of your health?
- Where do you go for healthcare?
- Does a doctor provide your healthcare?
- Does a nurse provide your healthcare?
- Does a healer associated with your culture or religion provide your healthcare?
- Do you have concerns about the people who will provide your healthcare?
- Are there special practices that need to be carried out by you or your family while you are receiving healthcare?
- Do you use cultural remedies for illness?
- Do you use any home remedies for illness?
- Where do you get information about healthcare?
- Have your healthcare practices changed over time?

The preceding questions and statements are used to elicit information about a client's health beliefs and practices. Many of them are closed questions and require follow-up if a client responds positively. For example, if a client responds that a faith healer is used or a cultural remedy is used, the nurse must follow up. Statements such as "Tell me about the healing" or "Tell me about the kinds of remedies you use" allow clients to describe the treatments or healing in their own words. These questions are included in a general cultural assessment as described in Box 10.2.

HEALTH PATTERNS. A **health pattern** is a set of related traits, habits, or acts that affect a client's health. The description of the client's health patterns plays a key role in the client's total health history because it is the "lifestyle thread" that, woven throughout the fabric of the health history, gives it depth, detail, and definition. For example, the number of hours a client sleeps, the time a client awakens and falls asleep, the number of times a client awakens during the night, and any dream activity are the behaviors that define a client's sleep patterns. Inadequate sleep can contribute to client stress, which in turn can be related to gastrointestinal symptoms, such as upset stomach.

The nurse compares a client's health behavior to predetermined standard health patterns. For example, most people sleep 7 to 9 hours per night, seldom awaken once asleep, and can recall some dream activity. When assessing a client's rest and sleep patterns, the nurse compares the client's behavior to the health pattern standard. Health pattern assessment includes information about diet and nutrition. Chapter 9 of this text provides details about nutritional assessment. ∞ The nurse usually collects information about a client's health patterns as a system or section of the body is assessed with which the health pattern is associated. For example, the nurse might collect information on patterns related to rest and sleep as the neurologic system is assessed, on activity and exercise as the musculoskeletal system is assessed, and on sexuality as the reproductive system is assessed.

Health patterns also refer to the types and frequency of healthcare in which a client participates. The nurse will ask questions related to the frequency of healthcare visits, preventive and screening measures used by the client including laboratory and other diagnostic testing, and the results if known. For example, the nurse will ask the client to give the dates of the last physical, dental, hearing, and eye examinations. In addition, the nurse will inquire about preventive measures such as flu or hepatitis immunization and ask the client about screening for health problems (e.g., mammography for breast cancer, stool examination for bleeding as a sign of rectal cancer, and laboratory screening of cholesterol and glucose levels because of the links with heart disease and diabetes, respectively).

MEDICATIONS. Information about the use of medications is obtained during this part of the health history. The information should include the use of prescription and over-the-counter (OTC) medications. The nurse should determine the name, dose, purpose, duration, frequency, and desired or undesired effects of each of the medications. When the client provides information about medications, the nurse is able to determine the level of knowledge about the medication regimen, whether the client has an understanding of the problem for which the medication has been prescribed, and if the client has noted or received information about the therapeutic effects of the medication. The source of the medication must be identified as well. For example, has the medication been obtained from another country? Has a cultural healer prepared the medication, or is the client using medication that was prescribed for someone else? Sharing of medication is common in some cultures. For instance, Cuban Americans and Chinese Americans often share medications based on the belief that if it helped one person or family member it will also help another. Medication sharing can have harmful effects. In an acute illness, such as a respiratory infection, medication is prescribed according to dose and duration (length of time the drug will be taken) to reduce symptoms and ultimately to cure the illness. When medication is shared, the appropriate dose for the intended duration cannot be achieved. As a result, the illness is ineffectively treated and may become worse. In addition, the medication shared with another may interact or interfere with drugs that the other individual is currently using.

The medication history includes the use of home remedies, folk remedies, herbs, teas, vitamins, dietary supplements, or other substances. The use of folk remedies and herbs is common among immigrant groups in the United States, and the use of vitamins is increasing in the nonimmigrant population. The use of herbal remedies, teas, vitamins, and folk remedies can interfere with the action of some prescribed medications and can in some instances be harmful. For example, exceeding the recommended daily allowance (RDA) of vitamins can result in side effects and toxicity. Large doses of vitamin E can result in increased levels of cholesterol, produce headaches or blurred vision, and increase the risk of bleeding in clients who are taking Coumadin. The nurse uses the medication history to identify any potential drug interactions and to determine if the client requires education about medications, dosing, side effects, and interactions.

When gathering information about medications, it is helpful to ask if the client has the container. Reading the name and dosage provides the specific information the nurse needs to make judgments about client data. It is also helpful to ask clients about categories of OTC medications. Categories may include laxatives; vitamins; herbs; pain relievers, including aspirin and nonsteroidal anti-inflammatory drugs (NSAIDs); dietary supplements; cold remedies; drops for the eyes, nose, or ears; enemas; allergy preparations; appetite stimulants or suppressants; sleeping aids; and medicated lotions, creams, or unguents. Asking about each category is an efficient method to obtain a comprehensive assessment of medication use.

Past History

The past history includes information about childhood diseases; immunizations; allergies; blood transfusions; major illnesses; injuries; hospitalizations; labor and deliveries; surgical procedures; mental, emotional, or psychiatric health problems; and the use of alcohol, tobacco, and other substances. Many health history forms include a checklist of the most commonly occurring illnesses or surgical procedures to help the client recall information. The nurse asks the client to recall all childhood diseases. A history of German measles, polio, chickenpox, streptococcal throat infections, or rheumatic fever is especially significant because these diseases have sequelae that may affect the client's health status and health concerns in adulthood. Also, the nurse ascertains a history of the client's immunizations. If the client is a child, the nurse checks whether the immunizations are up to date. If possible, the immunization data should be verified through immunization records. The nurse questions adult clients concerning the administration of recent tetanus immunizations or boosters, flu shots, or immunizations required for foreign travel. The complete immunization history includes the name of the immunization, the number of doses, and the date of each dose. Chapter 2 provides information about recommended immunization schedules across the age span. ∞

The nurse elicits information about any history of major illnesses, injuries, surgical procedures, hospitalizations, major outpatient care, or therapies. The client should describe each incident, including the date, treatment, healthcare provider, and any other pertinent information. If the client has had a surgical procedure, the nurse elicits specific information concerning the type of surgery and postoperative course. Complicated labor and deliveries are recorded here, as well as in the reproductive section of the review of the systems.

It is important to obtain a thorough history of any chronic illness and major health concerns. Disease processes such as diabetes, heart disease, or asthma are examples of illnesses in this category. The nurse records the onset, frequency, precipitating factors, signs and symptoms, method of treatment, and long-term effects so that this information can be used to meet the learning needs of the client and develop appropriate nursing interventions in the nursing care plan.

Information about the client's emotional, mental, or psychiatric health should include the description of the problem. The nurse asks the client to identify whether care was received through a healthcare provider, through a support group, from a clergyperson or pastor, or within the family or community.

The information should include a description of the therapy or remedy as well as the outcome of treatment. The nurse's questioning must reflect sensitivity to individual and cultural reluctance to describe problems of an emotional or psychiatric dimension. For example, mental or emotional illness is considered as a disgrace by many Asian cultures and as a stigma by those of Arab heritage.

The following questions or statements are used to obtain information about emotional and mental health.

- Have you ever had an emotionally upsetting experience?
- Tell me about any emotional upsets you have experienced.
- Have you ever sought assistance for an emotional problem?
- Where did you go to get assistance?
- Did the assistance help you with the problem?
- Have you ever been told that you have a mental illness or psychiatric disorder?
- What were the circumstances that led to the mental or psychiatric problem?
- What care did you receive for the mental or psychiatric problem?
- Has the care helped the problem?
- Do you take any medication for a mental or psychiatric problem?
- Are you experiencing problems now?
- What kind of help would you like to receive for the emotional, mental, or psychiatric problem?

Information about allergies and the use of illicit drugs, caffeine, alcohol, and tobacco is included in the health history. Information about allergies should include determination of the allergy as food, drug, or environmentally occurring as well as the symptoms, treatment, and personal adaptation. It is important to determine the extent of the client's knowledge about allergens, especially when exposure to allergens can result in anaphylactic reactions. The nurse should ask the client to describe the ways allergies are managed. The information should indicate if a client's allergies have been identified through testing, through confirmation of a cause by a healthcare professional, or by informal means. Eliciting information about adaptation includes identification of client practices such as avoidance of allergens, the use of environmental controls (e.g., filters, air conditioners, or other devices) in the home or work environment, and the use of ingested remedies or medications. The information enables the nurse to begin to identify educational needs about allergies. The learning needs may include general or specific details about avoidance of allergens, methods to manage allergy symptoms, and measures to employ in severe allergic reactions. For example, the nurse may suggest that a client obtain and wear a medic alert bracelet when an allergy to medications is identified.

When gathering information about the use of alcohol, tobacco, caffeine, and illicit drugs, the nurse will want to know the type, amount, duration, and frequency of use of each substance. The information is elicited whether the client is currently using any substances or reports that he or she has stopped using the products. Tobacco use includes cigarettes, cigars, and products that are chewed or inhaled as snuff. Use of any of these products

has an impact on the physical and emotional health of the client and family. Smoking is a causative factor in lung cancer and emphysema. Family members of smokers are at risk for asthma, emphysema, and cancer from secondhand smoke. Alcohol abuse promotes liver disease, increases risk of injury or death in accidents, and is associated with disruptions in families.

Family History

The family history is a review of the client's family to determine if any genetic or familial patterns of health or illness might shed light on the client's current health status. For example, if the client has a family history of type 1 diabetes, the nurse will question the client closely about signs of the disease. These signs include increased appetite, frequent urination, and weight loss. The family history begins with a review of the immediate family, parents, siblings, children, grandparents, aunts, uncles, and cousins. The nurse should encourage the client to recall as many generations as possible to develop a complete picture. If the client provides data about a genetic or familial disease, it is helpful to interview older members of the family for additional information. Adopted children, spouses, and other individuals living with the client may not be related by blood; however, their health history should be reviewed because the client's concern may have an environmental basis. For example, illnesses may be associated with secondhand smoke in the spouse or child of a smoker, or illness may be associated with exposure to toxins or fumes carried into the home on the clothing of a spouse or family member. The nurse documents information collected from the client and the family in a family genogram. A **genogram** is a pictorial representation of family relationships and medical history. The family genogram, also known as a pedigree or family tree, is the most effective method of recording the large amount of data gathered from a family's health history (see Figure 10.5 ●). More information about family history and constructing a pedigree is available through genetics intradisciplinary faculty training, which can be linked to through the Companion Website.

Psychosocial History

The psychosocial history includes information about the client's occupational history, educational level, financial background, roles and relationships, ethnicity and culture, family, spirituality, and self-concept. The information about occupation, education, and finances provides the nurse with cues about previous experiences that may impact current or future health. A client's occupational history can reveal risk factors for a variety of problems. For example, coal mining increases the risk for respiratory diseases, truck driving is associated with kidney disease, and exposure to asbestos in the shipbuilding and construction industries is associated with lung cancer. Determining the client's level of education establishes expectations related to the ability to comprehend verbal and written language. These abilities are significant during the assessment process, in discussion of health problems or needs, and in education of the client. The types of words that will be used and the choice of educational approaches and materials are influenced by the client's abilities to read, write, and in some cases perform calculations. The client's financial situation, that is, the ability to obtain health insurance or pay for health services, has an impact

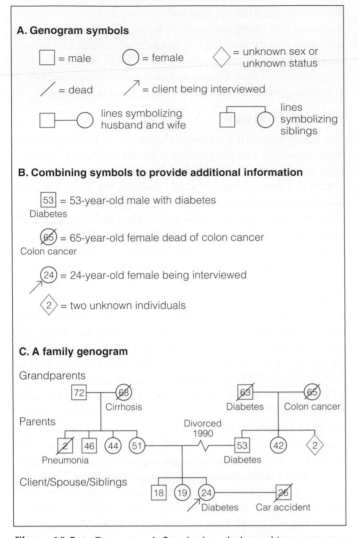

Figure 10.5 ● Genogram. A. Standard symbols used in constructing the family genogram. B. Combining symbols to provide additional information. C. A family genogram.

on health, health practices, and health-seeking behaviors. Low income is associated with a lowered health status and predisposition to illness. A client may report that he now enjoys a secure financial situation. However, he may have been born and raised in poverty. Poverty in youth is associated with poor nutrition and lack of regular medical and dental care. These deficiencies can have long-term consequences for the client.

The nurse will also gather information about the client's roles and relationships, family, ethnicity and culture, spirituality, and self-concept. The nurse will ask the client to identify a significant other and support systems. Support systems include family members, friends, neighbors, club members, clergy and church members, and members of the healthcare team. The information provides an initial impression of the family dynamics and informs the nurse of religious and spiritual needs of the client. Remember that culture influences roles and relationships within families and society. For example, the head of the Cuban household is the male. In Filipino households, the authority in the family is egalitarian, yet the decisions related to healthcare are made mostly by the women. In many Native American groups,

mothers and grandmothers are the decision makers. Determination of roles and relationships is important when planning healthcare and assisting the client to make healthcare decisions. The nurse must respect the practices of the client and prepare to include recognized decision makers in the planning process.

The following are questions and statements to elicit information about roles and relationships, family, and self-concept.

- Tell me about your family.
- How many people are in your family?
- Who is the head of the family?
- What is your role in the family?
- Who makes decisions about healthcare in your family?
- Who is involved in discussing health or emotional problems in your family?
- Are there certain roles for children in the family?
- Who is your significant other?
- Tell me about your support system.
- Tell me how you feel about yourself.
- How would you describe yourself to someone else?
- Tell me about your body image.

When conducting the assessment of culture, the nurse must be careful to avoid stereotyping. That is, the nurse must not assume because a client looks a certain way or has a certain name that he or she belongs to or identifies with a certain cultural or religious group. For example, Mexico is considered a Catholic country, but not all Mexican people are Catholics. In addition, even if the nurse is of the same cultural or ethnic background as the client, it cannot be assumed that the nurse's beliefs and practices are the same. The nurse and the client may identify themselves as Hispanic. However, if the nurse relates to a Colombian culture while the client is from Cuba, the nurse must recognize that aspects of the Latin or Hispanic cultures from those areas can be quite different. A nurse who was born and raised in the United States must avoid assuming that a client who states, "I'm all American" shares the same beliefs and values. The nurse should ask clients to describe what identification with a specific culture means to them. The use of open-ended questions helps to obtain information about the meaning of the client's statements about ethnic or cultural identity. Often the follow-up question about the family's cultural or ethnic identity can reveal areas to explore in relation to beliefs about illness or disease, about diet, and about relationships. For example, a client who states, "I'm all American," may reveal links with ethnic groups after further questioning by saying, "My parents are from Germany, and we eat lots of German foods, but I'm like all of my American friends."

Ethnic Identity and Culture

Information about ethnicity and culture is gathered because it enables the nurse to determine physical and social characteristics that influence healthcare decisions. Ethnicity or culture influences a number of health-related factors for the client. These factors include health beliefs, health practices, verbal and nonverbal methods of communication, roles and relationships in the family and society, perceptions of healthcare professionals, diet, dress and rituals, and rites associated with birth, marriage, child rearing, and death.

Information about the client's ethnicity and culture is obtained by asking the following questions.

- Do you identify with a specific ethnic group?
- How strong would you say that identity is?
- What language do you speak at home?
- Do you or members of your family speak a second language?
- Are you comfortable receiving information about your health in English?
- Would you like an interpreter during this interview?
- Would you like to have an interpreter during the physical examination?
- Are there rules in your culture about the ways an examination must be carried out?
- Are there rules about the gender of the person who is examining you?
- Do you need to have someone in your family participate in the interview or examination?

Information about health beliefs and practices, family, roles and relationships, cultural influences on diet, activity, emotional health, and other topics are included in other components of the health history including the review of systems. For example, when asking about the client's health patterns, the nurse will gather information about cultural healing or rituals associated with health and health maintenance. Further, when asking about nutrition, the nurse will gather information about cultural influences on food selection, preparation, and consumption.

Information about ethnicity and culture can be obtained by conducting a complete cultural assessment at this point in the health history. Box 10.2 includes the information to be obtained in a complete cultural assessment. For more information, review Chapter 4 of this text. ∞

Spirituality refers to the individual's sense of self in relation to others and a higher being, and what one believes gives meaning to life. Assessment of spirituality can be evaluated by asking the following questions.

- Tell me how you meet your spiritual needs.
- Do you have special objects of a religious or spiritual nature that you carry with you or are in your home?
- Are there any religious or spiritual objects that you would want with you if you were ill or hospitalized?
- Is there a member of the clergy you would want to contact if you were ill or hospitalized?
- Is there a person who you would want to contact to help you with prayer or spiritual practices if you were ill or hospitalized?
- Do you use spiritual healers?
- Are there rituals that are important to you when you are ill or have a health problem?
- Tell me about the rituals you use when you are ill or need healthcare.

Chapter 5 of this text provided information about spirituality and spiritual assessment. ∞

Review of Body Systems

The focus of this portion of the health history is to uncover current and past information about each body system and its organs. The nurse asks the client about system function and any abnormal signs or symptoms, paying special attention to gathering information about the functional patterns of each system. For example, when assessing the gastrointestinal system, the nurse should ask the client to describe digestive and elimination patterns ("How many bowel movements do you have each day?") as well as function ("Are your bowel movements usually hard or soft?"). Open-ended questions or statements are best for eliciting information about abnormal signs or symptoms: "Describe the abdominal pain you've been experiencing. What other symptoms are associated with the pain?" The nurse carefully explores characteristics and quality of each subjective symptom the client identifies to obtain a total picture of each system.

Some health history formats use a cephalocaudal or head-to-toe approach for collecting data. In this approach, one considers regions of the body rather than systems. Other formats use an approach related to a nursing theory. Regardless of the method, each area of the body must be reviewed until all systems are covered in each region.

Unit III of this text provides information related to the systems of the body. ∞ Each chapter provides suggestions for questions to gather data about a particular system. Focused interview questions are included and follow-up information is provided to elicit details when symptoms are reported. Examples of the types of information required for comprehensive system review are included in the sample documentation of the health history. Box 10.3 lists the systems included in this part of the health history.

DOCUMENTATION

The data collected during the interview is recorded in the nurse's health history. The type of recording is often influenced by the agency or facility in which the interview is carried out. Forms for documentation are varied and include checklists, fill-in forms, and narrative records. The nurse's health history becomes part of the client record and is a legal document. Principles of documentation must be applied.

Box 10.3	Review of Body Systems

- Skin, Hair, and Nails
- Head, Neck, and Related Lymphatics
- Eye
- Ear, Nose, Mouth, and Throat
- Respiratory System
- Breasts and Axillae
- Cardiovascular System
- Peripheral Vascular System
- Abdomen
- Urinary System
- Reproductive System
- Musculoskeletal System
- Neurologic System

The subjective data is recorded using quotes. The nurse uses communication skills to elicit as much detail as possible about each area and topic within the health history. The nurse should ask the client to explain his or her meaning of words such as good, average, okay, normal, and adequate. The nurse must be sure to record what the client intended by use of such terms.

When recording data, the information must be presented in a clear and concise manner. For example, the nurse would use dates and write them in descending order from present to past when providing details about events. Sample documentation of the health history is included in Boxes 10.4 and 10.5. Box 10.4 is a case study presented in narrative form. Box 10.5 represents a fill-in form for documentation of the health history. The fill-in form does not use quotation marks because all entries are as stated by the client.

Box 10.4	Narrative Recording of the Health History

Biographical Data Mrs. Amparo Bellisimo, age 31, comes to the health center for a health assessment. She is employed as an account representative for a large clothing retail establishment. Mrs. Bellisimo has insurance through Corporate Insurance Company, through her employer. It covers medical, dental, and eye care. She lives in a single-family residence at 22 Highland Avenue, Midland Park, New Jersey. Mrs. Bellisimo lives with her husband, who she names as her emergency contact. Mrs. Bellisimo was born on July 20, 1973, in Santa Clara, Cuba. She emigrated to the United States 9 years ago. She speaks English with an accent. Mrs. Bellisimo can read and write in English and Spanish. Mrs. Bellisimo has no immediate family in the United States. She completed 12 years of schooling in Cuba and took several accounting courses in a community college in New Jersey. She has no formal religious affiliations, because religious practice was not permitted in Cuba when she was there. Some of her family were "hidden" Catholics. She states, "I am happy with my life. I have made adjustments to being in the United States. I have many Cuban friends and have a close relationship with my husband's family. I like my job, except when it gets crazy."

Present Health Status: Reason for Seeking Health Care
Mrs. Bellisimo has no complaints except "weight gain and occasional headaches relieved with aspirin." The weight gain has occurred "over 3 years since I started dating my husband and more since we got married last year." The headaches occur "when I'm tired, stressed, or reading too much."

Health Beliefs and Practices Mrs. Bellisimo has no current health problem, except as stated above. She believes "health is important and you need to take care of yourself, but sometimes it's out of your control." When she was a child her mother used to tell her things like "no bathing when you have your period, no water at all" and she "prepared certain foods for certain illnesses and sometimes got medicines from a botanica for ailments." Since she has been covered by health insurance and encouraged by her husband, she has had regular physical, gynecologic, dental, and eye examinations, all of which have been completed annually for 3 years.

Mrs. Bellisimo states she "sleeps well most nights about 8 hours, unless I stay up and read." She "feels rested most mornings." She tries to exercise but finds it hard "after work and when it's cold out."

Mrs. Bellisimo would like to lose weight. She would "feel healthier, my clothes would fit and I'd feel good about myself." People in Cuba would not have a problem with this weight, but "I don't like it." Eating patterns include "fast foods at lunch, bread at every meal, and dessert or snacks at night."

Medications Mrs. Bellisimo uses oral contraceptives "for 4 years," without problems, and takes a multivitamin every day. She is not undergoing any therapy and "really have never needed any specific care."

Past Hisotry, Surgeries and Illnesses Mrs. Bellisimo had measles as a child. She received smallpox, polio, mumps, tetanus, and other "vaccines" as a child. She has had no major illnesses. She has never been hospitalized, received a blood transfusion, been pregnant, or had allergies. Mrs. Bellisimo cut her lower left leg on glass as a child and had sutures, and a scar remains. She had four wisdom teeth extracted 2 years ago with no complications, "no other surgery."

Emotional History Mrs. Bellisimo states, "I miss my family and get sad when I can't see them. I get frustrated when I don't understand some American ways. I'm pretty emotional. I cry over books and movies, but I haven't had a mental problem." She doesn't smoke, but her whole family smoked when she was in Cuba. "I drink some beer, wine, and tequila on weekends or at dinner with my in-laws. I have never used drugs or anything like that."

Family History Mrs. Bellisimo's father died at age 56 from "some cancer." "He didn't live with us, so I don't know for sure and my mother doesn't say." Her mother is 49 and well. She has a brother, 33, and a sister, 27. Both are "well." Her grandparents were not really known to her but were "old when they died."

Psychosocial History-Occupation Mrs. Bellisimo held jobs in hotels as a teenager in Cuba. "Since coming to America, I have worked in a factory making clothes, been a receptionist in a hair salon, and in some form of accounting for the past 5 years." She states, "I have not been poor but just okay almost all my life until the last 4 or 5 years. Things are really bad in Cuba, no proper food or medicine. They were better when I was there, but not like here."

Roles and Relationships She states, "I love my family, but I can't see them. I have friends here that are like my family. My friends were a big part of my wedding. One walked me down the aisle. I call home to Cuba, but it's hard to be far away. My husband is American and we dated for 2 years before we got engaged. He helped me a lot and we love each other a lot. His family are like my new family. We see them a lot, they help us, and they treat me like a daughter, so it's very good."

Ethnicity and Culture Mrs. Bellisimo says she will always consider herself Cuban, but "I am an American citizen now, and am so much more of a gringo than my friends. I have come to like American food, especially pasta, but still make my beans and rice and other Cuban foods. My husband likes it too but not every day. I laugh sometimes when I call my mother in Cuba and speak English sometimes."

Spirituality Mrs. Bellisimo states, "I have no real religion; family and honesty are important to me. I believe in God and sometimes pray, but really believe your family helps you when you are in need."

Self Concept Mrs. Bellisimo says of herself, "I am a good person. I worry about others. I want to have a family, with children who understand about being Cuban but who believe America is a good place. I was brainwashed and thought gringos were mean and selfish people. I have come to know better. I take care of myself and other than some extra pounds think I look pretty good."

Box 10.4	**Narrative Recording of the Health History** *(continued)*

Review of Systems

Skin, Hair, and Nails

No reported problems. "I use sunscreen, shower daily, use conditioner on my hair and lotion to prevent dry skin. I would like to have a professional manicure more often, but keep my nails looking nice."

Head and Neck

No reported problems except "occasional headache relieved by aspirin."

Eyes

Annual eye exam for 3 years. Glasses for "driving."

Ear, Nose, Mouth, and Throat

No problems with hearing, has "never had an official exam." Regular dental exams. Wisdom teeth extracted with no problems. No trouble eating or swallowing.

Respiratory

No reported problems. "A cold once a year." No exposure to pollutants. No history of tobacco use. Exposure to secondhand smoke from birth to 22 years of age at home. Denies cough, difficulty breathing.

Breasts and Axillae

"I have large breasts and have since I was 12. I don't like to examine my breasts; I get scared I might find something. I do get them checked every year by the doctor." No changes, discharge, discomfort.

Cardiac

No reported problems. No history of heart disease. Never has palpitations.

Peripheral Vascular

No reported problems. "The doctor says my blood pressure is fine. I have two veiny spots on my legs, but they don't hurt. They are flat and stringy."

Gastrointestinal

No reported problems. "My bowels move every day with no problem. I get diarrhea when I'm nervous sometimes."

Urinary

No reported problems. "I pass urine five or six times a day and more if I drink more."

Reproductive

Onset of menses age 11. "Regular every 28 days for 3 or 4 days. I take birth control pills." Denies pregnancy, abortion. "Relations are good with my husband."

Musculoskeletal

No reported problems. "I don't get enough exercise."

Neurologic

No history of head injury, seizure, tremor, loss of consciousness. "Other than headache, I'm okay."

Box 10.5	**Documentation of a Health History**

Health History

Date: June 30th

Name:	Amparo Bellisimo
Address:	22 Highland Avenue
	Midland Park, NJ 07432
Telephone:	201-555-0000
Age:	31
Date of birth:	July 20, 1974
Birthplace:	Santa Clara, Cuba. Came to U.S. 9 years ago.
	(Sixth largest city in Cuba, hospital, university, manufacturing. Three hours from Havana. Historical significance: Last battle site of Revolution, memorial to Che Guevara.)
Gender:	Female
Marital status:	Married (Chris, age 32, emergency contact)
Race:	Cuban
Religion:	None really, religious practice was forbidden in Cuba.
	Some family are hidden Catholics.
Occupation:	Account representative. Retail clothing establishment.
Health insurance:	Corporate insurance. Medical, dental, eye care.
Source:	Client
Reliability:	Reliable, alert, oriented, recall of information intact.
	(nursing assessment).

Present Health/Illness

Reason for seeking care

Scheduled health assessment. No complaints except weight gain and occasional headaches, relieved with aspirin. Weight gain of 20 pounds over 3 years since I started dating my husband, most since we got married last year. I get headaches when I'm stressed, tired, or read too much.

Health beliefs and practices

Health is important and you need to take care of yourself, but sometimes it's out of your control. When I was younger my mother would tell me no bathing when you have your period, no water at all. My mother prepared certain foods for certain illnesses and sometimes got medicine from a botanica for ailments. All medical care was done well because it was all free.

Health patterns

At first in America I didn't see doctors. Since I have health insurance and my husband reminds me to make appointments, I have medical, dentist, gynecologist, and eye doctor exams. I have had them all every year for the

(continued)

Box 10.5	Documentation of a Health History *(continued)*

last 3 years. I don't examine my breasts but the doctor does it each year. I haven't had any vaccines since I came here and I think my blood tests are okay. I sleep well most nights for about 8 hours, unless I stay up and read. I try to exercise but it is so hard after work and when it's cold out. Diet is crazy sometimes. I have coffee and toast in the morning. Lunch depends on my schedule, sometimes a sandwich, sometimes a salad. Dinner is probably pizza or fast food three or four times a week. I have a sweet at night.

I like all kinds of foods and I still like Cuban foods like beans, pork, and rice. I eat all kinds of American foods. I especially like pasta and I like bread, I have it at almost all meals.

Medications

I take birth control pills.

I have been on them for 4 years.

I have not had a problem.

I take a vitamin "one-a-day" every day, my doctor told me to.

I take aspirin for headaches but that's all.

I don't use stuff like my mother did in Cuba and that some of my friends do.

Health goals

To lose weight so my clothes fit and I feel better about myself. In Cuba people would not have a problem with this weight, but I don't like it.

Past History

Childhood Illnesses

Measles when I was little. I don't remember other illnesses.

Immunizations

Smallpox, polio, and other vaccines like tetanus as a child. I don't remember other specifically.

Medical Illnesses

A cold every year—but really no serious illnesses.

Hospitalization

I've never been in the hospital.

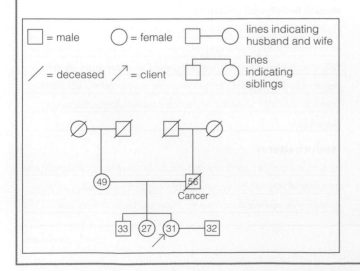

Surgery

Never had any except wisdom teeth. All four out 2 years ago because the dentist said they were packed in. I did okay.

Injury

Cut on my leg on glass, had stitches and have a scar by my knee.

Blood transfusion

Never had one.

Emotional/psychiatric problems

I miss my family and get sad when I can't see them. I get frustrated when I don't understand some American ways and I'm pretty emotional. I cry over books and movies, but I haven't had a mental problem.

Allergies

Food: None I know of.

Medication: I don't know of any.

Environment: No, I don't have a problem.

Use of tobacco

I don't smoke, never have, but my family smoked when I was in Cuba.

Use of alcohol

I have a glass of beer or wine or tequila on weekends or at dinner with my in-laws. One or two glasses maybe two times a week.

Use of illicit drugs

I have never used drugs or anything like that.

Family History

Father

He died at age 56 from "some cancer." He didn't live with us, so I don't know for sure and my mother doesn't say.

Mother

Her mother is 49 and well.

Siblings

She has a brother, 33, and a sister, 27. Both are "well."

Grandparents

Her grandparents were not really known to her but were "old" when they died.

Psychosocial History

Occupational history

Jobs in hotels as teenager in Cuba.

In America—a factory making clothes, a receptionist in a hair salon, and in some form of accounting for 5 years.

Educational level

Completed 12 years in Cuba.

A few courses in accounting in community college in America 6 years ago.

Speaks: English, Spanish

Reads: English, Spanish

Box 10.5	Documentation of a Health History *(continued)*

Financial background

I have not been poor but just okay for all my life until the last 4 or 5 years. Things are really bad in Cuba. No food or medicine. They were better when I was there but not like here.

Roles and relationships

I love my family but I can't see them. I have friends here that are like my family. My friends were a big part of my wedding. One walked me down the aisle. I call home to Cuba but it's hard to be far away.

Ethnicity and culture

I will always consider myself Cuban but I am an American citizen now and am so much more gringo than my friends. I like all American things, especially food. I still make beans and rice and other Cuban foods. My husband likes it too but not every day.

Family

My family is in Cuba. Oh, I miss them bad. Would like them to come here someday. My husband is American. We dated for 2 years before we got married. He helped me a lot and we love each other very much. His family is my new family. We see them a lot, they help us out, they treat me like a daughter so it's very good.

Spirituality

I have no real religion. Family and honesty are important to me. I believe in God and sometimes pray but I really believe your family helps you when you are in need.

Self-concept

I am a good person. I worry about others. I want to have a family with children who understand being Cuban but who believe America is a good place. I take care of myself and except for a few pounds I think I look pretty good.

Review of Systems

Skin, hair, nails

No changes, rashes, lesions, color changes, sweating. No birthmarks. Scar left knee. Shower daily, hair shampoo every other day. No use of hair dyes for 2 years. Would like professional manicure more often but keeps nails nice.

Head, neck, related lymphatics

Occasional headaches relieved by aspirin. No history of injury, seizure, tremor, dizziness. No neck swelling.

Eye

Annual exam—no change in 2 years.

Glasses for distance.

Next exam—3 months.

Ears, nose, mouth, and throat

No hearing problems, never had specific exam.

Nose patent, no injury, sense of smell intact, clear drainage with cold.

No trouble eating or swallowing.

Dental exam annually, last exam 1 month ago. Brushes and flosses twice daily.

Respiratory

No respiratory problems. A cold once a year. No exposure to pollutants.

No history of tobacco use. Exposure to secondhand smoke birth to 22 years. Denies cough, difficult breathing.

No history of respiratory problems.

Unsure of TB screening.

Breasts and axillae

Annual exam by physician.

No SBE.

Large breasts with no masses, lumps, or discharge.

Cardiovascula

No history of heart disease. Never has palpitations. No edema or cyanosis.

Peripheral vascular

The doctor says my blood pressure is fine. I have two veiny spots on my legs but they don't hurt.

Abdomen

No reported problems. My bowels move every day with no problem. I get diarrhea when I'm nervous sometimes.

Urinary

No reported problems. No history of UTI. I pass urine five or six times a day and more if I drink more.

Reproductive

On oral contraceptives. Onset menses age 11. Regular every 28 days for 3 to 4 days.

Para 0

Gravida 0

Relations are good with my husband.

Musculoskeletal

No problems.

I don't get enough exercise.

Range of motion—normal. No problems with strength.

Neurologic

Other than headache, I'm okay.

Denies falls, balance problems, memory problems.

Right-handed. Can sense touch and temperature.

NURSING CONSIDERATIONS

The professional nurse must consider the ability of the client to participate in the interview process. As stated previously, culture and language are important considerations in establishing a positive relationship. Additional factors that can affect the interview process are alterations in the senses, such as blindness or hearing deficits, developmental level, and pain. The nurse may have to develop written questions for use with clients with hearing deficits to overcome the difficulty.

It is important to consider the client's developmental level when conducting an interview. Word usage and overall communication will differ when interviewing children and adolescents. In addition, one may find that the developmental level of a client differs from that expected for a stated age. Clients who have experienced neurologic problems congenitally, as a result of injury or aging, may not be able to participate effectively in an interview. Last, when a client is experiencing unrelieved acute or chronic pain, the ability to participate in a lengthy interview is diminished. The nurse must then focus on the immediacy of the problem and gather in-depth information at another time.

The nurse uses the health history and interview in various healthcare settings to create a comprehensive account of the client's past and present health. The completed health history is a compilation of all the client data collected by the nurse, and it is combined with information obtained during the nursing physical assessment to form the total health database for the client. The nurse can use this database, which provides a total picture of the client's past and present physical, psychological, social, cultural, and spiritual health, to formulate nursing diagnoses and plan the client's care.

The process of interviewing to obtain a complete picture of the client can be uncomfortable. To obtain the required information the nurse will be asking clients to provide information about their physical and psychosocial well-being, family, personal habits, body functions, and lifestyle. The nurse may believe that clients will perceive questions about religion, culture, economic status, body functions, and sexuality as intrusive. The nurse may feel that he or she is prying or being nosy by asking certain questions. Remember that the nurse- client interaction is different from social interaction experienced in the past. When taking on the role of the nurse, the questions are intended to guide healthcare decisions. It is helpful to practice the communication techniques that were discussed earlier in the chapter. The nurse will also find it helpful to prepare a list of questions or statements for each category of the health history before conducting the interview. For example, when asking about the financial status of the client, the nurse may state, "Tell me about your financial situation" or "How would you classify your economic situation?" The nurse may want to use a list of categories in the following way. "Of the following economic levels—low, middle, or high income—how would you rate your current situation?" The nurse could add actual dollar amounts to be more specific.

The nurse should be prepared to address areas concerned with the client's self-esteem and emotional state. For example, clients may be asked to describe their image in a mirror. The nurse could ask each client to describe the following in a few sentences: self-perception of strengths and weaknesses, personality, or how a friend or loved one would describe him or her. Often, when addressing sensitive areas such as mental and emotional health, a straightforward question is the best approach. For example, "Have you ever experienced an emotional upset?" If the response is yes, the nurse should ask the client to describe it. The nurse might ask the client, "Have you ever had a strong emotional response to a person or situation?" If the response is yes, the nurse would ask the client to describe it. The nurse may also list a number of emotional behaviors and ask the client to respond yes or no to each item on the list. Examples of emotional behaviors include anxiety, depression, fear, grief, loneliness, or joy.

Questions about body functions, habits, adaptation, and lifestyle may be difficult for a novice in nursing. It is helpful to use the words and terms associated with parts of the body, body functions, and habits regularly when speaking and writing. The focused interview questions provided in each chapter of Unit III of this text are intended to guide the nurse in eliciting information about functions, practices, and behaviors associated with each of the body systems. ⬭ One should refer to these frequently and use them in preparation for client interviews.

Application Through Critical Thinking

CASE STUDY

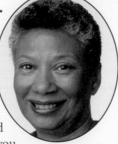

*T*he nurse conducted a health history interview with Mrs. Martha Washburn, a 67-year-old African American. The following are excerpts from the health history.

Mrs. Washburn, I am going to ask you a lot of questions before your physical. I need to have correct responses and I have to tell you, there will be a lot of them if we are to get to the root of your problem. I will use the information to develop a plan of care.

What are you here for? Did someone come with you? I see on your chart that you have some problems with urination; are you incontinent? How long have you had the problem?

The nurse included the following questions: What is your economic status? Do you go to church? What do you do when you are ill?

We need information about your family, so let's start out with your parents. Are they alive? Do you have siblings?

The nurse completed a review of symptoms and prepared the client for the physical examination by showing her into a room and telling her to get undressed.

▶ Critical Thinking Questions

1. Critique the nurse's actions in the initial interview phase of the case study.

2. Identify the types of information sought in the questions in the case study.
3. Create alternative approaches to the interview and questioning techniques in the case study.
4. Describe your preparation for an interview of Mrs. Washburn.

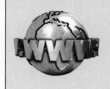

Please refer to the Companion Website at www.prenhall.com/damico and click on Chapter 10, the Application Through Critical Thinking module, to complete the following activities related to this case study:

▶ **Critical Thinking questions**

EXPLORE MediaLink

Additional resources for this chapter are found on the Student CD-ROM accompanying this textbook and on the Companion Website.

CD-ROM CONTENT

Content for this chapter includes:
Objectives
Key Concepts
NCLEX-RN® Review Questions
Model Documentation Forms
Audio Glossary
Head-to-Toe Physical Examination Video

COMPANION WEBSITE CONTENT

www.prenhall.com/damico

Content for this chapter includes:
Objectives
NCLEX-RN® Review Questions
Application Through Critical Thinking
    Case Study Teaching Plan Challenge

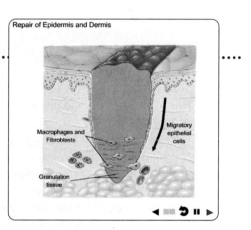

Repair of Epidermis and Dermis

Macrophages and Fibroblasts

Migratory epithelial cells

Granulation tissue

MediaLinks
MediaLink Application
Tool Box
    Cultural Assessment
    Review of Body Systems
    Health Promotion
        Healthy People 2010
        Client Education
New York Times

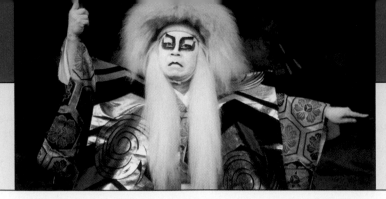

11
Skin, Hair, and Nails

CHAPTER OBJECTIVES

Upon completion of this chapter, you will be able to:

1. Identify the anatomy and physiology of the skin, hair, and nails.

2. Develop questions to be used when completing the focused interview.

3. Explain client preparation for assessment of the skin, hair, and nails.

4. Differentiate normal from abnormal findings in physical assessment.

5. Describe developmental, psychosocial, cultural, and environmental variations in assessment techniques and findings.

6. Discuss the focus areas related to overall health of the skin as presented in *Healthy People 2010* initiatives.

7. Apply critical thinking in selected simulations related to physical assessment of the skin, hair, and nails.

MEDIALINK

www.prenhall.com/damico

The CD-ROM in the back of this textbook and the Media-Link website contain NCLEX-RN® review questions, interactive exercises, case study challenges, animations, videos, documentation and checklist forms, and review materials. For a complete listing of the media content specific to Chapter 11, see the Explore MediaLink at the end of the chapter.

CHAPTER OUTLINE

The skin, hair, and nails are the major components of the integumentary system. The integumentary system consists of the skin and the accessory structures, the sweat and oil glands, the hair, and the nails. The largest organ of the body, the skin weighs approximately 9 lb (4.09 kg) and has a surface area of about 15 to 20 (4.5 to 6 m) ft in adults. Every square inch of the skin contains 10 to 15 ft (3 to 4.5 m) of blood vessels and nerves, hundreds of sweat and oil glands, and over 3 million cells that are constantly dying and being replaced. This complex shield protects the body against heat, ultraviolet rays, trauma, and invasion by bacteria. In addition, the skin works with other body systems to regulate body temperature, synthesize vitamin D, store blood and fats, excrete body wastes, and help humans sense the world around them.

A thorough assessment of the skin, hair, and nails provides valuable clues to a client's general health. The skin, hair, and nails can suggest the status of a client's nutrition, airway clearance, thermoregulation, and tissue perfusion. The skin, hair, and nails can also reveal alterations in activity, sleep and rest, level of stress, and self-care ability. A client's ancestry, cultural practices, and physical environment, both at home and at work, can greatly influence integumentary health and are an integral part of the assessment data. Identification and reduction of environmental risk factors for skin diseases including skin cancer and occupational skin disorders are among the objectives related to integumentary health as shown in the *Healthy People 2010* feature on page 229.

A client's developmental stage has a tremendous influence on the appearance and functioning of these structures. Skin is very thin at birth and thickens throughout childhood. Sweat and oil glands are activated during adolescence. The function of these glands diminishes in the older adult. The appearance of the skin, hair, and nails impacts the self-concept of the individual. Skin disorders may interfere with social relationships, roles, and sexuality. Stress may also trigger or exacerbate skin disorders. The type of soap or agents used as part of the cleansing routine may contribute to dry, oily, itchy skin, or rashes. Hair-styling methods, use of hair products, chemical curling, or bleaching may be factors in damage, breakage, or loss of hair.

ANATOMY AND PHYSIOLOGY REVIEW

The skin is composed of the epidermal, dermal, and subcutaneous layers. The cutaneous glands, which are located in the dermal layer, release secretions to lubricate the skin and to assist in temperature regulation. The hair and nails are composed of keratinized (hardened) cells and serve to protect the skin and the ends of the fingers and toes. Each of these anatomical structures is described in the following paragraphs.

SKIN AND GLANDS

The skin is composed of two distinct layers. The outer layer, called the **epidermis,** is firmly attached to an underlying layer called the **dermis.** Deep in the dermis is a layer of subcutaneous tissue that anchors the skin to the underlying body structures.

Epidermis

The epidermis is a layer of epithelial tissue that comprises the outermost portion of the skin. Where exposure to friction is greatest, such as on the fingertips, palms, and soles of the feet, the epidermis consists of five layers (or strata), as shown in Figure 11.1 ●. These five layers are, from deep to superficial, the stratum basale, stratum spinosum, stratum granulosum, stratum lucidum, and stratum corneum.

New skin cells are formed in the stratum basale, or basal layer, which is also known as the stratum germinativum (germinating layer). These new skin cells consist mostly of a fibrous protein called **keratin,** which gives the epidermis its tough, protective qualities. About 25% of the cells in the stratum basale are *melanocytes,* which produce the skin pigment called **melanin.** All humans have the same relative number of melanocytes, but the

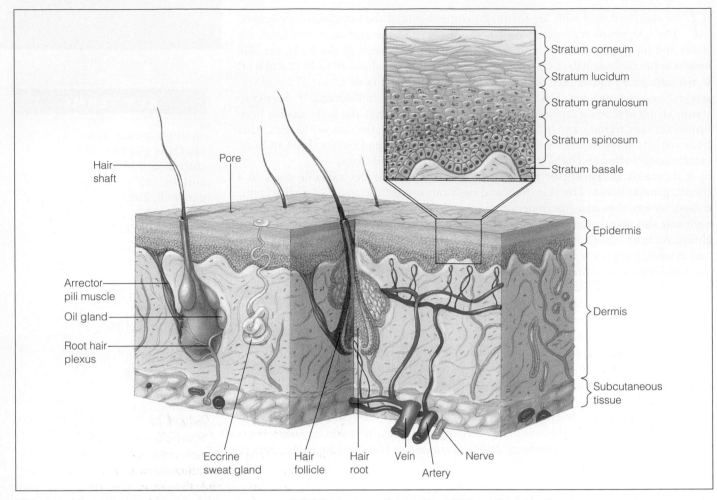

Figure 11.1 ● Skin structure. Three-dimensional view of the skin, subcutaneous tissue, glands, and hairs.

amount of melanin they produce varies according to genetic, hormonal, and environmental factors.

Cells produced in the stratum basale gradually move through the layers of the epidermis toward the stratum corneum, where they are sloughed off. The abundance of keratin in this tough "horny layer" protects against abrasion and trauma, repels water, resists water loss, and renders the body insensitive to a variety of environmental toxins.

Dermis

The dermis is a layer of connective tissue that lies just below the epidermis. The dermis consists mainly of two types of fibers: collagen, which gives the skin its toughness and enables it to resist tearing, and the elastic fibers, which give the skin its elasticity. The dermis is richly supplied with nerves, blood vessels, and lymphatic vessels, and it is embedded with hair follicles, sweat glands, oil glands, and sensory receptors.

SUBCUTANEOUS TISSUE

The subcutaneous tissue (or **hypodermis**) is a loose connective tissue that stores approximately half of the body's fat cells. Thus, it cushions the body against trauma, insulates the body from heat loss, and stores fat for energy.

CUTANEOUS GLANDS

The cutaneous glands are formed in the stratum basale and push deep into the dermis. They release their secretions through ducts onto the skin surface.

There are two types of sweat (or sudoriferous) glands: eccrine and apocrine. **Eccrine glands** are more numerous and more widely distributed. They produce a clear perspiration mostly made up of water and salts, which they release into funnel-shaped pores at the skin surface. **Apocrine glands** are found primarily in the axillary and anogenital regions. They are dormant until the onset of puberty. Apocrine glands produce a secretion made up of water, salts, fatty acids, and proteins, which is released into hair follicles. When apocrine sweat mixes with bacteria on the skin surface, it assumes a musky odor.

OIL GLANDS

Oil glands, or **sebaceous glands,** are distributed over most of the body except the palms of the hands and soles of the feet. They produce *sebum,* an oily secretion composed of fat and keratin that is usually released into hair follicles.

The major functions of the skin are the following:

● Perceiving touch, pressure, temperature, and pain via the nerve endings

- Protecting against mechanical, chemical, thermal, and solar damage
- Protecting against loss of water and electrolytes
- Regulating body temperature
- Repairing surface wounds through cellular replacement
- Synthesizing vitamin D
- Allowing identification through uniqueness of facial contours, skin and hair color, and fingerprints

The major functions of the cutaneous glands are the following:

- Excreting uric acid, urea, ammonia, sodium, potassium, and other metabolic wastes
- Regulating temperature through evaporation of perspiration on the skin surface
- Protecting against bacterial growth on the skin surface
- Softening, lubricating, and waterproofing skin and hair
- Resisting water loss from the skin surface in low-humidity environments
- Protecting deeper skin regions from bacteria on the skin surface

HAIR

A **hair** is a thin, flexible, elongated fiber composed of dead, keratinized cells that grow out in a columnar fashion (Figure 11.1). Each hair shaft arises from a follicle. Nerve endings in the follicle are sensitive to the slightest movement of the hair. Each hair follicle also has an arrector pili muscle that causes the hair to contract and stand upright when a person is under stress or exposed to cold.

The deep end of each follicle expands to form a hair bulb. New cells are produced at the hair bulb. Hair growth is cyclic; scalp hair typically has an active phase of about 4 years and a resting phase of a few months. Because these phases are not synchronous, only a small percentage of a person's hair follicles shed their hair at any given time.

Hair color is determined by the amount of melanin produced in the hair follicle. Black or brown hair contains the greatest amount of melanin.

The type and distribution of hair vary in different parts of the body. **Vellus hair,** a pale, fine, short strand, grows over the entire body except for the margins of the lips, the nipples, the palms of the hands, the soles of the feet, and parts of the external genitals. The **terminal hair** of the eyebrows and scalp is usually darker, coarser, and longer. At puberty, hormones signal the growth of terminal hair in the axillae, pubic region, and legs of both sexes, and on the face and chest of most males.

The major functions of the hair are to insulate against heat and cold, protect against ultraviolet and infrared rays, perceive movement or touch, protect the eyes from sweat, and protect the nasal passages from foreign particles.

NAILS

Nails are thin plates of keratinized epidermal cells that shield the distal ends of the fingers and toes (see Figure 11.2 ●). Nail growth occurs at the nail matrix, as new cells arise from the basal layer of the epidermis. As the nail cells grow out from the matrix, they form a transparent layer, called the body of the nail, which extends over the nail bed. The nail body appears pink because of the blood supply in the underlying dermis. A moon-shaped crescent called a **lunula** appears on the nail body over the thickened nail matrix. A fold of epidermal skin called a **cuticle** protects the root and sides of each nail. The major functions of the nails are to protect the tips of the fingers and toes and aid in picking up small objects, grasping, and scratching.

SPECIAL CONSIDERATIONS

Throughout the assessment process, the nurse gathers subjective and objective data reflecting the client's state of health. Using critical thinking and the nursing process, the nurse identifies many factors to be considered when collecting the data. Some of these factors include but are not limited to age, developmental level, race, ethnicity, work history, living conditions, social economics, and emotional well-being.

DEVELOPMENTAL CONSIDERATIONS

Growth and development are dynamic processes that describe change over time. Data collection, interpretation of these findings in relation to normative values, is important. The following discussion presents specific variations for different age groups.

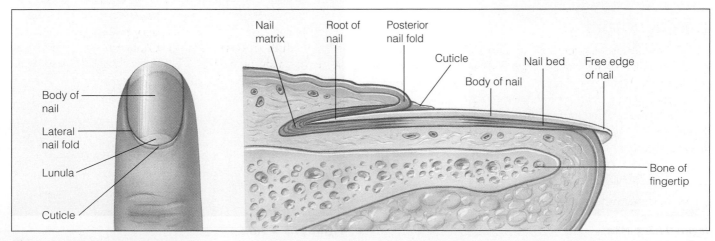

Figure 11.2 ● Structure of a nail.

Infants and Children

At birth, the newborn's skin typically is covered with **vernix caseosa,** a white, cheeselike mixture of sebum and epidermal cells. The skin color of newborns is often bright red for the first 24 hours of life and then fades. Some newborns develop physiological jaundice 3 to 4 days after birth, resulting in a yellowing of the skin, sclera, and mucous membranes. Jaundice can occur within the first 24 hours after birth or as late as 7 days postnatally. Physiological jaundice is a temporary condition treated with fluids and phototherapy. The skin of dark-skinned newborns normally is not fully pigmented until 2 to 3 months after birth. An infant's skin is very thin, soft, and free of terminal hair.

Many harmless skin markings are common in newborns. For example, they may have areas of tiny white facial papules. These are called **milia** and are due to sebum that collects in the openings of hair follicles (see Figure 11.3 ●). Milia usually disappear spontaneously within a few weeks of birth. Vascular markings are also common. These may include stork bites, which are irregular red or pink patches found most commonly on the back of the neck. Vascular markings disappear spontaneously within a year of birth. The newborn may also have transient mottling or other transient color changes such as harlequin color change, in which a side-lying infant becomes markedly pink on the lower side and pale on the higher side. **Mongolian spots** are gray, blue, or purple spots in the sacral and buttocks areas of newborns (see Figure 11.4 ●). Mongolian spots occur in about 90% of newborns of African ancestry and in about 80% of newborns of Asian or Native American ancestry. Mongolian spots fade during the first year of life. Because the subcutaneous fat layer is poorly developed in infants and the eccrine sweat glands do not secrete until the first few months of life, their temperature regulation is inefficient and absorption of topical medications is increased. The fine, downy hair of the newborn, called

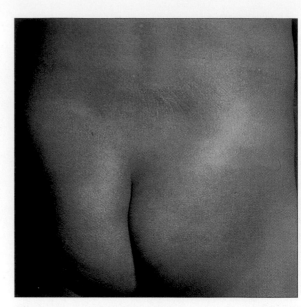

Figure 11.4 ● Mongolian spots.

lanugo, is replaced within a few months by vellus hair. Hair growth accelerates throughout childhood.

Throughout childhood, the epidermis thickens, pigmentation increases, and more subcutaneous fat is deposited, especially in females during puberty. During adolescence, both the sweat glands and the oil glands increase their production. Increased production of sebum by the oil glands predisposes adolescents to develop acne (see Figure 11.5 ●). Increased axillary perspiration occurs as the apocrine glands mature, and body odor may develop for the first time. Pubic and axillary hair appears during adolescence, and males may develop facial and chest hair.

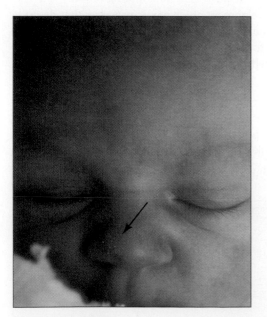

Figure 11.3 ● Milia.

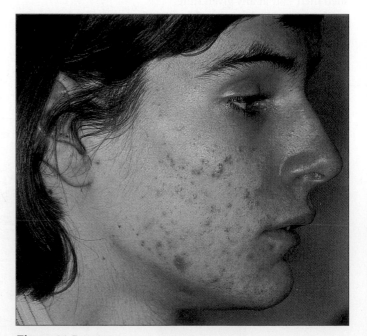

Figure 11.5 ● Acne.

Ch. 9 Nutrition

$$BMI = \text{weight (kg)} / \text{height}^2 \text{(m)}$$

17-18.49 = mild malnutrition
18.5-24.9 = normal
25-29.9 = overweight
30-34.9 = obese

excess centrally located abd fat →
risk for cardiovascular disease
males > 102 cm, females > 88 cm

Poor nutrition →
alopecia - dyspigmentation!
dry mucosa (xerophthalmia), yellow
subdermal fat deposits around lids
(xanthelasma), Bitot's spot
cracks of corners (angular) stomatitis
atrophic papillae

Ch. 11

lanugo = newborn's fine, dawny hair

~~chloa~~ chloasma/melasma = mask of
pregnancy, hyperpigmentation on
face

stria gravidium = stretch marks
acne in 1st trimester due to
hyperactive sweat glands →
↓ 3rd trimester

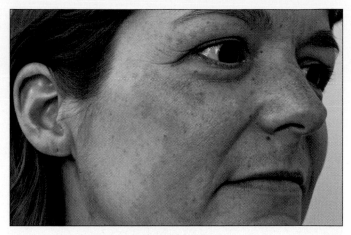

Figure 11.6 ● Melasma.

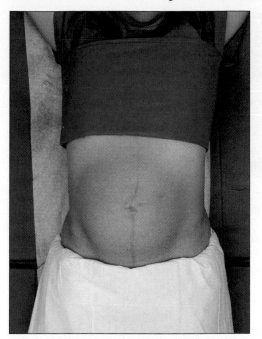

Figure 11.7 ● Linea nigra.

The Pregnant Female

Pigmentation of the skin commonly increases during pregnancy, especially in the areolae, nipples, vulva, and perianal area. Approximately 70% of pregnant women develop hyperpigmented patches on the face referred to as **chloasma,** melasma, gravidum, or "the mask of pregnancy" (see Figure 11.6 ●). This normal condition disappears after pregnancy in some women but may be permanent in others. Some pregnant clients may also have a dark line called a **linea nigra** running from the umbilicus to the pubic area (see Figure 11.7 ●), increased pigmentation of the areolae and nipples, and darkened moles and scars. These are all normal findings.

Many pregnant females develop striae gravidarum (stretch marks) across the abdomen. These usually fade after pregnancy but do not disappear entirely. Cutaneous tags are not uncommon, especially on the neck and upper chest.

Hormonal changes may cause the oil and sweat glands to become hyperactive during pregnancy. This increased secretion may in turn lead to a worsening of acne in the first trimester of pregnancy and an improvement in the third trimester. As more hairs enter the growth phase under hormonal influences in pregnancy, more than the usual number of hairs reach maturity and fall out in the postpartum period during months 1 to 5. Usually all hair grows back by 6 to 15 months postpartum.

The Older Adult

As the skin ages, the epidermis thins and stretches out, and collagen and elastin fibers decrease, causing decreased skin elasticity and increased skin wrinkling. The skin becomes slack and may hang loosely on the frame. It may sag, especially beneath the chin and eyes, in the breasts of females, and in the scrotum of males.

The older client's skin is also more delicate and more susceptible to injury. Decreased production of sebum leads to dryness of both the skin and the hair. The skin may appear especially thin on the dorsal surfaces of the hands and feet and over the bony prominences. Tenting of the skin is common

(see Figure 11.8 ●). The sweat glands also decrease their activity, and the older adult perspires less. Decreased melanin production leads to a heightened sensitivity to sunlight, and skin cancer rates increase with age.

Some light-skinned older clients may appear pale because of decreased vascularity in the dermis, even though they may be healthy and well oxygenated. The color of a dark-skinned elderly person may appear dull, gray, or darker for the same reason.

A variety of lesions are common in older adults. For example, the skin of many older clients may develop senile *lentigines* (liver spots), which look like hyperpigmented freckles, most commonly on the backs of the hands and the arms (see Figure 11.9 ●). Cherry angiomas are small, bright red spots common in older adults (see Figure 11.10 ●). They increase in number with age. Cutaneous tags may appear on the neck and upper chest (see Figure 11.11 ●), and cutaneous horns may occur on any part of the face (see Figure 11.12 ●).

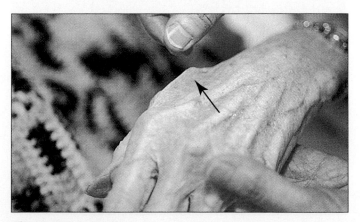

Figure 11.8 ● Tenting.

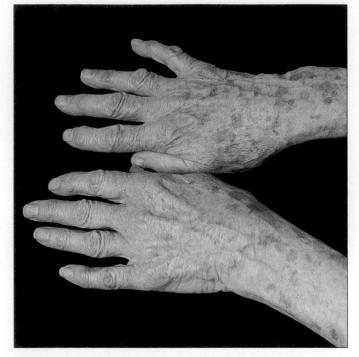

Figure 11.9 ● Senile lentigines.

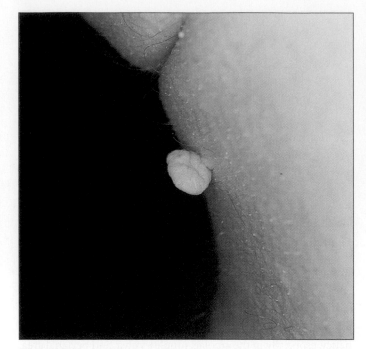

Figure 11.11 ● Cutaneous tag.

The hair becomes increasingly gray as melanin production decreases. Hair thins as the number of active hair follicles decreases. Facial hair may become more coarse.

The nails may show little change, or they may show the effects of decreased circulation in the body extremities, appearing thicker, harder, yellowed, oddly shaped, or opaque. They may be brittle and peeling, and may be prone to splitting and breaking.

PSYCHOSOCIAL CONSIDERATIONS

Stress may exacerbate certain skin conditions such as rashes or acne. Stress may also be a factor in compulsive behaviors such as hair twisting or plucking (trichotillomania) and nail biting, signaled by nails that have no visible free edge or that have short, jagged edges. A lack of cleanliness of the skin, hair, or nails also may result from emotional distress, poor self-esteem, or a disturbed body image. If appropriate, the nurse should re-

fer the client to social services or a mental health professional for assistance.

However, a visible skin disorder may trigger psychosocial health problems leading to social isolation, a body image disturbance, or a self-esteem disturbance. If appropriate, the client should be assessed further for the presence of emotional distress or anxiety related to a skin disorder.

CULTURAL AND ENVIRONMENTAL CONSIDERATIONS

A client's culture, socioeconomic status, home environment, and means of employment may affect the health of the skin, hair, and nails (see the Cultural Considerations feature). If the client's skin, hair, and nails appear unclean, the nurse should

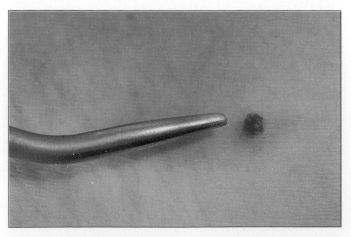

Figure 11.10 ● Cherry angioma.

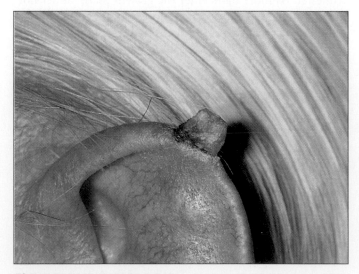

Figure 11.12 ● Cutaneous horn.

Cultural Considerations

- Skin color variations exist in all cultures. Assessment for oxygenation, jaundice, and petechiae in dark-skinned clients requires examination of nail bed refill, sclera, and mucous membranes, respectively.
- Caucasians are at greater risk for skin cancers than are darker-skinned clients.
- African Americans have an increased incidence of chronic inflammatory skin diseases.
- Sparse body hair is common in Asian Americans, especially those of Vietnamese descent.
- Asian males have less facial hair than males of other cultures.
- African Americans have a tendency to develop keloid formations.
- Chinese, Native American, and African American newborns have increased incidence of Mongolian spots on the sacral area.
- Pseudofolliculitis (razor bumps) is more frequent in African American males.
- Melasma (mask of pregnancy) occurs more frequently in dark-skinned African American women.
- Dark-skinned individuals may have pigmented streaks in the nails.

- Linguistic and cultural factors must be considered to avoid miscommunication and misinterpretation of information about diagnosis when caring for many immigrant populations.
- Indian females may have nose piercing.
- Arabic and Indian females use henna as a skin adornment.
- Sikhs are prohibited from removing or cutting hair on any part of the body.
- Religions or cultural practices of covering the head and hair are common in Muslims and Orthodox Jews.
- Touching the head is prohibited in the Vietnamese culture.
- Tattoos and body piercing can be part of cultural or religious practices.
- Tattoos and body piercing are increasing among adolescents in the American cultures.
- Females may require the presence of another female during physical assessment of the skin, especially when the examiner is not of the same sex.
- One must be sensitive to cultural issues about disrobing for the assessment of the skin.

consider the client's job, socioeconomic status, and living situation. A client who seems unkempt may have just come from a physically demanding job or may be ill, disabled, or depressed.

Changes in skin color may be difficult to evaluate in clients with dark skin. It is helpful to inspect areas of the body with less pigmentation, such as the lips, oral mucosa, sclerae, palms of the hands, and conjunctivae of the inner eyelids. The nurse must be careful not to mistake the normal deposition of melanin in the lips of some olive to dark-skinned people for cyanosis. Some individuals with dark skin have increased pigmentation in the creases of the palms and soles, and yellow or brown-tinged sclerae. These are normal findings (see Table 11.1 on page 190 for evaluating color variations in light and dark skin).

Dry skin does not necessarily indicate dehydration and in fact may be normal for the dark-skinned client. Additionally, since many clients use petroleum-based products to lubricate their skin, the nurse should ask about self-care before concluding that the client has oily skin.

The skin's response to stressors such as ultraviolet radiation is similar in all races. Dark-skinned clients tan, and their skin suffers the same damaging effects from the sun, although skin damage may take longer to occur. Therefore, assessment of color, texture, moles, and other lesions should be as thorough as for light-skinned clients.

Calluses (circumscribed, painless thickenings of the epidermis) tend to form on parts of the body that are regularly exposed to pressure, weight bearing, or friction. Common sites of calluses include the fingers, palms, toes, and soles of the feet.

Differences in hair color and texture are widely variable among cultural groups. Individuals of Asian origins tend to have long, straight, dark hair. Scandinavians typically have very light, blonde hair. African Americans may have straight, kinky, or long braided hair, and it can often be dry.

The client's occupation (e.g., gardener, mechanic) may make it difficult to keep the fingers and nails unstained. Chemicals used in certain occupations, and smoking tobacco may stain the nails. The client's occupation may require frequent or prolonged immersion of the hands in water, which may lead to paronychia. The nail plates of dark-skinned clients may show dark pigmented streaks, which are normal findings.

Clients from many cultures use therapies that are not part of standard Western treatment. Among many Asian cultures, coining and cupping are used in treatment for a variety of illnesses. These alternative therapies include using coins, cups, or pinching on areas of the body. The use of this therapy results in lesions including welts, and bruises. These lesions can suggest abuse. Therefore, one must inquire about cultural healing practices. Box 11.1 describes these therapies. For further information about cultural concerns in healthcare, consult the Office of Minority Health. Link to their Website through the Companion Website.

Box 11.1	Coining, Cupping, Pinching
Coining	Coining refers to rubbing the skin of the back, upper chest, neck, and arms with a coin in symmetrical patterns. Coining results in skin bruising.
Cupping	Cupping is sucking of the skin on the forehead, back, and upper chest. Glass cups are heated until air is removed. The heated cups are placed on the skin. Red circular lesions arise on the skin from cupping.
Pinching	When pinching, the first and second fingers pull upward on the skin of the neck, back, and chest, and between the eyebrows. The pinching produces bruises.

These treatments stimulate circulation and restore balance in children and adults with a variety of ailments.

Table 11.1	Color Variations in Light and Dark Skin		
COLOR VARIATION/ LOCALIZATION	**POSSIBLE CAUSES**	**APPEARANCE IN LIGHT SKIN**	**APPEARANCE IN DARK SKIN**
Pallor *Loss of color in skin due to the absence of oxygenated hemoglobin.* Widespread, but most apparent in face, mouth, conjunctivae, and nails.	May be caused by sympathetic nervous stimulation resulting in peripheral vasoconstriction due to smoking, a cold environment, or stress. May also be caused by decreased tissue perfusion due to cardiopulmonary disease, shock and hypotension, lack of oxygen, or prolonged elevation of a body part. May also be caused by anemia.	White skin loses its rosy tones. Skin with natural yellow tones appears more yellow; may be mistaken for mild jaundice.	Black skin loses its red undertones and appears ash-gray. Brown skin becomes yellow-tinged. Skin looks dull.
Absence of Color *Congenital or acquired loss of melanin pigment.* Congenital loss is typically generalized, and acquired loss is typically patchy.	Generalized depigmentation may be caused by albinism. Localized depigmentation may be due to vitiligo or tinea versicolor, a common fungal infection.	Albinism appears as white skin, white or pale blond hair, and pink irises. Vitiligo appears as patchy milk-white areas, especially around the mouth. Tinea versicolor appears as patchy areas paler than the surrounding skin.	Albinism appears as white skin, white or pale blond hair, and pink irises. Vitiligo is very noticeable as patchy milk-white areas. Tinea versicolor appears as patchy areas paler than the surrounding skin.
Cyanosis *Mottled blue color in skin due to inadequate tissue perfusion with oxygenated blood.* Most apparent in the nails, lips, oral mucosa, and tongue.	Systemic or central cyanosis is due to cardiac disease, pulmonary disease, heart malformations, and low hemoglobin levels. Localized or peripheral cyanosis is due to vasoconstriction, exposure to cold, and emotional stress.	The skin, lips, and mucous membranes look blue-tinged. The conjunctive and nail beds are blue.	The skin may appear a shade darker. Cyanosis may be undetectable except for the lips, tongue, and oral mucous membranes, nail beds, and conjunctivae, which appear pale or blue-tinged.
Reddish Blue Tone *Ruddy tone due to an increased hemoglobin and stasis of blood in capillaries.* Most apparent in the face, mouth, hands, feet, and conjunctivae.	Polycythemia vera, an overproduction of red blood cells, granulocytes, and platelets.	Reddish purple hue.	Difficult to detect. The normal skin color may appear darker in some clients. Check lips for redness.
Erythema *Redness of the skin due to increased visibility of normal oxyhemoglobin.* Generalized, or on face and upper chest, or localized to area of inflammation or exposure.	Hyperemia, a dilatation and congestion of blood in superficial arteries. Due to fever, warm environment, local inflammation, allergy, emotions (blushing or embarrassment), exposure to extreme cold, consumption of alcohol, dependent position of body extremity.	Readily identifiable over entire body or in localized areas. Local inflammation and redness are accompanied by higher temperature at the site.	Generalized redness may be difficult to detect. Localized areas of inflammation appear purple or darker than surrounding skin. May be accompanied by higher temperature, hardness, swelling.
Jaundice *Yellow undertone due to increased bilirubin in the blood.* Generalized, but most apparent in the conjunctivae and mucous membranes.	Increased bilirubin may be due to liver disease, biliary obstruction, or hemolytic disease following infections, severe burns, or resulting from sickle cell anemia or pernicious anemia.	Generalized. Also visible in sclerae, oral mucosa, hard palate, fingernails, palms of hands, and soles of the feet.	Visible in the sclerae, oral mucosa, junction of hard and soft palate, palms of the hands, and soles of the feet.
Carotenemia *Yellow-orange tinge caused by increased levels of carotene in the blood and skin.* Most apparent in face, palms of the hands, and soles of the feet.	Excess carotene due to ingestion of foods high in carotene such as carrots, egg yolks, sweet potatoes, milk, and fats. Also may be seen in clients with anorexia nervosa or endocrine disorders such as diabetes mellitus, myxedema, and hypopituitarism.	Yellow-orange seen in forehead, palms, soles. No yellowing of sclerae or mucous membranes.	Yellow-orange tinge most visible in palms of the hands and soles of the feet. No yellowing of sclerae or mucous membranes.

Table 11.1	Color Variations in Light and Dark Skin (continued)		
COLOR VARIATION/ LOCALIZATION	**POSSIBLE CAUSES**	**APPEARANCE IN LIGHT SKIN**	**APPEARANCE IN DARK SKIN**
Uremia *Pale yellow tone due to retention of urinary chromogens in the blood.* Generalized, if perceptible.	Chronic renal disease, in which blood levels of nitrogenous wastes increase. Increased melanin may also contribute, and anemia is usually present as well.	Generalized pallor and yellow tinge, but does not affect conjunctivae or mucous membranes. Skin may show bruising.	Very difficult to discern because the yellow tinge is very pale and does not affect conjunctivae or mucous membranes. Rely on laboratory and other data.
Brown *An increase in the production and deposition of melanin.* Generalized or localized.	May be due to Addison's disease or a pituitary tumor. Localized increase in facial pigmentation may be caused by hormonal changes during pregnancy or the use of birth control pills. More commonly due to exposure to ultraviolet radiation from the sun or from tanning booths.	With endocrine disorders, general bronzed skin. Hyperpigmentation in nipples, palmar creases, genitals, and pressure points. Sun exposure causes red tinge in pale skin, and olive-toned skin tans with little or no reddening.	With endocrine disorders, general deepening of skin tone. Hyperpigmentation in nipples, genitals, and pressure points. Sun exposure leads to tanning in various degrees from brown to black.

Gathering the Data

*A*ssessment of the integumentary system includes gathering subjective and objective data about the skin, hair, and nails. Subjective data collection occurs during the interview, before the actual physical assessment. The nurse will use a variety of communication techniques to elicit general and specific information about the condition of the client's skin, hair, and nails. Health records and the results of laboratory tests are important secondary sources to be reviewed and included in the data-gathering process. In physical assessment of the integumentary system, the techniques of inspection and palpation will be used. The questions in the focused interview form part of the subjective data and provide valuable information to meet the objectives related to integumentary health included in the *Healthy People 2010* feature on page 229.

FOCUSED INTERVIEW

The focused interview for the integumentary system concerns data related to the structures and functions of that system. Subjective data related to the condition of the skin, hair, and nails are gathered during the focused interview. The nurse must be prepared to observe the client and listen for cues related to the integumentary system. The nurse may use closed or open-ended questions to obtain information. A number of follow-up questions or requests for descriptions may be required to clarify data or gather missing information. Follow-up questions are used to identify the source of problems, determine the duration

of difficulties, identify measures to alleviate problems, and provide clues about the client's knowledge of his or her own health.

The focused interview guides the physical assessment of the integumentary system. The information is always considered in relation to norms and expectations about the function of the integument. Therefore, the nurse must consider age, gender, race, culture, environment, health practices, and past and concurrent problems and therapies when forming questions and using techniques to elicit information. In order to address all of the factors when conducting a focused interview, categories of questions related to the status and function of each part of the integumentary system have been developed. These categories include general questions that are asked of all clients; those addressing illness or infection; questions related to symptoms, pain, or behaviors; those related to habits or practices; questions that are specific to clients according to age; those for pregnant females; and questions that address environmental concerns.

The nurse must consider the client's ability to participate in the focused interview and physical assessment. Further, the nurse must consider that the appearance of the skin has an impact on self-image. A client with clear, healthy skin may have a heightened self-esteem. Clients with changes in the skin due to the normal aging process or from skin disorders may be anxious about the way they appear to others. Clients with visible skin disorders are often sensitive about the condition and their appearance. The nurse must select communication techniques that demonstrate caring and preserve the dignity of the client.

FOCUSED INTERVIEW QUESTIONS

RATIONALES

The following sections provide sample questions and bulleted follow-up questions in each of the categories for the skin. A rationale for each of the questions is provided. The list of questions is not all-inclusive but represents the types of questions required in a comprehensive focused interview related to the skin. Questions related to the hair and nails are included but are not divided into the previously mentioned categories of questions.

SKIN
GENERAL QUESTIONS

1. **Describe your skin today.**
   - How does it compare to 2 months ago? How does it compare to 2 years ago?

2. **Do you ever have trouble controlling body odor? If so, at what times?**

3. **How much and how easily do you sweat?**

4. **Have you had episodes of increased sweating that occur at certain times, especially at night?**

5. **Have you noticed any changes in the color of your skin?**
   - If so, did the change occur over your entire body or only in one area?

6. **Has your skin become either more oily or more dry recently?**
   - Have you noticed other changes in the way your skin feels?

7. **Is there a history of allergies, rashes, or other skin problems in your family?**

► This question give clients the opportunity to provide their own perceptions about the skin.

► Body odor becomes stronger during heavy activity because of increased excretion of uric acid. Body odor may also be related to diet. A change in body odor may indicate the presence of a systemic disorder.

► Profuse sweating is a significant avenue for sodium chloride loss and may indicate the presence of a systemic disorder. Increased sweating is a side effect of some medications. Decreased sweating increases the risk of heat stroke and may be a side effect of medications.

► Such episodes can suggest the presence of an infectious process.

► Widespread or localized color changes may indicate the presence of a disorder.

► Metabolic disorders or simple age-related changes in the production of sebum may produce changes in the texture of the skin.

► Some allergies and skin disorders are familial; thus, the client may be predisposed. Follow-up is required to obtain details about specific problems, their occurrence, treatments, and outcomes.

QUESTIONS RELATED TO ILLNESS OR INFECTION

1. **Have you ever had a skin problem?**
   - When were you diagnosed with the problem?
   - What treatment was prescribed for the problem?
   - Was the treatment helpful?
   - What kinds of things do you do to help with the problem?
   - Has the problem ever recurred (acute)?
   - How are you managing the disease now (chronic)?

2. **Have you had an illness recently? If so, please describe it.**

3. **An alternative to question 1 is to list possible skin problems or illnesses, such as lupus, psoriasis, lesions, burns, and trauma, and ask the client to respond yes or no as each is stated.**

► The client has an opportunity to provide information about specific skin problems or illnesses. If a diagnosed illness is identified, follow-up about the date of diagnosis, treatment, and outcomes is required. Data about each illness identified by the client is essential to an accurate health assessment. Illnesses can be classified as acute or chronic, and follow-up regarding each classification will differ.

► Some skin disorders are manifestations of systemic illness.

► This is a comprehensive and easy way to elicit information about all skin disorders. Follow-up would be carried out for each identified diagnosis as in question 1.

FOCUSED INTERVIEW QUESTIONS	RATIONALES

4. Do you have or have you had a skin infection?
- When were you diagnosed with the infection?
- What treatment was prescribed for the problem?
- Was the treatment helpful? What kinds of things do you do to help with the problem?
- Has the problem ever recurred (acute)?
- How are you managing the infection now (chronic)?

▶ If an infection is identified, follow-up about the date of infection, treatment, and outcomes is required. Data about each infection identified by the client is essential to an accurate health assessment. Infections can be classified as acute or chronic, and follow-up regarding each classification will differ.

5. An alternative to question 4 is to list possible skin infections, such as pruritus, warts, herpes simplex, herpes zoster, candida, and acne, and ask the client to respond yes or no as each is stated.

▶ This is a comprehensive and easy way to elicit information about all skin infections. Follow-up would be carried out for each identified infection as in question 3.

QUESTIONS RELATED TO SYMPTOMS OR BEHAVIORS

When gathering information about symptoms, many questions are required to elicit details and descriptions that assist in the analysis of the data. Discrimination is made in relation to the significance of a symptom, in relation to specific diseases or problems, and in relation to potential follow-up examination or referral. One rationale may be provided for a group of questions in this category.

The following questions refer to specific symptoms and behaviors associated with the skin. For each symptom, questions and follow-up are required. The details to be elicited are the characteristics of the symptom; the onset, duration, and frequency of the symptom; the treatment or remedy for the symptom including over-the-counter and home remedies; the determination if diagnosis has been sought; the effect of treatments; and family history associated with a symptom or illness.

QUESTIONS RELATED TO SYMPTOMS

1. Do you have any sores or ulcers on your body that are slow in healing?
- Where are these?
- Do you have frequent boils or skin infections?

▶ Delayed healing or frequent skin infections may be a sign of diabetes mellitus or inadequate nutrition.

2. Does your skin itch? If so, where?
- How severe is it?
- When does it occur?

▶ These questions may help in determining if the itching is due to an allergic reaction or eczema.

3. Have you noticed any rashes on your body? If so, please describe.
- Where on your body did the rash start? Where did it spread?
- When did you first notice it?
- Does the rash happen at the same time as any other symptoms, such as fever or chills?

▶ These factors may help in determining the cause.

4. If you have a rash, do you notice it more after wearing certain clothes or jewelry?
- After using certain skin products?
- Did it occur soon after starting a new medication?
- Does the rash happen during or after any other activities such as gardening or washing dishes?

▶ Rashes related to clothing, jewelry, or cosmetics may be due to contact dermatitis, a type of allergy. Many medications cause allergic skin reactions. A drug reaction can occur even after the client has taken the drug a long time. Aspirin, antibiotics, and barbiturates are a few of the drugs that fall into this category.

5. Have you noticed a change in the size, color, shape, or appearance of any moles or birthmarks?
- When did you first notice this?
- Describe the change.
- Are they painful? Do they itch? Bleed?

▶ Any changes in a mole or birthmark may signal a skin cancer.

6. Have you noticed any other lesions, lumps, bumps, tender spots, or painful areas on your body?
- If so, when did you first notice them? Where?
- Describe how they have spread and where they are located now.

▶ The time of onset and pattern of development may help determine the source of the problem. For instance, certain patterns of bruises may signal frequent falls or physical abuse.

FOCUSED INTERVIEW QUESTIONS

RATIONALES

7. Have you noticed any drainage from any skin region?
   - If so, where does the drainage come from? What does it look like? Does it have an odor?
   - Is the drainage accompanied by any other symptoms? If so, please describe.

8. Please describe anything you have done to treat your skin condition.
   - When did you begin this treatment? How has your skin responded to the treatment?

▶ Diagnostic cues such as pain, chills, or fever may aid in identifying the source of the problem.

QUESTIONS RELATED TO PAIN

1. Please describe any skin pain or discomfort.

2. Have you experienced any pain or discomfort in any body folds, for example, between the toes, under the breasts, between the buttocks, or in the perianal area?

3. Where is the pain?

4. How often do you experience the pain?

5. How long does the pain last?

6. How long have you had the pain?

7. How would you rate the pain on a scale of 1 to 10?

8. Is there a trigger for the pain?

9. What do you do to relieve the pain?

10. Is this treatment effective?

▶ Note that the warm, dark, moist environment in body folds may breed bacterial and fungal infections.

▶ Questions 3 through 7 are standard questions associated with pain to determine the location, frequency, duration, and intensity of the pain.

▶ Questions 9 and 10 are intended to determine if the client has selected a treatment based on past experience, knowledge of respiratory illness, or use of complementary and alternative care and its effectiveness.

QUESTIONS RELATED TO BEHAVIORS

1. Do you sunbathe?

2. Have you ever sunbathed?

3. Do you spend time in the sun exercising or playing sports?

4. Do you work outdoors?

5. How does your skin react to sun exposure?
   - Do you use a lotion with sun protection factor (SPF) when spending time in the sun?
   - What SPF lotion do you use? Do you reapply the lotion after several hours or after swimming?

6. Do you remember having a sunburn that left blisters?

7. How do you care for your skin?
   - What kind of soap, cleansers, toners, or other treatments do you use?
   - How do you clean your clothes?
   - What kind of detergent do you use?
   - How often do you bathe or shower?

8. Do you now have or have you ever had a tattoo(s)?
   - How long have you had the tattoo(s)? Have you had any problems with that area of the skin? Further follow-up would include questions related to treatment and outcomes if skin problems accompanied tattoos.

▶ Excessive exposure to the ultraviolet radiation of the sun thickens and damages the skin, depresses the immune system, and alters the DNA in skin cells, predisposing an individual to cancer.

▶ The ultraviolet radiation that accompanies a sunburn is capable of disabling cells that initiate the normal immune response. Individuals who burn easily or have a history of serious sunburns may have a greater risk for developing skin cancer.

▶ A history of blistering sunburn increases the risk for skin cancer, especially if it occurred in childhood.

▶ Some skin products and laundry detergents may affect the skin of some clients. Infrequent cleansing of the skin increases the likelihood of skin infections, whereas excessive bathing decreases protective skin oils.

▶ Tattoos can cause skin irritation, and the process of tattooing puts an individual at risk for infection, hepatitis C, and HIV.

FOCUSED INTERVIEW QUESTIONS | RATIONALES

9. **Do you now have or have you ever had piercing of any part of your body?**
   - Where are the sites of piercing?
   - How long have you had the piercing?
   - Have any piercing sites closed?
   - Have you ever had a problem at the piercing site?
   - What was the problem?
   - Did you seek treatment for the problem?
   - What was the outcome of the treatment?
   - What is the current condition of piercing sites?

▶ Piercing of any body part puts an individual at risk for infection and hepatitis C and can result in the development of scar tissue at the site.

QUESTIONS RELATED TO AGE

The focused interview must reflect the anatomical and physiological differences that exist along the age span. The following questions are presented as examples of those that would be specific for children, pregnant females, and older adults.

QUESTIONS REGARDING INFANTS AND CHILDREN

1. **Does the child have any birthmarks? If so, where are they?**

2. **Has the infant developed an orange hue in the skin?**

▶ Ingestion of large amounts of carotene in vegetables such as carrots, sweet potatoes, and squash can cause an orange hue.

3. **Does the child have a rash? If so, what seems to cause it?**
   - Have you introduced any new foods into your child's diet?
   - How do you clean the child's diaper area?
   - How do you wash the child's diapers?

▶ Many children may have allergic reactions to certain foods, especially milk, chocolate, and eggs. Infrequent changing of diapers may lead to diaper rash. Harsh detergents may cause skin reactions in some children.

QUESTIONS FOR THE PREGNANT FEMALE

1. **What changes have you noticed in your skin since you became pregnant?**

▶ The hormonal changes of pregnancy may cause various benign changes in skin pigmentation, moisture, texture, and vascularity that are entirely normal.

2. **Do you use any topical medications for problems with the skin, hair, or nails?**

▶ Topical medications that can result in birth defects include Retin-A for acne, antifungal agents, and minoxidil for hair growth.

3. **Do you use topical medications for other problems? If so, identify the medications.**

▶ Many medications that are absorbed through the skin may reach the baby through the bloodstream. Some of these medications may harm the developing fetus. Among the medications are antibiotics, steroids, and medications for muscle pain.

QUESTIONS FOR THE OLDER ADULT

1. **What changes have you noticed in your skin in the past few years?**

▶ The normal changes of aging, such as increased dryness and wrinkling of the skin, may cause distress for some clients.

2. **Does your skin itch?**

▶ **Pruritus** (itching) increases in incidence with age. It is usually due to dry skin, which may in turn be caused by excessive bathing or use of harsh skin cleansers.

3. **Do you experience frequent falls?**

▶ Older adults bruise easily. Multiple bruises may result from frequent falls.

FOCUSED INTERVIEW QUESTIONS	RATIONALES

QUESTIONS RELATED TO THE ENVIRONMENT

Environment refers to both the internal and external environments. Questions related to the internal environment include all of the previous questions and those associated with internal or physiological responses. Questions regarding the external environment include those related to home, work, or social environments.

INTERNAL ENVIRONMENT

1. **How would you describe your level of stress? Has it changed in the past few weeks? Few months? Describe.**

   ▶ Emotional stress may aggravate skin disorders.

2. **Are you now experiencing, or have you ever experienced, intermittent or prolonged anxiety or emotional upset?**
   - Describe the situation.
   - Can you determine precipitating factors?
   - Have you sought care or treatment for the problem?
   - What do you do when the problem arises?

3. **Are you taking any prescription or over-the-counter medications?**

   ▶ Clients may experience rashes or other skin eruptions in response to various drugs. Some drugs, such as antibiotics, antihistamines, antipsychotics, oral hypoglycemic agents, and oral contraceptives, can cause an adverse effect if the client is exposed to the sun.

4. **Have you changed your diet recently? Have you recently tried any unfamiliar types of food? Please describe.**

   ▶ Changes in diet or eating new foods may cause rashes and other skin reactions.

5. **Has the condition of your skin affected your social relationships in any way? Has it limited you in any way? If so, how?**

   ▶ Skin problems may affect a person's self-concept and body image, interfering with social relationships, roles, and sexuality. This is especially true for adolescents and young adults. Serious skin problems may also affect a person's ability to function and maintain a job.

6. **Female clients: Are you pregnant? If not, are you menstruating regularly? Describe your menstrual periods.**

   ▶ The skin may be affected by changes in hormonal balance.

EXTERNAL ENVIRONMENT

The following questions deal with substances and irritants found in the physical environment of the client. The physical environment includes the indoor and outdoor environments of the home and the workplace, those encountered for social engagements, and any encountered during travel.

1. **Have you been exposed recently to extremes in temperature?**
   - If so, when? How long was the exposure? Where did this occur?
   - Describe the temperature of your home environment. Of your work environment.

   ▶ Extremes in environmental temperature may exacerbate skin disorders.

2. **Do you work in an environment where radioisotopes or x-rays are used?**
   - If so, are you vigilant about following precautions and using protective gear?

   ▶ Excessive exposure to x-rays or radioisotopes may predispose a client to skin cancer.

3. **Do you wear gloves for work? If so, what types of gloves?**

   ▶ Certain types of gloves, especially latex, can cause mild to severe skin allergic reactions.

4. **How often do you travel?**
   - Have you traveled recently?
   - If so, where?
   - Have you come into contact with anyone who has a similar rash?

   ▶ The nurse should suspect unfamiliar foods, water, plants, or insects as potential causes of rashes and other skin problems if the client has traveled recently. In addition, some rashes, such as measles and impetigo, are contagious.

FOCUSED INTERVIEW QUESTIONS	RATIONALES

5. Does your job or hobby require you to perform repetitive tasks?
- To work with any chemicals?
- Does your job or hobby require you to wear a specific type of helmet, hat, goggles, gloves, or shoes?

▶ Regular work with certain tools or regular wear of ill-fitting helmets, hats, goggles, or shoes may cause skin abrasions. Additionally, the skin absorbs some organic solvents used in industry, such as acetone, dry-cleaning fluid, dyes, formaldehyde, and paint thinner. Excessive exposure to these and other types of irritants may contribute to rashes, skin cancers, or other skin reactions.

HAIR

GENERAL QUESTIONS

1. Describe your hair now.
- How does it compare to 2 months ago? How does it compare to 2 years ago?
- Have you ever had problems with your hair? If so, please describe the problem, including any treatment and resolution.

2. How often do you wash your hair?
- What kinds of shampoos do you use?
- Do you have excessive dandruff?
- Do you do anything to control it?

▶ Excessive washing or washing with harsh shampoos can remove protective oils and dry the hair. Removal of natural scalp oils through shampooing also encourages dandruff. Excessive dandruff may also occur with protein and vitamin B deficiencies as well as a decrease in some essential fatty acids.

3. Have you noticed an increased hair loss recently?
- If so, describe how the hair fell out.
- Have you been ill in the last few months?

▶ The scalp typically sheds about 90 hairs each day, and so some hair loss is normal. Progressive diffuse hair loss is natural in some men. Hair loss in women that follows a male pattern may be due to an imbalance of adrenal hormones. When patches of hair fall out, the nurse should suspect trauma to the scalp due to chemicals, infections, or blows to the head. Chemotherapeutic agents cause hair loss. Also, some people with nervous disorders pull or twist their hair, causing it to fall out. If hair loss is distributed over the entire head, it may be caused by a systemic disease or fungal infection. Abnormal hair loss sometimes follows a feverish illness. Thinning or shedding of the hair on the scalp (telogen effluvium) may occur in pregnancy. Hair shedding may last for several months and continue for up to 15 months after delivery.

4. Are you taking any prescription or over-the-counter medications?

▶ Certain medications can change the texture of the hair or lead to hair loss. For instance, oral contraceptives may change the hair texture or rate of hair growth in some women, and drugs used in the treatment of circulatory disorders and cancer may result in a temporary generalized hair loss over the entire body.

5. How do you style your hair?

▶ Use of styling products can dry or damage hair, as can use of hair dryers, curling irons, and heated rollers. Some methods of setting hair, and sleeping in hair rollers, may cause breakage and lead to patchy hair loss. Repeated tight braiding may damage hair and lead to patchy hair loss.

FOCUSED INTERVIEW QUESTIONS	**RATIONALES**

6. **Do you bleach, color, perm, or chemically straighten your hair?**
   - If so, how often? When did you last have this done?

▶ These chemical processes may damage the scalp and hair and may cause hair loss.

7. **Do you pluck your eyebrows or facial hair?**
   - Do you shave the hair on your face, on your legs, or under your arms?
   - Do you use chemical hair removers or electrolysis?

▶ Each of these hair removal methods can cause trauma to the skin. Use of unclean equipment can contaminate the skin. Plucking leaves an open portal for bacteria and may lead to infection if aseptic technique is not used.

8. **Do you swim regularly? How often? For how long? Where?**

▶ Swimming regularly in salt water or chlorinated pools can dry the scalp and hair and may cause increased dandruff.

QUESTIONS REGARDING INFANTS AND CHILDREN

1. **Has the child shared hair combs, brushes, or pillows with other children?**

▶ Sharing hair care implements or pillows may expose the child to head lice.

NAILS

GENERAL QUESTIONS

1. **Describe your nails now?**
   - How do they compare to 2 months ago? How do they compare to 2 years ago?
   - Have you ever had problems with your nails?
   - If so, please describe the problem, including any treatment and resolution.

▶ Ridged, brittle, split, or peeling fingernails may be caused by protein or vitamin B deficiencies. Changes in circulation may affect the nails. Newly acquired dark longitudinal lines may signal a nevus or melanoma in the nail root. Dark lines may be normal, especially in dark-skinned clients, or associated with some medications including antiretrovirals.

2. **Have you noticed any pain, swelling, or drainage around your cuticles?**
   - If so, when did you first notice this?
   - What do you think might have caused it?

▶ Infection of the cuticles could be due to an ingrown nail or to use of contaminated instruments during a manicure or pedicure.

3. **Have you been ill recently?**

▶ Cancer, heart disease, liver disease, anemia, and other illnesses can cause various changes in the nails such as grooves, ridges, or discoloration.

4. **Have you been taking any prescription or over-the-counter medications?**

▶ Some medication may cause nail changes in some clients. For example, clients who have been treated with the antiviral drug zidovudine (Retrovir, AZT) can develop dark, longitudinal lines on all of their fingernails.

5. **Do you wear nail enamel? Do you wear artificial fingernails, tips, or wraps?**

▶ Prolonged use of nail polish may dry or discolor the nails. Additionally, some clients may have an allergic reaction to nail polish. Use of artificial nails may encourage growth of fungi or damage the nail plate.

6. **Do you spend a great deal of time at work or at home with your hands in water?**

▶ Bacterial and fungal infections of the cuticles may occur in people who submerge their hands in water for long periods.

QUESTIONS REGARDING INFANTS AND CHILDREN

1. **Does the child have any habits such as pulling or twisting the hair, rubbing the head, or biting the nails?**

▶ These habits may signal anxiety or emotional distress. Nail biting may also lead to impaired skin integrity.

FOCUSED INTERVIEW QUESTIONS	**RATIONALES**

QUESTIONS FOR THE PREGNANT FEMALE

1. Have your nails changed? If so, what are the changes?

▶ Nail changes in pregnancy include brittleness, formation of grooves, or onycholysis (separation of the nail from the nail bed).

QUESTIONS FOR THE OLDER ADULT

1. Do you find it difficult to care for your skin, hair, and nails? If so, describe any difficulties you are experiencing.

▶ Older adults with impaired mobility may have difficulty cleansing or grooming their skin, hair, and nails. Some older adults may have trouble reaching down to their feet to groom their toenails

CLIENT INTERACTION

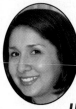

Ms. Tanish Thalia, age 32, reports to the Medi-Center with a chief complaint of pain, swelling, and redness at the nails of two fingers on her left hand. Following is an excerpt of the focused interview.

INTERVIEW

Nurse: Good morning. Ms. Thalia, I see from your information sheet that you have a problem with the fingernails of your left hand.

Ms. Thalia: Yes, I think it's my nails, but I'm not sure.

Nurse: The problem involves two digits of the left hand.

Ms. Thalia: Yes, the thumb and index finger are the only two. The other three seem to be okay.

Nurse: Looking at your nails, I see they are highly polished.

Ms. Thalia: Yes, I have them done professionally every 7 to 10 days. They were done 5 days ago.

Nurse: Are these your natural nails?

Ms. Thalia: Yes, I have silk wraps on all my nails to help make them stronger.

Nurse: Does the manicurist push and cut your cuticles?

Ms. Thalia: Yes, she does both. Do you think this is from having the manicure?

Nurse: It could be. I'm not sure. I need more information. When did you first notice the pain and swelling?

Ms. Thalia: It started several days after I had my nails done, and now it seems to be getting worse. What is causing this?

Nurse: Is this the first time the manicurist did your nails?

Ms. Thalia: Oh no, Sally has been doing my nails for 3 years. This is the first time I have had anything like this.

Nurse: How much time are your hands and nails in water?

Ms. Thalia: Not much. I use gloves when I do the dishes.

ANALYSIS

The nurse uses closed questions to obtain the necessary information from Ms. Thalia. The nurse seeks clarification regarding the fingers involved and also confirms the condition of the nails, the frequency of care, and the type of care regarding cutting of the cuticles. When asked, Ms. Thalia is able to provide specific information regarding date of last manicure, symptoms involved, and the relationship between these two factors. The nurse does not make a judgment, and indicates more information is needed.

Please refer to the Companion Website at **www.prenhall.com/damico** and click on Chapter 11, the **Client Interaction** module, to answer questions about this case. In addition, see other resources for this chapter including NCLEX review questions and other interactive exercises and materials.

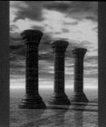

Physical Assessment

ASSESSMENT TECHNIQUES AND FINDINGS

Physical assessment of the skin, hair, and nails requires the use of inspection and palpation. Inspection includes looking at the skin, hair, and nails to determine color, consistency, shape, and hygiene-related factors. Knowledge of norms or expected findings is essential in determining the meaning of the data as the nurse performs the physical assessment.

The skin of the adult should be clean, free from odor, and consistent in color. It should feel warm and moist and should have a smooth texture. The skin should be mobile with blood vessels visible beneath the surfaces of the abdomen and eyelids. It should be free of lesions except for findings of freckles and birthmarks. The skin is sensitive to touch and temperature.

The scalp and hair in the adult should be clean. Hair color is determined by the amount of melanin. Gray hair can occur as a result of decreased melanin, genetics, or aging. Hair texture may be coarse or thin. Hair distribution is expected to be even over the scalp. Male pattern baldness is a normal finding.

Fine hair is distributed over the body with coarser, darker, longer hair in the axillae and pubic regions in adults. The nails should have a pink undertone and lie flat or form a convex curve on the nail bed.

Physical assessment of the skin, hair, and nails follows an organized pattern. It begins with a survey and inspection of the skin, followed by palpation of the skin. Inspection and palpation of the hair and nails is then carried out. When lesions are present, measurements are used to identify the size of the lesions and the location in relation to accepted landmarks.

EQUIPMENT

examination gown and drape	centimeter ruler
examination light	magnifying glass
examination gloves clean and nonsterile	penlight
	Wood's lamp (filtered ultraviolet light) for special procedures

HELPFUL HINTS

- A warm, private environment will reduce client anxiety.
- Provide special instructions and explain the purpose for removal of clothing, jewelry, hairpieces, nail enamel.
- Maintain the client's dignity by using draping techniques.
- Monitor one's verbal responses to skin conditions that already threaten the client's self-image.
- Be sensitive to cultural issues. In some cultures touching or examination by members of the opposite sex is prohibited.
- Covering the head, hair, face, or skin may be part of religious or cultural beliefs. Provide careful explanations regarding the need to expose these areas for assessment.
- Direct sunlight is best for assessment of the skin; if it is not available, lighting must be strong and direct. Tangential lighting may be helpful in assessment of dark skinned clients.
- Use Standard Precautions throughout the assessment.

TECHNIQUES AND NORMAL FINDINGS

ABNORMAL FINDINGS SPECIAL CONSIDERATIONS

SURVEY

A quick survey enables the nurse to identify any immediate problem and the client's ability to participate in the assessment. The nurse inspects the overall appearance of the client, notes hygiene and odor, and observes for signs of anxiety.

ALERT!

The nurse must be alert for the possibility of impending shock if the client has pallor accompanied with a drop in blood pressure, increased pulse and respirations, and marked anxiety. If these cues are present, a physician should be consulted immediately.

▶ Clients experiencing pain or discomfort may not be able to participate in the assessment. Severe pain or distress may require referral to an emergency care facility.

Clients experiencing anxiety may demonstrate pallor and diaphoresis. Acknowledgment of the problem and discussion of the procedures often provide relief.

TECHNIQUES AND NORMAL FINDINGS	**ABNORMAL FINDINGS SPECIAL CONSIDERATIONS**

INSPECTION OF THE SKIN

1. Position the client.

- The client should be in a sitting position with all clothing removed except the examination gown (see Figure 11.13 ●).

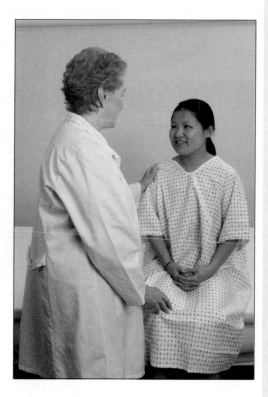

Figure 11.13 ● Positioning of client.

2. Instruct the client.

- Explain that you will be looking carefully at the client's skin.

3. Observe for cleanliness and use the sense of smell to determine body odor.

- Body odor is produced when bacterial waste products mix with perspiration on the skin surface. During heavy physical activity, body odor increases. Amounts of urea and ammonia are excreted in perspiration.

▶ Urea and ammonia salts are found on the skin of clients with kidney disorders.

4. Observe the client's skin tone.

- Evaluate any widespread color changes such as cyanosis, pallor, erythema, or jaundice. For example, always assess cyanotic clients for vital signs and level of consciousness.
  Use Table 11.1 to evaluate color variations in light and dark skin.

- The amount of melanin and carotene pigments, the oxygen content of the blood, and the level of exposure to the sun influence skin color. Dark skin contains large amounts of melanin, while fair skin has small amounts. The skin of most Asians contains a large amount of carotene, which causes a yellow cast.

▶ Cyanosis or pallor indicates abnormally low plasma oxygen, placing the client at risk for altered tissue perfusion. Pallor is seen in anemia.

<table>
<tr><td>

TECHNIQUES AND NORMAL FINDINGS

</td><td>

</td></tr>
</table>

5. Inspect the skin for even pigmentation over the body.

- In most cases, increased or decreased pigmentation is caused by differences in the distribution of melanin throughout the body. These are normal variations. For example, the margins of the lips, areolae, nipples, and external genitalia are more darkly pigmented. Freckles (see Figure 11.14 ●) and certain *nevi* (congenital marks; see Figure 11.15 ●) occur in people of all skin colors in varying degrees.

▶ For unknown reasons, some people develop patchy depigmented areas over the face, neck, hands, feet, and body folds. This condition is called **vitiligo** (see Figure 11.16 ●). Skin is otherwise normal. Vitiligo occurs in all races in all parts of the world but seems to affect dark-skinned people more severely. Clients with vitiligo may suffer a severe disturbance in body image.

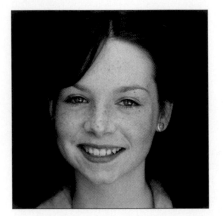

Figure 11.14 ● Freckles.

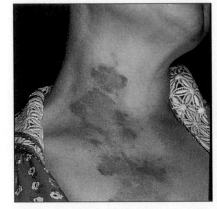

Figure 11.15 ● Nevus.

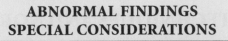

Figure 11.16 ● Vitiligo.

6. Inspect the skin for superficial arteries and veins.

- A fine network of veins or a few dilated blood vessels visible just beneath the surface of the skin are normal findings in areas of the body where skin is thin (e.g., the abdomen and eyelids).

PALPATION OF THE SKIN

1. Instruct the client.

- Explain that you will be touching the client in various areas with different parts of your hand.

2. Determine the client's skin temperature.

- Use the dorsal surface of your fingers, which is most sensitive to temperature. Palpate the forehead or face first. Continue to palpate inferiorly, including the hands and feet, comparing the temperature on the right and left side of the body (see Figure 11.17 ●).

▶ The temperature of the skin is higher than normal in the presence of a systemic infection or metabolic disorder such as hyperthyroidism, after vigorous activity, and when the external environment is warm.

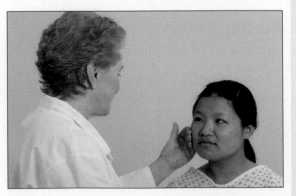

Figure 11.17 ●
Palpating skin temperature.

| TECHNIQUES AND NORMAL FINDINGS | ABNORMAL FINDINGS SPECIAL CONSIDERATIONS |

TECHNIQUES AND NORMAL FINDINGS

- Local skin temperature is controlled by the amount and rate of blood circulating through a body region. Normal temperatures range from mildly cool to slightly warm.

- The skin on both sides of the body is warm when tissue is perfused. Sometimes the hands and feet are cooler than the rest of the body, but the temperature is normally similar on both sides.

3. Assess the amount of moisture on the skin surface.

- Inspect and palpate the face, skin folds, axillae, palms, and soles of the feet, where perspiration is most easily detected.

- A fine sheen of perspiration or oil is not an abnormal finding, nor is moderately dry skin, especially in cold or dry climates.

4. Palpate the skin for texture.

- Use the palmar surface of fingers and finger pads when palpating for texture. Normal skin feels smooth, firm, and even.

5. Palpate the skin to determine its thickness.

- The outer layer of the skin is thin and firm over most parts of the body except the palms, soles of the feet, elbows, and knees, where it is thicker. Normally, the skin over the eyelids and lips is thinner.

6. Palpate the skin for elasticity.

- Elasticity is a combination of turgor (resiliency, or the skin's ability to return to its normal position and shape) and mobility (the skin's ability to be lifted).

    Using the forefinger and thumb, grasp a fold of skin beneath the clavicle or on the medial aspect of the wrist (see Figure 11.18 ●).

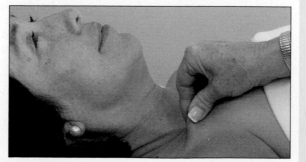

Figure 11.18 ●
Palpating for skin elasticity.

ABNORMAL FINDINGS SPECIAL CONSIDERATIONS

▶ The temperature of the skin is lower than normal in the presence of metabolic disorders such as hypothyroidism or when the external environment is cool. Localized coolness results from decreased circulation due to vasoconstriction or occlusion, which may occur from peripheral arterial insufficiency.

▶ A difference in temperature *bilaterally* may indicate an interruption in or lack of circulation on the cool side due to compression, immobilization, or elevation. If one side is warmer than normal, inflammation may be present on that side.

▶ **Diaphoresis** (profuse sweating) occurs during exertion, fever, pain, and emotional stress and in the presence of some metabolic disorders such as hyperthyroidism. It may also indicate an impending medical crisis such as a myocardial infarction.

▶ Severely dry skin typically is dark, weathered, and fissured. Pruritus frequently accompanies dry skin and may lead to abrasion and thickening if prolonged. Generalized dryness may occur in an individual who is dehydrated or has a systemic disorder such as hypothyroidism.
▶ Dry, parched lips and mucous membranes of the mouth are clear indicators of systemic dehydration. These areas should be checked if dehydration is suspected. Dry skin over the lower legs may be due to vascular insufficiency. Localized itching may indicate a skin allergy.

▶ The skin may become excessively smooth and velvety in clients with hyperthyroidism, whereas clients with hypothyroidism may have rough, scaly skin.

▶ Very thin, shiny skin may signal impaired circulation.

▶ When skin turgor is decreased, the skinfold "tents" (holds its pinched formation) and slowly returns to the former position. See Figure 11.8. Decreased turgor occurs when the client is dehydrated or has lost large amounts of weight.

    Increased skin turgor may be caused by scleroderma, literally "hard skin," a condition in which the underlying connective tissue becomes scarred and immobile.

TECHNIQUES AND NORMAL FINDINGS

- Notice the reaction of the skin both as you grasp and as you release. Healthy skin is mobile and returns rapidly to its previous shape and position.
- Finally palpate the feet, ankles, and sacrum. Edema is present if your palpation leaves a dent in the skin. See Chapter 18 for greater detail.
- Grade any edema on a four-point scale: 1 indicates mild edema, and 4 indicates deep edema (see Figure 11.19 ●).
- Note that because the fluid of edema lies above the pigmented and vascular layers of the skin, skin tone in the client with edema is obscured.

▶ **Edema** is a decrease in skin mobility caused by an accumulation of fluid in the intercellular spaces. Edema makes the skin look puffy, pitted, and tight. It may be most noticeable in the skin of the hands, feet, ankles, and sacral area (see Figure 11.20 ●).

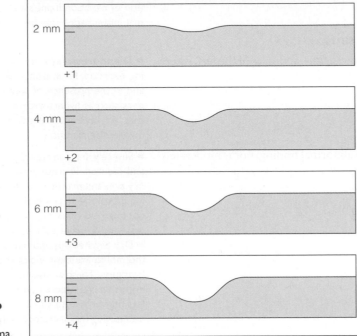

Figure 11.19 ●
Four-point scale
for grading edema.

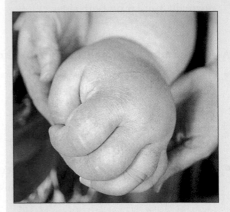

Figure 11.20 ● Edema of the hand.

7. Inspect and palpate the skin for lesions.

- Lesions of the skin are changes in normal skin structure. **Primary lesions** develop on previously unaltered skin. Lesions that change over time or because of scratching, abrasion, or infection are called **secondary lesions.**
- Carefully inspect the client's body, including skin folds and crevices, using a good source of light.
- When lesions are observed, palpate lesions between the thumb and index finger. Measure all lesion dimensions (including height, if possible) with a small, clear, flexible ruler.
- Document lesion size in centimeters. If necessary, use a magnifying glass or a penlight for closer inspection (see Figure 11.21 ●).

▶ The periumbilical and flank areas of the body should be observed for the presence of **ecchymosis** (bruising). Ecchymoses in the periumbilical area may signal bleeding somewhere in the abdomen (Cullen's sign). Ecchymoses in the flank area are associated with pancreatitis or bleeding in the peritoneum (Grey Turner's sign). Certain systemic disorders may produce characteristic patterns of lesions on particular body regions. Widespread lesions may indicate systemic or genetic disorders, or allergic reactions. Localized lesions may indicate physical trauma, chemical irritants, or allergic dermatitis. The nurse may wish to photograph the client's skin to document the presence, pattern, or spread of certain lesions.

| TECHNIQUES AND NORMAL FINDINGS | ABNORMAL FINDINGS SPECIAL CONSIDERATIONS |

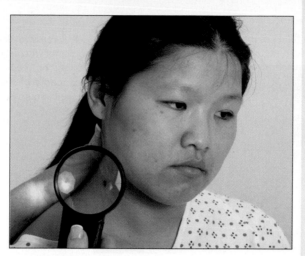

Figure 11.21 ●
Using a magnifying glass.

- Shine a Wood's lamp on the skin to distinguish fluorescing lesions.
- Assess any drainage for color, odor, consistency, amount, and location. If indicated, obtain a specimen of the drainage for culture and sensitivity.
- Some fungal infections including tinea capitis do not fluoresce.
- Healthy skin is typically smooth and free of lesions; however, some lesions, such as freckles, insect bites, healed scars, and certain birthmarks, are expected findings.

8. Palpate the skin for sensitivity.

- Palpate the skin in various regions of the body and ask the client to describe the sensations.
- Give special attention to any pain or discomfort that the client reports, especially when palpating skin lesions.
- Ask the client to describe the sensation as closely as possible, and document the findings.
- The client should not report any discomfort from your touch.

ALERT!

Localized hot, red, swollen painful areas indicate the presence of inflammation and possible infection. These areas should not be palpated, because the slightest disturbance may spread the infection deeper into skin layers.

INSPECTION OF THE SCALP AND HAIR

1. Instruct the client.

- Explain that you will be looking at the client's scalp and hair. Tell the client you will be parting the hair to observe the scalp.

2. Observe for cleanliness.

- Ask the client to remove any hairpins, hair ties, barrettes, wigs, or hairpieces and to undo braids. If the client is unwilling to do this, examine any strands of hair that are loose or undone.

▶ Physical abuse should be suspected if the client has any of the following: bruises or welts that appear in a pattern suggesting the use of a belt or stick; burns with sharply demarcated edges suggesting injury from cigarettes, irons, or immersion of a hand in boiling water; additional injuries such as fractures or dislocations; or multiple injuries in various stages of healing. A nurse must be especially sensitive if the client is fearful of family members, is reluctant to return home, and has a history of previous injuries. When any of these diagnostic cues are evident, it is important to obtain medical assistance and follow the state's legal requirements to notify the police or local protective agency.

The injection of drugs into the veins of the arms or other parts of the body results in a series of small scars called *track marks* along the course of the blood vessel. A nurse who sees track marks and suspects substance abuse should refer the client to a mental health or substance abuse professional.

TECHNIQUES AND NORMAL FINDINGS	ABNORMAL FINDINGS SPECIAL CONSIDERATIONS

- Part and divide the hair at 1-in. intervals and observe (see Figure 11.22 ●).
- A small amount of **dandruff** (dead, scaly flakes of epidermal cells) may be present.

▶ Excessive dandruff occurs on the scalp of clients with certain skin disorders, such as psoriasis or seborrheic dermatitis, in which large amounts of the epidermis slough away. Dandruff should be distinguished from head lice.

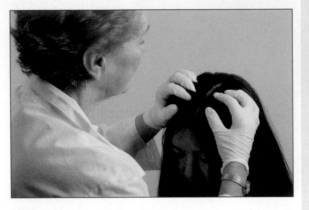

Figure 11.22 ●
Inspecting the hair and scalp.

3. **Observe the client's hair color.**
   - Like skin color, hair color varies according to the level of melanin production. Graying is influenced by genetics and may begin as early as the late teens in some clients.

▶ Graying of the hair in patches may indicate a nutritional deficiency, commonly of protein or copper.

4. **Assess the texture of the hair.**
   - Roll a few strands of hair between your thumb and forefinger.
   - Hold a few strands of hair taut with one hand while you slide the thumb and forefinger of your other hand along the length of the strand.
   - Hair may be thick or fine and may appear straight, wavy, or curly.

▶ Hypothyroidism and other metabolic disorders, as well as nutritional deficiencies, may cause the hair to be dull, dry, brittle, and coarse.

5. **Observe the amount and distribution of the hair throughout the scalp.**
   - The amount of hair varies with age, gender, and overall health. Healthy hair is evenly distributed throughout the scalp.

   - In most men and women, atrophy of the hair follicles causes hair growth to decline by the age of 50. Male pattern baldness (see Figure 11.23 ●), a genetically determined progressive loss of hair beginning at the anterior hairline, has no clinical significance. It is the most frequent reason for hair loss in men.

▶ When hair loss occurs in women, it is thought to be caused by an imbalance in adrenal hormones.

▶ Widespread hair loss may also be caused by illness, infections, metabolic disorders, nutritional deficiencies, and chemotherapy. Patchy hair loss (**alopecia areata**) may be due to infection.

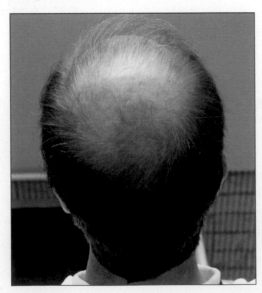

Figure 11.23 ●
Male pattern baldness.

TECHNIQUES AND NORMAL FINDINGS	ABNORMAL FINDINGS SPECIAL CONSIDERATIONS

- Remember to assess the amount, texture, and distribution of body hair. Some practitioners prefer to perform this assessment with the regions of the body.

6. Inspect the scalp for lesions.

- Dim the room light and shine a Wood's lamp on the client's scalp as you part the hair (see Figure 11.24 ●).

► Gray, scaly patches with broken hair may indicate the presence of a fungal infection such as ringworm. Regions of infection will fluoresce when exposed to the ultraviolet light of a Wood's lamp.

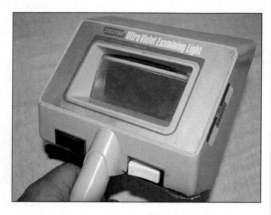

Figure 11.24 ●
Using a Wood's lamp.

- The healthy scalp is free from lesions and areas of fluorescent glow.

► Infestation by **pediculosis capitis** (head lice) is signaled by tiny, white, oval eggs (nits) that adhere to the hair shaft. Head lice usually cause intense itching. The scalp should be checked for excoriation from scratching.

ASSESSMENT OF THE NAILS

1. Instruct the client.

- Explain that you will be looking at and touching the client's nails and that you will ask the client to hold the hands and fingers in certain positions while you are inspecting the fingernails.

2. Assess for hygiene.

- Confirm that the nails are clean and well groomed.

► Dirty fingernails may indicate a self-care deficit but could also be related to a person's occupation.

3. Inspect the nails for an even, pink undertone.

- Small, white markings in the nail are normal findings and indicate minor trauma.

► The nails appear pale and colorless in clients with peripheral arteriosclerosis or anemia. The nails appear yellow in clients with jaundice, and dark red in clients with *polycythemia*, a pathological increase in production of red blood cells. Fungal infections may cause the nails to discolor. Horizontal white bands may occur in chronic hepatic or renal disease. A darkly pigmented band in a single nail may be a sign of a melanoma in the nail matrix and should be referred to a physician for further evaluation.

4. Assess capillary refill.

- Depress the nail edge briefly to blanch, and then release. Color returns to healthy nails instantly upon release.

► The nail beds appear blue, and color return is sluggish in clients with cardiovascular or respiratory disorders.

TECHNIQUES AND NORMAL FINDINGS

5. Inspect and palpate the nails for shape and contour.

- Perform the Schamroth technique to assess clubbing. Ask the client to bring the dorsal aspect of corresponding fingers together, creating a mirror image.

- Look at the distal phalanx and observe the diamond-shaped opening created by nails. When clubbing is present, the diamond is not formed and the distance increases at the fingertip (see Figure 11.25 ●).

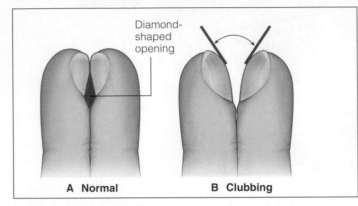

Diamond-shaped opening

A Normal   **B Clubbing**

Figure 11.25 ●
Schamroth technique.
A. Healthy nail.
B. Clubbing.

- The nails normally form a slight convex curve or lie flat on the nail bed. When viewed laterally, the angle between the skin and the nail base should be approximately 160 degrees (see Figure 11.27 ●).

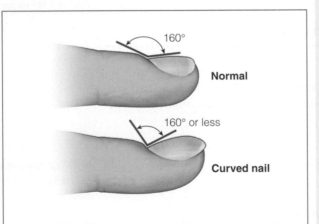

160°

Normal

160° or less

Curved nail

Figure 11.27 ●
Angle of fingernail.

6. Palpate the nails to determine their thickness, regularity, and attachment to the nail bed.

- Healthy nails are smooth, strong, and regular and are firmly attached to the nail bed, with only a slight degree of mobility.

7. Inspect and palpate the cuticles.

- The cuticles are smooth and flat in healthy nails.

▶ *Clubbing of the fingernails* occurs when there is hypoxia or impaired peripheral tissue perfusion over a long period of time. It may also occur with cirrhosis, colitis, thyroid disease, or long-term tobacco smoking. The ends of the fingers become enlarged, soft, and spongy, and the angle between the skin and the nail base is greater than 160 degrees (see Figure 11.26 ●).

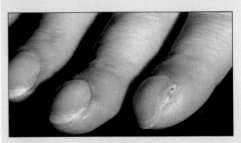

Figure 11.26 ● Clubbing of fingernails.

▶ *Spoon nails* form a concave curve and are thought to be associated with iron deficiency (see Figure 11.28 ●).

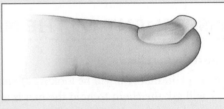

Figure 11.28 ● Spoon nail.

▶ Nails may be thickened in clients with circulatory disorders. **Onycholysis,** separation of the nail plate from the nail bed, occurs with trauma, infection, or skin lesions.

▶ *Hangnails* are jagged tears in the lateral skin folds around the nail. An untreated hangnail may become inflamed and lead to a **paronychia,** an infection of the cuticle.

Refer to the Companion Website at **www.prenhall.com/damico** and click on the **Documentation** module for documentation samples and documentation practice exercises.

*A*bnormal findings of the integumentary system include alterations in the skin, hair, or nails. Skin abnormalities include lesions, vascular lesions, and malignant lesions. Figures 11.29 through 11.75 depict these skin abnormalities. Abnormalities of the hair are depicted in Figures 11.76 through 11.81. Splinter hemorrhage, clubbing, and paronychia are among the abnormalities of the nail depicted in Figures 11.82 through 11.87.

VASCULAR LESIONS

Hemangioma

Hemangioma is a bright red, raised lesion about 2 to 10 cm in diameter. It does not blanch with pressure. It is usually present at birth or within a few months of birth. Typically, it disappears by age 3. The lesion pictured in Figure 11.29 ● is located on the dorsal surface on the hand.

Cause: A cluster of immature capillaries.

Localization/Distribution: Can appear on any part of the body.

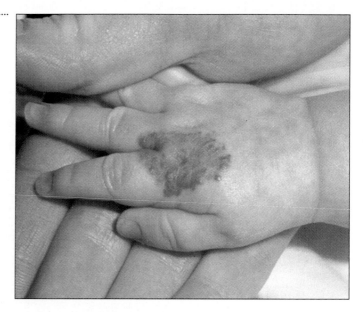

Figure 11.29 ● Hemangioma.

Port-Wine Stain

A port-wine stain is a flat, irregularly shaped lesion ranging in color from pale red to deep purple-red. Color deepens with exertion, emotional response, or exposure to extremes of temperature. It is present at birth and typically does not fade (see Figure 11.30 ●).

Cause: A large, flat mass of blood vessels on the skin surface.

Localization/Distribution: Most commonly appears on the face and head but may occur in other sites.

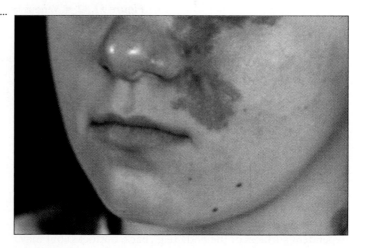

Figure 11.30 ● Port-wine stain (nevus flammeus).

Spider Angioma

Spider angioma is a flat, bright red dot with tiny radiating blood vessels ranging in size from a pinpoint to 2 cm. It blanches with pressure (see Figure 11.31 •).

Cause: A type of telangiectasis (vascular dilatation) caused by elevated estrogen levels, pregnancy, estrogen therapy, vitamin B deficiency, or liver disease, or may not be pathologic.

Localization/Distribution: Most commonly appears on the upper half of the body.

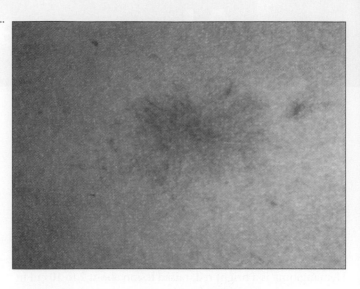

Figure 11.31 • Spider (star) angioma.

Venous Lake

Venous lake is a flat blue lesion with radiating, cascading, or linear veins extending from the center. It ranges in size from 3 to 25 cm (see Figure 11.32 •).

Cause: A type of telangiectasis (vascular dilatation) caused by increased intravenous pressure in superficial veins.

Localization/Distribution: Most commonly appears on the anterior chest and the lower legs near varicose veins.

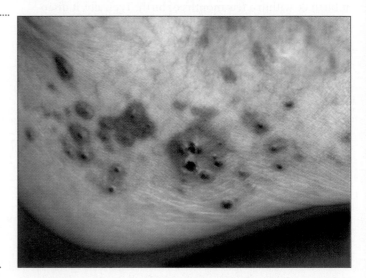

Figure 11.32 • Venous lake.

Petechiae

Petechiae are flat red or purple rounded "freckles" approximately 1 to 3 mm in diameter (see Figure 11.33 •).
They are difficult to detect in dark skin. Do not blanch.

Cause: Minute hemorrhages resulting from fragile capillaries, petechiae are caused by septicemias, liver disease, or vitamin C or K deficiency. They may also be caused by anticoagulant therapy.

Localization/Distribution: Most commonly appear on the dependent surfaces of the body (e.g., back, buttocks) but may occur elsewhere on the body. In the client with dark skin, may be seen in the oral mucosa and conjunctivae.

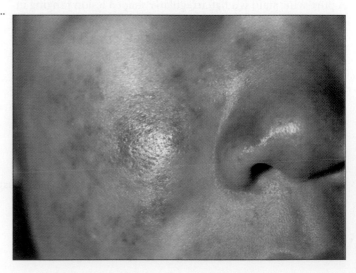

Figure 11.33 • Petechiae.

Purpura

Purpura are flat, reddish blue, irregularly shaped extensive patches of varying size (see Figure 11.34 ●).

Cause: Bleeding disorders, scurvy, and capillary fragility in the older adult (senile purpura).

Localization/Distribution: May appear anywhere on the body, but are most noticeable on the legs, arms, and backs of hands.

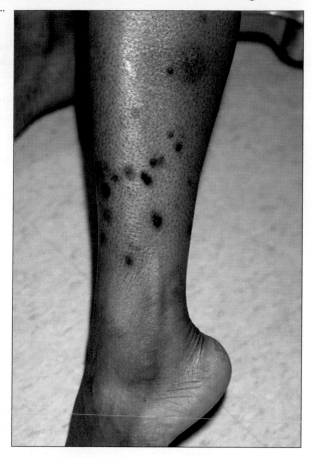

Figure 11.34 ● Purpura.

Ecchymosis

Ecchymosis is a flat, irregularly shaped lesion of varying size with no pulsation (see Figure 11.35 ●). It does not blanch with pressure. In light skin, it begins as a bluish purple mark that changes to greenish yellow. In brown skin, it varies from blue to deep purple. In black skin, it appears as a darkened area.

Cause: Release of blood from superficial vessels into surrounding tissue due to trauma, hemophilia, liver disease, or deficiency of vitamin C or K.

Localization/Distribution: Occurs anywhere on the body at the site of trauma or pressure.

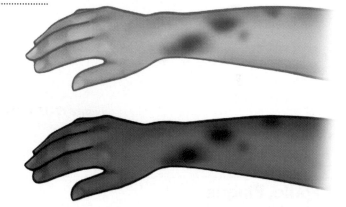

Figure 11.35 ● Ecchymosis (bruise).

Hematoma

A hematoma is a raised, irregularly shaped lesion similar to an ecchymosis except that it elevates the skin and looks like a swelling (see Figure 11.36 ●).

Cause: A leakage of blood into the skin and subcutaneous tissue as a result of trauma or surgical incision.

Localization/Distribution: May occur anywhere on the body at the site of trauma, pressure, or surgical incision.

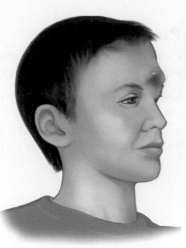

Figure 11.36 ● Hematoma.

PRIMARY LESIONS

Macule, Patch

A macule, patch is a flat, nonpalpable change in skin color. Macules are smaller than 1 cm, with a circumscribed border (see Figure 11.37 ●), and patches are larger than 1 cm and may have an irregular border.

Examples: Macules: freckles, measles, and petechiae. Patches: mongolian spots, port-wine stains, vitiligo, and chloasma.

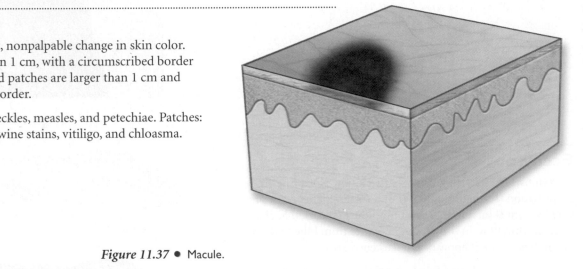

Figure 11.37 ● Macule.

Papule, Plaque

A papule, plaque is an elevated, solid palpable mass with circumscribed border (see Figure 11.38 ●). Papules are smaller than 0.5 cm; plaques are groups of papules that form lesions larger than 0.5 cm.

Examples: Papules: elevated moles, warts, and lichen planus. Plaques: psoriasis, actinic keratosis, and also lichen planus.

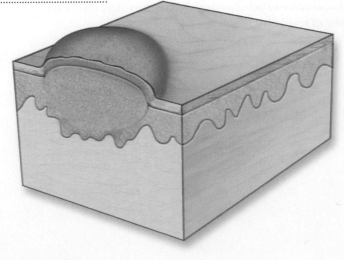

Figure 11.38 ● Papule, plaque.

Nodule, Tumor

A nodule, tumor is an elevated, solid, hard or soft palpable mass extending deeper into the dermis than a papule (see Figure 11.39 ●). Nodules have circumscribed borders and are 0.5 to 2 cm; tumors may have irregular borders and are larger than 2 cm.

Examples: Nodules: small lipoma, squamous cell carcinoma, fibroma, and intradermal nevi. Tumors: large lipoma, carcinoma, and hemangioma.

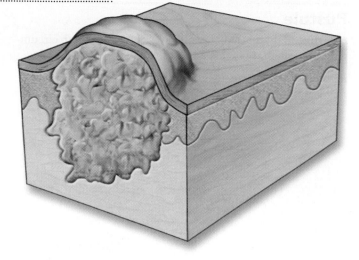

Figure 11.39 ● Nodule, tumor.

Vesicle, Bulla

A vesicle, bulla is an elevated, fluid-filled, round or oval-shaped, palpable mass with thin, translucent walls and circumscribed borders (see Figure 11.40 ●). Vesicles are smaller than 0.5 cm; bullae are larger than 0.5 cm.

Examples: Vesicles: herpes simplex/zoster, early chickenpox, poison ivy, and small burn blisters. Bullae: contact dermatitis, friction blisters, and large burn blisters.

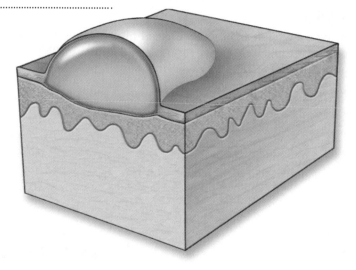

Figure 11.40 ● Vesicle, bulla.

Wheal

A wheal is an elevated, often reddish area with irregular border caused by diffuse fluid in tissues rather than free fluid in a cavity, as in vesicles (see Figure 11.41 ●). Size varies.

Examples: Insect bites and hives (extensive wheals).

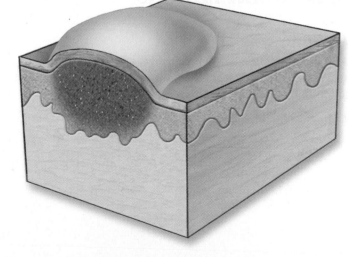

Figure 11.41 ● Wheal.

Pustule

A pustule is an elevated, pus-filled vesicle or bulla with circumscribed border (see Figure 11.42 ●). Size varies.

Examples: Acne, impetigo, and carbuncles (large boils).

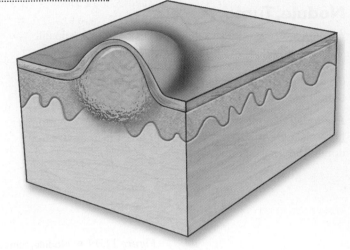

Figure 11.42 ● Pustule.

Cyst

A cyst is an elevated, encapsulated, fluid-filled or semisolid mass originating in the subcutaneous tissue or dermis, usually 1 cm or larger (see Figure 11.43 ●).

Examples: Varieties include sebaceous cysts and epidermoid cysts.

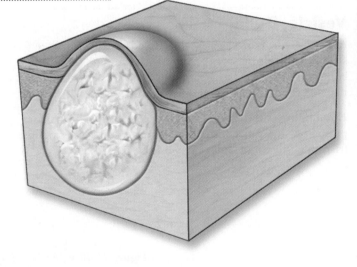

Figure 11.43 ● Cyst.

SECONDARY LESIONS

Atrophy

Atrophy is a translucent, dry, paperlike, sometimes wrinkled skin surface resulting from thinning or wasting of the skin due to loss of collagen and elastin (see Figure 11.44 ●).

Examples: Striae, aged skin.

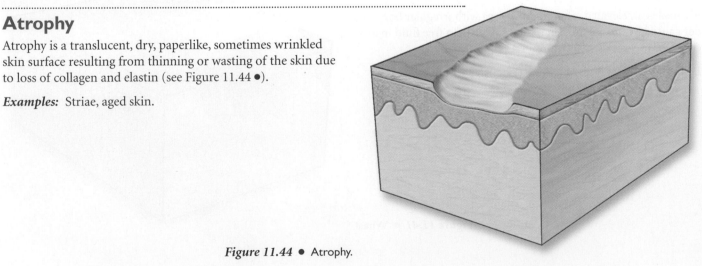

Figure 11.44 ● Atrophy.

Erosion

Erosion is wearing away of the superficial epidermis causing a moist, shallow depression. Because erosions do not extend into the dermis, they heal without scarring (see Figure 11.45 ●).

Examples: Scratch marks, ruptured vesicles.

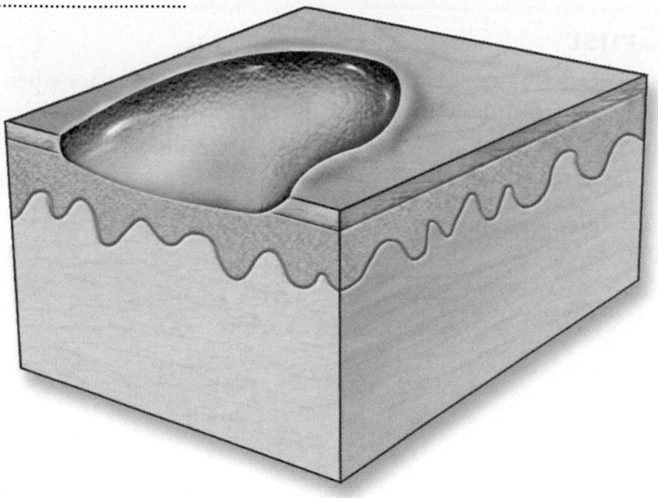

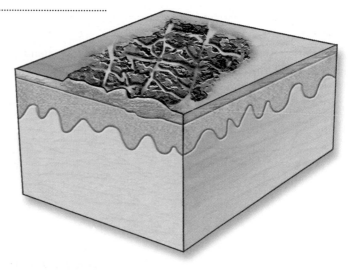

Figure 11.45 ● Erosion.

Lichenification

Lichenification is a rough, thickened, hardened area of epidermis resulting from chronic irritation such as scratching or rubbing (see Figure 11.46 ●).

Examples: Chronic dermatitis.

Figure 11.46 ● Lichenification.

Scales

Scales are shedding flakes of greasy, keratinized skin tissue. Color may be white, gray, or silver. Texture may vary from fine to thick (see Figure 11.47 ●).

Examples: Dry skin, dandruff, psoriasis, and eczema.

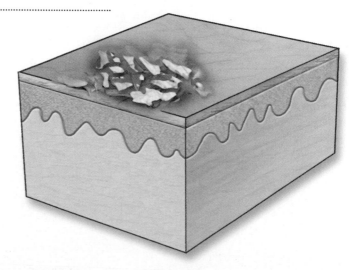

Figure 11.47 ● Scales.

Crust

Crust is dry blood, serum, or pus left on the skin surface when vesicles or pustules burst (see Figure 11.48 ●). It can be red-brown, orange, or yellow. Large crusts that adhere to the skin surface are called scabs.

Examples: Eczema, impetigo, herpes, or scabs following abrasion.

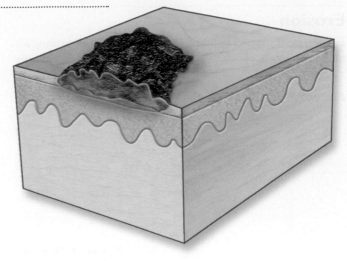

Figure 11.48 ● Crust.

Ulcer

An ulcer is a deep, irregularly shaped area of skin loss extending into the dermis or subcutaneous tissue (see Figure 11.49 ●). It may bleed or leave a scar.

Examples: Decubitus ulcers (pressure sores), stasis ulcers, chancres.

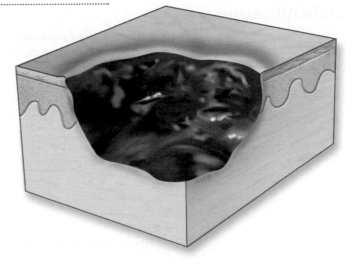

Figure 11.49 ● Ulcer.

Fissure

A fissure is a linear crack with sharp edges, extending into the dermis (see Figure 11.50 ●).

Examples: Cracks at the corners of the mouth or in the hands, athlete's foot.

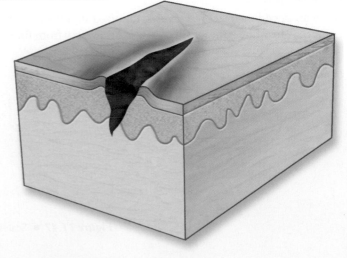

Figure 11.50 ● Fissure.

Scar

A scar is a flat, irregular area of connective tissue left after a lesion or wound has healed (see Figure 11.51 ●). New scars may be red or purple; older scars may be silvery or white.

Examples: Healed surgical wound or injury, healed acne.

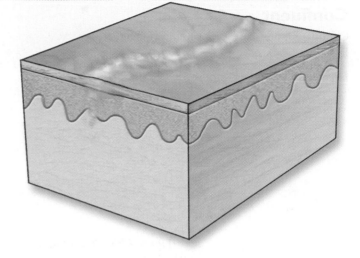

Figure 11.51 ● Scar.

Keloid

A keloid is an elevated, irregular, darkened area of excess scar tissue caused by excessive collagen formation during healing (see Figure 11.52 ●). It extends beyond the site of the original injury. There is higher incidence in people of African descent.

Examples: Keloid from ear-piercing or surgery.

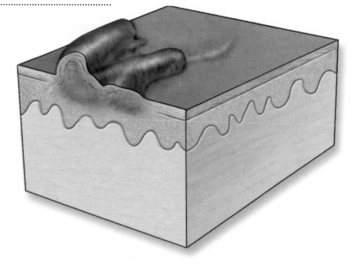

Figure 11.52 ● Keloid.

CONFIGURATIONS AND SHAPES OF LESIONS

Annular

Annular lesions are lesions with a circular shape (see Figure 11.53 ●).

Examples: Tinea corporis, pityriasis rosea.

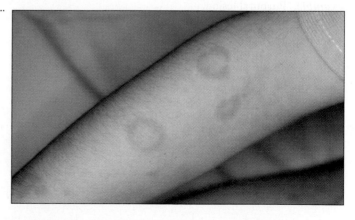

Figure 11.53 ● Annular lesions.

Confluent

Confluent lesions are lesions that run together (see Figure 11.54 ●).

Example: Urticaria.

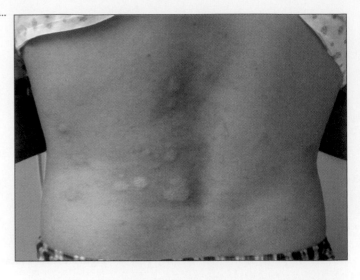

Figure 11.54 ● Confluent lesions.

Discrete

Discrete lesions are lesions that are separate and discrete (see Figure 11.55 ●).

Example: Malluscum.

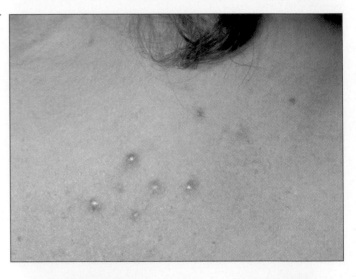

Figure 11.55 ● Discrete lesions.

Grouped

Grouped lesions are lesions that appear in clusters (see Figure 11.56 ●).

Example: Purpural lesion.

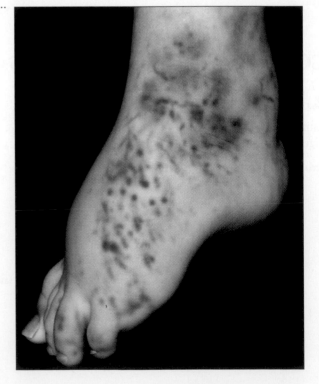

Figure 11.56 ● Grouped lesions.

Gyrate

Gyrate lesions are lesions that are coiled or twisted (see Figure 11.57 ●).

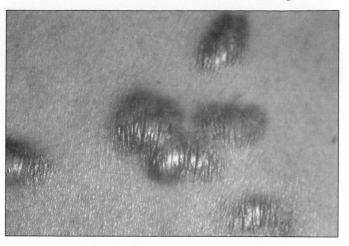

Figure 11.57 ● Gyrate lesions.

Target

Target lesions are lesions with concentric circles of color (see Figure 11.58 ●).

Example: Erythema multiforme.

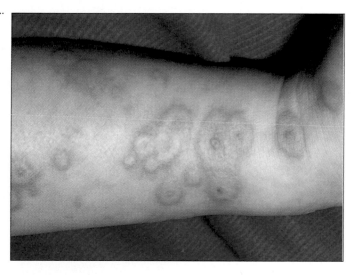

Figure 11.58 ● Target lesions.

Linear

Linear lesions are lesions that appear as a line (see Figure 11.59 ●).

Example: Scratches.

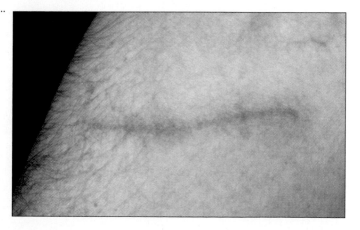

Figure 11.59 ● Linear lesions.

Polycyclic

Polycyclic lesions are lesions that are circular but united (see Figure 11.60 ●).

Example: Psoriasis.

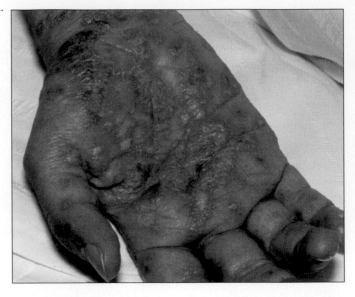

Figure 11.60 ● Polycyclic lesions.

Zosteriform

Zosteriform lesions are arranged in a linear manner along a nerve route (see Figure 11.61 ●).

Example: Herpes zoster.

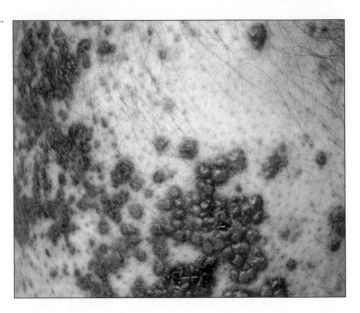

Figure 11.61 ● Zosteriform lesions.

COMMON SKIN LESIONS

Tinea

Tinea is fungal infection affecting the body (tinea corporis), the scalp (tinea capitis), or the feet (tinea pedis, also known as athlete's foot). Secondary bacterial infection may also be present. The appearance of the lesions varies, and they may present as papules, pustules, vesicles, or scales (see Figure 11.62 ●).

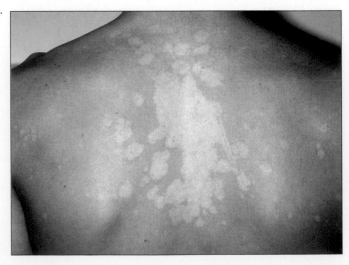

Figure 11.62 ● Tinea corporis.

Measles (Rubeola)

Measles is a highly contagious viral disease that causes a rash of red to purple macules or papules (see Figure 11.63 ●). The rash begins on the face, then progresses over the neck, trunk, arms, and legs. It does not blanch. It may be accompanied by tiny white spots that look like grains of salt (called Koplik's spots) on the oral mucosa. It occurs mostly in children.

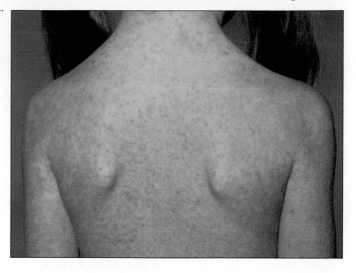

Figure 11.63 ● Measles (rubeola).

German Measles (Rubella)

German measles is a highly contagious disease caused by a virus. Typically it begins as a pink, papular rash that is similar to measles but paler (see Figure 11.64 ●). Like measles, it begins on the face, then spreads over the body. Unlike measles, it may be accompanied by swollen glands. It is not accompanied by Koplik's spots. It occurs mostly in children.

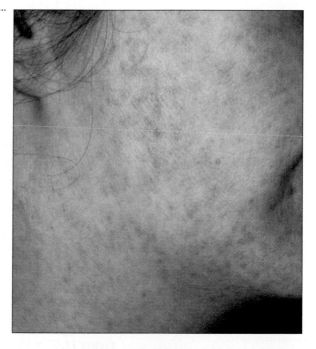

Figure 11.64 ● German measles (rubella).

Chickenpox (Varicella)

Chickenpox is a mild infectious disease caused by the herpes zoster virus. It begins as groups of small, red, fluid-filled vesicles usually on the trunk (see Figure 11.65 ●), and progresses to the face, arms, and legs. Vesicles erupt over several days, forming pustules, then crusts. The condition may cause intense itching. It occurs mostly in children.

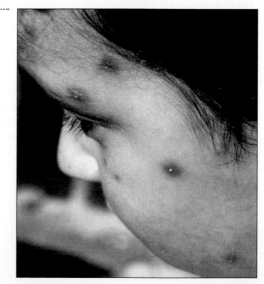

Figure 11.65 ● Chickenpox (varicella).

Herpes Simplex

Herpes simplex is a viral infection that causes characteristic lesions on the lips and oral mucosa (see Figure 11.66 ●). Lesions progress from vesicles to pustules, and then crusts. Herpes simplex also occurs in the genitals.

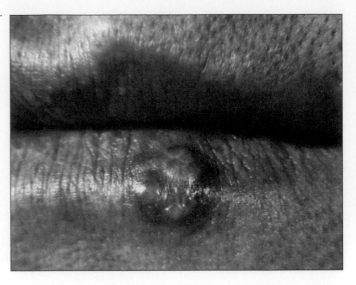

Figure 11.66 ● Herpes simplex.

Herpes Zoster

Herpes zoster is an eruption of dormant herpes zoster virus, which typically has invaded the body during an attack of chickenpox. Clusters of small vesicles form on the skin along the route of sensory nerves. Vesicles progress to pustules and then crusts (see Figure 11.67 ●). It causes intense pain and itching. The condition is more common and more severe in older adults.

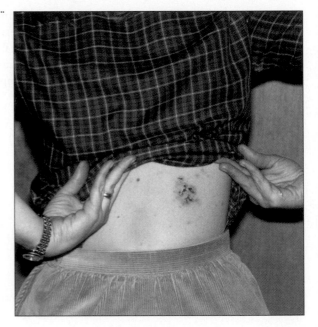

Figure 11.67 ● Herpes zoster (shingles).

Psoriasis

Psoriasis is thickening of the skin in dry, silvery, scaly patches (see Figure 11.68 ●). It occurs with overproduction of skin cells resulting in buildup of cells faster than they can be shed. It may be triggered by emotional stress or generally poor health. It may be located on scalp, elbows and knees, lower back, and perianal area.

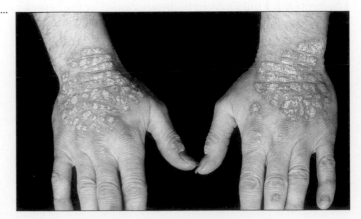

Figure 11.68 ● Psoriasis.

Contact Dermatitis

Contact dermatitis is inflammation of the skin due to an allergy to a substance that comes into contact with the skin, such as clothing, jewelry, plants, chemicals, or cosmetics. The location of the lesions may help identify the allergen. It may progress from redness to hives, vesicles, or scales (see Figure 11.69 ●), and is usually accompanied by intense itching.

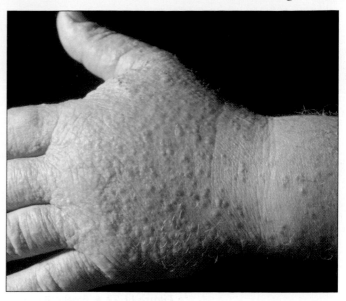

Figure 11.69 ● Contact dermatitis.

Eczema

Eczema is internally provoked inflammation of the skin causing reddened papules and vesicles that ooze, weep, and progress to form crusts (see Figure 11.70 ●). The lesions are usually located on the scalp, face, elbows, knees, forearms, torso, and wrists. Eczema usually causes intense itching.

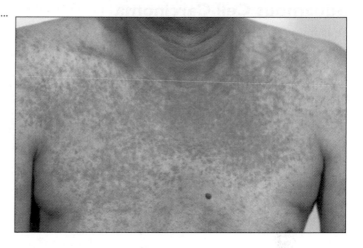

Figure 11.70 ● Eczema (atopic dermatitis).

Impetigo

Impetigo is a bacterial skin infection that usually appears on the skin around the nose and mouth (see Figure 11.71 ●). It is contagious and common in children. It may begin as a barely perceptible patch of blisters that breaks, exposing red, weeping area beneath. A tan crust soon forms over this area, and the infection may spread out of the edges.

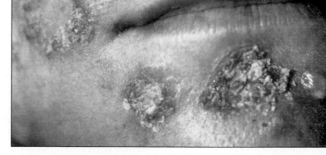

Figure 11.71 ● Impetigo.

MALIGNANT SKIN LESIONS

Basal Cell Carcinoma

Basal cell carcinoma is the most common but least malignant type of skin cancer. Basal cell carcinoma is a proliferation of the cells of the stratum basale into the dermis and subcutaneous tissue. The lesions begin as shiny papules that develop central ulcers with rounded, pearly edges (see Figure 11.72 ●). Lesions occur most often on skin regions regularly exposed to the sun.

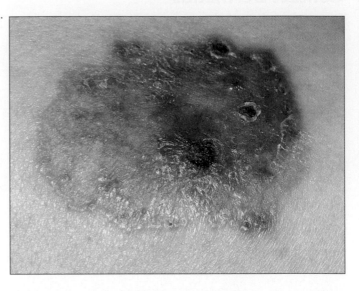

Figure 11.72 ● Basal cell carcinoma.

Squamous Cell Carcinoma

Squamous cell carcinoma arises from the cells of the stratum spinosum. It begins as a reddened, scaly papule, then forms a shallow ulcer with a clearly delineated, elevated border (see Figure 11.73 ●). It commonly appears on the scalp, ears, backs of the hands, and lower lip, and is thought to be caused by exposure to the sun. It grows rapidly.

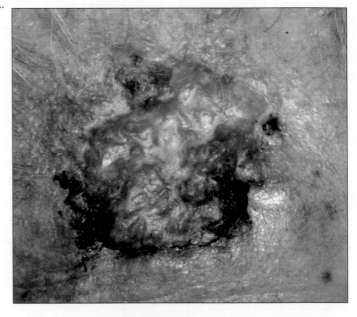

Figure 11.73 ● Squamous cell carcinoma.

Malignant Melanoma

Malignant melanoma is the least common but most serious type of skin cancer, because it spreads rapidly to lymph and blood vessels. The lesion contains areas of varied pigmentation from black to brown to blue or red. The edges are often irregular, with notched borders, and the diameter is greater than 6 mm (see Figure 11.74 ●).

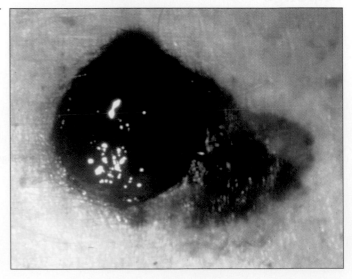

Figure 11.74 ● Malignant melanoma.

Kaposi's Sarcoma

Kaposi's sarcoma is a malignant tumor of the epidermis and internal epithelial tissues. Lesions are typically soft, blue to purple, and painless (see Figure 11.75 ●). Other characteristics are variable: they may be macular or papular and may resemble keloids or bruises. Kaposi's sarcoma is common in HIV-positive people.

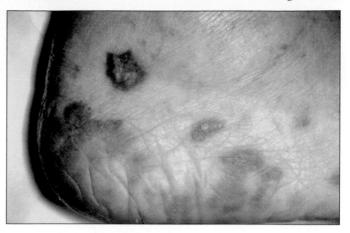

Figure 11.75 ● Kaposi's sarcoma.

ABNORMALITIES OF THE HAIR

Seborrheic Dermatitis

Seborrheic dermatitis is common in infants. It appears as eczema of yellow-white greasy scales on the scalp and forehead. It is also known as cradle cap (see Figure 11.76 ●).

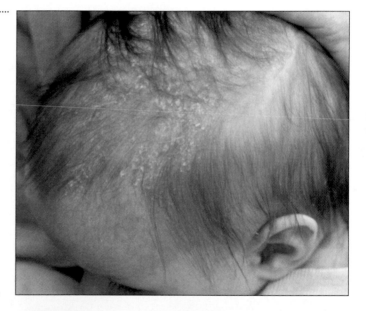

Figure 11.76 ● Seborrheic dermatitis (cradle cap).

Tinea Capitis

Tinea capitis is patchy hair loss on the head with pustules on the skin (see Figure 11.77 ●). This highly contagious fungal disease is transmitted from the soil, from animals, or from person to person.

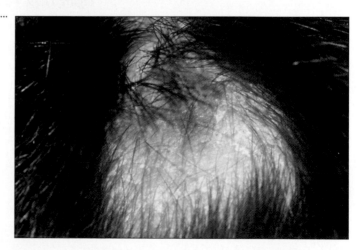

Figure 11.77 ● Tinea capitis (scalp ringworm).

Alopecia Areata

There is no known cause for the sudden loss of hair in a round balding patch on the scalp (see Figure 11.78 ●).

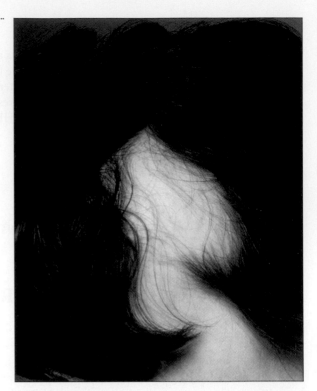

Figure 11.78 ● Alopecia areata.

Folliculitis

Folliculitis, infections of hair follicles, appears as pustules with underlying erythema (see Figure 11.79 ●).

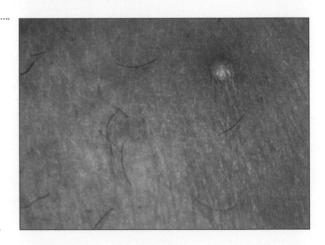

Figure 11.79 ● Folliculitis.

Furuncle/Abscess

Infected hair follicles give rise to furuncles (see Figure 11.80 ●). These are hard, erythematous, pus-filled lesions. Abscesses are caused by bacteria entering the skin. These are larger lesions than furuncles.

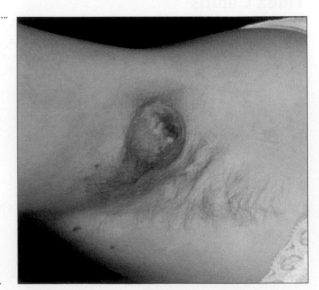

Figure 11.80 ● Furuncle/abscess.

Hirsutism

Hirsutism is excess body hair in females on the face, chest, abdomen, arms, and legs, following the male pattern. This example shows excessive hair on the female chin (see Figure 11.81 ●). It is typically due to endocrine or metabolic dysfunction, though it may be idiopathic.

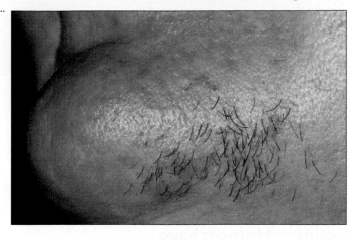

Figure 11.81 ● Hirsutism.

ABNORMALITIES OF THE NAILS

Spoon Nails

Concavity and thinning of the nails (see Figure 11.82 ●), which is commonly a congenital condition.

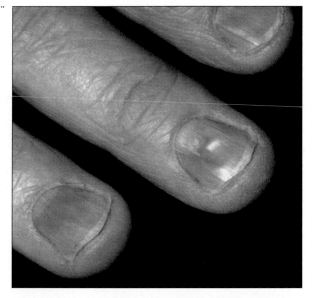

Figure 11.82 ● Spoon nails (Koilonychia).

Paronychia

Paronychia is an infection of the skin adjacent to the nail, usually caused by bacteria or fungi (see Figure 11.83 ●). The affected area becomes red, swollen, and painful, and pus may ooze from it.

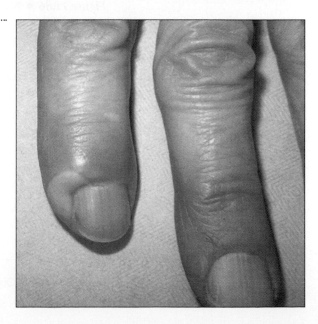

Figure 11.83 ● Paronychia.

Beau's Line

Beau's line occurs from trauma or illness affecting nail formation. A linear depression develops at the base and moves distally as the nail grows (see Figure 11.84 ●).

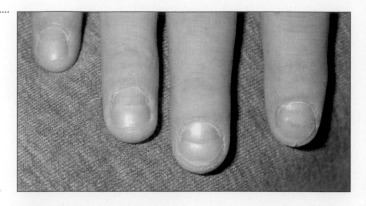

Figure 11.84 ● Beau's line.

Splinter Hemorrhage

Splinter hemorrhage can occur as a result of trauma or in endocarditis. These appear as reddish-brown spots in the nail (see Figure 11.85 ●).

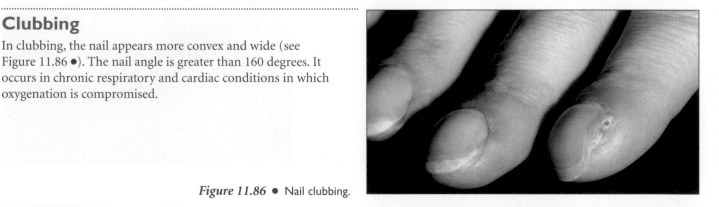

Figure 11.85 ● Splinter hemorrhages.

Clubbing

In clubbing, the nail appears more convex and wide (see Figure 11.86 ●). The nail angle is greater than 160 degrees. It occurs in chronic respiratory and cardiac conditions in which oxygenation is compromised.

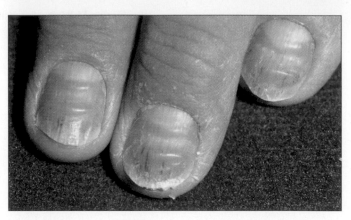

Figure 11.86 ● Nail clubbing.

Onycholysis

In onycholysis, the nail plate loosens from the distal nail and proceeds to the proximal portion (see Figure 11.87 ●).

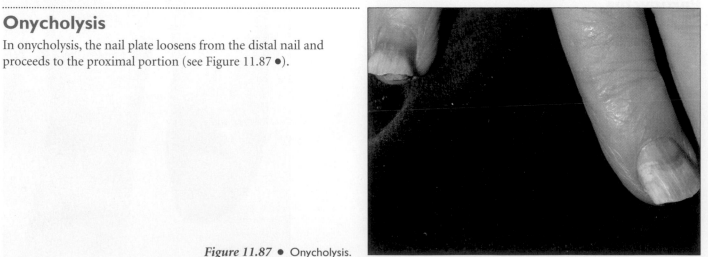

Figure 11.87 ● Onycholysis.

Health Promotion

HEALTHY PEOPLE 2010

FOCUS AREA	PREVALENCE	OBJECTIVES	ACTIONS
Occupational Skin Disorders	• Occupational skin disorders (OSDs) occur in agriculture, forestry, fishing, and manufacturing. • Allergic and irritant dermatitis are the most common OSDs. OSD is the most common non-trauma-related occupational disorder.	• Reduce OSD in full-time workers.	• Screening. • Reduction of allergens and irritants. • Education about personal protection (including the use of protective equipment), exposure, and hygiene.
Skin Cancer	• Melanoma is responsible for the highest number of skin cancer deaths. • Risk factors include personal or family history of melanoma. • Melanoma risk is highest in Caucasians, and males have death rates twice as high as females.	• Increase the number of persons using protective measures to reduce the risk of skin cancer.	• Education about risks. • Education about the use of protective products. • Education about skin screening and assessment.

CLIENT EDUCATION

The following are risk factors for physiological, behavioral, and cultural considerations that affect the health of the skin, hair, and nails. Several factors are cited in *Healthy People 2010*. The nurse provides advice and education to reduce risks associated with these factors and to promote and maintain the health of the skin, hair, and nails across the life span.

LIFE SPAN CONSIDERATIONS

RISK FACTORS

- Infants have permeable epidermis increasing the risk of fluid loss through the skin, and they have active sebaceous glands leading to milia and cradle cap.
- Infants' skin lacks the ability to contract. Therefore, they cannot shiver and do not perspire, limiting thermal regulation.

- Children's skin texture changes, but perspiration and sebaceous gland function is limited, resulting in dry skin.
- In adolescence, skin texture continues to change. Sebaceous gland activity increases in response to hormonal changes. Eccrine glands increase function, resulting in increased perspiration, especially in response to emotional changes.
- Children and adolescents are at risk for skin trauma associated with accidents, play, and sports activity.

CLIENT EDUCATION

- Teach parents and caregivers that infants require regular bathing and washing of the scalp and hair.

- Soap and shampoos should be mild and the skin should be thoroughly rinsed. Patting dry is recommended for sensitive young skin. Further, infants require clothing that is appropriate for the external temperature and environment since they have limited thermal regulation.
- Tell parents that children's dry skin needs to be monitored and mild lotions used when dryness is excessive.
- Teach adolescents that hygiene is important in relation to increasing oil production and perspiration and that soaps and deodorants are effective in controlling body odors.

- Provide information about recognition and levels of skin trauma to reduce risk of infection and damage and about when to seek assistance from healthcare providers for skin trauma and problems.

RISK FACTORS

- Aging results in thinning and graying of the hair and decreasing amounts of body hair. Aging skin repairs more slowly, sweat gland activity decreases, and the nails become thicker and ridged in aging.

CLIENT EDUCATION

- Teach all clients that nail care includes cleaning and drying the nails to prevent infectious material from collecting under the nails.
- Inform clients that unusual markings in the nails or change in the color or texture of the nails may indicate localized or systemic problems requiring healthcare.
- Tell older adults that they may require the use of lotions to maintain moisture and should limit the use of soaps to prevent increased dryness of the skin.
- Encourage older adults to "accident proof" their environments. Falls, slips, and bumps often result in tearing or injury to the increasingly fragile skin.

CULTURAL CONSIDERATIONS

RISK FACTORS

- African American males are prone to develop folliculitis.
- African Americans are more likely to have dry scalps and dry, fragile hair.

CLIENT EDUCATION

- Teach all clients how to examine their skin (see Box 11.2).
- Provide African American women with information about the risks associated with chemical treatments, excessive combing, and pulling to braid fragile hair.

ENVIRONMENTAL CONSIDERATIONS

RISK FACTORS

- Medication, both topical and ingested, can cause skin irritation or problems as a result of sensitivity or allergy and can exacerbate existing skin problems.

- Clients with diabetes, liver disease, or circulatory disease are at increased risk for problems with the skin and with healing of existing skin problems.
- Genetic predisposition and moles increase the risk of developing skin cancer.
- Sun exposure, particularly with repeated sunburn, increases the risk of skin cancer.

- Exposure to chemicals, allergens, and pollutants in the home, workplace, and environment can cause skin damage.

CLIENT EDUCATION

- Provide information about medications that may affect the skin, including side effects that may appear as skin changes. Further, information about when to seek assistance in the event of unexpected reactions to medications is essential.
  Instruct clients about exercise and its importance in skin maintenance across the age span and that the diet should include protein, fats, and vitamins to promote healthy skin, hair, and nails.
- Provide clients who have existing health problems such as diabetes with information about examination of and preventive care of the skin.
- Teach clients to monitor moles for changes in color, size, or texture.
- Tell clients that limiting sun exposure and using sunblock are important ways to decrease skin damage and reduce the risk of skin cancer.
  Teach all clients the steps for self-examination of the skin (Box 11.2).
- Provide information about the use of protective clothing, gloves, and other equipment to reduce exposure to risks associated with chemicals, pollutants, and irritants in the home and environment.

Box 11.2	Self-Examination of the Skin

1. Use a room that is well lit and has a full-length mirror. Have a handheld mirror and chair available. Remove all of your clothes.
2. Examine all of your skin surface, front and back. Begin with your hands, including the spaces between your fingers. Continue with your arms, chest, abdomen, pubic area, thighs, lower legs, and toes. Next examine your face and neck. Make sure you inspect your underarms, the sides of your trunk, the back of your neck, the buttocks, and the soles of your feet.

3. Next, sit down with one leg elevated. Use the handheld mirror to examine the inside of the elevated leg, from the groin area to the foot. Repeat on the other leg.
4. Use the handheld mirror to inspect your scalp.
5. Consult your physician promptly if you see any newly pigmented area or if any existing mole has changed in color, size, shape, or elevation. Also report sores that do not heal; redness or swelling around a growth or lesion; a change in sensation such as itching, pain, tenderness, or numbness in a lesion or the skin around it; and a change in the texture or consistency of the skin.

BEHAVIORAL CONSIDERATIONS

RISK FACTORS

- Hygiene and grooming practices influence the condition of the skin, hair, and nails.
- Proper nutrition and fluid intake influence the condition of the skin across the age span.
- Regular exercise and mobility are essential to promoting circulation to the skin and preventing problems of immobility.
- Tattooing and body piercing may be culturally based and are increasing in adolescents and young adults in the American culture, increasing risk for skin and systemic infection.

CLIENT EDUCATION

- Tell clients that hygiene, including regular bathing in adolescence and young adulthood, reduces risks of infection and decreases body odor.
- Provide individuals, adolescents, and parents with information about the risks associated with tattooing and body piercing including infection, scarring, and exposure to hepatitis C and HIV.
- Educate clients and their families about immediate and follow-up care of tattooed or pierced skin to prevent future problems.

Application Through Critical Thinking

CASE STUDY

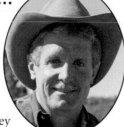

*M*r. Shelley is a 54-year-old grounds-keeper for a large corporation in the Southwest. Today, he visited the company's health and wellness office saying, "My wife told me to have someone check my leathery skin."

Julieta Caredenas, RN, asked Mr. Shelley how much time he spends outdoors. He revealed that he is outside from about 8:00 a.m. until 4:00 p.m. each day, except for his lunch break, which he usually takes in the cafeteria. He reported that he does not use sunscreen. In the summertime, he works in a short-sleeved shirt, shorts, and a hat. He doesn't recall ever having had a bad sunburn. He stated that he has a mole on his left thigh that has been present since birth, but to his knowledge it has not changed. He is not aware of any other birthmarks or skin lesions. He has never performed a skin self-assessment. He reported no family history of skin cancer. He stated that he never sunbathes or swims, and that he plays outdoor sports only at the annual family picnic. He showers each day before going home and uses deodorant soap. He admitted that his skin is often quite dry but said he feels that sunscreens and lotions "are for women."

The nursing assessment of Mr. Shelley's skin revealed the following data: His skin was clean. It was a ruddy brown color where frequently exposed to the sun and a pinkish tan elsewhere. His temperature was warm bilaterally, and he had a mild sheen of perspiration on his face, neck, and upper trunk. Where exposed to the sun, his skin was thick with decreased elasticity. There were no unexpected visible blood vessels or vascular lesions. There was a mole approximately 2 cm by 2 cm on the anterior surface of his left thigh. No drainage was noted. Mr. Shelley's scalp and hair appeared dry but clean and free of

lesions. Soil was embedded beneath the free edge of his nails. He stated that he had been transplanting cuttings.

▶ Complete Documentation

The following information is summarized from the case study. **SUBJECTIVE DATA:** Seeks checkup for "leathery skin." Works as groundskeeper. Outdoors 7 hours a day. No sunscreen, protective clothing. No recall of sunburn. Mole left thigh since birth, reports unchanged. No other lesions. No self-skin assessment. No family history of skin cancer. Denies sunbathing or swimming. Occasional outdoor baseball. Showers daily with deodorant soap. Feels skin is "dry." "Sunscreens and lotions are for women."

OBJECTIVE DATA: Skin clean, ruddy brown where exposed, pinkish tan in unexposed areas. Temperature warm, bilaterally, mild perspiration face, neck, upper trunk. Exposed skin thick, decreased elasticity. No unexpected vessels, vascular lesions. Mole 2 cm × 2 cm anterior (L) thigh, no drainage. Scalp and hair, no lesions. Nails, soil embedded beneath free edge.

A sample assessment form appears on page 232.

▶ Critical Thinking Questions

1. Describe the findings from the case study.
2. Identify the findings as normal or abnormal.
3. Determine the categories that emerge from clustering of the data.
4. Analyze the categories to identify the physical and psychosocial nursing care priorities for Mr. Shelley.

▶ Applying Nursing Diagnoses

1. The NANDA taxonomy includes the nursing diagnosis *risk for impaired skin integrity*. Do the data support this diagnosis? If so, identify the data.

2. Use the NANDA taxonomy (see Appendix A ∞) to formulate additional diagnoses for Mr. Shelley. For each diagnosis identify the following:
   a. Type of diagnosis
   b. Defining characteristics
   c. Risks or related factors

►Prepare Teaching Plan:

LEARNING NEED: The data from the case study reveal that Mr. Shelley is concerned about his "leathery skin." His skin condition is associated with unprotected skin exposure to the sun for long periods of the daytime. Mr. Shelley is at risk for skin cancer.

The case study provides data that is representative of risks, symptoms, and behaviors of many individuals. Therefore, the following teaching plan is based on the need to provide information to members of any community about skin cancer.

GOAL: The participants in this learning program will have increased awareness of risk factors and strategies to prevent skin cancer.

OBJECTIVES: At the completion of this learning session, the learner will be able to:

1. Identify risk factors associated with skin cancer.
2. List the symptoms of skin cancer.
3. Describe the types of skin cancer.
4. Discuss strategies to prevent skin cancer.

Following is an example of the teaching plan for Objective 1. After reviewing this sample teaching plan for Objective 1, go to the Companion Website for this text to complete the teaching plan for the other objectives.

ASSESSMENT FORM

HISTORY

Problems

Skin: *No family history, mole left thigh (unchanged) skin dry*

Hair: *N/A*

Nails: *N/A*

Hygiene: *Shower daily–deodorant soap*

Environment: *Works outdoors 7 hrs./day. No sunscreeen or protective clothing*

PHYSICAL FINDINGS

Skin

Color: *Ruddy brown where exposed, pinkish tan in unexposed areas*

Turgor: *Decreased in exposed areas*

Moisture: *Perspiration face, neck, and upper trunk*

Temperature: *Warm*

Odors: *None*

Lesions: *2 cm X 2 cm mole anterior (L) thigh, no drainage*

Hair

Distribution:

Texture:

Hygiene: *Dry scalp, no lesions*

Nails

Contour:

Nail bed:

Hygiene: *Soil under free edge*

APPLICATION OF OBJECTIVE I: Identify risk factors associated with skin cancer

Content	Teaching Strategy	Evaluation
• *Moles.* Usually harmless pigmented growth. Multiple moles or large moles indicate risk. • *Fair complexion.* Skin cancer risk is higher in those with fair skin, freckles, blue eyes, and blond hair. • *Family history of skin cancer.* • *Too much time in the sun or tanning booth.* Severe sunburn as child or teen. • *Age.* Half of skin cancer occurs after age 50.	• Lecture • Discussion • Audiovisual materials • Printed materials Lecture is appropriate when disseminating information to large groups. Discussion allows participants to bring up concerns and to raise questions. Audiovisual materials such as illustrations of the moles reinforce verbal presentation. Printed material, especially to be taken away with learners, allows review, reinforcement, and reading at the learner's pace.	• Written examination. May use short answer, fill-in, or multiple-choice items, or a combination of items. If these are short and easy to evaluate, the learner receives immediate feedback.

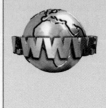

Please refer to the Companion Website at www.prenhall.com/damico and click on Chapter 11, the Application Through Critical Thinking module, to complete the following activities related to this case study:
► **Critical Thinking questions**
► **Extended Nursing Diagnosis challenge**
► **Documentation activity**
► **Teaching Plan for Objectives 2, 3, and 4**

EXPLORE MediaLink

Additional resources for this chapter are found on the Student CD-ROM accompanying this textbook and on the Companion Website.

CD-ROM MEDIA CONTENT

Content for this chapter includes:
Objectives
Key Concepts
NCLEX-RN® Review Questions
Model Documentation Forms
Audio Glossary
Animations
   Skin Wound Repair
   Pressure Ulcer Development
Games and Challenges
Clinical Spotlight Videos
   Eczema
   Skin Cancer
   Decubitus
Head-to-Toe Physical Examination Video

COMPANION WEBSITE CONTENT

www.prenhall.com/damico

Content for this chapter includes:
Objectives
NCLEX-RN® Review Questions

Client Interaction Case Study Challenge
Application Through Critical Thinking
   Case Study Teaching Plan Challenge
MediaLinks
MediaLink Application
Tool Box
   Chapter Documentation Form Example
   Color Variations in Light and Dark Skin
   Self-Examination of the Skin
   Health Promotion
      Healthy People 2010
      Client Education
New York Times

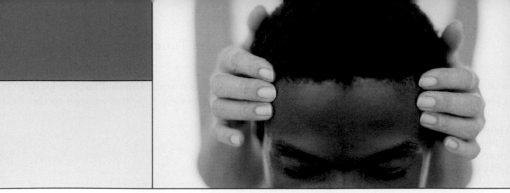

12

Head, Neck, and Related Lymphatics

CHAPTER OBJECTIVES

Upon completion of this chapter, you will be able to:

1. Identify the anatomy and physiology of the structures of the head and neck.

2. Develop questions to be used when completing the focused interview.

3. Describe the techniques required for assessment of the head and neck.

4. Differentiate normal from abnormal findings in physical assessment of the head, neck, and related structures.

5. Describe developmental, psychosocial, cultural, and environmental variations in assessment techniques and findings.

6. Discuss the focus areas related to the overall health of the head, neck, and related lymphatics as presented in *Healthy People 2010*.

7. Apply critical thinking in selected simulations related to physical assessment of the head, neck, and related structures.

MEDIALINK

www.prenhall.com/damico

The CD-ROM in the back of this textbook and the Media-Link website contain NCLEX-RN® review questions, interactive exercises, case study challenges, animations, videos, documentation and checklist forms, and review materials. For a complete listing of the media content specific to Chapter 12, see the Explore MediaLink at the end of the chapter.

he head and neck region is in many ways the most important region in the body. Several systems are integrated in the head and neck. For example, the musculoskeletal system permits movement of the neck and face, while the bones protect the brain, spinal cord, and eyes.

Several body systems overlap in the head and neck region. The nurse will be assessing several systems at the same time. For instance, the integumentary system provides covering and protection. Food is taken in through the mouth, which is the beginning of the gastrointestinal system. Air enters the lungs through the nose, mouth, and trachea, which make up the upper respiratory system. The cardiovascular system carries oxygen and other nutrients to the region and transports wastes. The nurse must consider this close interrelationship of systems when assessing the client's head and neck, where clues to the client's nutritional status, airway clearance, tissue perfusion, metabolism, level of activity, sleep and rest, level of stress, and self-care ability may be apparent.

When performing an assessment of the head and neck, one must be aware of psychosocial factors, such as stress and anxiety, that can influence the health of this body area. It is also important for the nurse to consider the client's self-care practices. Many clients spend a great deal of time caring for this area of the body, and alterations in health may affect their ability to provide this care. A client's ancestry, cultural practices, socioeconomic status, and physical environment both at home and at work can greatly influence the health of the head and neck, and are an integral part of the assessment data. Additionally, a client's developmental stage has a tremendous influence on the appearance and functioning of the region. A focus area described in *Healthy People 2010* is the prevention of injury and violence. The goal is to reduce the number of injuries, disabilities, and deaths from a multitude of causes including head injuries as described in the *Healthy People 2010* feature on page 259.

ANATOMY AND PHYSIOLOGY REVIEW

The structures of the head include the skull and facial bones. The vertebrae, hyoid bone, cartilage, muscles, thyroid gland, and major blood vessels are found within the neck. A large supply of lymph nodes is located in the head and neck region. Each of these structures is described in the following paragraphs.

HEAD

The skull is a protective shell made up of the bones of the cranium (see Figure 12.1 ●) and face. The major bones of the cranium are the frontal, parietal, temporal, and occipital bones. These bones are connected to each other by means of **sutures,** or nonmovable joints. The solidification process of the sutures is completed by the second year of life. The primary function of the skull is to protect the brain. The bones of the skull are covered by muscles and skin, which is commonly called the scalp. The bones provide landmarks for assessment. Fourteen bones form the anterior region of the skull, commonly called the face. These bones are the frontal, maxillae, zygomatic, nasal, ethmoid, lacrimal, sphenoid, and mandible. The intricate fusion of these bones provides structure for the face, and cavities for the eyes, nose, and mouth. It also allows movement of the mandible at the temporomandibular joint (TMJ). The TMJ is located anterior to the tragus of the ear and allows a person to open and close the mouth, protract and retract the chin, and slide the lower jaw from side to side. These actions are used for chewing and speaking.

The skin, muscles, and bones of the face provide landmarks for assessment, as do the bones of the skull. The eyebrows, appendages of the skin, are over the supraorbital margins of the skull. The lateral canthus of the eye forms a straight line with the pinna, and the nasolabial folds are equal (see Figure 12.2 ●).

KEY TERMS

acromegaly, 255
anterior triangle, 237
atlas, 236
axis, 236
Bell's palsy, 255
craniosynostosis, 254
Cushing's syndrome, 255
Down syndrome, 256
goiter, 241
hydrocephalus, 254
hyoid, 237
hyperthyroidism, 250
hypothyroidism, 258
lymphadenopathy, 252
posterior triangle, 237
sutures, 235
thyroid gland, 237
torticollis, 257

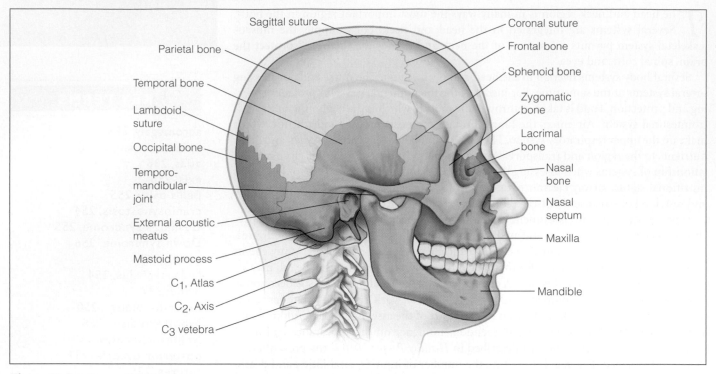

Figure 12.1 • Bones of the head.

Figure 12.3 • identifies the main muscles of the scalp, face, and neck. These muscles play a major role in expressing emotions through facial expressions. They also contribute to movement of the head and neck. Details regarding movement of the structures of the head and neck are discussed in Chapter 23 of this text. ⊙ Cranial nerve innervation of muscles, senses, and balance are discussed in detail in Chapter 24 of this text. ⊙

NECK

The neck is formed by the seven cervical vertebrae, ligaments, and muscles, which support the cranium. The first cervical vertebra (C_1), commonly called the **atlas,** carries the skull. The second cervical vertebra (C_2), commonly called the **axis,** allows for movement of the head (see Figure 12.1). The greatest mobility is at the level of C_4, C_5, and C_6. The seventh cervical vertebra (vertebra prominens) has the largest spinous process.

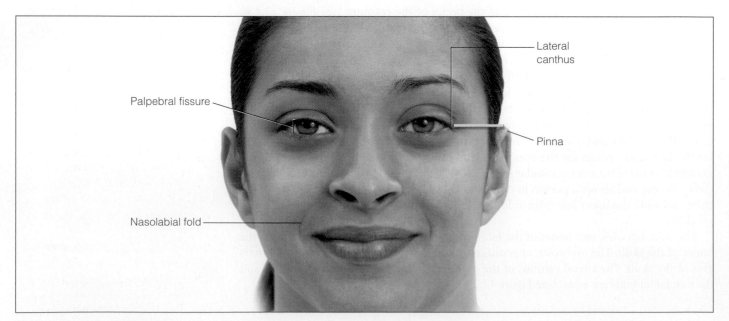

Figure 12.2 • Facial landmarks.

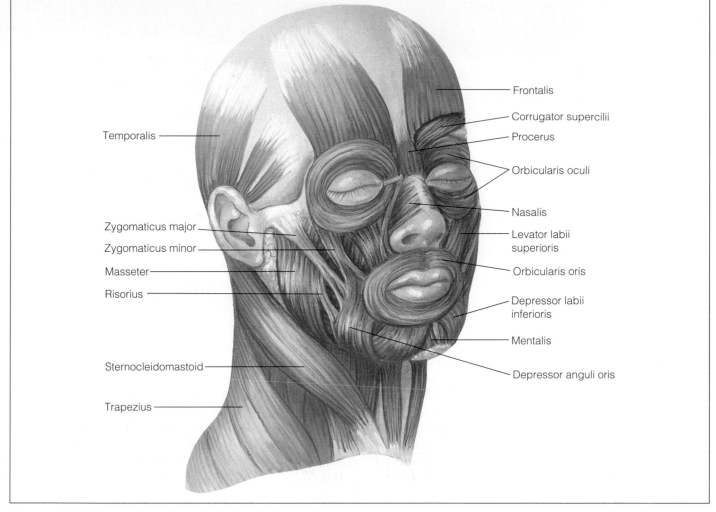

Temporalis

Zygomaticus major
Zygomaticus minor
Masseter
Risorius

Sternocleidomastoid

Trapezius

Frontalis
Corrugator supercilii
Procerus
Orbicularis oculi
Nasalis
Levator labii
superioris
Orbicularis oris
Depressor labii
inferioris
Mentalis
Depressor anguli oris

Figure 12.3 ● Muscles of the head and neck.

This vertebral process is visible and easily palpated, making it a definite landmark during client assessment.

The sternocleidomastoid and trapezius muscles are the primary muscles of the neck. The sternocleidomastoid muscles, innervated by cranial nerve XI, originate at the manubrium of the sternum and the medial portion of the clavicles. The insertion of this muscle is at the mastoid process of the temporal bones.

Each trapezius muscle, also innervated by cranial nerve XI, originates on the occipital bone of the skull and spine of several vertebrae. The insertion of these muscles is on the scapulae and lateral third of the clavicles.

These two muscle groups form the anterior and posterior triangles of the neck. The mandible, the midline of the neck, and the anterior aspect of the sternocleidomastoid muscles border the **anterior triangle.** The trapezius muscle, the sternocleidomastoid muscle, and the clavicle form the **posterior triangle** (see Figure 12.4 ●).

The hyoid bone is suspended in the neck (see Figure 12.5 ●) approximately 2 cm (1 in.) above the larynx. The **hyoid** is the only bone in the body that does not articulate directly with another bone. The base of the tongue rests on the curved body of

this bone. The curved shape of the bone produces a horn at each end that is palpable just inferior to the angle of the jaw. This serves as a landmark for assessing structures of the neck, especially the trachea and thyroid gland.

The thyroid cartilage is the largest cartilage of the larynx and is formed by the joining of two pieces of cartilage. This fusion forms a ridge called the Adam's apple. This ridge is significantly larger in males (Figure 12.5). The cricoid cartilage, C-shaped ring, is the first cartilage ring anchored to the trachea. The trachea, commonly called the windpipe, descends from the larynx to the bronchi of the respiratory system. The trachea has slight mobility and flexibility. The C-shaped rings help maintain the shape of the trachea and are palpable superior to the sternum at the midline of the neck (Figure 12.5).

The **thyroid gland,** the largest gland of the endocrine system, is butterfly shaped. It is located in the anterior portion of the neck. The isthmus of the thyroid connects the right and left lobes of the thyroid gland. The thyroid gland lies over the trachea, and the sternocleidomastoid muscles cover the lateral aspects of the lobes (Figure 12.5).

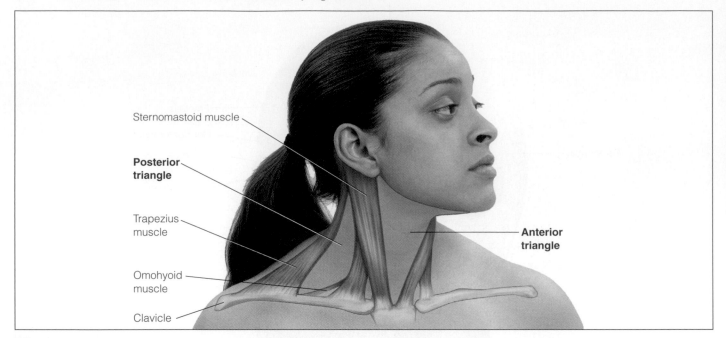

Figure 12.4 ● Triangles of the neck.

The carotid arteries and the jugular veins are located in the neck. The carotid artery is palpated in the groove between the trachea and the sternocleidomastoid muscle below the angle of the jaw. The external and internal jugular veins are also in the neck, in proximity to the common carotid artery. The external jugular veins are more superficial and lateral to the sternocleidomastoid muscle. The internal jugular veins are larger and not visible; however, a reflection of the undulation is seen (see Figure 12.6 ●). These vessels are deep and medial to the muscle. The carotid arteries and jugular veins are discussed in detail in Chapter 17 of this text. ⚭

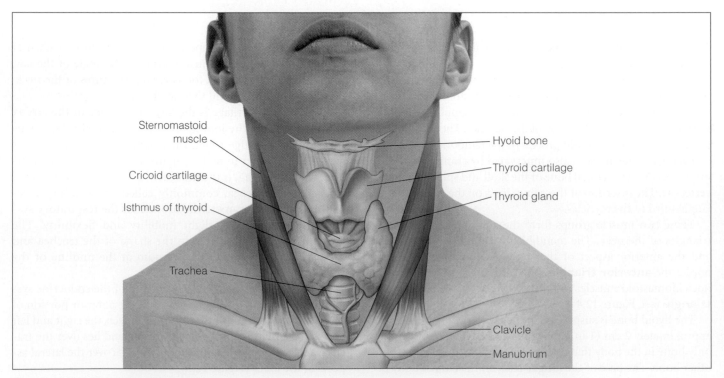

Figure 12.5 ● Structures of the neck.

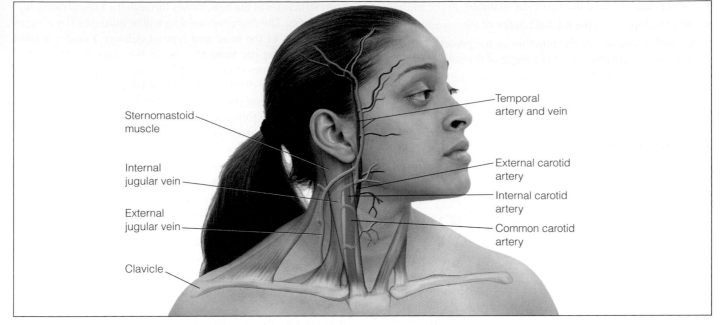

Figure 12.6 ● Vessels of the neck.

Labels on figure:
Sternomastoid muscle
Internal jugular vein
External jugular vein
Clavicle
Temporal artery and vein
External carotid artery
Internal carotid artery
Common carotid artery

LYMPHATICS

A large supply of lymph nodes is located in the head and neck region of the body. These nodes provide defense against invasion of foreign substances by producing lymphocytes and antibodies. The lymph nodes are clustered along lymphatic vessels that infiltrate tissue capillaries and pick up excess fluid called *lymph*. The nurse palpates various areas of the head and neck looking for lymph nodes. Normally, the nodes are nonpalpable. Occasionally, an isolated node is found on palpation. This is usually not considered an abnormal finding. Nodes are palpable when infected or enlarged. This finding may be significant in recognizing signs of early infection. The names of the nodes may vary depending on the author or practitioner; however, they usually correspond to adjacent anatomical structures or locations (see Figure 12.7 ●). The nodes most commonly assessed are the following:

- **Preauricular**—in front of the ear
- **Occipital**—at the base of the skull
- **Postauricular**—behind the ear, over the outer surface of the mastoid bone

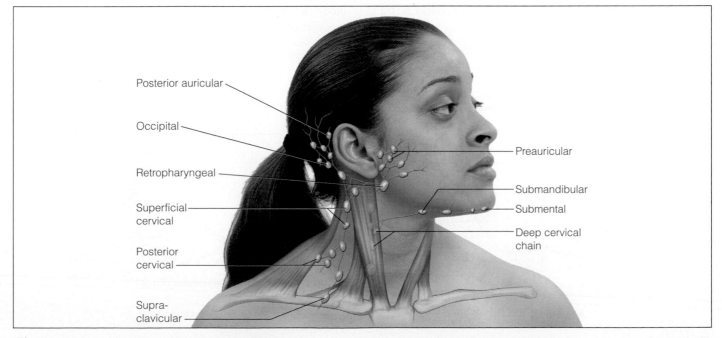

Figure 12.7 ● Lymph nodes of the head and neck.

Labels on figure:
Posterior auricular
Occipital
Retropharyngeal
Superficial cervical
Posterior cervical
Supra-clavicular
Preauricular
Submandibular
Submental
Deep cervical chain

- **Submental**—behind the tip of the mandible at the midline
- **Submaxillary**—on the medial border of the mandible
- **Retropharyngeal**—at the junction of the posterior and lateral walls of the pharynx at the angle of the jaw
- **Superficial cervical**—anterior to and over the sternocleidomastoid muscle
- **Deep cervical**—posterior to and under the sternocleidomastoid muscle
- **Supraclavicular**—above the clavicle

A detailed description of the lymphatic system is provided in Chapter 18 of this text. ⬭

SPECIAL CONSIDERATIONS

Throughout the assessment process, the nurse gathers subjective and objective data reflecting the client's state of health. Using critical thinking and the nursing process, the nurse identifies many factors to be considered when collecting the data. Some of these factors include but are not limited to age, developmental level, race, ethnicity, work history, living conditions, social economics, and emotional well-being.

DEVELOPMENTAL CONSIDERATIONS

Growth and development are dynamic processes that describe change over time. It is important to understand data collection and interpretation of findings regarding growth and development in relation to normative values. The following discussion presents specific variations in the head and neck for different age groups.

Infants and Children

An infant's head should be measured at each visit until 2 years of age. The newborn's head is about 34 cm (13 to 14 in.), and this is generally equal to the chest circumference. The shape of the head may indicate *molding*, the shaping of the head by pressure on the

bony structures as the head moves through the vaginal canal during delivery. The degree of molding will be influenced by the presenting part of the head and type of delivery. Usually, it takes several days for the head to take on the more normal round shape. Suture lines should be open as are the fontanels. The anterior fontanel is diamond shaped, and the posterior fontanel is triangular in shape (see Figure 12.8 ●). The fontanels should be firm and even with the skull. Slight pulsations are normal. The neck of the newborn is short with many skin folds and begins to lengthen over time. By about 4 months of age the infant begins to demonstrate control of the head. In toddlers, the head is relatively large and the muscles of the neck are underdeveloped compared to adults. The proportions change throughout the preschool years, and by school age the proportions are similar to those of adults.

The thyroid gland, located in the neck, plays an important role in growth and development. The thyroid is difficult to palpate on an infant, but it can be accomplished on a child using two or three fingers. Abnormalities in thyroid function are generally detected by assessment of growth and development and through laboratory testing. Further information related to the structures of the head and neck in infants and children is included in Chapter 25 of this text. ⬭

The Pregnant Female

The pregnant female may develop blotchy pigmented spots (melasma) on her face (see Figure 11.6 on page 187 ⬭), facial edema, and enlargement of the thyroid. All of these symptoms are considered normal and subside after childbirth. The pregnant female may also complain of headaches during the first trimester, which may be related to increased hormones; however, severe persistent headaches should be evaluated. Serious headaches, especially in late pregnancy, are associated with preeclampsia. Preeclampsia is a serious pregnancy-induced syndrome of high blood pressure, fluid retention, and protein excretion in the urine. Preeclampsia can result in restricted blood flow to the placenta and harm to the developing fetus.

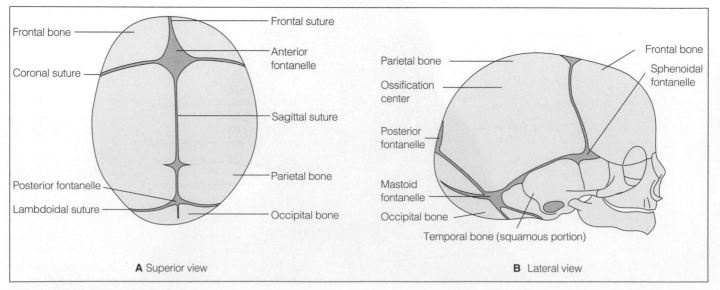

A Superior view

B Lateral view

Figure 12.8 ● The newborn's skull.

Cultural Considerations

- Covering of the hair or face is required in some cultures, such as Muslim and Sikh.
- Hypothyroidism occurs more frequently in Caucasians and Mexican Americans than in African Americans.
- Immigrants from countries in which millet is a staple food are more likely to have goiter.

- Facial malformations may occur in infants with fetal alcohol syndrome. Fetal alcohol syndrome (FAS) occurs more frequently in Native Americans, Alaska Natives, and African Americans than in other cultural groups.

The Older Adult

The older adult loses subcutaneous fat in the face. This increases the wrinkles in the skin, yielding an older appearance. A decrease in reproductive hormones results in the development of coarse, long eyebrows and nasal hair in males and coarse hair, usually on the chin, in females. Loss of teeth and improperly fitting dentures provide a change to facial expressions and symmetry. Rigidity of the cervical vertebrae is common, causing limited range of motion of the neck. The thyroid gland produces fewer hormones with age.

PSYCHOSOCIAL CONSIDERATIONS

A client who is under a great deal of stress may be prone to headaches, including tension headaches, neck pain, and mouth ulcers. Pain in the TMJ may be due to unconscious clenching of the jaw during stressful situations, such as driving in heavy traffic or taking an exam. It may also be caused by nighttime teeth grinding. Chronic TMJ syndrome may eventually result in a wearing down of the teeth, and the client may need to consult a dentist or orthodontist.

Other indications of psychosocial disturbances include tics (involuntary muscle spasms), hair twisting or pulling, lip biting, and excessive blinking. Relaxation techniques such as meditation and guided imagery may help relieve head and neck symptoms related to stress. If appropriate, the nurse should refer the client to a mental health professional for assistance.

CULTURAL AND ENVIRONMENTAL CONSIDERATIONS

Within some cultures, eye contact and smiling are considered rude or aggressive. Furthermore, sharing of personal information with strangers is not permitted. This makes obtaining a detailed health history or conducting a focused interview most difficult. Some cultures and religions such as Muslims and Sikhs require the individual to cover the head or face.

Facial malformations are a frequent occurrence in children with fetal alcohol syndrome (FAS). Some infants have a flat occipital prominence (plagiocephaly), which may result from putting them to sleep on their backs. Placing infants on their backs for sleep has become a common practice to reduce the incidence of sudden infant death syndrome (SIDS). Flattening of the head may also occur when infant boards are used, for example, in Central American cultures.

Thyroid disease is common in areas where iodine is limited. Iodine deficiency disorders including **goiter** (enlarged thyroid) and hypothyroidism are significant health problems in India and China. Iodine deficiencies occur in areas with soil poor in iodine. These areas include eastern Europe, parts of South America, Australia, and the western United States. Use of iodized salt has generally obliterated iodine deficiencies in the United States. The World Health Organization (WHO) is overseeing global programs to increase the use of iodized salt to prevent these deficiencies.

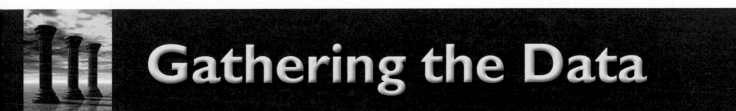

Gathering the Data

*H*ealth assessment of the head and neck includes gathering subjective and objective data. Recall that subjective data collection occurs during the client interview, before the physical assessment, with the collection of the objective data. During the interview, the nurse uses a variety of communication techniques to elicit general and specific information about the structures of the client's head and neck. Health records, the results of laboratory tests, and radiologic and imaging reports are important secondary sources to be reviewed and included in the data-gathering process. During physical assessment of the head and neck, the techniques of inspection, palpation, and auscultation will be used to gather the objective data.

FOCUSED INTERVIEW

The focused interview for the head and neck concerns data related to the head, the face, and structures of the neck including the thyroid, trachea, and lymph nodes. Subjective data is gathered during the focused interview. The nurse must be prepared to observe the client and listen for cues related to the functions of structures within the head and neck. The nurse may use open-ended or closed questions to obtain information. Follow-up questions or requests for descriptions are required to clarify data or gather missing information. Follow-up questions are intended to identify the source of problems, explain the duration of problems, discuss ways to alleviate problems, and provide clues about the client's knowledge about his or her own health. Remember, the subjective data collected and the questions asked during the health history and focused interview will provide information to help meet the goal of safety with reduced injuries and disabilities as described in *Healthy People 2010*.

The focused interview guides the physical assessment of the head and neck. The information is always considered in relation to normative values and expectations regarding function of the specific structure. Therefore, the nurse must consider age, gender, race, culture, environment, health practices, past and concurrent problems, and therapies when framing questions and using techniques to elicit information. In order to address all of the factors when conducting a focused interview, categories of questions related to status and function of the head and neck have been developed. These categories include general questions that are asked of all clients; those addressing acute and chronic illness or infections; questions related to symptoms, pain, or behaviors; those related to habits or practices; questions that are specific to clients according to age; those for pregnant females; and questions that address environmental concerns.

The nurse must consider the client's ability to participate in the focused interview and physical assessment of the head and neck. If a client is experiencing pain, stiffness, or anxiety that accompanies any of these problems, attention must focus on relief of symptoms.

FOCUSED INTERVIEW QUESTIONS

RATIONALES

The following section provides sample questions and follow-up questions in each of the previously mentioned categories. A rationale for each of the questions is provided. The list of questions is not inclusive, but rather represents the types of questions required in a comprehensive focused interview related to the head and neck. The follow-up bulleted questions are asked to seek clarification with additional information from the client to enhance the subjective database. The subjective data collected and the questions asked during the health history and the focused interview will provide data to help meet the goal of preventing head injuries and resulting disabilities.

GENERAL QUESTIONS

1. **Describe the condition of your scalp today.**
   - Is it different from 2 months ago? From 2 years ago?

   ▶ This question gives clients the opportunity to provide their own perceptions about the condition of the scalp.

2. **Do you have any problems that affect your scalp?**

   ▶ This question elicits information about problems or illnesses that may be localized or systemic that impact the scalp. If the client identifies any problems, follow-up is required to obtain descriptions and details about what, when, and how problems occur, and the duration of each problem.

3. **Is there anyone in your family who has had a problem with his or her scalp or a problem that affected his or her scalp?**

   ▶ This question may elicit information about illnesses with a familial or genetic predisposition. Follow-up is required to obtain details about specific problems related to occurrence, treatment, and outcomes.

4. **Questions 1, 2, and 3 would be repeated for the skull, face, trachea, thyroid, and lymph nodes.**

FOCUSED INTERVIEW QUESTIONS	RATIONALES

QUESTIONS RELATED TO ILLNESS, INFECTION, OR INJURY

1. **Have you ever been diagnosed with an illness affecting your head, face, or neck?**
   - When were you diagnosed with the problem?
   - What treatment was prescribed for the problem?
   - What kinds of things do you do to help with the problem?
   - Has the problem ever recurred (acute)?
   - How are you managing the disease now (chronic)?

   ▶ The client has an opportunity to provide information about specific illnesses. If a specific disease or illness is identified, follow-up about the date of diagnosis, treatment, and outcomes is required. Data about each illness identified by the client is essential to an accurate health assessment. Illnesses are classified as acute or chronic, and follow-up regarding each classification will differ.

2. **Do you now have or have you ever had an infection affecting your head, face, or neck?**

   ▶ The client has an opportunity to provide information about infectious processes. Follow-up would be carried out as in question 1.

3. **Have you ever had any problem with your thyroid gland? Have you had thyroid surgery? Are you currently taking thyroid medication?**

   ▶ Over- or undersecretion by the thyroid gland may cause rapid weight gain or loss, erratic temperature regulation, fatigue, dyspnea (painful breathing), mood swings, and other alterations in health.

4. **Describe any recent or past injury to your head.**
   - Did you have any symptoms afterwards? Describe them.
   - How and where were you treated for this injury?
   - How did it occur?
   - Did you lose consciousness?
   - How long were you unconscious?
   - Have problems recurred (acute)?
   - How are you managing the problem now (chronic)?

   ▶ Head injury can result in acute or chronic neurologic problems.

QUESTIONS RELATED TO SYMPTOMS OR BEHAVIORS

When gathering information about symptoms, many questions are required to elicit details and descriptions. Questions are asked in relation to the significance of a symptom, specific diseases or problems, and potential follow-up examination or referral. One rationale may be provided for a group of questions in this category.

QUESTIONS RELATED TO SYMPTOMS

The following questions refer to specific symptoms associated with the head and neck. For each symptom, questions and follow-up are required. The details to be elicited are the characteristics of the symptom; the onset, duration, and frequency of the symptom; the treatment or remedy for the symptom, including over-the-counter and home remedies; the determination if diagnosis has been sought; the effect of treatments; and family history associated with a symptom or illness.

1. **Have you had any dizziness, loss of consciousness, seizures, or blurred vision? When did each symptom occur? How long did the symptom last? What did you do to relieve the symptom? Does the treatment help?**

   ▶ These symptoms may indicate problems with carotid arteries, cerebral clots or bleeding, recent head injury, or neurologic disease.

2. **Have you noticed any swelling, lumps, bumps, or skin sores on your head that did not heal?**

   ▶ Swellings, masses, and lesions that do not heal may indicate cancer.

3. **Have you noticed any lumps or swellings on your neck?**

   ▶ Lateral neck masses are usually due to enlargement of the cervical lymph nodes, indicative of infection or malignancy.

FOCUSED INTERVIEW QUESTIONS	RATIONALES

QUESTIONS RELATED TO PAIN

1. **Do you have headaches? If so, please tell me about them.**
   - **Frequency:** How often?
   - **Onset:** How long have you been bothered with this type of headache? When does the headache begin?
   - **Duration:** How long does a typical headache last?
   - **Location:** Where is the pain? On one side of the head? Behind the eyes? In the sinus area?
   - **Character:** Is the pain throbbing, steady, dull, sharp? On a scale of 1 to 10 with 10 being the strongest, how severe is the pain?
   - **Associated symptoms:** Do you experience any nausea, vomiting, sensitivity to light or noise, muscle pain, or other symptoms along with the headache?
   - **Precipitating factors:** Do you feel that the headaches usually are triggered by stress, alcohol intake, anxiety, menstrual cycle, allergies, or any other factors? Please describe.
   - **Treatment:** What seems to relieve the symptoms? Resting? Medication? Exercise?

2. **Do you experience any problems that precede the headache, such as visual problems?**

3. **Do your headaches occur in episodes? If so, describe the episodes.**
   - Do your headaches increase in severity with each episode?

4. **Have you recently had an infection or cold?**

5. **Has your neck been weak, sore, or stiff?**

▶ Questions 1, 2, and 3 encourage the client to provide a detailed description of the headache necessary to help determine the cause, and possible treatments.

▶ These conditions may be accompanied by headaches.

▶ Neck symptoms may indicate problems with the muscles of the neck or the cervical spinal cord, or an infectious problem such as meningitis.

QUESTIONS RELATED TO BEHAVIORS

1. **Do you now use or have you ever used alcohol, recreational drugs, tobacco products, or caffeine?**
   - How much of the product do you use?
   - When did you start using the product?
   - How long have you used the product?
   - Have you had problems associated with the product?
   - What have you done to deal with the problem?

▶ Use of alcohol, tobacco, street drugs, and large amounts of caffeine can affect neurologic function and increase headaches.

QUESTIONS RELATED TO AGE

The focused interview must reflect the anatomical and physiological differences that exist along the age span. The following questions are examples of those that would be specific for infants and children, the pregnant female, and the older adult.

QUESTIONS REGARDING INFANTS AND CHILDREN

1. **Did you use alcohol or recreational drugs during your pregnancy?**

2. **Have you noticed any depression or bulging over the infant's "soft spots" (fontanels)?**

▶ Fetal alcohol syndrome causes some deformities of the face. Use of cocaine during pregnancy can result in neurologic problems in the infant.

▶ A depressed fontanel can indicate dehydration, and a bulging fontanel can indicate an infection.

FOCUSED INTERVIEW QUESTIONS	RATIONALES

QUESTIONS FOR THE PREGNANT FEMALE

1. Do you have frequent headaches?

▶ Headaches are common during the first trimester, but it is important to rule out other possible complications of pregnancy such as preeclampsia.

2. Have you noticed changes in the skin on your face? If yes, what changes have occurred?

▶ Increasing hormonal changes can result in melasma or chloasma, pigmented areas on the face. In addition the hormonal changes cause increased secretions of oils in the skin, which may result in acne.

3. Do you have a history of thyroid disease? If yes, what is the disease and treatment?

▶ Thyroid diseases can result in problems with the developing fetus. Existing thyroid problems require careful monitoring of medications.

QUESTIONS FOR THE OLDER ADULT

1. Do you carry out safety precautions in your home? When driving or away from home?

▶ Safety precautions can reduce the risk for falls and injuries to the head and neck. Older adults are at increased risk for falls.

QUESTIONS RELATED TO THE ENVIRONMENT

Environment refers to both the internal and external environments. Questions related to the internal environment include all of the previous questions and those associated with internal or physiological responses. Questions regarding the external environment include those related to home, work, or social environments.

INTERNAL ENVIRONMENT

1. Are you now experiencing or have you ever had an experience of intermittent or prolonged anxiety or emotional upset?

▶ Anxiety and situations of emotional upset impact the sympathetic nervous system, producing hormonal responses that affect vascular function. The vasoconstriction can contribute to headache, hypertension, and risk for neurologic problems. Stress and tension precipitate and increase neck pain or stiffness.

2. Do you now use or have you used prescribed or over-the-counter (OTC) medications, home remedies, cultural treatments, or therapies for problems with your head and neck or for any other purpose?

▶ Medications can have side effects and interactions that exacerbate or enhance symptoms. Knowledge of medication usage provides information that assists in analysis of client situations and determination of the significance of findings in a comprehensive assessment.

EXTERNAL ENVIRONMENT

The following questions deal with substances and irritants found in the physical environment of the client. These include the indoor and outdoor environments of the home and the workplace, and those encountered during travel.

1. Have you ever had irradiation of the head or neck?

▶ Radiation exposure increases the risk for thyroid tumors.

2. Are you exposed to chemicals or toxins in your home or work environment?

▶ Environmental chemicals and toxins can be precipitating factors for headache and neurologic problems.

CLIENT INTERACTION

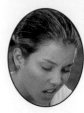

Ms. Dowd, a 20-year-old college sophomore, reports to the university health office with a "very bad headache." Following is part of the focused interview taken by the nurse.

INTERVIEW

Nurse: Ms. Dorothy Dowd, you have already told me you have a headache, and I would like to know more about it. On a scale of 1 to 10 with 10 being the worst pain, please rate your headache.

Ms. Dowd: Right now my headache is an 8.

Nurse: During the interview, should you need to stop, close your eyes, and relax for a few minutes, let me know.

Ms. Dowd: Okay, but I should be all right.

Nurse: Tell me about your headaches.

Ms. Dowd: I have had this for 2 to 3 weeks, on and off. Now it feels like it is all the time, but it is not always 8. Sometimes it is 5.

Nurse: Using one or two words, can you describe the pain?

Ms. Dowd: It is usually a dull, constant ache.

Nurse: Describe the location of this dull ache in your head.

Ms. Dowd: It always seems to start at the top of my neck. As it gets worse, it moves up to the top of my head.

Nurse: Are you talking about the right or left side?

Ms. Dowd: Right now it is both sides. That's why I'm here. I can't stand it anymore. Sometimes it's only one side. Sometimes it stays low (pointing to the occipital region) and doesn't come high.

Nurse: Have you always had headaches?

Ms. Dowd: I would have an occasional headache. Sometimes a day or two before my period and then it would go away. Nothing like this though.

Nurse: What do you think is causing your headaches?

Ms. Dowd: I don't know. I have not been sleeping very well lately. I'm worried about this one course. I can't seem to "get it" and I'm afraid it will kill my GPA. If that happens I will lose my scholarship. I'm working so hard in this course that some of my other work is beginning to slide.

ANALYSIS

The nurse begins the interview with confirmation of the reason for seeking help and then asks the client to confirm the severity of the pain. The nurse acknowledges Ms. Dowd's pain before seeking more specific subjective data from the client. Using an open-ended approach encourages Ms. Dowd to communicate more openly.

Please refer to the Companion Website at **www.prenhall.com/damico** and click on Chapter 12, the **Client Interaction** module, to answer questions about this case. In addition, see other resources for this chapter including NCLEX review questions and other interactive exercises and materials.

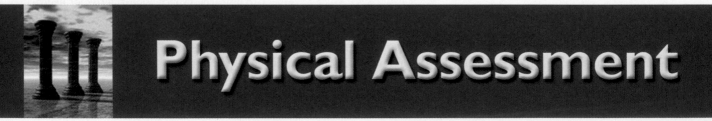

Physical Assessment

ASSESSMENT TECHNIQUES AND FINDINGS

Physical assessment of the head and neck requires the use of inspection, palpation, and auscultation. During each of the procedures, the nurse is gathering objective data related to the structures of the head and neck, and the functions of the structures within them. Inspection includes looking at skin color, the scalp, the skull, and the face for symmetry of bones and structure. The trachea is palpated for position. The thyroid is palpated for movement, texture, and identification of size or abnormalities. The lymph nodes of the head and neck are palpated. The temporal artery is auscultated. Knowledge of normal

parameters and expected findings is essential to interpreting data as the nurse performs the assessment.

In adults, the skull should be normocephalic, that is, a rounded and symmetrical shape. The frontal parietal and occipital prominences are present and symmetrical. The scalp is clear and free of lesions; the hair is evenly distributed. The face is symmetrical in shape; the eyes, ears, nose, and mouth are symmetrically placed. The facial movements are smooth, are coordinated, and demonstrate a variety of expressions. The temporal artery feels smooth and firm with no tenderness to palpation and without bruits. The TMJ has nonpainful, full, and smooth range of motion. The head is held erect without tremors. The neck is symmetrical without swelling and has full range of motion. Carotid artery pulsation is visible bilaterally. The trachea is midline, and the hyoid bone and tracheal cartilage move with swallowing. The thyroid is not enlarged and is without palpable nodules. The lymph nodes of the head and neck are non-palpable in adults.

EQUIPMENT

examination gown	glass of water
clean, nonsterile	stethoscope
examination gloves	

HELPFUL HINTS

- Explain what is expected of the client for each step of the assessment.
- Tell the client the purpose of each procedure and when and if discomfort will accompany any examination.
- Identify and remedy language or cultural barriers at the outset of the client interaction.
- Explain to the client the need to remove any items that would interfere with the assessment, including jewelry, hats, scarves, veils, hairpieces, and wigs.
- Use Standard Precautions.

TECHNIQUES AND NORMAL FINDINGS	ABNORMAL FINDINGS SPECIAL CONSIDERATIONS

THE HEAD

1. Position the client.

- Ask the client to sit comfortably on the examination table (see Figure 12.9 ●).

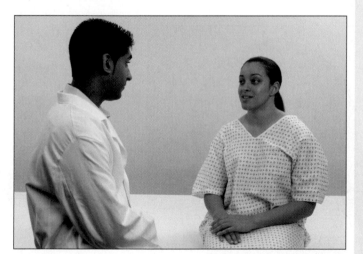

Figure 12.9 ●
Client is positioned.

2. Instruct the client.

- Explain that you will be looking at the client and touching the head, hair, and face. Explain that no discomfort should occur, but if the client experiences pain or discomfort you will stop that part of the examination.

3. Inspect the head and scalp.

- Note size, shape, symmetry, and integrity of the head and scalp. Identify the prominences—frontal, parietal, and occipital—that determine the shape and symmetry of the head.
- Part the hair and look for scaliness of the scalp, lesions, or foreign bodies. (Refer to Figure 11.22 on page 206. ∞)
- Check hair distribution and hygiene.

TECHNIQUES AND NORMAL FINDINGS	ABNORMAL FINDINGS SPECIAL CONSIDERATIONS

4. Inspect the face.

- Note the facial expression and symmetry of structures. The eyes, ears, nose, and mouth should be symmetrically placed. The nasolabial folds should be equal. The palpebral fissures should be equal. The top of the ear should be equal to the canthi of the eyes (see Figure 12.2 on page 236).

5. Observe movements of the head, face, and eyes.

- All movements should be smooth and with purpose. Cranial nerves III, IV, and VI control movement of the eye. Cranial nerve V stimulates movement for mastication. Cranial nerve VII controls movement of the face. A detailed discussion of the cranial nerves is found in Chapter 24. ∞

▶ Jerky movements or tics may be the result of neurologic or psychological disorders.

6. Palpate the head and scalp.

- Note contour, size, and texture. Ask the client to report any tenderness as you palpate. Normally there is no tenderness with palpation.

▶ Note any tenderness, swelling, edema, or masses, which require further evaluation.

7. Confirm skin and tissue integrity.

- The skin should be intact.

▶ Note any alteration in skin or tissue integrity related to ulcerations, rashes, discolorations, or swellings.

8. Palpate the temporal artery.

- Palpate between the eye and the top of the ear (see Figure 12.10 ●). The artery should feel smooth.

▶ Any thickening or tenderness could indicate inflammation of the artery.

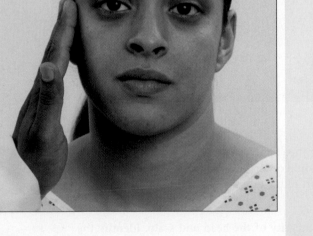

Figure 12.10 ●
Palpating the temporal artery.

9. Auscultate the temporal artery.

- Use the bell of the stethoscope to auscultate for a bruit (a soft blowing sound). Bruits are not normally present.

▶ A bruit is indicative of stenosis (narrowing) of the vessel.

TECHNIQUES AND NORMAL FINDINGS	ABNORMAL FINDINGS SPECIAL CONSIDERATIONS

10. Test the range of motion of the TMJ.

- Place your fingers in front of each ear and ask the client to open and close the mouth slowly. There should be no limitation of movement or tenderness. You should feel a slight indentation of the joint. (For more detail on assessment of the TMJ, see Chapter 23 ⊙⊙).

  Soft clicking noises on movement are sometimes heard and are considered normal.

▶ Any limitation of movement or tenderness on movement requires further evaluation.

▶ Crepitation, a crackling sound on movement, may indicate joint problems.

THE NECK

1. Instruct the client.

- Explain that you will be looking at and touching the front and sides of the client's neck. Tell the client that you will provide specific instructions for special tests. Advise the client to inform you of any discomfort.

2. Inspect the neck for skin color, integrity, shape, and symmetry.

- Observe for any swelling of the lymph nodes below the angle of the jaw and along the sternocleidomastoid muscle.
- The head should be held erect with no tremors.

▶ Excessive rigidity of the neck may indicate arthritis. Inability to hold the neck erect may be due to muscle spasms. Swelling of the lymph nodes may indicate infection and requires further assessment.

3. Test range of motion of the neck.

- Ask the client to slowly move the chin to the chest, turn the head right and left, then touch the left ear to left shoulder and the right ear to right shoulder (without raising the shoulders). Then ask the client to extend the head back.

  There should be no pain and no limitation of movement (for further discussion, see Chapter 23 ⊙⊙).

▶ Any pain or limitation of movement could indicate arthritis, muscle spasm, or inflammation. Rapid movement and compression of cerebral vertebrae may cause dizziness.

4. Observe the carotid arteries and jugular veins.

- The carotid artery runs just below the angle of the jaw, and its pulsations can frequently be seen. Assessment of the carotid arteries and jugular veins is discussed fully in Chapter 18. ⊙⊙

▶ Any distention or prominence may indicate a vascular disorder.

5. Palpate the trachea.

- Palpate the sternal notch. Move the finger pad of the palpating finger off the notch to the midline of the neck. Lightly palpate the area. You will feel the C rings (cricoid cartilage) of the trachea.

  Move the finger laterally, first to the right and then to the left. You have now identified the lateral borders of the trachea (see Figure 12.11 ●).
- The trachea should be midline, and the distance to the sternocleidomastoid muscles on each side should be equal. Place the thumb and index finger on each side of the trachea and slide them upward. As the trachea begins to widen, you have now identified the thyroid cartilage. Continue to slide your thumb and index finger high into the neck. Palpate the hyoid bone. The greater horns of the hyoid bone are most prominent. Confirm that the hyoid bone and tracheal cartilages move when the client swallows.

▶ Tracheal displacement is the result of masses in the neck or mediastinum, pneumothorax, or fibrosis.

TECHNIQUES AND NORMAL FINDINGS	ABNORMAL FINDINGS SPECIAL CONSIDERATIONS

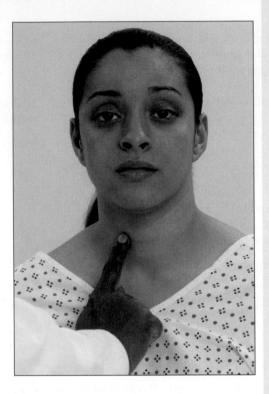

Figure 12.11 ●
Palpating the trachea.

6. Inspect the thyroid gland.

- The thyroid is not observable normally until the client swallows. Give the client a cup of water.

- Distinguish the thyroid from other structures in the neck by asking the client to drink a sip of water.

- The thyroid tissue is attached to the trachea, and, as the client swallows, it moves superiorly. You may want to adjust the lighting in the room if possible so that shadows are cast on the client's neck. This may help you to visualize the thyroid.

▶ If the client has any enlargement of the thyroid or masses near the thyroid, they appear as bulges when the client swallows.

7. Palpate the thyroid gland from behind the client.

- Normally, the thyroid gland is nonpalpable, and so you need to be patient as you learn this technique.

- Stand behind the client.

- Ask the client to sit up straight, lower the chin, and turn the head slightly to the right.

- This position causes the client's neck muscles to relax.

- Using the fingers of your left hand, push the trachea to the right. Use light pressure during palpation, to avoid obliterating findings.

- With the fingers of the right hand, palpate the area between the trachea and the sternocleidomastoid muscle. Slowly and gently retract the sternocleidomastoid muscle, then ask the client to drink a sip of water. Palpate as the thyroid gland moves up during swallowing (see Figure 12.12 ●). Normally, you will not feel the thyroid gland, although in some clients with long, thin necks, you may be able to feel the isthmus. Reverse the procedure for the left side.

▶ An enlarged thyroid gland may be due to a metabolic disorder such as **hyperthyroidism.** Palpable masses of 5 mm or larger are alterations in health. Their location, size, and shape should be documented, and the client should be evaluated further. In pregnancy, a slightly enlarged thyroid can be a normal finding. Most pathologic hyperthyroidism in pregnancy is caused by Graves' disease, an autoimmune disorder that causes increased production of thyroid hormones.

TECHNIQUES AND NORMAL FINDINGS	ABNORMAL FINDINGS SPECIAL CONSIDERATIONS

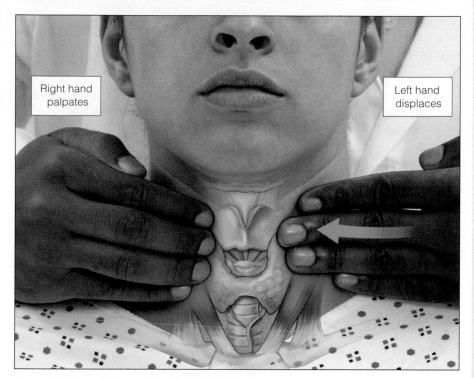

Figure 12.12 ● Palpating the thyroid using a posterior approach.

8. Palpate the thyroid gland from in front of the client.

- This is an alternative approach. Stand in front of the client. Ask the client to lower the head and turn slightly to the right. Using the thumb of your right hand, push the trachea to the right (see Figure 12.13 ●).

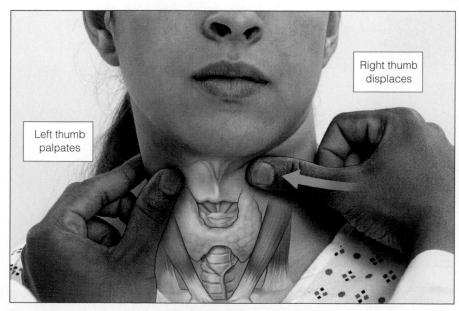

Figure 12.13 ● Alternative technique for palpating the thyroid.

TECHNIQUES AND NORMAL FINDINGS	ABNORMAL FINDINGS SPECIAL CONSIDERATIONS

- Place your left thumb and fingers over the sternocleidomastoid muscle and feel for any enlargement of the right lobe as the client swallows. Have water available to make swallowing easier. Reverse the procedure for the left side.

9. Auscultate the thyroid.

- If the thyroid is enlarged, the area over the thyroid is auscultated to detect any bruits. In an enlarged thyroid, blood flows through the arteries at an accelerated rate, producing a soft, rushing sound. This sound can best be detected with the bell of the stethoscope.

▶ The presence of a bruit is abnormal and is an indication of increased blood flow.

10. Palpate the lymph nodes of the head and neck.

- Palpate the lymph nodes by exerting gentle circular pressure with the finger pads of both hands. It is important to avoid strong pressure, which can push the nodes into the muscle and underlying structures, making them difficult to find. It is also important to establish a routine for examination; otherwise, it is possible to omit one or more of the groups of nodes. The following is one suggested order of examination (see Figure 12.14 ●).

    1. Preauricular
    2. Postauricular
    3. Occipital
    4. Retropharyngeal
    5. Submaxillary
    6. Submental (with one hand)
    7. Superficial cervical chain
    8. Deep cervical chain
    9. Supraclavicular

▶ Enlargement of lymph nodes is called **lymphadenopathy** and can be due to infection, allergies, or a tumor.

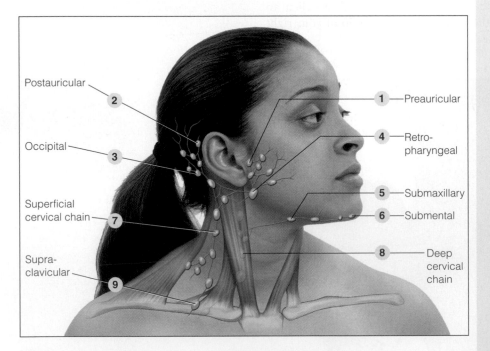

Figure 12.14 ● Suggested sequence for palpating lymph nodes.

TECHNIQUES AND NORMAL FINDINGS	ABNORMAL FINDINGS SPECIAL CONSIDERATIONS

- Ask the client to bend the head toward the side being examined to relax the muscles and make the nodes easier to palpate. If any lymph nodes are palpable, make a note of their location, size, shape, fixation or mobility, and tenderness (see Figure 12.15 ●).

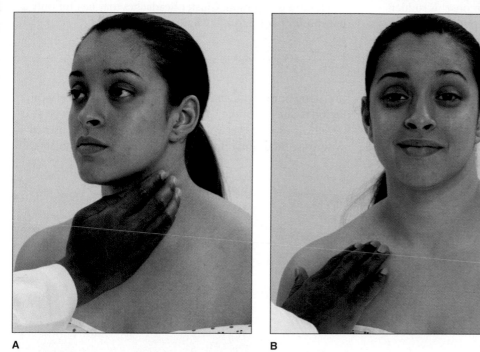

A   **B**

Figure 12.15 ● Palpating lymph nodes. A. Cervical. B. Supraclavicular.

 Refer to the Companion Website at **www.prenhall.com/damico** and click on the **Documentation** module for documentation samples and documentation practice exercises.

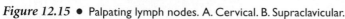

Abnormal Findings

Abnormal findings in the head and neck include headaches, abnormalities in the size and contour of the skull, malformations or abnormalities of the face and neck, and thyroid disorders. Examples of common abnormalities of the head and neck are presented in the following pages.

HEADACHES

Classic Migraine

A classic migraine is usually preceded by an aura during which the client may feel depressed, restless, or irritable; see spots or flashes of light; feel nauseated; or experience numbing or tingling in the face or extremities. The pain of the migraine itself may be mild or debilitating, requiring the client to lie down in the darkness in silence. It is usually a pulsating pain that is localized to the side, front, or back of the head and may be accompanied by nausea, vertigo, tremors, and other symptoms. The acute phase of a classic migraine typically lasts from 4 to 6 hours.

Cluster Headache

A cluster headache is so named because numerous episodes occur over a period of days or even months and then are followed by a period of remission during which no headaches occur. Cluster headaches have no aura. Their onset is sudden and may be associated with alcohol consumption, stress, or emotional distress. They often begin suddenly at night with an excruciating pain on one side of the face spreading upward behind one eye. The nose and affected eye water, and nasal congestion is common. Cluster headaches may last for only a few minutes or up to a few hours.

Tension Headache

A tension headache, also known as a muscle contraction headache, is due to sustained contraction of the muscles in the head, neck, or upper back. The onset is gradual, not sudden, and the pain is usually steady, not throbbing. The pain may be unilateral or bilateral and typically ranges from the cervical region to the top of the head. Tension headaches may be associated with stress, overwork, dental problems, premenstrual syndrome, sinus inflammation, and other health problems.

ABNORMALITIES OF THE SKULL AND FACE

Hydrocephalus

Hydrocephalus is enlargement of the head caused by inadequate drainage of cerebrospinal fluid, resulting in abnormal growth of the skull (see Figure 12.16 ●).

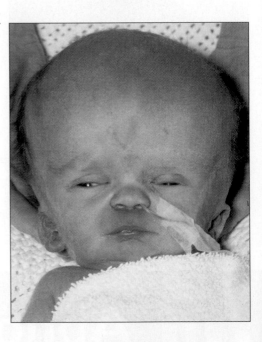

Figure 12.16 ● Hydrocephalus.

Craniosynostosis

Craniosynostosis is early closure of sutures (see Figure 12.17 ●). With early closure of the sagittal sutures, the head elongates. With early closure of the coronal sutures, the head, face, and orbits are altered.

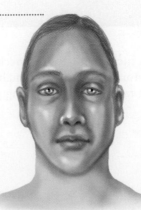
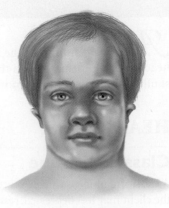

Figure 12.17 ● Craniosynostosis.

Acromegaly

Acromegaly is enlargement of the bones, and facial features due to increased growth hormone (see Figure 12.18 ●).

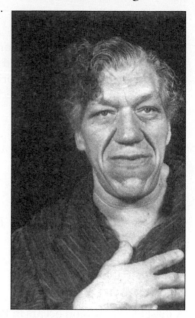

Figure 12.18 ● Acromegaly.

Bell's Palsy

Bell's palsy is a temporary disorder affecting cranial nerve VII and producing a unilateral facial paralysis (see Figure 12.19 ●). It may be caused by a virus. Its onset is sudden, and it usually resolves spontaneously in a few weeks without residual effects.

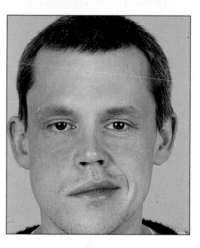

Figure 12.19 ● Bell's palsy.

Cushing's Syndrome

Cushing's syndrome is increased adrenal hormone production leading to a rounded "moon" face, ruddy cheeks, prominent jowls, and excess facial hair (see Figure 12.20 ●).

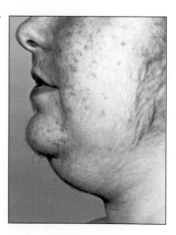

Figure 12.20 ● Cushing's syndrome.

Down Syndrome

Down syndrome is a chromosomal defect causing varying degrees of mental retardation and characteristic facial features such as slanted eyes, a flat nasal bridge, a flat nose, a protruding tongue, and a short, broad neck (see Figure 12.21 ●).

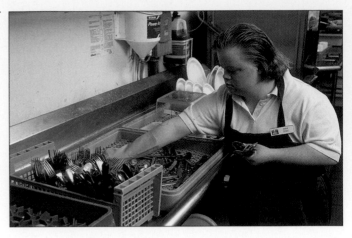

Figure 12.21 ● Down syndrome.

Parkinson's Disease

A masklike expression occurs in Parkinson's disease (see Figure 12.22 ●). The disease is the result of a decrease in dopamine, a neurotransmitter.

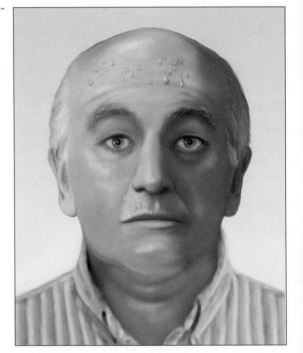

Figure 12.22 ● Parkinson's disease.

Brain Attack

A brain attack, stroke, or cerebrovascular accident (CVA) can result in neurologic deficits that include facial paralysis (see Figure 12.23 ●).

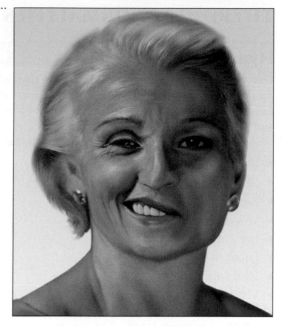

Figure 12.23 ● Brain attack.

Fetal Alcohol Syndrome

Fetal alcohol syndrome is a disorder characterized by epicanthal folds, narrow palpebral fissures, a deformed upper lip below the septum of the nose, and some degree of mental retardation (see Figure 12.24 ●). FAS is seen in infants of mothers whose intake of alcohol during pregnancy was significant.

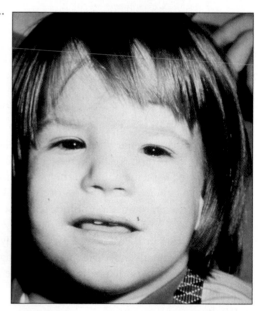

Figure 12.24 ● Fetal alcohol syndrome.

Torticollis

Torticollis is spasm of the sternocleidomastoid muscle on one side of the body, which often results from birth trauma (see Figure 12.25 ●). If left untreated, the muscle becomes fibrotic and permanently shortened.

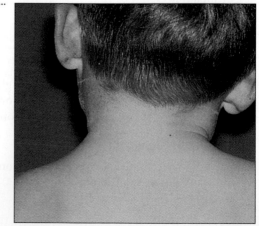

Figure 12.25 ● Torticollis.

THYROID ABNORMALITIES

Hyperthyroidism

Hyperthyroidism is excessive production of thyroid hormones. Hyperthyroidism results in enlargement of the gland, exophthalmos (bulging eyes), fine hair, weight loss, diarrhea, and other alterations.

Symptoms of hyperthyroidism include the following:

- Irritability/nervousness
- Muscle weakness or tremors
- Amenorrhea
- Weight loss
- Insomnia
- Enlarged thyroid
- Heat sensitivity
- Visual disturbances

Goiter

A goiter is an enlargement of the thyroid gland.

Graves' Disease

Graves' disease is the most common type of hyperthyroidism. There is no known cause. Graves' disease may be an autoimmune response or related to hereditary factors.

Thyroid Adenoma

Thyroid adenoma refers to benign thyroid nodules that occur most frequently in older adults. There is no known cause for thyroid adenomas.

Thyroid Carcinoma

Thyroid carcinoma can occur following radiation of the thyroid, chronic goiter, or as a result of hereditary factors. Thyroid carcinomas are malignant tumors in hormone-producing cells or supporting cells. Excess thyroid hormone is produced in the tumors.

Hyperthyroidism and Medication

Excessive iodine in some medications may cause oversecretion of thyroid hormones.

Hypothyroidism

Hypothyroidism occurs when there is a decrease in production of thyroid hormones. The decrease in thyroid hormones results in lowered basal metabolism. The most common occurrence in hypothyroidism is loss of thyroid tissue as a result of iodine deficiency or an autoimmune response. It may be a result of decreased pituitary stimulation of the thyroid gland or lack of hypothalamic thyroid-releasing factor. Hypothyroidism occurs most frequently in females between the ages of 30 and 50.

Symptoms of hypothyroidism include the following:

- Fatigue
- Weakness
- Weight gain
- Constipation
- Memory impairment
- Intolerance to cold
- Depression

Congenital Hypothyroidism

In congenital hypothyroidism, the thyroid is nonfunctioning at birth. If untreated it results in retardation of physical and mental growth.

Myxedema

This severe form of hypothyroidism causes nonpitting edema throughout the body and thickening of facial features. Complications of this disease affect major organ systems. Myxedema coma results in cardiovascular collapse, electrolyte disturbances, respiratory depression, and cerebral hypoxia.

Thyroiditis

Thyroiditis is an inflammation of the thyroid gland. This inflammation may cause release of stored hormones, resulting in temporary hyperthyroidism of weeks or months.

Postpartum Thyroiditis

Postpartum thyroiditis is a temporary condition occurring in 5% to 9% of females postpartum.

Hashimoto's Thyroiditis

Hashimoto's thyroiditis is an autoimmune disease that is thought to be hereditary and results in primary hypothyroidism.

Health Promotion

HEALTHY PEOPLE 2010

FOCUS AREA	PREVALENCE	OBJECTIVES	ACTIONS
Head Injury	• Motor vehicle crashes, bicycling, and falls contribute to the numbers of fatal and nonfatal head injuries in the United States. • Cyclist death rates from head injuries are twice as high in states where there are no helmet laws or in which they only apply to young riders when compared to states in which helmets are required by all riders. • In children under 14 years of age, deaths and severe injury from head trauma are mainly caused by falls. • Falls are the second leading cause of brain injury in those over 65 years of age.	• Reduce hospitalization for nonfatal head injuries. • Reduce deaths caused by motor vehicle crashes. • Increase the use of safety belts. • Increase the use of helmets by cyclists. • Reduce deaths by falls.	• Educational programs about safety including helmets, seat belts, and child restraints. • Community programs to improve safety in playground and schoolyard equipment. • Education about fall-proofing homes for the elderly.

CLIENT EDUCATION

The following are physiological, behavioral, and cultural factors that affect the head and neck across the age span. Several of these factors reflect trends cited in *Healthy People 2010*. The nurse provides advice and education to reduce risks associated with these factors and to promote and maintain health and function of the structures of the head and neck.

LIFE SPAN CONSIDERATIONS

RISK FACTORS

- Alcohol use during pregnancy can result in facial deformities in the newborn.
- Congenital hypothyroidism can result in physical and mental retardation.
- Thyroid disease occurs with greater frequency in females than in males.
- The development of thyroid dysfunction occurs more frequently in males and females after age 60.

- Production of thyroid hormone decreases with age.

CLIENT EDUCATION

- Encourage prenatal care to pregnant females and stress cessation of alcohol consumption during pregnancy.
- Teach parents the signs of hypothyroidism in newborns.

- Advise females of all ages to have thyroid screening performed if there is a family history of thyroid disease.
- Depression in old age may be associated with hypothyroidism. Advise clients and families to consult with healthcare providers if the symptom arises.
- Advise older adults to have thyroid screening and annual monitoring of thyroid hormone levels.

CULTURAL CONSIDERATIONS

RISK FACTOR

- Iodine deficiency leads to thyroid dysfunction and may occur in immigrant populations.

CLIENT EDUCATION

- Advise immigrants to include iodized salt in their diet if they are at risk for thyroid dysfunction.

ENVIRONMENTAL CONSIDERATIONS

RISK FACTORS

- Medications with iodine can cause hyperthyroidism.

- Thyroid diseases such as Hashimoto's (an autoimmune disorder causing hypothyroidism) are genetic disorders.

CLIENT EDUCATION

- Provide information about potential side effects of medications, especially those with iodine.

- Teach at-risk clients (those with a family history of Hashimoto's) about the signs and symptoms of the disorder.

Application Through Critical Thinking

CASE STUDY

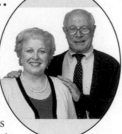

A married couple has come to the clinic for renewal of prescriptions and annual flu shots. During the encounter, the husband mentions to the nurse that he is concerned about his 69-year-old wife. He tells the nurse she has become very forgetful. She eats very little, but has seemed to gain weight. She seems "down" all the time. When questioned, the wife states she "just hasn't been herself." She admits she doesn't have much of an appetite. She explains that she has not been as active as she used to be and as a result her bowels are not as regular. She thinks those are the reasons she feels "out of sorts." She chides her husband that his memory "isn't so hot either." He insists that she is forgetting simple things while he has always forgotten to write down phone messages and birthdays and such.

The nurse is concerned about this client and carries out a further interview, which reveals the following findings: The client is generally cold, feels tired all of the time, and really doesn't have the energy to do much around the house. She finds the thought of going out exhausting. She tells the nurse that her tongue feels thick and she thinks her voice has changed.

The client agrees to a physical examination. The findings include a weight gain of 10 lb from her last clinic visit, 6 months ago. Her thyroid is enlarged and palpable. Her skin is dry, she has edema of the lower extremities, and her speech is slow. Her abdomen is distended with bowel sounds in all quadrants.

The nurse recommends that this woman have laboratory testing for thyroid dysfunction and arranges for consultation with a physician. The nurse schedules a follow-up appointment and makes some recommendations for this client that include increasing fluid intake and fiber to improve bowel function. The client is advised to wear warm clothing and to rest frequently. The nurse explains the functions of the thyroid and that medication can improve all aspects of her current condition when taken regularly.

▶ Complete Documentation

The following information is summarized from the case study. **SUBJECTIVE DATA:** "Just haven't been myself." Loss of appetite, decreased activity, irregular bowel function. Generally cold, tired, lack of energy, thick tongue, and change in voice. Husband states that wife is forgetful, eats very little, has gained weight, and seems "down."

OBJECTIVE DATA: BP 120/76—P 64—T 98.4. Alert and oriented. Unable to repeat list of five words after 5 minutes. Weight gain 10 lb over 6 months. Thyroid enlarged and palpable. Skin cool, dry, edema lower extremities. Slow speech. Abdomen distended. Bowel sounds present all quadrants.

A sample assessment form appears on page 261.

► Critical Thinking Questions

1. What may be responsible for the findings about this 69-year-old female?
2. What further data should the nurse collect?
3. What aspects of physical assessment and what tests are important in arriving at a diagnosis for this client?

► Applying Nursing Diagnoses

1. *Activity intolerance* is a diagnostic statement in the NANDA taxonomy (see Appendix A ⚭).
2. Do the data in the case study support this diagnosis? If so, identify the data.
3. Use the NANDA taxonomy to formulate additional diagnoses for the female client in the case study. Identify the data required for the PES (problem, etiology, signs or symptoms) statements.

► Prepare Teaching Plan

LEARNING NEED: The case study includes subjective and objective data indicative of a thyroid dysfunction. The nurse provides for diagnostic studies, follows up with a physician, and provides information about the thyroid gland and medication as treatment for the problem. The nurse's actions are based on determination that the client needs suggestions to ease current symptoms, information that will reassure her and assist her in decision making about the diagnosis and treatment of her problem.

The client is representative of a population at risk for hypothyroidism, that is, female and over 50 years of age. Aging individuals could benefit from education about hypothyroidism. The following teaching plan is intended to provide information about hypothyroidism for a group of learners.

ASSESSMENT FORM

Vital Signs: *BP 120/76—P 64—T 98.4*

Neurologic: *Alert and oriented*

Speech: *Slow, slurred, unable to recall list of words at 5 minutes*

Skin: *Cool, dry, edema lower extremities*

Nutrition: *Lack of appetite, weight gain 10 lbs in 6 months*

Neck: *Thyroid enlarged, palpable*

Abdomen: *Distended, BS+ X 4*

GOAL: The participants will acquire information of value in promotion of thyroid health.

OBJECTIVES: Upon completion of the learning session, the participants will be able to:

1. Discuss thyroid function.
2. Describe hypothyroidism.
3. List symptoms of hypothyroidism.
4. Identify diagnostic tests for hypothyroidism.
5. Discuss treatment for hypothyroidism.

Following is an example of the teaching plan for Objective 2. After reviewing this sample teaching plan for Objective 2, go to the Companion Website for this text to complete the teaching plan for other objectives.

APPLICATION OF OBJECTIVE 2: Describe hypothyroidism

Content	Teaching Strategy	Evaluation
• Hypothyroidism occurs when the thyroid does not produce enough of the thyroid hormones.	• Lecture	• Written examination.
• Hypothyroidism can occur as a result of inflammation of the thyroid leading to failure of parts of the gland.	• Discussion	May use short answer, fill-in, or multiple-choice items or a combination of items.
• Hashimoto's disease is an autoimmune disease that leads to thyroid failure. The immune system attacks the thyroid.	• Printed materials	If these are short and easy to evaluate, the learner receives immediate feedback.
• Other causes include surgical removal of part of the gland, irradiation of the gland, or other inflammatory processes.	Lecture is appropriate when disseminating information to large groups.	
• Hypothyroidism occurs more frequently in females and after 50 years of age.	Discussion allows participants to bring up concerns and to raise questions.	
• Risk factors include obesity, x-ray exposure in the neck area, or radiation treatment of the thyroid.	Printed material, especially to be taken away with learners, allows review, reinforcement, and reading at the learner's pace.	

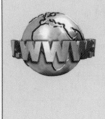

Please refer to the Companion Website at www.prenhall.com/damico and click on Chapter 12, the Application Through Critical Thinking module, to complete the following activities related to this case study:
► Critical Thinking questions
► Extended Nursing Diagnosis challenge
► Documentation activity
► Teaching Plan for Objectives 1, 3, 4, and 5

EXPLORE MediaLink

Additional resources for this chapter are found on the Student CD-ROM accompanying this textbook and on the Companion Website.

CD-ROM CONTENT

Content for this chapter includes:
Objectives
Key Concepts
NCLEX-RN® Review Questions
Model Documentation Forms
Audio Glossary
Animations
   Head and Neck Anatomy
Games and Challenges
Head-to-Toe Physical Examination Video

COMPANION WEBSITE CONTENT

www.prenhall.com/damico

Content for this chapter includes:
Objectives
NCLEX-RN® Review Questions
Client Interaction Case Study Challenge

Application Through Critical Thinking
   Case Study Teaching Plan Challenge
MediaLinks
MediaLink Application
Tool Box
   Chapter Documentation Form Example
   Health Promotion
     Healthy People 2010
     Client Education
New York Times

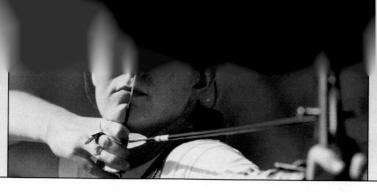

13

Eye

*T*he eyes are located in the orbital cavities of the skull. Only the anterior aspect of the eye is exposed. The eyes are the sensory organs responsible for vision. Vision is a major mechanism for experiencing the world. *Healthy People 2010* describes vision as "an essential part of everyday life, depended on constantly by people at all ages. Vision affects development, learning, communicating, working, health and quality of life" (USDHHS, 2000, pp. 28–33). Therefore, a goal has been created to improve visual health through prevention, early diagnosis, prompt treatment, and rehabilitation as described in the *Healthy People 2010* feature on page 299.

ANATOMY AND PHYSIOLOGY REVIEW

The eye is the structure through which light is gathered to produce vision. Layers and membranes serve several purposes. The accessory structures of the eye provide protection and are responsible for movement of the eye. Each anatomical structure is described in the following section.

EYE

The eye, commonly called the eyeball, is a fluid-filled sphere having a diameter of approximately 2.5 cm (1 in.). The eye receives light waves and transmits these waves to the brain for interpretation as visual images. Only a small portion of the eye is seen. Most of the eye is set into and protected by the bony orbit of the skull (see Figure 13.1 ●).

The eye is composed of three layers: the sclera, the choroids, and the retina. The **sclera,** the outermost layer, is an extremely dense, hard, fibrous membrane that helps to maintain the shape of the eye. It is the white fibrous part of the eye that is seen anteriorly. Its primary function is to support and protect the structures of the eye (see Figure 13.2 ●).

The **cornea** is the clear, transparent part of the sclera and forms the anterior one sixth of the eye. It is considered to be the window of the eye, allowing light to enter. The extensive nerve endings in the cornea are responsible for the blink reflex, increase the secretion of tears for protection, and are most sensitive to pain.

The **choroid,** the middle layer, is the vascular-pigmented layer of the eye. The **iris** is the circular, colored muscular aspect of this layer of the eye and is located in the anterior portion of the eye. The center of the iris is opened and is called the pupil. The iris responds to light by making the pupil larger or smaller, thereby controlling the amount of light that enters the eye. A dim light will cause the iris to respond, enlarging the pupil size (**miosis**). This increases the amount of light entering the eye, enhancing distant vision (**hydiasis**). A bright light causes the iris to respond by decreasing pupil size (miosis), thus decreasing the

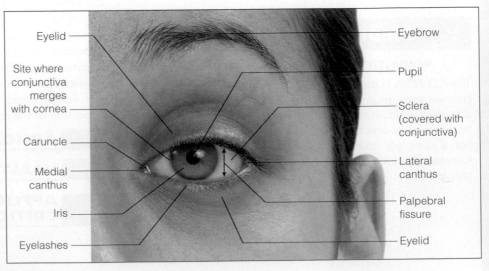

Figure 13.1 ● Structures of the external eye.

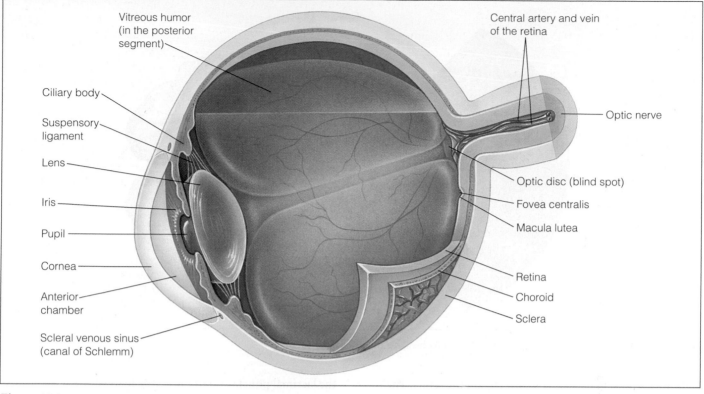

Figure 13.2 ● Interior of the eye.

amount of light entering the eye, accommodating near vision. The third cranial nerve controls pupillary constriction and dilation. The parasympathetic branch of this nerve stimulates pupillary constriction while the sympathetic branch stimulates dilation of the pupil.

The third and innermost membrane, the **retina,** is the sensory portion of the eye. The retina, a direct extension of the optic nerve, helps to change light waves to neuroimpulses for interpretation as visual impulses by the brain. The retina contains many rods and cones. The rods function in dim light and are also considered to be peripheral vision receptors. The cones function in bright light, are central vision receptors, and provide color to sight.

The **optic disc,** on the nasal aspect of the retina, is round with clear margins. It is usually creamy yellow and is the point at which the optic nerve and retina meet. The color of the disc and the retinal background differ according to skin color. The color is lighter in persons with light skin and darker in individuals with darker skin color. The center of this disc, the physiologic cup, is the point at which the vascular network enters the eye.

The **macula** is responsible for central vision. The macula, with its yellow pitlike center called the *fovea centralis,* appears as a hyperpigmented spot on the temporal aspect of the retina.

REFRACTION OF THE EYE

Light rays travel in a straight line. The light rays must change direction or refract as they pass from one source to another source for vision to occur. Each structure in the pathway of light

has a different density. Several structures of the eye help with the deflection or refraction of the light rays. The structures responsible for refraction include the cornea, aqueous humor, crystalline lens, and vitreous humor.

Refraction allows the light rays to enter the eye and be aimed (reflected) to the correct part of the retina for most accurate vision. **Emmetropia** is the normal refractive condition of the eye. **Myopia** (nearsightedness) is a condition in which the light rays focus in front of the retina. In **hyperopia** (farsightedness) the light rays focus behind the retina.

The **aqueous humor** is a clear, fluidlike substance found in the anterior segment of the eye that helps maintain ocular pressure. The aqueous humor is a refractory medium of the eye that is constantly being formed and is always flowing through the pupil and draining into the venous system. The **vitreous humor,** another refractory medium, is a clear gel located in the posterior segment of the eye. This gel helps maintain the intraocular pressure and the shape of the eye, and transmits light rays through the eye.

The **lens,** situated directly behind the pupil, is a biconvex (convex on both surfaces), transparent, and flexible structure. It separates the anterior and posterior segments of the eye. The ability of the lens to accommodate or change its shape permits light to focus properly on the retina and enhances fine focusing of images.

VISUAL PATHWAYS

An object external to the body creates an image. Via light waves, this image is transported to the brain for interpretation as vision.

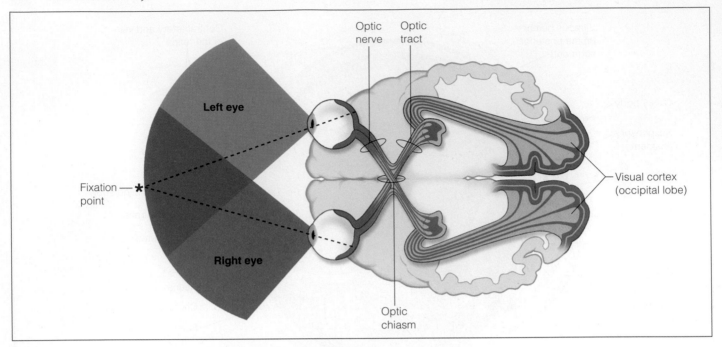

Figure 13.3 ● Visual fields of the eye and the visual pathway to the brain.

Light waves must bend to focus correctly on the retina. The refractory structures—the cornea, aqueous humor, anterior and posterior chambers, lens, and vitreous humor—help bend the light waves onto the retina. This retinal image, via the nerve fibers, is conducted to the optic nerve (cranial nerve II). At the optic chiasm, the optic fibers of the nerves cross over and join the temporal fibers from the opposite eye. Optic tracts encircle the brain and the impulse is transmitted to the occipital lobe of the brain for interpretation (see Figure 13.3 ●).

ACCESSORY STRUCTURES OF THE EYE

The eye has several external accessory structures. The eyebrows are the coarse short hairs that are located on the lower portion of the forehead at the orbital margins. The primary function of the eyebrow is to protect the eye (Figure 13.1).

The eyelids, or **palpebrae,** are the movable folds of skin that cover and protect the eyes. The opening between the upper and lower eyelids is called the **palpebral fissure.** The eyelids meet medially and laterally to form the medial canthus and the lateral canthus. The meibomian glands, embedded in the eyelids, are modified sebaceous glands that produce an oily substance to help lubricate the eyes and eyelids. The eyelashes are hairs which projected from the eyelids and curl outward. The high supply of nerve fibers help support the blink reflex, thereby protecting the eye.

The conjunctiva, a thin mucous membrane, lines the interior of the eyelids and continues over the anterior portion of the eye, meeting the cornea but not covering it. The conjunctiva protects the eye by preventing foreign objects from entering the eye. The conjunctiva also produces a lubricating fluid that prevents the eyes from drying.

The lacrimal apparatus consists of the lacrimal glands and ducts. Lacrimal secretions, commonly called tears, are secreted and spread over the conjunctiva when blinking. The tears enter the lacrimal puncta and drain via the many ducts into the posterior nasal passage (see Figure 13.4 ●).

Each eye has six extrinsic or extraocular muscles. They help hold the eye in place within the bony orbit. These muscles are the lateral rectus, medial rectus, superior rectus, inferior rectus, inferior oblique, and superior oblique (see Figure 13.5 ●). With the coordination of these muscles, the individual experiences one image sight. These muscles are innervated by cranial nerves III, IV, and VI. Figure 13.6 ● depicts the correlation of eye movement with eye muscle and cranial nerve.

SPECIAL CONSIDERATIONS

Throughout the assessment process, the nurse gathers subjective and objective data reflecting the client's state of health. Using critical thinking and the nursing process, the nurse identifies many factors to be considered when collecting the data. Vision and eye health are influenced by a number of factors including age, developmental level, race, ethnicity, occupation, socioeconomics, and emotional well-being. The nurse must consider these factors when gathering subjective and objective data during a comprehensive health assessment.

DEVELOPMENTAL CONSIDERATIONS

Comprehensive health assessment includes interpretation of findings in relation to normative values. The following sections describe normal variations in structures and functions of the eye for different age groups.

Infants and Children

At birth, the eyes of the neonate should be symmetrical. The pupils are equal and respond to light. The iris is generally brown in dark-skinned neonates, and slate gray-blue in light-

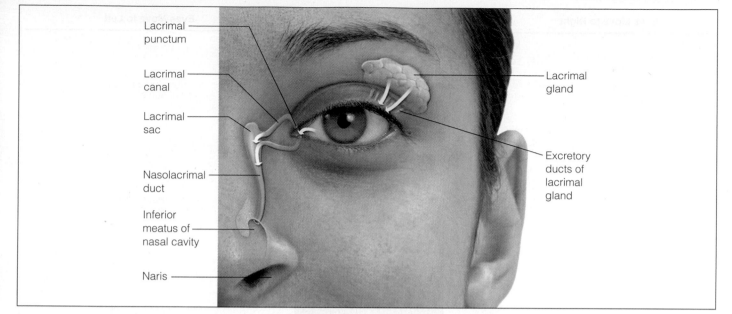

Figure 13.4 ● Lacrimal glands of the eye.

skinned neonates. By about the third month of age, the color of the eyes begins to change to a more permanent shade. Many times the eyelids are edematous at birth. Little to no tears are present at birth but begin to appear by the fourth week. Binocular vision (vision in both eyes) begins to develop by 6 weeks of age. Before this time, neonates will fixate on a bright or moving object. The eyes reach adult size by 8 years of age. The *red reflex,* a glowing red color that fills the pupil as light from the ophthalmoscope reflects off the retina, should be elicited from birth. Peripheral vision may be assessed by confrontation in children older than 3 years of age. It is important to assess extraocular muscle function as early as possible in young children because delay can lead to permanent visual damage. The corneal light reflex, Hirschberg's test, can be used to determine symmetry of muscle function. Lateral deviations of the eye (disconjugate gaze) are normal findings until 4 months of age.

The Pregnant Female

The pregnant female may complain of dry eyes and may discontinue wearing contact lenses during her pregnancy. The pregnant client may also describe visual changes due to shifting fluid in the cornea. These symptoms are usually not significant and disappear after childbirth. Changes in eyesight such

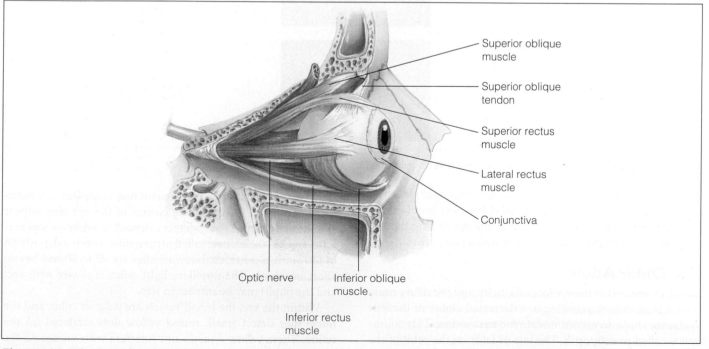

Figure 13.5 ● Extraocular muscles.

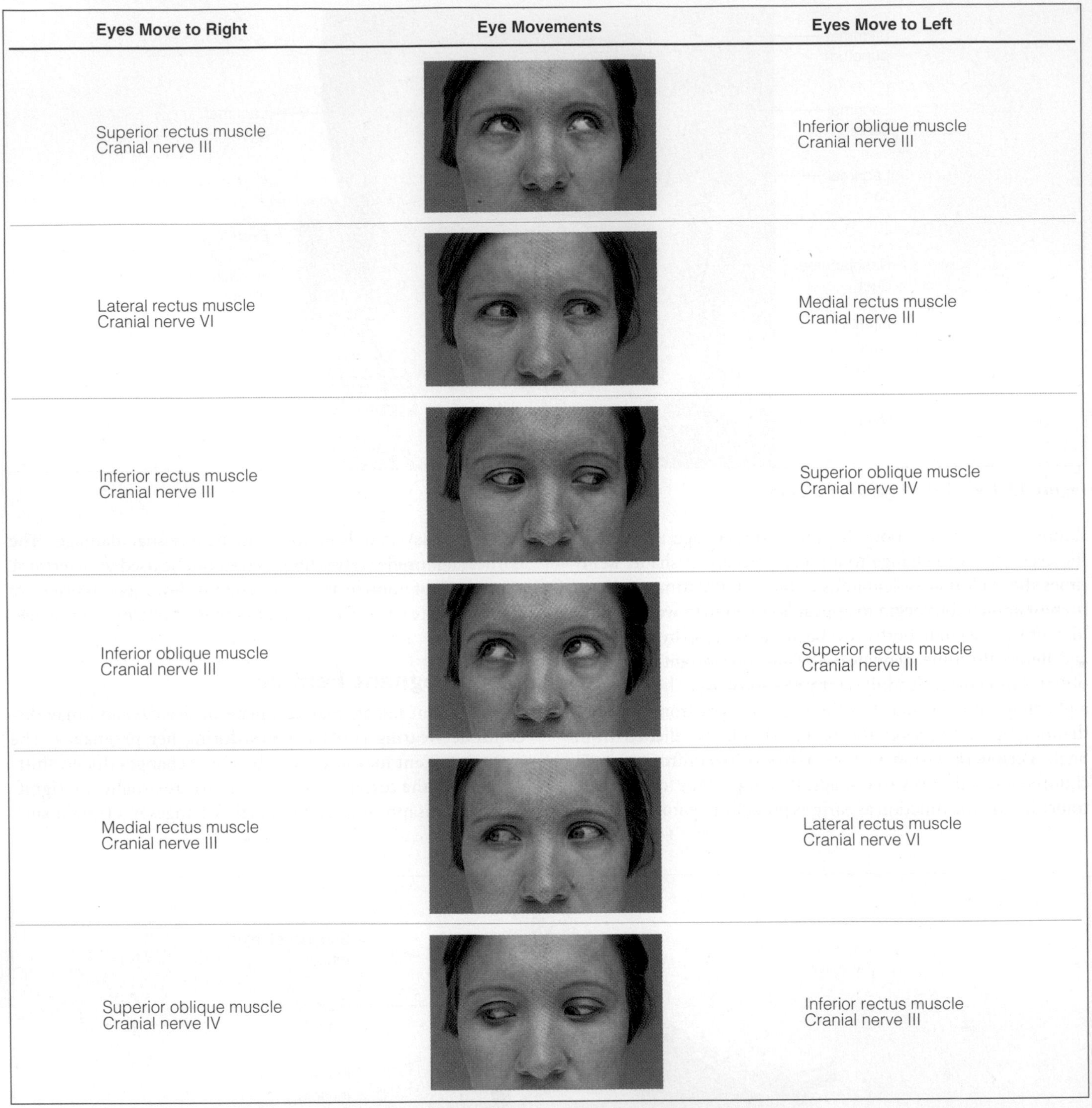

Eyes Move to Right	Eye Movements	Eyes Move to Left
Superior rectus muscle Cranial nerve III		Inferior oblique muscle Cranial nerve III
Lateral rectus muscle Cranial nerve VI		Medial rectus muscle Cranial nerve III
Inferior rectus muscle Cranial nerve III		Superior oblique muscle Cranial nerve IV
Inferior oblique muscle Cranial nerve III		Superior rectus muscle Cranial nerve III
Medial rectus muscle Cranial nerve III		Lateral rectus muscle Cranial nerve VI
Superior oblique muscle Cranial nerve IV		Inferior rectus muscle Cranial nerve III

Figure 13.6 ● Eye movements with muscle and nerve coordinclon.

as refraction changes requiring a new prescription for glasses or contact lenses, blurriness, or distorted vision can occur because of temporary changes in the shape of the eye during the last trimester of pregnancy and the first 6 weeks postpartum.

The Older Adult

By age 45, the lens of the eye loses elasticity, and the ciliary muscles become weaker, resulting in a decreased ability of the lens to change shape to accommodate for near vision. This condition is called **presbyopia.** The loss of fat from the orbit of the eye produces a drooping appearance. The lacrimal glands de-

crease tear production, and the client may complain of a burning sensation in the eyes. The cornea of the eye may appear cloudy, and the nurse may detect a deposit of white-yellow material around the cornea, called *arcus senilis.* This is a deposition of fat, but it is considered normal after age 45 to 50 and has no effect on vision. The pupillary light reflex is slower with age, and the pupils may be smaller in size.

Within the eye, the blood vessels are paler in color, and the nurse may detect small, round yellow dots scattered on the retina. These yellow dots do not interfere with vision. As the client ages, the lens continues to thicken and yellow, forming a

Cultural Considerations

- Prevalence rates of age-related macular degeneration are higher in Caucasians than in other groups over 75 years of age.
- African American females have a higher incidence of age-related macular degeneration than males until the age of 75.
- Cataracts occur more frequently in Caucasian females than in other races.
- Glaucoma occurs more frequently in African Americans than in Hispanics and Caucasians.
- Hispanics have higher rates of visual impairments than other races.
- The prevalence of myopia is related to national origin and ethnicity. Myopia occurs more frequently in industrialized nations.

- Asians, Alaska Natives, and some Native American tribes have higher rates of myopia than other cultural groups.
- Individuals from underdeveloped nations have higher rates of blindness than those from other nations. The cause of blindness is associated with trachoma, vitamin A deficiency, river blindness, and other infectious diseases.
- Blindness can occur as a result of diabetic retinopathy. Rates of type 2 diabetes are higher in African Americans, Hispanic Americans, Asian Americans, Pacific Islanders, and Native Americans.

dense area that reduces lens clarity. This condition is the beginning of a **cataract** formation. Macular degeneration can occur in the older client, resulting in a loss of central vision. The ophthalmoscopic examination may reveal narrowed blood vessels with a granular pigment in the macula.

PSYCHOSOCIAL CONSIDERATIONS

Decreased visual acuity and visual impairment can impact individuals across the age span. Visually impaired children may have developmental delays and may require special assistive social and educational services into adulthood. Adults with visual impairments may lose some personal independence, may experience decreased quality of life, and may find it difficult to obtain or maintain employment. Visual impairment results in stress for individuals and families as they adapt to alterations in activities of daily living (ADLs) and as they navigate the healthcare and social service systems for diagnosis, treatment, and assistance.

Eye contact with other people varies, especially during the communication process. Age, gender, and culture influence the type and amount of eye contact people make with others.

CULTURAL AND ENVIRONMENTAL CONSIDERATIONS

Asian clients have prominent epicanthic folds (a vertical fold of skin) covering the inner canthus of the eye. Dark-skinned individuals may have dark pigmented spots on the sclera, and their retinae may appear darker. People with light-colored eyes typically have lighter retinae and better night vision, but are more sensitive to bright sunlight and artificial light.

Excessive sun exposure without the use of sunglasses may promote cataract formation. A deficiency of vitamin A may cause night blindness. Some medications have side effects that may cause excessive corneal dryness, vision changes, or increased intraocular pressure. When assessing a client who wears contact lenses, it is important to determine what type of contact lens is worn (hard versus soft, extended wear versus daily change) and evaluate the client's cleansing routine. Makeup and applicators should be discarded after 3 months, and makeup should not be shared to reduce the risk of infection. Trauma or damage to the eye can occur in work, recreational, and social environments. Safety glasses or protective goggles are recommended when the eye is at risk. For example, protective eyewear is used in carpentry, welding, and chemical laboratories to prevent debris or splashes from entering the eye.

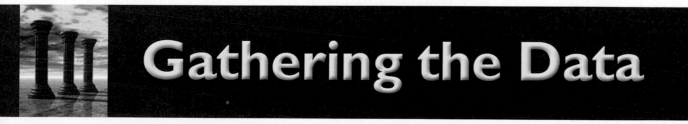

Gathering the Data

*H*ealth assessment of the eye includes the gathering of subjective and objective data. The subjective data is collected during the interview in which the professional nurse uses a variety of communication techniques to elicit general and specific information about the health of the eye. Health records combine subjective and objective data. The results of laboratory tests and radiologic studies are important secondary sources of objective data. Physical assessment of the eye, during which objective data is collected, includes the technique of inspection, the application of specific tests of vision and structures of the eye, and the use of the ophthalmoscope to assess the inner eye.

FOCUSED INTERVIEW

The focused interview for assessment of the eye concerns data related to the structures of the internal and external eye, and those data concerned with vision. The nurse will observe the client and listen for cues that relate to the status and function of the eye. The nurse may use closed or open-ended questions to obtain information. Follow-up bulleted questions or requests for descriptions are required to clarify data or to supply missing information. Follow-up questions are used to identify the source of problems, duration of difficulties, measures to alleviate problems, and cues about the client's knowledge of his or her own health and health practices.

The focused interview guides the physical assessment of the eye. The information obtained is considered in relation to norms and expectations about the function of the eye and structures of the eye. Therefore, the nurse must consider age, gender, race, culture, environment, health practices, past and current problems, and therapies when framing questions and using techniques to elicit information. Remember, the subjective data collected and the questions asked during the health history and focused interview will provide data to help meet the goal of promoting visual acuity as stated in *Healthy People 2010*. In order to address all of the factors, categories of questions related to status and functions

of the eye have been developed. These categories include general questions that are asked of all clients, those addressing illness or infection, questions related to symptoms or behaviors, those related to habits or practices, questions that are specific to clients according to age, those for the pregnant female, and questions to address environmental concerns.

The nurse must consider the client's ability to participate in the focused interview and physical assessment of the eye. The ability to communicate is essential to the focused interview. If language barriers exist, a translator must be used. If the client is experiencing discomfort or anxiety, efforts to address those problems have priority over other aspects of health assessment.

FOCUSED INTERVIEW QUESTIONS

RATIONALES

The following section provides sample questions and bulleted follow-up questions in each of the previously mentioned categories. A rationale for each of the questions is provided. The list of questions is not all-inclusive, but rather represents the types of questions required in a comprehensive focused interview related to the eye.

GENERAL QUESTIONS

1. **Describe your vision today. Please describe any changes in your vision in the past few months.**

   ▶ These questions provide an opportunity for clients to describe their own perceptions about vision.

2. **What was the date of your last eye examination? What were the results of that examination?**
   - What medications were prescribed or measures taken to relieve the problem?
   - Have the medications or measures been effective in relieving the problem?
   - Has the problem affected your activities of daily living?

   ▶ These questions provide specific information about healthcare practices and identify any known visual problems.

   Follow-up questions would be required when a problem with vision or with the structures of the eye have been identified as results of an eye examination.

3. **Do you wear glasses or contact lenses?**
   - How long have you used glasses or contact lenses?
   - Describe your vision with and without the use of glasses or contact lenses.

   ▶ These questions elicit information about vision correction and the effectiveness of the correction.

4. **Have you or any member of your family been diagnosed with hypertension, diabetes, or glaucoma?**

   ▶ This question may reveal information about diseases associated with genetic or familial predisposition. Each of the diseases mentioned can lead to vision problems. Hypertension can cause arteriosclerosis of the retina. Diabetes can cause bleeding in the capillaries of the retina.

QUESTIONS RELATED TO ILLNESS OR INFECTION

1. **Have you ever been diagnosed with a disease of the eye?**
   - When were you diagnosed with the problem?
   - What treatment was prescribed for the problem?
   - Was the treatment helpful?
   - What kinds of things do you do to help with the problem?
   - Has the problem ever recurred (acute)?
   - How are you managing the disease now (chronic)?

   ▶ The client has an opportunity to provide information about a specific eye disease or problem. If a diagnosed illness is identified, follow-up about the date of diagnosis, treatment, and outcomes is required. Data about each illness identified by the client is essential to an accurate health assessment. Illnesses can be classified as acute or chronic, and follow-up about each classification will differ.

FOCUSED INTERVIEW QUESTIONS	**RATIONALES**

2. An alternative to question 1 is to list possible eye diseases, such as glaucoma, cataracts, corneal injury, Horner's syndrome, and exophthalmos, and ask the client to respond yes or no as each is stated.

▶ This is a comprehensive and efficient way to elicit information about all eye-related diseases. Follow-up would be carried out for each identified diagnosis as in question 1.

3. Do you now have or have you had an infection of the eye?

▶ If an infection is identified, follow-up about the date of the infection, treatment, and outcomes is required. Data about each infection identified by the client is essential to an accurate health assessment. Infections can be classified as acute or chronic, and follow-up about each classification will differ.

4. An alternative to question 3 is to list possible eye infections, such as conjunctivitis, iritis, uveitis, blepharitis, dacryocystitis, stye (hordeolum), and episcleritis, and ask the client to respond yes or no as each is stated.

▶ This is a comprehensive and efficient way to elicit information about all eye infections. Follow-up would be carried out for each identified infection as in question 3.

5. Have you had an injury to the eye?

6. Have you had eye surgery?

▶ Questions 5 and 6 require follow-up regarding the type of injury or surgery, the causes and treatments, and the adaptations the individual has made to overcome visual or other deficits as a result of the injury or surgery.

QUESTIONS RELATED TO SYMPTOMS OR BEHAVIORS

When gathering information about symptoms, many questions are required to elicit details and descriptions that assist in analysis of the data. Discrimination is made in relation to the significance of the symptom associated with a specific disease or problem, or in association with the need for referrals and follow-up. One rationale may be provided for a group of questions about symptoms.

The following questions refer to specific symptoms and behaviors associated with the eyes and vision. For each symptom, questions and follow-up are required. The details to be elicited are the characteristics of the symptom; the onset, duration, and frequency of the symptom; the treatment or remedy for the symptom, including over-the-counter and home remedies; the determination if diagnosis has been sought; the effect of treatments; and family history associated with a symptom or illness.

Questions 1 through 14 refer to blurred vision as a symptom. The rationales and follow-up questions provide examples of the number and types of questions required in a focused interview when symptoms exist. The remaining questions refer to other symptoms associated with problems with the eyes or vision. Follow-up is included only when required for clarification.

QUESTIONS RELATED TO SYMPTOMS

1. Have you ever experienced blurred vision?

2. How long have you had blurred vision?

▶ Determining the duration of symptoms is helpful in determining the significance of symptoms in relation to specific diseases and problems. Blurred vision can be an indication of a neurologic, cardiovascular, or endocrine problem; a need for corrective lenses; or cataracts.

3. Is your vision blurred all of the time?

▶ It is important to determine if a symptom is constant or intermittent.

FOCUSED INTERVIEW QUESTIONS	**RATIONALES**

4. Do you know what causes the blurred vision?

▶ This question permits clients to identify whether an actual diagnosis has been made in regard to the symptom or to express their beliefs or perceptions about the cause of the symptom.

5. Describe your blurred vision.

▶ Descriptions provide information about symptoms in the client's own words. The descriptions often provide cues for further follow-up questions.

6. Have you sought treatment for the blurred vision?

7. When was that treatment sought?

8. What occurred when you sought treatment?

9. Was something recommended or prescribed to help with the blurred vision?

10. What was the effect of the treatment?

▶ Questions 6 through 10 provide information about the need for diagnosis, referral, or continued evaluation of the symptom as well as information about the client's knowledge of a current diagnosis and the response to intervention.

11. Do you use any over-the-counter or home remedies for the blurred vision?

12. What are the remedies that you use?

13. How often do you use them?

14. How much of them do you use?

▶ Questions 11 through 14 provide information about drugs and/or remedies that may relieve symptoms or provide comfort. Conversely, some remedies may interfere with the effect of prescribed treatments or medications and may harm the client.

15. Have you ever experienced double vision?

▶ Double vision can be caused by muscle or nerve complications and some medications.

16. Are you now or have you ever been sensitive to light?

17. Do you experience burning or itching of the eyes?

▶ Burning and itching of the eyes are often associated with altered tear production and allergies.

18. Do you ever see small black dots that seem to move when you are looking at something?

▶ Black dots or spots are known as floaters. Floaters are considered normal unless they obstruct vision.

19. Do you see halos around lights?

20. Do you have trouble seeing at night?

21. Do you have trouble driving at night?

▶ Halos around lights are associated with glaucoma, a disease marked by increased intraocular pressure.

▶ If the client responds affirmatively to any of these, follow-up is required. Follow-up would include determination of onset, duration, and frequency of the symptom; identification of treatment and the effectiveness of the treatment; and determination of a diagnosis for the problem.

QUESTIONS RELATED TO PAIN

1. Have you had any eye pain?

▶ Eye pain can be superficial, affecting the outer eye only, or deep and throbbing, possibly associated with glaucoma. Any sudden onset of eye pain should be referred immediately to a physician.

2. Where is the pain?

3. How often do you experience the pain?

4. How long does the pain last?

5. How long have you had the pain?

6. How would you rate the pain on a scale of 1 to 10?

▶ Questions 2 through 6 are standard questions associated with pain to determine the duration, location, frequency, and intensity of the pain.

FOCUSED INTERVIEW QUESTIONS	RATIONALES

7. Is there a trigger for the pain?

8. Can you describe the pain?

9. Does the pain radiate to any other areas?

10. What do you do to relieve the pain?

11. Is this treatment effective?

QUESTIONS RELATED TO BEHAVIORS

1. How do you clean and care for your eyes?

2. If you use eye makeup, how do you apply it and remove it? How often do you replace the makeup and applicators?

3. How do you clean and care for contact lenses if used?

► Some eye care products, facial cleansers, and skin care products can be irritating to the eyes. Products used in applying makeup to the eyes and improper care of contact lenses can irritate the eye or cause infection if they are not cleaned or changed frequently.

QUESTIONS RELATED TO AGE

The focused interview must reflect the anatomical and physiological differences that exist along the age span. The following questions are presented as examples of those that would be specific for children, the pregnant female, and the older adult.

QUESTIONS REGARDING INFANTS AND CHILDREN

1. Did the mother have any vaginal infections at the time of delivery?

2. Did the baby get eye ointment after birth?

3. Was the infant preterm or full term?

4. Does the infant look directly at you? Does your infant follow objects with the eyes?

5. Do you have concerns about the child's ability to see? Does the school-age child like to sit at the front of the classroom?

6. Has the child had a vision examination? When was the last eye examination?
   - How often has the child's vision been checked?
   - By whom?
   - What were the results?

7. Does the child rub his or her eyes frequently?

► Vaginal infections in the mother can cause eye infections in the newborn.

► If the infant was born preterm, resuscitation and oxygen may have been required, which can damage the eyes.

► The infant may have crossed eyes or eyes that move in different directions normally until 4 months of age; then the findings may be associated with weakness of the eye muscles.

► Poor eyesight may necessitate sitting at the front of the room.

► Rubbing of the eyes can be associated with infection, allergy, or visual problems. Some children rub their eyes when fatigued.

QUESTIONS FOR THE PREGNANT FEMALE

1. Have you had any changes in your eyesight during your pregnancy?

► Changes in vision should be referred to an ophthalmologist.

FOCUSED INTERVIEW QUESTIONS	RATIONALES

QUESTIONS FOR THE OLDER ADULT

1. Do you experience dryness or burning in your eyes?

2. Do you have problems seeing at night?

3. Do bright lights bother you?

4. Are you routinely tested for glaucoma?

5. What was the date of your last eye examination?

▶ Dryness is usually due to decreased tear production, which occurs with aging.

▶ Night blindness is associated with cataracts and some retinal diseases.

▶ The lens of the eye thickens with aging; therefore, accommodation to light is not as rapid.

QUESTIONS RELATED TO THE ENVIRONMENT

Environment refers to both the internal and external environments. Questions related to the internal environment include all of the previous questions and those associated with internal or physiological responses. Questions regarding the external environment include those related to home, work, or social environments.

INTERNAL ENVIRONMENT

1. What medications are you taking?

2. Are you taking any medications specifically for the eyes?

3. Have you or any family member had diabetes, hypertension, or glaucoma?

▶ Some medications have side effects that impact the eye.

▶ All of these diseases can be hereditary and can cause visual difficulties. Hypertension can cause arteriosclerosis of the retina. Diabetes can cause bleeding of the capillaries of the retina eventually affecting vision.

EXTERNAL ENVIRONMENT

The following questions deal with substances, irritants, and other factors found in the physical environment of the client that could impact the eyes or vision. The physical environment includes the indoor and outdoor environments of the home and the workplace, those encountered for social engagements, and any encountered during travel.

1. Have you been exposed to inhalants such as dust, pollen, chemical fumes, or flying debris that caused eye irritation?

▶ Prolonged work under bright lights or at a computer screen can cause eyestrain. Use of equipment at work or at home may require the use of safety glasses to prevent eye injury from debris. Some athletic activities put the client at risk for eye injury, and shields or masks are recommended to prevent or reduce the risk for injury.

2. What were those irritants?

3. What was the effect on your eyes?

4. What have you done to remedy the eye problem?

5. What have you done to decrease the exposure to the irritant?

6. What kind of activities do you perform at work?

FOCUSED INTERVIEW QUESTIONS

7. **Do you need or wear safety glasses at work?**

8. **How many hours in the workday are you using a computer?**

9. **What sports or hobbies do you participate in?**

10. **Do you routinely wear sunglasses when outside in bright light?**
    - Follow-up questions would include all of the questions previously mentioned that address symptoms and problems.

RATIONALES

CLIENT INTERACTION

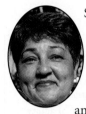 Sophia Rodriguez, a 62-year-old Mexican immigrant, is employed as a sewing machine operator at the local shirt factory. The operators are paid based on work production. Sophia has always received a monthly bonus for her production. Lately, her productivity has decreased and her supervisor tries to help determine the reason. Sophia tells the supervisor she needs a better, stronger light on the sewing machine since it is very hard to see the stitches and thread. Sophia is directed to the local eye clinic. Following is an excerpt of the focused interview.

INTERVIEW

Nurse: Mrs. Rodriguez, tell me your reason for coming to the eye clinic today.

Mrs. Rodriguez: I can't see the thread or the stitches like I used to. I don't sew as many sleeves like I used to. I make mistakes now, and that slows me down.

Nurse: Have you ever had your eyes examined?

Mrs. Rodriguez: Yes, several years ago. They told me everything was okay. No glasses.

Nurse: Describe your vision.

Mrs. Rodriguez: I don't know what you want me to say. I just can't see like I used to.

Nurse: Can you see to read the newspaper?

Mrs. Rodriguez: Yes.

Nurse: Do you need to hold the newspaper closer to your eyes or farther away when reading?

Mrs. Rodriguez: A little farther away. But I can't read it at night unless I'm next to the light in the room.

Nurse: Can you see the street signs when you are driving?

Mrs. Rodriguez: Yes, that is not a problem.

Nurse: Is your vision blurred?

Mrs. Rodriguez: Sometimes, especially if I'm tired.

Nurse: Do you ever see black spots floating in your eyes?

Mrs. Rodriguez: No.

Nurse: Are your eyes sensitive to light?

Mrs. Rodriguez: No.

Nurse: Do you see halos or rings around lights?

Mrs. Rodriguez: No.

Nurse: Do you have any pain or burning in your eyes?

Mrs. Rodriguez: No.

ANALYSIS

The nurse knows presbyopia is a common change of the eye associated with aging. The nurse begins the interview using open-ended statements to gather data associated with presbyopia and other medical diagnoses. Using open-ended statements, the nurse obtains clear baseline data. When the client indicates she is not clear how to respond, the nurse proceeds using closed-ended statements. This allows the client to respond yes or no. The nurse must be sure to present the many questions in a non-threatening manner.

 Please refer to the Companion Website at **www.prenhall.com/damico** and click on Chapter 13, the **Client Interaction** module, to answer questions about this case. In addition, see other resources for this chapter including NCLEX review questions and other interactive exercises and materials.

Physical Assessment

ASSESSMENT TECHNIQUES AND FINDINGS

Physical assessment of the eyes requires the use of inspection, palpation, and tests of the function of the eyes. The ophthalmoscope is used to assess the internal eye. During each of the assessments the nurse is gathering data related to the client's vision, the internal and external structures, and functions of the eye. Inspection includes looking at the size, shape, and symmetry of the eye, eyelids, eyebrows, and eye movements. Knowledge of the norms and expectations related to the eye and vision according to age and development is essential in determining the meaning of the data.

In adults and children over 6 years of age, normal visual acuity is 20/20. Normal vision for children under 6 years of age varies. Further information about vision in children is included in Chapter 25 of this text. ⚭ Presbyopia, the inability to accommodate for near vision, is common in clients over the age of 45. The size, shape, and position of the eyes should be symmetrical. The sclerae are white, the cornea is clear, and the pupils are round and symmetrical in size and respond briskly to light. The eyebrows are located equally above the eyes; the eyelashes are full and everted. The eyes are moist, indicating tear production. The movements of the eye are smooth and symmetrical. Upon ophthalmoscopic examination, the red reflex is visible in each eye and the retinae are a uniform yellowish pink with a sharply defined disc and visible vessels.

Physical assessment of the eyes follows an organized pattern. It begins with assessment of visual acuity and is followed by assessments of visual fields, muscle function, and external eye structures. The assessment of the eye concludes with the ophthalmoscopic examination.

EQUIPMENT

visual acuity charts (Snellen or E for distant vision, Rosenbaum for near vision)
opaque card or eye cover
penlight
cotton-tipped applicator
ophthalmoscope

HELPFUL HINTS

- Provide specific instructions about what is expected of the client. This would include telling the client clearly which eye to cover when conducting an assessment of visual acuity.
- The ability to read letters will determine the type of acuity chart to be used. Children and non-English-speaking clients can use the E chart or a chart with figures and images for visual acuity.
- An opaque card or eye cover is used for covering the eye in several assessments. The client must be instructed not to close or apply pressure to the covered eye.
- Several types of lighting are required. Visual acuity requires bright lighting, while the room is darkened to assess pupillary responses and the internal eye.
- The room must provide 20 feet from the Snellen chart.
- The assessment may be conducted with the client seated or standing. The nurse stands or sits at eye level with the client.
- Use Standard Precautions.

TECHNIQUES AND NORMAL FINDINGS	ABNORMAL FINDINGS SPECIAL CONSIDERATIONS

TESTING VISUAL ACUITY

DISTANT VISION

1. **Position the client.**

   - Position the client exactly 20 ft, or 6.1 meters (m), from the Snellen chart. The client may be standing or seated. The chart should be at the client's eye level.

2. **Instruct the client.**

   - Explain that you are testing distant vision. Explain that the client will read the letters from the top of the chart down to the smallest line of letters that the client can see, reading each line left to right. Explain that each line of the chart has a number that indicates what the client's vision is in relation to that of a person with normal vision (see Figure 13.7 ●).

| **TECHNIQUES AND NORMAL FINDINGS** | **ABNORMAL FINDINGS**
SPECIAL CONSIDERATIONS |

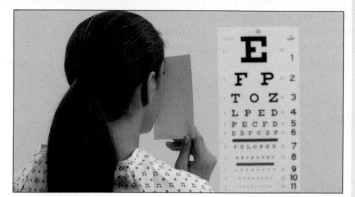

Figure 13.7 •
Testing distant vision.

TEST DISTANCE VISION

1. **Ask the client to cover one eye with the opaque card or eye cover. Tell the client to read, left to right, from the top of the chart down to the smallest line of letters that the client can see.**

2. **Ask the client to cover the other eye and to read from the top of the chart down to the smallest line of letters that the client can see.**

3. **Ask the client to read from the top of the chart down to the smallest line of letters that the client can see with both eyes uncovered.**

4. **If a client uses corrective lenses for distance vision, test first with eyeglasses or contact lenses. Then test without glasses or contact lenses.**

   • The results are recorded as a fraction. The numerator indicates the distance from the chart (20 ft). The denominator indicates the distance at which a person with normal vision can read the last line.

   • Normal vision is 20/20; therefore, at 20 ft the client can read the line numbered 20. If a client's vision is 20/30, the client reads at 20 ft what a person with normal vision reads at 30 ft. Observe while the client is reading the chart.

   • If the client is unable to read more than one half of the letters on a line, record the number of the line above.

THE SNELLEN E CHART

The Snellen E chart has Es pointing in different directions (see Figure 13.8 •).

▶ Frowning, leaning forward, and squinting indicate visual or reading difficulties.

  Inability to see objects at a distance is myopia. The smaller the fraction, the worse the vision. Vision of 20/200 is considered legal blindness.

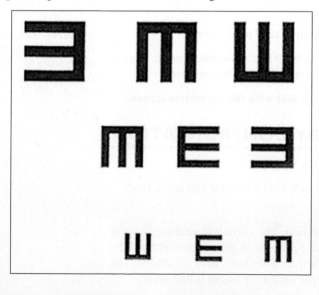

Figure 13.8 •
E chart for testing distant vision.

TECHNIQUES AND NORMAL FINDINGS

- The letter E becomes smaller as one proceeds from the top to the bottom of the chart. Numbers on each line correspond to the client's vision in relation to that of a person with normal vision that would be seen testing distant vision with the E chart.
- Repeat steps 1 to 4 as previously noted but ask the client to start at the top of the chart and to point in the direction the letter faces on each line until the client can no longer see the Es.
- Observe while the client is reading the chart.

NEAR VISION

1. Position the client.

- The client is sitting with a Rosenbaum chart held at a distance of 12 to 14 in. (30.5 to 35.5 cm) from the eyes.

2. Instruct the client.

- Explain that you are testing near vision, and the client will read the letters from the top of the card down to the smallest line the client can see. Tell the client to hold the card at the same distance throughout the test. Explain that each line on the card has a number that indicates what the client's vision is in relation to that of a person with normal vision (see Figure 13.9 ●).

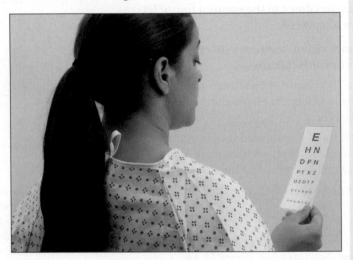

Figure 13.9 ●
Testing near vision.

TESTING NEAR VISION

1. Ask the client to cover one eye with the opaque card or eye cover.

2. Repeat the test with the other eye and then with both eyes uncovered. The results are recorded as a fraction. A normal result is 14/14 in each eye.

3. If a client uses corrective lenses for reading, test with the corrective lenses.

TESTING VISUAL FIELDS BY CONFRONTATION

1. Position the client.

- The client should be sitting 2 to 3 ft (0.6 to 0.9 m) from you and at eye level.

2. Instruct the client.

- Explain that you are testing peripheral vision. The client will alternately cover an eye and must look directly into your open eye. A pen or penlight will be moved into the client's field of vision, sequentially from four directions. The client is to indicate by saying "now" or "yes" when the object is first seen.

▶ Inability to see objects at close range is called hyperopia. Presbyopia, the inability to accommodate for near vision, is common in persons over 45 years of age.

TECHNIQUES AND NORMAL FINDINGS	ABNORMAL FINDINGS SPECIAL CONSIDERATIONS

3. Ask the client to cover one eye with a card while you cover your opposite eye with a card.

4. Holding a penlight in one hand, extend your arm upward, and advance it in from the periphery to the midline point (see Figure 13.10 ●).

▶ If the client is not able to see the object at the same time that the examiner does, there may be some peripheral vision loss. The client should be evaluated further.

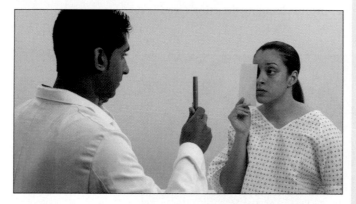

Figure 13.10 ●
Testing visual fields by confrontation.

5. Be sure to keep the penlight equidistant between the client and yourself.

6. Ask the client to report when the object is first seen. Repeat the procedure upward, toward the nose, and downward. Then repeat the entire procedure with the other eye covered. This test assumes the examiner has normal peripheral vision.

TESTING THE SIX CARDINAL FIELDS OF GAZE

1. **Position the client.**
   - The client is sitting in a comfortable position. You are at eye level with the client.

2. **Instruct the client.**
   - Explain that you will be testing eye movements and the muscles of the eye. Explain that the client must keep the head still while following a pen or penlight that you will move in several directions in front of the client's eyes.

3. **Stand about 2 ft (0.6 m) in front of the client.**

4. **Letter "H" method.**
   - Starting at midline, move the penlight to the left, then straight up, then straight down.
   - Drop your hand. Position the penlight against the midline.
   - Now move the penlight to the right, then straight up, then straight down (see Figure 13.11 ●).

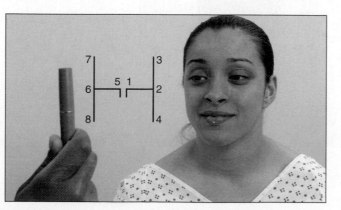

Figure 13.11 ●
Testing cardinal field of gaze.

TECHNIQUES AND NORMAL FINDINGS	ABNORMAL FINDINGS SPECIAL CONSIDERATIONS

5. Wagon wheel method.

- Start at midline move the pen or light in the direction to form a star or wagon wheel.
- Use random direction pattern to create the movement.
- Always return the light or pen to the center before changing direction (see Figure 13.12 ●).

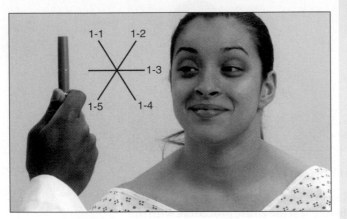

Figure 13.12 ●
Alternative method of testing cardinal field of gaze.

6. Assess the client's ability to follow your movements with the eyes (see Figure 13.11 ●). Nystagmus, rapid fluttering of the eyeball, occurs at completion of rapid lateral eye movement.

► If nystagmus occurs during testing, there could be a weakness in the extraocular muscles or cranial nerve III.

ASSESSMENT OF CORNEAL LIGHT REFLEX

1. Position the client.

- You will sit at eye level with the client.

2. Instruct the client.

- Explain that you are examining the cornea of the eyes. Instruct the client to stare straight ahead while you hold a penlight 12 in. (30.5 cm) from both eyes.

3. Shine the light into the eyes from a distance of 12 inches (see Figure 13.13 ●).

► If the reflection of light is not symmetrical, there could be a weakness in the extraocular muscles.

Figure 13.13 ●
Testing the corneal light reflex.

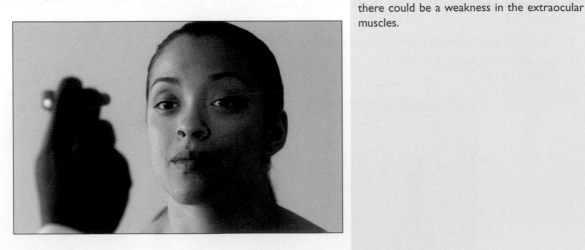

- The reflection of light should appear in the same spot on both pupils. This appears as a "twinkle" in the eye.

| **TECHNIQUES AND NORMAL FINDINGS** | **ABNORMAL FINDINGS SPECIAL CONSIDERATIONS** |

PERFORM THE COVER TEST

1. **Position the client.**
   - You should be sitting at eye level with the client.

2. **Instruct the client.**
   - Explain that this test determines the balance mechanism (fusion reflex) that keeps the eyes parallel. Explain that the client will look at a fixed point while covering each eye. You will observe the eyes.

3. **Cover one eye with a card and observe the uncovered eye, which should remain focused on the designated point.**

4. **Remove the card from the covered eye and observe the newly uncovered eye for movement. It should focus straight ahead.**

5. **Repeat the procedure with the other eye.**

▶ If there is a weakness in one of the eye muscles, the fusion reflex is blocked when one eye is covered and the weakness of the eye can be observed.

INSPECTION OF THE PUPILS

1. **Position the client.**
   - In this and all subsequent tests, you will sit at eye level with the client.

2. **Instruct the client.**
   - Explain that you will be looking at the client's eyes to assess the size and shape of the pupils.

3. **Inspect the pupils.**
   - The pupils should be round, equal in size and shape, and in the center of the eye. This is controlled by cranial nerve III.

▶ Pupils that are not round and symmetrical may indicate previous ocular surgery, increased intracranial pressure, or cranial nerve pathology.

EVALUATION OF PUPILLARY RESPONSE

1. **Instruct the client.**
   - Explain that you are testing the pupil's response to light. Tell the client that the room light must be dimmed. Explain that you will shine a light directly at each eye and that the client must stare straight ahead.

2. **Moving your penlight in from the client's side, shine light directly into one eye.**

3. **Observe the constriction in the illuminated pupil.**
   - Also observe the simultaneous reaction (**consensual constriction**) of the other pupil. The direct reaction should be faster and greater than the consensual reaction.

▶ If the illuminated pupil fails to constrict, there is a defect in the direct pupillary response. If the unilluminated pupil fails to constrict, there is a defect in the consensual response, controlled by cranial nerve III (oculomotor).

| TECHNIQUES AND NORMAL FINDINGS | ABNORMAL FINDINGS SPECIAL CONSIDERATIONS |

TESTING FOR ACCOMMODATION OF PUPIL RESPONSE

1. **Instruct the client.**
   - Explain that you are testing muscles of the eye. Tell the client to shift the gaze from the far wall to an object held 4 to 5 in. (10 to 12 cm) from the client's nose.

2. **Ask the client to stare straight ahead at a distant point.**

▶ Lack of **convergence** (turning inward of the eye) and failure of the pupils to constrict indicates dysfunction of cranial nerves III, IV, and VI.

3. **Hold a penlight about 4 to 5 in. (10 to 12 cm) from the client's nose; then ask the client to shift the gaze from the distant point to the penlight.**
   - The eyes should converge (turn inward) and the pupils should constrict as the eyes focus on the penlight. This pupillary change is **accommodation**, a change in size to adjust vision from far to near.
   - A normal response to pupillary testing is recorded as PERRLA (pupils equal, round, react to light, and accommodation).

TESTING OF THE CORNEAL REFLEX

1. **Instruct the client.**
   - Explain that you will be testing nerve stimulation to the cornea. Tell the client that you will be touching each eye gently and quickly with a wisp of cotton. The client will react by blinking the eyes. The client may experience tearing of the eyes.

2. **Take a sterile cotton ball and twist it into a very thin strand.**

3. **Using a lateral approach, gently touch the cornea on the outer aspect of each eye (see Figure 13.14 ●).**

▶ If one or both eyes fail to respond, there could be a problem with cranial nerve V, VII, or both, since cranial nerve V is sensory for this reflex, and cranial nerve VII is motor. Note that long-term use of contact lenses can diminish the corneal reflex.

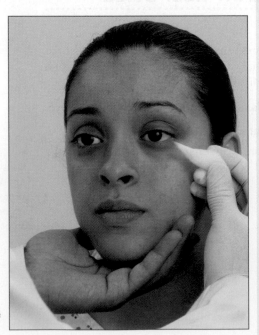

Figure 13.14 ● Approaching the eye for testing the corneal reflex.

| TECHNIQUES AND NORMAL FINDINGS | ABNORMAL FINDINGS SPECIAL CONSIDERATIONS |

4. Confirm that both eyes blink when either cornea is touched. Be sure not to touch the eyelashes or conjunctiva.

INSPECTION OF THE EXTERNAL EYE

1. Instruct the client.

- Explain that you will be examining the client's eye. You will be looking at the client's eyes and touching them to see inside the lids. Explain that you will provide specific instructions before each test.

2. Stand directly in front of the client and focus on the external structures of the eye. The eyebrows should be symmetrical in shape and the eyelashes similar in quantity and distribution. The eyebrows and eyelashes should be free of flakes and drainage.

3. With the client's eyes open, confirm that the distances between the palpebral fissures are equal. Confirm that the upper eyelid covers a small arc of the iris.

4. Confirm that the eyelids symmetrically cover the eyeballs when closed. The eyeball should be neither protruding nor sunken.

5. Gently separate the eyelids and ask the client to look up, down, and to each side. The conjunctiva should be moist and clear, with small blood vessels. The lens should be clear, and the sclera white. The irises should be round and both of the same color, although irises of different colors can be a normal finding.

6. Inspect the cornea by shining a penlight from the side across the cornea. The cornea should be clear with no irregularities. The pupils should be round and equal in size (see Figure 13.15 ●).

▶ Absence of the lateral third of the eyebrow is associated with hypothyroidism. Absent eyelashes may indicate pulling or plucking associated with obsessive-compulsive behavior.

One eyelid drooping (**ptosis**) can be caused by a dysfunction of cranial nerve III (oculomotor). Eyes that protrude beyond the supraorbital ridge can indicate a thyroid disorder; however, this trait may be normal for the client. Edema of the eyelids can be caused by allergies, heart disease, or kidney disease. Inability to move the eyelids can indicate dysfunction of the nervous system, including facial nerve paralysis.

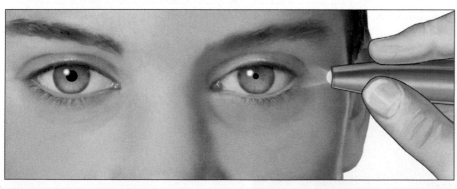

Figure 13.15 ● Inspecting the cornea.

PALPATION OF THE EYE

1. Ask the client to close both eyes.

2. Using the first two or three fingers, gently palpate the lacrimal sacs, the eyelids, and the eyeballs.

3. Confirm that there is no swelling or tenderness and that the eyeballs feel firm.

▶ Swelling may be a symptom of infection, cardiovascular problems, or renal problems.

▶ Less than firm eyeballs can be an indication of dehydration.

TECHNIQUES AND NORMAL FINDINGS

EXAMINATION OF THE CONJUNCTIVA AND SCLERA UNDER THE LOWER EYELID

1. **Evert the lower eyelid by asking the client to look down, pressing the lower lid against the lower orbital rim, then asking the client to look up (see Figure 13.16 ●).**

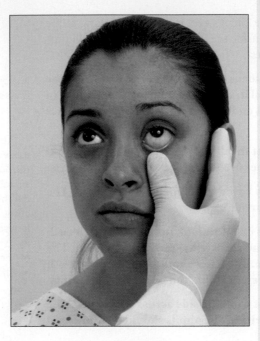

Figure 13.16 ● Inspecting the conjunctiva of the lower lid.

- The conjunctiva should be clear showing pink of the underlying tissue with no tenderness or irregularities. If you find any abnormality, examine the conjunctiva under the upper eyelid.

2. **Ask the client to close the eyes.**

3. **Evert the upper eyelid by placing a cotton-tipped applicator against the upper lid (see Figure 13.17 ●).**

▶ Inflammation and edema of the conjunctiva indicate an infection or possible foreign body.

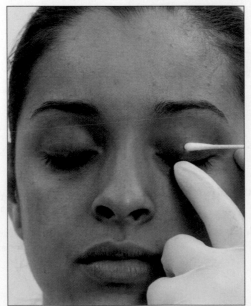

Figure 13.17 ● Step 1 of upper eyelid eversion.

TECHNIQUES AND NORMAL FINDINGS	ABNORMAL FINDINGS SPECIAL CONSIDERATIONS

4. Grasp the eyelashes and pull the eyelid downward, forward, and up over the applicator (see Figure 13.18 ●). Inspect the conjunctiva.

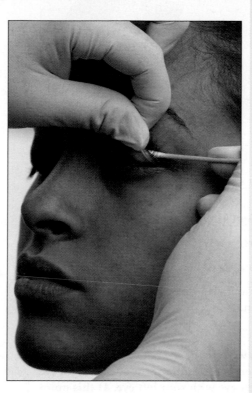

Figure 13.18 ● Step 2 of upper eyelid eversion.

5. Gently release and return the eyelid to the normal position when finished.

INSPECTION OF THE FUNDUS WITH THE OPHTHALMOSCOPE

1. Instruct the client.

- Explain that you will be using the ophthalmoscope to look into the inner deep part of the eye (**fundus**) and that the lights in the room will be dimmed. Explain that the client must stare ahead at a fixed point while you move in front with the ophthalmoscope. Tell the client to maintain a fixed gaze, as if looking through you. Explain that you will place your hand on the client's head so you both remain stable. (Refer to Chapter 6 to review the parts of the ophthalmoscope.) ○○

2. To examine the right eye, hold the ophthalmoscope in your right hand with the index finger on the lens wheel.

3. Begin with the lens on the 0 diopter. With the light on, place the ophthalmoscope over your right eye (see Figure 13.19 ●).

TECHNIQUES AND NORMAL FINDINGS

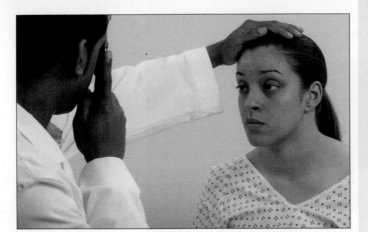

Figure 13.19 •
Approaching the
client for the
ophthalmoscopic
exam.

4. **Stand at a slight angle lateral to the client's line of vision.**

5. **Approach the client at about a 15-degree angle toward the client's nose.**

6. **Place your left hand on the client's shoulder or head.**

7. **Hold the ophthalmoscope against your head, directing the light into the client's pupil. Keep your other eye open.**

8. **Advance toward the client.**

9. **As you look into the client's pupil, you will see the *red reflex*, which is the reflection of the light off the retina. Remember to examine the client's right eye with your right eye, and the client's left eye with your left eye. At this point you may need to adjust the lens wheel to bring the ocular structures into focus. Normally, you will see no shadows or dots interrupting the red reflex. If the light strays from the pupil, you will lose the red reflex. Adjust your angle until you see the red reflex again.**

   ▶ Persistent absence of the red reflex may indicate a cataract, an opacity of the lens.

10. **Keep advancing toward the client until the ophthalmoscope is almost touching the client's eyelashes (see Figure 13.20 •).**

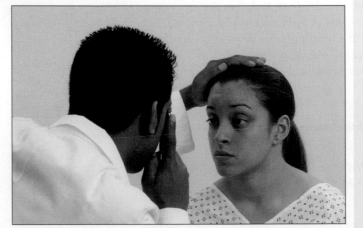

Figure 13.20 •
Examining the
eye using the
ophthalmoscope.

11. **Rotate the diopter wheel if necessary to bring the ocular fundus into focus.**

12. **If the client's vision is myopic, you will need to rotate the wheel into the minus numbers (see Figure 13.21 •).**

TECHNIQUES AND NORMAL FINDINGS	ABNORMAL FINDINGS SPECIAL CONSIDERATIONS

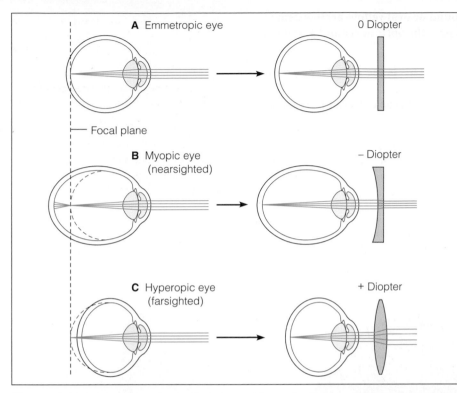

Figure 13.21 ● Use of diopter to adjust for problems of refraction. A. In the emmetropic (normal) eye, light is focused properly on the retina, and the 0 diopter is used. B. In the myopic eye, light from a distant source converges to a focal point before reaching the retina. Negative diopter numbers are used. C. In the hyperopic eye, light from a near source converges to a focal point past the retina. Positive diopter numbers are used.

13. If the client's vision is hyperopic, rotate the wheel into the plus numbers.

14. Begin to look for the optic disc by following the path of the blood vessels. As they grow larger, they lead to the optic disc on the nasal side of the retina (see Figure 13.22 ●).

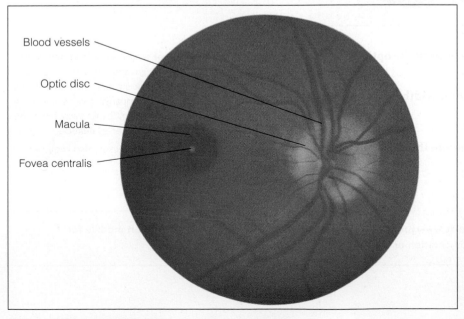

Figure 13.22 ● The optic disc.

TECHNIQUES AND NORMAL FINDINGS	ABNORMAL FINDINGS SPECIAL CONSIDERATIONS

The optic disc normally looks like a round or oval yellow-orange depression with a distinct margin. It is the site where the optic nerve and blood vessels exit the eye.

15. Follow the vessels laterally to a darker circle. This is the *macula,* or area of central vision.

    The *fovea centralis,* a small white spot located in the center of the macula, is the area of sharpest vision.

    ▶ Degeneration of the macula is common in older adults and results in impaired central vision. It may be due to hemorrhages, cysts, or other alterations.

16. Systematically inspect these structures. A crescent shape around the margin of the optic disc is a normal finding. A *scleral crescent* is an absence of pigment in the choroid and is a dull white color. A *pigment crescent,* which is black, is an accumulation of pigment in the choroid.

    ▶ Abnormalities of the retinal structures present as dark or opaque spots on the retina, an irregularly shaped optic disc, and lesions or hemorrhages on the fundus.

17. Use the optic disc as a clock face for documenting the position of a finding, and the diameter of the disc (DD) for noting its distance from the optic disc. For instance, "at 2:00, 2 DD from the disc" describes the finding in Figure 13.23 ●.

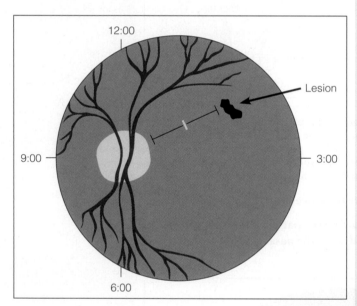

Figure 13.23 ●
Documenting a finding from the ophthalmoscopic examination.

18. Trace the path of a paired artery and vein from the optic disc to the periphery in the four quadrants of the eyeball.

19. Note the number of major vessels, color, width, and any crossing of the vessels.

20. Repeat the preceding procedure to examine the client's left eye, using your left hand and left eye.

▶ An absence of major vessels in any of the four quadrants is an abnormal finding. Constricted arteries look smaller than two thirds the diameter of accompanying veins. Crossing of the vessels more than 2 DD away from the optic disc requires further evaluation.

▶ Extremely tortuous vessels also require further evaluation.

Refer to the Companion Website at **www.prenhall.com/damico** and click on the **Documentation** module for documentation samples and documentation practice exercises.

*A*bnormalities of the eye arise for a variety of reasons and can be associated with vision, eye movement, and the internal and external structures of the eye. The following sections address abnormal findings associated with the functions and structures of the eye.

Visual Acuity

Visual acuity is dependent upon the ability of the eye to refract light rays and focus them upon the retina. The shape of the eye is one determinant in the refractive and focusing processes of vision.

Emmetropia is the normal refractive condition of the eye in which light rays are brought into sharp focus on the retina (see Figure 13.24 ●).

Myopia (nearsightedness) is generally inherited and occurs when the eye is longer than normal. As a result, light rays focus in front of the retina (see Figure 13.25 ●).

Hyperopia (farsightedness) is also an inherited condition in which the eye is shorter than normal. In hyperopia the light rays focus behind the retina (see Figure 13.26 ●).

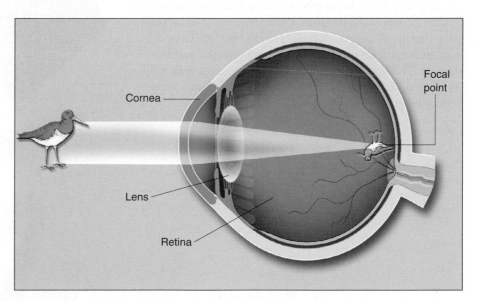

Figure 13.24 ● Emmetropia.

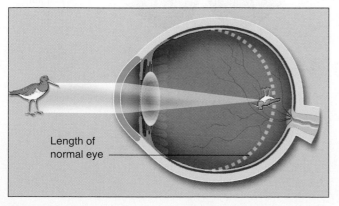

Figure 13.25 ● Myopia.

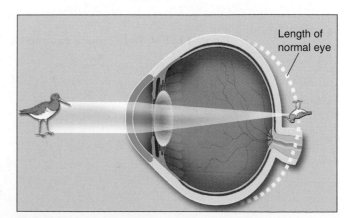

Figure 13.26 ● Hyperopia.

Astigmatism is often a familial condition in which the refraction of light is spread over a wide area rather than on a distinct point on the retina. In the normal eye, the cornea is round in shape, whereas in astigmatism the cornea curves more in one direction than another. As a result, light is refracted and focused on two focal points on or near the retina. Vision in astigmatism may be blurred or doubled (see Figure 13.27 ●).

Presbyopia is an age-related condition in which the lens of the eye loses the ability to accommodate. As a result, light is focused behind the retina, and focus on near objects becomes difficult.

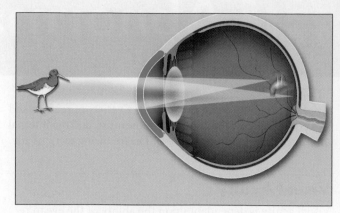

Figure 13.27 ● Astigmatism.

Visual Fields

The **visual field** refers to the total area in which objects can be seen in the periphery while the eye remains focused on a central point. Testing visual fields enables the examiner to detect and map losses in peripheral vision. The mapping aids in determination of the problem. Changes in visual fields accompany damage to the retina, lesions in the optic nerve or chiasm, increased intraocular pressure, and retinal vascular damage. The normal visual pathways and loss of visual fields in relation to the previously-mentioned conditions are depicted in Figures 13.28 ● and 13.29 ●, respectively.

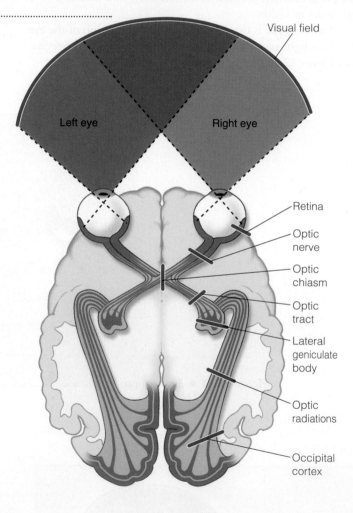

Figure 13.28 ● Visual pathway abnormalities.

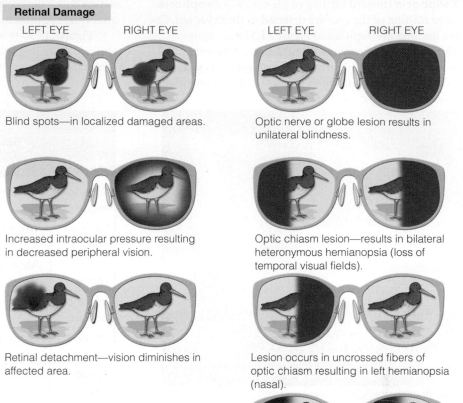

Retinal Damage

LEFT EYE   RIGHT EYE

Blind spots—in localized damaged areas.

Increased intraocular pressure resulting in decreased peripheral vision.

Retinal detachment—vision diminishes in affected area.

LEFT EYE   RIGHT EYE

Optic nerve or globe lesion results in unilateral blindness.

Optic chiasm lesion—results in bilateral heteronymous hemianopsia (loss of temporal visual fields).

Lesion occurs in uncrossed fibers of optic chiasm resulting in left hemianopsia (nasal).

Right optic tract or optic radiation lesion resulting in loss of right nasal and left temporal fields. Homonymous hemianopsia.

Figure 13.29 ● Client's view with visual field loss.

Cardinal Fields of Gaze

Eye movement is controlled by six extraocular muscles and by cranial nerves III, IV, and VI. Muscle weakness or dysfunction of a cranial nerve can be identified by assessing the fields of gaze, assessing corneal light reflex, and performing the cover test.

Strabismus is a condition in which the axes of the eyes cannot be directed at the same object. Strabismus can be classified as convergent (esotropia) in which the eye deviates inward, and divergent (exotropia) in which the deviation is outward. In strabismus, light can be seen to reflect in different axes (see Figure 13.30 ●).

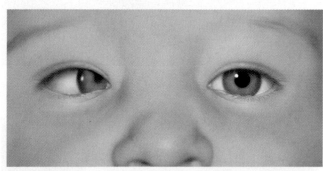

Esotropia

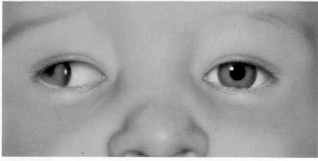

Figure 13.30 ● Strabismus.   Exotropia

Esophoria (inward turning of the eye) and **exophoria** (outward turning of the eye) are detected in the cover test. Esotropic findings are depicted in Figure 13.31 ●.

Nonparallel eye movements and failure of the eyes to follow in a certain direction are indicative of problems with extraocular muscles or cranial nerves. Figure 13.32 ● provides details about the specific muscles and nerves associated with abnormal eye movement.

Figures 13.33 through 13.53 ● include information about abnormalities in pupillary response, structures of the external eye, and the fundus of the eye.

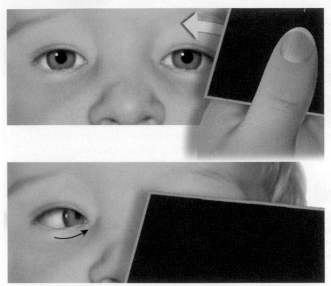

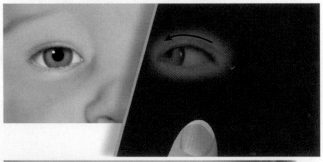

A Right, or uncovered eye, is weaker.

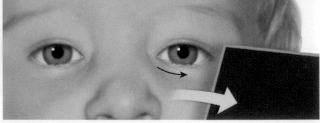

B Left, or covered eye, is weaker.

Figure 13.31 ● Cover test.

	Disruption of Function	
Muscle	**Cranial Nerve**	**Results**
Superior rectus	Oculomotor	Inability to move eye upward or temporally
Superior oblique	Trochlear	Inability to move eye down or nasally
Lateral rectus	Abducens	Inability to move eye temporally
Inferior oblique	Oculomotor	Inability to move eye upward or temporally
Inferior rectus	Oculomotor	Inability to move eye downward or temporally
Medial rectus	Oculomotor	Inability to move eye nasally

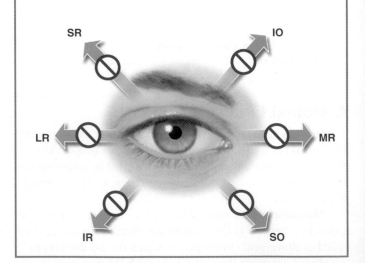

Figure 13.32 ● Extraocular muscle abnormalities.

ABNORMAL PUPILLARY RESPONSE

Adie's Pupil

Also known as tonic pupil, Adie's pupil is unilateral and slug-gish pupillary response (see Figure 13.33 ●).

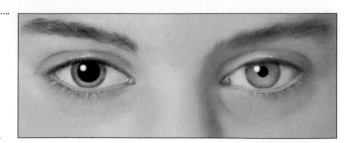

Figure 13.33 ● Tonic pupil (Adie's pupil).

Argyll Robertson Pupils

Argyll Robertson pupils exist bilaterally and are small, irregu-lar, and nonreactive to light (see Figure 13.34 ●). These occur with central nervous system disorders including tumor, syphilis, and narcotic use.

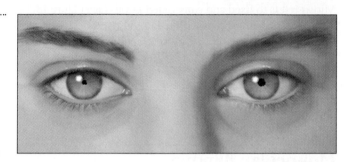

Figure 13.34 ● Argyll Robertson pupils.

Anisocoria

Anisocoria is unequal pupillary size, which may be a normal finding or may indicate central nervous system disease (see Figure 13.35 ●).

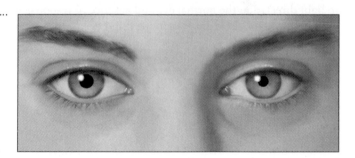

Figure 13.35 ● Anisocoria.

Cranial Nerve III Damage

Cranial nerve III damage results in a unilaterally dilated pupil (see Figure 13.36 ●). There is no reaction to light. Ptosis may be seen.

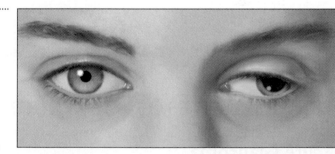

Figure 13.36 ● Cranial nerve III damage.

Horner's Syndrome

Horner's syndrome is a result of blockage of sympathetic nerve stimulation. Findings include unilateral, small regular pupil that is nonreactive to light (see Figure 13.37 ●). Ptosis and anhidrosis of the same side accompany the pupillary signs.

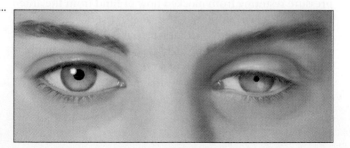

Figure 13.37 ● Horner's syndrome.

Mydriasis

Mydriasis refers to fixed and dilated pupils (see Figure 13.38 ●). This condition may occur with sympathetic nerve stimulation, glaucoma, central nervous system damage, or deep anesthesia.

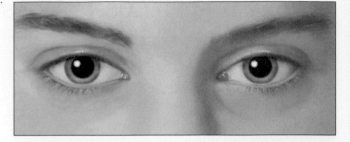

Figure 13.38 ● Mydriasis.

Miosis

Miosis refers to fixed and constricted pupils (see Figure 13.39 ●). This condition may occur with the use of narcotics, with damage to the pons, or as a result of treatment for glaucoma.

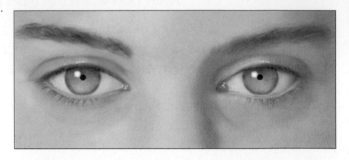

Figure 13.39 ● Miosis.

Monocular Blindness

Monocular blindness results in direct and consensual response to light directed in the normal eye and absence of response in either eye when light is directed in the blind eye (see Figure 13.40 ●).

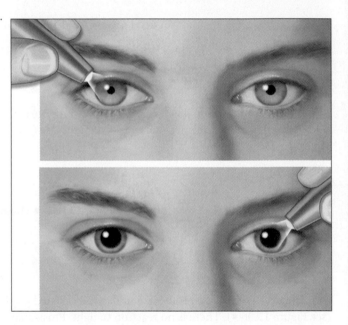

Figure 13.40 ● Monocular blindness.

ABNORMALITIES OF THE STRUCTURES OF THE EXTERNAL EYE

Acute Glaucoma

Acute glaucoma is a result of sudden increase in intraocular pressure resulting from blocked flow of fluid from the anterior chamber. The pupil is oval in shape and dilated (see Figure 13.41 ●). There is circumcorneal redness. The cornea appears cloudy and steamy. Pain is sudden in onset and is accompanied by decrease in vision and halos around lights. Acute glaucoma requires immediate intervention.

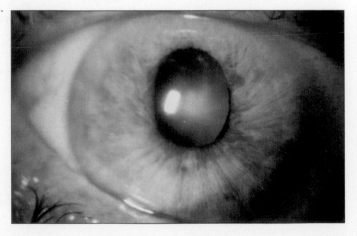

Figure 13.41 ● Acute glaucoma.

Basal Cell Carcinoma

Basal cell carcinoma has a papular appearance (see Figure 13.42 ●). This form of cancer is usually seen on the lower lid and medial canthus.

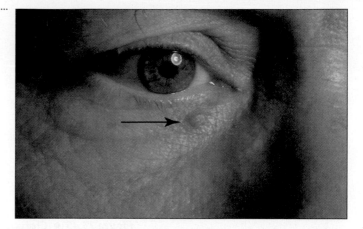

Figure 13.42 ● Basal cell carcinoma.

Blepharitis

Blepharitis is inflammation of the eyelids (see Figure 13.43 ●). Staphylococcal infection leads to red, scaly, and crusted lids. The eye burns, itches, and tears.

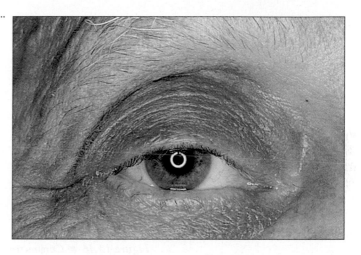

Figure 13.43 ● Blepharitis.

Cataract

A cataract is an opacity in the lens (see Figure 13.44 ●). It usually occurs in aging.

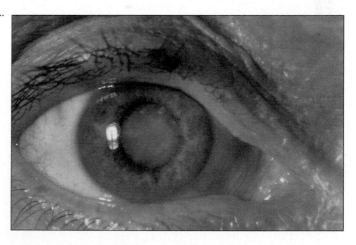

Figure 13.44 ● Cataract.

Chalazion

A chalazion is a firm, nontender nodule on the eyelid, arising from infection of the meibomian gland (see Figure 13.45 ●). It is not painful unless inflamed.

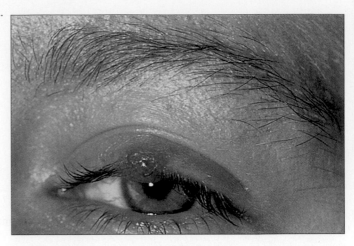

Figure 13.45 ● Chalazion.

Conjunctivitis

Conjunctivitis is an infection of the conjunctiva usually due to bacteria or virus but which may result from chemical exposure (see Figure 13.46 ●).

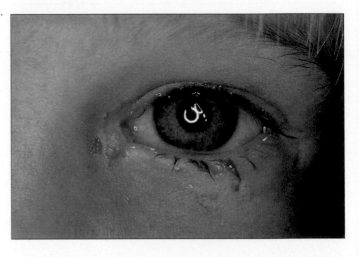

Figure 13.46 ● Conjunctivitis.

Ectropion

Ectropion is eversion of the lower eyelid caused by muscle weakness. The palpebral conjunctiva is exposed (see Figure 13.47 ●).

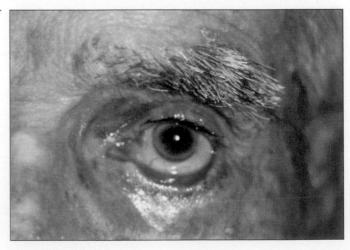

Figure 13.47 ● Ectropion.

Entropion

Entropion is inversion of the lid and lashes caused by muscle spasm of the eyelid (see Figure 13.48 ●). Friction from lashes can cause corneal irritation.

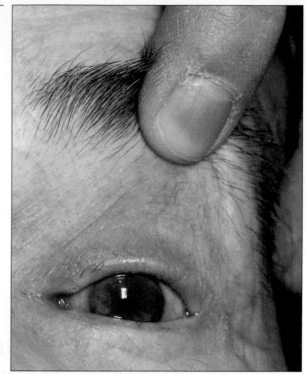

Figure 13.48 ● Entropion.

Hordeolum (Stye)

A hordeolum or stye is a result of a staphylococcal infection of hair follicles on the margin of the lids (see Figure 13.49 ●). The affected eye is swollen, red, and painful.

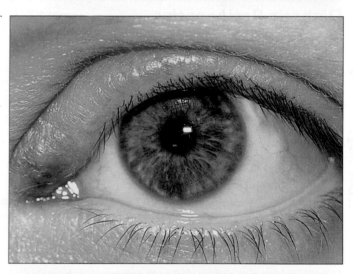

Figure 13.49 ● Hordeolum (stye).

Iritis

Iritis is a serious disorder characterized by redness around the iris and cornea (see Figure 13.50 ●). The pupil is often irregular. Vision is decreased and the client experiences deep aching pain.

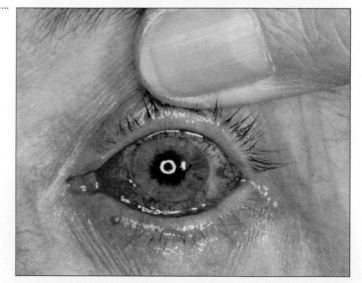

Figure 13.50 ● Iritis.

Periorbital Edema

Periorbital edema refers to swollen, puffy lids (see Figure 13.51 ●). Periorbital edema occurs with crying, infection, and systemic problems including kidney failure, heart failure, and allergy.

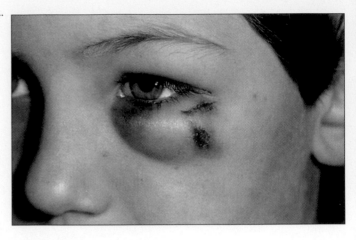

Figure 13.51 ● Periorbital edema.

Ptosis

Ptosis refers to drooping of the eyelid. This occurs with cranial nerve damage or systemic neuromuscular weakness.

ABNORMALITIES OF THE FUNDUS

Diabetic Retinopathy

Diabetic retinopathy refers to the changes that occur in the retina and vasculature of the retina including microaneurysms, hemorrhages, macular edema, and retinal exudates (see Figure 13.52 ●).

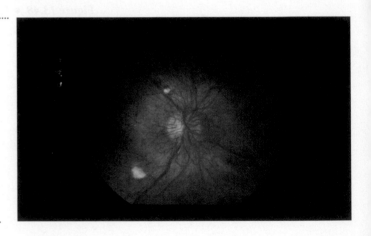

Figure 13.52 ● Diabetic retinopathy.

Hypertensive Retinopathy

Hypertensive retinopathy refers to the changes in the retina and vasculature of the retina in response to elevations in blood pressure that accompany atherosclerosis, heart disease, and kidney disease. The changes include flame hemorrhages, nicking of vessels, and "cotton wool" spots that arise from infarction of the nerve fibers.

Macular Degeneration

Age-related macular degeneration (ARMD) is a degenerative condition of the macula, the central retina (see Figure 13.53 ●). Central vision is lost gradually while peripheral vision remains intact. The eyes are affected at different rates.

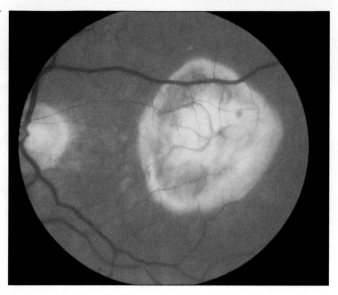

Figure 13.53 ● Macular degeneration.

Health Promotion

HEALTHY PEOPLE 2010

FOCUS AREA	PREVALENCE	OBJECTIVES	ACTIONS
Visual Impairment	• Eighty million people in the United States have diseases leading to blindness. • Three million people in the United States have low vision. • Impaired vision is a frequent cause of disability. • The most frequent causes of visual impairment are diabetic retinopathy, cataracts, glaucoma, and age-related macular degeneration (ARMD). • Blindness in African Americans is most frequently caused by glaucoma. • Almost 25% of the population in the United States has myopia.	• Increase the number of persons who have dilated eye exams. • Increase vision screening in preschool children. • Reduce visual impairment due to disease.	• Screening. • Education about eye health and eye examination. • Early detection and treatment programs. • Education about risks. • Diabetes education and treatment.

CLIENT EDUCATION

The following are physiological, behavioral, and cultural factors that affect the health of the eye across the life span. Several factors related to the eye are cited in *Healthy People 2010*. The nurse provides advice and education to promote and maintain health and reduce risks associated with the aforementioned factors that impact the eye across the life span.

LIFE SPAN CONSIDERATIONS

RISK FACTORS

- Children with fetal alcohol syndrome experience changes in the structure of the eye, ptosis, and visual disturbances including reduced visual acuity, nystagmus, cataracts, and strabismus.
- Visual disturbances in children are often discovered as a result of learning or behavioral problems.

- Presbyopia, the gradual decrease in near vision, occurs in all individuals with an onset at around age 45.
- Older adults experience a decrease in lacrimal secretions resulting in a dryness of the eyes.
- Senile ptosis and ectropion or entropion accompany loss of muscle tone in older adults.

CLIENT EDUCATION

- Discuss risks of alcohol abuse with females of childbearing age.
- Provide information about support services and agencies to assist those with alcohol addiction.
- Provide information to parents about the development of vision from infancy to adolescence.
- Guide parents to recognize symptoms of problems with the structures of the eye or neuromuscular functions.
- Provide information about lubricating agents for older adults with drying of the eyes.
- Provide information about recommendations for eye examinations across the life span.

CULTURAL CONSIDERATIONS

RISK FACTORS

- African Americans are at higher risk for glaucoma than other racial groups.
- Diabetic retinopathy is the leading cause of blindness in the United States. Retinal changes occur in diabetes types 1 and 2.
- Type 2 diabetes occurs more frequently in African Americans, Asian Americans, Hispanic Americans, and Native Americans than in Caucasians.

CLIENT EDUCATION

- Instruct clients with diabetes or those with a family history of diabetes to have a vision and retinal examination annually.

ENVIRONMENTAL CONSIDERATIONS

RISK FACTORS

- Environmental factors including pollutants and ultraviolet light can affect the health of the eye and vision.
- Medications can affect the integrity and function of the eye.

CLIENT EDUCATION

- Advise clients to use sunglasses to avoid environmental hazards.
- Instruct the client regarding prescription and over-the-counter (OTC) medications in terms of proper instillation of eye medications as well as side effects and potential interactions between and among medications.

BEHAVIORAL CONSIDERATIONS

RISK FACTOR

- Trauma to the eye can occur during recreational activities, in the workplace, and in the home.

CLIENT EDUCATION

- Provide information about eye safety in the home, in the workplace, and during recreational activity including the use of protective eyewear.
- Instruct the client in emergency eye care for substances in the eye, chemical splash, cuts in or near the eye, and blunt injury to the eye.

Application Through Critical Thinking

CASE STUDY

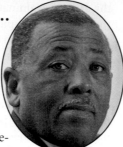

John Jerome is a 45-year-old African American male who made an appointment for an annual employment physical examination. Mr. Jerome completed a written questionnaire in preparation for his meeting with a healthcare professional. He checked "none" for all categories of family history of disease except diabetes. He indicated that he knew of no changes in his health since his last examination.

The following observations were made during the initial encounter with Mr. Jerome. A tall, African American male wearing eyeglasses entered the room. He turned his head to the left and right and looked about the room before sitting across from the examiner. The client had some redness in the sclera of both eyes. During the interview, the client revealed that his last eye examination occurred 6 months ago, and he received a prescription for new glasses. He stated that he was still having a problem with the new glasses and needed to have them checked. When asked to describe the problem, Mr. Jerome replied, "I just don't feel right with these glasses, and these are the second pair in a little over a year." He fur-

ther stated, "I just think I am overworking my eyes lately. I need to rest them more than ever and I have had some headaches. I thought the glasses would help, but it hasn't gotten better." The client denied any other problems. In response to inquiries about family history, he reported that his mother had diabetes but had no problems with her eyes. He didn't know of any other eye problems in his family, except his mother had told him that an aunt of hers had been blind for some time. He reiterated that his only problem of late had been "this thing with my glasses, otherwise I feel fine."

The physical examination revealed the following:

- Vital signs: BP 128/84—P 88—RR 22
- Height 6′3″, weight 188 lb
- Eyeball firm to palpation
- Moderately dilated pupils
- Cupping of the optic disc

▶ Complete Documentation

The following information is summarized from the case study. **SUBJECTIVE DATA:** Visit for annual employment physical examination. Negative family history except diabetes. No changes in health since last examination. Last eye examination 6 months ago—result prescription for new glasses. Stated he

ASSESSMENT FORM

HISTORY	No	Yes	Describe
Visual disorder		X	(glasses) see below—aunt blind
Diabetes		X	(mother)
Hypertension	X		
Glaucoma	X		
Correction	Eyeglasses—"I just don't feel right"		
Last exam	6 months ago		
Other	"Headache"		
PHYSICAL FINDINGS			
VS	BP 128/84—P 88—RR 22		
	Ht. 6′3″ Wt. 188lb		
Eyeball	Firm		
Pupils	Dilated		
Optic disc	Cupping		

was having a problem with the new glasses. "I don't feel right with them." Stated, "I think I'm overworking my eyes lately. I thought the new glasses would help, but it hasn't gotten better." History of aunt with blindness.

OBJECTIVE DATA: Turns head to left and right and looked around room before sitting across from examiner. Scleral redness bilaterally. Eyeball firm to palpation. Pupils moderate dilation. Cupping of optic disc. Height 6′3″, weight 188 lb. VS: BP 128/84—P 88—RR 22.

▶ Critical Thinking Questions

1. What conclusions would the nurse reach based on the data?
2. How was this conclusion formulated?
3. What information is missing?
4. Describe the priority for this client and the options that would apply.
5. Create a plan to address the problem.

▶ Applying Nursing Diagnoses

1. *Disturbed visual sensory perception* is a nursing diagnosis in the NANDA taxonomy (see Appendix A ⚭). Identify the data in the case study for John Jerome that supports this diagnosis.
2. *Anxiety* and *denial* are included as nursing diagnoses in the NANDA taxonomy (see Appendix A ⚭). Is there data in the case study to support these diagnoses? If so, identify the data.

3. Use the NANDA taxonomy in Appendix A to identify additional diagnoses for John Jerome. ⚭

▶ Prepare Teaching Plan

LEARNING NEED: The data in the case study revealed that Mr. Jerome was experiencing eye problems and had a family history of diabetes and blindness. Because of his history, he would be tested for diabetes and screened for diabetic retinopathy. His eye examination revealed cupping of the optic disc and slightly dilated pupils, both of which are associated with glaucoma. Blindness can occur with glaucoma and may have caused his aunt's blindness. Mr. Jerome will be referred for further evaluation of two suggested problems.

The case study provides data that is representative of risks, symptoms, and behaviors of many individuals. Therefore, the following teaching plan is based on the need to provide information to members of any community about glaucoma.

GOAL: The participants in this learning program will have increased awareness about glaucoma and follow recommendations for eye care.

OBJECTIVES: At the completion of this learning session, the participants will be able to:

1. Discuss glaucoma.
2. Identify risk factors associated with glaucoma.
3. List the diagnostic tests for glaucoma.
4. Describe recommendations for eye care.

APPLICATION OF OBJECTIVE 2: Identify risk factors associated with glaucoma

Content	Teaching Strategy	Evaluation
• African Americans. Glaucoma is six to eight times more common in African Americans.	• Lecture	• Written examination.
• Age. Individuals over the age of 60 are six times more likely to get glaucoma than younger people.	• Discussion	May use short answer, fill-in, or multiple-choice items or a combination of items.
• Heredity. Individuals with a family history, especially immediate family, of glaucoma are at greater risk. Family history increases risk four to nine times.	• Audiovisual materials • Printed materials Lecture is appropriate when disseminating information to large groups.	If these are short and easy to evaluate, the learner receives immediate feedback.
• Steroid use. Some evidence links glaucoma with steroid use. It is associated with high doses of steroids, for example, that would be used for severe asthma.	Discussion allows participants to bring up concerns and to raise questions. Audiovisual materials such as illustrations of the structures of the eye reinforce verbal presentation.	
• Eye injury. Blunt trauma such as occurs with a blow to the head or blunt trauma to the eye in baseball or boxing can cause glaucoma immediately or years later.	Printed material, especially to be taken away with learners, allows review, reinforcement, and reading at the learner's pace.	

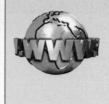

Please refer to the Companion Website at www.prenhall.com/damico and click on Chapter 13, the Application Through Critical Thinking module, to complete the following activities related to this case study:
▶ **Critical Thinking questions**
▶ **Extended Nursing Diagnosis challenge**
▶ **Documentation activity**
▶ **Teaching Plan for Objectives 1, 3, and 4**

EXPLORE MediaLink

Additional resources for this chapter are found on the Student CD-ROM accompanying this textbook and on the Companion Website.

CD-ROM CONTENT

Content for this chapter includes:
Objectives
Key Concepts
NCLEX-RN® Review Questions
Model Documentation Forms
Audio Glossary
Animations
  Eye Orbit Anatomy
Games and Challenges
Head-to-Toe Physical Examination Video

COMPANION WEBSITE CONTENT

www.prenhall.com/damico

Content for this chapter includes:
Objectives
NCLEX-RN® Review Questions
Client Interaction Case Study Challenge

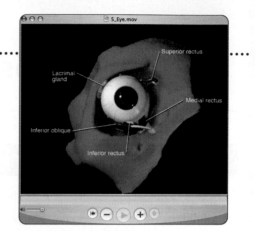

Application Through Critical Thinking
  Case Study Teaching Plan Challenge
MediaLinks
MediaLink Application
Tool Box
  Chapter Documentation Form Example
  Health Promotion
    Healthy People 2010
    Client Education
New York Times

14

Ears, Nose, Mouth, and Throat

MEDIALINK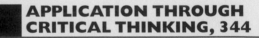

www.prenhall.com/damico

The CD-ROM in the back of this textbook and the Media-Link website contain NCLEX-RN® review questions, interactive exercises, case study challenges, animations, videos, documentation and checklist forms, and review materials. For a complete listing of the media content specific to Chapter 14, see the Explore MediaLink at the end of the chapter.

*T*he structures of the ear, nose, mouth, and throat are responsible for the senses of hearing, smell, and taste. Each of these body systems will be discussed in this chapter and again when describing the neurologic assessment in Chapter 24. ⊕

The interrelationships of the senses, and their structures, provide data for several body systems. For example, the sense of smell in the nose also impacts the respiratory and digestive systems. Hearing and oral health are two of the focus areas in *Healthy People 2010*. Goals within these focus areas include improvement in hearing and the prevention and control of oral diseases and conditions as discussed in the *Healthy People 2010* feature on page 343.

ANATOMY AND PHYSIOLOGY REVIEW

The anatomical structures of the ear, nose, mouth, and throat include the internal and external ear, the nose and sinuses, the oral cavity, and the pharynx (throat). Each of the structures will be described in the following sections.

EAR

The ear is the sensory organ that functions in hearing and equilibrium. It is divided into the external, middle, and inner ear. The external portion, or what most people think of as the ear, is called the **auricle** or **pinna**. It has a shell of cartilage covered with skin that funnels sound into the meatus (opening) of the external auditory canal.

External Ear

Figure 14.1 ● depicts the surface anatomy of the external ear. The external large rim of the auricle is called the **helix**. The **tragus** is a stiff projection that protects the anterior meatus of the auditory canal. The **lobule** of the ear is a small flap of flesh at the inferior end

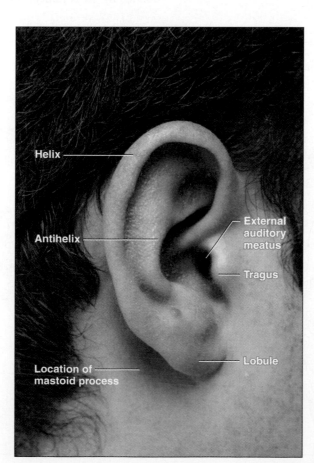

Helix

Antihelix

External auditory meatus

Tragus

Lobule

Location of mastoid process

Figure 14.1 ● External ear.

of the auricle. The external auditory canal is about 1 in. in length, is S-shaped, and leads to the middle ear. It is lined with glands that secrete a yellow-brown wax called **cerumen.** These secretions lubricate and protect the ear. The functions of chewing and talking help move the cerumen in the canal. The mastoid process, part of the temporal bone of the skull, is adjacent to the cavity of the middle ear. It contains many air cells and is assessed with the ear. This process has no role in hearing or balance. The mastoid process may become infected following ear infections in the adult.

Middle Ear

The external ear and middle ear are separated by the **tympanic membrane** or eardrum (see Figure 14.2 ●). This thin, translucent membrane is pearly gray in color and lies obliquely in the canal. Sound waves entering the auditory canal strike the membrane, causing it to vibrate. The vibrations are transferred to the **ossicles,** or bones of the middle ear: the malleus, the incus, and the stapes. The ossicles, in turn, transfer the vibration to the oval window of the inner ear. Note that the malleus projects inferiorly and laterally and can be seen through the translucent tympanic membrane when viewed with the otoscope. The **eustachian tube** or auditory tube connects the middle ear with the nasopharynx. These tubes help to equalize air pressure on both sides of the tympanic membrane. The middle ear functions to conduct sound vibrations from the external ear to the inner ear. It also protects the inner ear by reducing loud sound vibrations.

Inner Ear

The inner ear contains the bony labyrinth, which consists of a central cavity called the vestibule, three semicircular canals responsible for the sense of equilibrium, and the **cochlea,** a spiraling chamber that contains the receptors for hearing. Impulses from the equilibrium receptors of the inner ear are sent via the eighth cranial nerve to the brain. Responses are then initiated to activate the eyes and muscles of the body to maintain balance. The cochlea transmits sound vibrations to the auditory nerve (cranial nerve VIII), which in turn carries the impulse to the auditory cortex in the temporal lobe of the brain for interpretation as hearing.

The major functions of the ears are collecting and transporting sound vibrations to the brain and maintaining the sense of equilibrium.

NOSE AND SINUSES

The nose is a triangular projection of bone and cartilage situated midline on the face (see Figure 14.3 ●). It is the only externally visible organ of the respiratory system. During inspiration, air enters the nasal cavity where it is filtered, warmed, and moistened before it moves toward the trachea and lungs.

The nose consists of external and internal structures. Externally, the bridge of the nose is on the superior aspect of the nose, medial to each orbit of the eyes. Inferior to the bridge and free of attachment to the face is the tip of the nose. The nares, two oval external openings at the base of the nose, are surrounded by the columella and ala structures of cartilage. Each

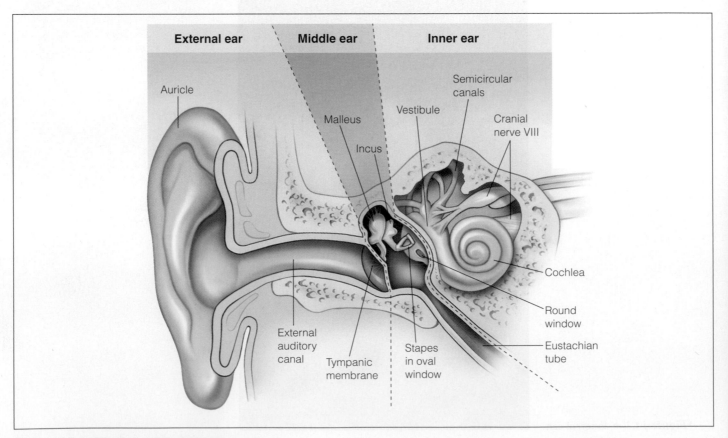

Figure 14.2 ● The three parts of the ear.

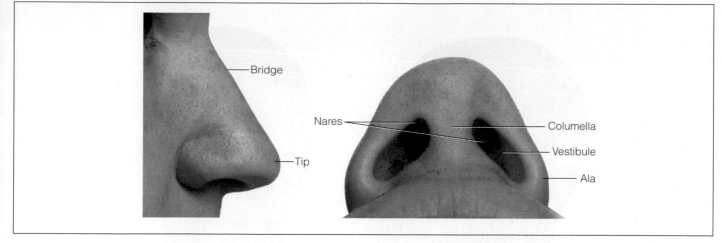

Figure 14.3 ● The nose.

nare widens into the internal vestibule and nasal cavity. The nasal septum is a continuation of the columella dividing the nose into a right and left side.

The nasal mucosa with its rich blood supply helps filter inspired air and has a redder appearance than the oral mucosa. Three turbinates (superior, middle, and inferior) project from the medial wall into each side of the nasal cavity. These bony projections, covered with nasal mucosa, add surface area for cleaning, moistening, and warming air entering the respiratory tract. Each side of the posterior nasal cavity opens into the nasopharynx (see Figure 14.4 ●).

The olfactory cells located in the roof of the nasal cavity form filaments that connect to the olfactory nerve (cranial nerve I) and are responsible for the sense of smell.

The **paranasal sinuses** are mucous-lined, air-filled cavities that surround the nasal cavity and perform the same air-processing functions of filtration, moistening, and warming.

They are named for the bones of the skull in which they are contained: sphenoid, frontal, ethmoid, and maxillary. The frontal and maxillary sinuses are accessible to examination and are discussed later in this chapter (see Figure 14.5 ●).

The major functions of the nose and sinuses are the following:

- Providing an airway for respiration
- Filtering, warming, and humidifying air flowing into the respiratory tract
- Providing resonance for the voice
- Housing the receptors for olfaction

MOUTH

The oral cavity, an oval-shaped cavity, is the beginning of the alimentary canal and digestive system (see Figure 14.6 ●). The oral cavity is divided into two parts by the teeth: the vestibule and the mouth. The vestibule, the anterior and smaller of the two regions,

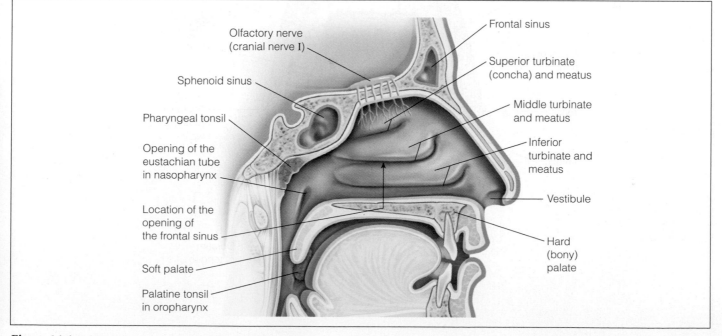

Figure 14.4 ● Internal structure of the nose—lateral view.

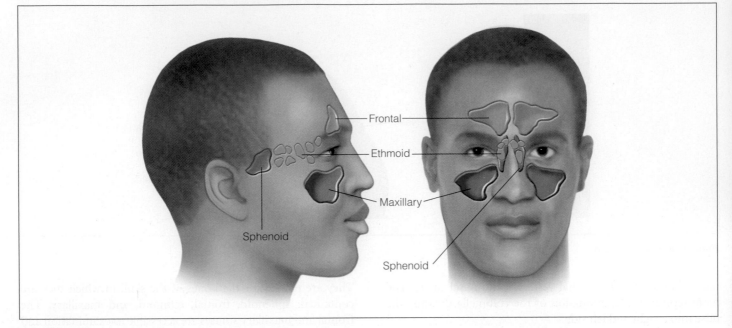

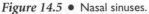
Figure 14.5 ● Nasal sinuses.

is composed of the lips, the buccal mucosa, the outer surface of the gums and teeth, and the cheeks. At the posterior aspect of the teeth, the mouth is formed and includes the tongue, the hard and soft palate, the **uvula**, and the mandibular arch and maxillary arch.

The lips are folds of skin that cover the underlying muscle. They help keep food in place when chewing and play a role in speech.

The cheeks form the side of the face and are continuous with the lips. Like the lips, the skin covers the underlying muscle. Both the lips and cheeks are lined internally with mucous membranes.

The gingivae or gums are bands of fibrous tissue that surround each tooth. The gums cover the mandibular and maxillary arches.

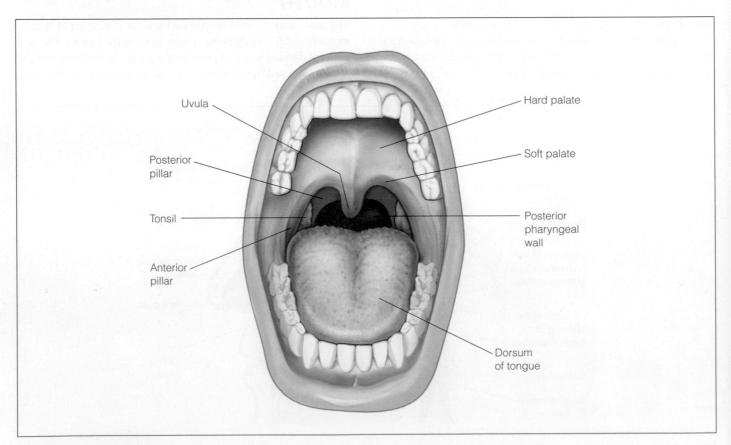

Figure 14.6 ● Oral cavity.

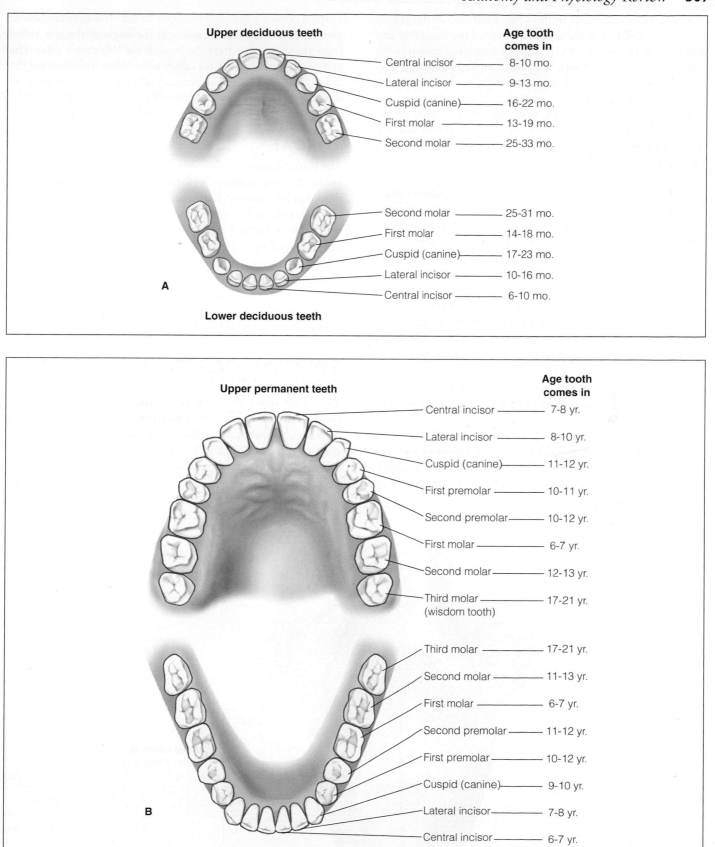

Upper deciduous teeth

	Age tooth comes in
Central incisor	8-10 mo.
Lateral incisor	9-13 mo.
Cuspid (canine)	16-22 mo.
First molar	13-19 mo.
Second molar	25-33 mo.

	Age tooth comes in
Second molar	25-31 mo.
First molar	14-18 mo.
Cuspid (canine)	17-23 mo.
Lateral incisor	10-16 mo.
Central incisor	6-10 mo.

A

Lower deciduous teeth

Upper permanent teeth

	Age tooth comes in
Central incisor	7-8 yr.
Lateral incisor	8-10 yr.
Cuspid (canine)	11-12 yr.
First premolar	10-11 yr.
Second premolar	10-12 yr.
First molar	6-7 yr.
Second molar	12-13 yr.
Third molar (wisdom tooth)	17-21 yr.

	Age tooth comes in
Third molar	17-21 yr.
Second molar	11-13 yr.
First molar	6-7 yr.
Second premolar	11-12 yr.
First premolar	10-12 yr.
Cuspid (canine)	9-10 yr.
Lateral incisor	7-8 yr.
Central incisor	6-7 yr.

B

Lower permanent teeth

Figure 14.7 ● Deciduous and permanent teeth.

Thirty-two permanent teeth in the adult and 20 deciduous teeth in the child sit in the alveoli sockets of the mandible and maxilla (see Figure 14.7 ●). The enamel-covered crown is the visible portion of the tooth. The root, embedded in the jawbone, helps hold the tooth in place. Teeth are used for biting and chewing of food.

The tongue, the organ for taste, sits on the floor of the mouth. Its base sits on the hyoid bone. The anterior portion of the tongue is attached to the floor of the mouth by the frenulum. The ventral surface (undersurface) of the tongue is smooth with visible vessels. The dorsal (top) surface of the tongue is rough and supports the papillae. Papillae contain the taste buds and assist with moving food in the mouth. Taste buds are distributed throughout the tongue and are innervated by the facial and glossopharyngeal nerves (see Figure 14.8 ●). The tongue also assists with speech and swallowing. These actions are stimulated by the hypoglossal nerve (cranial nerve XII).

Hard and soft palates form the roof of the mouth. The hard **palate**, formed by bones, is the anterior portion of the roof of the mouth. The soft palate, formed by muscle, does not have a bony structure and is the posterior and somewhat mobile aspect of the roof of the mouth. The uvula hangs from the free edge of the soft palate. The uvula and soft palate move with swallowing, breathing, and phonation and are innervated by cranial nerves IX and X.

Parotid, submandibular, and sublingual salivary glands are responsible for the production of saliva (see Figure 14.9 ●). The parotid glands are situated anterior to the ear within the cheek. Saliva enters the mouth via Stensen's duct located in the buccal mucosa opposite the second upper molar. The submandibular glands sit beneath the mandible at the angle of the jaw. Saliva from these glands enters the mouth via Wharton's duct. The orifice of these ducts is on either side of the frenulum on the floor of the mouth. The sublingual salivary glands, the smallest of the glands, are situated in the floor of the mouth and have many ducts that empty into the floor of the mouth.

THROAT

The throat, known as the pharynx, connects the nose, mouth, larynx, and esophagus. The three sections of the throat are the nasopharynx (behind the nose), the oropharynx (behind the mouth), and the laryngopharynx (behind the larynx). The nasopharynx is behind the nose and above the soft palate. The adenoids and openings of the eustachian tubes are located in the nasopharynx.

The oropharynx is behind the mouth and below the nasopharynx. It extends to the epiglottis and serves as a passageway for air and food. The tonsils are located behind the pillars (palatopharyngeal folds) on either side.

SPECIAL CONSIDERATIONS

The nurse must be aware that variations in findings from health assessment occur in relation to age, developmental level, race, ethnicity, work history, living conditions, socioeconomics, and emotional well-being. The following sections describe some factors to consider when collecting subjective and objective data.

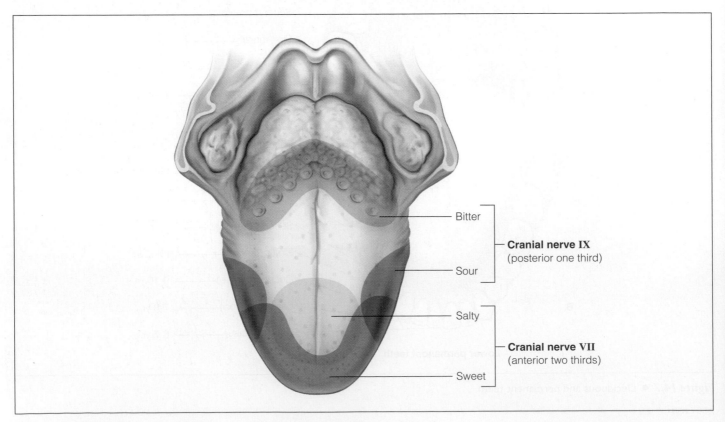

Figure 14.8 ● Taste buds of the tongue.

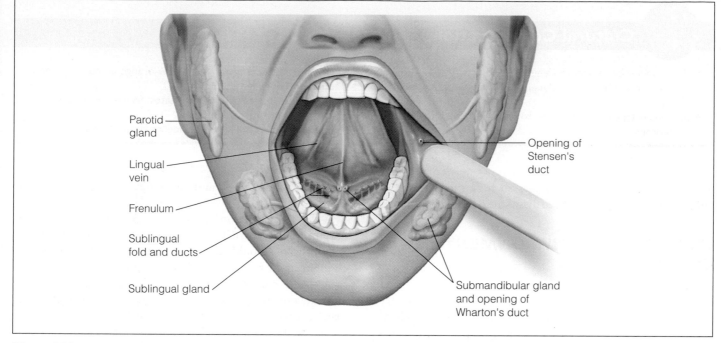

Figure 14.9 ● Salivary glands.

DEVELOPMENTAL CONSIDERATIONS

Changes in anatomy and physiology occur during growth and development. The ability to interpret data in relation to the normative values at various ages is important in the assessment process. Specific variations for different age groups are presented in the following sections.

Infants and Children

The infant's auditory canal is shorter than the adult's and has an upward curve, which persists until about 3 years of age. Children have a more horizontal auditory tube than adults, which leads to easier migration of organisms from infection in the throat to the middle ear. The nose of a child is too small to examine with a speculum. True development of the nose begins in the pubertal period with the development of secondary sex characteristics. Both sets of teeth develop before birth. Deciduous (baby) teeth begin to erupt between 6 months and 2 years of age. Eruption of permanent teeth begins at around age 6 and continues through adolescence. Salivation begins at 3 months of age. Drooling of saliva occurs for several months until swallowing saliva is learned.

The Pregnant Female

Changes in estrogen levels cause increased vascularity throughout the body in pregnancy. Vessel changes of the middle ear may cause a feeling of fullness or earaches. Increased blood flow (hyperemia) to the sinuses can cause rhinitis (inflammation of the nasal cavity) and epistaxis (nosebleed). The sense of smell is heightened in pregnancy. Edema of the vocal cords may cause hoarseness or deepening of the voice. Hyperemia of the throat can lead to an increase in snoring. Small blood vessels and connective tissue increase in the mouth. As a result, gingivitis or inflammation of the gums occurs in many females, which leads to bleeding and discomfort with brushing of the teeth and eating. Occasionally, a hyperplastic overgrowth forms a mass on the gums called *epulis,* which bleeds easily and recedes after birth.

The Older Adult

The older adult may have coarse hairs at the opening of the auditory meatus. The ears may appear more prominent, because cartilage formation continues throughout life. The tympanic membrane becomes paler in color and thicker in appearance with aging. Assessment of hearing may reveal a loss of high-frequency tones, which is consistent with aging. Over time, this loss often progresses to lower-frequency sounds as well. Gradual hearing loss with age is called **presbycusis**.

As the adult ages, many changes occur inside the mouth. The lips and buccal mucosa of the mouth become thinner and less vascular. Gums are paler in color. The tongue develops more fissures, and motor function may become impaired, resulting in problems with swallowing. Senile tremors may cause slight protrusion of the tongue. A decreased sense of taste and smell may contribute to a decreased appetite and poor nutrition. There may also be a decreased production of saliva. This may be due to atrophy of the salivary glands or a side effect of a medication. Gums begin to recede, and some tooth loss may occur due to osteoporosis. If teeth are lost, the remaining teeth may drift. Lesions of the mouth may also develop from ill-fitting dentures.

PSYCHOSOCIAL CONSIDERATIONS

A client who is under a great deal of stress may be prone to mouth ulcers and lip biting. Tics (involuntary muscle spasms) and unconscious clenching of the jaw may indicate psychosocial

Cultural Considerations

- Otitis media occurs more frequently and with greater severity in Hispanics and Native Americans than in other cultural groups.
- Cerumen appears dry and gray to brown in Asians and Native Americans.

- Cerumen appears moist and yellow-orange in African Americans and Caucasians.
- Cleft lip and palate occur with greatest frequency in Asians and least often in African Americans.
- Caucasians have the highest incidence of tooth decay.

disturbances. Relaxation techniques such as meditation and guided imagery may help relieve these stress-related behaviors.

CULTURAL AND ENVIRONMENTAL CONSIDERATIONS

Dark-skinned clients may have darker cerumen in the ear, and their oral mucosa may be darker. People of European ancestry tend to have more tooth decay and tooth loss than people of African ancestry. The size of the teeth varies with cultural ancestry. People of European descent have the smallest teeth;

Asians, Alaska Natives, and Australian Aborigines have the largest.

A client's occupation may increase the risk for hearing loss. For example, construction workers, welders, groundskeepers, and musicians should be evaluated and use earplugs. Noise levels in the home may also need to be evaluated.

A client's socioeconomic status may affect the appearance and function of the structures of the mouth. For example, many clients do not have dental insurance and cannot afford regular dental care. Referral to a low-cost dental clinic or a dental school offering free care may be appropriate.

Gathering the Data

*H*ealth assessment of the ears, nose, mouth, and throat includes gathering subjective and objective data. Recall that subjective data collection occurs during the client interview, before the actual physical assessment. During the interview the nurse uses a variety of communication techniques to elicit general and specific information about the state of health or illness of the client's ears, nose, mouth, and throat. Health records, the results of laboratory tests, and x-rays are important secondary sources to be reviewed and included in the data-gathering process. In physical assessment of the ears, nose, mouth, and throat, the techniques of inspection, palpation, and percussion will be used. Before proceeding, it may be helpful to review the information about each of the data-gathering processes and practice the techniques of health assessment. Some special equipment and assessments will be included—for example, the use of the otoscope.

FOCUSED INTERVIEW

The focused interview concerns data related to the structures and functions of the ears, nose, mouth, and throat. Subjective data related to these structures is gathered during the focused interview. The nurse must be prepared to observe the client and listen for cues related to the functions of these structures. The nurse may use open- or closed-ended questions to obtain in-

formation. Follow-up questions or requests for descriptions are required to clarify data or gather missing information. Follow-up questions identify the source of problems, duration of difficulties, and measures to alleviate problems. They also provide clues about the client's knowledge about his or her own health.

The focused interview guides the physical assessment of the ears, nose, mouth, and throat. The information is always considered in relation to normative parameters and expectations about function. Therefore, the nurse must consider age, gender, race, culture, environment, health practices, past and concurrent problems, and therapies when framing questions and using techniques to elicit information. In order to address all of the factors when conducting a focused interview, categories of questions have been developed. These categories include general questions that are asked of all clients; those addressing illness or infection; questions related to symptoms, pain, or behaviors; those related to habits or practices; questions that are specific to clients according to age; those for the pregnant female; and questions that address environmental concerns.

The nurse must consider the client's ability to participate in the focused interview and physical assessment of the ears, nose, mouth, and throat. If a client is experiencing pain, discomfort, or anxiety, attention must focus on relief of symptoms.

FOCUSED INTERVIEW QUESTIONS	RATIONALES

The following section provides sample questions and bulleted follow-up questions in each of the previously identified categories. For assessment of the ears, a rationale for each of the questions is provided. The list of questions is not all-inclusive but represents the types of questions required in a comprehensive focused interview related to the ears. Questions for the nose, mouth, and throat are included. These questions would follow the same format and be categorized as those for the ear. The bulleted follow-up questions are asked to seek clarification. This additional information from the client expands the subjective database. Remember the subjective data collected and the questions asked during the health history and the focused interview will provide information to help meet the goals of improving hearing and preventing and controlling oral diseases as described in Healthy People 2010.

GENERAL QUESTIONS

1. **Describe your hearing. Have you noticed any change in your hearing? If so, tell me about:**
   - *Onset:* Gradual or sudden?
   - *Character:* Just certain sounds or tones, or all hearing?
   - *Situations:* When using a telephone? Watching television? During conversations?

▶ The client's failure to respond to questions, or asking the nurse to repeat questions, may indicate a hearing loss. Hearing acuity decreases gradually with age. Any sudden loss of hearing should be investigated.

2. **When was your last hearing test?**
   - What were the results?
   - Does your hearing seem better in one ear than the other?
   - Which ear?

▶ Hearing tests should be conducted annually for children, middle adults, and older adults who live or work in noisy environments. Hearing loss in one ear could indicate an obstruction with cerumen or a ruptured tympanic membrane.

3. **Has any member of your family had ear problems or hearing loss?**

▶ Hearing loss can be hereditary.

QUESTIONS RELATED TO ILLNESS OR INFECTION

1. **Have you ever been diagnosed with a disease affecting the ears?**
   - When were you diagnosed with the problem?
   - What treatment was prescribed for the problem?
   - What kinds of things do you do to help with the problem?
   - Has the problem ever recurred (acute)?
   - How are you managing the disease now (chronic)?

▶ The client has an opportunity to provide information about specific illnesses affecting the ears. If a diagnosed illness is identified, follow-up about the diagnosis, treatment, and outcomes is required. Data about each illness identified by the client is essential to an accurate health assessment. Illnesses are classified as acute or chronic, and follow-up regarding each classification will differ.

2. **An alternative to question 1 is to list possible illnesses of the ears, such as Meniere's disease, vertigo, and acoustic neuroma, and ask the client to respond yes or no as each is stated.**

▶ This is a comprehensive and easy way to elicit information about all diagnoses related to the ear. Follow-up would be carried out for each identified diagnosis as in question 1.

3. **Do you now have or have you had an ear infection?**
   - When were you diagnosed with the infection?
   - What treatment was prescribed for the problem?
   - Was the treatment helpful?
   - What kinds of things do you do to help with the problem?
   - Has the problem ever recurred (acute)?
   - How are you managing the infection now (chronic)?

▶ If an infection is identified, follow-up about the date of infection, treatment, and outcomes is required. Data about each infection identified by the client is essential to an accurate health assessment. Infections can be classified as acute or chronic, and follow-up regarding each classification will differ.

4. **An alternative to question 3 is to list possible ear infections, such as external otitis, otitis media, labyrinthitis, and mastoiditis, and ask the client to respond yes or no as each is stated.**

▶ This is a comprehensive and easy way to elicit information about all ear infections. Follow-up would be carried out for each identified infection as in question 3.

FOCUSED INTERVIEW QUESTIONS	RATIONALES

QUESTIONS RELATED TO SYMPTOMS OR BEHAVIORS

When gathering information about symptoms, many questions are required to elicit details and descriptions that assist in the analysis of the data. Discrimination is made in relation to the significance of a symptom, in relation to specific diseases or problems, and in relation to potential follow-up examination or referral. One rationale may be provided for a group of questions in this category.

The following questions refer to specific symptoms and behaviors associated with the ear. For each symptom, questions and follow-up are required. The details to be elicited are the characteristics of the symptom; the onset, duration and frequency of the symptom; the treatment or remedy for the symptom including over-the-counter and home remedies; the determination if diagnosis has been sought; the effect of treatments; and family history associated with a symptom or illness.

QUESTIONS RELATED TO SYMPTOMS

1. **Have you had any ear drainage? If so, describe it.**

   ▶ Ear drainage may indicate an infection. Bloody or purulent drainage could indicate otitis media, infection of the middle ear. Serous drainage could indicate allergic reaction. Clear drainage could be cerebral spinal fluid following trauma.

2. **Have you had dizziness, nausea, vomiting, or ringing in your ears?**

   ▶ These symptoms could indicate a problem with the inner ear, could be related to a neurologic problem, or could be drug related.

QUESTIONS RELATED TO PAIN

1. **Do you have any pain in your ears?**
   - If so, describe it. If yes, have you recently had a cold or sore throat?
   - Have you had any problems lately with your sinuses or your teeth?
   - Have you had any ear trauma or surgery?

   ▶ Pain in one or both ears may be caused by a cold, ear or sinus infection, trauma, dental problems, or cerumen blockage.

QUESTIONS RELATED TO BEHAVIORS

1. **How do you clean your ears?**

   ▶ Many people use cotton-tipped applicators to remove cerumen. This practice can cause trauma to the eardrum and cause cerumen to become impacted. Ear canals should never be cleaned. Cerumen moves to the outside naturally. Commercial cerumen removal products are available, but should be used with the guidance of a healthcare provider.

2. **Do you either own or use a hearing aid?**

   ▶ Some clients have hearing aids but will not use them because of increased background noise, because of embarrassment, or because they cannot pay for the batteries for the hearing aid.

QUESTIONS RELATED TO THE ENVIRONMENT

Environment refers to both the internal and external environments. Questions related to the internal environment include all of the previous questions and those associated with internal or physiological responses. Questions regarding the external environment include those related to home, work, or social environments.

FOCUSED INTERVIEW QUESTIONS	RATIONALES

INTERNAL ENVIRONMENT

1. **Are you taking any medications?**
   - What are they?
   - How often?

► Certain medicines affect the ears. Aspirin can cause ringing in the ears (tinnitus). Some antibiotics can cause hearing loss and dizziness.

EXTERNAL ENVIRONMENT

The following questions deal with substances and irritants found in the physical environment of the client. The physical environment includes the indoor and outdoor environments of the home and workplace, those encountered for social engagements, and any encountered during travel.

1. **Are you frequently exposed to loud noise?**
   - When?
   - How often?
   - Are protective devices available and do you use them?

► Long-term exposure to loud noise can result in hearing loss. Clients at risk are those with jobs in noisy factories; jobs at airports; jobs requiring the use of explosives, firearms, jackhammers, or other loud equipment; and jobs in nightclubs. Frequent exposure to loud music, either live or from stereos or headphones, can also contribute to hearing loss.

2. **Do you experience ear infections or irritations after swimming or being exposed to dust or smoke? If so, describe them.**

► Contaminated water left in the ear may cause **otitis externa**, or swimmer's ear. Irritation of the ear after exposure to certain substances may indicate an allergy to such substances.

QUESTIONS RELATED TO AGE

The focused interview must reflect the anatomical and physiological differences that exist along the age span. The following questions are presented as examples of those that would be specific for infants and children, pregnant females, and older adults.

QUESTIONS REGARDING INFANTS AND CHILDREN

1. **Does the child have recurrent ear infections?**
   - How many ear infections has the child had in the last 6 months?
   - How were they treated?
   - Has the child had any ear surgery such as insertion of ear tubes?
   - When?
   - What were the results?
   - Does the child attend day care?

2. **Does the child tug at his or her ears?**

► Tugging at the ears can be an early sign of infection.

3. **Does the child respond to loud noises?**

► A lack of response could indicate hearing loss.

4. **If the child is over 6 months of age, does the child babble?**

► A child who does not babble may have a hearing impairment.

5. **Have you ever had the child's hearing tested?**
   - What were the results?

6. **Has the child had measles, mumps, or any disease with a high fever?**
   - Has the child been treated recently with any antibiotics such as streptomycin or neomycin?

► High fevers and certain drugs can cause hearing loss.

7. **How do you clean the child's ears?**

► The nurse should ascertain whether the procedure is harmful, such as cleaning ears with cotton swabs, which may cause impacted cerumen.

FOCUSED INTERVIEW QUESTIONS	RATIONALES

QUESTIONS FOR THE PREGNANT FEMALE

1. Have you ever experienced a humming in your ears?

▶ Humming in the ears during pregnancy may occur with hypertension associated with preeclampsia (a serious condition that can threaten maternal and fetal health).

2. Have you experienced an earache or a feeling of fullness in your ears?

▶ Changes in estrogen produce increased vascularity throughout the systems of the body during pregnancy. The vascularity may cause a feeling of fullness or an aching in the ears.

QUESTIONS FOR THE OLDER ADULT

1. Do you wear a hearing aid?
   - If so, is it effective?
   - How often do you wear your hearing aid?

▶ Many older adults have a hearing loss but cannot adjust to using a hearing aid, or cannot afford batteries for the hearing aid.

2. Do you have any difficulty operating the hearing aid?
   - How do you clean the hearing aid?

▶ Some clients forget to clean the tubes of the hearing aid periodically.

NOSE AND SINUSES

1. Are you having any problems with your nose or sinuses? If so, describe them. Are you able to breathe through your nose?
   - Can you breathe through both nostrils?
   - Is one side obstructed?
   - Describe any problems you have had breathing in the last few days. In the last few weeks.

▶ A history of frequent respiratory problems may indicate an underlying respiratory problem such as allergies or recurring infections.

2. Do you have nasal discharge?
   - If so, is it continuous or occasional?
   - Describe it.

▶ A thin, watery discharge is the result of acute rhinitis from either a viral infection, such as the common cold, or an allergic reaction. Allergies that cause nasal discharge can also produce postnasal drip, sore throats, ear infections, or headaches. Some allergies are seasonal; others are constant.

3. Do you have nosebleeds?
   - How often?
   - What is your usual blood pressure?
   - Do you use nasal sprays?
   - How do you treat your nosebleeds?

▶ Nosebleeds can occur as a result of high blood pressure, overuse of nasal sprays, and certain blood disorders.

4. Have you ever had any nose injury or nose surgery?
   - If so, describe it.
   - How was the injury treated?
   - Do you have any residual problems from the injury or surgery?

5. Describe your sense of smell.
   - Are there any circumstances, objects, places, or activities that affect your sense of smell? If so, describe them.

▶ Anosmia, the inability to smell, may be neurologic, hereditary, or due to a deficiency of zinc in the diet.

6. What prescribed or over-the-counter drugs do you take to relieve your nasal symptoms?
   - Do you use a nasal inhalant, oxygen, or a humidifier to help you breathe?
   - What other medications do you take regularly?

▶ Certain medications can produce unpleasant side effects in the nose such as nasal stuffiness or nosebleeds. Many drugs administered by nasal inhalers may irritate the nasal mucosa and cause nosebleeds. Steroid inhalers can cause growth of *Candida* in the nose, mouth, or throat.

7. Do you use recreational drugs?
   - If so, what drugs? How often?

▶ Some inhaled drugs, such as cocaine, gradually break down the nasal lining by vasoconstriction. A very pale color of the nasal septum, or holes in the septum, may indicate drug sniffing.

FOCUSED INTERVIEW QUESTIONS	**RATIONALES**

QUESTIONS REGARDING INFANTS AND CHILDREN

1. Does the child put objects into his or her nose?

   ▶ Foreign objects can cause trauma to nasal tissues.

2. Does the child frequently have drainage from the nose?

   ▶ Frequent drainage can indicate an infection or allergies.

QUESTIONS FOR THE PREGNANT FEMALE

1. Have you had nosebleeds during your pregnancy? If so, how often?

   ▶ Nosebleeds and nasal congestion are common during pregnancy because of increased vascularity in the nasal passages.

MOUTH AND THROAT

1. How would you describe the condition of your mouth and teeth?
   - Have you noticed any changes in the last few months?

2. Do you have any problems swallowing?

   ▶ Dysphagia, or difficulty in swallowing, may be due to a neurologic or gastrointestinal problem, or it may be related to ill-fitting dentures or malocclusion. Achalasia, a chronic difficulty in swallowing caused by constriction of the esophagus, may be related to anxiety or stress. Finally, painful or difficult swallowing could be related to cancer of the throat or esophagus.

3. Do you have any sores or lesions in your mouth or on your tongue?
   - If so, describe them.
   - Are they present constantly or do they come and go periodically?

   ▶ Lesions of the mouth or tongue may be cold sores or mouth ulcers. They may also accompany viral infections and gum infections. Some lesions may be caused by ill-fitting dentures. Finally, any lesion of the mouth that does not heal should be evaluated for oral cancer.

4. Do your gums bleed frequently?

   ▶ Gum diseases such as gingivitis and periodontitis may cause gums to bleed easily. Gums may also bleed easily with ill-fitting braces or dentures.

5. Have you noticed a change in your sense of taste recently?

   ▶ Loss of the sense of taste commonly accompanies colds. A foul taste in the mouth may signal a gum infection or inadequate care of teeth or dentures.

6. What dental problems, surgeries, or procedures have you had in the past?
   - Describe them.

7. Do you wear dentures, partial plates, retainers, or any other removable or permanent dental appliance?
   - Does it fit well? Is it comfortable?
   - Why are you wearing the appliance?
   - Does it help resolve the problem?
   - Are any of your teeth capped?
   - Which ones?

8. How often do you brush your teeth or dentures?
   - Do you use floss regularly?

   ▶ Regular mouth care is important in maintaining healthy teeth and gums and preventing gum diseases such as gingivitis and periodontitis.

9. When was your last dental examination?
   - Are you unable to eat some foods because of problems with your teeth?
   - Do you have any pain in one or more teeth?

10. Do you have frequent sore throats?

    ▶ A sore throat may be the result of irritation from sinus drainage, viral or bacterial infection, or the first sign of throat cancer.

FOCUSED INTERVIEW QUESTIONS

RATIONALES

11. Have you noticed any hoarseness or loss of your voice?

▶ Hoarseness is a common finding in disorders of the throat. Recurrent or persistent hoarseness may indicate cancer of the larynx. Hoarseness may also be due to anxiety, overuse of the voice, or a cold. Smoking and drinking alcohol can lead to inflammation of the vocal cords and result in hoarseness.

12. Do you now or did you ever smoke a pipe, cigarettes, or cigars?
    • Chew tobacco or dip snuff?
    • How much? How often?

▶ Smoking, dipping snuff, or chewing tobacco may result in cancer of the lips, mouth, and throat.

QUESTIONS REGARDING INFANTS AND CHILDREN

1. Does the child suck his or her thumb or a pacifier?

▶ These behaviors can interfere with alignment of secondary teeth.

2. When did the child's teeth begin to erupt?

▶ Late eruption of teeth could indicate delayed development.

3. Does the child go to bed with a bottle at night?
   • What is in the bottle?

▶ Frequent use of a bottle with milk or juice at night can cause decay of teeth.

4. Does the child know how to brush teeth?
   • Does the child brush daily?

5. How often does the child go to the dentist?

▶ Children should begin annual visits to the dentist between the ages of 3 and 4 years.

6. Is the child's drinking water fluoridated?

▶ Fluoride in the water supply helps prevent tooth decay.

QUESTIONS FOR THE OLDER ADULT

1. Are you able to chew all types of food?

▶ If teeth are missing or dentures fit improperly, the client may not be able to chew meat or certain vegetables, resulting in undernutrition.

2. Do you experience dryness in your mouth?

▶ Certain medications may cause dryness, which may interfere with the client's appetite or digestion.

3. Do you wear dentures?
   • If so, do they fit properly?

▶ Ill-fitting dentures can interfere with proper nutrition and can cause various problems in the mouth, such as lesions and bleeding gums.

CLIENT INTERACTION

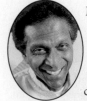

Mr. Sanji, age 65, comes to the Medi-Center with a chief complaint of "having trouble hearing." The intake sheet that Mr. Sanji completed reveals a slow progressive loss of hearing with no pain in the ears or head. Following is an excerpt of the focused interview.

INTERVIEW

Nurse: Good morning Mr. Sanji. Please have a seat and tell me about your deafness.

The nurse and Mr. Sanji sit down across the desk from each other. During the interview, the nurse's head is down. The nurse maintains some eye contact by looking over the rim of the eye glasses.

Mr. Sanji: I'm not deaf. I can't hear like before.

Nurse: How long have you noticed this progressive loss of hearing?

Mr. Sanji: I'm not sure, a while, but I'm not deaf.

Nurse: Have you had any purulent drainage from your ears?

Mr. Sanji: Hum!

Nurse: Do you have a history of having otitis media or a tympanoplasty?

Mr. Sanji does not answer the question.

Nurse: Would you like me to repeat the question?

Mr. Sanji: Yeah, louder and in simple language!

ANALYSIS

In this situation the nurse has utilized several strategies that act as a hindrance to effective communication. The first problem is the nurse's body position and lack of eye contact. Keeping the head down muffles the sound for any person, especially one with a hearing deficit. The nurse should look up, speak directly to the client, and maintain eye contact. Twice the client says he is not deaf and the nurse does not seek clarification. Using language and terminology the individual does not understand is another obstacle. Mr. Sanji tells the nurse to speak louder and in simple terms.

Please refer to the Companion Website at **www.prenhall.com/damico** and click on Chapter 14, the **Client Interaction** module, to answer questions about this case. In addition, see other resources for this chapter including NCLEX review questions and other interactive exercises and materials.

Physical Assessment

ASSESSMENT TECHNIQUES AND FINDINGS

Physical assessment of the ears, nose, mouth, and throat requires the use of inspection, palpation, percussion, and transillumination of sinuses. In addition, special examination techniques include the use of the otoscope, tuning fork, and nasal speculum. These techniques are used to gather objective data. Knowledge of normal or expected findings is essential in determining the meaning of data as the nurse proceeds.

Adults have binaural hearing; the ears are symmetrical in size, shape, color, and configuration. The external auditory canal is patent and free of drainage. The external ear and mastoid process are free of lesions, and the tragus is movable. Under otoscopic examination the external ear canal is open, is nontender, and is free of lesions, inflammation, or foreign substances. Cerumen, if present, is soft and in small amounts. The tympanic membrane is flat, gray, and translucent without lesions. The malleolar process and reflected light are visible on the tympanic membrane. The tympanic membrane flutters with the Valsalva maneuver. During hearing tests, air conduction is longer than bone conduction. Adults are able to maintain balance.

The external nose is free of lesions, the nares are patent, and the mucosa of the nasal cavity is dark pink and smooth. The nasal septum is midline, straight, and intact. The sinuses are nontender and transilluminate. The lips are smooth, symmetrical, and lesion-free. The adult has 32 permanent teeth that are white with smooth edges. The tongue is mobile, is pink, and has papillae on the dorsum. The oral mucosa is pink, moist, and smooth. Salivary ducts are visible and not inflamed. The membranes and structures of the throat are pink and moist. The uvula is midline and, like the soft palate, rises when the client says "ah."

Physical assessment of the ears, nose, mouth, and throat follows an organized pattern. It begins with instruction of the client and proceeds through inspection, palpation, and otoscopic examination of the ears, followed by hearing assessment and the Romberg test. The nose is inspected and the internal aspect visualized while using a speculum. The sinuses are palpated, percussed, and transilluminated. The assessment concludes with inspection of the external mouth, the internal structures of the mouth, and assessment of the throat.

EQUIPMENT

examination gown	nasal speculum
clean, nonsterile exam gloves	penlight
otoscope	gauze pads
tuning fork	tongue blade

HELPFUL HINTS

- Provide specific instructions about what is expected of the client. The nurse would state whether the head must be turned or the mouth opened.
- Consider the age of the client. Response to directions varies across the life span.
- Pay attention to nonverbal cues throughout the assessment.
- Hearing difficulties may affect the data gathering process. Clarify problems and possible remedies before beginning the assessment. The client may use sign language, hearing aids, lip reading, or written communication.
- Explain the use of each piece of equipment throughout the assessment.
- Use Standard Precautions.

TECHNIQUES AND NORMAL FINDINGS	ABNORMAL FINDINGS SPECIAL CONSIDERATIONS

EAR

1. **Position the client.**
   - The client should be in a sitting position. Lighting must be adequate to detect skin color changes, discharge, and lesions.

2. **Instruct the client.**
   - Explain that you will be carrying out a variety of assessments of the ear. Tell the client you will be touching the ear areas, that it should cause no discomfort, and that any pain or discomfort should be reported.

3. **Note that you will have begun to evaluate the client's hearing while taking the health history.**
   - Did the client hear the questions you asked?
   - Did the client answer appropriately?
   - Generally, the formal evaluation of hearing is performed after otoscopic examination so that physical barriers to hearing, such as large amounts of cerumen, can be identified.

4. **Inspect the external ear for symmetry, proportion, color, and integrity.**
   - Confirm that the external auditory meatus is patent with no drainage. The color of the ear should match that of the surrounding area and the face, with no redness, nodules, swelling, or lesions.

▶ Any discharge, redness, or swelling may indicate an infection or allergy.

5. **Palpate the auricle and push on the tragus (see Figure 14.10 ●).**
   - Confirm that there are no hard nodules, lesions, or swelling. The tragus should be movable.
   - This technique should not cause pain.

▶ Pain could be the result of an infection of the external ear (otitis externa). Pain could also indicate temporomandibular joint dysfunction with pressure on the tragus. Hard nodules (tophi) are uric acid crystal deposits, which are a sign of gout.

Lesions accompanied by a history of long-term exposure to the sun may be cancerous.

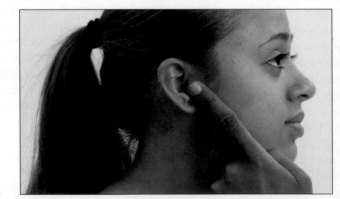

Figure 14.10 ●
Palpating the tragus.

6. **Palpate the mastoid process lying directly behind the ear (see Figure 14.11 ●).**
   - Confirm that there are no lesions, pain, or swelling.

▶ **Mastoiditis** is a complication of either a middle ear infection or a throat infection. Mastoiditis is very difficult to treat. It spreads easily to the brain since the mastoid area is separated from the brain by only a thin, bony plate.

TECHNIQUES AND NORMAL FINDINGS	ABNORMAL FINDINGS SPECIAL CONSIDERATIONS

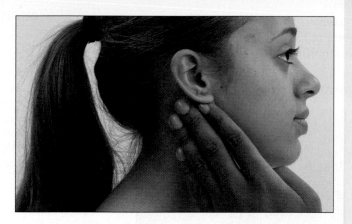

Figure 14.11 ●
Palpating the
mastoid process.

7. **Inspect the auditory canal using the otoscope.**
   - For the best visualization, use the largest speculum that will fit into the auditory canal.
   - Ask the client to tilt the head away from you toward the opposite shoulder.
   - Hold the otoscope between the palm and first two fingers of the dominant hand. The handle may be positioned upward or downward (see Figure 14.13 on page 322).
   - Use your other hand to straighten the canal.
   - In the adult client, pull the pinna up, back, and out to straighten the canal (see Figure 14.12 ●).

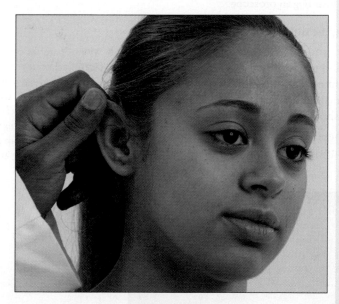

Figure 14.12 ●
Pulling the pinna to
straighten the canal.

   - Be sure to maintain this position until the speculum is removed.
   - Instruct the client to tell you if any discomfort is experienced but not to move the head or suddenly pull away.

ALERT!

One must use care when inserting the speculum of the otoscope into the ear. The inner two thirds of the ear are very sensitive, and pressing the speculum against either side of the auditory canal will cause pain.

TECHNIQUES AND NORMAL FINDINGS

- With the light on, use the upward or downward position of the handle to insert the speculum into the ear (see Figures 14.13A and B ●). The external canal should be open and without tenderness, inflammation, lesions, growths, discharge, or foreign substances.

- Note the amount of cerumen that is present, the texture, and the color.

▶ If the ear canal is occluded with cerumen, it must be removed. Most cerumen can be removed with a cerumen spoon. If the cerumen is dry, the external canal should be irrigated using a bulb syringe and a warmed solution of mineral oil and hydrogen peroxide, followed by warm water.

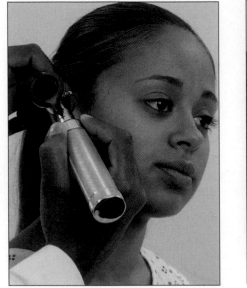 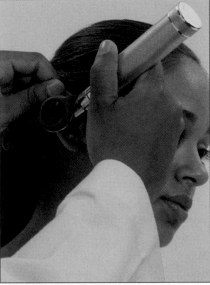

Figure 14.13 ● Two techniques for holding and inserting an otoscope.

8. Examine the tympanic membrane using the otoscope.

- The membrane should be flat, gray, and translucent with no scars (see Figure 14.14 ●). A cone-shaped reflection of the otoscope light should be visible at the 5-o'clock position in the right ear and the 7-o'clock position in the left ear. The short process of the malleus should be seen as a shadow behind the tympanic membrane. The membrane should be intact.

- If you cannot visualize the tympanic membrane, remove the otoscope, reposition the auricle, and reinsert the otoscope. Do not reposition the auricle with the otoscope in place.

▶ White patches on the tympanic membrane indicate scars from prior infections. If the membrane is yellow or reddish, it could indicate an infection of the middle ear. A bulging membrane may indicate increased pressure in the middle ear, whereas a retracted membrane may indicate a vacuum in the middle ear, due to a blocked eustachian tube.

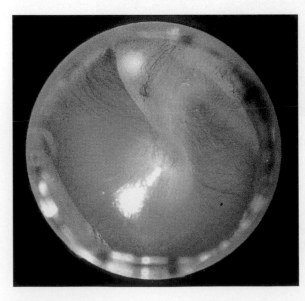

Figure 14.14 ●
Normal tympanic membrane with cone of light and process of malleus.

TECHNIQUES AND NORMAL FINDINGS	ABNORMAL FINDINGS SPECIAL CONSIDERATIONS

9. While looking through the otoscope, instruct the client to perform the Valsalva maneuver.

- Have the tympanic membrane in clear view.
- Ask the client to close the lips, pinch the nose, and gently blow the nose.
- This maneuver lets you assess the mobility of the tympanic membrane and the patency of the eustachian tubes. The tympanic membrane should flutter toward the otoscope slightly as the client performs this maneuver.

▶ Rigidity of the tympanic membrane may be due to a variety of alterations and requires further evaluation.

ALERT!

An older client should not be asked to perform the Valsalva maneuver because it may result in dizziness. This maneuver is also dangerous if the client has an upper respiratory infection, because it could force pathogenic organisms into the middle ear.

10. Perform the whisper test.

- This test evaluates hearing acuity of high-frequency sounds.
- Ask the client to occlude the left ear.
- Cover your mouth so that the client cannot see your lips.
- Standing at the client's side at a distance of 1 to 2 ft, whisper a simple phrase such as, "The weather is hot today." Ask the client to repeat the phrase. Then do the same procedure to test the right ear using a different phrase. The client should be able to repeat the phrases correctly (see Figure 14.15 ●).

▶ Inability to repeat the phrases may indicate a loss of the ability to hear high-frequency sounds.

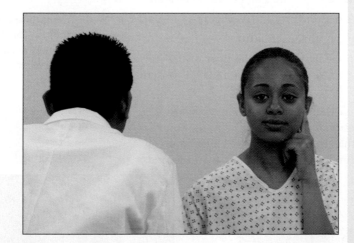

Figure 14.15 ●
Performing the whisper test.

- Tuning forks are used to evaluate auditory acuity. The tines of the fork, when activated, produce sound waves. The frequency, or cycles per second (cps), is the expression used to describe the action of the instrument. A fork with 512 cps vibrates 512 times per second and is the size of choice for auditory evaluations. The tines are set into motion by squeezing, stroking, or lightly tapping against your hand. The fork must be held at the handle to prevent interference with the vibration of the tines (see Figure 14.16 ●).

TECHNIQUES AND NORMAL FINDINGS	ABNORMAL FINDINGS SPECIAL CONSIDERATIONS

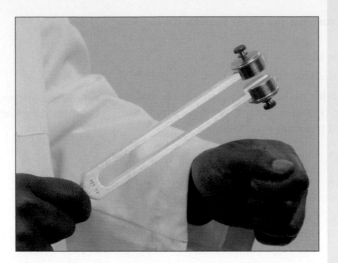

Figure 14.16 ●
Activating the tuning fork.

- The following tests use a tuning fork primarily to evaluate conductive versus perceptive hearing loss. **Air conduction (AC)** is the transmission of sound through the tympanic membrane to the cochlea and auditory nerve. **Bone conduction (BC)** is the transmission of sound through the bones of the skull to the cochlea and auditory nerve.

11. Perform the Rinne test.

- The Rinne test compares air and bone conduction. Hold the tuning fork by the handle and gently strike the fork on the palm of your hand to set it vibrating.
- Place the base of the fork on the client's mastoid process (see Figure 14.17A ●).
- Ask the client to tell you when the sound is no longer heard.
- Note the number of seconds. Then immediately move the tines of the still-vibrating fork in front of the external auditory meatus. It should be 1 to 2 cm (about 1/2 in.) from the meatus.
- Ask the client to tell you again when the sound is no longer heard (see Figure 14.17B ●). Again note the number of seconds. Normally, the sound is heard twice as long by air conduction than by bone conduction after bone conduction stops. For example, a normal finding is AC 30 seconds, BC 15 seconds.

▶ If the client hears the bone-conducted sound as long as or longer than the air-conducted sound, the client may have some degree of conductive hearing loss.

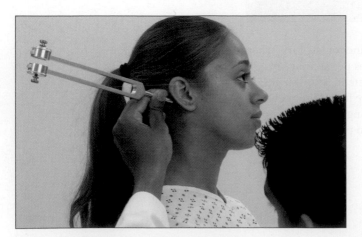

Figure 14.17A ● Rinne test. Bone conduction.

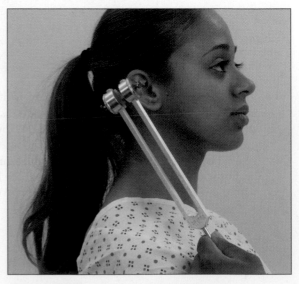

Figure 14.17B ● Rinne test. Air conduction.

TECHNIQUES AND NORMAL FINDINGS

ABNORMAL FINDINGS
SPECIAL CONSIDERATIONS

12. Perform the Weber test.

- The Weber test uses bone conduction to evaluate hearing in a person who hears better in one ear than in the other. Hold the tuning fork by the handle and strike the fork on the palm of the hand. Place the base of the vibrating fork against the client's skull. The midline of the anterior portion of the frontal bone is used. The midline of the forehead is an alternative choice (see Figure 14.18 ●).

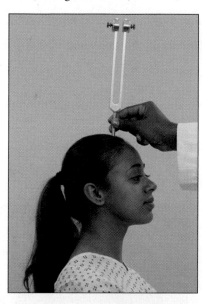

Figure 14.18 ● Weber test.

- Ask the client if the sound is heard equally on both sides, or better in one ear than the other. The normal response is bilaterally equal sound, which is recorded as "no lateralization." If the sound is lateralized, ask the client to tell you which ear hears the sound better.

13. Perform the Romberg test.

- The Romberg test assesses equilibrium. Ask the client to stand with feet together and arms at sides, first with eyes opened and then with eyes closed (see Figure 14.19 ●).

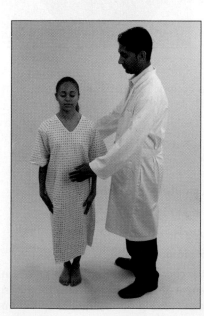

Figure 14.19 ● Romberg test.

▶ If the client hears the sound in one ear better than the other ear, the hearing loss may be due to either poor conduction or nerve damage. If the client has poor conduction in one ear, the sound is heard better in the impaired ear because the sound is being conducted directly through the bone to the ear, and the extraneous sounds in the environment are not being picked up. Conductive loss in one ear may be due to impacted cerumen, infection, or a perforated eardrum. If the client has a hearing loss due to nerve damage, the sound is referred to the better ear, in which the cochlea or auditory nerve is functioning better.

▶ The abnormal findings are recorded as "sound lateralizes to (right or left) ear."

TECHNIQUES AND NORMAL FINDINGS

- Wait about 20 seconds. The person should be able to maintain this position, although some mild swaying may occur. Mild swaying is documented as a negative Romberg. It is important to stand nearby and prepare to support the client if there is a loss of balance. Hearing and balance are functions of cranial nerve VIII and are discussed in Chapter 24. ⚭

▶ If the client is unable to maintain balance or needs to have the feet farther apart, there may be a problem with functioning of the vestibular apparatus.

NOSE AND SINUSES

Note: The sense of smell and function of cranial nerve I is evaluated with the neurologic assessment presented in Chapter 24. ⚭

1. **Instruct the client.**
   - Explain that you will be looking at and touching the client's nose. Tell the client to inform you of discomfort.

2. **Inspect the nose for symmetry, shape, skin lesions, or signs of infection.**
   - Confirm that the nose is straight, the nares are equal in size, the skin is intact, and no drainage is present (see Figure 14.20 ●).

▶ If breathing is noisy or a discharge is present, the client may have an obstruction or an infection.

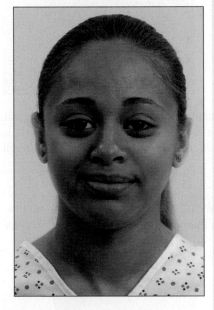

Figure 14.20 ● Inspection of the nose.

3. **Test for patency.**
   - Press your finger on the client's nostril to occlude one naris, and ask the client to breathe through the opposite side.
   - Repeat with the other nostril.
   - The client should be able to breathe through each naris.

▶ If the client cannot breathe through each naris, severe inflammation or an obstruction may be present.

▶ Ineffective breathing patterns or mouth breathing may be related to nasal swelling or trauma.

4. **Palpate the external nose for tenderness, swelling, and stability.**
   - Using two fingers, palpate the nose.
   - Note the smoothness and stability of the underlying soft tissue and cartilage.

5. **Inspect the nasal cavity using a nasal speculum.**
   - With your nondominant hand, stabilize the client's head. With the speculum in your dominant hand, insert the speculum with blades closed into the naris. Then separate the blades, dilating the naris (see Figure 14.21). The speculum

| **TECHNIQUES AND NORMAL FINDINGS** | **ABNORMAL FINDINGS SPECIAL CONSIDERATIONS** |

should be in the dominant hand for better control at the time of insertion to avoid hitting the sensitive septum.

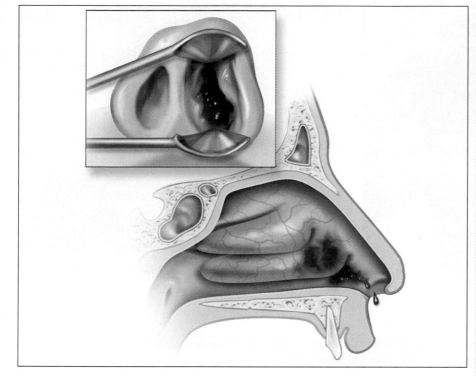

Figure 14.21 ● Using the nasal speculum.

- With the client's head erect, inspect the inferior turbinates (Figure 14.21 ●).
- With the client's head tilted back, inspect the middle meatus and middle turbinates. Mucosa should be dark pink and smooth without swelling, discharge, bleeding, or foreign bodies. The septum should be midline, straight, and intact.
- When finished with inspection, close the blades of the speculum and remove. Again, do not hit the sensitive septum.
- Repeat on other side.

6. **Palpate the sinuses.**
- Begin by pressing your thumbs over the frontal sinuses below the superior orbital ridge. Palpate the maxillary sinuses below the zygomatic arches of the cheekbones (see Figures 14.22A and B ●).
- Observe the client for signs of discomfort. Ask the client to inform you of pain.

▶ If the mucosa is swollen and red, the client may have an upper respiratory infection. If mucosa is pale and boggy or swollen, the client may have chronic allergies. A *deviated septum* appears as an irregular lump in one nasal cavity. Slight deviations do not present problems for most clients. **Nasal polyps** are smooth, pale, benign growths found in many clients with chronic allergies.

▶ Tenderness upon palpation may indicate chronic allergies or sinusitis.

TECHNIQUES AND NORMAL FINDINGS	ABNORMAL FINDINGS SPECIAL CONSIDERATIONS

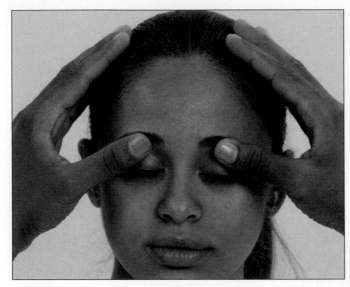

Figure 14.22A ● Palpating the frontal sinuses.

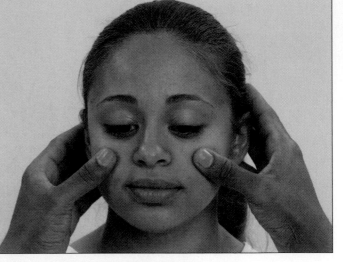

Figure 14.22B ● Palpating the maxillary sinuses.

7. **Percuss the sinuses.**

- To determine if there is pain in the sinuses, directly percuss over the maxillary and frontal sinuses by lightly tapping with one finger (see Figures 14.23A and B ●).

▶ Pain may indicate sinus fullness, allergies, or infection.

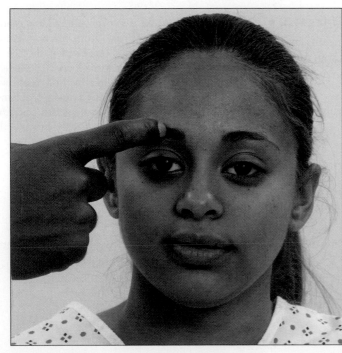

Figure 14.23A ● Percussion of frontal sinuses.

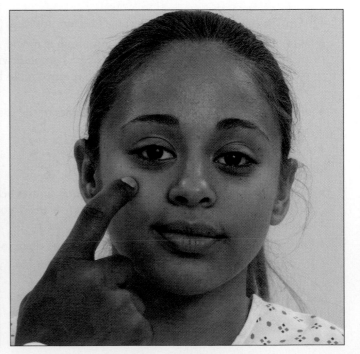

Figure 14.23B ● Percussion of maxillary sinuses.

TECHNIQUES AND NORMAL FINDINGS	ABNORMAL FINDINGS SPECIAL CONSIDERATIONS

8. Transilluminate the sinuses.

- If you suspect a sinus infection, the maxillary and frontal sinuses may be transilluminated.
- To transilluminate the frontal sinus, darken the room and hold a penlight under the superior orbit ridge against the frontal sinus area (see Figure 14.24A ●).

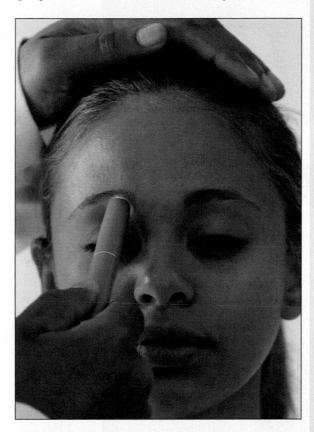

Figure 14.24A ●
Transillumination of the frontal sinuses.

- Cover it with your hand. There should be a red glow over the frontal sinus area (see Figure 14.24B ●).

▶ If the sinus is filled with fluid, it will not transilluminate.

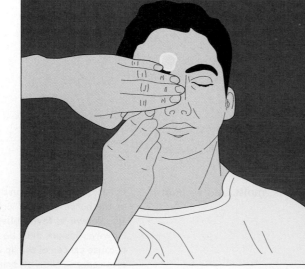

Figure 14.24B ●
Observing transillumination of the frontal sinuses.

TECHNIQUES AND NORMAL FINDINGS

ABNORMAL FINDINGS
SPECIAL CONSIDERATIONS

- To test the maxillary sinus, place a clean penlight in the client's mouth and shine the light on one side of the hard palate, then the other.
- There should be a red glow over the cheeks (see Figure 14.25A ●). Make sure the penlight is cleaned before using it again.

▶ If there is no red glow under the eyes, the sinuses may be inflamed.

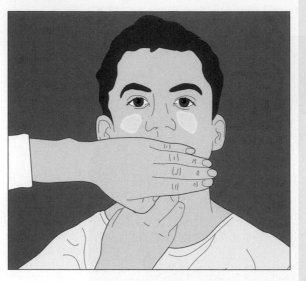

Figure 14.25A ●
Transillumination of the maxillary sinuses.

- An alternate technique is to place the penlight directly on the cheek and observe the glow of light on the hard palate (see Figure 14.25B ●).

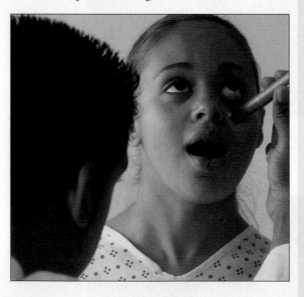

Figure 14.25B ●
Transillumination of the maxillary sinuses using alternate technique.

MOUTH AND THROAT

Note: Be sure to wear clean, nonsterile examination gloves for this part of the assessment.

1. **Inspect and palpate the lips.**
   - Confirm that the lips are symmetrical, smooth, pink, moist, and without lesions. Makeup or lipstick should be removed.

▶ Lesions or blisters on the lips may be caused by the herpes simplex virus. These lesions are also known as **fever blisters** or **cold sores**. However, lesions must be evaluated for cancer, because cancer of the lip is the most common oral cancer. Pallor or cyanosis of the lips may indicate hypoxia.

| TECHNIQUES AND NORMAL FINDINGS | ABNORMAL FINDINGS SPECIAL CONSIDERATIONS |

2. Inspect the teeth.

- Observe the client's dental hygiene. Ask the client to clench the teeth and smile while you observe occlusion.

- Note dentures and caps at this time.

- The teeth should be white, with smooth edges, and free of debris. Adults should have 32 permanent teeth (see Figure 14.26 ●), if wisdom teeth are intact.

▶ Loose, painful, broken, misaligned teeth, mal-occlusion, and inflamed gums need further evaluation.

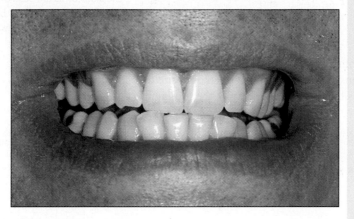

Figure 14.26 ● Inspecting the teeth.

3. Inspect and palpate the buccal mucosa, gums, and tongue.

- Look into the client's mouth under a strong light.

- Confirm that the tongue is pink and moist with papillae on the dorsal surface.

- Ask the client to touch the roof of the mouth with the tip of the tongue. The ventral surface should be smooth and pink. Palpate the area under the tongue.

- Check for lesions or nodules. Using a gauze pad, grasp the client's tongue and inspect for any lumps or nodules (see Figure 14.27 ●). The tissue should be smooth.

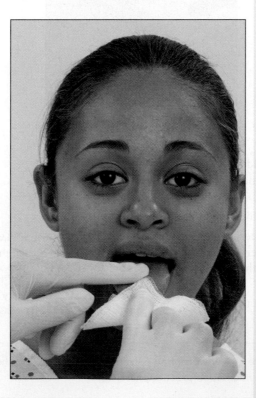

Figure 14.27 ● Palpating the tongue.

TECHNIQUES AND NORMAL FINDINGS	ABNORMAL FINDINGS SPECIAL CONSIDERATIONS

- Use a tongue blade to hold the tongue aside while you inspect the mucous lining of the mouth and the gums.
- Confirm that these areas are pink, moist, smooth, and free of lesions.
- Confirm the integrity of both the soft and the hard palate.
- The sense of taste (cranial nerves VII and IX) and movement of the tongue (cranial nerve XII) are discussed in detail in Chapter 24. ∞

▶ A smooth, coated, or hairy tongue is usually related to dehydration or disease. A small tongue may indicate undernutrition. Tremor of the tongue may indicate a dysfunction of the hypoglossal nerve (cranial nerve XII). Persistent lesions on the tongue must be evaluated further. Cancerous lesions occur most commonly on the sides or at the base of the tongue. The gums are diseased if there is bleeding, retraction, or overgrowth onto the teeth.

4. Inspect the salivary glands.

- The salivary glands open into the mouth. Wharton's ducts (submandibular) open close to the lingual frenulum. Stensen's ducts (parotid) open opposite the second upper molars. Both ducts are visible, whereas the ducts of the sublingual glands are not visible.
- Confirm that all salivary ducts are visible, with no pain, tenderness, swelling, or redness.
- Touch the area close to the ducts with a sterile applicator, and confirm the flow of saliva.

▶ Pain or the lack of saliva can indicate infection or an obstruction.

5. Inspect the throat.

- Use a tongue blade and penlight to inspect the throat (see Figure 14.28 ●).

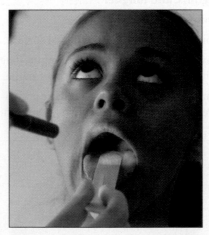

Figure 14.28 ● Inspecting the throat.

- Ask the client to open the mouth wide, tilt the head back, and say "aah." The uvula should rise in the midline.
- Use the tongue blade to depress the middle of the arched tongue enough so that you can clearly visualize the throat, but not so much that the client gags. Ask the client to say "aah" again.
- Confirm the rising of the soft palate, which is a test for cranial nerve X.
- Confirm that the tonsils, uvula, and posterior pharynx are pink and are without inflammation, swelling, or lesions. Observe the tonsils behind the anterior tonsillar pillar. The color should be pink with slight vascularity present. Tonsils may be partially or totally absent.
- As you inspect the throat, note any mouth odors.
- Discard the tongue blade.

▶ Viral pharyngitis may accompany a cold. Tonsils may be bright red and swollen, and may have white spots on them.

Clients with diabetic acidosis have a sweet, fruity breath. The breath of clients with kidney disease smells of ammonia.

 Refer to the Companion Website at **www.prenhall.com/damico** and click on the **Documentation** module for documentation samples and documentation practice exercises.

bnormal findings in the ears, nose, mouth, and throat include lesions, deformities, infectious processes, and dental problems. Figures 14.29 through 14.52 depict common abnormal findings in these structures.

EAR

Hemotympanum

Hemotympanum is a bluish tinge to the tympanic membrane indicating the presence of blood in the middle ear (see Figure 14.29 ●). It is usually caused by head trauma.

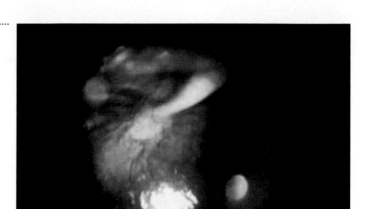

Figure 14.29 ● Hemotympanum.

Otitis Externa

Otitis externa is infection of the outer ear, often called "swimmer's ear." Otitis externa causes redness and swelling of the auricle and ear canal (see Figure 14.30 ●). Drainage is usually scanty. It may be accompanied by itching, fever, and enlarged lymph nodes.

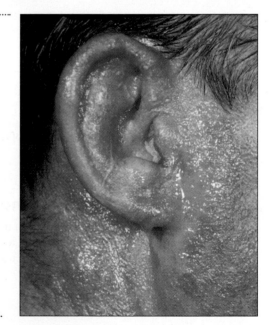

Figure 14.30 ● Otitis externa.

Otitis Media

Otitis media is infection of the middle ear producing a red, bulging eardrum, fever, and hearing loss (see Figure 14.31 ●). The otoscopic examination reveals absent light reflex. Otitis media is more common in children, whose auditory tubes are wider, shorter, and more horizontal than those of adults, thus allowing easier access for infections ascending from the pharynx.

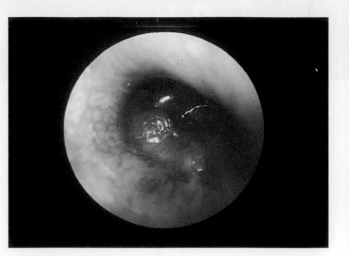

Figure 14.31 ● Otitis media.

Perforation of the Tympanic Membrane

Perforation of the tympanic membrane is a rupturing of the eardrum due to trauma or infection. During otoscopic inspection, the perforation may be seen as a dark spot on the eardrum (see Figure 14.32 ●).

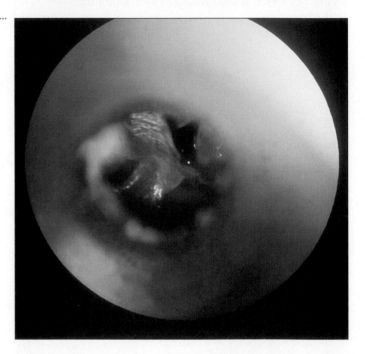

Figure 14.32 ● Perforation of tympanic membrane.

Scarred Tympanic Membrane

A scarred tympanic membrane is a condition in which the eardrum has white patches of scar tissue due to repeated ear infections (see Figure 14.33 ●).

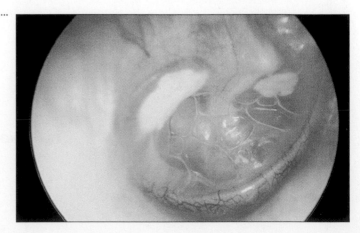

Figure 14.33 ● Scarred tympanic membrane.

Tophi

Tophi are small white nodules on the helix or antihelix (see Figure 14.34 ●). These nodules contain uric acid crystals and are a sign of gout.

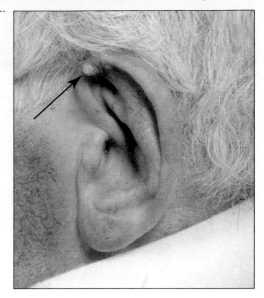

Figure 14.34 ● Tophi.

Tympanostomy Tubes

Tympanostomy tubes are ear tubes inserted to relieve middle ear pressure and allow drainage from repeated middle ear infections (see Figure 14.35 ●).

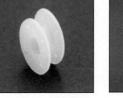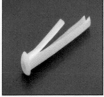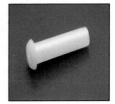

Figure 14.35 ● Tympanostomy tubes.

NOSE AND SINUSES

Epistaxis

Epistaxis is a nosebleed. This may follow trauma, such as a blow to the nose, or it may accompany another alteration in health, such as rhinitis, hypertension, or a blood coagulation disorder (see Figure 14.36 ●).

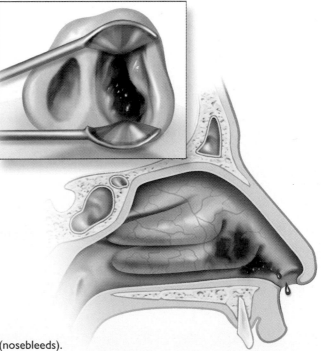

Figure 14.36 ● Epistaxis (nosebleeds).

Rhinitis

Rhinitis is a nasal inflammation usually due to a viral infection or allergy. It is accompanied by a watery and often copious discharge, sneezing, and congestion (stuffy nose). Acute rhinitis (see Figure 14.37 ●) is caused by a virus, whereas allergic rhinitis (see Figure 14.38 ●) results from contact with allergens such as pollen and dust.

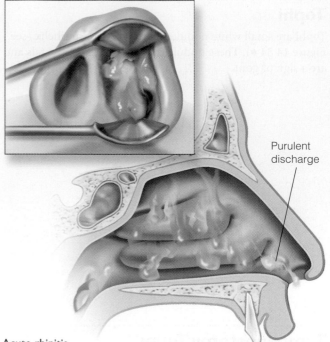

Purulent discharge

Figure 14.37 ● Acute rhinitis.

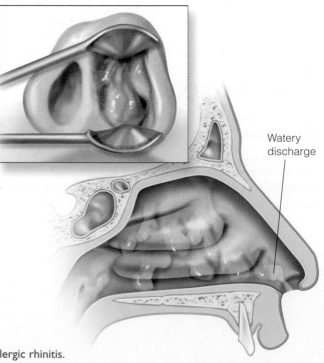

Watery discharge

Figure 14.38 ● Allergic rhinitis.

Sinusitis

Sinusitis is inflammation of the sinuses usually following an upper respiratory infection. It causes facial pain, inflammation, and discharge (see Figure 14.39 ●). Fever, chills, frontal headache, or a dull, pulsating pain in the cheeks or teeth may accompany sinusitis.

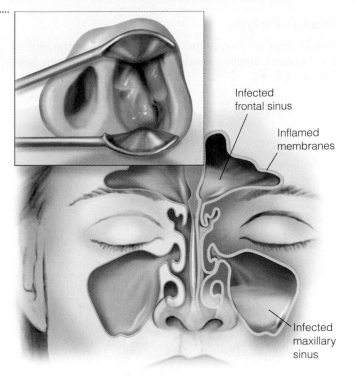

Infected
frontal sinus

Inflamed
membranes

Infected
maxillary
sinus

Figure 14.39 ● Sinusitis.

Deviated Septum

A deviated septum is a slight ingrowth of the lower nasal septum (see Figure 14.40 ●). When viewed with a nasal speculum, one nasal cavity appears to have an outgrowth or shelf.

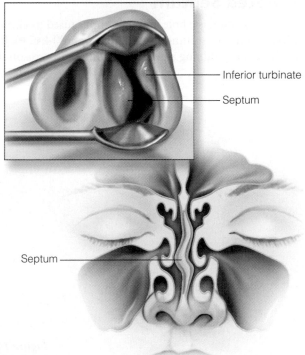

Inferior turbinate

Septum

Septum

Figure 14.40 ● Deviated septum.

Nasal Polyps

Nasal polyps are pale, round, firm, nonpainful overgrowth of nasal mucosa usually caused by chronic allergic rhinitis (see Figure 14.41 ●).

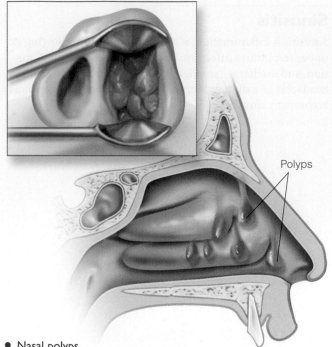

Figure 14.41 ● Nasal polyps.

Perforated Septum

A perforated septum is a hole in the septum caused by chronic infection, trauma, or sniffing cocaine (see Figure 14.42 ●). It can be detected by shining a penlight through the naris on the other side.

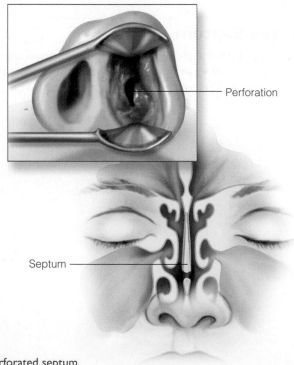

Figure 14.42 ● Perforated septum.

MOUTH AND THROAT

Ankyloglossia

Ankyloglossia is a fixation of the tip of the tongue to the floor of the mouth due to a shortened lingual frenulum (see Figure 14.43 ●). The condition is usually congenital and may be corrected surgically.

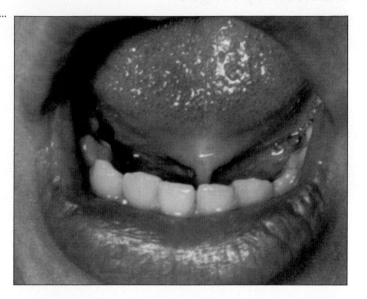

Figure 14.43 ● Ankyloglossia.

Aphthous Ulcers

Apthous ulcers, commonly called *canker sores,* are small, round, white lesions occurring singularly or in clusters on the oral mucosa (see Figure 14.44 ●). The lesions are acutely painful when they come in contact with the tongue, a toothbrush, or food. They commonly result from oral trauma, such as jabbing the side of the mouth with a toothbrush, but they are also associated with stress, exhaustion, and allergies to certain foods.

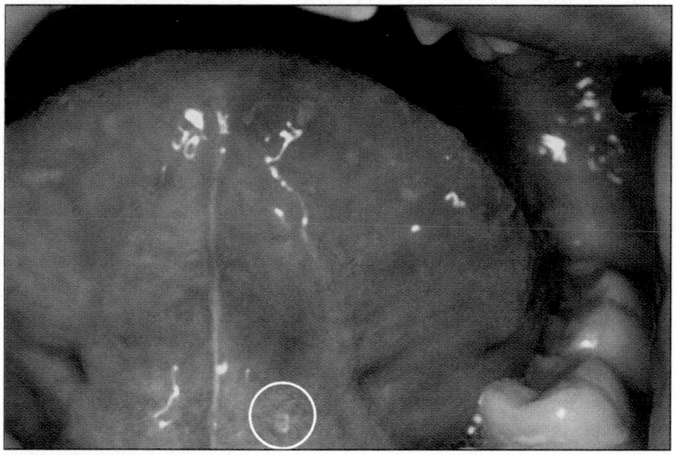

Figure 14.44 ● Aphthous ulcers.

Black Hairy Tongue

Black hairy tongue is a temporary condition caused by the inhibition of normal bacteria and the overgrowth of fungus on the papillae of the tongue (see Figure 14.45 ●). It is usually associated with the use of antibiotics.

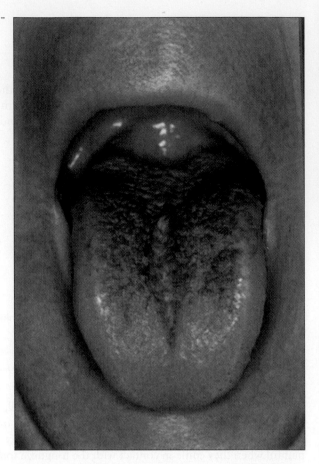

Figure 14.45 ● Black hairy tongue.

Gingival Hyperplasia

Gingival hyperplasia is an enlargement of the gums (see Figure 14.46 ●) frequently seen in pregnancy, in leukemia, or after prolonged use of phenytoin (Dilantin).

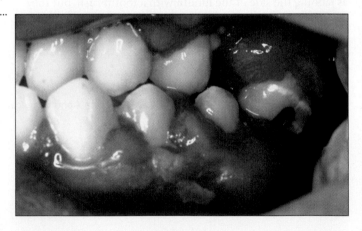

Figure 14.46 ● Gingival hyperplasia.

Gingivitis

Gingivitis is inflammation of the gums (see Figure 14.47 ●). It may be caused by poor dental hygiene or a deficiency of vitamin C. If left untreated, gingivitis may progress to periodontal disease and tooth loss.

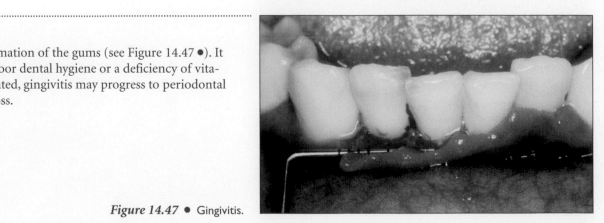

Figure 14.47 ● Gingivitis.

Tonsillitis

Tonsillitis is inflammation of the tonsils. The throat is red and the tonsils are swollen and covered by white or yellow patches or exudate (see Figure 14.48 ●). Lymph nodes in the cervical chain may be enlarged. Tonsillitis may be accompanied by a high fever.

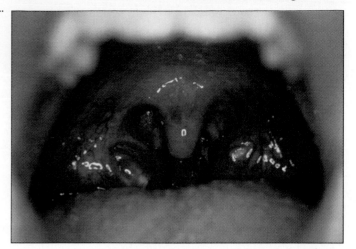

Figure 14.48 ● Tonsillitis.

Smooth Tongue

Smooth tongue is a condition occurring as a result of vitamin B and iron deficiency. The surface of the tongue is smooth and red with a shiny appearance (see Figure 14.49 ●).

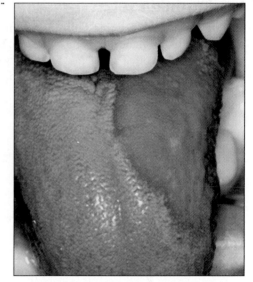

Figure 14.49 ● Smooth, glossy tongue (atrophic glossitis).

Herpes Simplex

Herpes simplex is a virus that is often accompanied by clear vesicles commonly called *cold sores* or *fever blisters,* usually at the junction of the skin and the lip (see Figure 14.50 ●). The vesicles erupt, then crust and heal within 2 weeks. They usually recur, especially after heavy exposure to bright sunlight (e.g., after a day at the beach).

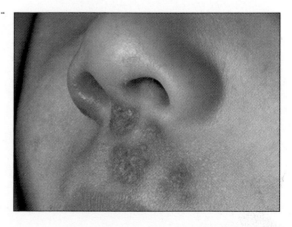

Figure 14.50 ● Herpes simplex.

Carcinoma

Oral cancers are most commonly found on the lower lip or the base (underside) of the tongue (see Figure 14.51 ●). Cancer is suspected if a sore or lesion does not heal within a few weeks. Heavy smoking, especially pipe smoking, and chewing tobacco increase the risk of oral cancer, as does chronic heavy use of alcohol.

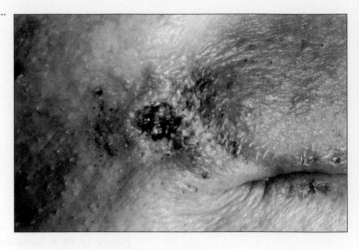

Figure 14.51 ● Carcinoma.

Leukoplakia

Leukoplakia is a whitish thickening of the mucous membrane in the mouth or tongue (see Figure 14.52 ●). It cannot be scraped off. Most often associated with heavy smoking or drinking, it can be a precancerous condition.

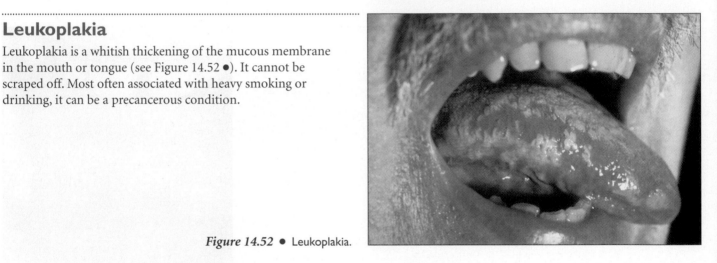

Figure 14.52 ● Leukoplakia.

Health Promotion

HEALTHY PEOPLE 2010

FOCUS AREA	PREVALENCE	OBJECTIVES	ACTIONS
Hearing	• Almost 28 million people in the United States have hearing deficits. • Bilateral deafness exists in approximately 1.5 million people over the age of 3 years. • Hearing loss is associated with genetic factors, noise, infection, or sensitivity to medication. • Noise-induced hearing loss (NIHL) is the most common occupational disorder. • About half of adults over 75 years of age experience loss of hearing. • Hearing loss impacts language development, literacy, and social interaction.	• Increase the number of people screened for hearing loss. • Reduce otitis media in children. • Increase the use of hearing protection. • Reduce NIHL.	• Education about screening at all ages. • Education about the treatment of ear infections. • Education about ear protection at all ages in schools, occupational areas, homes, and social areas.
Oral Health	• Dental caries is the most frequent chronic illness in children. • Tooth loss and endentulism is decreasing in the United States. • Endentulism occurs most frequently in low-income groups and is associated with periodontal disease. • People with less than high school education experience more tooth decay than those with more education. • African Americans have lower survival rates in cases of oropharyngeal cancer than Caucasians.	• Decrease the number of people with dental caries and decay. • Decrease the incidence of periodontal disease. • Increase the early detection of oropharyngeal cancers. • Increase the number of people receiving dental and oral care.	• Education regarding hygiene and treatment. • Education regarding regular oral and dental examinations. • Community or clinic access and referral.

CLIENT EDUCATION

The following are physiological, behavioral, and cultural factors that affect the health of the ears, nose, mouth, and throat across the age span. Several factors reflect trends cited in *Healthy People 2010*. The nurse provides advice and education to reduce risks associated with the previously mentioned factors and to promote and maintain health of the ears, nose, mouth, and throat.

LIFE SPAN CONSIDERATIONS

RISK FACTORS

- Bottles at bedtime or propped in the crib with infants increase the risk for dental disease and ear infection.
- Children are likely to introduce foreign objects into the nose and ears.
- Hearing acuity diminishes with aging.
- The sense of smell diminishes with aging.

CLIENT EDUCATION

- Provide information about bottles at bedtime in relation to dental health and prevention of ear problems.
- Teach parents about safety in relation to toys and objects that may have small parts or easily loosened small parts. Advise them to seek assistance from healthcare providers to remove foreign bodies from the ears or nose.
- Advise adults to have annual hearing tests after age 55 and provide information about use of hearing aids for older adults.
- Advise clients with decreased sense of smell about the use of smoke alarms in the home and to establish the practice of monitoring pilot lights or dials of gas appliances.

ENVIRONMENTAL CONSIDERATIONS

RISK FACTORS

- Loud noise from machinery and music in the workplace or home can result in diminished hearing.
- Respiratory infections are easily transmissible through diffusion of droplets and spraying of nasal and oral secretions.
- Some medications including Dilantin and steroids in infants may promote problems with the gums or oral mucosa.

CLIENT EDUCATION

- Educate clients across the age span that noise in the work, home, and social environments can increase the risk of hearing loss. Provide advice about safety.
- Instruct all clients about use of tissues and hand washing to reduce the risk of spread of respiratory infections.
- Inform clients about medications. Teach self-assessment regarding side effects that affect the gums and mouth including gingivitis and fungal infections.

BEHAVIORAL CONSIDERATIONS

RISK FACTOR

- Smoking and the use of oral tobacco products increase the risk for oral cancer.

CLIENT EDUCATION

- Advise clients about smoking cessation. Inform individuals and parents about recommendations for dental examination and hygiene measures.

Application Through Critical Thinking

CASE STUDY

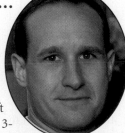

Harold Chandler is a 35-year-old executive in a computer firm who comes to the employees' wellness center complaining of a marked loss of hearing in his left ear. He says that he woke up yesterday with a "feeling of fullness" in his left ear but no pain. He further relates that his 3-year-old daughter has a "bad cold and an earache," and he wonders if he has "the same thing." He denies any other symptoms of infection, has had no discharge from either ear, and is not taking any medicine at this time. He has not had an audiometric examination since his last physical 3 years ago. He

further volunteers that he has just returned from a business trip to Europe and wonders whether the pressurized atmosphere of the airplane "created a problem with his hearing."

Nurse Michael Navarro's focused assessment of Mr. Chandler reveals normal vital signs. His left ear's external canal is of a uniform pink color, with no redness, swelling, lesions, or discharge. The Weber test reveals lateralization to the left ear. The otoscopic examination reveals a left ear impacted with brown-gray cerumen, and the tympanic membrane cannot be visualized. Examination of the right ear shows the external canal is of a uniform pink color with no redness, swelling, lesions, or discharge. During the otoscopic examination, the tympanic membrane is easily visualized. It is translucent and pearl-gray with the cone of light at the 5-o'clock position. No perforations are noted.

To visualize the tympanic membrane of the left ear, Mr. Navarro prepares a solution of mineral oil and hydrogen peroxide and instills the solution into the left ear canal to soften the cerumen. Then he irrigates the canal with warm water using a bulb syringe. After Mr. Navarro completes the irrigation, Mr. Chandler is surprised to discover that his hearing has returned in his left ear. Now Mr. Navarro completes the otoscopic examination. He is able to visualize the tympanic membrane, which is translucent and pearl-gray with the cone of light at the 7-o'clock position. No perforations are noted.

To be sure that Mr. Chandler's hearing has been restored, Mr. Navarro performs a screening evaluation of his auditory function. He is able to hear a low whisper at 2 ft. His Rinne test is positive, and his Weber test indicates equal lateralization.

► Complete Documentation

The following is sample documentation for Harold Chandler.
SUBJECTIVE DATA: 35-year-old c/o hearing loss (L) ear. Woke up yesterday with fullness, no pain (L) ear. His 3-year-old daughter has "bad cold and earache," wonders if he has the same. Denies signs of infection, no discharge, and no medication. Audiometric examination 3 years ago. Recent air travel, wonders if pressurized atmosphere created hearing problem.
OBJECTIVE DATA: Ears, equal in size, shape. Tragus mobile, nontender bilaterally. Left ear canal pink, no redness, edema, lesions, discharge. Weber—lateralization to left. Otoscopic exam-

ination: Left ear impacted—brown-gray cerumen, no visualization tympanic membrane. Right ear—canal pink, clear, no edema, tympanic membrane gray with no lesions.

► Critical Thinking Questions

1. Describe the application of critical thinking to the situation.
2. How was information clustered to guide decision making?
3. What recommendations should the nurse provide for this client?

► Applying Nursing Diagnoses

1. *Disturbed sensory perception* is a nursing diagnosis in the NANDA taxonomy. Do the data for Mr. Chandler support this diagnosis? If so, identify the data.
2. Use the NANDA taxonomy in Appendix A to develop a diagnosis for Mr. Chandler. ∞ Identify the data required for the PES (problem, etiology, signs or symptoms) statement.

► Prepare Teaching Plan

LEARNING NEED: Mr. Chandler experienced a hearing problem and sought treatment because he was unsure of the cause. The data revealed his concern that the hearing loss and ear discomfort he experienced were from "a cold, like my daughter" or "pressure changes due to air travel." After examination, it was determined that the cause of Mr. Chandler's problem was impacted cerumen.

ASSESSMENT FORM

EXTERNAL EAR:

Size	L = R	_x_ yes	___ no							
Shape	L = R	_x_ yes	___ no							
Lesions	L	_x_ yes	___ no							
	R	_x_ yes	___ no							
Tragus	L	Mobile	_x_ yes	___ no	Tender	_x_ no	___ yes			
	R	Mobile	_x_ yes	___ no	Tender	_x_ no	___ yes			
Meatus	L	Patent	_x_ yes	___ no	Discharge	_x_ no	___ yes			
	R	Patent	_x_ yes	___ no	Discharge	_x_ no	___ yes			

INTERNAL EAR:

Canal	L	Clear	___ yes	_x_ no	*Impacted cerumen*		
	R	Clear	_x_ yes	___ no			
Cerumen	L	Present	_x_ small	___ medium	___ large	_x_	
	R	Present	_x_ small	_x_ medium	___ large		
	L	Soft	___ yes	_x_ no	Color	*Brown-gray*	
	R	Soft	_x_ yes	___ no	Color	*Orange*	
Tympanic	L	Gray	___ yes	___ no	*(unknown)*		
	R	Gray	_x_ yes	___ no			
	L	Lesions	___ no	___ yes	*(unknown)*		
	R	Lesions	_x_ no	___ yes			
Weber	L = R		___ yes	_x_ no	*Lateralizes left*		

APPLICATION OF OBJECTIVE 3: Describe measures for care of the ear

Content	Teaching Strategy and Rationale	Evaluation

• An old adage: Never put anything smaller than your elbow in your ear.
 • Ear canals should never have to be cleaned. The cerumen moves to the outside naturally.
 • Sometimes, the cerumen is excreted in large amounts or it is not effectively cleared.
 • Do's and Don'ts
   • Do consult your physician when you have ear symptoms.
   • Do follow the instructions for use of commercial ear wax removal products.
   • Don't use cotton swabs, hairpins, or paper clips to attempt to remove cerumen. You may perforate the eardrum or merely push the cerumen farther into the canal.
	• Lecture
	 • Discussion
	 • Audiovisual materials
	 • Printed materials
	 Lecture is appropriate when disseminating information to large groups.
	 Discussion allows participants to bring up concerns and to raise questions.
	 Audiovisual materials, such as illustrations of the structures of the ear, reinforce verbal presentation.
	 Printed material, especially to be taken away with learners, allows review, reinforcement, and reading at the learner's own pace.
		• Written examination. May use short answer, fill-in, or multiple-choice items or a combination of items.
		 • If these are short and easy to evaluate, the learner receives immediate feedback.

The case study provides data that is representative of symptoms and behaviors of a variety of hearing and ear problems. Individuals and groups could benefit from education about the ear, hearing loss, and care of the ear. The following teaching plan is intended for a group of learners and focuses on ear care.

GOAL: The participants will practice safe care of the ear.

OBJECTIVES: Upon completion of this educational session, the participants will be able to:

1. Identify the structures of the ear.
2. Discuss common problems with the ear.
3. Describe measures for care of the ear.

Circle **T** for true and **F** for false, fill in the blank, or select the correct answer(s) for the following statements:

1. The outer ear funnels sound.   T   F

2. Cerumen is made in the ear canal.   T   F

3. The eardrum separates the outer and inner ear.   T   F

4. The eustachian tube helps equalize pressure in the ear.   T   F

5. Structures of the ear regulate balance.   T   F

6. The purposes of cerumen are to _____ and _____ .

7. Hearing loss can occur in which of the following problems:

    a. infection

    b. neurologic problems

    c. perforated eardrum

    d. cerumen buildup

8. The symptoms of cerumen blockage are _____
_____ .

9. You should not use cotton swabs in the ear canal because _____
_____ .

10. Always follow the directions when using _____ .

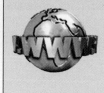

Please refer to the Companion Website at www.prenhall.com/damico and click on Chapter 14, the Application Through Critical Thinking module, to complete the following activities related to this case study:
► **Critical Thinking questions**
► **Extended Nursing Diagnosis challenge**
► **Documentation activity**
► **Teaching Plan for Objectives 1 and 2**

EXPLORE MediaLink

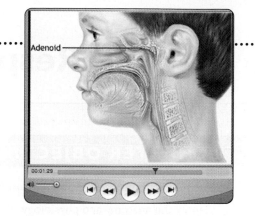

Additional resources for this chapter are found on the Student CD-ROM accompanying this textbook and on the Companion Website.

CD-ROM CONTENT

Content for this chapter includes:
Objectives
Key Concepts
NCLEX-RN® Review Questions
Model Documentation Forms
Audio Glossary
Animations
   The Middle Ear
   Ear Anatomy
   Caries of the Teeth
Games and Challenges
Clinical Spotlight Videos
   Allergic Rhinitis
   Otitis Media
   Sleep Apnea
Head-to-Toe Physical Examination Video

Client Interaction Case Study Challenge
Application Through Critical Thinking
   Case Study Teaching Plan Challenge
MediaLinks
MediaLink Application
Tool Box
   Chapter Documentation Form Example
   Health Promotion
     Healthy People 2010
     Client Education
New York Times

COMPANION WEBSITE CONTENT

www.prenhall.com/damico

Content for this chapter includes:
Objectives
NCLEX-RN® Review Questions

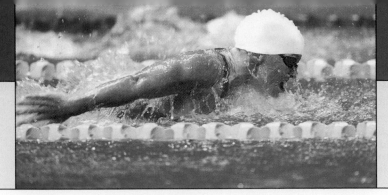

15

Respiratory System

MEDIALINK

www.prenhall.com/damico

The CD-ROM in the back of this textbook and the Media-Link website contain NCLEX-RN® review questions, interactive exercises, case study challenges, animations, videos, documentation and checklist forms, and review materials. For a complete listing of the media content specific to Chapter 15, see the Explore MediaLink at the end of the chapter.

The primary responsibility of the respiratory system is the exchange of gases in the body. Exchange of oxygen and carbon dioxide is essential to the homeostatic and hemodynamic process of the body. The intake of oxygen needed for metabolism and the release of carbon dioxide, which is the waste product of metabolism, occurs with each respiratory cycle. This delicate balance of gas exchange is influenced by the nervous system, the cardiovascular system, and the musculoskeletal system. The central nervous system, influenced by the amount of gases in the blood, regulates the rate and depth of each respiratory cycle. The cardiovascular system is responsible for transporting the gases throughout the body. The musculoskeletal system provides the bones to protect the structures of the respiratory system, and the muscular activity allows for the rhythmic movement of the thoracic cavity. This coordinated movement with pressure changes in the thoracic cavity leads to the exchange of the oxygen and carbon dioxide.

The respiratory system has a major role in helping the body to maintain acid-base balance. The amount of carbon dioxide in the blood directly influences the amount of carbonic acid and hydrogen ion concentration in the blood. The respiratory system responds to the needs of the body to either retain or excrete carbon dioxide. This action will help maintain the delicate balance of carbonic acid and bicarbonate ions at the 1:20 ratio keeping the plasma pH between 7.35 and 7.45, the normal range.

The respiratory system is also influential in the production of vocal sounds. As air moves out of the lungs and passes over the vocal cords, the individual produces sounds commonly called speech. The length of the vocal cords, the tension of the vocal cords, the movement of the glottis, and the force of the air across the vocal cords influence the pitch and volume of one's speech. The quality of the voice is further influenced by other structures including the pharynx, tongue, palate, mouth, and lips.

Assessment of respiratory function is an integral aspect of the total client assessment performed by the professional nurse. Developmental factors are considered during assessment of the respiratory system. Newborns have a high respiratory rate. Respirations of a child are abdominal in nature. As the uterus enlarges during pregnancy for the pregnant female, the pressure in the abdominal cavity also increases. As a result, diaphragmatic excursion is limited and can result in more rapid and shallow respirations.

Environmental factors also contribute to respiratory difficulty and pathology, which ultimately can affect respiratory function. Assessment must identify exposure to irritants such as dust, tobacco, smoke, pollen, smog, asbestos, and vapors from household cleaners. Tobacco use is one of the leading health indicators described in *Healthy People 2010*. A goal of *Healthy People 2010* is to promote respiratory health through prevention, detection, treatment, and education (see *Healthy People 2010* feature on page 392). The nurse must be cognizant of factors that influence respiratory health as questions for the focused interview are formulated and physical assessment is performed.

ANATOMY AND PHYSIOLOGY REVIEW

The thorax, commonly called the chest, is a closed cavity of the body, containing structures needed for respirations. The thorax, or thoracic cavity, is surrounded by ribs and muscles and extends from the base of the neck to the diaphragm. It has three sections: the mediastinum and the right and left pleural cavities. The **mediastinum** contains the heart, trachea, esophagus, and major blood vessels of the body. Each pleural cavity contains a lung (see Figure 15.1 ●).

The major structures of the respiratory system are situated in the thoracic cavity. The major function of the respiratory system is to supply the body with oxygen and expel carbon dioxide. Air moves in and out of the lungs with each **respiratory cycle.** A complete respiratory cycle consists of an inspiratory phase and an expiratory phase of breathing. The exchange of oxygen and carbon dioxide at the alveoli level of the lung is *external respiration*. Gases are transported from the lungs via the blood to the cells of the body. As the gases move across the systemic capillaries, exchange of oxygen and carbon dioxide occurs at the cellular level and *internal respiration* occurs.

KEY TERMS

adventitious sounds, 378
angle of Louis, 353
bronchial sounds, 377
bronchophony, 379
bronchovesicular sounds, 377
dullness, 375
dyspnea, 353
egophony, 379
eupnea, 353
fremitus, 373
landmarks, 353
manubrium, 353
mediastinum, 349
rales, 378
resonance, 374
respiratory cycle, 349
rhonchi, 378
tracheal sounds, 377
vesicular sounds, 377
wheezes, 378
whispered pectoriloquy, 379

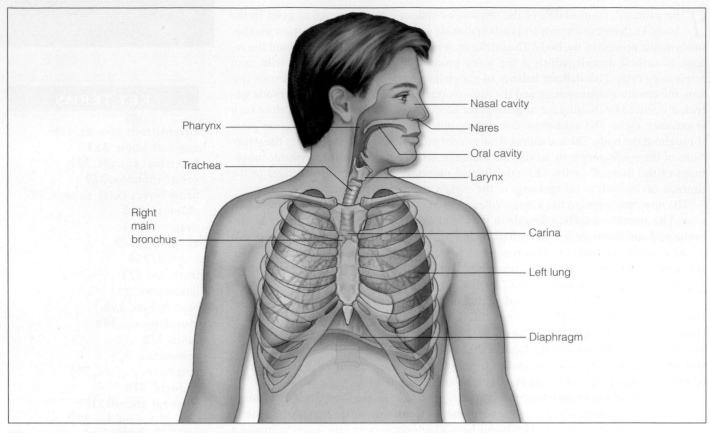

Figure 15.1 • Anatomy of the respiratory system.

The respiratory system consists of the upper and lower respiratory tracts. The structures of the upper respiratory tract consist of the nose, the mouth, the sinuses, the pharynx, the larynx, and a portion of the trachea. The lower respiratory tract includes the distal portion of the trachea, bronchi, and lungs. Pleural membranes, the muscles of respiration, and the mediastinum complete the lower respiratory tract.

The anatomy and physiology review and assessment of the structures of the upper respiratory tract were discussed in Chapter 12 on pages 235–253. ⊙⊙ Before proceeding, it may be helpful to review this information.

LOWER RESPIRATORY TRACT

The lower respiratory tract includes the trachea, bronchi, and lungs. Additional structures of the pleural membranes, the mediastinum, and the muscles of respiration are also discussed at this time. Consideration must be given to all structures during the assessment process.

Trachea

The trachea, located in the mediastinum, descends from the larynx in the neck to the main bronchi at the distal point. It is approximately 10 to 12 cm (4 in.) long and 2.5 cm (1 in.) in diameter. The trachea is a very flexible and mobile structure, bifurcating anteriorly at about the sternal angle and posteriorly at about the vertebrae T_3 to T_5. The trachea contains 16 to 20 rings of hyaline cartilage. These C-shaped rings help maintain the shape of the trachea and prevent its collapse during inspiration

and expiration. Just above the point of bifurcation, the last tracheal cartilage, known as the carina, is expanded. The carina separates the openings of the two main bronchi. The trachea, like other structures of the respiratory tract, is lined with a mucous-producing membrane that traps dust, bacteria, and other foreign bodies. This membrane at the level of the carina is most sensitive to foreign substances. Coughing and cilia, hairlike projections of the membrane, help sweep debris toward the mouth for removal.

Bronchi

Anteriorly, the trachea bifurcates at about the level of the sternal angle forming the right and left main bronchi (see Figure 15.2 •). The main bronchus enters each lung at the hilus (medial depression) and maintains an oblique position in the mediastinum. The right main bronchus is shorter, wider, and more vertical than the left bronchus; therefore, aspirated objects are more likely to enter the right lung. The bronchi continue to divide within each lobe of the lung. The terminal bronchioles are less than 0.5 mm in diameter. The bronchi and the many branches continue to warm and moisten air as it moves along the respiratory tract to the alveoli in the lungs.

Lungs

The lungs are cone-shaped, elastic, spongy, air-filled structures that are situated in the pleural cavities of the thorax on either side of the mediastinum (see Figure 15.3 •). The apex of each lung is slightly superior to the inner third of the clavicle, and

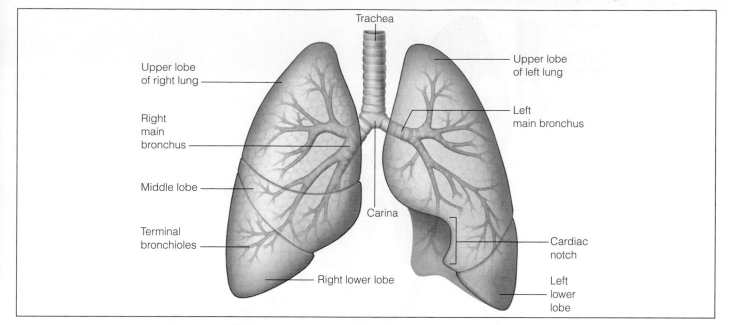

Figure 15.2 ● Respiratory passages.

the base of each lung is at the level of the diaphragm. The left lung has two lobes (upper and lower) and tends to be longer and narrower than the right lung. The left lung accommodates the heart at the medial surface. The oblique fissure separates the two lobes of this lung. The right lung has three lobes (upper, middle, and lower) and is slightly larger, wider, and shorter than the left lung. The horizontal and oblique fissures separate the lobes of the right lung. Within each lung, the numerous terminal bronchioles branch into the alveolar ducts, which lead into alveolar sacs and alveoli. The single-layered cells of the alveoli permit simple diffusion and gas exchanges to occur (see Figure 15.4 ●).

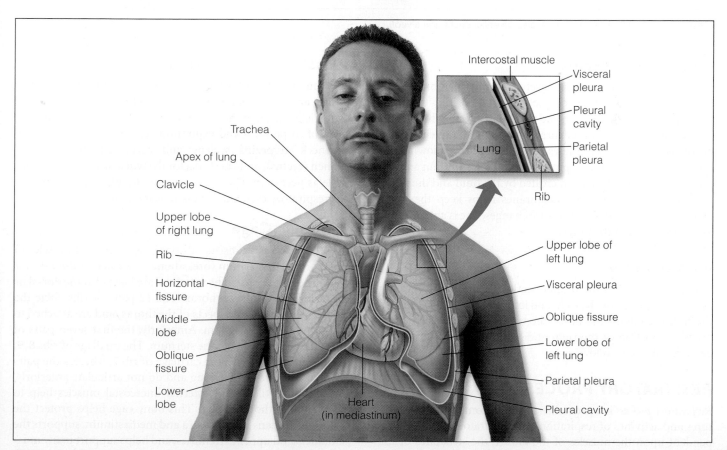

Figure 15.3 ● Anterior view of thorax and lungs.

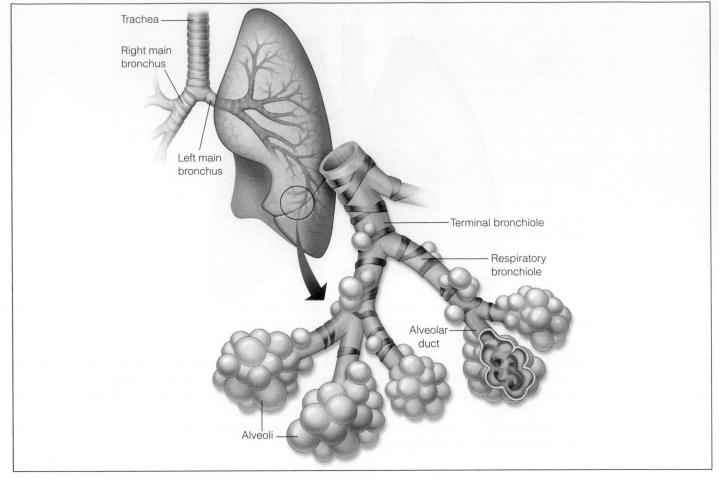

Figure 15.4 ● Respiratory bronchioles, alveolar ducts, and alveoli.

Pleural Membranes

The pleura is a thin, double-layered, serous membrane that lines each pleural cavity. The parietal membrane lines the superior aspect of the diaphragm and the thoracic wall. The visceral membrane covers the outer surface of the lung. A pleural fluid produced by these membranes acts as a lubricant allowing the lung to glide during the respiratory cycle of inspiration and expiration. The surface tension created by the fluid and the negative pressure between the membranes helps keep the lungs expanded. As the negative pressure changes, one is able to move air into and out of the lungs.

Mediastinum

The mediastinum is the middle section of the thoracic cavity and is surrounded by the right and left pleural cavities. The mediastinum contains the heart, the trachea, the esophagus, the proximal portion of the right and left main bronchi, and the great vessels of the body.

RESPIRATORY PROCESS

Respiratory process is a general term that encompasses the structures and activities of respiration. The respiratory process is dependent upon the muscles of the thorax, the structures of the thoracic cage, and the ability of air to move in and out of the body.

Muscles of Respiration

The muscles of the thoracic cage (internal and external intercostal) and the diaphragm assist in the breathing process. The synergistic action of these muscle groups aids in the respiratory cycle of inspiration and expiration. The accessory muscles of the neck (trapezius, scalene, and sternocleidomastoid), abdomen (rectus), and chest (pectorals) will assist the respiratory cycle as necessary. The accessory muscles play a major role in the respiratory cycle during distress and pathology.

Thoracic Cage

The thoracic cage consists of bones, cartilage, and muscles of the thorax. The sternum (breastbone) is located in the anterior midline of the thorax. The vertebrae are located at the dorsal or posterior aspect of the thorax. The 12 pairs of ribs circle the body, form the lateral aspects of the thorax, and are attached to the vertebrae and sternum. Anteriorly, the first seven pairs of ribs articulate directly to the sternum. The cartilage of ribs 8, 9, and 10 articulates with the cartilage of rib 7, whereas the pairs of 11 and 12 are free floating and do not articulate anteriorly. The costal cartilage and external intercostal muscles help to complete the thoracic cage. This bony cage helps protect the many vital organs of the pleura and mediastinum, supports the shoulders and upper extremities, and helps support many muscles of the upper part of the body.

Respiratory Cycle

Respiratory cycle, respirations, and *breathing* are terms used interchangeably to indicate the movement of air in and out of the body. Breathing consists of two phases: inspiration and expiration, thus, the term *respiratory cycle.* Inspiration is considered to be the active aspect of the respiratory cycle. For air to enter the body, respiratory muscles contract, the chest expands, alveolar pressure decreases, and the negative intrapleural pressure increases. These combined activities allow air to enter the expanded lungs. During expiration, the passive phase of the process, the activities reverse themselves, the lungs recoil, and air leaves the body. The regular, even-depth, rhythmic pattern of inspiration and expiration describes **eupnea:** normal breathing. A change in this pattern, producing shortness of breath or difficulty in breathing, is **dyspnea.**

LANDMARKS

Identification and location of **landmarks** helps the professional nurse develop a mental picture of the structures being assessed. Thoracic reference points and specific anatomical structures are used as landmarks (see Figure 15.5). They help provide an exact location for the assessment findings and an accurate orientation for documentation of findings. Landmark identification for the thorax includes bony structures, horizontal and vertical lines, and the division of the thorax.

The thorax may be divided into two or three sections for assessment. Two sections include the anterior and posterior thorax, while three sections include the anterior, lateral, and posterior aspects. This text uses the former option: The lateral areas are incorporated into the anterior and posterior sections. The bony structures include the sternum, clavicles, ribs, and vertebrae. At the horizontal plane, the landmarks are the clavicles, the ribs, and the corresponding intercostal spaces. Anteriorly, the vertical lines start at the sternum and are strategically drawn parallel to this structure. Posteriorly, the vertical lines start at the vertebral column and additional lines are drawn parallel to this reference point.

The first bony landmark to be considered is the sternum, commonly called the breastbone. It is a flat, elongated bone located in the midline of the anterior thoracic cage and consists of three parts: the manubrium, body, and xiphoid process. The clavicles and some of the pairs of ribs articulate with the sternum. The **manubrium** is the superior portion of the sternum. The depression at the superior border is called the suprasternal notch or jugular notch. This becomes a primary landmark used to identify and locate other landmarks. The manubrium joins the body of the sternum. As these structures meet, a horizontal ridge is formed, referred to as the sternal angle or **angle of Louis.** The second rib and the second intercostal space are at this level of the sternum. The sternum terminates at the xiphoid process. This process and the inferior borders of the seventh ribs form a triangle referred to as the costal angle. The inferior border of the ribs and the costal angle help identify the level of the diaphragm, the base of the lungs, and the separation of the thoracic cavity from the abdomen (Figure 15.5A ●).

The clavicles are long, slender, curved bones that articulate with the manubrium at the medial aspect. The lateral aspects help form the shoulder joint with the acromion of the scapula. The clavicles act as a shock absorber protecting the upper portion of the thoracic cage and the delicate underlying structures. Lung tissue will be assessed above and below the clavicles. Findings above the clavicle are considered supraclavicular, while findings below the clavicle are infraclavicular.

The 12 pairs of ribs are another bony landmark used in respiratory assessment. The ribs circle the body and help form horizontal reference points. Posteriorly, each rib attaches to a thoracic vertebra. The ribs curve downward and forward as they become anterior (Figure 15.5B ●). Bilaterally, the first seven ribs attach to the sternum and are called true ribs. Ribs 8, 9, and 10 attach to cartilage of the superior rib, while ribs 11 and 12 are free floating anteriorly. A number identifies each rib. Each intercostal space, the space between the ribs, takes the number of the superior rib. The first rib and the first intercostal space, being obscured by the clavicle, are not palpable. Anteriorly, ribs 2 to 7 and the corresponding intercostal spaces are easily palpated along the sternal border. Posteriorly, the ribs are best palpated and counted close to the vertebral column. Each rib and intercostal space form a horizontal line used as a landmark.

The vertebral column, commonly called the spine, is located at the midline of the posterior portion of the thoracic cage. Twelve vertebrae are thoracic, and a pair of ribs articulates with each. The vertebral column contributes to the vertical lines to be discussed later in this chapter. The seventh cervical vertebra (C_7) is most visible at the base of the neck. The much larger spinous process contributes to the uniqueness of the vertebrae. This prominent vertebra (C_7) is used to count and locate other spinous processes. When two spinous processes are equally prominent, they are C_7 and T_1 (see Figure 15.6 ●).

Five imaginary vertical lines are identified on the anterior aspect of the thoracic cage (see Figure 15.7 ●). These lines are the sternal line, the right and left midclavicular lines, and the right and left anterior axillary lines. The sternal or midsternal line (SL) starts at the sternal notch and descends through the xiphoid process. It divides the sternum in half and ultimately identifies the right and left thoracic cage. The right and left midclavicular lines are parallel to the sternal line. The midclavicular line begins at the midpoint of the clavicle and descends to the level of the twelfth rib. The nipples of the breast are slightly lateral to this line. This line subdivides the right and left thoracic cage into two equal parts. The anterior axillary line (AAL) is another line drawn parallel to the sternal line. It begins at the anterior fold of the axillae and descends along the anterior lateral aspect of the thoracic cage to the twelfth rib.

Five imaginary lines are located on the posterior aspect of the thoracic cage (see Figure 15.8 ●). The vertebral line, the right and left scapular lines, and the right and left posterior axillary lines are used as landmarks on the posterior aspect of the thoracic cage. The vertebral or midspinous line commences at C_7 and descends through the spinous process of each thoracic vertebra. It divides the vertebral column in half, forming the posterior right and left thoracic cage.

The scapular line, parallel to the vertebral line, is drawn from the inferior angle of the scapula to the level of the twelfth rib. This line subdivides the right and left thoracic cage into

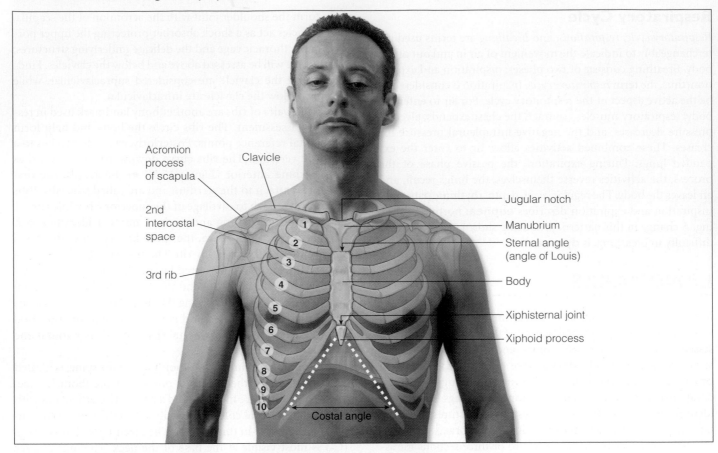

Figure 15.5A ● Landmarks of the anterior thorax, anterior view.

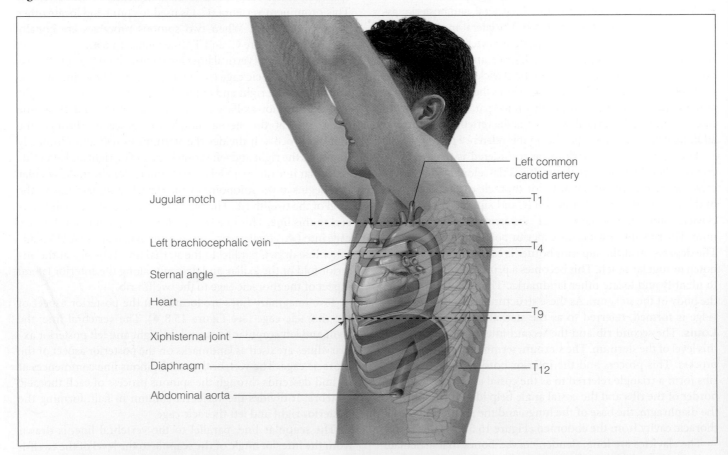

Figure 15.5B ● Landmarks of the anterior thorax, left lateral view, showing relationship of anterior landmarks to the vertebral column.

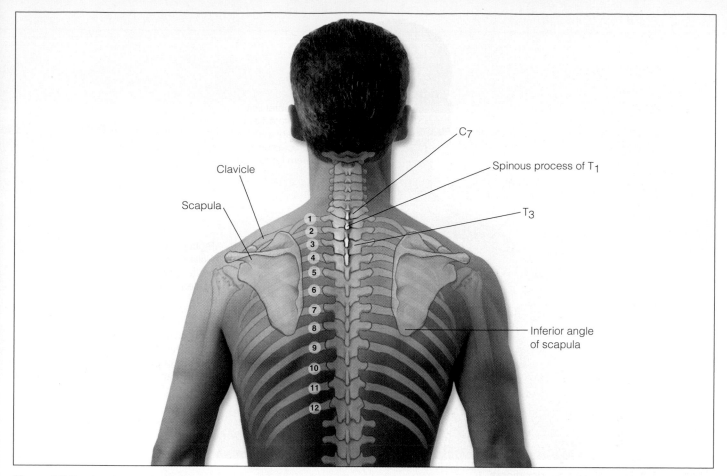

Figure 15.6 ● Landmarks: Posterior thorax.

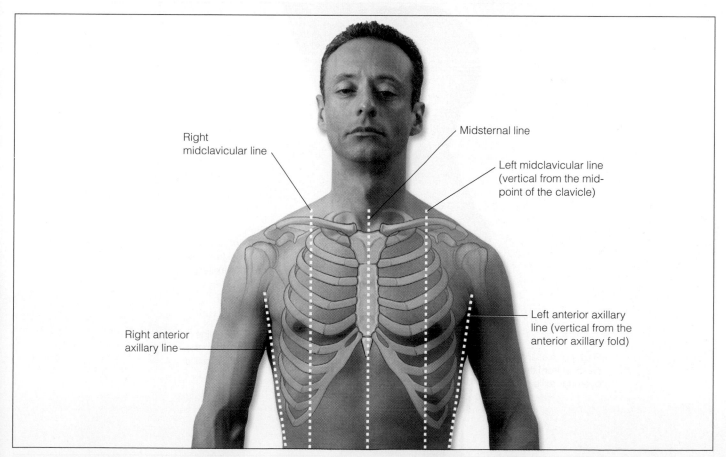

Figure 15.7 ● Lines of the anterior thorax.

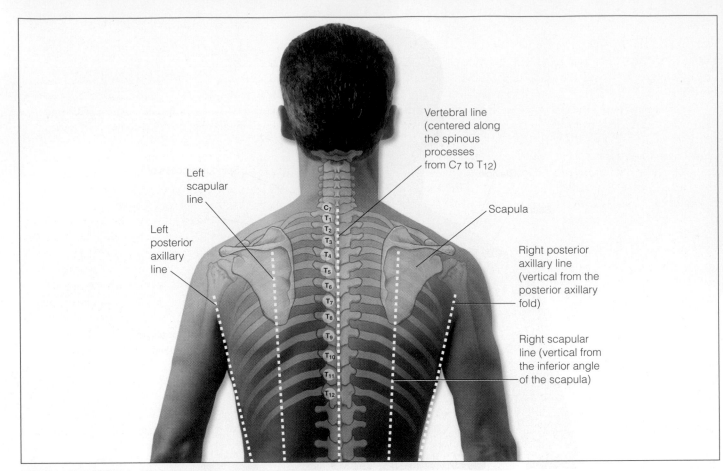

Figure 15.8 ● Lines of the posterior thorax.

Vertebral line
(centered along
the spinous
processes
from C7 to T12)

Left
scapular
line

Left
posterior
axillary
line

Scapula

Right posterior
axillary line
(vertical from the
posterior axillary
fold)

Right scapular
line (vertical from
the inferior angle
of the scapula)

C7
T1
T2
T3
T4
T5
T6
T7
T8
T9
T10
T11
T12

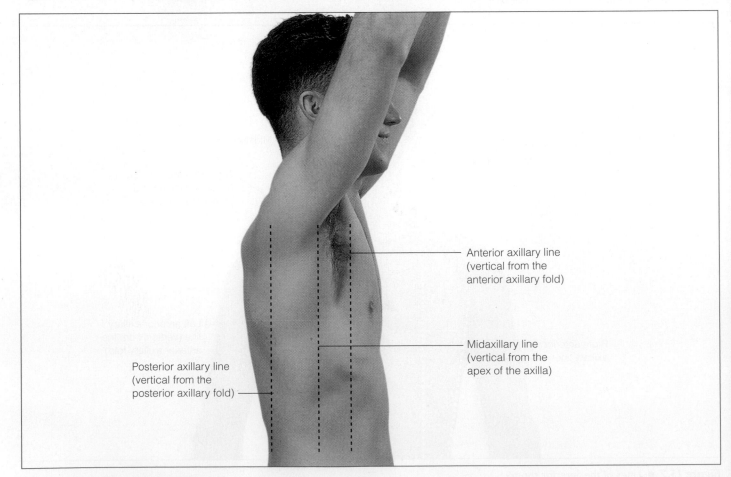

Figure 15.9 ● Lines of the lateral thorax.

Anterior axillary line
(vertical from the
anterior axillary fold)

Midaxillary line
(vertical from the
apex of the axilla)

Posterior axillary line
(vertical from the
posterior axillary fold)

two equal parts. The posterior axillary line (PAL) is parallel to the vertebral line. It starts at the posterior axillary fold and descends along the lateral aspect of the thoracic cage to the twelfth rib.

The lateral aspect of the thoracic cage is the third section to be considered. Three imaginary lines are identified in this section (see Figure 15.9 ●). They are the anterior, posterior, and midaxillary lines. Two of these lines, the anterior and posterior lines, have been described. The midaxillary line is parallel to the anterior and posterior axillary lines. This line descends from the middle of the axillae to the level of the twelfth rib. It forms the frontal plane dividing the thorax into the anterior and posterior portions.

The described landmarks serve as a reference point for internal structures of the respiratory system. Recall that the trachea bifurcates, forming the right and left main bronchus. Anteriorly, this occurs at the level of the angle of Louis or sternal angle. Posteriorly, this bifurcation occurs between the third and fifth thoracic vertebrae.

The apices of the lung extend 2 to 4 cm above the inner third of the clavicle anteriorly. Posteriorly, the apices of the lungs are located superior to the scapula between the vertebral line and midscapular line. The base of the lung has three reference points. The lung is cone shaped, and the base of the lung is located at the sixth intercostal space at the midclavicular line. At the midaxillary line the base of the lung is at the eighth intercostal space. At

the scapular line on the posterior thorax, the base of the lung is at the tenth intercostal space.

Using external landmarks and drawing imaginary lines can also identify the five lobes of the lungs. Remember that the right lung has three lobes and the left lung has two lobes. The right and left oblique fissure divides the lung into upper and lower lobes. Starting at C_7 identify T_3. Draw an imaginary line from T_3 at the vertebral line to the fifth intercostal space at the midaxillary line. This line follows the border of the scapula when the arms are extended over the head. It reflects the oblique fissure on the posterior wall of the thorax (see Figure 15.10 ●). On the left side continue this line to the sixth intercostal at the left midclavicular line. The two lobes of the left lung have been identified at the posterior, lateral, and anterior aspects of the left thorax.

Anteriorly, on the right side, draw two lines from the fifth intercostal space at the midaxillary line. One line descends to the sixth intercostal space at the right midclavicular line. The second line transverses the right thorax to the sternal border inferior to the fourth rib. These lines identify the oblique fissure and the horizontal fissure forming the three lobes of the right lung (see Figure 15.11 ● and Figures 15.12A ● and B ●).

The clavicle, the scapula, and the lateral base of the neck form a triangle at the superior aspect of the thorax. This triangle, also known as Kronig's area, will be used for palpation of muscles and lymph nodes and for percussion and auscultation of the apex and the lungs.

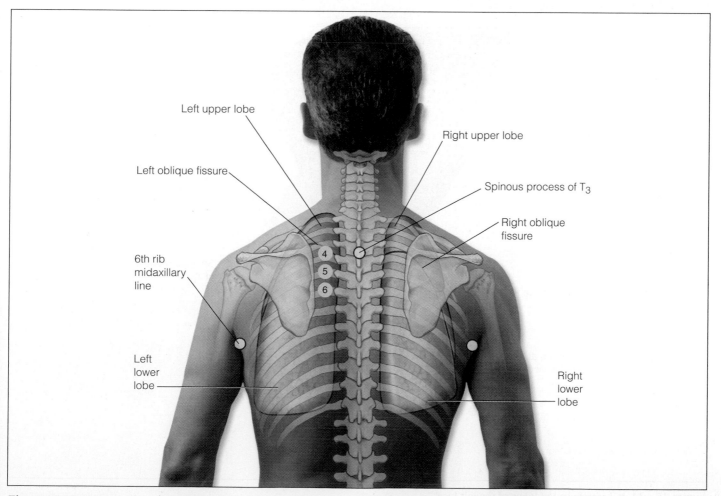

Figure 15.10 ● Lobes of the lungs: Posterior view.

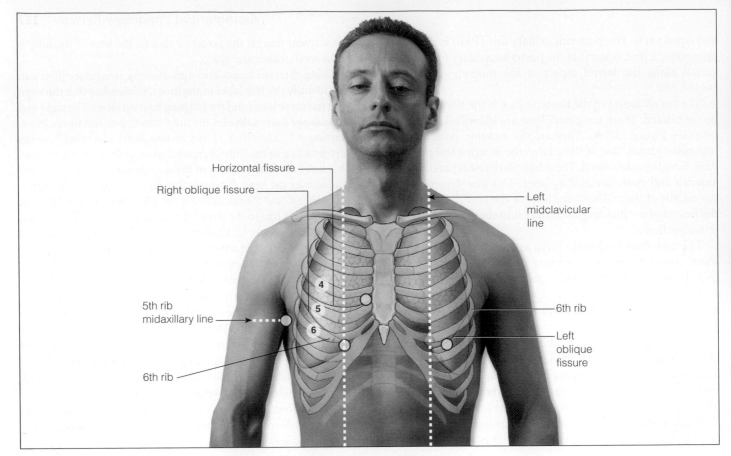

Horizontal fissure

Right oblique fissure

Left
midclavicular
line

5th rib
midaxillary line

4

5

6

6th rib

6th rib

Left
oblique
fissure

Figure 15.11 ● Lobes of the lungs: Anterior view.

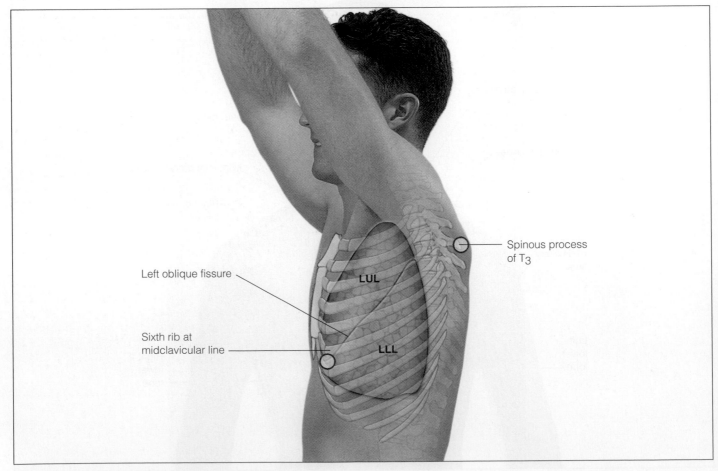

Spinous process
of T₃

Left oblique fissure

LUL

Sixth rib at
midclavicular line

LLL

Figure 15.12A ● Lateral view of lobes of the left lung.

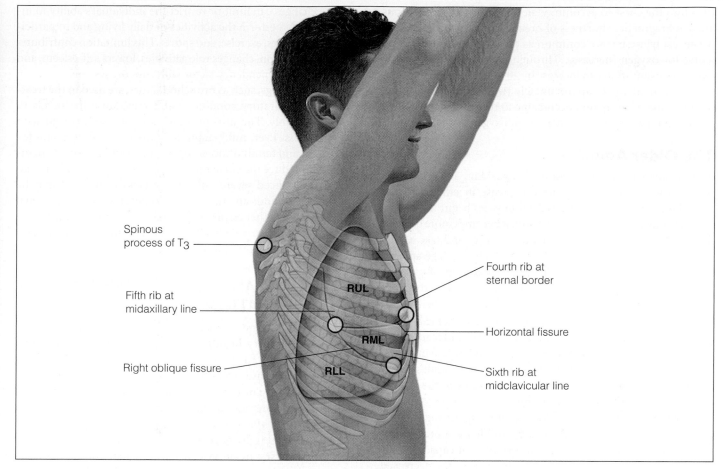

Spinous process of T₃

Fifth rib at midaxillary line

Right oblique fissure

RUL

RML

RLL

Fourth rib at sternal border

Horizontal fissure

Sixth rib at midclavicular line

Figure 15.12B ● Lateral view of lobes of the right lung.

SPECIAL CONSIDERATIONS

Throughout the assessment process the nurse gathers subjective and objective data reflecting the client's state of health. Using critical thinking and the nursing process, the nurse identifies many factors to be considered when collecting the data. Some of these factors include but are not limited to age, developmental level, race, ethnicity, work history, living conditions, socioeconomic status, and emotional wellness.

DEVELOPMENTAL CONSIDERATIONS

Growth and development are dynamic processes that describe change over time. The collection of data and interpretation of findings in relation to normative values is important. This data will reflect the growth and developmental stages of the individual. The following discussion presents specific variations for different age groups.

Infants and Children

During fetal development, respirations are passive and gas exchange occurs at the placenta. At birth, rapid changes occur in the respiratory system as fetal circulation closes. One significant change that occurs is a marked increase in pulmonary blood flow. Other changes include the closure of the foramen ovale and

ductus arteriosus and the increase in chest expansion. Gaseous exchanges now take place via the respiratory system and atmosphere. During the first several hours of extrauterine life, the respiratory rate of the newborn is rapid (40 to 80 per minute) and irregular. During the neonatal and infant period, the respiratory rate decreases and becomes more regular. By 5 years of age, the respiratory rate is about 35 breaths per minute.

At birth, the circumference of the chest is slightly less than the circumference of the head. During childhood, chest circumference exceeds head size by about 5 to 7 cm. The chest is usually round with the lateral and anterior-posterior diameters being almost equal. Bony structures of the chest are more prominent during infancy since skin and musculature are thin. Neonates have a respiratory rate and depth likely to be irregular. At this age, breathing involves use of abdominal muscles; therefore, inspection of the abdomen will yield a more accurate respiratory rate. Abdominal breathing continues during childhood until about 5 to 7 years of age. Costal breathing is the expected pattern after 7 years of age.

The Pregnant Female

The hormonal changes of pregnancy and the growing fetus produce changes in the respiratory system of the pregnant female. The ligaments of the thorax relax, the horizontal diameter expands, and the costal angle increases. At rest, the diaphragm rises into the chest to accommodate the fetus and respirations are diaphragmatic. Shortness of breath and dyspnea, especially in the last trimester, are common as the maternal and fetal demand for oxygen increases. Throughout pregnancy, the total oxygen consumption can increase by 20% and the maternal respiratory rate increases approximately two breaths per minute. Maternal hyperventilation occurs due to the increase in minute ventilation that exceeds the increase in oxygen consumption.

The Older Adult

As individuals age, body functions change. Many activities of the respiratory system demonstrate a decrease in efficiency. The lungs lose their elasticity, the skeletal muscles begin to weaken, and bones lose their density. As a result, it becomes more difficult for the older adult to expand the thoracic cage and take a deep breath. The diameters of the thoracic cage change. The appearance of a barrel chest (kyphosis) and calcification of cartilage contribute to the decrease in thoracic excursion. Thus, the older adult inhales and exhales smaller amounts of air. There is less oxygen for body use, and more carbon dioxide is retained. This is related to the loss of elasticity of the alveoli. The older adult also experiences an increase in residual volume and hypoventilation. Weakening of the chest muscles hinders the older adult's ability to cough. Dry mucous membranes decrease cilia in the system, and the inability to cough compromises airway clearance.

Rate of respirations in the older adult is slightly higher than in the middle-aged adult. The older adult has a more shallow respiratory cycle because of the decreased vital capacity. Auscultatory sounds may be less audible because of the decreased pulmonary function. The trapping of air in the alveoli will produce a sound of hyperresonance upon percussion.

The older adult may tire more easily and may need frequent rest periods during the assessment process. Deep mouth breathing during auscultation may increase the fatigue of the older adult. As with any client, the nurse must prevent hyperventilation at this time.

PSYCHOSOCIAL CONSIDERATIONS

Stress, anxiety, pain, and fatigue may exacerbate respiratory problems. Clients experiencing acute or chronic respiratory problems will have a physiological alteration with gas exchange.

These changes can limit or restrict the individual's ability to independently perform the activities of daily living and to participate in activities, exercise, and sports. This limitation contributes to social isolation, changes role activities, lowers self-esteem, and increases the dependency factor with support systems.

Certain drugs, such as bronchodilators, are used in the treatment of respiratory conditions and may cause the hands to tremble visibly. The nurse should not confuse this sign with nervousness. Even mild respiratory distress is frightening for the client and family. Proceeding in a calm and reassuring manner helps reduce the client's fear. Parents of young children who have experienced severe asthmatic attacks in the past may be extremely anxious any time the child develops a cold, seasonal allergy, or any other respiratory problem. A calm and careful assessment of the current health status helps to decrease the anxiety level of all involved individuals.

CULTURAL AND ENVIRONMENTAL CONSIDERATIONS

Race, ethnicity, and socioeconomic status are significant factors in respiratory health. The incidence of respiratory diseases, such as tuberculosis, asthma, chronic obstructive pulmonary disease, and obstructive sleep apnea, is greater in the non-Caucasian populations in the United States, in poor rural populations, and in recent immigrant groups. Thorough assessment of the respiratory system is best accomplished when the client is disrobed and the surfaces of the anterior and posterior chest can be visualized, touched, and auscultated. Some cultural or religious practices, including the wearing or prohibition of removal of symbolic icons, jewelry, undergarments, or clothing, may interfere with physical examination. Additionally, the requirement of a same-sex examiner or the presence of a companion during the assessment are issues that must be addressed. Careful questioning of the client, with the assistance of a translator when necessary, during the interview will allow for clarification, negotiation, and decision making about the assessment process.

Clients with allergies or asthma should be encouraged to explore the possibility of allergens in their work or home environment. For example, pets, dust, and molds are common allergens found in the home. Secondhand smoke in the home

Cultural Considerations

- Chest volumes differ according to culture. Chest volume, vital capacity, and forced expiratory volume are greatest in Caucasians, followed by African Americans, Asians, and Native Americans.
- Asthma occurs more frequently in African Americans than in Caucasians.
- Obstructive sleep apnea (OSA) is twice as likely to be experienced by young African Americans compared to young Caucasians.
- Contracting TB is eight times more likely in African Americans than in Caucasians.
- African Americans are more likely to be exposed to occupational hazards that contribute to respiratory disease than are Caucasians.

- Sarcoidosis occurs more frequently and with greater severity in African Americans than in Caucasians.
- Asian, Pacific Islander, Hispanic, Native American, and migrant and farm worker populations have a higher risk for and greater incidence of TB.
- African Americans report symptoms of asthma in different terms than do Caucasians.
- Linguistic and cultural factors must be considered to avoid miscommunication and misinterpretation of information about diagnoses when caring for many immigrant populations.
- Children in urban areas and from low socioeconomic groups have a higher incidence of asthma.

or work environment can also lead to respiratory distress. Research has established a link between exposure to secondhand smoke and the development of lung cancer.

In some industries workers may be exposed to substances that are hazardous to their respiratory health, such as caustic fumes, fungi, asbestos, coal tar, nickel, silver, textile fibers, chromate, and vinyl chlorides. All of these substances are known carcinogens. Exposure to large amounts of dust in a granary or mine may lead to the development of silicosis. Coal miners are susceptible to pneumoconiosis, a form of black lung disease. People working in an office building may need to be concerned with air conditioners and forced hot air heat. The ducts of the cooling and heating systems can carry airborne organisms increasing the risk for respiratory infections.

The geographic location of an individual's environment will also influence respiratory health. Factors to be considered are temperature, moisture, altitude, and pollution. A cold environment encourages vasoconstriction and ultimately a decreased need for oxygen. An environment with increased moisture or humidity has heavy air. Individuals will tire easily, increasing the need for oxygen. As the altitude increases, the partial pressure of oxygen decreases. The individual must adapt by increasing the rate and depth of the respiratory cycle. Air pollution with smog, industrial wastes, or exhaust fumes contributes to respiratory problems in all people.

Factors within the home and social environment will influence respiratory health. Forced hot air heat is very drying to the membranes of the body. Individuals are encouraged to add moisture or use a humidifier to keep the air moist and support respiratory health. In the hot, humid, hazy days of summer an air conditioner or dehumidifier may be necessary to help lessen the moisture in the air. Secondhand smoke, foods, dust, pets, and stress will also contribute to respiratory changes.

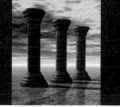

Gathering the Data

*R*espiratory health assessment includes the gathering of subjective and objective data. Recall that subjective data collection occurs during the client interview, before the actual physical assessment. During the interview the nurse uses a variety of communication techniques to elicit general and specific information about the client's state of respiratory health or illness. Health records, the results of laboratory tests, and x-rays are important secondary sources to be reviewed and included in the data-gathering process. In physical assessment of the respiratory system, the techniques of inspection, palpation, percussion, and auscultation will be used. Before proceeding, it may be helpful to review the information about each of the data-gathering processes and practice the techniques of health assessment.

FOCUSED INTERVIEW

The focused interview for the respiratory system concerns data related to the structures and functions of that system. Subjective data related to respiratory status is gathered during the focused interview. The nurse must be prepared to observe the client and listen for cues related to the function of the respiratory system. The nurse may use open-ended or closed questions to obtain information. Often a number of follow-up questions or requests for descriptions are required to clarify data or gather missing information. The subjective data collected and the questions asked during the health history and focused interview will provide information to help meet the goal of promoting respiratory health as stated in *Healthy People 2010* (see the *Healthy People 2010* feature on page 392). Follow-up questions are intended to identify the source of problems, the duration of difficulties, and measures to alleviate problems. Follow-up questions also provide clues about the client's knowledge of his or her own health.

The focused interview guides the physical assessment of the respiratory system. The information is always considered in relation to norms and expectations about respiratory function. Therefore, the nurse must consider age, gender, race, culture, environment, health practices, past and concurrent problems, and therapies when framing questions and using techniques to elicit information. In order to address all of the factors when conducting a focused interview, categories of questions related to respiratory status and function have been developed. These categories include general questions that are asked of all clients: those addressing illness or infection; questions related to symptoms, pain, or behaviors; those related to habits or practices; questions that are specific to clients according to age; those for pregnant females; and questions that address environmental concerns.

The nurse must consider the client's ability to participate in the focused interview and physical assessment of the respiratory system. If a client is experiencing dyspnea, cyanosis, difficulty with speech, and the anxiety that accompanies any of these problems, attention must focus on relief of symptoms and restoration of oxygenation.

FOCUSED INTERVIEW QUESTIONS	RATIONALES

The following sections provide sample questions and bulleted follow-up questions in each of the previously mentioned categories. A rationale for each of the questions is provided. The list of questions is not all-inclusive but rather represents the types of questions required in a comprehensive focused interview related to the respiratory system.

GENERAL QUESTIONS

1. **Describe your breathing today. Is it different from 2 months ago? From 2 years ago?**

▶ These questions give clients the opportunity to provide their own perceptions about breathing.

2. **Do you breathe through your mouth or nose?**
   - Have you always breathed through your mouth?
   - Do you have a problem with your nose?
   - How long have you had the problem?
   - Have you received any treatment for the problem?
   - Did the treatment help?

▶ Nose breathing allows inhaled air to be warmed, moistened, and filtered before entering the lung and is considered the norm. Clients who identify themselves as mouth breathers require follow-up. Mouth breathing is associated with problems in the nose, habit, or air hunger.

3. **Are you able to carry out all of your regular activities without a change in your breathing?**
   - Describe the change in your breathing.
   - Do you know what causes the change?
   - What do you do when this occurs?
   - How long has this been happening?
   - Have you discussed this with a healthcare professional?

▶ This provides an opportunity to elicit information about typical breathing patterns and changes related to normal activities of daily living. A yes would be considered the norm. Any other response requires follow-up questions to determine the type of change and factors that contribute to or predispose the client to changes in breathing.

4. **Describe your breathing when you are engaged in exercise or vigorous activity.**
   - Describe the breathing problem that occurs when you are exercising or very active.
   - How long has this been happening?
   - What do you do when it happens?
   - Do your actions relieve the problem?

▶ A normal expectation is that the client will describe his or her breathing as becoming more rapid or deeper with activity but quickly returning to normal upon completion of the exercise or activity. Follow-up is required when the client describes dyspnea during or slow recovery from exercise or activity.

5. **When you sleep do you lie down flat, prop yourself up with pillows, or sit up?**
   - Tell me why you prefer to sit up.
   - How many pillows do you use?
   - Does the position or number of pillows help with your breathing?
   - How long have you slept like this?
   - Have you discussed this with a healthcare professional?
   - What treatment was recommended?
   - Did the treatment help?

▶ The norm is for a client to sleep fully reclined with a pillow. The number of pillows for propping up oneself should be determined. Clients who must prop themselves up or sit up while sleeping may have orthopnea, that is, dyspnea when lying down. It is important to determine if the propping up or sitting up is simply a preference or because of breathing problems or some other cause.

6. **Do you have any physical problems that affect your breathing?**
   - Describe the way your breathing is affected.
   - How long has this been occurring?
   - Have you sought treatment for the problem?
   - What was the treatment?
   - Did the treatment help?

▶ This is a general question to elicit information about respiratory or other problems that impact breathing. For example, pain from an injury to the upper body may impact breathing but not be directly related to respiratory structures. If the client identifies any problems that affect breathing, follow-up is required. The nurse should ask for clear descriptions and details about what, when, and how problems occur and impact breathing, as well as the duration of the problems.

FOCUSED INTERVIEW QUESTIONS	**RATIONALES**

7. **Is there anyone in your family who has had a respiratory disease or problem?**
   - What is/was the disease or problem?
   - Who in the family has had the disease?
   - When was it diagnosed? How has it been treated?
   - How has it been treated?
   - How effective has the treatment been?

▶ This information may reveal information about respiratory diseases associated with familial or genetic predisposition. Follow-up is required to obtain details about specific problems, their occurrence, treatment, and outcomes.

QUESTIONS RELATED TO ILLNESS OR INFECTION

1. **Have you ever been diagnosed with a respiratory disease?**
   - When were you diagnosed with the problem?
   - What treatment was prescribed for the problem?
   - Was the treatment helpful?
   - What kinds of things do you do to help with the problem?
   - Has the problem ever recurred (acute)?
   - How are you managing the disease now (chronic)?

▶ The client has an opportunity to provide information about specific respiratory illnesses. If a diagnosed illness is identified, follow-up about the date of diagnosis, treatment, and outcomes is required. Data about each illness identified by the client is essential to an accurate health assessment. Illnesses can be classified as acute or chronic, and follow-up regarding each classification will differ.

2. **An alternative to question 1 is to list possible respiratory illnesses, such as asthma, COPD, and emphysema, and ask the client to respond yes or no as each is stated.**

▶ This is a comprehensive and easy way to elicit information about all respiratory diagnoses. Follow-up would be carried out for each identified diagnosis as in question 1.

3. **Do you now have or have you had a respiratory infection?**
   - When were you diagnosed with the infection?
   - What treatment was prescribed for the problem?
   - Was the treatment helpful?
   - What kinds of things do you do to help with the problem?
   - Has the problem ever recurred (acute)?
   - How are you managing the infection now (chronic)?

▶ If an infection is identified, follow-up about the date of infection, treatment, and outcomes is required. Data about each infection identified by the client is essential to an accurate health assessment. Infections can be classified as acute or chronic, and follow-up regarding each classification will differ.

4. **An alternative to question 3 is to list possible respiratory infections, such as bronchitis, pneumonia, and pleurisy, and ask the client to respond yes or no as each is stated.**

▶ This is a comprehensive and easy way to elicit information about all respiratory infections. Follow-up would be carried out for each identified infection as in question 3.

QUESTIONS RELATED TO SYMPTOMS OR BEHAVIORS

When gathering information about symptoms, many questions are required to elicit details and descriptions that assist in the analysis of the data. Discrimination is made in relation to the significance of a symptom, specific diseases or problems, and potential follow-up examination or referral. One rationale may be provided for a group of questions in this category.

The following questions refer to specific symptoms and behaviors associated with the respiratory system. For each symptom, questions and follow-up are required. The details to be elicited are the characteristics of the symptom; the onset, duration, and frequency of the symptom; the treatment or remedy for the symptom, including over-the-counter (OTC) and home remedies; the determination if diagnosis has been sought; the effect of treatments; and family history associated with a symptom or illness.

Questions 1 through 23 refer to coughing as a symptom associated with respiratory diseases or problems and are comprehensive enough to provide an example of the number and types of questions required in a focused interview when a symptom exists. The remaining questions refer to other symptoms associated with respiratory problems. The number and types of questions are limited to identification of the symptom. Follow-up is included only when required for clarification.

FOCUSED INTERVIEW QUESTIONS	RATIONALES

QUESTIONS RELATED TO SYMPTOMS

1. Do you have a cough?

2. How long have you had the cough?

3. How often are you coughing?

4. Do you know what causes the cough?

5. Is there a difference in the cough at different times of the day?

6. Describe your cough.

7. Is it dry, hacking, hoarse, moist, barking?

8. Are you coughing up mucus or phlegm?

9. What does the mucus look like?

10. Does the mucus have any odor?

11. Has the amount of mucus changed?

12. Has the consistency or thickness of the mucus changed?

13. Do you have pain when you cough?
   - Describe the type, severity, and location of the pain.
   - What do you do for the cough or the pain?
   - Is the remedy effective?

14. Have you sought treatment for the cough?

15. When was that treatment sought?

16. What occurred when you sought that treatment?

17. Was something prescribed or recommended to help with the cough?

18. What was the effect of the remedy?

19. Do you use over-the-counter or home remedies for the cough?

20. What are those over-the-counter medications or remedies that you use?

21. How often do you use them?

▶ Question 1 identifies the existence of a symptom, and questions 2 through 5 add knowledge about the symptom.

▶ Determining the duration of symptoms is helpful in determining the significance of symptoms in relation to specific diseases and problems.

▶ The type of cough may indicate a symptom associated with a specific disease or problem. For example, wet or moist coughs are most often associated with lung infection.

▶ The color and odor of any mucus or phlegm (sputum) is associated with specific diseases or problems. For example, rust-colored mucus is associated with tuberculosis, while green or yellow mucus often signals lung infection.

▶ A change in the amount or character of sputum is often a sign of a respiratory disease.

▶ Painful coughing may occur because of muscle pain or may be indicative of an underlying lung disease. Follow-up elicits details that assist in data analysis.

▶ These questions provide information about need for diagnosis, referral, or continued evaluation of the symptom; information about the client's knowledge of a current diagnosis or underlying problem; and information about the client's response to intervention.

FOCUSED INTERVIEW QUESTIONS	RATIONALES
22. How much of them do you use?	▶ These questions provide information about drugs and substances that may relieve symptoms or provide comfort. Some substances may mask symptoms, interfere with the effect of prescribed medications, or harm the client.
23. Do you now have or have you ever had any wheezing?	
24. Have you had a change in your weight recently? • How much weight have you gained or lost? • Over what period of time did this change occur? • Was the change purposeful? • Can you associate the change with any event or problem?	▶ Weight loss or gain may be associated with lung or cardiac diseases.
25. Describe your diet. Do you use any nutritional supplements?	▶ Questions about nutritional intake are important to determine the contribution to production of red blood cells (erythropoiesis) and hemoglobin, which are essential to oxygenation.
26. Do you ever become light-headed or dizzy? • When did or does that occur? • How often? • Do you associate this with any event or activity? • What do you do when this happens?	▶ Light-headedness or dizziness may be associated with hypoxia.

QUESTIONS RELATED TO PAIN

1. Do you have pain anywhere in your chest?	▶ Chest pain may be related to cardiac or respiratory problems.
2. Where is the pain?	▶ Questions 2 through 6 are standard questions associated with pain to determine the location, frequency, duration, and intensity of the pain.
3. How often do you experience the pain?	
4. How long does the pain last?	
5. How long have you had the pain?	
6. How would you rate the pain on a scale of 1 to 10, with 10 being the worst?	
7. Does the pain affect your breathing? • Are you short of breath? • Are you able to take a deep breath? • What do you do when this happens?	▶ Follow-up questions would relate to the ways in which breathing is affected. ▶ Questions 7 through 11 are intended to discriminate characteristics of pain associated with underlying acute or chronic respiratory disease from muscular pain that can occur with cough or maintaining a posture to ease breathing.
8. Does the pain occur when you are taking a breath, when you are exhaling, or both?	
9. Is there a trigger for the pain, such as cough or movement?	
10. Can you describe the pain?	
11. Does the pain radiate to other areas?	
12. What do you do to relieve the pain?	▶ Questions 12 and 13 are intended to determine if the client has selected a treatment based on past experience, knowledge of respiratory illness, or use of complementary care and its effectiveness.
13. Is this treatment effective?	

FOCUSED INTERVIEW QUESTIONS	RATIONALES

QUESTIONS RELATED TO BEHAVIORS

1. Do you now smoke or have you ever smoked tobacco products?

2. What type of tobacco product do/did you smoke?

3. How much of the product do/did you smoke?

4. When did you start smoking?

5. When did you stop smoking?

6. Have you tried to stop smoking?

7. What did you do to stop smoking?

8. Do you have any symptoms related to smoking?

▶ Smoking tobacco products is associated with respiratory diseases including emphysema and lung cancer. Tobacco products include cigarettes, cigars, and pipe tobacco. If the client exhibits or affirms that respiratory symptoms exist, questions for any symptom as previously described would be asked.

9. Do you smoke or inhale marijuana, other herbal products, or chemical preparations such as glue or spray paint? Have you done so in the past?
   - What is the substance you inhale?
   - How much do you use?
   - How often do you inhale the substance?
   - For those clients who state they have inhaled substances in the past, ask: When did you stop using the substance?

▶ Inhalation of marijuana, herbal substances, and/or chemicals may result in respiratory problems associated with incidental or continuous irritation of the linings of the respiratory organs.

10. Have you received immunization for respiratory illnesses such as flu or pneumonia?
   - What immunizations have you had?
   - When was each given? Were there any adverse effects?

▶ Immunization reduces the risk of infection from flu or pneumonia.

QUESTIONS RELATED TO AGE

The focused interview must reflect the anatomical and physiological differences that exist along the age span. The following questions are presented as examples of those that would be specific for infants and children, pregnant female, and older adults.

QUESTIONS REGARDING INFANTS AND CHILDREN

1. Is the child taking solid foods?
   - When were they started?
   - What types of food are taken?
   - Does the child have difficulty chewing or swallowing?

▶ Introduction of solid foods puts infants at risk for aspiration.

2. How many colds has the child had in the past 12 months?
   - What was the course of the cold?
   - Was any treatment provided?
   - Was medical care sought?
   - What was the effect of the treatment?

▶ Children may experience as many as six uncomplicated respiratory infections in a year. More than this number of complicated infections may indicate chronic disease.

3. Has the child been immunized against respiratory illnesses?
   - What immunization did your child have?
   - When was it given?
   - Were there any adverse effects?

▶ This question identifies risk reduction and assists in discrimination of symptoms if and when they occur. Infants are at greater risk for complications from flu and pneumonia.

FOCUSED INTERVIEW QUESTIONS	**RATIONALES**

QUESTIONS FOR THE PREGNANT FEMALE

1. **Do you experience any shortness of breath or dyspnea?**
   - When does it occur?
   - How long have you experienced this?
   - Have you sought a remedy?

▶ The enlarged uterus puts pressure on the diaphragm and can decrease lung expansion, which may result in shortness of breath.

QUESTIONS FOR THE OLDER ADULT

1. **Describe any changes in breathing you have experienced.**

2. **Have you had any difficulty performing activities that you once found easy?**

3. **Do you find that you are more tired than you have been in the past?**

▶ Older adults may experience symptoms associated with reduced oxygenation as a result of changes in posture and muscle strength that may contribute to reduced lung expansion. Fatigue may be associated with anemia and other chronic problems such as COPD, asthma, and cancer.

4. **Have you received any immunization for respiratory illnesses?**
   - What immunization did you receive?
   - When was it given?
   - Were there any adverse effects?

▶ Older adults are at greater risk for flu and pneumonia.

QUESTIONS RELATED TO THE ENVIRONMENT

Environment refers to both the internal and the external environments. Questions related to the internal environment include all of the previous questions and those associated with internal or physiological responses. Questions regarding the external environment include those related to home, work, or social environments.

INTERNAL ENVIRONMENT

1. **Are you now experiencing or have you ever had an experience of intermittent or prolonged anxiety or emotional upset?**
   - Describe the situation.
   - Can you determine precipitating factors?
   - Have you sought care or treatment for the problem?
   - What do you do when the problem arises?

▶ Anxiety, emotional situations, and stress impact the sympathetic nervous system, producing hormonal responses that affect respiratory function.

2. **Do you use now or have you ever used medications or devices to alter or improve your respiratory function?**

▶ Medications such as inhalers and steroids for respiratory symptoms can have cascading side effects that result in exacerbation of problems or enhancement of symptoms. Devices for treatment of respiratory ailments include oxygen therapy, devices to relieve sleep apnea, and others. Knowledge of the medications and devices helps the nurse to analyze client situations and determine the significance of findings in the comprehensive assessment.

EXTERNAL ENVIRONMENT

The following questions deal with substances and irritants found in the client's physical environment. The physical environment includes the indoor and outdoor environments of the home and the workplace, those surroundings encountered for social engagements, and any encountered during travel.

FOCUSED INTERVIEW QUESTIONS	RATIONALES

1. Have you had allergy testing?

2. Do you have any allergies?

3. Do those allergies impact respiratory function?

4. What are the allergens?

5. When were these allergies diagnosed?

6. How do you address exposure to the allergen?

7. What are the respiratory symptoms you experience?

8. What remedies do you use to take care of the symptoms?

9. Have the remedies been effective?

▶ Allergies often result in respiratory problems including asthma and bronchitis. It is important to determine if specific allergens have been identified and if the client uses appropriate measures to address the problems. Remedies may include avoidance of the allergen.

10. Are you now or have you ever been exposed to respiratory irritants (gases, fumes, dust, lint, smoke, chemical exhaust)?

11. Were the irritants identified?

12. Where are/were the irritants? In the home, in the workplace, in the community, or outside of the community?

13. What is or was your respiratory response to irritants?

14. Have you ever experienced an illness related to exposure to an irritant?

15. How have you dealt with that illness?

16. How does the illness impact your life now?
   • Follow-up questions would include all of the questions previously mentioned that address symptoms and problems of the respiratory system.

▶ Irritants, pollutants, and chemicals in the environment can result in acute and/or chronic respiratory disease (i.e., mesothelioma, asbestosis, and psittacosis). Acute and chronic problems with respiratory function can have devastating effects on the ability to function. Identification of the place of exposure or possible exposure through travel, military, or employment service may assist in identifying probable causes for new or ongoing respiratory problems.

CLIENT INTERACTION

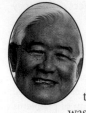

Mr. Loi is a 78-year-old with a history of COPD who recently moved from another state to live with his daughter, Anita. His daughter scheduled an appointment for Mr. Loi with her healthcare group. When Anita called to arrange the appointment she explained that her father was widowed 3 years ago and had been doing well in his own home, but he seemed lonely and was not participating in activities in his neighborhood and community as he had been. He also didn't say much when she phoned. Anita stated that he has COPD. Although it didn't seem to affect his activity in the past, she was concerned about him. She visited him and suggested he move in with them and was relieved that he agreed. Since the move, he has been quiet and resting in his room most of the time. His breathing seems okay. He has had a cough once in a while, but she thought she had better get him set up with a doctor just in case something happened.

Mr. Loi completed several forms before his health interview. These forms included biographical information, personal

and family health history, and information about his current diagnosis and medications.

INTERVIEW

Because Mr. Loi's only diagnosed health problem is COPD, the nurse begins the interview with questions related to his respiratory system. The nurse greets Mr. Loi, offers him a seat, and explains the interview process. Mr. Loi takes a seat, smiles, and nods.

Nurse: Tell me about your breathing.

Mr. Loi: I'm doing fine. I take all my medications.

Nurse: Has your breathing changed in the last 2 months?

Mr. Loi: Oh, I moved here to be with my daughter a month ago. *The nurse realizes that Mr. Loi has not answered the question. It is not clear if Mr. Loi did not hear the question, misunderstood the question, or is seeking an opportunity to discuss his move. The nurse uses an open-ended statement to allow him to discuss the move.*

Nurse: Tell me a little about your move.

Mr. Loi leans forward and focuses on the nurse's lips while listening to the question.

Mr. Loi: Well, my daughter wanted me here. She worries that I don't get out and see people. You know I have COPD, but it's been okay as long as I take my pills.

Mr. Loi's posture and focus while the nurse spoke suggests that Mr. Loi is having difficulty hearing. Further, Mr. Loi's daughter was concerned about her father's diminished social contact and decreasing phone communication, which are additional signs of hearing deficit.

In order to complete the health assessment, the nurse will use techniques appropriate for those clients with hearing impairment.

The nurse faces Mr. Loi, uses a low-pitched voice at normal loudness, and speaks in short sentences to conduct the interview.

The nurse pauses after each statement so Mr. Loi can interpret the statement.

Nurse: What do you think of the move?

Mr. Loi: So far, so good. She's been great and so has her family. It's all pretty different but I think I'll be okay. I don't want her to worry so I agreed to come and get checked out here. You know . . . my COPD and all.

Nurse: Tell me about the COPD.

Mr. Loi: Well, it started about 5 years ago. I was getting winded with just a little work around the house. Then I got bronchitis and it just took off from there.

Please refer to the Companion Website at **www.prenhall.com/damico** and click on Chapter 15, the **Client Interaction** module, to answer questions about this case. In addition, see other resources for this chapter, including NCLEX review questions and other interactive exercises and materials.

Physical Assessment

ASSESSMENT TECHNIQUES AND FINDINGS

Physical assessment of the respiratory system requires the use of inspection, palpation, percussion, and auscultation. During each of the procedures, the nurse is gathering data related to the client's breathing and level of oxygenation. The nurse inspects skin color, structures of the thoracic cavity, chest configuration, and respiratory rate rhythm and effort. Knowledge of norms or expected findings is essential in determining the meaning of the data as one proceeds.

Adults normally breathe at a rate of 12 to 20 breaths per minute. Infants and children have higher rates, up to 40 breaths per minute in newborns. The respiratory cycle includes full inspiration and expiration. The ratio of the length of inspiration to expiration is about 1:2 (I:E). Breathing should be even, regular, and coordinated. Chest movement should be uniform; the structures of the thorax should be aligned and the thorax should be symmetrical. The sternum is midline and flat. The costal angle is less than 90 degrees in an adult. The vertebrae are midline and follow the pattern of cervical, thoracic, and lumbar

curves. The anterior to posterior diameter of the chest should be half of the lateral diameter. Pink skin or pink undertones indicate normal oxygenation. Assessment for pink-colored tongue or oral mucous membranes may be required in dark-skinned individuals. The color of the skin of the thorax should be consistent with that of the rest of the body.

Physical assessment of the respiratory system follows an organized pattern. It begins with a client survey followed by inspection of the anterior thorax and complete assessment of the posterior thorax. The assessment ends with palpation, percussion, and auscultation of the anterior thorax. The nurse includes the anterior, posterior, and lateral aspects of the thorax when conducting each of the assessments.

HELPFUL HINTS
- Provide an environment that is comfortable and private.
- Explain each step of the procedure.
- Provide specific instructions about what is expected of the client, for example whether deep or regular breathing will be required.
- Tell client the purpose of each procedure and when and if discomfort will accompany any examination.
- Pay attention to nonverbal cues that may indicate discomfort and ask client to indicate if he or she experiences any difficulties or discomforts.
- An organized and professional approach goes a long way toward putting the client at ease.

EQUIPMENT

examination gown and drape	skin marker
examination gloves	metric ruler
examination light	tissues
stethoscope	face mask

TECHNIQUES AND NORMAL FINDINGS	ABNORMAL FINDINGS SPECIAL CONSIDERATIONS

SURVEY

A quick survey of the client enables the nurse to identify any immediate problems as well as the client's ability to participate in the assessment.

> **ALERT!**
>
> *Individuals experiencing pain and dyspnea, who are restless, anxious, and unable to follow directions, may need immediate medical assistance.*

Inspect the overall appearance, posture, and position of the client. Note the skin color and respiratory effort. Observe for signs of anxiety or distress.

INSPECTION OF THE ANTERIOR THORAX

> **ALERT!**
>
> *Be sensitive to the client's privacy, and limit exposure of body parts.*

1. Position the client.

- The client should be in a sitting position with clothing removed except for an examination gown and drape (see Figure 15.13 ●).

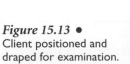

Figure 15.13 ●
Client positioned and draped for examination.

- Stand in front of the client. Lighting must be adequate to detect color differences, lesions, and chest movement.

2. Instruct the client.

- Explain that you are going to be looking at the client's chest structures. Tell the client to breathe normally.

3. Observe skin color.

- Skin color varies among individuals, but pink undertones indicate normal oxygenation. Skin color of the thorax should be consistent with that of the rest of the body.

▶ Clients experiencing anxiety may demonstrate pallor and shallow breathing. Acknowledgment of the problem and discussion of the procedures often provide some relief. If a client is in obvious respiratory distress, the problem must be addressed. The client may require referral to a medical care provider or emergency care facility.

Circumoral cyanosis may be present in clients with respiratory distress or hypoxia.

▶ Pigments and levels of oxygenation influence skin color. Pallor, cyanosis, rubor, erythema, or grayness requires further evaluation.

TECHNIQUES AND NORMAL FINDINGS	ABNORMAL FINDINGS SPECIAL CONSIDERATIONS

4. Inspect the structures of the thorax.

- The clavicles should be at the same height. The sternum should be midline. The costal angle should be less than 90 degrees.

▶ Misalignment of clavicles may be caused by deviations in the vertebral column such as scoliosis. Increase in the costal angle in an adult may indicate COPD. The thorax of children is rounder than that of adults.

5. Inspect for symmetry.

- The structures of the chest and chest movement should be symmetrical.

▶ Asymmetry may indicate postural problems or underlying respiratory dysfunction.

6. Inspect chest configuration.

- The adult transverse diameter is approximately twice that of the anteroposterior diameter (AP:T = 1:2).

▶ A change in the ratio requires further evaluation. Remember: Older adults have a decreased ratio.

7. Count the respiratory rate.

- Count the number of respiratory cycles per minute. Normal adult respiratory rate is 12 to 20.
  - Observe chest movement.
  - Observe the muscles of the chest and neck, including the intercostal muscles and sternocleidomastoids.
- Do not tell the client that you are counting respirations—it may alter the normal breathing pattern.
  - Respirations should be even and smooth. Chest movement should be symmetrical.
- Males tend to breathe abdominally.
  - Females breathe more costally.

▶ Intercostal muscle retraction and prominent sternocleidomastoids may be seen in respiratory distress.

INSPECTION OF THE POSTERIOR THORAX

1. Instruct the client.

- Explain to the client that you will be performing several assessments and that you will provide instructions as you move from one step to the next. Tell the client to try to relax and breathe normally to begin the examination.

2. Observe skin color.

- Skin color of the posterior thorax should be consistent with that of the rest of the body.

3. Inspect the structures of the posterior thorax.

- The height of the scapulae should be even; the vertebrae should be midline.

▶ Lateral deviation of the spine and elevation of one scapula is indicative of scoliosis.

4. Inspect for symmetry.

- The structures of the chest and chest movement should be symmetrical.

▶ Asymmetry may indicate postural problems or underlying respiratory problems.

5. Observe respirations.

- Respirations should be smooth and even.

TECHNIQUES AND NORMAL FINDINGS	ABNORMAL FINDINGS SPECIAL CONSIDERATIONS

PALPATION OF THE POSTERIOR THORAX

1. Instruct the client.

- Explain that you will be touching the client's back to determine if there are any areas of tenderness. Tell the client to breathe normally during this part of the examination and to tell you if pain or discomfort is felt at any area.

2. Lightly palpate the posterior thorax.

- Use the finger pads to lightly palpate symmetrical areas on the posterior thorax. Include the entire thorax by starting at the areas above each scapula and move from side to side to below the twelfth rib and laterally to the midaxillary line on each side (see Figure 15.14 ●).
- Assess muscle mass.
- Assess for growths, nodules, and masses.
- Assess for tenderness.
- Muscle mass should be firm and underlying tissue smooth. The chest should be free of lesions or masses. The area should be nontender to palpation.

► Pain may occur with inflammation of fibrous tissue or underlying structures such as the pleura. Crepitus is a crunching feeling under the skin caused by air leaking into subcutaneous tissue.

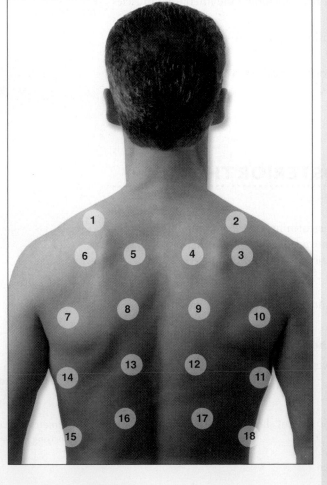

Figure 15.14 ●
Pattern for palpating the posterior thorax.

3. Palpate and count ribs and intercostal spaces.

- Instruct the client to flex the neck, round the shoulders, and lean forward. Tell the client you will be applying light pressure to the spine and rib areas. Instruct the client to breathe normally and to tell you of pain or discomfort.

| TECHNIQUES AND NORMAL FINDINGS | ABNORMAL FINDINGS SPECIAL CONSIDERATIONS |

- When the neck is flexed, the spinous process of C_7 is most prominent. When two spinous processes are equally prominent, they are C_7 and T_1. Use the finger pads to palpate each spinous process. The spinous processes should form a straight line. Further assessment is discussed in Chapter 23. ◯◯ Move to the left and right to identify ribs and intercostal spaces from C_7 through T_{12}.

▶ Lateral deviation of the thoracic spinous processes indicates a scoliosis.

4. **Palpate for respiratory expansion.**
   - Explain that you will be assessing the movement of the chest during breathing by placing your hands on the lower chest and asking the client to take a deep breath.
   - Place the palmar surface of your hands, with thumbs close to the vertebrae, on the chest at the level of T_{10}. Pinch up some skin between your thumbs. Ask the client to take a deep breath (see Figure 15.15 ●).

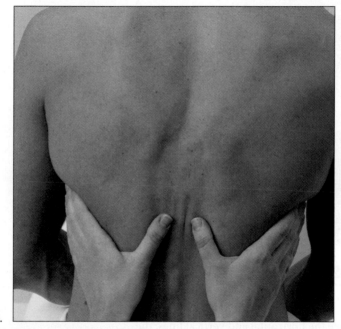

Figure 15.15 ●
Palpation for
respiratory expansion.

- The movement and pressure of the chest against your hands should feel smooth and even. Your thumbs should move away from the spine and the skin should move smoothly as the chest moves with inspiration.

▶ Unilateral decrease or delay in expansion may indicate underlying fibrotic or obstructive lung disease or may result from splinting associated with pleural pain or pneumothorax.

5. **Palpate for tactile fremitus.**
   - **Fremitus** is the palpable vibration on the chest wall when the client speaks. Fremitus is strongest over the trachea, diminishes over the bronchi, and becomes almost nonexistent over the alveoli of the lungs.
   - Explain that you will be feeling for vibrations on the chest while the client speaks. Tell the client you will be placing your hands on various areas of the chest while he or she repeats "ninety-nine" or "one, two, three" in a clear, loud voice.
   - Use the ulnar surface of the hand or the palmar surface of the hand at the base of the metacarpophalangeal joints when palpating. Palpate and compare symmetrical areas of the lungs by moving from side to side from apices to bases. Using one hand to palpate for fremitus is believed to increase accuracy of findings. Two-handed methods may, however, increase speed and facilitate identification of asymmetry (see Figure 15.16 ●).

▶ Decreased or absent fremitus may result from a soft voice, from a very thick chest wall, or from underlying diseases including COPD, pleural effusion, fibrosis, or tumor. Increased fremitus occurs with fluid in the lungs or in infection.

TECHNIQUES AND NORMAL FINDINGS	ABNORMAL FINDINGS SPECIAL CONSIDERATIONS

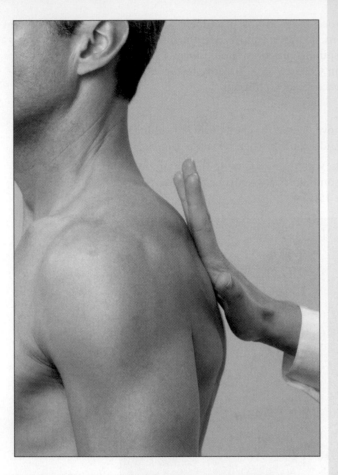

Figure 15.16 ●
Palpation for tactile fremitus using metacarpophalangeal joint area.

PERCUSSION OF THE POSTERIOR THORAX

1. **Visualize the landmarks.**
   - Observe the posterior thorax and visualize the horizontal and vertical lines, the level of the diaphragm, and the fissures of the lungs.

2. **Recall the expected findings.**
   - Percussion allows assessment of underlying structures. The usual sound in the thorax when over lung tissue is **resonance,** a long, low-pitched hollow sound.

   ▶ An unexpected finding would be hyperresonance, which is heard in conditions of overinflation of the lungs as in emphysema, or with pneumothorax.

3. **Instruct the client.**
   - Explain to the client that you will be tapping on the chest in a variety of areas.
   - Tell the client to breathe normally through this examination. Ask the client to lean forward and round the shoulders. This position moves the scapulae laterally, permitting more area at the upper vertebral borders, and widens the intercostal spaces for percussion.
   - Position the client so that your arms are almost fully extended throughout the percussion.

TECHNIQUES AND NORMAL FINDINGS	ABNORMAL FINDINGS SPECIAL CONSIDERATIONS

4. Percuss the lungs.

- Place the pleximeter in the intercostal space parallel to the ribs during percussion. Standing slightly to the side of the client allows the pleximeter finger to lie more firmly on the chest as you move through all thoracic areas.
- Percuss the apex of the left lung, then the apex of the right lung. Percuss from side to side, comparing sounds, in the intercostal spaces as you percuss to the bases of the lungs and laterally to each midaxillary line (see Figure 15.17 ●).

▶ Percussion will yield dull sounds over solidified or fluid-filled areas, as may exist in pleural effusion. Percussion over bone will yield flat sounds. Be sure to check that finger placement is correct.

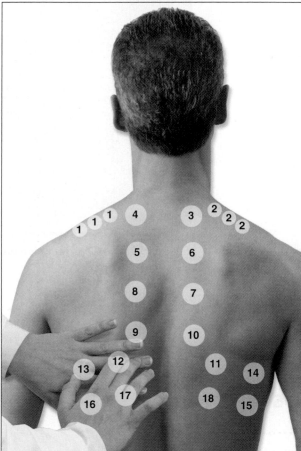

Figure 15.17 ●
Pattern for percussion:
Posterior thorax.

5. Percuss for movement of the diaphragmatic excursion.

- This assessment requires the use of a skin marker and a ruler. The client remains in the position previously described for percussion. Explain that you will be doing more tapping on the chest and at two points you will ask the client to exhale and inhale. Determine the level of the diaphragm during quiet respiration by placing the pleximeter finger above the expected level of diaphragmatic **dullness** (T_7 or T_8) at the midscapular line. Percuss in steps downward until dullness replaces resonance on both sides of the chest. Mark those areas. These marks should be at approximately the level of T_{10}.
- The marks should be parallel.
- Measure diaphragmatic movement by asking the client to fully exhale. Starting at the previous skin marking on the left chest, percuss upward from dullness to resonance. Mark that area. Then ask the client to inhale fully and hold it as you

▶ An asymmetrical diaphragm may indicate diaphragmatic paralysis or pleural effusion of the elevated side.

TECHNIQUES AND NORMAL FINDINGS	ABNORMAL FINDINGS SPECIAL CONSIDERATIONS

begin to percuss from the level of the diaphragm downward, moving from resonance to dullness. Mark that area and repeat on the right side of the chest. Use the ruler to measure the difference between the marks for exhalation and inhalation (see Figure 15.18 ●).

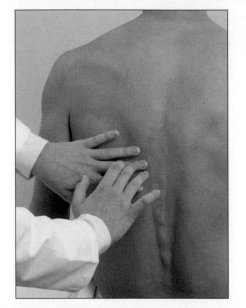

Figure 15.18A ● Diaphragmatic movement, percussion.

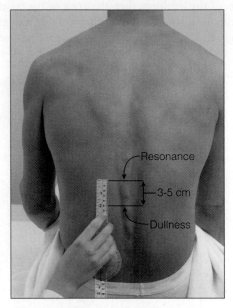

Figure 15.18B ● Diaphragmatic movement, measurement.

- The distance between the marks should be 3 to 5 cm (1 1/4 to 2 in.) and even on each side. The right side may be 1 to 2 cm higher because of the location of the liver.
- Anticipate a greater distance on a physically fit client.

▶ Shortened excursion indicates that the lungs are not fully expanding. Pain or abdominal pressure can inhibit full expansion. The diaphragmatic movement is shortened in emphysema, atelectasis, and respiratory depression.

AUSCULTATION OF THE POSTERIOR THORAX

Auscultation of the respiratory system refers to listening to the sounds of breathing through the stethoscope. The sounds are produced by air moving through the airways. Sounds change as the airway size changes or with the presence of fluid or mucus.

The pattern for auscultation of the respiratory system is the same as that for percussion (see Figure 15.19 ●).

Use the diaphragm of the stethoscope and listen through the full respiratory cycle. When auscultating, classify each sound according to intensity, location, pitch, duration, and characteristic.

▶ Auscultation through clothing or coarse chest hair may produce deceptive sounds. Thick, coarse chest hair may be matted with a damp cloth or lotion to prevent interference with auscultation.

ALERT!

It is important to monitor the client's breathing to prevent hyperventilation.

TECHNIQUES AND NORMAL FINDINGS	ABNORMAL FINDINGS SPECIAL CONSIDERATIONS

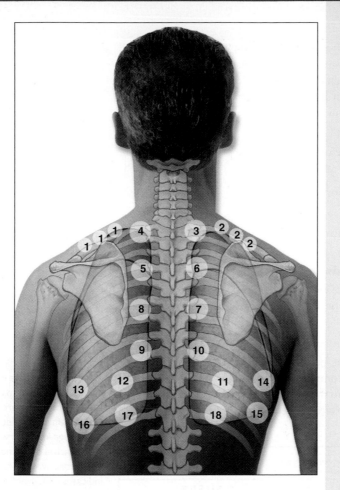

Figure 15.19 •
Pattern for auscultation:
Posterior thorax.

Four normal breath sounds are heard during respiratory auscultation. **Tracheal sounds** are harsh, high-pitched sounds heard over the trachea when the client inhales and exhales. **Bronchial sounds** are loud, high-pitched sounds heard next to the trachea and are longer on exhalation. **Bronchovesicular sounds** are medium in loudness and pitch. They are heard between the scapula, posteriorly and next to the sternum, and anteriorly upon inhalation and exhalation. **Vesicular sounds** are soft and low-pitched and heard over the remainder of the lungs. Vesicular sounds are longer on inhalation than exhalation (see Table 15.1).

Table 15.1	Normal Breath Sounds		
SOUND	**LOCATION**	**RATIO INSPIRATION TO EXPIRATION**	**QUALITY**
Tracheal	Over trachea	I < E	Harsh, high-pitched
Bronchial	Next to trachea	E > I	Loud, high-pitched
Bronchovesicular	Sternal border between scapula	I = E	Medium loudness, medium pitch
Vesicular	Remainder of lungs	I > E	Soft, low-pitched

TECHNIQUES AND NORMAL FINDINGS

1. **Instruct the client.**
   - Explain that you will be listening to the client's breathing with the stethoscope.
   - The client will be in the same position as during percussion. Ask the client to breathe deeply through the mouth each time the stethoscope is placed on a new spot. Tell the client to let you know if he or she is becoming tired or short of breath and if so you will stop and allow time to rest.

2. **Visualize the landmarks.**
   - Visualize the landmarks as you did before percussing the posterior thorax.

3. **Auscultate for tracheal sounds.**
   - Auscultate at the vertebral line superior to C_7.

4. **Auscultate for bronchial sounds.**
   - Start at the vertebral line at C_7 and move the stethoscope down toward T_3. The sound will be bronchial.

5. **Auscultate for bronchovesicular sounds.**
   - The right and left primary bronchi are located at the level of T_3 and T_5. Auscultate at the right and left of the vertebrae at those levels. The breath sounds will be bronchovesicular.

6. **Auscultate for vesicular sounds.**
   - Auscultate the lungs by following the pattern used for percussion. Move the stethoscope from side to side while comparing sounds. Start at the apices and move to the bases of the lungs and laterally to the midaxillary line. The breath sounds over most of the posterior surface are vesicular.

▶ Auscultation of diminished but normal breath sounds in both lungs may indicate emphysema, atelectasis, bronchospasm, or shallow breathing. Breath sounds heard in just one lung indicate pleural effusion, pneumothorax, tumor, or mucous plugs in the airways in the other lung. Finding bronchial or bronchovesicular sounds in areas where one would normally hear vesicular sounds indicates that alveoli and small bronchioles are affected by fluid or exudate. Fluid and exudate decrease the movement of air through small airways and result in loss of vesicular sounds.

▶ Added or adventitious sounds are superimposed on normal breath sounds and often indicative of underlying airway problems or diseases of the cardiovascular or respiratory systems.

Adventitious sounds are classified as discontinuous or continuous. Discontinuous sounds are crackles, which are intermittent, nonmusical, and brief. These sounds are commonly referred to as **rales.** Fine rales are soft, high-pitched, and very brief. Coarse rales/crackles are louder, lower in pitch, and longer. Continuous sounds are musical and longer than rales but do not necessarily persist through the entire respiratory cycle. The two types are wheezes/sibilant wheezes and rhonchi (sonorous wheezes). **Wheezes** (sibilant) are high-pitched with a shrill quality. **Rhonchi** are low-pitched with a snoring quality (see Table 15.2).

Table 15.2	**Adventitious Sounds**		
SOUND	**OCCURRENCE**	**QUALITY**	**CAUSES**
Rales/ Crackles			
Fine	End inspiration, don't clear with cough	High-pitched, short, crackling	Collapsed or fluid-filled alveoli open
Coarse	End inspiration, don't clear with cough	Loud, moist, low-pitched, bubbling	Collapsed or fluid-filled alveoli open
Ronchi			
Wheezes (sibilant)	Expiration Inspiration when severe	High-pitched, continuous	Blocked airflow as in asthma, infection, foreign body obstruction
Ronchi (sonorous)	Expiration/inspiration Change/disappear with cough	Low-pitched, continuous, snoring, rattling	Fluid-blocked airways
Stridor	Inspiration	Loud, high-pitched crowing heard without stethoscope	Obstructed upper airway
Friction rub	Inhalation/exhalation	Low-pitched grating, rubbing	Pleural inflammation

TECHNIQUES AND NORMAL FINDINGS	ABNORMAL FINDINGS SPECIAL CONSIDERATIONS

ASSESSMENT OF VOICE SOUNDS

The spoken voice can be heard over the chest wall. The sound is produced by vibrations as the client speaks.

1. **Instruct the client.**
   - The client will remain in the same position as for percussion and auscultation. Explain that you will be listening to the chest while the client says certain words, letters, or numbers.

2. **Auscultation of voice sounds.**
   - Use the same pattern for evaluating voice sounds as for auscultation of the lungs. This sequence will be followed for three different findings.
   - **Bronchophony.** Ask the client to say "ninety-nine" each time you place the stethoscope on the chest. In normal lung tissue the sound will be muffled.
   - **Egophony.** Ask the client to say "E" each time you place the stethoscope on the chest. In normal lung tissue you should hear "eeeeee" through the stethoscope.
   - **Whispered pectoriloquy.** Ask the client to whisper "one, two, three" each time you place the stethoscope on the chest. In normal lung tissue the sound will be faint, almost indistinguishable.
   - Voice sounds are heard as muffled sounds in the normal lung.

► The words sound loud and more distinct over areas of lung consolidation.

► The "E" sounds like "aaaaay" over areas of lung consolidation.

► The numbers sound loud and clear over areas of lung consolidation.

ASSESSMENT OF THE ANTERIOR THORAX

Inspection of the anterior thorax was conducted prior to the entire assessment of the posterior thorax. That assessment included a survey and inspection of chest structures, skin color, and respiratory rate and pattern.

PALPATION OF THE ANTERIOR THORAX

1. **Position the client.**
   - The client is usually in a supine position for palpation, percussion, and auscultation of the anterior thorax. If the client is experiencing discomfort or dyspnea, a sitting position may be used, or the client may be in a Fowler's position. The breasts of female clients normally flatten when in a supine position. Large and pendulous breasts may have to be moved to perform a complete assessment. Explain this to the client and inform her that she may move and lift her own breasts if that will make her more comfortable.

2. **Instruct the client.**
   - Explain to the client that you will be performing several assessments and that you will continue to provide explanations as you move from one assessment to the next. Tell the client to breathe normally throughout this initial examination and to tell you if pain or discomfort is felt at any area.

3. **Palpate the sternum, ribs, and intercostal spaces.**
   - Locate the suprasternal notch; palpate downward to the sternal angle (angle of Louis) where the manubrium meets the body of the sternum. Palpate laterally to the left and right to locate the second rib and second intercostal space. Continue palpating the sternum to the xiphoid process and to the left and right of the sternum to count the ribs.

TECHNIQUES AND NORMAL FINDINGS	ABNORMAL FINDINGS SPECIAL CONSIDERATIONS

- The sternum should feel flat except for the ridge of the sternal angle and should taper to the xiphoid. The ribs should feel smooth and the spacing of ribs and intercostal spaces should be symmetrical.

4. Lightly palpate the anterior thorax.

- Use the finger pads to lightly palpate the anterior thorax. Include the entire thorax by starting at the areas above each clavicle and move from side to side to below the costal angle and laterally to the midaxillary line (see Figure 15.20 ●).

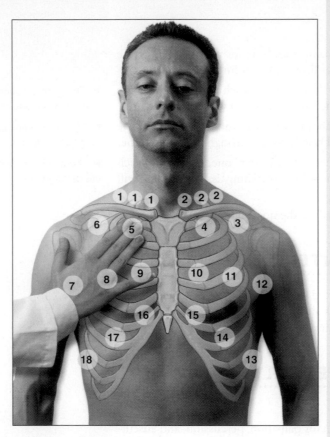

Figure 15.20 ●
Pattern for palpation:
Anterior thorax.

- Assess muscle mass.
- Assess for growths, nodules, and masses.
- Assess for tenderness.
- Muscle mass should be firm and underlying tissue smooth. The chest should be free of lesions or masses. The area should be nontender to palpation.

5. Palpate for respiratory expansion.

- Explain that you will be assessing movement of the chest during breathing by placing your hands on the lower chest and asking the client to take a breath.

▶ Pain may occur with inflammation of fibrous tissue or underlying structures. Crepitus may be felt if there is air in the subcutaneous tissue.

TECHNIQUES AND NORMAL FINDINGS

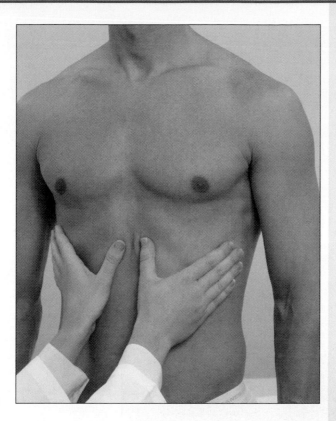

Figure 15.21 ●
Palpation for respiratory
expansion: Anterior view.

- Place the palmar surface of your hands along each costal margin with thumbs close to the midsternal line. Pinch up some skin between your thumbs. Ask the client to take a deep breath (see Figure 15.21 ●).

- The movement of the chest beneath your hands should feel smooth and even. Your thumbs should move apart and the skin move smoothly as the chest expands with inspiration.

▶ Unilateral decrease or delay in expansion may indicate fibrotic or obstructive lung disease or may result from splinting associated with pleural pain.

6. Palpate for tactile fremitus.

- Explain that you will be feeling for vibrations on the chest wall while the client speaks. Explain that you will be placing your hands on various areas of the chest while the client repeats "ninety-nine" or "one, two, three" in a clear, loud voice.

- Use the ulnar surface of the hand or the palmar surface of the hand at the base of the metacarpophalangeal joints when palpating for fremitus. Palpate and compare symmetrical areas of the lungs by moving from side to side from apices to bases (see Figure 15.22 ●). Displace female breasts as required.

- Fremitus normally diminishes as you move from large to small airways and is decreased or absent over the precordium.

▶ Absent or decreased fremitus in other areas may result from underlying diseases including emphysema, pleural effusion, or fibrosis.

TECHNIQUES AND NORMAL FINDINGS	ABNORMAL FINDINGS SPECIAL CONSIDERATIONS

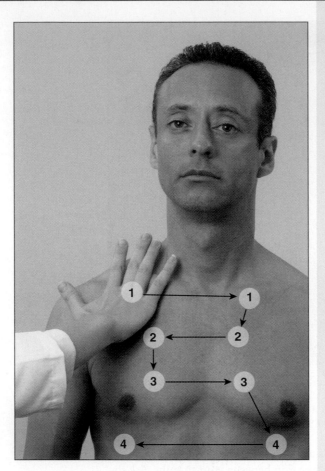

Figure 15.22 ●
Palpation for tactile
fremitus: Anterior thorax.

PERCUSSION OF THE ANTERIOR THORAX

1. Visualize the landmarks.

- Observe the anterior thorax and visualize the horizontal and vertical lines, the level of the diaphragm, and the lobes of the lungs.

2. Recall the expected findings.

- Percussion allows assessment of underlying structures. The usual sound in the thorax is resonance.

► An unexpected sound would be hyperresonance, which is heard in conditions of overinflation of the lungs.

3. Instruct the client.

- Explain that you will be tapping on the client's chest in a variety of areas. Tell the client to breathe normally throughout this examination.

4. Percuss the lungs.

- Begin at the apices of the lungs. Ask the client to turn the head to the opposite side of percussion to increase the size of the surface required for placing your pleximeter finger and to avoid interference from the clavicle. Move to the chest wall and place the pleximeter in the intercostal space parallel to the ribs during percussion. Percuss the anterior chest from side to side, comparing sounds, in the intercostal spaces. Percuss to the bases and laterally to the midaxillary line (see Figure 15.23 ●).

► Percussion of the anterior thorax will yield dull sounds over solidified or fluid-filled areas, as may exist in pleural effusion, consolidation, or tumor.

TECHNIQUES AND NORMAL FINDINGS	ABNORMAL FINDINGS SPECIAL CONSIDERATIONS

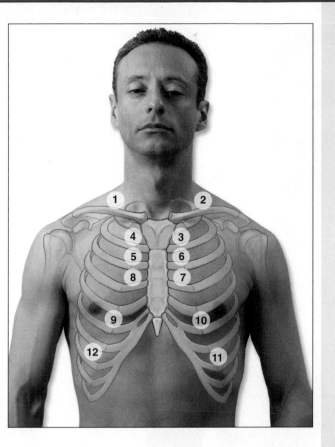

Figure 15.23 ●
Pattern for percussion:
Anterior thorax.

- Percussion over bone or organs will yield flat or dull sounds. Avoid percussion over the clavicles, sternum, and ribs. Percussion over the heart will produce dullness to the left of the sternum from the third to fifth intercostal spaces. Percuss the left lung lateral to the midclavicular line. Percussion sounds in the lower left thorax change from resonance to tympany over the gastric air bubble. Percussion sounds in the right lower thorax change from resonance to dullness at the upper liver border.

AUSCULTATION OF THE ANTERIOR THORAX

Auscultation is used to identify and discriminate between and among normal and adventitious breath sounds. Listen to the full respiratory cycle with each placement of the stethoscope (see Figure 15.24 ●).

1. **Instruct the client.**
   - Explain that you will be listening to the client's breathing with the stethoscope. Ask the client to breathe deeply through the mouth each time the stethoscope is placed on the chest and to let you know if the client is becoming short of breath or tired.

2. **Auscultate the trachea.**
   - Place the stethoscope over the trachea above the suprasternal notch. You will hear tracheal breath sounds. Move the stethoscope to the left, then the right side of the trachea, just above each sternoclavicular joint. You will hear bronchial breath sounds.

TECHNIQUES AND NORMAL FINDINGS

ABNORMAL FINDINGS SPECIAL CONSIDERATIONS

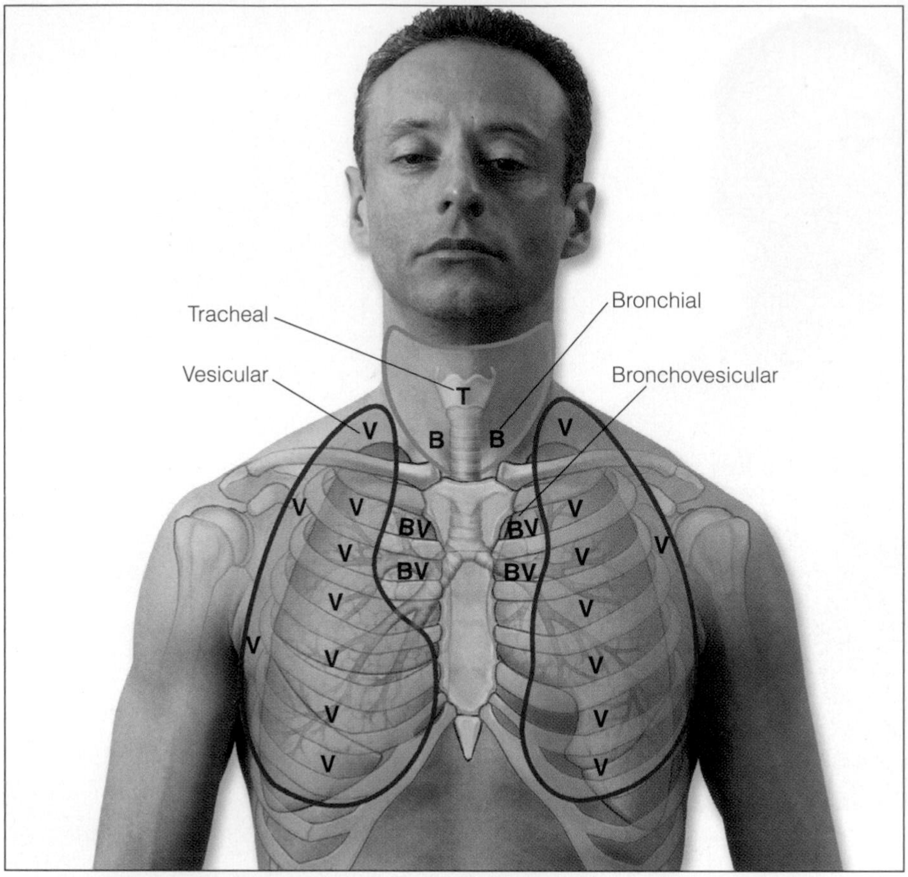

Figure 15.24 • Auscultatory sounds: Anterior thorax.

3. Auscultate the apices.

- Place the stethoscope in the triangular areas just superior to each clavicle. You will hear vesicular sounds.

4. Auscultate the bronchi.

- The bronchi are auscultated at the second and third intercostal spaces at the left and right sternal borders. You will hear bronchovesicular sounds.

5. Auscultate the lungs.

- Auscultate the lungs by following the pattern for percussion. Move the stethoscope from side to side as you compare sounds. Move down to the sixth intercostal space and laterally to the midaxillary line. You will hear vesicular sounds.

6. Interpret the findings.

- Refer to the descriptions and interpretations of normal and adventitious breath sounds described in auscultation of the posterior thorax.

Box 15.1	Normal and Abnormal Respiratory Rates and Patterns

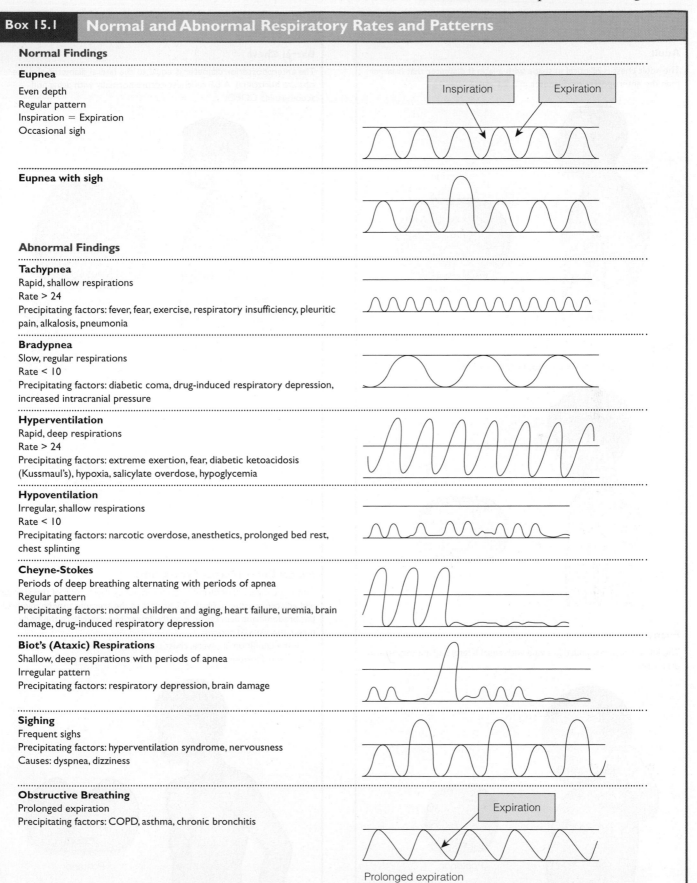

Normal Findings

Eupnea

Even depth
Regular pattern
Inspiration = Expiration
Occasional sigh

Inspiration   Expiration

Eupnea with sigh

Abnormal Findings

Tachypnea
Rapid, shallow respirations
Rate > 24
Precipitating factors: fever, fear, exercise, respiratory insufficiency, pleuritic pain, alkalosis, pneumonia

Bradypnea
Slow, regular respirations
Rate < 10
Precipitating factors: diabetic coma, drug-induced respiratory depression, increased intracranial pressure

Hyperventilation
Rapid, deep respirations
Rate > 24
Precipitating factors: extreme exertion, fear, diabetic ketoacidosis (Kussmaul's), hypoxia, salicylate overdose, hypoglycemia

Hypoventilation
Irregular, shallow respirations
Rate < 10
Precipitating factors: narcotic overdose, anesthetics, prolonged bed rest, chest splinting

Cheyne-Stokes
Periods of deep breathing alternating with periods of apnea
Regular pattern
Precipitating factors: normal children and aging, heart failure, uremia, brain damage, drug-induced respiratory depression

Biot's (Ataxic) Respirations
Shallow, deep respirations with periods of apnea
Irregular pattern
Precipitating factors: respiratory depression, brain damage

Sighing
Frequent sighs
Precipitating factors: hyperventilation syndrome, nervousness
Causes: dyspnea, dizziness

Obstructive Breathing
Prolonged expiration
Precipitating factors: COPD, asthma, chronic bronchitis

Expiration

Prolonged expiration

Box 15.2	Normal Chest Configurations

Adult

The adult chest is elliptical in shape with a lateral diameter that is larger than the anteroposterior diameter in a 2:1 ratio.

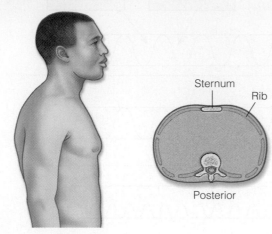

Sternum
Rib
Posterior

Child

The chest of a child is of adult proportion by age 6.

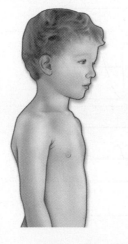
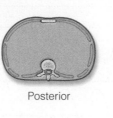

Posterior

Infant

The infant chest is rounded in shape with equal lateral and anteroposterior diameters.

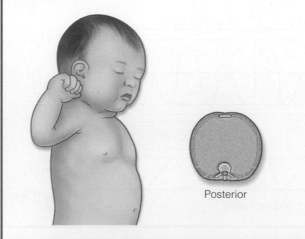

Posterior

Box 15.3	Abnormal Chest Configurations

Barrel Chest

The anteroposterior diameter is equal to the lateral diameter, and the ribs are horizontal. A barrel chest occurs normally with aging and accompanies COPD.

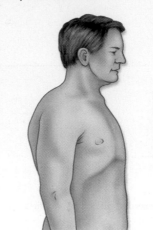
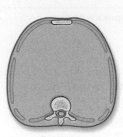

Posterior

Funnel Chest (Pectus Excavatum)

This is a congenital deformity characterized by depression of the sternum and adjacent costal cartilage. All or part of the sternum may be involved but predominant depression is at the lower portion where the body meets the xiphoid process.

If the condition is severe, chest compression may interfere with respiration. Murmurs may be present with cardiac compression.

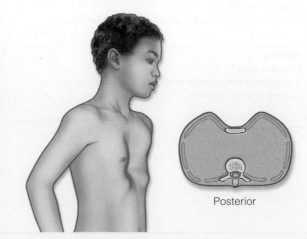

Posterior

Box 15.3 **Abnormal Chest Configurations** *(continued)*

Scoliosis

Scoliosis is a condition in which there is lateral curvature and rotation of the thoracic and lumbar spine. It occurs more frequently in females. Scoliosis may result in elevation of the shoulder and pelvis.

Deviation greater than 45° may cause distortion of the lung, which results in decreased lung volume or difficulty in interpretation of findings from physical assessment.

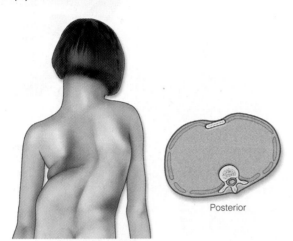

Posterior

Kyphosis

Kyphosis is exaggerated posterior curvature of the thoracic spine. It is associated with aging. Severe kyphosis may decrease lung expansion and increase cardiac problems.

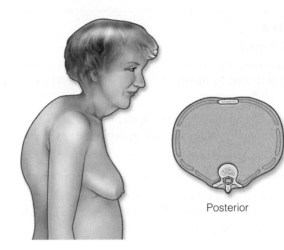

Posterior

Pigeon Chest (Pectus Carinatum)

This congenital deformity is characterized by forward displacement of the sternum with depression of the adjacent costal cartilage. This condition generally requires no treatment.

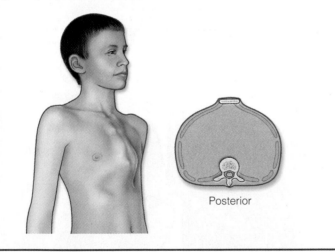

Posterior

Refer to the Companion Website at **www.prenhall.com/damico** and click on the **Documentation** module for documentation samples and documentation practice exercises.

RESPIRATORY DISORDERS

Asthma

A chronic hyperreactive condition resulting in bronchospasm, mucosal edema, and increased mucous secretion. Usually occurs in response to inhaled irritants or allergens (see Figure 15.25 ●).

Inspection: Dyspnea, increased respiratory rate, use of accessory muscles, anxiety, audible wheeze, prolonged expiration.

Palpation: Decreased tactile fremitus.

Percussion: Resonance. Hyperresonance when chronic.

Auscultation: Breath sounds obscured by wheezes. Decreased voice sounds. In severe asthma, air movement may be so limited that no breath sounds are heard.

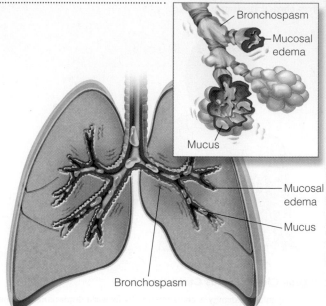

Figure 15.25 ● Asthma.

Atelectasis

A condition in which there is an obstruction of airflow. The alveoli or an entire lung may collapse from airway obstruction, such as a mucous plug, lack of surfactant, or a compressed chest wall (see Figure 15.26 ●).

Inspection: Decreased lung expansion on the affected side, increased respiratory rate, dyspnea, cyanosis. If severe, the trachea shifts to the affected side.

Palpation: Lack of tactile fremitus.

Percussion: Dullness over the affected area.

Auscultation: Decreased or absent breath sounds and voice sounds.

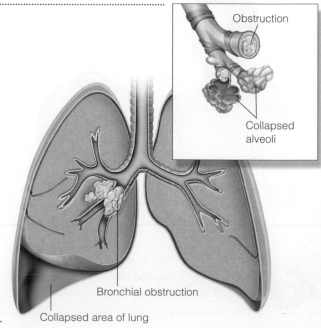

Figure 15.26 ● Atelectasis.

Chronic Bronchitis

Chronic inflammation of the tracheobronchial tree leads to increased mucous production and blocked airways. A productive cough is present (see Figure 15.27 ●).

Inspection: Dyspnea, chronic productive cough, tachypnea, use of accessory muscles.

Palpation: Normal tactile fremitus.

Percussion: Resonance.

Auscultation: Wheezes and rhonchi may be present.

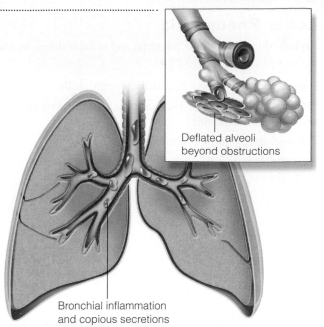

Deflated alveoli beyond obstructions

Bronchial inflammation and copious secretions

Figure 15.27 ● Chronic bronchitis.

Emphysema

A condition in which chronic inflammation of the lungs leads to destruction of alveoli and decreased elasticity of the lungs. As a result, air is trapped and lungs hyperinflate (see Figure 15.28 ●).

Inspection: Shortness of breath, especially on exertion, barrel chest, pursed lip breathing, use of accessory muscles, cyanosis, clubbing of fingers, tripod posture.

Palpation: Decreased chest expansion, decreased tactile fremitus.

Percussion: Hyperresonance.

Auscultation: Decreased vesicular sounds and possible wheeze.

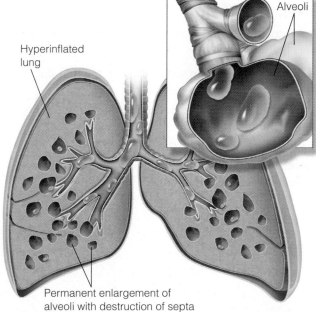

Hyperinflated lung

Alveoli

Permanent enlargement of alveoli with destruction of septa

Figure 15.28 ● Emphysema.

Lobar Pneumonia

An infection causes fluid, bacteria, and cellular debris to fill the alveoli (see Figure 15.29 ●).

Inspection: Tachypnea, productive cough, chills.

Palpation: Increased tactile fremitus. Decreased chest expansion of the affected side.

Percussion: Dullness over the affected area.

Auscultation: Bronchophony, egophony, whispered pectoriloquy. Bronchial breath sounds and crackles.

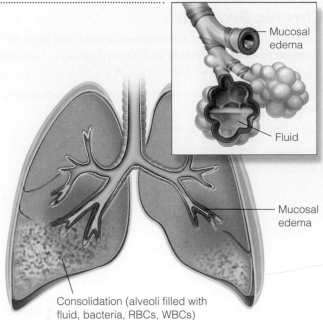

Figure 15.29 ● Lobar pneumonia.

Pleural Effusion

In this condition fluid accumulates in the pleural space (see Figure 15.30 ●).

Inspection: Dyspnea. In severe effusion, tracheal shift to the unaffected side.

Palpation: Decreased tactile fremitus and chest expansion on the affected side.

Percussion: Dullness over the fluid.

Auscultation: Breath sounds and voice sounds decreased or absent. Possible pleural rub.

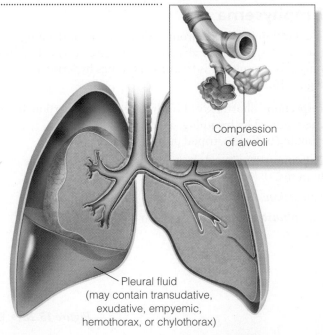

Figure 15.30 ● Pleural effusion.

Pneumothorax

A condition in which air moves into the pleural space and causes partial or complete collapse of the lung. Pneumothorax can be spontaneous, traumatic, or tension (see Figure 15.31 ●).

Inspection: Tachypnea, decreased expansion of the chest wall on the affected side, tracheal shift to the unaffected side.

Palpation: Decreased tactile fremitus.

Percussion: Hyperresonance.

Auscultation: Breath sounds and voice sounds are decreased or absent.

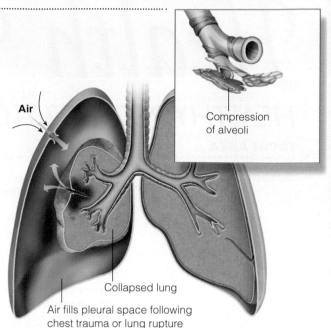

Figure 15.31 ● Pneumothorax.

Congestive Heart Failure

Increased pressure in the pulmonary veins causes interstitial edema around the alveoli and may cause edema of the bronchial mucosa (see Figure 15.32 ●).

Inspection: Increased respiratory rate, shortness of breath (especially on exertion), orthopnea, peripheral edema, pallor.

Palpation: Normal tactile fremitus. Skin cool and clammy.

Percussion: Resonance.

Auscultation: Normal breath sounds and voice sounds. Wheezes or crackles at the bases of the lungs.

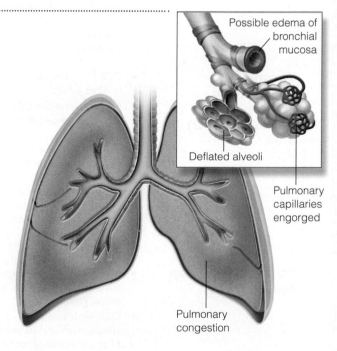

Figure 15.32 ● Congestive heart failure.

Health Promotion

HEALTHY PEOPLE 2010

FOCUS AREA	PREVALENCE	OBJECTIVES	ACTIONS
Asthma	• Nearly 14.9 million people in the United States have asthma. • Each year, asthma accounts for 500,000 hospitalizations, 5,000 deaths, and 134 million days of restricted activity. • More cases of asthma are diagnosed in adults but the rate of asthma in preschool-age children is growing. • African Americans and Hispanics are 2 to 6 times more likely to die from asthma than are Caucasians.	• Reduce the number of asthma deaths. • Reduce the number of hospitalizations for asthma. • Increase the number of asthmatics who receive appropriate care. • Reduce activity limitations.	• Patient education. • Identification and tracking of environmental triggers. • Development of asthma action plans (when and how to take medications and what to do when asthma worsens). • Long-term management strategies.
Chronic Obstructive Pulmonary Disease (COPD)	• COPD occurs most often in older adults. • Ninety percent of COPD is attributable to cigarette smoking. • COPD can occur as a result of exposure to occupational and environmental toxins. • Death from COPD is more common in males than females.	• Reduce the number of COPD deaths. • Reduce the number of adults who have limited activity because of COPD.	• Screening for COPD. • Counseling and treatment. • Smoking cessation.
Obstructive Sleep Apnea (OSA)	• OSA affects all races, ages, socioeconomic groups, and ethnic groups. • OSA most frequently affects men over 50 years of age and postmenopausal women. • Young African Americans experience symptoms of OSA twice as frequently as Caucasians. • Infants who have siblings or relatives with OSA are at increased risk for SIDS.	• Increase the number of persons with symptoms of OSA that are medically managed. • Reduce vehicular accidents related to excessive sleepiness.	• Education about OSA. • Identify persons at risk.

FOCUS AREA	PREVALENCE	OBJECTIVES	ACTIONS
Tobacco Use	• More deaths are attributable to cigarette smoking than to AIDS, alcohol, heroin, homicide, suicide, motor vehicle accidents, and fires combined. • Adolescent smoking increased in the 1990s with the greatest increase in Caucasians. • Smoking occurs most frequently in low socioeconomic groups and those with less than 12 years of education. • Smoking rates are slightly higher in men than women. • The highest rates of smoking are found in American Indians, Alaska Natives, blue-collar workers, and military personnel.	• Reduce tobacco use by adults and adolescents. • Increase the numbers of adults and adolescents who participate in smoking cessation programs. • Decrease exposure to secondhand smoke.	• Education about hazards. • Programs to prevent initiation of smoking. • Programs to assist with smoking cessation. • Education about the avoidance of environmental tobacco smoke.

CLIENT EDUCATION

The following are risk factors for physiological, behavioral, cultural, and life span considerations that affect respiratory health. Several factors are cited as trends in *Healthy People 2010*.

The nurse provides advice and education to reduce risks associated with the factors and to promote and maintain respiratory health.

LIFE SPAN CONSIDERATIONS

RISK FACTOR(S)

- Infants have small, delicate respiratory structures leaving them susceptible to infection.

- There has been an increase in the incidence of sudden infant death syndrome (SIDS), theorized to be associated with problems of the respiratory system or suffocation.
- The activities, environments, and hygiene practices of preschool and early school-age children put them at increased risk for respiratory infections.
- Suffocation and aspiration occur with greater frequency in infants and preschool children and are associated with plastic bags, toys, and household objects.

- Middle adults are at risk from respiratory illness and problems with oxygenation because of decreased elasticity of the lung and decrease in lung capacity by 25% to 30%.

- Older adults experience skeletal, muscular, and organic changes that result in decreased respiratory expansion and effectiveness, which increases the risk for respiratory problems.

CLIENT EDUCATION

- Teach that immunization is important across the age span. Recommended schedules should be followed. For example: Infants should receive immunizations for DPT and *H. influenzae* type b.
- Teach caregivers to place infants on their back for sleep to reduce the incidence of SIDS.

- Teach hygiene measures including hand washing, use of tissues, and covering the mouth when coughing to prevent the spread of infection.
- Teach caregivers that toys for infants and children must be age appropriate and without small inhalable parts and that plastic bags must not be used in bedding or left within reach of children.
- Teach that regular exercise strengthens the musculoskeletal system, maintains the efficiency of the respiratory system, and contributes to weight loss, all of which impact respiratory health.
- Instruct older adults that regular exercise strengthens the musculoskeletal system, maintains the efficiency of the respiratory system, and contributes to weight loss, all of which impact respiratory health.

CULTURAL CONSIDERATIONS

RISK FACTOR(S)

- The incidence of TB has increased and has been attributed to existence of the disease in immigrant populations, crowded conditions in urban areas, increased international travel, and decreased immune response in individuals with AIDS.

CLIENT EDUCATION

- Teach travelers to update immunizations and to have TB testing. Immigrant populations require TB testing and treatment.

BEHAVIORAL CONSIDERATIONS

RISK FACTOR(S)

- Smoking and experimentation with drugs (especially inhalants) are increasing, and the use of gaseous substances can result in permanent damage to the lungs.

- Experimental sexual activity, sexual activity with multiple partners, and drug use are on the rise in adolescents and young adults. These activities increase the risk of contracting AIDS and the associated respiratory diseases such as *Pneumocystis carinii* pneumonia.

- In the United States, obesity has become increasingly prevalent across the age span. Obesity can alter respiratory effort, can compromise function, and is associated with an increase in OSA.

CLIENT EDUCATION

- Provide information about support for not smoking. Can be addressed within families in schools and healthcare settings.
- Advise parents, adolescents, and young adults about drug use in relation to respiratory health problems, how to recognize behaviors associated with drug use, and about prevention programs and addiction services that are aimed at reducing inhalation injuries and contraction of AIDS.
- Provide information about abstinence or protected sexual activity to reduce the incidence of AIDS.

- Teach clients that regular exercise strengthens the musculoskeletal system, maintains the efficiency of the respiratory system, and contributes to weight loss, all of which impact respiratory health.
- Teach that healthy eating from infancy to old age prevents obesity and contributes to improved oxygenation.

ENVIRONMENTAL CONSIDERATIONS

RISK FACTOR(S)

- Asthma and other allergic and chronic respiratory diseases are increasing in all populations, but particularly children of low socioeconomic status. The increase is attributed to urbanization and increased exposure to pollutants and chemicals in cities and rural farm areas.

CLIENT EDUCATION

- Teach clients to limit exposure to allergens, pollutants, and irritants in the home and workplace. Assist clients to identify allergens and irritants as an important first step in preventing problems and promoting respiratory health. Provide information about filters, masks, and other protective equipment for use in the home or work environments.

Application Through Critical Thinking

CASE STUDY

*T*anisha Robinson, a 14-year-old female, has been seen regularly in the clinic for chronic asthma. Today, Tanisha's mother has accompanied her for a checkup. Tanisha has required two visits to the emergency room (ER) for severe wheezing in the month since her last clinic visit.

The physical assessment revealed that the client was in no distress and breath sounds were clear. Her vital signs were BP 126/82—P 84—RR 20. Her skin was warm, dry, and pink in color. Tanisha could speak clearly and seemed relaxed.

During the interview the nurse learned that the client has been following her prescribed treatments and has done well except for the two ER visits.

The nurse learned that each ER visit occurred after school hours. The client experienced severe shortness of breath and wheezing that was unrelieved by rest or use of her inhalers. ER treatment consisted of injection of epinephrine and administration of oxygen, IV fluids, Benadryl, and steroids. Each ER visit lasted approximately 6 hours. The client's breathing was restored to nearly normal at discharge and she was given a prescription for a course of prednisone.

When asked if she could identify any precipitating factors, Tanisha replied, "I know they happened on days that we had gym, but I don't usually have a problem with that." The nurse asked if she had any changes in her routines, activities, or environments. She said, "No, not that I can think of." Her mother stated, "We're so upset. She's been out twice this month." The client then added, "Yes, I hate to have to miss school and get behind and now my friend and I have to work twice as hard as before to get our project done."

The nurse asked about the project and the client said, "We are working on an art project—collecting materials and doing a thing on textures. It's pretty cool. We collected old clothes from the Salvation Army and a garage sale and we've been cutting them up sort of in a collage." The nurse asked if the work on the project coincided with her recent attacks. The client said, "Gee, I don't know, I never thought about it." Her mother stated, "Oh, we never even thought about that, but on both days, she had been working on the project after school with her friend and really got bad as the evening wore on."

► Complete Documentation

The following is a sample documentation from assessment of Tanisha Robinson.

SUBJECTIVE DATA: Visit to clinic for a checkup, 14-year-old female asthmatic. Required two ER visits for severe wheezing in month since last clinic visit. Following prescribed treatments. Doing well except ER visits. ER visits occurred on school days when client had gym, but usually no problem with physical activity. ER visits associated with work on art project—a textile collage from old clothes. Wheezing started after work on project and increased in severity requiring epinephrine, IV, Benadryl, and steroids. Client is discharged with course of oral steroids after each visit. Resumed normal treatment and activity after episodes.

OBJECTIVE DATA: Breath sounds clear. Skin warm, dry, and pink. Clear speech, relaxed. VS: BP 126/82—P 84—RR 20.

► Critical Thinking Questions

1. Describe the nurse's thoughts and actions as the nurse applies the steps of the critical thinking process in this situation.
2. In interpreting the data, how would it be clustered?

ASSESSMENT FORM

REASON FOR VISIT

Scheduled monthly checkup.

HISTORY

Chronic asthma, follows prescribed treatment

Two recent ER visits R/T severe wheezing

Epinephrine, IV, Benadryl, steroids—6 hr. stay

Discharges—prednisone—recovery—resume normal routine

Episodes R/T work with "old" clothes for school project.

ASSESSMENT

BP: *126/82*   **P** *84*   **RR** *20*

Skin: *Pink, warm, dry*

Lungs: *Clear—all fields*

Affect: *Relaxed*

Speech: *Clear*

---

3. What are the options that could be developed for this 14-year-old and her mother?

► Applying Nursing Diagnoses

1. Identify two nursing diagnoses that could be derived from the data in this case study.
2. Is the data in the case study supportive of the diagnosis *ineffective breathing pattern?* Provide examples of the definition, defining characteristics, and risks or related factors of the diagnoses.

► Prepare Teaching Plan

LEARNING NEED: Data reveals two episodes of respiratory distress following the construction of a textile collage for a school project. Tanisha needs to learn more about environmental allergens as causing her respiratory distress.

GOAL: Tanisha will decrease the number of acute respiratory distress episodes.

OBJECTIVES: At the end of the lesson, Tanisha will be able to:

1. Identify locations of known allergens in her environment.
2. Identify strategies to decrease her exposure to allergens.

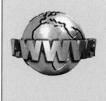

Please refer to the Companion Website at www.prenhall.com/damico and click on Chapter 15, the Application Through Critical Thinking module, to complete the following activities related to this case study:
- ► **Critical Thinking questions**
- ► **Extended Nursing Diagnosis challenge**
- ► **Documentation activity**
- ► **Teaching Plan for Objective 1**

EXAMPLE OF TEACHING PLAN FOR OBJECTIVE 2: Identify strategies to decrease her exposure to allergens (cognitive)

Content	Teaching Strategy and Rationale	Evaluation
You have been able to recall your allergens and have identified environmental placement. Now you need to look for alternatives to prevent future exposure and distress.	• One-to-one discussion to provide recall and reinforcement of learner's knowledge	Name three alternative strategies to be used when completing the school project.
Alternative strategies could include the following:	• Printed material to provide review and reinforcement of material	

• Work in a well-ventilated area.
• Plan all activities to decrease exposure to allergens:
  • Use clean and dry materials.
  • Select other substances for texture—wood, stone, plastic.
  • Wash material before handling.
• Read all labels to be sure allergens are not in the product being used.
• Use objects that are allergen-free.		

EXPLORE MediaLink

Additional resources for this chapter are found on the Student CD-ROM accompanying this textbook and on the Companion Website.

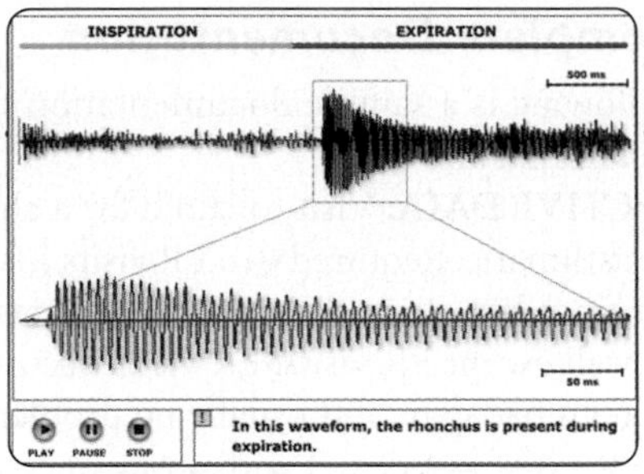

CD-ROM CONTENT

Content for this chapter includes:
Objectives
Key Concepts
NCLEX-RN® Review Questions
Model Documentation Forms
Audio Glossary
Lung Sounds
    Bronchial Breath Sounds
    Vesicular Breath Sounds
    Bronchovesicular Breath Sounds
    Fine Crackles
    Coarse Crackles
    Wheezes
    Rhonchi
    Pleural Friction Rub
    Stridor
Animations
    Respiratory System
    Gas Exchange
    Oxygen Transport
    Asthma
Games and Challenges
Clinical Spotlight Videos
    Tuberculosis
    Asthma
Head-to-Toe Physical Examination Video

INSPIRATION   EXPIRATION

In this waveform, the rhonchus is present during expiration.

PLAY   PAUSE   STOP

COMPANION WEBSITE CONTENT

www.prenhall.com/damico

Content for this chapter includes:
Objectives
NCLEX-RN® Review Questions
Client Interaction Case Study Challenge
Application Through Critical Thinking
    Case Study Teaching Plan Challenge
MediaLinks
MediaLink Application
Tool Box
    Documentation Form Example
    Normal Breath Sounds
    Adventitious Sounds
    Normal and Abnormal Respiratory Rates and Patterns
    Health Promotion
        Healthy People 2010
        Client Education
New York Times

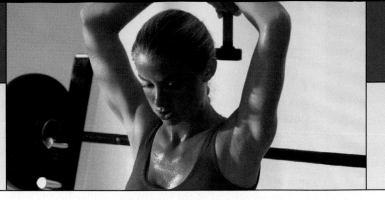

16
Breasts and Axillae

MEDIALINK

www.prenhall.com/damico

The CD-ROM in the back of this textbook and the Media-Link website contain NCLEX-RN® review questions, interactive exercises, case study challenges, animations, videos, documentation and checklist forms, and review materials. For a complete listing of the media content specific to Chapter 16, see the Explore MediaLink at the end of the chapter.

S tatistics compiled by the American Cancer Society (2004) indicate that breast cancer is the most common cancer among females, accounting for one of every three cancers diagnosed in females. Breast cancer incidence rates have increased by 0.5% per year since the late 1990s. However, breast cancer mortality has declined. The decline has been attributed to the benefits of mammography screening and improved treatments for breast cancer. Use of screening programs that detect tumors before they become clinically apparent is beneficial in detecting breast changes and tumors. A thorough breast examination is a part of that screening process.

The assessment of the breasts and axillae begins with a thorough health history. During the focused interview, the nurse gathers additional information by asking pertinent questions relating to the client's general health and breast and lymph nodes in particular. The physical assessment of the breasts may be incorporated into the total body assessment along with the heart and lung assessment when the client is sitting and again when supine. Although the majority of the material in this chapter assumes that the client is female, it is important to incorporate assessment of the male client's breasts during the physical assessment, usually when assessing the thorax.

Cancer is considered to be a focus area as described in *Healthy People 2010* on page 420. The goal is to promote health with the reduction of the new cases of cancer as well as the related illnesses, disabilities, and deaths. This includes breast and cervical cancer in the female. Therefore, the nurse must be cognizant of these factors as questions for the focused interview are formulated and the physical assessment is performed.

Accurate knowledge of the structure and function of the breasts and lymphatic system is necessary to carry out the assessment activities related to the breasts and axillae. It is also important that the nurse understand the interrelationships of the various body systems that contribute to this region. For example, the musculoskeletal system supports the overlying integument, and the lymphatic system drains the region. In addition, while performing the assessment, one must keep in mind the normal variations for the client's developmental stage. An understanding and acceptance of different individuals' feelings, beliefs, and practices regarding the breasts and breast care are also essential.

ANATOMY AND PHYSIOLOGY REVIEW

The breasts are located on the anterior chest and supported by muscles and ligaments. The breast includes the areola and nipple, as well as the glandular, adipose, and fibrous tissue. A system of lymph nodes drains lymph from the breasts and axillae. These tissues and structures are described in the following paragraphs.

BREASTS

The breasts are paired mammary glands located on the anterior chest wall. Breast tissue extends from the second or third rib to the sixth or seventh rib and from the sternal margin to the midaxillary line, depending on body shape and size (see Figure 16.1 ●). The breasts lie anterior to the pectoralis major and serratus anterior muscles. The nipple is centrally located within a circular pigmented field of wrinkled skin called the **areola.** The surface of the areola is speckled with tiny sebaceous glands known as **Montgomery's glands** (Montgomery's tubercles; see Figure 16.2 ●). Hair follicles are normally seen around the periphery of the areola. Commonly, breast tissue extends superiolaterally into the axilla as the **axillary tail** (tail of Spence). The internal and lateral thoracic arteries and cutaneous branches of the posterior intercostal arteries provide an abundant supply of blood to the breasts.

Breasts are composed of glandular, fibrous, and adipose (fat) tissue. The glandular tissue is arranged into 15 to 20 lobes per breast that radiate from the nipple (see Figure 16.3 ●). Each lobe is composed of 20 to 40 lobules that contain the **acini cells** (or alveoli) that produce milk. These cells empty into the lactiferous ducts, which carry milk from each lobe to the nipple. The fibrous tissue provides support for the glandular tissue. **Suspensory ligaments** (Cooper's ligaments) extend from the connective tissue layer, through the breast, and attach to the fascia underlying the breast. Subcutaneous and retromammary adipose tissue

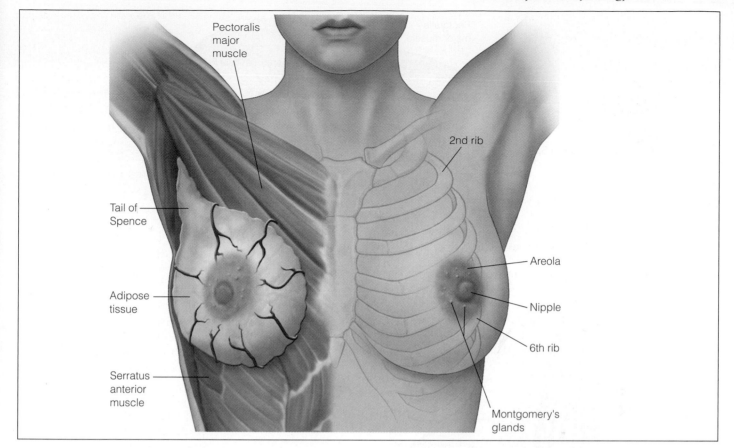

Figure 16.1 ● Anatomy of the breast.

make up the remainder of the breast. The proportions of these three components vary with age, the general state of the client's health, menstrual cycle, pregnancy, lactation, and other factors. Supernumerary nipples or breast tissue may be present along the **mammary ridge,** or "milk line," which extends from each axilla to the groin (see Figure 16.4 ●). Usually this tissue atrophies during development, but occasionally a nipple persists and is visible. It needs to be differentiated from a mole (see

Figure 16.5 ●). For the purpose of documenting assessment findings, the breast is divided into four quadrants defined by a vertical line and a horizontal line that intersect at the nipple (see Figure 16.6 ●). The location of clinical findings may be described according to clock positions, for example, at the 2-o'clock position, 5 cm from the nipple. The male breast is composed of a small nipple and flat areola. These are superior to a thin disk of undeveloped breast tissue that may not be distinguishable from the surrounding tissues. The major functions of the breasts include producing, storing, and supplying milk for the process of lactation. Breasts also provide a mechanism for sexual arousal.

AXILLAE AND LYMPH NODES

A complex system of lymph nodes drains lymph from the breasts and axillae and returns it to the blood. Superficial lymph nodes drain the skin, and deep lymph nodes drain the mammary lobules. Figure 16.7 ● depicts the groups of nodes that drain the breasts and axillae.

The lymph nodes are usually nonpalpable. The following nodes are palpated during the assessment.

1. Internal mammary nodes
2. Supraclavicular nodes
3. Subclavicular (infraclavicular) nodes
4. Interpectoral nodes
5. Central axillary nodes
6. Brachial (lateral axillary) nodes

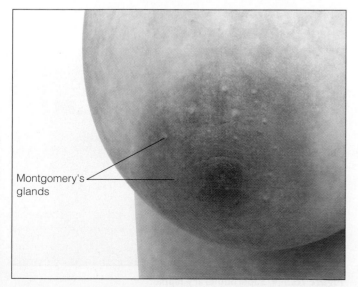

Figure 16.2 ● Montgomery's glands.

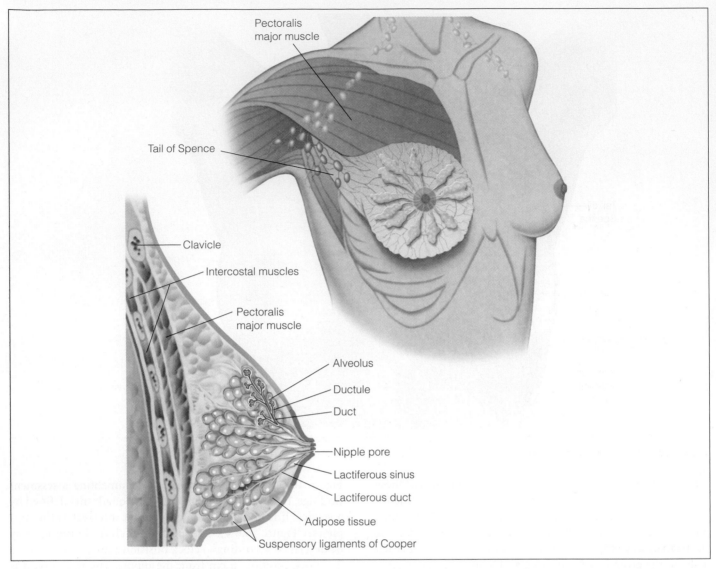

Pectoralis major muscle

Tail of Spence

Clavicle

Intercostal muscles

Pectoralis major muscle

Alveolus

Ductule

Duct

Nipple pore

Lactiferous sinus

Lactiferous duct

Adipose tissue

Suspensory ligaments of Cooper

Figure 16.3 ● Anterior and lateral views of breast anatomy.

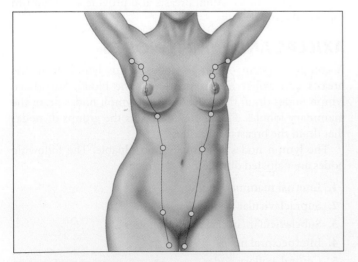

Figure 16.4 ● Mammary ridge.

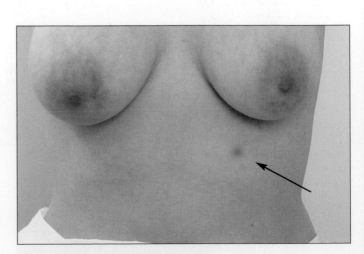

Figure 16.5 ● Supernumerary nipple.

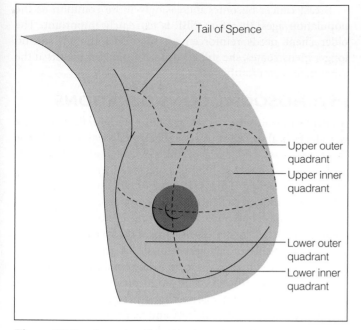

Figure 16.6 ● Breast quadrants.

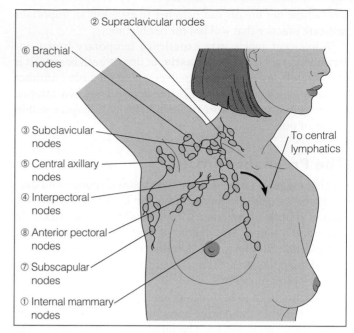

Figure 16.7 ● Lymphatic drainage of the breast.

7. Subscapular (posterior axillary) nodes
8. Pectoral (anterior axillary) nodes

The internal mammary nodes drain toward the abdomen and the opposite breast. Most of the lymph from the rest of the breast drains toward the axilla and subclavicular region. Thus, a cancerous lesion can spread via the lymphatic system to the subclavicular nodes, into deep channels within the chest or abdomen, and even to the opposite breast. The male breast has the same potential and needs to be examined as well. The major functions of the lymphatic system include returning water and proteins from the interstitial spaces to the blood, thus helping to maintain blood osmotic pressure and body fluid balance. It also helps filter out microorganisms and other body debris.

MUSCLES OF THE CHEST WALL

The major muscles of the chest wall, which support the breast and contribute to its shape, are the pectoralis major and serratus anterior muscles (see Figure 16.1). The overall contour of the breasts is determined by the suspensory ligaments, which provide support. The major function of the muscles of the chest wall is to support breast and lymphatic tissue.

SPECIAL CONSIDERATIONS

Age, developmental level, race, ethnicity, work history, living conditions, socioeconomics, and emotional well-being are among the factors that influence breast health. These factors must be considered when collecting subjective and objective data during the comprehensive health assessment. The nurse applies critical thinking to assess the client's state of health and to identify the factors that may influence breast health.

DEVELOPMENTAL CONSIDERATIONS

Growth and development are dynamic processes that describe change over time. The following discussion presents specific variations of the breasts for different age groups.

Infants and Children

The breast tissue of newborns is sometimes swollen because of the hyperestrogenism of pregnancy. Some infants may produce a thin discharge called "witch's milk." This secretion subsides as the infant's body eliminates maternal hormones.

Breast tissue starts to enlarge in females with the onset of puberty, usually between the ages of 9 and 13. At first there is only a bud around the nipple and areola, which may be tender initially. The ductile system matures, extensive fat deposits occur, and the areola and nipples grow and become pigmented. These changes are correlated with an increased level of estrogen and progesterone in the body as sexual maturity progresses. Growth of the breasts is not necessarily steady or symmetrical. This may be frustrating or embarrassing to some girls. Because a female's primary sexual organs cannot be observed, breast development provides visual confirmation that the adolescent is becoming a woman. For the developing adolescent, her breasts are a visible symbol of her feminine identity and an important part of her body image and self-esteem. The nurse can reassure girls that the rate of breast tissue growth is dependent upon changing hormone levels and is uniquely individual, as are the eventual size and shape of the breasts.

Benign fibroadenomas in adolescent females are not uncommon. The nurse should reassure the girl and her parents or caregivers that no correlation has been established between fibroadenomas and malignant cancers. Although the American Cancer Society recommends that females begin self-breast examination (SBE) at age 20, teaching the adolescent female how to examine her breasts can help her to establish an important self-care practice that will last for her lifetime.

Adolescent males may experience temporary breast enlargement, called **gynecomastia,** in one or both breasts. It is usually self-limiting and resolves spontaneously. Another concern to adolescent males is transient masses beneath one areola or both. These "breast buds" usually disappear within a year of onset.

The Pregnant Female

During pregnancy, breast tissue enlarges as glandular and ductal tissue increases in preparation for lactation. During the second month of pregnancy, nipples and areolae darken in color and enlarge. The degree of pigmentation varies with complexion. Nipples may leak **colostrum** in the month prior to childbirth. As breast tissue enlarges, venous networks may be more pronounced.

SBE also needs to be done during pregnancy. The procedure is the same, even though the breast tissue will be firmer, larger, and possibly more tender. The lobules are more distinct. The areolae and nipples are usually darker. Cancer of the breast during pregnancy needs to be identified as soon as possible and is treated on an individual basis. SBE of the lactating breast (in females who are breast-feeding) should be after the child has completed breast-feeding.

The Older Adult

More time may be required for the focused interview of an older client. Many people have a difficult time talking about something as private as the breasts, and older adults may be even less comfortable with this topic. They may be modest and self-conscious, or they may feel that the nurse is too young to understand. There may also be cultural taboos about such private matters. The nurse should acknowledge that talking about the breasts may be somewhat uncomfortable but explain that sharing this information will promote the client's health.

Older adults may have limited range of motion. If so, the client should be asked to raise her arms to a height that does not cause discomfort. Because the older adult may have failing eyesight, the nurse may want to provide large mirrors, additional lighting, and a magnifying glass for close inspection when teaching SBE. Pamphlets and handouts with large print may be provided.

As menopause approaches, there is a decrease in glandular tissue, which is replaced by fatty tissue. The lobular texture of glandular tissue is replaced by a finer, granular texture. Breasts are less firm and tend to be more pendulous. As the suspensory ligaments relax, breast tissue hangs more loosely from the chest wall. The nipples become smaller and flatter and lose some erectile ability. The inframammary ridge thickens and can be palpated more easily.

Gynecomastia may occur in older adult males as a result of hormonal changes due to disease or medication. The nurse must be sensitive to possible embarrassment during the exam.

Breast cancer becomes increasingly more common as the population ages; therefore, SBE is extremely important. The older client needs reinforcement that even though she no longer menstruates, she still needs to examine her breasts at the same time each month.

PSYCHOSOCIAL CONSIDERATIONS

A client's overall sense of self-esteem may be reflected in the way she feels about her breasts. In fact, some women may view their breasts as a badge of femininity. Media portrayal of idealized images of "perfect" breasts, especially by advertisers, may increase this feeling. Thus, clients whose breasts are smaller or larger than average, clients with asymmetrical breasts, and clients who have had a mastectomy or other breast surgery or trauma are at an increased risk for body image disturbance, self-esteem disturbance, and dysfunctional grieving.

Many females do not perform SBE even after receiving instruction in the procedure. In addition, many do not seek medical attention after discovering a breast lump. These behaviors may be related to anxiety and fear of cancer or surgery, a body image change, or a change in significant relationships. Other factors may include denial, feelings of powerlessness, or a lack of knowledge about breast disorders. During the assessment of the breasts and axillae, the nurse needs to encourage the client to share her fears and concerns. Research indicates that a high-fat diet may increase a female's risk of developing breast cancer. Alcohol intake in excess of nine drinks a week has also been implicated.

The efficacy of SBE in prevention of breast cancer has been questioned as a result of recent research (Freund, 2004). However, the United States Preventive Services Task Force (USPSTF) concluded in 2002 that there is insufficient evidence to recommend for or against clinical breast examination alone for screening. The American Cancer Society (2004, p. 1) reviewed much of the current research and stated that "breast self-examination is prudent and is worth the time to teach and use."

CULTURAL AND ENVIRONMENTAL CONSIDERATIONS

The nurse must be aware of variations in breast development related to ethnicity. For example, females of African ancestry may develop secondary sexual characteristics earlier than females of European ancestry. The time of appearance, texture, and distribution of axillary and pubic hair also vary according to race and ethnicity. Feelings of embarrassment may differ among clients of various cultural or religious groups. Breast cancer rates vary across different cultural groups, but this variation may be due partly to differences in diet or alcohol consumption.

Socioeconomic factors may influence a client's access to screening mammography and regular physical examinations. As mentioned earlier, although most of the information in this chapter assumes a female client, assessment of the male breasts and axillae is also important.

Cultural Considerations

- Caucasian females over 40 years of age have a higher incidence of breast cancer than any other racial or ethnic group.
- African American females under 40 have a slightly higher incidence of breast cancer than Caucasians.
- Hispanics and Asians have the lowest rates of breast cancer; however, breast cancer is the leading cause of cancer deaths in Hispanic females.
- Minority females, who are not well educated, are more inclined to fear that a diagnosis of breast cancer means certain mortality; therefore, they avoid diagnostic procedures.
- Hispanic females put themselves last in terms of family healthcare. As a result, they may not seek preventive care nor seek help until symptoms appear.

- Asian females often exhibit stoicism and do not seek preventive care, but only seek help when symptoms are severe.
- Females in many immigrant cultures were raised in environments in which looking at or touching oneself is prohibited. As a result they do not conduct self-breast examinations.
- Females in immigrant cultures often distrust "medicine" and seek help from cultural healers.
- Language is a barrier for many females of immigrant cultures. Lack of information about breast health in native languages prevents them from seeking preventive services and healthcare for breast disease.
- Females in many cultures have concerns about disrobing and being examined by others, especially when the examiner is of the opposite sex.

Gathering the Data

*B*reast health assessment includes the gathering of subjective and objective data. Subjective data collection occurs during the client interview, before the actual physical assessment. During the interview the nurse uses a variety of communication techniques to elicit general and specific information about the client's state of breast health or illness. Health records, the results of laboratory tests, mammography, and magnetic resonance imaging (MRI) are important secondary sources to be reviewed and included in the data-gathering process. During physical assessment of the breasts and axillae, the techniques of inspection and palpation will be used. Before proceeding, it may be helpful to review the information about each of the data-gathering processes and practice the techniques of health assessment.

FOCUSED INTERVIEW

The focused interview for the breasts and axillae concerns data related to the structures and functions of the breasts and lymphatic system. Subjective data related to breast health is gathered during the focused interview. The nurse must be prepared to observe the client and listen for cues related to the breasts and axillae. The nurse may use open- or closed-ended questions to obtain information. Often a number of follow-up questions or requests for descriptions are required to clarify data or gather

missing information. Follow-up questions are aimed at identifying the source of problems, duration of difficulties, measures to alleviate problems, and clues about the client's knowledge of his or her own health. The subjective data collected and the questions asked during the health history and focused interview provide information to help meet the goals of improving breast health and preventing and controlling breast disease as described in the *Healthy People 2010* feature on page 420.

The focused interview guides physical assessment of the breasts and axillae. The information is always considered in relation to norms and expectations about breast and lymphatic function. Therefore, the nurse must consider age, gender, race, culture, environment, and health practices as well as past and concurrent problems and therapies when framing questions and using techniques to elicit information. In order to address all of the factors when conducting a focused interview, categories of questions related to the breasts and axillae have been developed. These categories include general questions that are asked of all clients, those addressing illness or infection, questions related to symptoms or behaviors, those related to habits or practices, questions that are specific to clients according to age, those for the pregnant female, and questions that address environmental concerns. The nurse must consider the client's ability to participate in the focused interview and physical assessment of the breasts and axillae. If a client is experiencing discomfort, pain, or anxiety related to the breast, attention must focus on relief of the problems.

FOCUSED INTERVIEW QUESTIONS	RATIONALES

The following section provides sample questions and bulleted follow-up questions in each of the categories previously mentioned. A rationale for each of the questions is provided. The list of questions is not all-inclusive but represents the types of questions required in a comprehensive focused interview related to the breasts and axillae.

GENERAL QUESTIONS

1. Describe your breasts today. How do they differ, if at all, from 3 months ago? From 3 years ago?

▶ This question gives the client the opportunity to share her perception of her breasts and any changes she has experienced that may be related to breast health.

2. Are you still menstruating?
   - If so, have you noticed any changes in your breasts that seem to be related to your normal menstrual cycle, such as tenderness, swelling, pain, or enlarged nodes? If so, please describe.

▶ These changes may occur with changing hormone levels, or they may be related to the use of oral, transdermal, and injectable contraceptives. "Lumpy breasts" occurring monthly prior to the onset of menses and resolving at the end of menstruation may be due to a benign condition called physiologic nodularity.

3. What was the date of your last menstrual period?

▶ This information, if applicable, helps correlate the current status of the breasts to the cycle.

QUESTIONS RELATED TO ILLNESS OR INFECTION

1. Have you ever had any breast disease such as cancer, fibrocystic breast disease, benign breast disease, or fibroadenoma?

▶ A history of breast cancer poses the risk of recurrence. Both fibroadenoma and the general lumpiness of fibrocystic breast disease need to be differentiated from cancer.

2. Have you ever had breast surgery?
   - If so, what type and when?
   - How do you feel about it?
   - How has it affected you?
   - Has it affected your sex life? If so, how?

▶ Previous breast surgery has implications for physical and psychological well-being. Breast surgery includes lumpectomy, mastectomy, breast reconstruction, breast reduction, and breast augmentation.

3. Have you had cancer in any other region of your body such as the uterus, ovaries, or colon?

▶ A history of these cancers increases the risk for breast cancer.

4. Has your mother or sister had breast cancer?

▶ If so, the client is at greater risk, especially if the relative's cancer occurred before menopause.

5. Has one of your grandmothers or an aunt had breast cancer?

▶ If so, the client is at slightly greater risk.

QUESTIONS RELATED TO SYMPTOMS OR BEHAVIORS

When gathering information about symptoms, many questions are required to elicit details and descriptions that assist in analysis of the data. The questions are intended to determine the significance of a symptom in relation to specific diseases and problems and to identify the need for follow-up examination or referral.

The following questions refer to specific symptoms and behaviors associated with the breasts and axillae. For each symptom, questions and follow-up are required. The details to be elicited are the characteristics of the symptom; the onset, duration, and frequency of the symptom; the treatment or remedy for the symptom, including home remedies; the determination if a diagnosis has been sought; the effects of treatments; and family history associated with a symptom or illness.

FOCUSED INTERVIEW QUESTIONS	**RATIONALES**

QUESTIONS RELATED TO SYMPTOMS

1. **Have you noticed any changes in breast characteristics, such as size, symmetry, shape, thickening, lumps, swelling, temperature, color of skin or vessels, or sensations such as tingling or tenderness?**
   - If so, how long have you had them? Please describe them.

▶ Pain and tenderness can be caused by physiologic nodularity, pregnancy, lactation, cancer, or other disorders. A lump may indicate a benign cyst, a fibroadenoma, fatty necrosis, or a malignant tumor. Skin irritation may be due to friction from a bra or to pendulous breasts. In older clients, decreased estrogen levels may cause the breasts to sag.

2. **Have you noticed any changes in nipple and areola characteristics, such as size, shape, open sores, lumps, pain, tenderness, discharge, skin changes, or retractions?**
   - If so, how long have you had them? Please describe them.

▶ Nipple discharge resulting from medication is usually clear. A bloody drainage is always a concern and needs to be further evaluated, especially in the presence of a lump. Eczematous changes of the skin of the nipples and areola may indicate Paget's disease, a rare form of breast cancer. Dimpling of skin or retraction of the nipple also suggests cancer.

3. **Have you ever experienced any trauma to your breasts?**

▶ Contact sports, automobile accidents, and physical abuse can cause bruising of the breast and tissue changes.

QUESTIONS RELATED TO BEHAVIORS

1. **Do you exercise?**
   - If so, describe your routine.
   - What kind of bra do you wear when you exercise?

▶ Firm support is recommended during exercise to prevent loss of tissue elasticity.

2. **Have you ever had a mammogram?**
   - If so, when was your most recent one?

▶ Mammography can detect a cancer before it is detectable by palpation. The USPSTF (2002) has made the following recommendations: ages 20 to 39, a clinical breast examination every 3 years; mammography and a clinical breast examination every year in females over 40 years of age.

3. **Do you see your healthcare provider regularly for a physical examination?**

▶ Clients from lower socioeconomic brackets may have reduced access to healthcare.

4. **Do you perform self-breast examination?**
   - If so, how often?
   - At what time of your menstrual cycle do you perform this exam?
   - Describe the procedure you use.

▶ The answer indicates the client's knowledge level and the importance placed on SBE. The nurse may use this opportunity to share information about the importance of SBE, but waiting until after the physical examination is completed for actual demonstration and teaching may allow for better learning.

QUESTIONS RELATED TO AGE

The following questions address breast health across the age span. Breast development begins in preadolescence, and changes continue into older adulthood.

QUESTIONS REGARDING PREADOLESCENTS

1. **Have you noticed any changes in the size or shape of your breasts?**
   - If so, tell me about these changes.

▶ Growth of the breasts is not necessarily steady or symmetrical. This may be frustrating or embarrassing to some girls. The nurse should reassure the client that her breast development is normal, if appropriate.

FOCUSED INTERVIEW QUESTIONS	**RATIONALES**

2. **How do you feel about your breasts and the way they are changing?**

▶ Breast development provides visual confirmation that the pubescent female is becoming a woman. For the developing pubescent female, her breasts are a visible symbol of her feminine identity and an important part of her body image and self-esteem. Girls should be reassured that the rate of growth of breast tissue depends on changing hormone levels and is uniquely individual, as are the eventual size and shape of the breasts. The nurse can reassure males that breast enlargement is generally temporary and in response to hormonal changes.

QUESTIONS FOR THE PREGNANT FEMALE

1. **What changes in your breasts have you noticed since your last examination?**

▶ The breasts continue to change throughout pregnancy. Some expected changes are increased size, sense of fullness or tingling, prominent veins, darkened areolae, and a more erect nipple. A thick, yellowish discharge called colostrum may be expressed from the breasts in the final weeks of pregnancy. The client should be reassured that all of these signs are normal.

QUESTIONS FOR THE OLDER ADULT

All of the preceding questions apply to the menopausal and postmenopausal client.

▶ It is important to obtain information from the older client because the incidence of breast cancer and mortality rates increase with age.

QUESTIONS RELATED TO THE ENVIRONMENT

Environment refers to both internal and external environments. Questions related to the internal environment include all of the previous questions and those associated with internal or physiological responses. Questions regarding the external environment include those related to home, work, or social environments.

INTERNAL ENVIRONMENT

1. **What medications are you presently taking?**

▶ Hormone replacement therapy is associated with an increased risk of cancer. Females taking these drugs need to be monitored very carefully.

2. **How do you feel about your breasts?**

▶ Answers to this question may reveal a body image disturbance, self-esteem disturbance, dysfunctional grieving (in a female who has had a mastectomy), or ineffective breast-feeding (in a lactating female).

3. **How old were you when you started to menstruate?**

▶ Clients with a history of menarche before age 12 are at greater risk for breast cancer.

4. **Do you have children?**
   ● How old were you when they were born?

▶ Females who have never had children or who had their first child after the age of 30 are at greater risk for breast cancer.

5. **Have you gone through menopause?**
   ● If so, at what age?
   ● Were there any residual problems?

▶ Females who undergo menopause after the age of 55 are at greater risk for breast cancer. Postmenopausal weight gain may increase risk of breast cancer. After menopause, decreased estrogen levels may result in decreased firmness of breast tissue. The client should be reassured that this is normal.

FOCUSED INTERVIEW QUESTIONS

6. **Have you been treated with hormone therapy during or since menopause?**

7. **Describe your weight from childhood up until now.**
   - Describe your dietary intake.

EXTERNAL ENVIRONMENT

1. **Have you been exposed to any environmental carcinogens such as benzene or asbestos, or to excessive radiation such as frequent repeated x-rays?**

RATIONALES

▶ Combined hormone replacement therapy places clients at increased risk for breast cancer.

▶ Obesity is considered a predisposing factor in breast cancer.

▶ Such exposures increase the risk of breast cancer.

CLIENT INTERACTION

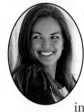

Miranda Cowan, a 22-year-old college student, makes an appointment with her gynecologist for a routine examination. Ms. Cowan indicates she is concerned since breast cancer seems to run in her family. Following is part of the focused interview taken by the nurse working in the office.

INTERVIEW

Nurse: Hello. Ms. Cowan, I see you are here for your routine examination.

Ms. Cowan: Yes, that is correct.

Nurse: Before the physical examination, I need to get some information from you, and I will be asking you questions. You indicated a concern regarding breast cancer in your family. Would you like to begin with your concern?

Ms. Cowan: No. I just don't know where to begin. You ask your questions first. I'm sure we will talk about my concerns.

Nurse: Describe your breasts today.

Ms. Cowan: They are small, firm, and equal in size.

Nurse: Have your breasts changed in the past several months?

Ms. Cowan: No, I think they are the same. Maybe a little fuller before my period but that's it.

Nurse: Describe your nipples and the skin around them.

Ms. Cowan: They are small, equal in size, and stick out a little. The skin around my nipples is round and pink, almost the same color as my nipple.

Nurse: Have you noticed any changes to your nipples or areolae (the skin around the nipples)?

Ms. Cowan: No, no changes.

Nurse: Do you do self-breast examination?

Ms. Cowan: Yes, every month 5 days after my period. You taught me last year and I follow the card from the American Cancer Society.

Nurse: Tell me about your family and breast cancer.

Ms. Cowan: My grandmother (maternal) and my aunt (paternal) both have been diagnosed and it worries me.

Nurse: What about your mother, your older sister, and your maternal aunt?

Ms. Cowan: No, they are fine. No problems.

Nurse: Your grandmother, do you know how old she was when diagnosed?

Ms. Cowan: No I don't. I guess she was in her late 60s. She was diagnosed 3 or 4 years ago and now she is 73 years old. She had surgery and seems to be doing all right.

ANALYSIS

The nurse sets the tone and sequence of events for Ms. Cowan's visit. Ms. Cowan declines the offer from the nurse to begin with her concerns of familial cancer. The nurse knows it will be beneficial to reduce any anxiety the client may have regarding her concern. Taking the lead from Ms. Cowan, the nurse proceeds with the focused interview using open-ended statements and introduces the family questions later in the interview.

Please refer to the Companion Website at **www.prenhall.com/damico** and click on Chapter 16, the **Client Interaction** module, to answer questions about this case. In addition, see other resources for this chapter including NCLEX-RN® review questions and other interactive exercises and materials.

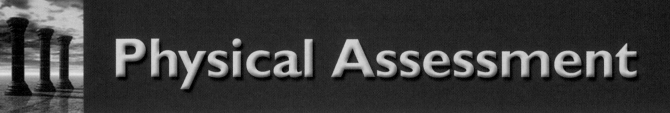

Physical Assessment

ASSESSMENT TECHNIQUES AND FINDINGS

Physical assessment of the breasts and axillae requires the use of inspection and palpation. During each of the procedures, the nurse is gathering data related to the breasts and axillae. Inspection includes looking at skin color, structures of the breast, and the appearance of the axillae. Knowledge of norms or expected findings is essential in determining the meaning of the data.

Adult breasts are generally symmetrical, although one breast is typically slightly larger than the other. The areolae should be round or oval and nearly equal in size. The nipples are the same color as the areolae. The nipples are in the center of the breast, point outward and upward, and are free of discharge, ulcerations, and crust. The breasts should move away from the chest wall with ease and symmetrically. The texture of the skin is smooth and the breast tissue is slightly granular. The axillae are clean and hair is present or removed. The skin is moist. Lymph nodes are nonpalpable.

Physical assessment of the breasts and axillae follows an organized pattern. It begins with a client survey followed by inspection of the breasts while the client assumes a variety of positions. Palpation includes the entire surface of each breast including the tail of Spence, and the lymph nodes of the axillae.

EQUIPMENT

examination gown and drape
clean, nonsterile examination gloves
small pillow or rolled towel
metric ruler

HELPFUL HINTS

- Provide an environment that is warm, comfortable, and private to relieve client anxiety.
- Provide specific instructions to the client; state whether the client must sit, stand, or lie down during a procedure.
- Exposure of the breasts is uncomfortable for many females. Use draping techniques to maintain the client's dignity.
- Explore cultural and language barriers at the onset of the interaction.
- In many Hispanic cultures, touching of the breasts is considered inappropriate. Explain the reasons for the examination and provide education about self breast examination.
- Nonsterile examination gloves may be required to prevent infection when clients have lesions or drainage in and around the breasts.
- Use Standard Precautions.

TECHNIQUES AND NORMAL FINDINGS	ABNORMAL FINDINGS SPECIAL CONSIDERATIONS

INSPECTION OF THE BREAST

1. **Instruct the client.**
   - Explain to the client that you will be examining her breasts in a variety of ways. First, you will have the client sit and then assume several positions that move the breasts away from the chest wall so that differences in size, shape, symmetry, contour, and color can be detected. Inform the client that she will then lie down and you will examine each breast by palpating the breast tissue and nipple. Also be sure to examine her axillae. Explain the purpose of each examination in terms the client will understand. Tell the client that none of the examinations should be painful; however, she must inform you of any tenderness or discomfort as the examination proceeds.

2. **Position the client.**
   - The client should sit comfortably and erect, with the gown at the waist so both breasts are exposed (see Figure 16.8 ●).

| **TECHNIQUES AND NORMAL FINDINGS** | **ABNORMAL FINDINGS SPECIAL CONSIDERATIONS** |

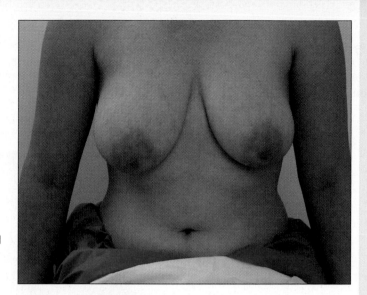

Figure 16.8 ●
The client is seated at the beginning of the breast examination.

3. Inspect and compare size and symmetry of the breasts.

  ● One breast may normally be slightly larger than the other.

▶ Obvious masses, flattening of the breast in one area, dimpling, or recent increase in the size of one breast may indicate abnormal growth or inflammation.

4. Inspect for skin color.

  ● Color should be consistent with the rest of the body. Observe for thickening, tautness, redness, rash, or ulceration.

▶ Inflamed skin is red and warm. Edema from blocked lymphatic drainage in advanced cancer causes an "orange peel" appearance called **peau d'orange** (see Figure 16.9 ●).

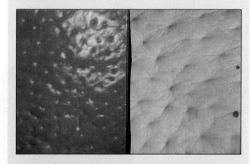

Figure 16.9 ● Left, Orange peel; Right, Peau d'orange sign.

5. Inspect for venous patterns.

  ● Venous patterns are the same bilaterally. Venous patterns may be more predominant in pregnancy or obesity.

▶ Pronounced unilateral venous patterns may indicate increased blood flow to a malignancy.

6. Inspect for moles or other markings.

  ● Moles that are unchanged, nontender, and long-standing are of no concern. Striae that are present in pregnancy or recent weight loss or gain may appear purple in color. Striae become silvery white over time.

▶ Moles that have changed or appear suddenly require further evaluation. A mole along the milk line may be a supernumerary nipple (see Figure 16.5).

7. Inspect the areolae.

  ● The areolae are normally round or oval and almost equal in size. Areolae are pink in light-skinned people and brown in dark-skinned people. The areolae darken in pregnancy.

▶ Peau d'orange associated with cancer may be first seen on the areolae.
    Redness and fissures may develop with breast-feeding.

TECHNIQUES AND NORMAL FINDINGS

8. **Inspect the nipples.**

- Nipples are normally the same color as the areolae and are equal in size and shape. Nipples are generally everted but may be flat or inverted. Nipples should point in the same direction outward and slightly upward. Nipples should be free of cracks, crust, erosions, ulcerations, pigment changes, or discharge.

▶ Recent retraction or inversion of a nipple or change in the direction of the nipple is suggestive of malignancy. Discharge requires cytologic examination. A red, scaly eczema-like area over the nipple could indicate Paget's disease, a rare type of breast cancer. The area may exude fluid, scale, or crust (see Figure 16.10 ●).

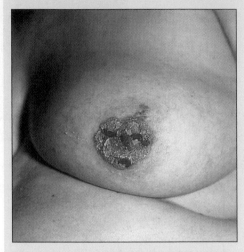

Figure 16.10 ●   Paget's disease of the nipple.

9. **Observe the breasts for shape, surface characteristics, and bilateral pull of suspensory ligaments.**

- Ask the client to assume the following positions while you continue to inspect the breasts.

10. **Inspect with the client's arms over the head (see Figure 16.11 ●).**

▶ Dimpling of the skin over a mass is usually a visible sign of breast cancer. Dimpling is accentuated in this position. Variations in contour and symmetry may also indicate breast cancer.

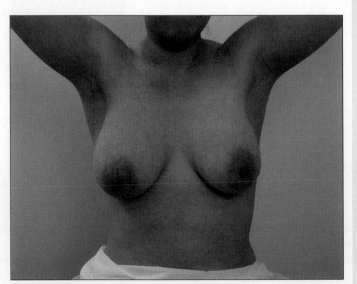

Figure 16.11 ●
Inspection of the breasts with the client's arms above her head.

TECHNIQUES AND NORMAL FINDINGS	ABNORMAL FINDINGS SPECIAL CONSIDERATIONS

11. **Inspect with the client's hands pressed against her waist (see Figure 16.12 ●).**

▶ Tightening of the pectoral muscles may help to accentuate dimpling.

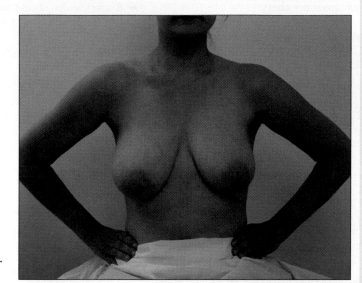

Figure 16.12 ●
Inspection of the breasts with the client's hands pressed against her waist.

12. **Inspect with the client's hands pressed together at the level of the waist (see Figure 16.13 ●).**

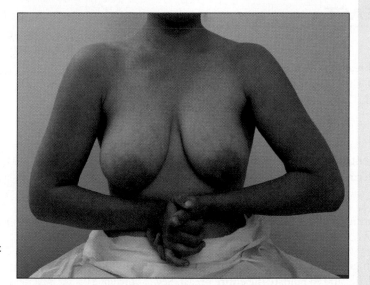

Figure 16.13 ●
Inspection of the breasts with the client's hands pressed together at the level of her waist.

TECHNIQUES AND NORMAL FINDINGS	ABNORMAL FINDINGS SPECIAL CONSIDERATIONS

13. Inspect with the client leaning forward from the waist (see Figure 16.14 ●).

- The breasts normally fall freely and evenly from the chest.

▶ Breast cancer should be suspected if the breasts do not fall freely from the chest.

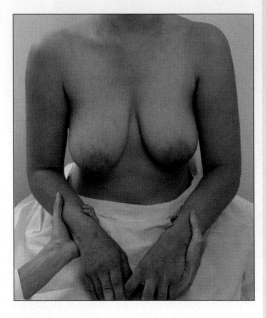

Figure 16.14 ●
Assisting the client to lean forward for inspection.

PALPATION OF THE BREAST

1. Position the client.

- Ask the client to lie down. Cover the breast that is not being examined. Place a small pillow or rolled towel under the shoulder of the side to be palpated and position the client's arm over her head. This maneuver flattens the breast tissue over the chest wall.

2. Instruct the client.

- Explain that you will be touching the entire breast and nipple. Tell the client to inform you of any discomfort or tenderness.

3. Palpate skin texture.

- Skin texture should be smooth with uninterrupted contour.

▶ Thickening of the skin suggests an underlying carcinoma.

4. Palpate the breast.

- Use the finger pads of the first three fingers in a slightly rotary motion to press the breast tissue against the chest wall. Be sure to palpate the entire breast. Several patterns may be used, but the most common is the concentric circle pattern (see Figure 16.15 ●).

▶ The incidence of breast cancers is highest in the upper outer quadrant, including the axillary tail of Spence. Masses in the tail must be distinguished from enlarged lymph nodes.

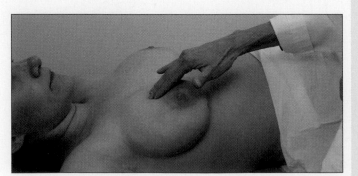

Figure 16.15 ●
Palpating the breast.

TECHNIQUES AND NORMAL FINDINGS	ABNORMAL FINDINGS SPECIAL CONSIDERATIONS

- Start at the periphery of the breast and palpate in to small circles until you reach the nipple. Try not to lift the finger pads off the breast as you move from one area to another.
- An alternative pattern used during palpation is the back and forth technique (see Figure 16.16 ●).

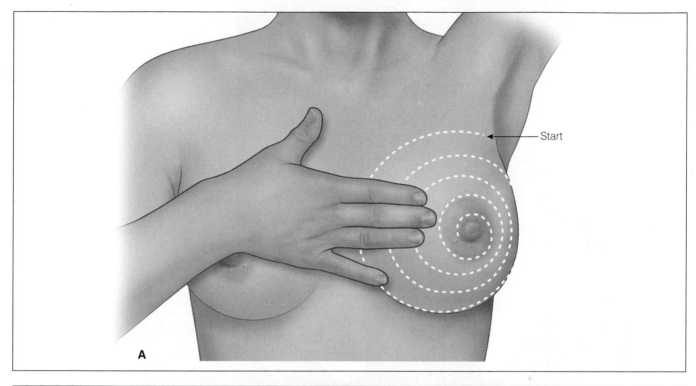

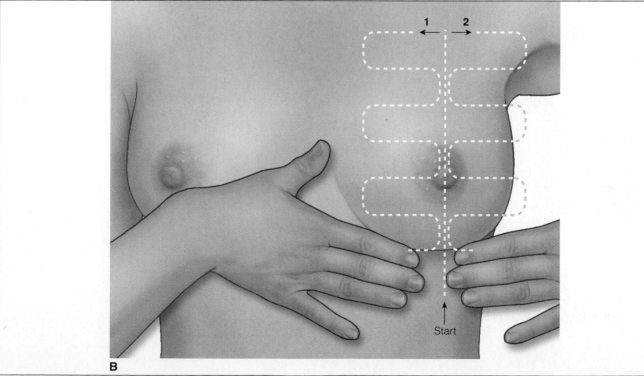

Figure 16.16 ● Alternative patterns for palpation. A. Concentric circles. B. Back and forth technique.

TECHNIQUES AND NORMAL FINDINGS

- In female clients with pendulous breasts, palpate with one hand under the breast to support it and the other hand pushing against breast tissue in a downward motion (see Figure 16.17 ●).

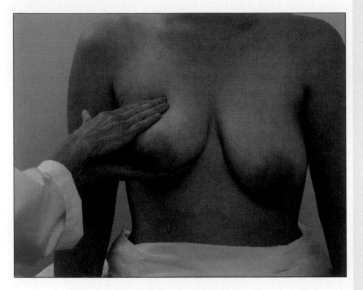

Figure 16.17 ●
Palpating a
pendulous breast.

- Palpation then continues into the tail of Spence (see Figure 16.18 ●).

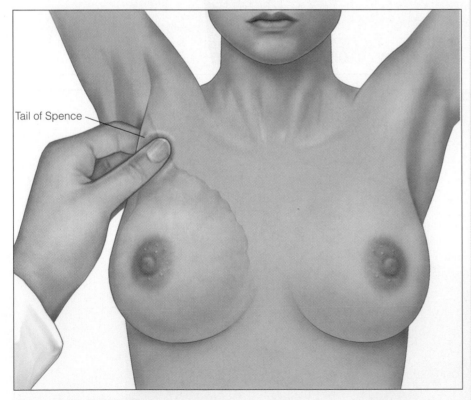

Tail of Spence

Figure 16.18 ● Palpating the tail of Spence.

TECHNIQUES AND NORMAL FINDINGS	ABNORMAL FINDINGS SPECIAL CONSIDERATIONS

5. Palpate the nipple and areolae.

- Compress the tissue between the thumb and forefinger (see Figure 16.19 ●) to observe for drainage. Confirm that the nipple is free of discharge, that it is nontender, and that the areola is free of masses.

- Repeat steps 1 through 5 on the other breast.

▶ Lactation not associated with childbearing is called **galactorrhea.** It occurs most commonly with endocrine disorders or medications including some antidepressants and antihypertensives.

  Unilateral discharge from the nipple is suggestive of benign breast disease, an intraductal papilloma, or cancer.

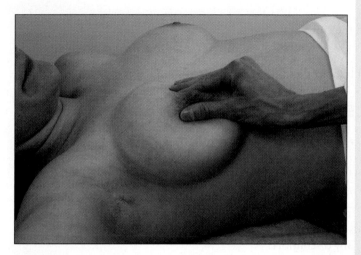

Figure 16.19 ●
Palpating the nipple.

EXAMINATION OF THE AXILLAE

1. Instruct the client.

- Explain that you will be examining the axillae by looking and palpating. Tell the client that she will sit for this examination and you will support the arm while palpating with the other hand. Explain that relaxation will make the examination more comfortable. Tell the client to inform you of any discomfort.

2. Position the client.

- Ask the client or assist the client to assume a sitting position. Flex the arm at the elbow and support it on your arm. Note the presence of axillary hair. Confirm that the axilla is free of redness, rashes, lumps, or lesions. With the palmar surface of your fingers, reach deep into the axilla (see Figure 16.20 ●). Gently palpate the anterior border of the axilla (anterior or subpectoral nodes), the central aspect along the rib cage (central nodes), the posterior border (subscapular/posterior nodes), and along the inner aspect of the upper arm (lateral nodes).

▶ Infections of the breast, arm, and hand cause enlargement and tenderness of the axillary lymph nodes. Hard, fixed nodes are suggestive of cancer or lymphoma. Clients who have had a wide local excision (removal of tumor and narrow margin of normal tissue) or mastectomy (removal of tumor and extensive areas of surrounding tissue) need to be examined carefully. The remaining tissue on the chest wall should be palpated as it would be for nonsurgical clients.

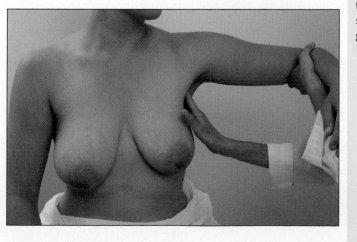

Figure 16.20 ●
Palpating the axilla. Note that the nurse is supporting the woman's arm with her own nondominant arm.

TECHNIQUES AND NORMAL FINDINGS	ABNORMAL FINDINGS SPECIAL CONSIDERATIONS

INSPECTION OF THE MALE BREAST

1. **Instruct the client.**
   - Explain all aspects of the procedure and the purpose for each part of the examination.

2. **Position the client.**
   - The client is in the sitting position with the gown at the waist.

3. **Inspect the male breasts.**
   - Observe that breasts are flat and free of lumps or lesions.

PALPATION OF THE MALE BREAST AND AXILLAE

1. **Position the client.**
   - Place the client in a supine position.

2. **Instruct the client.**
   - Explain that you will be using the pads of your fingers to gently palpate the breast area. Instruct the client to report any discomfort.

3. **Palpate the male breasts.**
   - Using the finger pads of the first three fingers, gently palpate the breast tissue, using concentric circles until you reach the nipple. The male breast feels like a thin disk of tissue under a flat nipple and areola (see Figure 16.21 ●).

▶ Gynecomastia (breast enlargement in males) is a temporary condition seen in infants, at puberty, and in older males. In older males it may accompany hormonal treatment for prostate cancer. Breast cancer in the male is usually identified as a hard nodule fixed to the nipple and underlying tissue. Nipple discharge may be present.

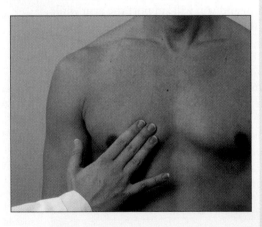

Figure 16.21 ●
Palpation of the male breast.

4. **Palpate the nipple.**
   - Compress the nipple between your thumb and forefinger.
   - The nipple should be free of discharge.

5. **Repeat on the other breast.**

6. **Palpate the axillae.**
   - Palpate axillary nodes in the male as you would for the female.

Refer to the Companion Website at **www.prenhall.com/damico** and click on the **Documentation** module for documentation samples and documentation practice exercises.

*S*ome of the problems identified during the physical assessment are entirely within the realm of nursing and are addressed with appropriate nursing interventions. Some problems, however, require collaborative management. Benign breast disease, fibroadenoma, intraductal papilloma, mammary duct ectasia, and breast cancer are the most common breast conditions that will challenge the nurse and the rest of the healthcare team. These common abnormalities are discussed in this section.

Benign Breast Disease

One of the most common benign breast problems is benign breast disease (also called fibrocystic breast disease). It is typically first seen in females in their 20s and is characterized by lumps, breast pain or tenderness, and nipple discharge. These symptoms are a result of *fibrosis,* a thickening of the normal breast tissue, which may be accompanied by cyst formation. Usually located in the upper outer quadrant, the cysts probably are a result of fluctuating hormones in the body that cause excessive cell growth in the ducts and lobules and inhibit the draining of normal secretions. The breasts usually become painful just prior to the onset of menses, and pain resolves at the end of menstruation. Upon palpation, the masses feel soft, well demarcated, and freely movable; they are almost always bilateral (see Figure 16.22 ●). Discharge from the nipples may be clear, straw colored, milky, or green. This is a disease of the reproductive years, and symptoms usually resolve after menopause because of a lack of estrogen.

Benign breast disease is not usually clinically significant, and there is no direct link between fibrocystic tissue changes and the incidence of cancer. In some cases, however, it may result in ductal hyperplasia and dysplasia, which may eventually develop into noninvasive intraductal, lobular, or intraepithelial carcinoma. This can be a potential focus for invasive carcinoma. Additionally, the presence of nodular tissue in the breast makes the early detection of malignant nodules more challenging. The physician monitors fibrocystic breast disease through periodic mammography and determines if an aspiration or biopsy is necessary.

Pharmacologic hormones and diuretics may be used in the medical management to relieve symptoms. Some studies suggest that limiting caffeine may help relieve symptoms, but the evidence is inconclusive. The nurse might suggest that the female client try eliminating caffeine, especially in the premenstrual period, and determine for herself if this action brings relief. The nurse may also suggest decreasing salt intake and taking mild analgesics. Wearing a supportive bra decreases discomfort. The nurse reinforces the need for regular SBE as well as regular mammography and physical examination.

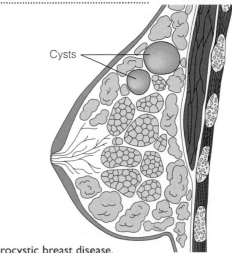

Cysts

Figure 16.22 ● Fibrocystic breast disease.

Fibroadenoma

Fibroadenoma is a common benign tumor of the glandular tissue of the breast. It is most common in females in their teens and early 20s. Its development in adolescents appears to be linked to breast hypertrophy, which may occur during the growth spurt of puberty. Fibroadenomas are well-defined, round, firm tumors, about 1 to 5 cm in diameter, which can be moved freely within the breast tissue (see Figure 16.23 ●). They usually occur as a single tumor near the nipple or in the upper outer quadrant. Because they are asymptomatic, they are often not discovered until SBE or examination by a physician. Careful observation over time is the usual treatment. Biopsy or excision of the lump, performed on an outpatient basis, is indicated if the findings are inconclusive. No relationship has been established between fibroadenomas and malignant neoplasms.

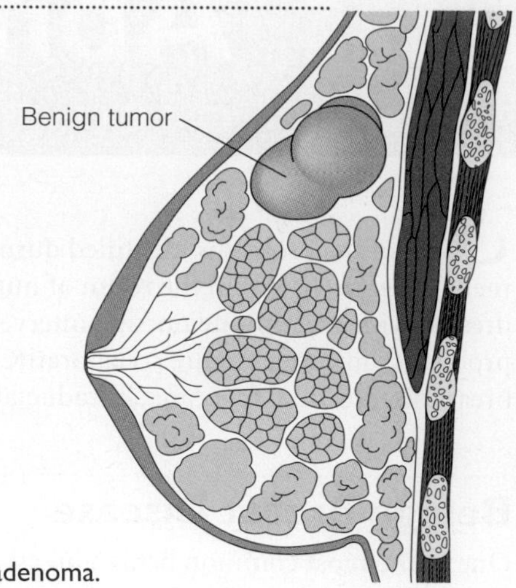

Benign tumor

Figure 16.23 ● Fibroadenoma.

Intraductal Papilloma

Intraductal papillomas (see Figure 16.24 ●) are tiny growths of epithelial cells that project into the lumen of the lactiferous ducts. These growths are fragile, and even minimal trauma causes leakage of blood or serum into the involved duct and subsequent discharge. Intraductal papillomas are the primary cause of nipple discharge in females who are not pregnant or lactating. They are more commonly found in menopausal females but may occur at any age.

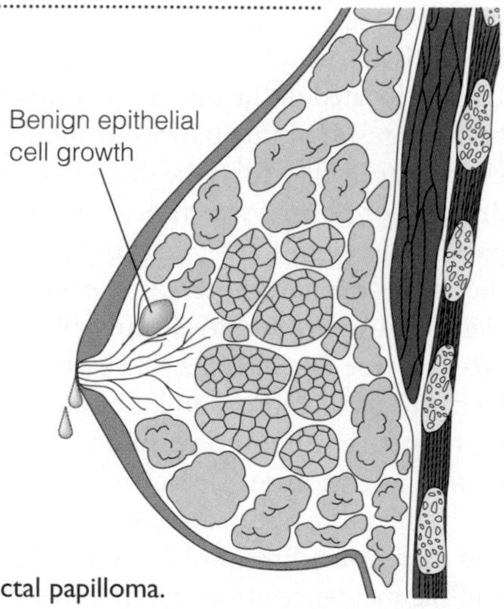

Benign epithelial cell growth

Figure 16.24 ● Intraductal papilloma.

Mammary Duct Ectasia

Mammary duct ectasia (see Figure 16.25 ●) is an inflammation of the lactiferous ducts behind the nipple. As cellular debris and fluid collect in the involved ducts, they become enlarged and form a palpable, painful mass. A thick, sticky discharge from the nipple is common. Because there may be some nipple retraction, a careful assessment is required to distinguish the condition from breast cancer. Although the disorder is painful, it is not associated with cancer and usually resolves spontaneously.

Enlarged ducts

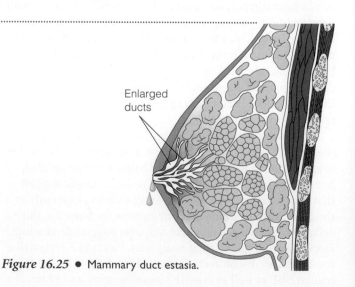

Figure 16.25 ● Mammary duct estasia.

Carcinoma of the Breast

The common signs of carcinoma of the breast (see Figure 16.26 ●) include the following:

- *Dimpling of the skin over the tumor caused by a retraction or pulling inward of breast tissue.* This results primarily from tissue fibrosis. Retraction is also caused by fat necrosis and mammary duct ectasia (described in the previous section).

- *Deviation of the breast or nipple from its normal alignment.* Deviation is also caused by retraction. The nipple typically deviates toward the underlying cancer.

- *Nipple retraction.* The nipple flattens or even turns inward. Retraction is also caused by tissue fibrosis.

- *Irregular shape of one breast as compared to the other, such as a flattening of one quadrant.* Irregularity of shape is also caused by retraction.

- *Edema, which may result in a peau d'orange appearance, especially near the nipple.* Edema is caused by blockage of the lymphatic ducts that normally drain the breast.

- *Discharge, which may be bloody or clear.*

The screening examination and studies for breast cancer are physical examination and mammography. A positive diagnosis of cancer is made by histologic examination following an open or closed (needle) biopsy. The tumor is then staged to determine characteristics of the tumor, nodal involvement, and the presence or absence of distant metastasis. The outcome of this staging determines which protocol is used for treatment. Treatment may consist of surgery, radiation therapy, chemotherapy, or a combination of these modalities.

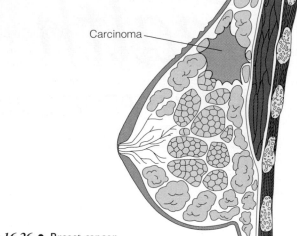

Carcinoma

Figure 16.26 ● Breast cancer.

Abnormalities of the Male Breast

Male breast tissue is similar to that of the female. Therefore, changes in relation to hormone secretion and disease occur. The following sections describe abnormalities in the male breast.

Gynecomastia

Gynecomastia is enlargement of the breast tissue in the male. This can occur at birth in response to maternal hormones. Additionally, at the onset of puberty more than 30% of males have enlargement of one or both breasts in response to hormonal changes. This can be a cause of embarrassment or shame if it occurs before puberty or continues for longer than 18 months. Gynecomastia may also occur in males over 50 due to pituitary or testicular tumors and in males taking estrogenic medication for prostate cancer. Gynecomastia may occur in cirrhosis of the liver and with adrenal and thyroid diseases (see Figure 16.27 ●).

Carcinoma

Male breast cancer is rare. Less than 1% of all breast cancer occurs in men. Predisposing factors include radiation exposure, cirrhosis, and estrogen medications. Increased rates have been seen in males with a familial history of breast cancer in primary female relatives (see Figure 16.28 ●).

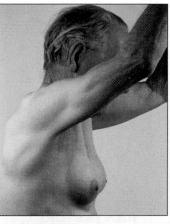

Figure 16.27 ● Gynecomastia.

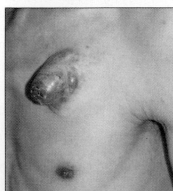

Figure 16.28 ● Carcinoma of the breast.

Health Promotion

HEALTHY PEOPLE 2010

FOCUS AREA	PREVALENCE	OBJECTIVE	ACTIONS
Breast Cancer	• Breast cancer is the most common form of cancer in women in the United States. • Obesity is a risk for postmenopausal women.	• Reduce death rate from breast cancer.	• Education about and promotion of screening for breast cancer. • Weight reduction programs.

CLIENT EDUCATION

The following are physiological, behavioral, and cultural factors that influence breast health across the life span. Several factors reflect trends cited in *Healthy People 2010*. The nurse provides advice and education to reduce risks associated with these factors and to promote and maintain breast health.

LIFE SPAN CONSIDERATIONS

RISK FACTORS

- Cyclic breast pain occurs in young females in association with the onset and continuation of the menstrual cycle.
  Cysts are the most common breast lumps in menstruating females.

- Fibroadenomas are benign lumps found in females in the late teens and early 20s.

- Physiologic nodularity and benign cysts occur in about 30% of females of all ages.

- The risk of breast cancer increases with aging, especially after 35 to 40 years of age.

CLIENT EDUCATION

- Instruct teenage girls to chart breast pain to determine if it is associated with the menstrual cycle.

- Tell teenage and young adult females that healthcare screening is required to diagnose fibroadenomas, which are usually surgically removed.

- Instruct clients that the discomfort associated with physiologic nodularity or cystic breasts may be alleviated with reduction in the ingestion of caffeine, chocolate, saturated fats, and salt. The addition of vitamins E and A to one's diet is recommended by some to reduce symptoms.

- Tell all clients that the recommendations for early detection of breast cancer include monthly SBE in females beginning at age 20, a physical examination of the breast by a healthcare provider every 3 years between the ages of 20 and 39, and mammography and physical examination of the breast by a healthcare provider every year in females over 40. See Box 16.1 for instructions for SBE.

CULTURAL CONSIDERATIONS

RISK FACTORS

- Caucasian females have a higher incidence of breast cancer after age 40 than do females in other racial and ethnic groups.
- Breast cancer is the leading cause of cancer death in Hispanic females.

- Male breast cancer is rare but occurs in men with a familial history of female breast cancer in a primary relative, and in men with radiation exposure, estrogen administration, and cirrhosis.

- Many Hispanic females and females from many immigrant cultures are brought up believing that looking at or touching themselves is prohibited.

CLIENT EDUCATION

- Tell all clients that the recommendations for early detection of breast cancer include monthly SBE in females beginning at age 20, a physical examination of the breast by a healthcare provider every 3 years between the ages of 20 and 39, and mammography and physical examination of the breast by a healthcare provider every year in females over 40. See Box 16.1 for instructions for SBE.

- Advise males with risk factors to have breast examination included as part of routine health examinations.

- Advise and encourage female clients who have uneasiness with touching their breasts to perform SBE and to seek care regularly for breast examination.

ENVIRONMENTAL CONSIDERATIONS

RISK FACTORS

- There is a genetic predisposition to breast cancer in approximately 10% of females in Western countries, and there is a higher incidence of breast cancer in Western countries, especially in North America.

- The risk of breast cancer is increased in females with a familial history, in those who have not had children, in females who use combined estrogen and progesterone or hormone replacement therapy, in females who use alcohol, and in obese females and those with a high-fat diet.

- Low income contributes to a lack of screening for breast disease.

CLIENT EDUCATION

- Tell all clients that the recommendations for early detection of breast cancer include monthly SBE in females beginning at age 20, a physical examination of the breast by a healthcare provider every 3 years between the ages of 20 and 39, and mammography and physical examination of the breast by a healthcare provider every year in females over 40. See Box 16.1 for instructions for SBE.

- Refer clients to the American Cancer Society or link to the breast cancer education website through the Companion Website.

- Tell all clients that the recommendations for early detection of breast cancer include monthly SBE in females beginning at age 20, a physical examination of the breast by a healthcare provider every 3 years between the ages of 20 and 39, and mammography and physical examination of the breast by a healthcare provider every year in females over 40. See Box 16.1 for instructions for SBE.

- Inform uninsured female clients of low-cost breast cancer screening available through the National Breast and Cervical Cancer Early Detection Program (NBCCEDP).

Box 16.1   **Teaching Self-Breast Examination (SBE)**

1. Teach the client to observe her breasts in front of a mirror and in good lighting. Tell her to observe her breasts in four positions:
   - With her arms relaxed and at her sides
   - With her arms lifted over her head
   - With her hands pressed against her hips
   - With her hands pressed together at the waist, leaning forward

   Instruct her to look at each breast individually, and then to compare them. She should observe for any visible abnormalities, such as lumps, dimpling, deviation, recent nipple retraction, irregular shape, edema, discharge, or asymmetry.

2. Teach the client to palpate both breasts while standing or sitting, with one hand behind her head (see Figure 16.29A ●). Tell her that many women palpate their breasts in the shower because water and soap make the skin slippery and easier to palpate. Show the client how to use the pads of her fingers to palpate all areas of her breast, using the concentric circles technique (see Figure 16.29B ●). Tell her to press the breast tissue gently against the chest wall and to be sure to palpate the axillary tail.

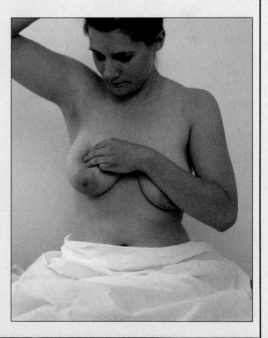

Figure 16.29A ● Self-breast examination. A. The female palpates her breasts while standing or sitting upright.

(continued)

Box 16.1 | **Teaching Self-Breast Examination (SBE)** *(continued)*

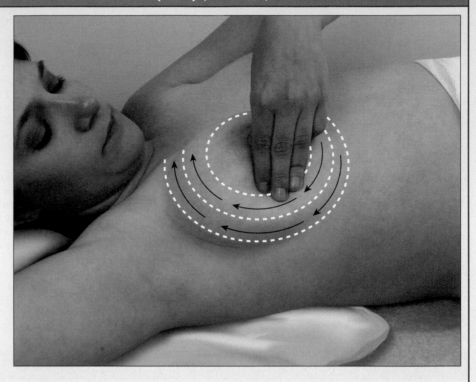

Figure 16.29B • Self-breast examination. B. The concentric circles approach.

3. Instruct the client to palpate her breasts again while lying down, as described in step 2. Suggest that she place a folded towel under the shoulder and back on the side to be palpated. The arm on the examining side should be over her head, with the hand under the head (see Figure 16.29C ●).
4. Teach the client to palpate the areolae and nipples next. Show her how to compress the nipple to check for discharge (see Figure 16.29D ●).

5. Remind the client to use a calendar to keep a record of when she performs SBE. Teach her to perform SBE at the same time each month, usually 5 days after the onset of menses, when there is less hormonal influence on tissues.
6. Remind clients who are postmenopausal to continue monthly SBE. They should perform the exam at the same time each month.

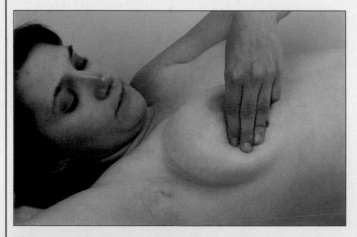

Figure 16.29C • Self-breast examination. C. The female client palpates her breasts while lying down.

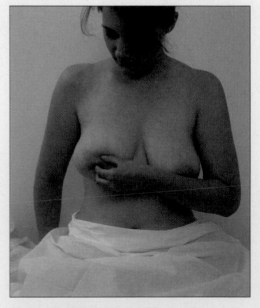

Figure 16.29D • Self-breast examination. D. The woman palpates her nipples.

Application Through Critical Thinking

CASE STUDY

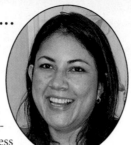

*T*he following information was gathered during a comprehensive health assessment of Carol Jenkins, a 29-year-old female.

The client stated that she has had breast tenderness associated with her periods for most of her adult life. The tenderness has increased over the past several months. Her breasts seem swollen and heavy, and what used to hurt in the outer portion of the breast has changed to discomfort all over. The physical examination revealed round, tender, mobile masses with smooth borders in all quadrants. The nipples are everted, round, and free of lesions. The breasts are symmetrical in shape and contour.

▶ Complete Documentation

The following is sample documentation for Carol Jenkins.

SUBJECTIVE DATA: Breast tenderness "with periods" for most of her adult life. Tenderness increasing over past several months. Breasts seem "swollen and heavy." Discomfort in outer breast now "discomfort all over."

OBJECTIVE DATA: Round, mobile masses with smooth borders in all quadrants bilaterally. Nipples everted, round, free of lesions. Breasts symmetrical in shape and contour.

ASSESSMENT FORM

REASON FOR VISIT
Increasing breast tenderness over past several months.

Findings

Breasts: Symmetrical shape, contour

Nipples: Round, everted, no lesions

Palpation: Round mobile masses, smooth borders—all
quadrants

▶ Critical Thinking Questions

1. What is most likely the cause of the client's symptoms?
2. Identify several differential diagnoses.
3. What information is required to validate the diagnoses?
4. What recommendations should the nurse make for this client?

▶ Applying Nursing Diagnoses

1. *Pain (chronic)* is a nursing diagnosis in the NANDA taxonomy. Do the data for Carol Jenkins support this diagnosis? If so, provide supporting data.
2. Identify additional nursing diagnoses from the NANDA taxonomy (see Appendix A ⚭) for Carol Jenkins. Identify the data that support the PES (problem, etiology, signs or symptoms) statements.

▶ Prepare Teaching Plan

LEARNING NEED: The data from the case study reveal that Carol Jenkins is concerned about her breast discomfort. Her symptoms indicate benign (fibrocystic) breast disease. Education about this disorder and methods to monitor breast health will be provided to this client.

The case study provides data that is representative of concerns about breast disease, especially cancer, of many individuals. Therefore, the following teaching plan is based on the need to provide information to members of any community about measures to detect breast cancer.

GOAL: The participants in this learning program will have increased awareness of recommendations for screening for breast cancer.

OBJECTIVES: At the completion of this learning session, the participants will be able to:

1. Identify the recommended schedule for breast cancer screening.
2. Describe methods for breast cancer screening.

APPLICATION OF OBJECTIVE 1: Identify the recommended schedule for breast cancer screening

Content	Teaching Strategy	Evaluation
• Self-breast examination (SBE) once a month from age 20. • Clinical examination by nurse or physician every 3 years between the ages of 20 and 40. Over 50 years of age, annual clinical examination. • Mammography first at age 40. Ages 40 to 49 mammography every 1 to 2 years. Annual mammogram after 50.	• Lecture • Discussion • Audiovisual materials • Printed materials Lecture is appropriate when disseminating information to large groups. Discussion allows participants to bring up concerns and to raise questions. Audiovisual materials such as illustrations of the breast and techniques reinforce verbal presentation. Printed material, especially to be taken away with learners, allows review, reinforcement, and reading at the learner's pace.	• Written examination. May use short answer, fill-in, or multiple-choice items, or a combination of items. If these are short and easy to evaluate, the learner receives immediate feedback.

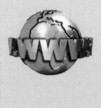

Please refer to the Companion Website at www.prenhall.com/damico and click on Chapter 16, the Application Through Critical Thinking module, to complete the following activities related to this case study:
► **Critical Thinking questions**
► **Extended Nursing Diagnosis challenge**
► **Documentation activity**
► **Teaching Plan for Objective 2**

EXPLORE MediaLink

Additional resources for this chapter are found on the Student CD-ROM accompanying this textbook and on the Companion Website.

CD-ROM CONTENT

Content for this chapter includes:
Objectives
Key Concepts
NCLEX-RN® Review Questions
Model Documentation Forms
Audio Glossary
Games and Challenges
Clinical Spotlight Videos
   Breast Self-examination
   Breast Cancer
Head-to-Toe Physical Examination Video

COMPANION WEBSITE CONTENT

www.prenhall.com/damico

Content for this chapter includes:
Objectives
NCLEX-RN® Review Questions

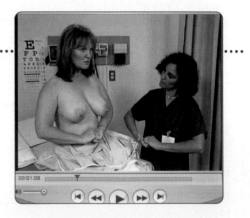

Client Interaction Case Study Challenge
Application Through Critical Thinking
   Case Study Teaching Plan Challenge
MediaLinks
MediaLink Application
Tool Box
   Documentation Form Example
   Health Promotion
      Healthy People 2010
      Client Education
   Health Promotion—Teaching Self-Breast Examination
New York Times

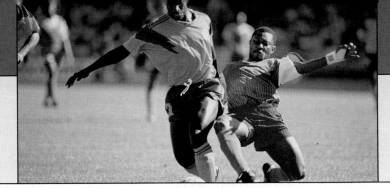

17

Cardiovascular System

MEDIALINK

www.prenhall.com/damico

The CD-ROM in the back of this textbook and the Media-Link website contain NCLEX-RN® review questions, interactive exercises, case study challenges, animations, videos, documentation and checklist forms, and review materials. For a complete listing of the media content specific to Chapter 17, see the Explore MediaLink at the end of the chapter.

The cardiovascular system circulates blood continuously throughout the body to deliver oxygen and nutrients to the body's organs and tissues and to dispose of their excreted wastes. The health of the cardiovascular system may be promoted throughout the life span by means of self-care habits such as eating a low-fat diet, exercising, and not smoking. Still, the delicate balance of this system is vulnerable to stress, trauma, and a variety of pathologic mechanisms that may impair its ability to function. Inadequate tissue perfusion results in both a diminished supply of nutrients necessary for metabolic functions and a buildup of metabolic wastes.

To perform an accurate cardiovascular assessment, a solid understanding of cardiovascular anatomy and physiology, reviewed in the next section, is necessary. By asking appropriate questions during the focused interview, the nurse uncovers clues to the client's health status and any cardiovascular problems. Assessment of the client's psychosocial health, self-care habits, family, culture, and environment is a major part of the focused interview. It is important to keep these findings in mind while conducting the physical assessment and to recognize that the health of the cardiovascular system affects and is affected by the health of all other body systems.

During the physical assessment, the nurse assesses and evaluates the sometimes ambiguous cues of actual and potential cardiac disease. A plan of collaborative or independent nursing care is then developed. Finally, the nurse plays a key role in teaching the healthy client the facts about preventing cardiovascular disease. For the client with cardiovascular disease, the nurse provides teaching to promote optimum health according to the client's individual needs. These actions by the nurse are consistent with the goals in the *Healthy People 2010* feature. The improvement of cardiovascular health that are described in the *Healthy People 2010* feature on page 471 with prevention, early diagnosis, and the reduction of risk factors is imperative.

ANATOMY AND PHYSIOLOGY REVIEW

The cardiovascular system is composed of the heart and the vascular system. The heart includes the cardiac muscle, atria, ventricles, valves, coronary arteries, cardiac veins, electrical conducting structures, and cardiac nerves. The vascular system is composed of the blood vessels of the body: the arteries, arterioles, veins, venules, and capillaries. In this chapter, only the coronary blood vessels are considered in detail. The peripheral vascular system is discussed in Chapter 18. ⊙⊙ The major functions of the cardiovascular system are transporting nutrients and oxygen to the body, removing wastes and carbon dioxide, and maintaining adequate perfusion of organs and tissues.

PERICARDIUM

The **pericardium** is a thin sac composed of a fibroserous material that surrounds the heart (see Figure 17.1 ●). Its tougher outer layer, called the *fibrous pericardium*, protects the heart and anchors it to the adjacent structures such as the diaphragm and great vessels. The inner layer is called the *serous pericardium*. The pericardium is also composed of two layers: parietal and visceral. The parietal layer is the outer layer. The **visceral layer of pericardium** is the inner layer, which lines the surface of the heart. Fluid between the fibrous and serous pericardium lubricates the layers and allows for a gliding motion between them with each heartbeat.

HEART

The **heart** is an intricately designed pump composed of a meticulous network of synchronized structures. It lies behind the sternum and typically extends from the second rib to the fifth intercostal space (see Figure 17.2 ●). The heart sits obliquely within the thoracic cavity between the lungs and above the diaphragm in an area called the **mediastinal space.** Ventrally, the right side of the heart is more forward than the left. The heartbeat is most easily palpated over the apex; thus, this point is referred to as the point of maximum impulse (PMI).

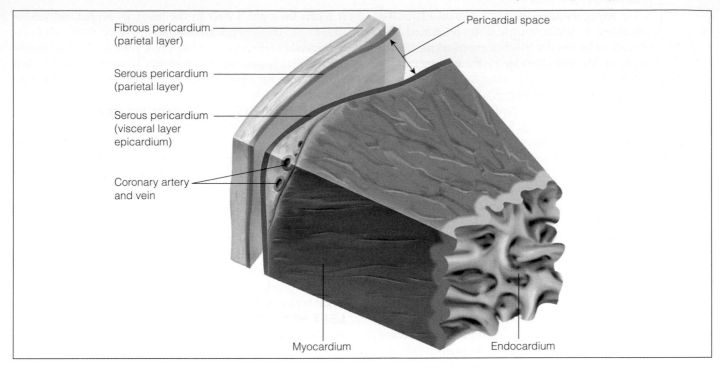

Figure 17.1 ● Layers of the heart.

The heart is approximately 12.8 cm (5 in.) long, 9 cm (3.5 in.) across, and 6.4 cm (2.5 in.) thick. It is slightly larger than the client's clenched fist. The heart of the female typically is smaller and weighs less than the heart of the male.

Heart Wall

The heart wall is composed of three layers: epicardium, myocardium, and endocardium (Figure 17.1). The outer layer, called the **epicardium,** is anatomically identical to the visceral

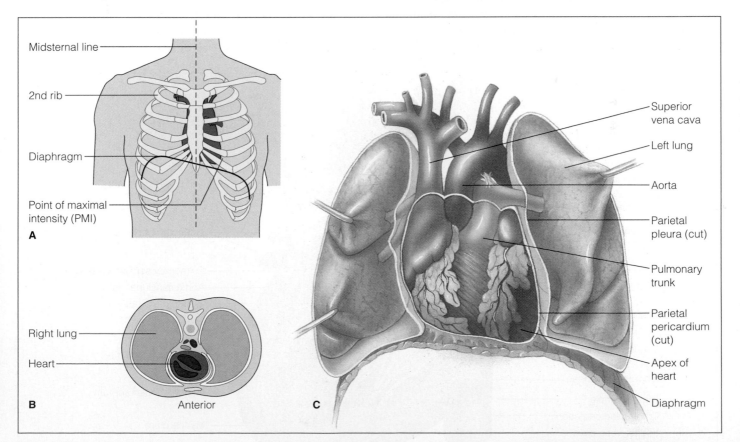

Figure 17.2 ● Location of the heart in the mediastinum of the thorax. A. Relationship of the heart to the sternum, ribs, and diaphragm. B. Cross-sectional view showing relative position of the heart in the thorax. C. Relationship of the heart and great vessels to the lungs.

pericardium. The **myocardium** is the thick, muscular layer. It is made up of bundles of cardiac muscle fibers reinforced by a branching network of connective tissue fibers called the fibrous skeleton of the heart. The innermost layer is the **endocardium,** a smooth layer that provides an inner lining for the chambers of the heart. The endocardium is continuous with the linings of the blood vessels that enter and leave the cardiac chambers.

Cardiac muscle is quite different from skeletal muscle. The muscle cells are shorter, interconnected, branched structures. Mitochondria, the cell's energy-producing organelles, compose about 25% of cardiac muscle fibers versus only about 2% of skeletal muscle fibers. This higher ratio is related to the much higher energy requirements of cardiac muscle. Unlike the independently functioning fibers of skeletal muscle, the fibers of cardiac muscle are interconnected by special junctions that provide for the conduction of impulses across the entire myocardium. This property allows the heart to contract as a single unit.

Heart Chambers

The heart is composed of four chambers: two smaller, superior chambers called atria, and two larger, inferior chambers called ventricles (see Figure 17.3 ●). One atrium is located on the right side of the heart and one on the left side. These serve as receiving chambers for blood returning to the heart from the major blood vessels of the body. The atria then pump the blood into the right and left ventricles, which lie directly below them. The ventricles also are located on each side of the heart. They eject blood into the vessels leaving the heart. A longitudinal partition separates the heart chambers. The *interatrial septum* separates the two atria, and the *interventricular septum* divides the ventricles.

RIGHT ATRIUM. The **right atrium** is a thin-walled chamber located above and slightly to the right of the right ventricle.

It forms the right border of the heart. Deoxygenated venous blood from the systemic circulation enters the right atrium via the inferior and superior venae cavae (two main structures of the venous system), and the coronary sinus. The blood is then ejected from the right atrium through the tricuspid valve into the right ventricle.

RIGHT VENTRICLE. The **right ventricle** is formed triangularly and comprises much of the anterior or sternocostal surface of the heart. After receiving deoxygenated blood from the right atrium, the right ventricle ejects it through the trunk of the pulmonary arteries so that the blood may be oxygenated within the lungs. Its wall is much thinner than that of the left ventricle, reflecting the relative low vascular pressure in the vessels of the lungs.

LEFT ATRIUM. The **left atrium** forms the posterior aspect of the heart. Its muscular structure is slightly thicker than that of the right atrium. It receives oxygenated blood from the pulmonary vasculature via the pulmonary veins. From here, the blood is pumped into the left ventricle.

LEFT VENTRICLE. The **left ventricle** is located behind the right ventricle and forms the left border of the heart. The left ventricle, which is egg shaped, is the most muscular chamber of the heart. The thick wall of ventricular muscle permits the pumping of blood into the aorta against high systemic vascular resistance. This causes the left ventricle to develop more mass than the right ventricle. The left ventricle of a female has about 10% less mass compared to that of a male.

VALVES

The valves of the heart are structures through which blood is ejected either from one chamber to another or from a chamber into a blood vessel. The flow of blood in a healthy individual

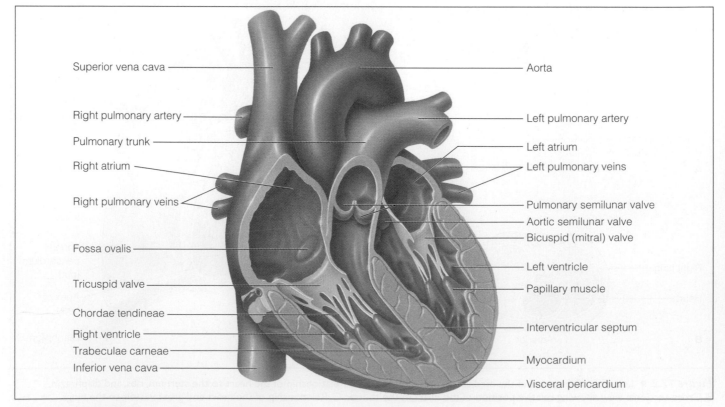

Figure 17.3 ● Structural components of the heart.

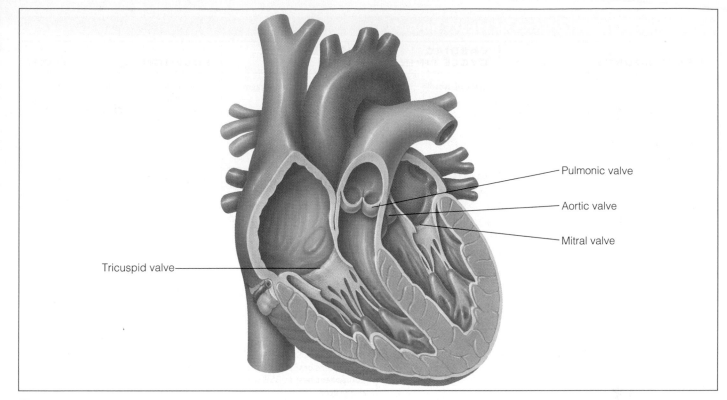

Figure 17.4 • Valves of the heart.

with competent valves is mostly unidirectional. When valves are diseased, forward blood flow is restricted, resulting in regurgitation (backflow) of blood into the chambers of the heart. The regurgitation is assessed as murmurs. Valves are classified by their location as either atrioventricular or semilunar.

Atrioventricular Valves

The **atrioventricular (AV) valves** separate the atria from the ventricles. The tricuspid valve lies between the right atrium and the right ventricle, whereas the thicker mitral (bicuspid) valve lies between the left atrium and left ventricle.

The AV valves open as a direct result of atrial contraction and the concomitant buildup of pressure within the atria. This pressure forces the valvular leaflets to open. When the ventricles contract, the increased ventricular pressure forces the valvular leaflets shut, thus preventing the blood from flowing back into the atria.

Semilunar Valves

The **semilunar valves** separate the ventricles from the vascular system. The pulmonary semilunar valve separates the right ventricle from the trunk of the pulmonary arteries, whereas the aortic semilunar valve separates the left ventricle from the aorta.

The semilunar valves open in response to rising pressure within the contracting ventricles. When the pressure is great enough, the cusps open, allowing blood to be ejected into either the pulmonary trunk or the aorta. Upon relaxation of the ventricles, the valves close, allowing for ventricular filling and preventing backflow into the chambers.

HEART SOUNDS

Closure of the valves of the heart gives rise to heart sounds (see Figure 17.4 •). Normal heart sounds include **S₁** and **S₂.** These are

heard as the *lub-dub* of the heart when auscultated over the precordium, the area of the chest that lies over the heart. The first heart sound, S_1 (*lub*), is heard when the AV valves close. Closure of these valves occurs when the ventricles have been filled. The second heart sound, S_2 (*dub*), occurs when the aortic and pulmonic valves close. These semilunar valves close when the ventricles have emptied their blood into the aorta and pulmonary arteries.

The heart sounds are associated with the contraction and relaxation phases of the heart. **Systole** refers to the phase of ventricular contraction. In the systolic phase the ventricles have been filled, then contract to expel blood into the aorta and pulmonary arteries. Systole begins with the closure of the AV valves (S_1) and ends with the closure of the aortic and pulmonic valves (S_2).

Diastole refers to the phase of ventricular relaxation. In the diastolic phase the ventricles relax and are filled as the atria contract. Diastole begins with the closure of the aortic and pulmonic valves (S_2) and ends with the closure of the AV valves (S_1) (see Figure 17.5 •).

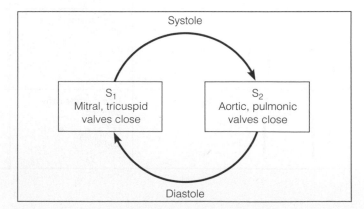

Figure 17.5 • Heart sounds in systole and diastole.

Table 17.1 Characteristics of Heart Sounds

HEART SOUNDS		CARDIAC CYCLE TIMING	AUSCULTATION SITE	POSITION	PITCH
S_1 S_2 LUB — dub	S_1	Start of systole	Best at apex with diaphragm	Position does not affect the sound	High
S_1 S_2 lub — DUB	S_2	End of systole	Both at 2nd ICS; pulmonary component best at LSB; aortic component best at RSB with diaphragm	Sitting or supine	High
S_1 S_2 T	Split S_1	Beginning of systole	If normal, at 2nd ICS, LSB; abnormal if heard at apex	Better heard in the supine position	High
S_1 S_2	Fixed Split S_2	End of systole	Both at 2nd ICS; pulmonary component best at LSB; aortic component best at RSB with diaphragm	Better heard in the supine position	High
Expiration S_1 S_2 $P_2 A_2$	Paradoxical Split S_2	End of systole	Both at 2nd ICS; pulmonary component best at LSB; aortic component best at RSB with diaphragm	Better heard in the supine position	High
Expiration S_1 S_2 Inspiration S_1 S_2	Wide Split S_2	End of systole	Both at 2nd ICS; pulmonary component best at LSB; aortic component best at RSB with diaphragm	Better heard in the supine position	High
S_1 S_2 S_3	S_3	Early diastole right after S_2	Apex with the bell	Auscultated better in left lateral position or supine	Low
S_1 S_2 S_4	S_4	Late diastole right before S_1	Apex with the bell	Auscultated in almost a left lateral position or supine	Low

Splitting of S_2 occurs toward the end of inspiration in some individuals. This results from a slight difference in the time in which the semilunar valves close. The increase in intrathoracic pressure during inspiration is a normal splitting of S_2. The aortic valve closes just slightly faster than the pulmonic valve. As a result, a split sound is heard (instead of *dub*, one hears *t-dub*). The valves close at the same time during expiration, and the sound of S_2 is *dub*.

Two other heart sounds that may be present in some healthy individuals are S_3 and S_4. S_3 may be heard in children, in young adults, or in pregnant females in their third trimester. It is heard after S_2 and is termed a *ventricular gallop*. When the AV valves open, blood flow into the ventricles may cause vibrations. These vibrations create the S_3 sound during diastole. The S_4 may also be heard in children, well-conditioned athletes, and even healthy elderly individuals without cardiac disease. It is caused by atrial contraction and ejection of blood into the ventricles in late diastole. S_4 is heard before S_1 and is termed an *atrial gallop*. S_3 and S_4 may be associated with pathologic conditions such as myocardial infarction (MI) or heart failure.

Heart sounds are interpreted according to the characteristics of pitch, duration, intensity, phase, and location on the precordium. Table 17.1 provides information about the characteristics of heart sounds.

ADDITIONAL HEART SOUNDS

The valves of the heart open without sound unless the tissue has been damaged. Clicks and snaps may be heard in clients with valvular disease. An opening snap may be heard in mitral stenosis. Ejection clicks occur in damaged pulmonic and aortic valves, and nonejection clicks are heard in prolapse of the mitral valve.

Friction rubs result from inflammation of the pericardial sac. The surfaces of the parietal and visceral layers of the pericardium cannot slide smoothly and produce the rubbing or grating sound. Table 17.2 includes information regarding interpretation of additional heart sounds.

Heart murmurs are harsh, blowing sounds caused by disruption of blood flow into the heart, between the chambers of the heart, or from the heart into the pulmonary or aortic systems. Methods to distinguish murmurs and classification of heart murmurs are provided in Tables 17.3 and 17.4, respectively.

CORONARY ARTERIES

The word *coronary* comes from the Latin word meaning crown, which accurately describes this extensive network of arteries supplying the heart (see Figure 17.6 ●). The coronary arteries

Table 17.2 Additional Heart Sounds

CLICKS	HEART SOUNDS	CARDIAC CYCLE TIMING	AUSCULTATION SITE	POSITION	PITCH
	Aortic Click	Early systole	2nd ICS, RSB for aortic click and apex with diaphragm	Sitting or supine position may increase sound	High
	Pulmonic	Early systole	2nd ICS, LSB for pulmonic click with diaphragm	Sitting	High
	Opening Snap	Early diastole	3rd to 4th ICS, LSB with diaphragm	Sitting or supine position may increase the sound	High
	Friction Rub	Can occur at any time	Best heard with the diaphragm, location variable	May be heard in any position, but best when the client sits forward	High, harsh in sound, grating

Table 17.3 Distinguishing Heart Murmurs

ASK YOURSELF	INFORMATION
1. How loud is the murmur?	Murmurs are graded on a rather subjective scale of 1–6: • Grade 1: Barely audible with stethoscope, often considered physiologic not pathologic. Requires concentration and a quiet environment. • Grade 2: Very soft but distinctly audible. • Grade 3: Moderately loud; there is no thrill or thrusting motion associated with the murmur. • Grade 4: Distinctly loud, in addition to a palpable thrill. • Grade 5: Very loud, can actually hear with part of the diaphragm of the stethoscope off the chest; palpable thrust and thrill present. • Grade 6: Loudest, can hear with the diaphragm off the chest; visible thrill and thrust.
2. Where does it occur in the cardiac cycle: systole, diastole, or both?	Location in cardiac cycle: • Systole: early systole, midsystole, late systole • Diastole: early diastole, mid-diastole, late diastole • Both
3a. Is the sound continuous throughout systole, diastole, or only heard for part of the cycle?	Duration of murmur: • Continuous through systole only • Continuous through diastole only • Continuous through systole and diastole *Systolic murmurs* may be of two types: • Midsystolic: Murmur is heard after S_1 and stops before S_2. • Pansystolic/holosystolic: Murmur begins with S_1 and stops at S_2. *Diastolic murmurs* may be one of three types: • Early diastolic: Murmur auscultated immediately after S_2 and then stops. There is a gap where this murmur stops and S_1 is heard. • Mid-diastolic: Murmur begins a short time after S_2 and stops well before S_1 is auscultated. • Late diastolic: This murmur starts well after S_2 and stops immediately before S_1 is heard.
3b. What does the configuration of the sound look like? *Potential configurations:*	 **Pansystolic/holosystolic:** **Continuous** **Crescendo (Systolic represented)** **Decrescendo (Diastolic represented)** **Crescendo Decrescendo (Systole represented)** **Rumble**
4. What is the quality of the sound of the murmur?	• Blowing • Harsh • Musical • Raspy • Rumbling
5. What is the pitch or frequency of the sound?	• Low • Medium • High
6. In which landmark(s) do you best hear the murmur?	Use the five landmarks for auscultation: • Pulmonic areas 1 and 2 • Aortic area • Tricuspid area • Mitral area • Apex

Table 17.3	Distinguishing Heart Murmurs (*continued*)

ASK YOURSELF	INFORMATION
7. Does it radiate?	• To the throat? • To the axilla?
8. Is there any change in pattern with respirations?	• Increases/decreases with inspiration • Increases/decreases with expiration
9. Is it associated with variations in heart sounds?	• Associated with split S_1? • Associated with split S_2? • Associated with S_3? • Associated with S_4? • Associated with a click or ejection sound?
10. Does intensity of murmur change with position?	• Increases/decreases with squatting? • Increases/decreases with client in the left lateral position? (Do not have the client perform the Valsalva maneuver or any abrupt positional changes, because some clients do not tolerate position changes well.)

Table 17.4	Classifications of Heart Murmurs

MURMUR	CARDIAC CYCLE TIMING	AUSCULTATION SITE	CONFIGURATION OF SOUND	CONTINUITY
Aortic stenosis	Midsystolic	RSB, 2nd ICS	S_1 — S_2	Crescendo-decrescendo, continuous
Pulmonary stenosis	Midsystolic	LSB, 2nd to 3rd ICS	S_1 — S_2	Crescendo-decrescendo, continuous
Mitral regurgitation	Systole	Apex	S_1 — S_2	Holosystolic, continuous
Tricuspid regurgitation	Systole	4th ICS, LSB	S_1 — S_2	Holosystolic, continuous
Mitral stenosis	Diastole	Apical	S_2 — S_1	Rumble that increases in sound toward the end, continuous
Tricuspid stenosis	Diastole	Lower LSB	S_2 — S_1	Rumble that increases in sound toward the end, continuous
Ventricular septal defect (left-to-right shunt)	Systole	3rd, 4th, 5th ICS, LSB	S_1 — S_2	Holosystolic, continuous
Aortic regurgitation	Diastole (early)	3rd ICS, LSB	S_2 — S_1	Decrescendo, continuous
Pulmonic regurgitation	Diastole (early)	3rd ICS, LSB	S_2 — S_1	Decrescendo, continuous

(*continued*)

Table 17.4	Classifications of Heart Murmurs *(continued)*			
MURMUR	**QUALITY**	**PITCH**	**RADIATION**	**CHANGES WITH RESPIRATIONS**
Aortic stenosis	Usually harsh, coarse	Medium	Most commonly into neck into carotid area and down left sternal border, possibly apex	Expiration may intensify the murmur
Pulmonary stenosis	Usually harsh	Medium	Toward the left upper neck and shoulder areas	Inspiration may intensify the murmur
Mitral regurgitation	Blowing and can be harsh in sound quality	High	Usually to left axilla, LSB, and base	Expiration may intensify the murmur
Tricuspid regurgitation	Blowing	High	May radiate to LSB and MCL but not to axilla	Inspiration may intensify the murmur
Mitral stenosis	Rumbling	Low and best heard with bell	Rare	Expiration may intensify the murmur
Tricuspid stenosis	Rumbling	Low	Rare	Inspiration may intensify the murmur
Ventricular septal defect (left-to-right shunt)	Harsh	High	May radiate across precordium but not to axilla	Expiration may intensify the murmur
Aortic regurgitation	Blowing	High, best auscultated with diaphragm unless client is sitting up and leaning forward	May radiate to 2nd ICS, RSB and may proceed to apex	Expiration may intensify the murmur if the client leans forward and sits up
Pulmonic regurgitation	Blowing	High, best auscultated with diaphragm	May radiate to 2nd ICS, RSB and may proceed to apex	Inspiration may intensify the murmur

are visible initially on the external surface of the heart but descend deep into the myocardial tissue layers. Their function is to transport blood bringing nutrients and oxygen to the myocardial muscle. The coronary arteries fill during diastole.

The main coronary arteries are the left main coronary artery, the right coronary artery, the left anterior descending coronary artery, and the circumflex coronary artery. These arteries and those that branch from them may vary in size and configuration among individuals. The coronary arteries are located above the aortic valve. The right and left main coronary arteries originate from the aorta and then diverge to provide blood to different surfaces. Atherosclerotic plaque in these arteries as well as in their branches contributes significantly to the development of ischemic and injury processes and the potential for death.

CARDIAC VEINS

The venous system of the heart is composed of the great cardiac vein, oblique vein, anterior cardiac vein, small cardiac vein, middle cardiac vein, cordis minimae veins, and posterior cardiac vein. The great cardiac vein serves as the tributary for the majority of venous blood drainage and empties into the coronary sinus. The small venae cordis minimae drain into the cardiac chambers.

CARDIAC CONDUCTION SYSTEM

The heart has its own conduction system, which can initiate an electrical charge and transmit that charge via cardiac muscle fibers throughout the myocardial tissue. This electrical charge stimulates the heart to contract, causing the propulsion of blood throughout the heart chambers and vascular

system. The main structures of the **cardiac conduction system** are the sinoatrial node (SA node), the intra-atrial conducting pathways, the atrioventricular (AV node) node, the bundle of His, the right and left bundle branches, and the Purkinje fibers (see Figure 17.7 ●).

Sinoatrial Node

The **Sinoatrial (SA) node** initiates the electrical impulse. For this reason, it has been called the pacemaker of the heart. The SA node is located at the junction of the superior vena cava and right atrium. The autonomic nervous system feeds into the SA node and can influence it to either speed up or slow down the discharge of electrical current. In the healthy individual, the SA node discharges an average of 60 to 100 times a minute.

Intra-Atrial Conduction Pathway

These loosely organized conducting fibers assist in the propagation of the electrical current emitted from the SA node through the right and left atrium. The network is composed of three main pathways: anterior, middle, and posterior.

Atrioventricular Node and Bundle of His

The **Atrioventricular (AV) node** and **bundle of His** are intricately connected and function to receive the current that has finished spreading throughout the atria. Here the impulse is slowed for about 0.1 second before it passes onto the bundle branches. The AV node is also capable of initiating electrical impulses in the event of SA node failure. The intrinsic rate of firing is slower and averages about 60 per minute.

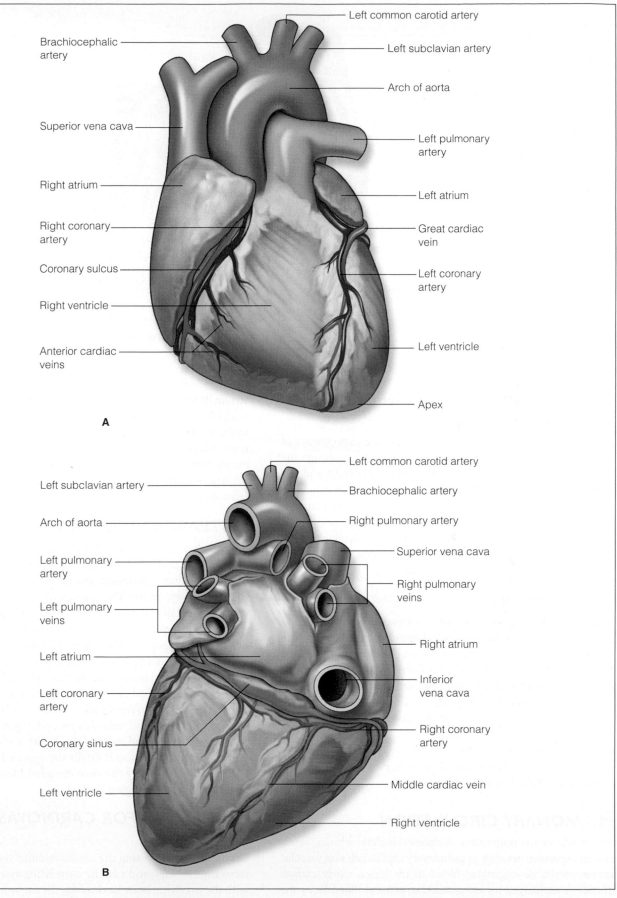

Figure 17.6 ● Vessels of the heart. A. Anterior. B. Posterior.

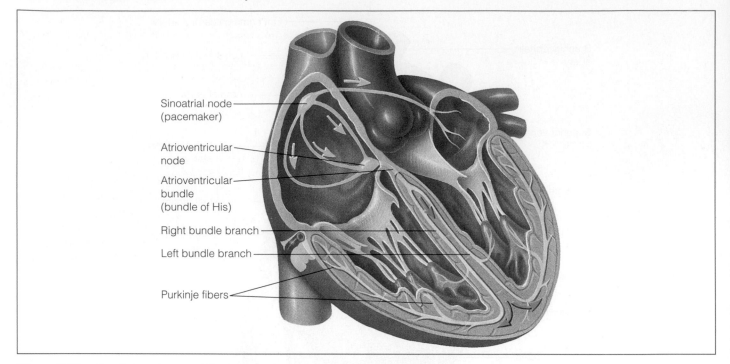

Sinoatrial node
(pacemaker)

Atrioventricular
node

Atrioventricular
bundle
(bundle of His)

Right bundle branch

Left bundle branch

Purkinje fibers

Figure 17.7 • Conduction system of the heart.

Right and Left Bundle Branches and Purkinje Fibers

The right and left **bundle branches** are like expressways of conducting fibers that spread the electrical current through the ventricular myocardial tissue. Arising from the right and left bundle branches are the **Purkinje fibers.** These fibers fan out and penetrate into the myocardial tissue to spread the current into the tissues themselves.

The bundle branches are also capable of initiating electrical charges in case both the SA node and AV node fail. Their intrinsic rate averages 40 to 60 per minute.

Cardiac Nerves

Just as there is an extensive network of vessels transporting oxygen and nutrients to the myocardial tissue and removing waste products, an equally important network of autonomic nerves is present. Both sympathetic nervous fibers and parasympathetic nervous fibers interact with the myocardial tissue. The sympathetic fibers stimulate the heart, increasing the heart rate, force of contraction, and dilation of the coronary arteries. Conversely, the parasympathetic fibers, such as the vagus nerve, exercise the opposite effect. The central nervous system influences the activation and interaction of these nerves through the information supplied by the cardiac plexus.

PULMONARY CIRCULATION

The vessels of the pulmonary circulation include arteries, veins, and an expansive network of pulmonary capillaries. This vascular system carries deoxygenated blood to the lungs, where carbon dioxide is exchanged for oxygen. Deoxygenated blood from the veins of the body enters this network by passing into the right atrium. It is then ejected through the tricuspid valve into the right ventricle and passes through the pulmonic valve into the pulmonary artery and pulmonary circulation. The pulmonary artery is the only artery to carry unoxygenated blood. After going through the pulmonary capillary network, oxygenated blood returns to the left atrium via the pulmonary veins (see Figure 17.8 •). Pulmonary veins are the only veins to carry oxygenated blood.

SYSTEMIC CIRCULATION

The vessels of the systemic circulation also include arteries, veins, and capillaries. This vascular system supplies freshly oxygenated blood to the body's periphery and returns deoxygenated blood to the pulmonary circuit. The arteries of the systemic circulation are composed of elastic tissue and smooth muscle, which allows their walls to stretch during systole. During systole, the elasticity of the walls propels the blood forward into the systemic circulation. The left ventricle propels freshly oxygenated blood into the aorta. As the blood moves toward the body periphery, the major arteries of the body subdivide into arterioles, which carry the nutrients and oxygen to the smallest blood vessels of the body, the capillaries. Oxygen and nutrients are exchanged in the capillaries for carbon dioxide and metabolites, which are then carried into the venules, then veins, and finally the superior and inferior venae cavae, which carry the deoxygenated blood into the right atrium of the heart (Figure 17.8).

LANDMARKS FOR CARDIOVASCULAR ASSESSMENT

Landmarks for assessing the cardiovascular system include the sternum, clavicles, and ribs. By correlating assessment findings with the overlying body landmarks, the nurse may gain vital information concerning underlying pathologic mechanisms.

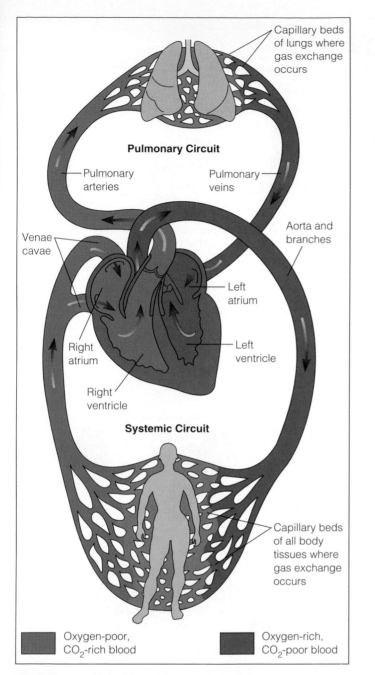

Pulmonary Circuit

Pulmonary arteries — Pulmonary veins —

Capillary beds of lungs where gas exchange occurs

Aorta and branches

Venae cavae —

Left atrium

Right atrium

Left ventricle

Right ventricle

Systemic Circuit

Capillary beds of all body tissues where gas exchange occurs

Oxygen-poor, CO_2-rich blood

Oxygen-rich, CO_2-poor blood

Figure 17.8 ● Pulmonary and systemic circulation. The left side of the heart pumps oxygenated blood (indicated in red) into the arteries of the systemic circulation, which provides oxygen and nutrients to the cells. Deoxygenated blood (indicated in blue) returns via the venous system into the right side of the heart, where it is transported to the pulmonary arterial system to be reoxygenated.

Many landmarks identified during the respiratory assessment are utilized also when performing a cardiac assessment. These include but are not limited to the sternum and the second through fifth intercostal spaces. It may be helpful to review the landmarks in Chapter 15 before proceeding. ⟳

The **sternum** is the flat, narrow center bone of the upper anterior chest (see Figure 17.9 ●). There are three portions of the adult sternum. The upper sternum is called the manubrium, the middle part is the body, and the inferior piece is the xiphoid process. The average sternal length in an adult is 18 cm (7 in.).

During cardiovascular assessment, the sternum is used as a vertical landmark, and the angle of Louis is used to locate the second intercostal space.

The clavicles are bones that attach at the top of the manubrium of the sternum above the first rib (Figure 17.9). The midclavicular line (MCL) is used as a landmark for cardiovascular assessment.

The ribs are flat, arched bones that form the thoracic cage. There are 12 pairs of ribs. Between each rib is an intercostal space (ICS). The first ICS lies between the first and the second rib, and each remaining ICS is numbered successively (Figure 17.9). The intercostal spaces, horizontal landmarks for cardiac assessment, are used to locate the base of the heart and the apex of the heart, and to auscultate the valvular sounds. The second ICS is located by feeling the angle of Louis, sliding the finger laterally to the second rib, and then sliding the finger down below the rib to the intercostal space. Each succeeding ICS is located by sliding the finger over the rib into the ICS. Additional landmarks are identified later in this chapter.

CARDIAC CYCLE

The **cardiac cycle** describes the events of one complete heartbeat—that is, the contraction and relaxation of the atria and ventricles. A healthy individual's heart averages about 72 beats per minute (bpm); thus, the average time for each cardiac cycle to be completed is 0.8 second. Synchrony between the mechanical and electrical events of the cycle is imperative. Any interruption in this balance affects the ability of the heart to provide oxygen and nutrients to the body. Significant disruptions in synchrony can be fatal.

Electrical and Mechanical Events

The cardiac cycle can be divided into three periods (see Figure 17.10 ●): the period of ventricular filling, ventricular systole, and isovolumetric relaxation.

PERIOD OF VENTRICULAR FILLING. This is the start of the cardiac cycle. Blood enters passively into the ventricles from the atria. About 70% of the blood that eventually ends up in the ventricles enters at this time. As this blood is entering the ventricles, the atria are stimulated to contract by the electrical current emanating from the SA node. Another 30% volume of blood exits the atria into the ventricles. This extra 30% volume is termed the *atrial kick*.

VENTRICULAR SYSTOLE. The electrical current stimulates the ventricles, and they respond by contracting. The force of contraction increases the pressure within both ventricles. The mitral and tricuspid valves respond to this increased pressure by snapping shut (S_1). The ventricular pressure continues to increase until it causes the aortic and pulmonic valves to open. Blood rushes out of the ventricles into the systemic and pulmonary circulation.

ISOVOLUMETRIC RELAXATION. Once the majority of blood is ejected, the pressure in the aorta and pulmonary artery becomes higher than in the ventricles, causing the aortic and pulmonic valves to shut (S_2). During ventricular systole, the atria have been filling with blood returning from the systemic and pulmonary circulation. When the pressure in the atria becomes higher than in the ventricles, the mitral and tricuspid valves open, and the cycle begins again.

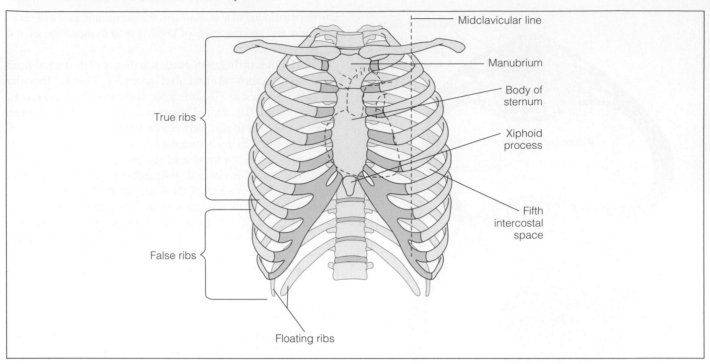

Figure 17.9 ● Landmarks for cardiovascular assessment.

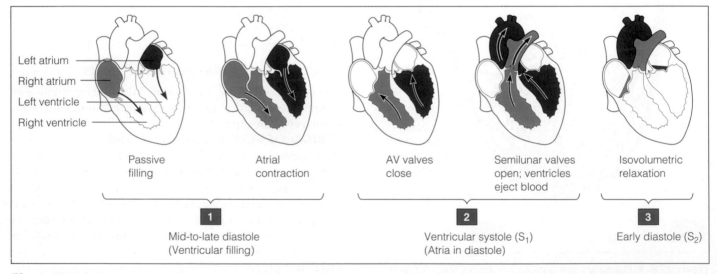

Figure 17.10 ● The cardiac cycle.

Electrical Representation of the Cardiac Cycle

Electrical representations of the cardiac cycle are documented by deflections on recording paper. A straight horizontal line means the absence of electrical activity. Deflections representing the flow of electrical current toward or away from an electrode record the timing of the electrical events in the cardiac cycle. The terms describing the electrical deflections are P wave, PR interval, QRS interval, and T wave. They are recorded as an **electrocardiogram (ECG)** (see Figure 17.11 ●). When the cardiac cell is in a resting state, it is more positively charged on the outside of the cell and more negatively charged on the inside of the cell. This spread of electrical current, called *depolarization*, causes the in-

side of the cardiac cell to become more positively charged. Depolarization occurs when the electrical current normally initiated in the SA node spreads across the atria. Contraction of the atria follows after stimulation by the electrical current. After contraction, the cardiac cells experience *repolarization*, during which the inside of the cell returns to its more negatively charged state. The same process occurs in the ventricles.

P WAVE. The P wave represents part of atrial depolarization. The pacemaker of the heart, the SA node, emits an electrical charge that initially spreads throughout the right and left atria. As a result of the electrical stimulation, the myocardial cells contract. The initial P wave deflection is caused by the initiation of the electrical current and atrial response to the current. It lasts an average 0.08 second.

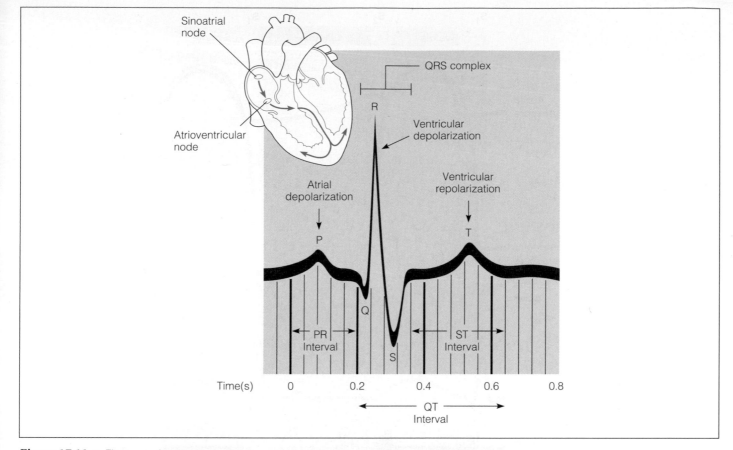

Figure 17.11 ● Electrocardiogram wave.

PR INTERVAL. The PR interval represents the time needed for the electrical current to travel across both atria and arrive at the AV node. The normal PR interval averages 0.12 to 0.20 second.

QRS INTERVAL. The QRS interval represents ventricular depolarization. Atrial repolarization is hidden in the QRS interval. The ventricular myocardial cells also respond to the spread of electrical current by becoming more positively charged. This change in polarity is ventricular depolarization. The QRS interval should be 0.08 to 0.11 second.

T WAVE. The T wave represents ventricular repolarization. Once the ventricular myocardial cells have been stimulated by the electrical current and contract, they return to their original electrical potential state. This change in polarity is repolarization. The atria also repolarize, but it is not recorded because it occurs at the same time as ventricular repolarization; therefore, the QRS covers it.

QT INTERVAL. The QT interval represents the period from the beginning of ventricular depolarization to the moment of repolarization. Thus, it represents ventricular contraction. Electrical events in the heart occur slightly ahead of the mechanical events. Figure 17.12 ● illustrates the events of the cardiac cycle in relation to heart sounds, pressure waves, and the ECG.

MEASUREMENTS OF CARDIAC FUNCTION

When the heart is functioning at optimal level, the synchrony of the events of the cardiac cycle produces an outflow of blood with oxygen and nutrients to every cell in the body. The terms that describe the effectiveness of the action of the cardiac cycle are stroke volume, cardiac output, and cardiac index.

Stroke volume describes the amount of blood that is ejected with every heartbeat. Normal stroke volume is 55 to 100 ml/beat. The formula for calculating stroke volume is:

stroke volume = cardiac output/heart rate for 1 minute

Cardiac output describes the amount of blood ejected from the left ventricle over 1 minute. Normal adult cardiac output is 4 to 8 liters/minute. The formula for calculating cardiac output is:

cardiac output = stroke volume × heart rate for 1 minute

The cardiac index is a valuable diagnostic measurement of the effectiveness of the pumping action of the heart. The cardiac index takes into consideration the individual's weight, which is a significant factor in judging the effectiveness of the pumping action. For example, suppose a cardiac output of 4 is obtained for two clients: an elderly female who weighs 60 kg and a middle-aged male who weighs 130 kg. The elderly female's cardiac index is significantly higher than that of the male, whose pumping effectiveness is significantly compromised. The formula for calculating cardiac index is:

cardiac index = cardiac output/body surface area

The body surface area (BSA) measurement is obtained and determined from published tables.

There are two strong influences on pumping action: preload and afterload. Preload is influenced by the volume of the blood

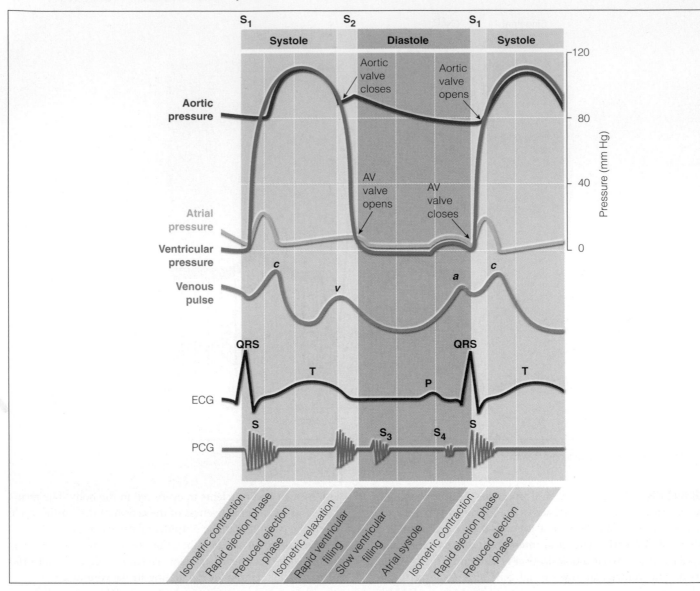

Figure 17.12 ● Events of the cardiac cycle.

in the ventricles and relates to the length of ventricular fiber stretch at the end of diastole. The Frank-Starling law states that an increasingly greater contractile ability is provided with greater stretching of the ventricular muscle fibers. Thus, the greater the stretch, the greater the contractile force, and the greater the volume of blood ejected with each contraction. Afterload is the amount of stress or tension present in the ventricular wall during systole. It is interrelated to the pressure in the aorta, because the pressure in the ventricular wall must be greater than that in the aorta and pulmonary trunk for the semilunar valves to open (see Figure 17.13 ●).

SPECIAL CONSIDERATIONS

Many factors influence the client's health status. Among these are age, developmental level, race, ethnicity, work history, living conditions, socioeconomics, and emotional well-being. Each of the factors must be addressed while gathering subjective and objective data during comprehensive health assessment.

DEVELOPMENTAL CONSIDERATIONS

Anatomy and physiology change as individuals grow and develop. It is important to understand these normal changes when interpreting findings in health assessment. Variations in the cardiovascular system for different age groups are presented in the following sections.

Infants and Children

During development, the fetus receives its nutrients and oxygen from its mother. The lungs are nonfunctional, and oxygen is carried in blood from the placenta to the right side of the heart. The majority of this blood passes through the foramen ovale to the left side of the heart, then into the aorta to enter the systemic circulation. The *foramen ovale* is a passageway for blood between the right and left atria. The rest of the blood passes through the pulmonary artery and ductus arteriosus and enters the aorta (Figure 17.14 ●). The *ductus arteriosus* is an opening between the pulmonary artery and the descending aorta.

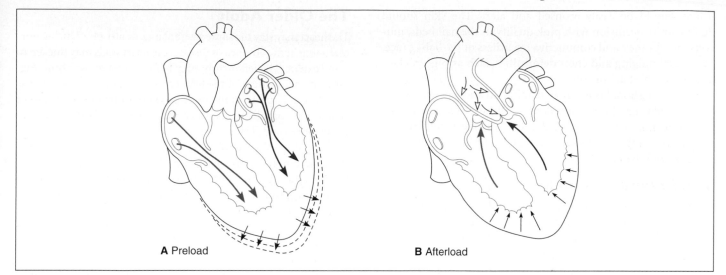

Figure 17.13 ● A. Preload is related to the amount of blood and stretching of the ventricular myocardial fibers. B. Afterload is the pressure that the ventricles must overcome in order to open the aortic and pulmonic valvular cusps.

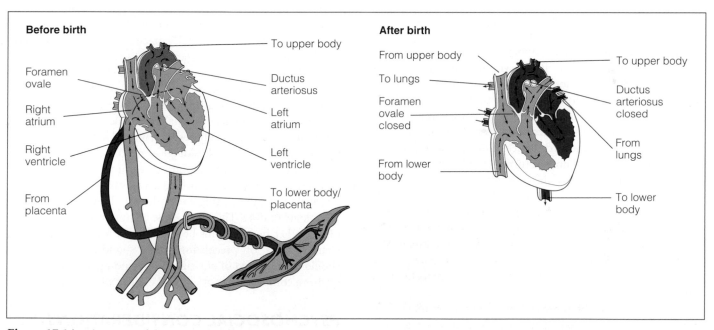

Figure 17.14 ● Location of the main structures and vessels present in the fetal and post-partal cardiovascular anatomy.

Inflation of the lungs at birth causes the pulmonary vasculature to dilate. Oxygenation occurs for the first time within the newborn's lungs. The foramen ovale closes shortly after birth because of increased pulmonary vascular return and decreased pressure in the right side of the heart. The ductus arteriosus closes within 24 to 46 hours in response to multiple physiological events, including decreased pulmonary resistance and decreased pressure in the right atrium versus increased pressure in the left atrium. Murmurs may be auscultated if these openings remain patent. However, if a ventricular septal defect is present, the murmur it causes may not be auscultated until the 4th to 6th week after delivery.

The infant's arterial pressure rises at birth, and the systemic vascular resistance increases significantly when the umbilical

cord is cut. Over time, the left ventricle increases in size and mass as it works to pump blood into the aorta against increasingly elevating systemic vascular resistance. The blood pressure of the full-term infant may average 70/50 mm Hg, and 10 mm Hg less in both systolic and diastolic readings in the preterm newborn. For more information, go to the chart for pediatric vital signs in Chapter 25. ◯◯ Weight significantly influences blood pressure.

The heart rate of the newborn initially may be as high as 175 to 180 bpm. Over the first 6 to 8 hours, it gradually decreases to an average of 115 to 120 bpm. Stimulation that causes crying, screaming, or coughing may cause the heart rate to rise temporarily to 180 bpm.

A newborn's cardiovascular system undergoes tremendous changes at birth and during the first several days of life. The infant should be easily aroused and alert. The skin should demonstrate perfusion with pink quality in the nail beds, mucous membranes, and conjunctiva regardless of the baby's race. Precordial bulging and chest deformities such as pigeon chest and barrel chest are of concern.

The nurse should use a small diaphragm and bell with an infant or child for optimal auscultation of heart sounds. Pathologic murmurs of a congenital cause include patent ductus arteriosus, tetralogy of Fallot, and septal defects. A complete assessment of infants and children is provided in Chapter 25. ∞

The Pregnant Female

During pregnancy, a female's body undergoes phenomenal adaptations, especially in the cardiovascular system. Usually these adaptations do not place her life at risk; however, if preexisting cardiovascular or other disease is present, her health may be significantly compromised. The heart is displaced to the left and upward, and the apex is pushed laterally and to the left. This anatomical shift may be seen when examining the electrical axis on the female's 12-lead ECG. The axis is rotated to the left. The physical strength of the female's abdominal muscles, the shape of the fetus, the gestational age, and the structural anatomy of the uterus influence the extent of this shift.

The cardiovascular system undergoes many physiological changes during pregnancy. Blood volume may increase as much as 30 to 50%. Red blood cell genesis is dramatically stimulated, and plasma volume increases by as much as 50%. Plasma albumin, conversely, decreases. Cardiac output increases 30 to 50% in just the first trimester. Dilation of surface veins, together with the low resistance of the uteroplacental circulation, increases the venous return to the heart. Stroke volume increases 30. Because of the substantial increase in volume and the resultant increased workload, the heart may appear as much as 10% larger on chest radiography. Systolic blood pressure may decrease by 2 to 3 mm Hg and diastolic blood pressure by 5 to 10 mm Hg during the first half of the pregnancy. These values return to their previous levels as the pregnancy progresses. Last, the great vessels may become more tortuous in appearance.

There may be a slight increase in resting pulse by about 10 to 15 bpm, although not every client experiences this increase. Because of the increased volume, preexisting murmurs may become louder. Murmurs may even be auscultated for the first time. Systolic murmurs are the most common (90% incidence), whereas diastolic murmurs occur less frequently (20% incidence). Heart tones may also change. The S_1 may split, and a prominent S_3 may be heard.

The position of the client may influence the cardiovascular dynamic state. Cardiac output may decrease when she lies on her back because of compression of the vena cava and aorta. The brachial pressure is highest when the client is sitting, then decreases when she is supine. Pressure is lowest when she is in the lateral recumbent position. Monitoring a client's blood pressure and pattern of the pressures is crucial. A blood pressure of 140/90 or greater may indicate preeclampsia and needs further assessment and monitoring. A complete assessment of the pregnant female is provided in Chapter 26. ∞

The Older Adult

The heart may stay the same size, enlarge, or atrophy. During normal aging in the absence of disease, the heart walls may thicken to some extent. The left atrium may increase in size over time. Significant enlargement of the left ventricle can be attributed to the influence of hypertension. Aging can also contribute to the loss of ventricular compliance as the cardiac valves and large vessels become more rigid. The aorta may dilate and lengthen.

Physiologically, systolic blood pressure may increase; however, there may be no significant change in resting heart rate. Diastolic filling time and pressure may increase to maintain a cardiac output adequate for physiological needs. Upon auscultation, the older client may have an S_4. Last, the electrical conduction system may experience a loss of automaticity when the SA node and conducting pathways become fibrotic and lose cellular integrity.

In the healthy older adult, cardiac output may remain stable. Stroke volume may increase just slightly when the client is at rest. The healthy client may tolerate exercise well. The healthy older adult may actually show a decreased heart rate, maximum oxygen consumption, and an increase in stroke volume during exercise. A client who has been physically active most of his or her life may have twice the work capacity of a client who has not.

The nurse should assess the older client in a position that is comfortable and be careful not to have the client make any sudden movements such as suddenly sitting, standing up, or lying down after standing or sitting. Systolic murmurs become more common as people age, especially because of aortic stenosis. These murmurs are usually best auscultated in the aortic area or base of the heart. Nonphysiological murmurs are not normal findings. However, an S_4 sound is a common finding in older adults who do not have identified cardiovascular disease. In individuals with preexisting heart disease, however, an S_4 is a pathologic finding. The nurse must be mindful of the presence of any other heart sounds beyond S_1 and S_2 or any change in characteristics of preexisting heart sounds. The physician should be informed of any significant findings. Chapter 27 describes a complete assessment of the older adult. ∞

PSYCHOSOCIAL CONSIDERATIONS

Stress causes an individual to experience longer periods of sympathetic stimulation, which increases the workload on the heart. Systemic vascular resistance may be elevated for longer periods of time, especially in situations of excessive stress. An individual who exhibits type A behavior may be driven to succeed, to excel, and to be the best regardless of the cost. For many years, type A behavior has been thought to contribute to the development of heart disease. Counseling, relaxation, yoga, meditation, and biofeedback techniques are usually helpful to reduce stress level.

CULTURAL AND ENVIRONMENTAL CONSIDERATIONS

Individuals whose blood-related parents, aunts, uncles, or siblings demonstrate atherosclerotic heart disease before the age of 50 are considered at risk for diabetes, hypertension, or high lipid levels.

In some cultures, "overfat" individuals are considered healthier than those who are leaner. The selection and preparation of food may also reflect cultural influences. The use of lard and other forms of saturated fat is common in some cultures and may contribute to the development of hypertension and diabetes. African Americans have a significantly higher percentage of hypertension than Caucasians. Cardiovascular disease contributes to a significant percentage of deaths in individuals from varied cultural backgrounds. Individuals of Cuban, Filipino, and Mexican heritage have a higher incidence of hypertension. The correlation of diet and heritage is also significant, as demonstrated by the low incidence of heart disease in Japanese individuals adhering to a traditional Japanese diet and the increasing incidence of heart disease in Japanese individuals who have adopted the Western diet of red meat and saturated fats.

Some data suggests that a low socioeconomic bracket is correlated with a higher incidence of hypertension, especially among adult females. There may be a correlation between this situation and the effect of stress related to lower incomes, limited exercise, diets containing saturated fats, or lack of access to quality healthcare.

Diet is one factor that may significantly influence the development of cardiovascular disease. Intake of fat, especially saturated fat, contributes significantly to cardiovascular disease. "Couch potato" is a popular term that describes a lifestyle of inactivity. Studies on individuals who perform continuous aerobic exercise for at least 30 to 45 minutes at least three times a week have shown a significant correlation to a slower progression of atherosclerosis. Exercise also helps to diffuse the effects of stress and, in most individuals, provides a feeling of relaxation. Smoking is a well-known contributor to the development of cardiovascular disease. In fact, it is one of the most devastating. The chemicals inhaled in cigarette smoke alter and injure the linings of the arteries, especially in areas of bifurcation (division into branches). Inhalation of passive smoke is also detrimental to the cardiovascular system.

Cocaine, especially crack cocaine, causes increased oxygen demands on the heart. Ventricular ectopy, electrical impulses that originate in the ventricles and cause early contraction of the ventricles, has been linked to cocaine use. Coronary artery spasm, myocardial infarction, malignant hypertension, and ruptured aorta also have been attributed to cocaine.

Alcoholism is associated with the development of many cardiovascular complications, such as cardiomyopathy (discussed later in the chapter). Alcohol consumption may also cause ventricular ectopy, which contributes to decreased cardiac output and may be life threatening.

Cultural Considerations

- Hypertension is a risk factor for coronary heart disease. Hypertension occurs more frequently in African Americans and Hispanics than in other cultural groups.
- Obesity contributes to cardiovascular disease. Obesity is increasing in all populations in the United States but is seen in greatest numbers in Hispanic females and African American youths.
- Diabetes is a risk factor for cardiovascular disease and is increasing in incidence in Native Americans, Hispanics, and African Americans.
- Smoking contributes to cardiovascular disease. Smoking is most prevalent in African American and Hispanic males.

- Native Americans under the age of 35 have twice the heart disease mortality of other groups.
- African American females between the ages of 25 and 54 have greater risk for coronary heart disease than other groups of the same age.
- Caucasian females between the ages of 65 and 74 years have a higher incidence of cardiovascular disease than African American females.
- African Americans with heart failure have higher mortality rates than Caucasians.
- High serum cholesterol levels increase the risk for heart disease. Caucasians have higher serum cholesterol levels than African Americans.

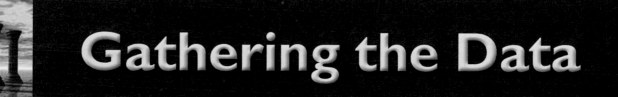

Gathering the Data

Cardiovascular assessment includes the gathering of subjective and objective data. Subjective data collection occurs during the client interview, before the actual physical assessment. During the interview the nurse uses a variety of communication techniques to elicit general and specific information about the client's state of cardiovascular health or illness. Health records, the results of laboratory tests, cardiograms, and other tests are important secondary sources to be reviewed and included in the data-gathering process. In physical assessment of the cardiovascular system, the techniques of inspection, palpation, percussion, and auscultation will be used. Before proceeding, it may be helpful to review the information about each of the data-gathering processes and practice the techniques of health assessment.

FOCUSED INTERVIEW

The focused interview for the cardiovascular system concerns data related to the structures and functions of that system. Subjective data related to cardiac status is gathered during the focused interview. The nurse must be prepared to observe the client and listen for cues related to the function of the cardiovascular system. The nurse may use open-ended or closed questions to obtain information. Often a number of follow-up questions or requests for descriptions are required to clarify data or gather missing information.

The focused interview guides the physical assessment of the cardiovascular system. The information is always considered in relation to normal parameters and expectations about cardiovascular function. Therefore, the nurse must consider age, gen-der, race, culture, environment, health practices, past and concurrent problems, and therapies when framing questions and using techniques to elicit information. In order to address all of the factors when conducting a focused interview, categories of questions related to cardiovascular status and function have been developed. These categories include general questions that are asked of all clients; those addressing illness or infection; questions related to symptoms, pain, or behaviors; those related to habits or practices; questions that are specific to clients according to age; those for the pregnant female; and questions that address internal and external environmental concerns.

As these questions are asked and subjective data is obtained during the focused interview, the data will be used to help meet the goal of improving cardiovascular health as indicated in *Healthy People 2010*. The nurse must consider the client's ability to participate in the focused interview and physical assessment of the cardiovascular system. If a client is experiencing pain, dyspnea, cyanosis, difficulty with speech, and the anxiety that accompanies any of these problems, attention must focus on relief of symptoms and improvement of oxygenation.

FOCUSED INTERVIEW QUESTIONS	RATIONALES
The following section provides sample questions and bulleted follow-up questions in each of the previously mentioned categories. A rationale for each of the questions is provided. The list of questions is not all-inclusive but represents the types of questions required in a comprehensive focused interview related to the cardiovascular system.	
1. **Describe how you are feeling. Has your sense of well-being changed in the last 2 months? Is your sense of well-being different than it was 2 years ago?** • Describe the changes. • How long have you experienced the change? • Do you know what caused the change? • Have you seen a healthcare provider? • Was a diagnosis made? • Was treatment prescribed? • What have you done to deal with the change?	▶ This gives clients the opportunity to provide their own perceptions about their health. Statements about fatigue, weakness, dizziness, or shortness of breath, especially after activity, may indicate problems with cardiovascular health.
2. **Are you able to perform all of the activities needed to meet your personal and work-related responsibilities?** • Describe the changes in your abilities. • Do you know what is causing the difficulty? • How long have you had this problem? • What have you done about the problem? • Have you discussed this with a healthcare professional?	▶ Inability to carry out or perform personal or work-related activities can be indicative of problems in the cardiovascular system.
3. **Is there anyone in your family who has had a cardiovascular problem or disease?** • What is the disease or problem? • Who in the family now has or ever had the problem? • When was it diagnosed? • How has the problem been treated? • What was the outcome?	▶ This may reveal information about cardiovascular diseases associated with familial predisposition. Follow-up is required to obtain details about specific problems, occurrence, treatment, and outcomes.
4. **What is your weight? Have you experienced a change in your weight?** • How much weight have you gained or lost? • Over what period of time did the change occur? • Do you know what caused the change? • Have you done anything to address the change in your weight? • Have you discussed the change with a healthcare provider?	▶ Obesity and high percentage of body fat are risk factors for cardiovascular disease. Weight gain or loss may accompany physical problems including systemic diseases such as diabetes, which increases risk for cardiovascular disease. Psychosocial problems including stress can affect weight gain or loss and also contribute to cardiovascular problems.

FOCUSED INTERVIEW QUESTIONS	**RATIONALES**

QUESTIONS RELATED TO ILLNESS

1. **Have you ever been diagnosed with a cardiovascular disease?**
   - When were you diagnosed with the problem?
   - What treatment was prescribed for the problem?
   - Was the treatment helpful?
   - What kinds of things do you do to help with the problem?
   - Has the problem ever recurred (acute)?
   - How are you managing the disease now (chronic)?

▶ The client has an opportunity to provide information about specific cardiovascular illnesses. If a diagnosed illness is identified, follow-up about the date of diagnosis, treatment, and outcomes is required. Data about each illness identified by the client is essential to an accurate health assessment. Illnesses can be classified as acute or chronic, and follow-up regarding each classification will differ.

2. **An alternative to question 1 is to list possible cardiovascular problems, such as myocardial infarction, congestive heart failure, arteriosclerosis, coronary artery disease, angina, arrhythmia, and valvular disease, and ask the client to respond yes or no as each is stated.**

▶ This is a comprehensive and easy way to elicit information about all diagnoses. Follow-up would be carried out for each identified diagnosis as in question 1.

3. **Do you now have or have you ever had an infection or viral illness affecting the cardiovascular system?**
   - When were you diagnosed with the infection?
   - What treatment was prescribed?
   - Has the treatment helped?
   - What kind of things do you do to help with the problem?
   - Has the infection recurred (acute)?
   - How are you managing the problem now (chronic)?

▶ If an infection is identified, follow-up about the date of infection, treatment, and outcome is required.

4. **An alternative to question 3 is to list possible infections, such as rheumatic fever, viral illness, endocarditis, and pericarditis, and ask the client to respond yes or no as each is stated.**

▶ This is a comprehensive and easy way to elicit information about all infections related to the cardiovascular system. Follow-up would be required as in question 3.

5. **Have you ever had a diagnostic test, such as an electrocardiogram, stress test, or echocardiogram, or a surgical procedure for a cardiovascular problem?**

▶ The client has the opportunity to provide information about diagnostic testing or surgical procedures related to cardiovascular problems. If a surgical procedure is identified, follow-up about the date of surgery, outcome, and effectiveness is required.

6. **An alternative to question 5 is to list possible surgical procedures, such as coronary artery bypass graft, angioplasty, pacemaker insertion, insertion of a defibrillator, and valve replacement, and ask the client to respond yes or no as each is stated.**

▶ This is a comprehensive and easy way to elicit information about surgeries. Follow-up would be required as in question 5.

7. **Do you have hypertension, diabetes, or thyroid disorders?**

▶ Medical conditions such as diabetes, hypertension, or thyroid dysfunction can contribute to cardiovascular problems.

8. **Do you know your cholesterol and triglyceride levels?**

▶ Elevated cholesterol and triglyceride levels are associated with cardiovascular disease.

QUESTIONS RELATED TO SYMPTOMS OR BEHAVIORS

When gathering information about symptoms, many questions are required to elicit details and descriptions that assist in the analysis of the data. Discrimination is made in relation to the significance of a symptom, in relation to specific diseases or problems, and in relation to potential follow-up examination or referral. One rationale may be provided for a group of questions in this category.

FOCUSED INTERVIEW QUESTIONS	**RATIONALES**

The following questions refer to specific symptoms and behaviors associated with the cardiovascular system. For each symptom, questions and follow-up are required. The details to be elicited are the characteristics of the symptom; the onset, duration, and frequency of the symptom; the treatment or remedy for the symptom, including over-the-counter and home remedies; the determination if diagnosis has been sought; the effect of treatments; and family history associated with a symptom or illness.

QUESTIONS RELATED TO SYMPTOMS

1. **Have you experienced any symptoms that may suggest the presence of cardiovascular disease: activity intolerance, loss of appetite, bloody sputum (mucous), changes in sexual activities or performance, confusion or difficulty with thinking or concentrating, chest discomfort, coughing, dizziness, dyspnea (difficulty breathing), fatigue, fever, hoarseness, frequent urination at night, leg pains after activity, sleeping pattern alteration, syncope (fainting), palpitations, or swelling?**

▶ For any of these symptoms, the nurse should gather objective information on the specific characteristics and ask clients to describe their own subjective experience. If the nurse prompts the client, valuable clues may be missed.

2. **Does a change in position increase, decrease, or do nothing to change the symptoms?**
   - Can you identify precipitating factors for the symptoms?

▶ The nurse should look for activity, emotion, stress, or drugs as a precipitating factor. However, heart symptoms may have no precipitating factors.

3. **Describe the quality of the symptom.**
   - Does it feel sharp, dull, or like pressure, piercing, or ripping?

▶ The description of the quality offers clues to the potential origin of the disease, especially when chest discomfort is present.

4. **Does the feeling radiate to other parts of the body?**

▶ Radiation of pain may occur with chest discomfort.

5. **Where do you feel the symptom on the body?**

▶ If the symptom or one of the symptoms is chest discomfort, the client should be asked to show the nurse the location on the body. Often, the client identifies chest discomfort of cardiac origin by placing a clenched fist over the precordium. When the client points one or more fingers to a limited area on the chest wall, it is generally more indicative of pain of a pulmonary or muscular origin. Females may experience less severe cardiac pain over the precordium, back pain, or fatigue.

6. **What relieves the symptoms?**

7. **Rate the severity of the symptoms on a scale of 1 to 10, with 1 being hardly noticeable and 10 being the worst discomfort you have ever experienced.**
   - What is the timing of the symptoms?
   - Is the timing predictable?
   - What is the duration of the symptoms?
   - Is it constant during that time or does it wax and wane?
   - Are the symptoms isolated or do they occur in combinations?
   - Have you seen your healthcare provider about these symptoms?
   - What is being done for these symptoms?

▶ This technique leaves the nurse's opinion on the degree of discomfort out of the picture.

QUESTIONS RELATED TO BEHAVIORS

1. **Describe your diet.**
   - What types of food do you eat? How often? How much?

2. **Do you keep track of the amount of fat, protein, and carbohydrates you eat?**

3. **Do you know the difference between saturated and unsaturated fat?**
   - How much daily fiber do you consume?

▶ Diet is one of the key interventions that a client can control when working to minimize the effects of aging, slow the progression of disease, or maintain optimum health while experiencing cardiac disease. Supplementing the diet with vitamins under proper supervision may be beneficial. Unfortunately, without

FOCUSED INTERVIEW QUESTIONS	RATIONALES

4. **Do you add salt or other flavor enhancers to your food? If so, how much and how often?**
   - Do you taste the food before adding these flavor enhancers?

5. **Do you eat differently when you travel, when at social functions, when under stress, or when on vacation?**

6. **Have you tried to lose weight? If so, describe type of diet, duration of diet, and diet supplements you take.**
   - Do you diet under the care of a healthcare provider?
   - Do you supplement your diet with vitamins, protein supplements, or antioxidants?
   - Do you use weight loss supplements or medications?
   - What type of nonalcoholic liquids do you drink? How much, and how often?
   - Do you exercise to lose weight?

7. **Do you smoke or are you frequently exposed to secondhand smoke?**
   - If you smoke, what type of product (cigarette, cigar, pipe) do you use?
   - How long have you smoked?
   - How many packs per day and what brand?
   - If you are exposed to secondhand smoke, where and for how long each day?
   - Did you ever smoke? When did you quit?

8. **Do you take any drugs such as cocaine?**
   - Do you drink alcohol? If so, describe the type, amount, frequency, and duration of use.

9. **Do you exercise? What type of exercise do you perform?**
   - How many times a week?
   - What is the duration of exercise?
   - The intensity?
   - What is your total exercising time?
   - Is the exercise continuous or interspersed with breaks?
   - What amount of aerobic exercise versus nonaerobic do you do?
   - Do you exercise with a partner or alone? Is the exercise pattern regular or sporadic?
   - What is your understanding about the benefits of exercise and the type of exercise selected?
   - What was your reason for choosing the specific exercise routines and patterns?
   - Is your exercise tolerance increasing, staying the same, or decreasing?
   - *If it is decreasing,* how has the tolerance decreased?
   - What were you able to do before versus now?
   - How rapidly has this change occurred?
   - What symptoms contribute to the decreased tolerance?
   - Do you know the causes?

RATIONALES

proper supervision, the poorly informed client may ingest an unbalanced proportion of supplements and compromise a healthy state. The nurse must be alert if the client has been dieting to reduce weight. Many diets deplete valuable electrolytes and subject the client to potential complications. Muscle wasting may occur if the diet is deficient in protein. Lack of protein may compromise cardiac function.

▶ Smoking has been linked to hypertension and is strongly suspected of contributing to injury in the walls of arteries, thus accelerating the development of atherosclerotic plaques. It is believed that the chemical contained in the cigarette smoke injures the inner wall of arterial vessels, thus contributing to the subsequent development of a coronary artery plaque.

▶ Substance abuse, especially of cocaine, is associated with coronary artery spasm and potential development of ischemia or injury of myocardial tissue.

▶ The benefits of exercise are well documented, yet the type, duration, and frequency of the exercise regimen produce variable results. It is important for the client to have a basic understanding of the benefits of aerobic versus nonaerobic exercise. One is not better than the other, and ultimately a blending of routines is invaluable whether the client is a well-conditioned athlete or an individual trying to stay healthy. Studies suggest that both aerobic exercise and resistance or weight training may increase high-density lipoprotein (HDL) levels in adult females.

QUESTIONS RELATED TO AGE

The focused interview must reflect the anatomical and physiological differences that exist along the age span. The following questions are examples of those that would be specific for children, the pregnant female, and the older adult.

FOCUSED INTERVIEW QUESTIONS	**RATIONALES**

QUESTIONS REGARDING INFANTS AND CHILDREN

1. **What was the pregnancy with this child like?**
   - During pregnancy, did you have any complications such as fever? If so, what were they?
   - What was done about them?
   - How was the infant affected?
   - How were the infant's complications treated?
   - Have the interventions helped?

▶ Complications during pregnancy may contribute to malformation in the infant or child.

2. **Did you smoke, take drugs, or drink alcohol during pregnancy? If so, describe substance, frequency, and amount.**
   - Did you take the substance early in pregnancy?
   - Did you take it right up to delivery?

▶ Smoking, recreational drugs such as cocaine, and alcohol may have significant effects on the development of the fetal cardiovascular system, especially in the first trimester.

3. **What is the child's energy level?**
   - HIs the child easily fatigued?
   - Does the child's nap seem to be longer than you would expect?

▶ Reduced energy levels and easy fatigability may suggest underlying cardiovascular abnormalities, such as atrial septal defect and large ventricular septal defect.

4. **Does the infant take a long time to feed?**
   - Does the infant seem tired after eating?
   - Does the child ever become short of breath? If so, what causes it?

▶ Fatigue can be related to congenital heart disease. It is especially noticeable during feeding.

5. **Does the infant or child favor squatting rather than sitting up straight?**

▶ The infant or child will squat when short of breath. It is currently believed that the squatting position decreases venous return to the right atrium from the legs.

6. **Does the child have symptoms of joint pain, headaches, fever, or respiratory infections?**

▶ Rheumatic fever may follow a respiratory infection with group A beta-hemolytic *streptococcus pyogenes* (strep throat) and produce symptoms of fever, swollen and painful joints, and headaches.

7. **Do you feel that the infant or child is gaining weight and growing as normal?**

▶ Failure to grow is associated with congenital heart disease, such as ventricular septal defect.

QUESTIONS FOR THE PREGNANT FEMALE

1. **Do you have any history of heart disease?**

▶ The changes of pregnancy can place the client with preexisting heart disease at risk.

2. **Has hypertension been apparent during this pregnancy?**
   - Is there a history of hypertension?

▶ Hypertension is a symptom of preeclampsia and places the mother and infant at risk.

3. **Have you observed any swelling in your face and hands?**
   - Have you experienced headaches or dizziness?

▶ Swelling can indicate a preeclamptic condition. Headaches and dizziness are associated with hypertension and preeclampsia. Preeclampsia can also be accompanied by chest pain, visual changes, and abdominal pain.

QUESTIONS FOR THE OLDER ADULT

All of the questions listed in the general section can offer significant data. In addition to the routine questions, the nurse should ask the following ones.

1. **Have you noticed any change—no matter how subtle—in your ability to concentrate, to remember things, or to perform simple mental tasks such as writing a letter or balancing your checkbook?**

▶ In the older adult, a change in mentation suggests inadequate perfusion and can be seen in clients with myocardial ischemia and infarction or increasingly severe congestive heart failure.

2. **Have you experienced reactions to any medications you are currently taking? These may include palpitations, rashes, vision changes, mentation changes, fatigue, or loss of previous sexual desire or function.**

▶ Many cardiovascular medications interact with medications for other diseases and may either potentiate or reduce their effects.

FOCUSED INTERVIEW QUESTIONS

RATIONALES

QUESTIONS RELATED TO THE ENVIRONMENT

Environment refers to both the internal and external environments. Questions related to the internal environment include all of the previous questions and those associated with internal or physiological responses. Questions regarding the external environment include those related to home, work, or social environments.

INTERNAL ENVIRONMENT

1. **What medications do you take?**
   - Are they prescribed or self-ordered?
   - What are the dose and brand of each medication?
   - How often do you take them?

   ► It is important to assess the client's knowledge, compliance, and ability to administer medication accurately, whether ordered by a physician or not. Medication actions may vary depending upon the mix of medications, diet, and additional supplementation.

2. **Why do you take these drugs?**

3. **Do you take these medications as prescribed?**
   - If you miss a dose, do you double up the next time?

4. **Who ordered these medications?**
   - If more than one person, does each know what the others have ordered?

5. **Do you know how the medications you are taking react with each other?**

6. **Do you know the side effects of the medications?**

7. **Are you experiencing any side effects that you think might be related to medications?**

8. **How would you describe your personality?**
   - How many hours do you work in a typical week? Do you work on weekends?
   - What do you do to unwind?
   - Describe the major stressors in your life.
   - What do you do to relieve stress?

   ► Having a type A personality is often associated with heart disease. It is not so much the behaviors, but the effect of constant sympathetic stimulation upon the cardiovascular system and the constant stress and drain on the rejuvenation process after a stressful event that may contribute to decompensation and vulnerability to disease processes. Excessive stress, no matter what the client's personality type, is a risk factor for cardiovascular disease.

The nurse should ask female clients the following questions.

1. **Do you take oral contraceptives?**

   ► If the client is over 35, takes oral contraceptives containing high doses of synthetic estrogen and progesterone, and smokes, the risk of developing cardiovascular disease increases significantly.

2. **Are you still menstruating?**
   - If not, at what age did menopause start?
   - Did you have a hysterectomy?
   - Were your ovaries removed?

   ► The earlier that menopause starts, the greater the risk for development of heart disease. New data suggests that coronary artery disease may be increased eightfold in the client who has had her ovaries removed before menopause.

EXTERNAL ENVIRONMENT

The following questions deal with substances and irritants found in the physical environment of the client. That includes the indoor and outdoor environments of the home and the workplace, those encountered for social engagements, and any encountered during travel.

FOCUSED INTERVIEW QUESTIONS

RATIONALES

1. **What is your present occupation?**

   ▶ Jobs with long hours, stress, deadlines, and tension are thought to contribute to the development of cardiovascular disease.

2. **What were your previous occupations?**
   - What is your work environment like?

3. **Have you been exposed to passive smoking in your environment?**

   ▶ Inhalation of secondhand cigarette smoke in a closed environment is currently thought to contribute to the development of coronary artery plaque.

4. **Have you been exposed to chemicals or other hazardous substances?**

   ▶ Such exposure may correlate to stress, alterations in eating habits and exercise habits, recreational drug use, and alterations in sleep patterns.

CLIENT INTERACTION

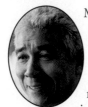

Mr. Ameen Abo-Hamzy reports to the office of his internist for his yearly physical examination. He is 53 years old and has worked for the same company for 22 years. At this time, he is part of the management team and is concerned regarding company layoffs and general downsizing. He tells the nurse, "I feel fine. I think I'm in good health. I have an occasional gas bubble or pressure right here [pointing to the xiphoid process on his chest] and then I can sometimes feel my heart beat real fast." The following is an excerpt from the focused interview with Mr. Abo-Hamzy:

INTERVIEW

Nurse: Good morning, Mr. Abo-Hamzy. I see from the record you were last here a year ago for your physical.

Mr. Abo-Hamzy: Yes, that is right.

Nurse: Let's talk about your state of health.

Mr. Abo-Hamzy: I consider myself a really healthy person. I haven't missed a day of work all year. I never got a cold when everybody at work seemed to catch one this past winter. It is just the pressure that I get right here.

Again, Mr. Abo-Hamzy points to the xiphoid process on his chest.

Nurse: Tell me more about this pressure.

Mr. Abo-Hamzy: It is just here, and not all the time.

Nurse: Does the pressure get worse before or after you eat?

Mr. Abo-Hamzy: I have not noticed any change when I eat.

Nurse: When do you notice the change?

Mr. Abo-Hamzy: I'm usually at work. I can always count on the pressure starting either during or after our management meetings.

Nurse: Do you find work stressful these days?

Mr. Abo-Hamzy: I guess you could call it that. Somebody is always getting a pink slip, you know being let go. I don't know what I will do if it happens to me. I have a family, a mortgage, and I carry the health insurance for all of us. My wife tells me I worry too much.

Nurse: And you? Do you think you worry too much?

ANALYSIS

Throughout the interview the nurse used open-ended and closed statements to collect detailed subjective data from Mr. Abo-Hamzy. The client mentioned subxiphoid pressure several times. The nurse picked up on this cue, sought clarification, ruled out gastrointestinal involvement, and ascertained the source of the pressure as being stress related before discussing another concern. The nurse used open-ended statements allowing Mr. Abo-Hamzy to discuss pertinent information about his chest discomfort. The nurse stayed with one topic before directing the response to another area of concern.

Please refer to the Companion Website at **www.prenhall.com/damico** and click on Chapter 17, the **Client Interaction** module, to answer questions about this case. In addition, see other resources for this chapter including NCLEX review questions and other interactive exercises and materials.

ASSESSMENT TECHNIQUES AND FINDINGS

Physical assessment of the cardiovascular system requires the use of inspection, palpation, percussion, and auscultation. During each of the procedures, the nurse is gathering objective data related to the function of the heart as determined by the heart rate and the quality and characteristics of the heart sounds. In addition, the nurse observes for signs of appropriate cardiac function in relation to oxygen perfusion by assessing skin color and temperature, abnormal pulsations, and the characteristics of the client's respiratory effort. Knowledge of normal parameters and expected findings is essential in determining the meaning of the data during a physical health assessment.

Adults have uniform skin color on the face, trunk, and extremities. The eyes are symmetrical. The periorbital area is flat, and the eyes do not bulge. The sclera of the eye should be white, the cornea clear, and the conjunctiva pink. The lips should be smooth and noncyanotic. The head should be steady and the skull proportional to the face. The earlobe should be smooth and without creases. The jugular veins are not visible when the chest is upright. Further, the jugular veins distend only 3 cm above the sternal angle when the client is at a 45-degree angle. Carotid pulsations are visible bilaterally. The fingers should be round and even with flat pink nails. The respiratory pattern is even, regular, and unlabored. Intercostal spaces and clavicles are visible; chest veins are evenly distributed and flat; no bulges or masses are visible. Pulsations over the pericardium are absent; however, aortic pulsations in the epigastric area are visible in thin clients. The lower extremities are of uniform color and temperature with even hair distribution. The skeleton should be free of deformity and the neck and extremities in proportion to the torso. Palpation over the pericardium reveals slight vibration at the apical area only. Carotid pulses are palpable and equal in intensity. Dullness to percussion should extend to the midclavicular line at the fifth intercostal space. S_2 is louder than S_1 at the aortic and pulmonic auscultatory areas. S_1 and S_2 are heard equally at Erb's point (third left intercostal space). S_1 is louder than S_2 at the tricuspid and apical areas. Murmurs are absent. The carotid pulse is synchronous with the apical pulse.

Physical assessment of the cardiovascular system follows an organized pattern. It begins with inspection of the client's head and neck, including eyes, ears, lips, face, skull, and neck vessels. The upper extremities, chest, abdomen, and lower extremities are also inspected. Palpation includes the precordium and carotid pulses. Percussion of the chest is conducted to determine the cardiac borders. Auscultation includes the heart in five areas with the diaphragm and the bell of the stethoscope. The carotid arteries and the apical pulse are auscultated.

EQUIPMENT

examination gown	metric rulers
examination drape	doppler
stethoscope	lamp

HELPFUL HINTS

- Provide specific instructions throughout the assessment. Explain what is expected of the client and state that he or she will be able to breathe regularly throughout the examination.
- Assessment of the heart will require several position changes; the nurse should assist the client if necessary; allow time for movement if the client is uncomfortable; and explain the purpose of the position change.
- The nurse's hands and the stethoscope should be warmed before beginning the examination.
- The room should be quiet so that subtle sounds may be heard.
- Provide adequate draping to prevent unnecessary exposure of the female breasts.
- Use Standard Precautions.

TECHNIQUES AND NORMAL FINDINGS

ABNORMAL FINDINGS SPECIAL CONSIDERATIONS

INSPECTION

1. **Instruct the client.**

   - Explain that you will be looking at the head, neck, and extremities to provide clues to cardiac function.

TECHNIQUES AND NORMAL FINDINGS	ABNORMAL FINDINGS SPECIAL CONSIDERATIONS

- Explain that you will ask the client to sit up and lie down as part of the examination and that you will provide specific instructions and assistance as required throughout the examination. Explain that you will be touching the neck and chest, as well as tapping on the chest and listening with the stethoscope. Tell the client that none of the procedures should cause discomfort but assure the client that you will stop any time if discomfort occurs or the examination is causing fatigue.

2. **Position the client.**

- Begin the examination with the client seated upright with the chest exposed (see Figure 17.15 ●).

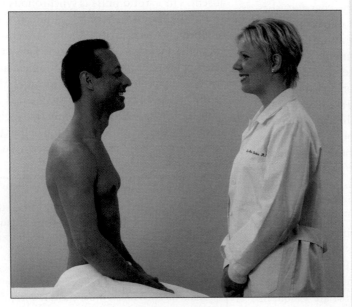

Figure 17.15 ●
The client is positioned for the examination.

3. **Inspect the client's face, lips, ears, and scalp.**

- These structures can provide valuable clues to the client's cardiovascular health. Begin with the facial skin. The skin color should be uniform.

  ▶ Flushed skin may indicate rheumatic heart disease or presence of a fever. Grayish undertones are often seen in clients with coronary artery disease or those in shock. A ruddy color may indicate *polycythemia*, a condition in which there is a significantly increased number of red blood cells, or *Cushing's syndrome*, which is excessive secretion of adrenocorticotropic hormone (ACTH) by the pituitary gland.

- Examine the eyes and the tissue surrounding the eyes (periorbital area). The eyes should be uniform and not have a protruding appearance.

  ▶ Protruding eyes are seen in *hyperthyroidism*. In hyperthyroidism, excessive hormone secretion results in high cardiac output, a tendency toward tachycardia (rapid heart rate), and potential for congestive heart failure.

- The periorbital area should be relatively flat. No puffiness should be present.

  ▶ Periorbital puffiness may result from fluid retention (edema) or valvular disease.

TECHNIQUES AND NORMAL FINDINGS	ABNORMAL FINDINGS SPECIAL CONSIDERATIONS

- The sclera should be whitish in color. The cornea should be without an *arcus*, which is a ringlike structure.

▶ A blue color in the sclera is often associated with **Marfan's syndrome,** a degenerative disease of the connective tissue, which over time may cause the ascending aorta to either dilate or dissect, leading to abrupt death. An arcus in a young person may indicate hypercholesterolemia; however, in people of African descent it may be normal.

- The conjunctiva should be clear, while underlying tissue is pinkish in color. The eyelid should be smooth. For information on how to examine the conjunctiva, see Chapter 13. ⬭

▶ **Xanthelasma** are yellowish cholesterol deposits seen on the eyelids and are indicative of premature atherosclerosis.

- Inspect the lips. They should be uniform in color without any underlying tinge of blueness. The buccal mucosa, gums, and tongue are also inspected for cyanosis.

▶ Blue-tinged lips may indicate cyanosis, which is often a late sign of inadequate tissue perfusion.

- Assess the general appearance of the face. It should be symmetrical with uniform contours.

▶ Clients with *Down syndrome* may exhibit a large protruding tongue, low-set ears, and an underdeveloped mandible. Children with Down syndrome often have congenital heart disease. Wide-set eyes may be seen in a child with *Noonan's syndrome*, which is accompanied by pulmonic stenosis (narrowing).

- Examine the head. Look first for the ability of the client to hold the head steady. Rhythmic head bobbing should not be present.

▶ Head bobbing up and down in synchrony with the heartbeat is characteristic of severe aortic regurgitation. This bobbing is created by the pulsatile waves of regurgitated blood, which reverberate upward toward the head.

- Assess the structure of the skull and the proportion of the skull to the face.

▶ A protruding skull is seen in *Paget's disease*, a rare bone disease characterized by localized loss of calcium from the bone and replacement with a porous bone formation, which leads to distorted, thickened contours. Paget's disease is also characterized by a high cardiac output, which may lead to heart failure.

- Examine the client's earlobes. The earlobes should be relatively smooth without the presence of creases unless an injury has been sustained.

▶ Bilateral earlobe creases, especially in the young adult, are often associated with coronary artery disease.

4. **Inspect the jugular veins.**

- Examination of the jugular veins can provide essential information about the client's central venous pressure and the heart's pumping efficiency.
- With the client sitting upright, adjust the gooseneck lamp to cast shadows on the client's neck. Tangential lighting is effective in visualizing the jugular vessels.
- Be sure that the client's head is turned slightly away from the side you are examining. Look for the external and internal jugular veins.
- Note that the jugular veins are not normally visible when the client sits upright. The external jugular vein is located over the sternocleidomastoid muscle. The internal jugular vein, which is the best indicator of central venous pressure, is located behind this muscle, medial to the external jugular and lateral to the carotid artery.

TECHNIQUES AND NORMAL FINDINGS

ABNORMAL FINDINGS SPECIAL CONSIDERATIONS

- If you are able to visualize the jugular veins, measure their distance superior to the clavicle. (Be sure not to confuse the carotid pulse with pulsations of the jugular veins.) The carotid pulse is lateral to the trachea. If jugular vein pulsations are visible, palpate the client's radial pulse and determine if these pulsations coincide with the palpated radial pulse.

- Next, have the client lie at a 45-degree angle if the client can tolerate this position without pain and is able to breathe comfortably.

- Place the first of the metric rulers vertically at the angle of Louis. Place the second metric ruler horizontally at a 90-degree angle to the first ruler. One end of this ruler should be at the angle of Louis and the other end in the jugular area on the lateral aspect of the neck (see Figure 17.16 ●).

▶ Obvious pulsations that are present during inspiration and expiration and coincide with the arterial pulse are commonly seen with severe congestive heart failure.

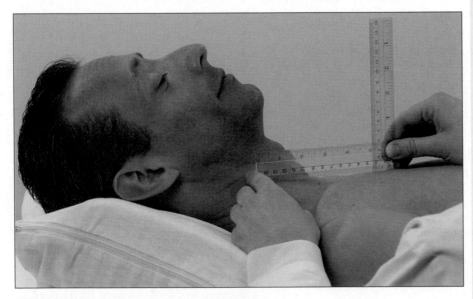

Figure 17.16 ● Assessment of central venous pressure.

- Inspect the neck for distention of the jugular veins. Raise the lateral portion of the horizontal ruler until it is at the top of the height of the distention and assess the height in centimeters of the elevation from the vertical ruler.

- The jugular veins normally distend only 3 cm above the sternal angle when the client is lying at a 45-degree angle (Figure 17.16). You need to measure the distention only on one side.

▶ Distention of the neck veins indicates elevation of central venous pressure commonly seen with congestive heart failure, fluid overload, or pressure on the superior vena cava.

5. **Inspect the carotid arteries.**
   - The carotid arteries are located lateral to the client's trachea in a groove that is medial to the sternocleidomastoid muscle.
   - With the client still lying at a 45-degree angle, using tangential lighting, inspect the carotid arteries for pulsations. Pulsations should be visible bilaterally.
   - When you finish, help the client back to an upright sitting position.

▶ Bounding pulses are not normal findings and may indicate fever. The absence of a pulsation may indicate an obstruction either internal or external to the artery.

| TECHNIQUES AND NORMAL FINDINGS | ABNORMAL FINDINGS SPECIAL CONSIDERATIONS |

TECHNIQUES AND NORMAL FINDINGS

6. Inspect the client's hands and fingers.

- Help the client to resume a sitting position. Confirm that the fingertips are rounded and even. The fingernails should be relatively pink, with white crescents at the base of each nail.

- Assess for Marfan's syndrome. Ask the client to make a fist by wrapping the fingers over the thumb. You can also assess for this syndrome by having the client wrap the thumb and little finger around the opposite wrist.

7. Inspect the client's chest.

- Observe the respiratory pattern, which should be even, regular, and unlabored, with no retractions.

- Observe the veins on the chest, which should be evenly distributed and relatively flat.

- Inspect the entire chest for bulges and masses. The intercostal spaces and clavicles should be even.

- Inspect the entire chest for pulsations. Observe the client first in an upright position and then at a 30-degree angle, which is a low- to mid-Fowler's position. In particular, observe for pulsations over the five key landmarks (see Figure 17.18 ●).

ABNORMAL FINDINGS SPECIAL CONSIDERATIONS

▶ Fingertips and nails that are clubbed bilaterally are characteristic of congenital heart disease. Clubbing may be associated with cyanosis or long-term tobacco smoking. Thin red lines or splinter hemorrhages in the nail beds are associated with **infective endocarditis** (see Figure 17.17 ●), a condition caused by bacterial infiltration of the lining of the heart's chambers.

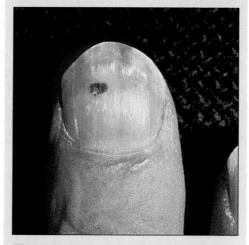

Figure 17.17 ● Splinter hemorrhage.

Fingernails and tips may be stained yellow when the client is a smoker. Smoking is one of the main contributors to the development of atherosclerosis.

▶ If the thumb is readily visible outside of the clenched fist or if the little finger extends at least 1 cm beyond the thumb, Marfan's syndrome should be suspected.

▶ Respiratory distress may be precipitated by various disorders. Pulmonary edema is often a severe complication of cardiovascular disease.

▶ Dilated, distended veins on the chest indicate an obstructive process, as seen with obstruction of the superior vena cava.

▶ Bulges are abnormal and may indicate obstructions or aneurysms. Masses may indicate obstructions or presence of tumors.

▶ If the entire *precordium* (anterior chest) pulsates and shakes with every heartbeat, extreme valvular regurgitation or shunting may be present.

TECHNIQUES AND NORMAL FINDINGS	ABNORMAL FINDINGS SPECIAL CONSIDERATIONS

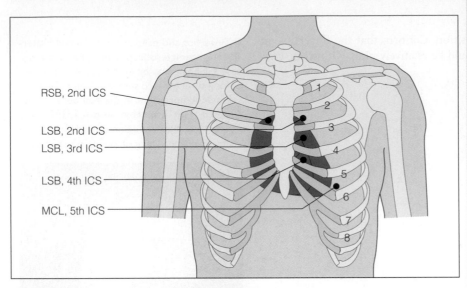

Figure 17.18 ● Landmarks in precordial assessments.

- Start by observing the right sternal border (RSB), second ICS. Next, observe the left sternal border (LSB), second ICS.

- Then observe the LSB, third to fifth ICS.
  - Move on to the apex: fifth ICS, midclavicular line (MCL).
  - Finish with the epigastric area, below the xiphoid process.

- Confirm that the apical impulse/*point of maximum impulse* (PMI) is located at the fifth ICS in the left MCL.

- Inspect the entire chest for heaves or lifts while the client is sitting upright and again with the client at a 30-degree angle.
  - *Heaves* or *lifts* are forceful risings of the landmark area.

- In particular, make sure you observe over the five key landmarks previously listed.

8. **Inspect the client's abdomen.**
   - Have the client lie flat, if possible.
     - Be mindful of any discomfort or difficulty in breathing.
   - Look for pulsations in the abdominal area over the areas where the major arteries are located. These sites include:
     - The *aorta*, which is located superior to the umbilicus to the left of the midline.
     - The *left renal artery*, which is located to the left of the umbilicus in the left upper quadrant.
     - The *right renal artery*, which is located to the right of the umbilicus in the right upper quadrant.
     - The *right iliac artery*, which is located to the right of the umbilicus in the right lower quadrant.
     - The *left iliac artery*, which is located to the left of the umbilicus in the left lower quadrant.

▶ Pulsations present in the LSB, second ICS indicate pulmonary artery dilation or excessive blood flow.

▶ Pulsations present in the LSB, third to fifth ICS may indicate right ventricular overload.

▶ If left ventricular hypertrophy is present, the PMI is displaced laterally from the fifth ICS, LMCL.

▶ A heave or lift found in the LSB, third to fifth ICS may indicate right ventricular hypertrophy or respiratory disease, such as pulmonary hypertension.

▶ Pulsations may be visible in lean clients. These are usually normal if seen in the epigastric area. Peristaltic waves may also be seen in thin individuals. They must not be confused with vascular pulsations. Prominent pulsations that are located in areas outside of the gastric area and are readily visible may be potentially life threatening.

▶ Abnormal pulsations usually indicate the presence of aortic aneurysm, which is a ballooning due to a weakness in the walls of arteries. These findings require immediate physician referral.

| TECHNIQUES AND NORMAL FINDINGS | ABNORMAL FINDINGS SPECIAL CONSIDERATIONS |

- (Chapter 19 of this text reviews abdominal arteries and abdominal quadrants.) ⚭
- Note the pattern of fat distribution.

▶ Males usually deposit fat in the abdominal area. This distribution pattern is thought to be associated with the development of coronary artery disease. Females usually deposit fat in the buttocks and thighs.

9. **Inspect the client's legs.**
   - Help the client to a sitting position.
   - Inspect the legs for skin color. The skin color should be even and uniform.
   - Inspect the legs for hair distribution. The distribution should be even without bare patches devoid of hair.

▶ Patches of lighter color may indicate compromised circulation. Mottling indicates severe hemodynamic compromise.
▶ Patchy hair distribution is often a sign of circulatory compromise that has occurred over time. The client should be asked if the hair distribution on the legs has changed over time.

10. **Inspect the client's skeletal structure.**
    - Ask the client to stand.
    - Observe the skeletal structure, which should be free of deformities.
    - Observe the neck and extremities, which should be in proportion to the torso.

▶ *Scoliosis* is associated with prolapsed mitral valve.
▶ A client who is tall and thin with an elongated neck and extremities should be evaluated further for the presence of Marfan's syndrome.

PALPATION

Palpate the chest in the six areas. Palpate each area with the client exhaling, and finally with the client holding the breath (if the client is able to do so). Note that palpation may be performed with the client sitting upright, reclining at a 45-degree or 30-degree angle, or lying flat. Start by palpating with the client sitting upright and then in the lowest position that the client can comfortably tolerate (see Figure 17.19 ●)

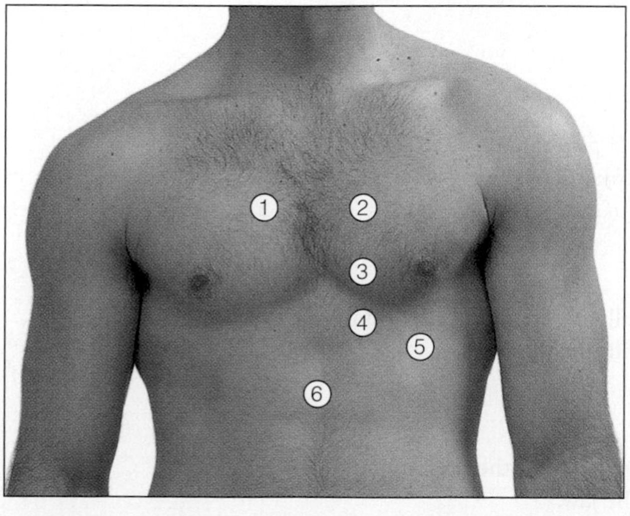

Figure 17.19 ●
Landmarks for palpation of the chest.

TECHNIQUES AND NORMAL FINDINGS	ABNORMAL FINDINGS SPECIAL CONSIDERATIONS

1. Palpate the chest.

- Place your right hand over the RSB, second ICS. Palpate with the base of your fingers.

  ▶ Pulsations or heaves in the RSB, second ICS, indicate the presence of ascending aortic enlargement or aneurysm, aortic stenosis, or systemic hypertension.

- You should not feel any pulsation, heave, or vibratory sensation against your palm in this location.
- Place your hand on the LSB, second ICS.

  ▶ Pulsations or heaves in the LSB, second ICS, are associated with pulmonary hypertension, pulmonary stenosis, right ventricular enlargement, atrial septal defect, enlarged left atrium, and large posterior left ventricular aneurysm.

- You should not feel any pulsation, heave, or vibratory sensation against your palm in this location except in some very thin clients who are nervous about the examination.
- Move your hand to the LSB, third then fourth ICS. No pulsations, heaves, or vibratory sensations should be felt.

  ▶ Pulsations or heaves over the LSB, third or fourth ICS, may indicate right ventricular enlargement or pressure overload on this ventricle, pulmonary stenosis, or pulmonary hypertension.

- Place your right hand over the apex: MCL, fifth ICS.
- When palpating over the MCL, fifth ICS, you should feel a soft vibration, a tapping sensation, with each heartbeat. The vibration felt in this location should be isolated to an area no more than 1 cm in diameter.

  ▶ The presence of a heave, which is a forceful thrust over the fifth ICS, MCL, indicates the potential presence of increased right ventricular stroke volume or pressure and mild to moderate aortic regurgitation. If vibration is felt in a downward and lateral position from where the normal PMI should be palpated, or if it can be palpated in an area greater than 1 cm in diameter, these conditions may be present: left ventricular hypertrophy, severe left ventricular volume overload, or severe aortic regurgitation.

- Palpate the epigastric area, below the xiphoid process.

  ▶ The presence of heaves or thrills in the subxiphoid area suggests the presence of elevated right ventricular volume or pressure overload. **Thrills** are soft vibratory sensations best assessed with either the fingertips or the palm flattened on the chest.

- Repeat the palpation technique, with the client at either a 30-degree angle or lying flat.

ALERT!

Some clients are unable to lie flat. The client should be placed in the lowest angle that is comfortably tolerated. It is necessary to be alert to any physical distress experienced by the client during examination and stop activity immediately if distress is experienced.

- Palpation with the client lying flat normally reveals either no pulsation or very faint taps in a very localized area. No thrills, heaves, or lifts should be palpated in any of the five locations.

2. Palpate the client's carotid pulses.

- The carotid artery is located in the groove between the trachea and sternocleidomastoid muscle beneath the angle of the jaw.
- It is important to palpate carotid pulses to assess their presence, strength, and equality. The client may remain supine, or you may help the client to sit upright.
- Ask the client to look straight ahead and keep the neck straight (see Figure 17.20 ●).

| TECHNIQUES AND NORMAL FINDINGS | ABNORMAL FINDINGS SPECIAL CONSIDERATIONS |

TECHNIQUES AND NORMAL FINDINGS

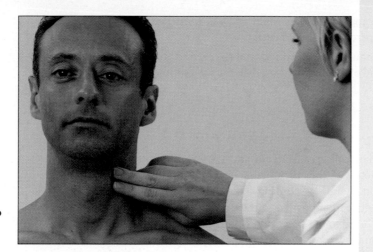

Figure 17.20 ●
Palpating the
carotid artery.

- Palpate each carotid pulse separately. Normal findings bilaterally should demonstrate equality in intensity and regular pattern. The pulses should be strong but not bounding. If the pulse is difficult to palpate, ask the client to turn the head slightly to the examining side.

ALERT!

The carotid pulses must never be palpated simultaneously since this may obstruct blood flow to the brain, resulting in severe bradycardia *(slow heart rate) or* asystole *(absent heart rate).*

PERCUSSION

1. **Percuss the client's chest to determine the cardiac border.**
   - Help the client to a reclining position at the lowest angle the client can tolerate.
   - Place the middle finger of your nondominant hand (pleximeter) in the fifth ICS at the left anterior axillary line.
   - Tap this finger at the distal phalanx, using the plexor of your dominant hand (see Figure 17.21 ●). You should hear resonance because you are over lung tissue.

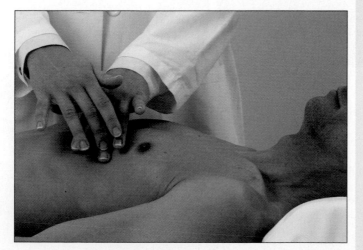

Figure 17.21 ●
Percussing the
chest.

▶ Diminished or absent carotid pulses may be found in clients with carotid disease or dissecting ascending aneurysm. Absence of both pulses indicates *asystole* (absent heart rate). If the client is in critical care and has an arterial line, a printout of the arterial waveform should be obtained.

▶ An enlarged heart emits a dull sound on percussion over a larger area than a heart of normal size. An x-ray film of the chest provides the most accurate information about the size of the client's heart.

- Continue to percuss in the fifth ICS toward the left MCL and the LSB. The sound will change to dullness as you percuss over the heart.
- Repeat the previous percussion technique in the third ICS and the second ICS on the left side of the thorax. The sound of resonance heard over the lung should change to dullness over the heart.

AUSCULTATION

The position of the client affects objective data collected from auscultatory examination. A full examination includes auscultation with the client sitting upright, leaning forward when upright, supine, and in the left lateral position. Have the client breathe normally initially. If you recognize the presence of abnormal sounds, have the client slow down the respirations so that you may listen to the effects of inspirations and expiratory efforts on the heart sounds. You may want to have some clients perform a forced expiration. When preparing to auscultate a child's chest, you may want to let the child listen to the parent's heart sounds with the stethoscope to reduce or prevent fear of this unfamiliar object. Use a stethoscope with a smaller bell and diaphragm when you examine a child.

1. **Auscultate the client's chest with the diaphragm of the stethoscope.**
   - Start the auscultation with the client sitting upright.
   - Inch the stethoscope slowly across the chest and listen over each of the five key landmarks (see Figure 17.22 ●).

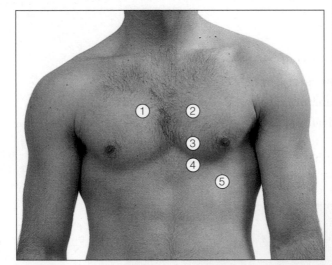

Figure 17.22 ●
Auscultating the chest over five key landmarks.

- Listen over the RSB, second ICS.
- In this location, the S_2 sound should be louder than the S_1 sound, because this site is over the aortic valve.
- Listen over the LSB, second ICS.
- Also in this location the S_2 sound should be louder than the S_1 sound, because this site is over the pulmonic valve.

TECHNIQUES AND NORMAL FINDINGS	ABNORMAL FINDINGS SPECIAL CONSIDERATIONS

TECHNIQUES AND NORMAL FINDINGS

- Listen over the LSB, third ICS, also called Erb's point.
- You should hear both the S_1 and S_2 heart tones, relatively equal in intensity.
- Listen at the LSB at the fourth ICS.
- In this location the S_1 sound should be louder than the S_2 sound, because the closure of the tricuspid valve is best auscultated here.
- Listen over the apex: fifth ICS, LMCL.
- In this location the S_1 sound should also be louder than the S_2 sound, because the closure of the mitral valve is best auscultated here.

2. Auscultate the client's chest with the bell of the stethoscope.
- Place the bell of the stethoscope lightly on each of the five key landmark positions shown with step 1.
- Listen for softer sounds over the five key landmarks. Start with the bell and listen for the S_3 and S_4 sounds. Then listen for murmurs.

3. Auscultate the carotid arteries.
- Listen with the diaphragm and bell of the stethoscope. Have the client hold the breath briefly. You may hear heart tones. This finding is normal.
- You should not hear any turbulent sounds like murmurs.

4. Compare the apical pulse to a carotid pulse.
- Auscultate the apical pulse.
- Simultaneously palpate a carotid pulse.
- Compare the findings. The two pulses should be synchronous. The carotid artery is used because it is closest to the heart and most accessible (see Figure 17.23 ●).

ABNORMAL FINDINGS / SPECIAL CONSIDERATIONS

▶ Low-pitched sounds are best auscultated with light application of the bell. Sounds such as S_3, S_4, murmurs (originating from stenotic valves), and gallops are best heard with the bell.

▶ A **bruit,** a loud blowing sound, is an abnormal finding. It is most often associated with a narrowing or stricture of the carotid artery usually associated with atherosclerotic plaque.

▶ An apical pulse greater than the carotid rate indicates a pulse deficit. The rate, rhythm, and regularity must be evaluated.

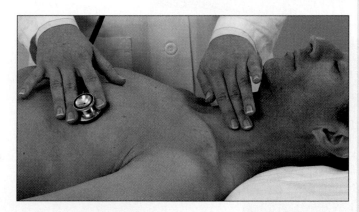

Figure 17.23 ● Comparing the carotid and apical pulses.

5. Repeat the auscultation of the client's chest.
- This time have the client lean forward, then lie supine, and finally lie in the left lateral position. Remember, not all clients will be able to tolerate all positions. In such cases, do not perform the technique (see Figure 17.24 A-C ●).

TECHNIQUES AND NORMAL FINDINGS

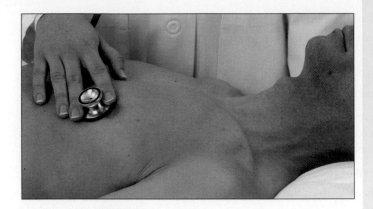

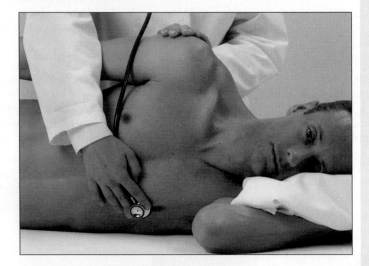

Figure 17.24A ●
Positions for
auscultation of the
heart. A. Supine.

Figure 17.24B ●
Positions for
auscultation of the
heart. B. Lateral.

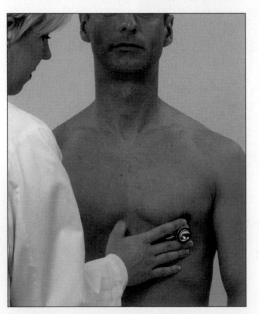

Figure 17.24C ●
Positions for
auscultation of the
heart. C. Sitting.

 Refer to the Companion Website at **www.prenhall.com/damico** and click on the **Documentation** module for documentation
samples and documentation practice exercises.

Abnormal findings in the cardiovascular system include murmurs (see Table 17.4), diseases of the myocardium and pumping capacity, valvular heart disease, septal defects, congenital heart disease, and electrical rhythm disturbances.

DISEASES OF THE MYOCARDIUM AND PUMPING CAPACITY OF THE HEART

Myocardial Ischemia

Ischemia is a common problem where the oxygen needs of the body are heightened, thus increasing the work of the heart. Unfortunately, the oxygen needs of the heart are not met as it works harder, and an ischemic process ensues. Ischemia is usually due to the presence of an atherosclerotic plaque. A blood clot may be associated with the plaque.

Myocardial Infarction

During infarction, there is complete disruption of oxygen and nutrient flow to the myocardial tissue in the area below a total occlusion. Infarction leads to the death of the myocardial tissue unless flow of blood is reestablished.

Congestive Heart Disease

This condition is the inability of the heart to produce a sufficient pumping effort. Most commonly, both right-sided and left-sided heart failure are present. Left-sided heart failure causes blood to back up into the pulmonary system and results in pulmonary edema. Right-sided heart failure causes backup of the blood into the systemic circulation and leads to distended neck veins, liver congestion, and peripheral edema.

left = lungs
right = edema

Ventricular Hypertrophy

Ventricular hypertrophy occurs in response to pumping against high pressures. Right ventricular hypertrophy occurs with pulmonary hypertension, congenital heart disease, pulmonary disease, pulmonary stenosis, and right ventricular infarction.

Left ventricular hypertrophy occurs in the presence of systemic hypertension, congenital heart disease, aortic stenosis, or myocardial infarction to the left ventricle.

VALVULAR DISEASE

Valvular Heart Disease

Disease of the valves denotes either narrowing (stenosis) of the valve leaflets or incompetence (regurgitation) of these same leaflets. Valvular disease may be caused by rheumatic fever, congenital defects, myocardial infarction, and normal aging.

Mitral Stenosis

Mitral stenosis is a narrowing of the left mitral valve (see Figure 17.25 ●).

Etiology: Rheumatic fever or cardiac infection.

Findings: Murmur heard at the apical area with the client in left lateral position.

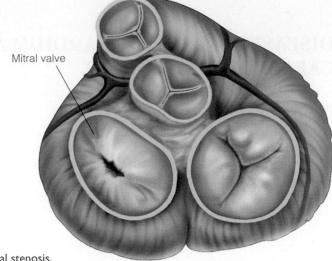

Figure 17.25 ● Mitral stenosis.

Aortic Stenosis

Aortic stenosis is a narrowing of the aortic valve (see Figure 17.26 ●).

Etiology: Congenital bicuspid valves, rheumatic heart disease, atherosclerosis.

Findings: Murmur at aortic area, RSB, second ICS.

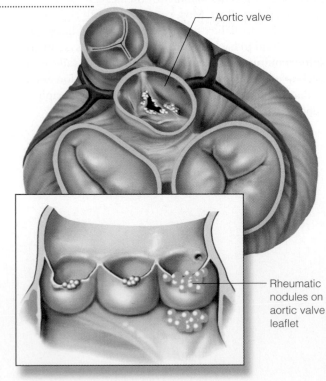

Figure 17.26 ● Aortic stenosis.

Mitral Regurgitation

Mitral regurgitation is the backflow of blood from the left ventricle into the left atrium (see Figure 17.27 ●).

Etiology: Rheumatic fever, myocardial infarction, rupture of chordae tendineae.

Findings: Murmur at apex. Sound is transmitted to (L) axillae.

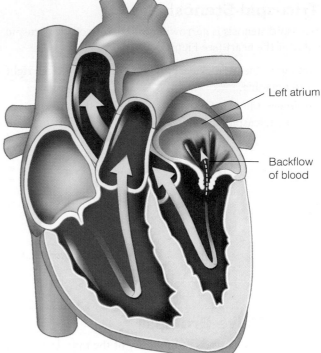

Figure 17.27 ● Mitral regurgitation.

Pulmonic Stenosis

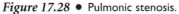

Pulmonic stenosis is narrowing of the opening between the pulmonary artery and the right ventricle (see Figure 17.28 ●).

Etiology: Congenital.

Findings: Murmur at pulmonic area radiates to neck. Thrill in (L) second and third ICS.

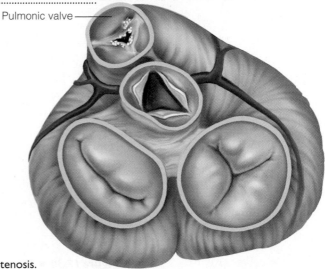

Figure 17.28 ● Pulmonic stenosis.

Tricuspid Stenosis

Tricuspid stenosis is narrowing or stricture of the tricuspid value of the heart (see Figure 17.29 ●).

Etiology: Rheumatic heart disease, congenital defect, right atrial myxoma.

Findings: Murmur heard with the bell of the stethoscope over the tricuspid area.

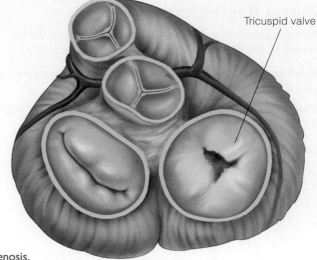

Tricuspid valve

Figure 17.29 ● Tricuspid stenosis.

Mitral Valve Prolapse

Mitral valve prolapse is redundancy of the mitral valve leaflets so they prolapse into the left atrium (see Figure 17.30 ●).

Etiology: May occur with pectus excavatum often unknown.

Findings: Murmur heard (L) lower sternal border in upright position.

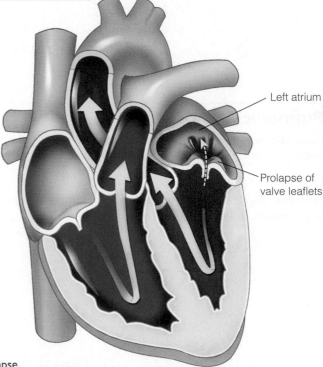

Left atrium

Prolapse of valve leaflets

Figure 17.30 ● Mitral valve prolapse.

Aortic Regurgitation

Aortic regurgitation is the backflow of blood from the aorta into the left ventricle (see Figure 17.31 ●).

Etiology: Rheumatic heart disease, endocarditis, Marfan's syndrome, syphilis.

Findings: Murmur with client leaning forward. Click in second ICS.

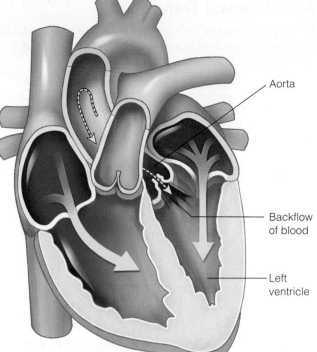

Figure 17.31 ● Aortic regurgitation.

SEPTAL DEFECTS

An atrial septal defect is an opening between the right and left atria, whereas a ventricular septal defect is an opening between the right and left ventricles. Both of these septal defects may result from congenital heart disease and myocardial infarction.

Ventricular Septal Defect

Regurgitation occurs through the defect resulting in a holosystolic murmur (see Figure 17.32 ●). The murmur is loud, coarse, high-pitched, and heard at the LSB, third to fifth ICS.

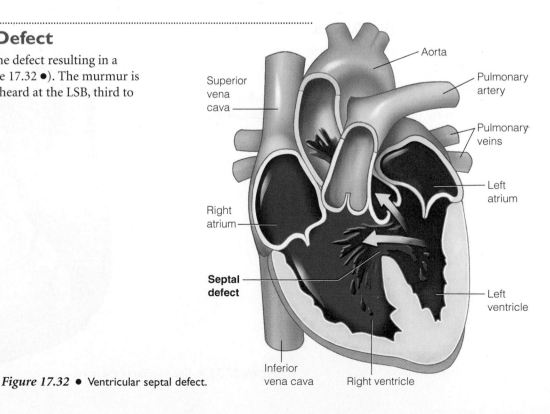

Figure 17.32 ● Ventricular septal defect.

Atrial Septal Defect

Regurgitation occurs through the defect resulting in a harsh, loud, high-pitched murmur heard at the LSB, second ICS (see Figure 17.33 ●).

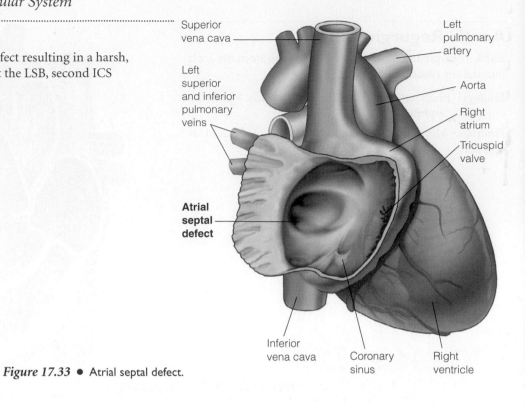

Figure 17.33 ● Atrial septal defect.

CONGENITAL HEART DISEASE

There are many forms of congenital heart disease, which is related to developmental defects. Most often valves and septal structures are affected.

Coarctation of the Aorta

In this condition, the aorta is severely narrowed in the region inferior to the left subclavian artery (see Figure 17.34 ●). The narrowing restricts blood flow from the left ventricle into the aorta and out into the systemic circulation, thus contributing to the development of congestive heart failure in the newborn. It can be surgically treated.

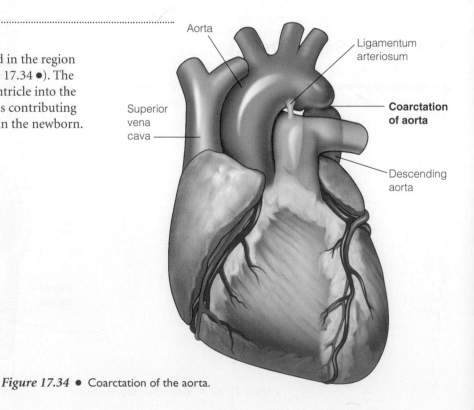

Figure 17.34 ● Coarctation of the aorta.

Patent Ductus Arteriosus

The ductus arteriosus is an opening between the aorta and pulmonary artery that is present in the fetus. This opening should spontaneously close permanently between 24 and 48 hours after delivery. If this closure does not occur completely, a condition called patent ductus arteriosus exists (see Figure 17.35 ●). It may be treated medically, through pharmacologic therapy, and surgically.

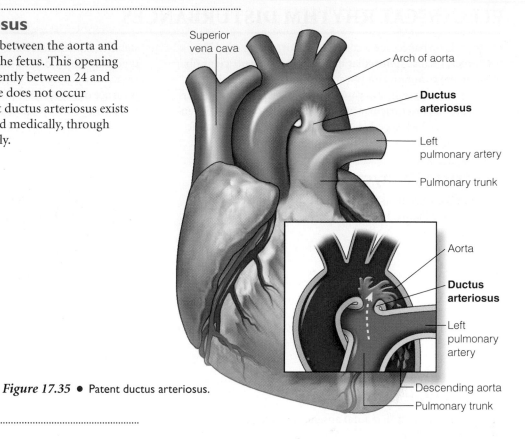

Figure 17.35 ● Patent ductus arteriosus.

Tetralogy of Fallot

The condition involves four cardiac defects: dextroposition of the aorta, pulmonary stenosis, right ventricular hypertrophy, and ventricular septal defect (see Figure 17.36 ●). This condition is life threatening for the newborn but can be treated surgically.

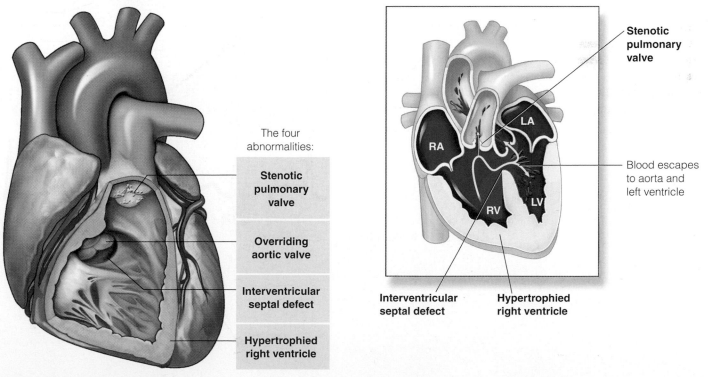

Figure 17.36 ● Tetralogy of Fallot.

ELECTRICAL RHYTHM DISTURBANCES

Rhythm disturbances are a common occurrence. Lethal dysrhythmias, such as ventricular tachycardia and ventricular fibrillation, are common complications of myocardial ischemia, myocardial infarction, and cardiomegaly. Heart blocks, such as first-degree atrioventricular block and second-degree atrioventricular heart block type 1, rarely compromise hemodynamic stability. However, second-degree atrioventricular heart block type 2 and third-degree atrioventricular heart block can significantly compromise hemodynamic stability, especially in the presence of myocardial infarction. Young individuals, mostly males, may suffer from tachycardias when extraconducting structures are present. These may be fatal in some cases.

Ventricle Tachycardia

Ventricle tachycardia is rapid, regular heartbeat as high as 200 bpm (see Figure 17.37 ●).

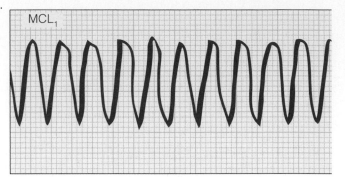

Figure 17.37 ● Ventricle tachycardia.

Ventricular Fibrillation

Ventricular fibrillation is total absence of regular heart rhythm (see Figure 17.38 ●).

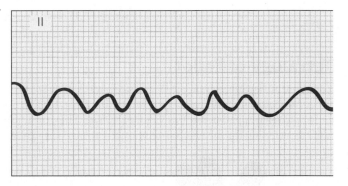

Figure 17.38 ● Ventricular fibrillation.

Heart Block

Slow heart rate can be as low as 20 to 40 bpm (see Figure 17.39 ●). Conduction between the atria and ventricles is disrupted.

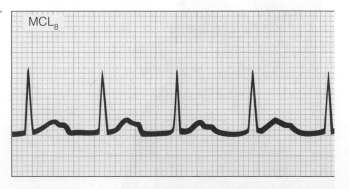

Figure 17.39 ● Heart block.

Atrial Flutter

The atrial rate can be as high as 200 bpm and exceeds the ventricular response and rate (see Figure 17.40 ●).

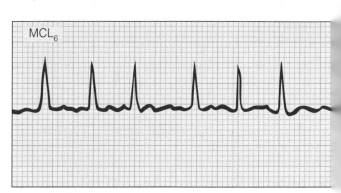

Figure 17.40 ● Atrial flutter.

Atrial Fibrillation

Atrial fibrillation is dysrhythmic atrial contraction with no regularity or pattern (see Figure 17.41 ●).

Figure 17.41 ● Atrial fibrillation.

Health Promotion

HEALTHY PEOPLE 2010

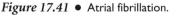

FOCUS AREA	PREVALENCE	OBJECTIVES	ACTIONS
Coronary Heart Disease (CHD)	• Approximately 12 million people in the United States have CHD. • Higher rates are found in males than females. • African Americans have higher rates of CHD than whites. • Obesity and limited physical activity are increasing in the United States and contribute to the development of CHD. • Smoking is a risk factor for CHD.	• Reduce CHD deaths. • Increase awareness of symptoms of heart attack and the need for rapid emergency care. • Increase the numbers of adults who can administer CPR. • Reduce the number of obese individuals. • Increase physical activity. • Increase the number of adults who are aware of risk factors and take action to reduce risks.	• Screening for risk factors. • Individual, community, culturally and linguistically appropriate education and counseling. • Weight reduction programs. • Programs to increase physical activity. • Education about symptoms and emergency care. • Smoking cessation programs.
High Blood Cholesterol	• Major risk factor for CHD. • Over 50 million people have cholesterol levels requiring treatment. • Approximately 90 million have cholesterol levels higher than recommended.	• Reduce the number of adults with elevated cholesterol levels. • Increase the number of adults who have cholesterol levels measured.	• Education about risks. • Education about diet and exercise.

CLIENT EDUCATION

The following are physiological, behavioral, and cultural factors that affect cardiovascular health across the age span. Several of these factors are cited as trends in *Healthy People 2010*. The nurse provides advice and education to reduce risks associated with the factors and to promote and maintain cardiovascular health.

LIFE SPAN CONSIDERATIONS

RISK FACTORS

- Congenital heart defects occur in 1 out of every 125 to 150 infants born in the United States.

- Rheumatic fever can result in cardiac problems. Though uncommon in the United States, it occurs with the greatest frequency in school-age children. It is caused by untreated strep infection.

- The incidence of cardiovascular disease increases with aging. Almost 80% of clients with coronary artery disease are 65 years of age or older.

CLIENT EDUCATION

- Support and provide education for parents of infants with congenital defects as they make decisions about surgical and other treatments for those problems.

- Educate pregnant females about the role of disease, medication, and personal habits in the development of congenital heart defects. Pregnant females who have not had or been immunized against rubella must avoid contraction of the virus during the first trimester of pregnancy. The use of Accutane, lithium, and some antiseizure medications may increase the risk of congenital heart defects. Females who are planning to become pregnant must discuss the use of medications with their healthcare provider. Alcohol and cocaine have been linked with congenital heart defects, and advice about avoiding these substances during pregnancy is warranted. Females with diabetes mellitus have an increased risk of having a child with a heart defect. Careful regulation of the diabetes before and in early pregnancy can reduce the risk.

- Parents of school-age children need to be advised to seek healthcare for pharyngeal infections. Untreated strep throat can result in rheumatic fever.

- Encourage older adults to participate in regular screening for risks associated with cardiovascular disease. Explain the association of age-related changes with cardiovascular health.

CULTURAL CONSIDERATIONS

RISK FACTORS

- Hypertension is a risk factor for coronary artery disease. Hypertension occurs more frequently in African Americans and Hispanics than in other groups.

- Obesity contributes to cardiovascular disease. Obesity is increasing in all age groups in the United States, but occurs most frequently in Hispanic females and African American children.

- Diabetes increases the risk of cardiovascular disease. The incidence of diabetes is highest in Native Americans, Hispanics, and African Americans.

CLIENT EDUCATION

- Tell clients that hypertension is often referred to as the silent killer because it is asymptomatic in most individuals. Clients need to participate in blood pressure screening, especially African Americans and Hispanics, who are at greater risk.

- Advise clients with a diagnosis of hypertension to be monitored regularly and to take medication as prescribed to decrease risks associated with hypertension.

- Provide information about diet to maintain healthy body weight and body fat percentage to clients of all ages. Recommendations for weight reduction and exercise programs should be provided to obese clients.

- Provide education about diet and exercise to assist clients with diabetes to avoid the risks for cardiovascular disease.

ENVIRONMENTAL CONSIDERATIONS

RISK FACTORS

- Family history of heart disease increases the risk for developing cardiovascular disease.

- Elevated cholesterol and triglyceride levels increase the risk for development of cardiovascular disease.

- Stress is associated with the development of cardiovascular disease.

CLIENT EDUCATION

- Provide clients who have a family history of heart disease with information about regular examinations, and encourage them to develop habits to avoid the risks.

  Refer clients to the American Heart Association for information and tips about heart disease and ways to reduce risks.

- Encourage clients to have cholesterol and triglyceride screening, explain the significance of elevated levels as risks for heart disease, educate clients about dietary habits to reduce cholesterol, and explain how to interpret the laboratory results.

- Support clients in stressful events and provide information about stress reduction techniques as methods to reduce risks for cardiovascular disease.

BEHAVIORAL CONSIDERATIONS

RISK FACTORS

- Smoking is a risk factor in development of cardiovascular disease. Smokers have double the mortality rate from myocardial infarction than nonsmokers.
- Lack of physical activity increases the risk for developing diseases that predispose one to cardiovascular disease such as diabetes, obesity, and hypertension.

CLIENT EDUCATION

- Participate in education to prevent smoking and assist clients who are looking for ways to stop smoking.

- Encourage regular exercise in clients of all ages. Exercise can reduce the risks for cardiovascular disease by promoting healthy weight, maintaining healthy blood pressure, and reducing the risk for development of diabetes.

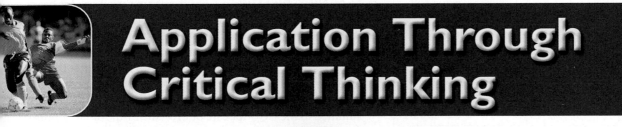

Application Through Critical Thinking

CASE STUDY

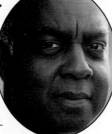

Jason Tibbs, a 56-year-old African American male, presents to the emergency room with a history of hypertension and juvenile-onset diabetes mellitus, which he controls with diet and insulin injections. Today, when taking his morning walk, he fatigued quickly, had difficulty catching his breath, felt a little nauseated, and experienced some unusual tingling in his left arm. Mr. Tibbs states that his wife noticed that he was back from his walk early and saw that he did not look right. He felt it was not something to worry about. "It will go away if I rest," he said. His wife insisted that he go to the hospital.

First, the nurse must determine if Mr. Tibbs is in acute distress by gathering objective and subjective data. The nurse will look for chest pain, pallor or cyanosis, respiratory effort, vital signs changes, and anxiety. If any of these are present, the nurse's goal is to maintain oxygen perfusion.

The nurse knows that hypertension and diabetes are risk factors for cardiovascular disease and that the symptoms of nausea, breathlessness, and numbness in the arm are indicators of a myocardial infarction.

The nurse must avoid assumptions without evidence. Assumptions one could make are that the client has not followed his diabetes treatment regimen and is affected by hyper- or hypoglycemia, that medications have been ineffective or not monitored for hypertension, or that some event of an emotional nature gave rise to the client's symptoms.

Using an organized approach, the nurse begins the assessment. The physical assessment reveals that Mr. Tibbs is diaphoretic and his skin is gray-tinged, especially around the eyes. His vital signs are B/P 89/52—P 102—RR 34.

Mr. Tibbs is in acute distress. Rapid interpretation of data is required. His skin color suggests altered tissue perfusion

He is hypotensive, is tachycardic, and has an elevated respiratory rate. All of the findings are indicative of an acute cardiovascular problem.

The goal is to restore tissue perfusion and prevent further systemic compromise.

Mr. Tibbs is placed on a cardiac monitor, and administration of O_2 via nasal cannula is begun. Atropine as ordered by the ER physician is administered.

Following the atropine administration, the client's B/P is 110/70 and heart rate (HR) is 70.

Mr. Tibbs occasionally rubs his chest and shakes his left arm, but denies pain. He has occasional belching and states, "This is all probably from something I ate or an insulin reaction. I'd like to go home."

Mr. Tibbs is to be admitted to the hospital and will go to the coronary care unit (CCU).

► *Complete Documentation*

The following is sample documentation for Jason Tibbs.
SUBJECTIVE DATA: History of hypertension and type 1 diabetes, controlled with diet and insulin. Fatigued quickly during morning walk, difficulty catching his breath, nausea, unusual tingling in left arm. He felt it was nothing to worry about and "it will go away if I rest." Wife stated Mr. Tibbs came home from walk "early" and he "did not look right."
OBJECTIVE DATA: 56-year-old African American male. Diaphoresis, gray-tinged skin, especially around eyes. VS: B/P 89/52—P 102—RR 34.

ASSESSMENT FORM

Chief Complaint: *Fatigue, difficulty breathing during walk, nausea, tingling left arm.*

History: *Hypertension, diabetes (type 1)—control diet, insulin*

Vital Signs: *B/P 89/52—P 102—RR 34*

Skin: *Diaphoresis, gray (especially eyes)*

► *Critical Thinking Questions*

1. What additional information will be required to formulate a plan of care for Mr. Tibbs in the CCU?
2. How should the nurse interpret the client's desire "to go home" and statement that "This is all probably from something I ate or an insulin reaction"?
3. What evidence has been provided or is required to support or refute the possible assumptions about Mr. Tibbs?
4. Explain the following conclusions about the client's physical condition.
   a. Decreased cardiac output
   b. Impaired gas exchange
   c. Fatigue
   d. Nausea

► *Applying Nursing Diagnoses*

1. *Cardiac output, decreased* is a nursing diagnosis in the NANDA taxonomy (see Appendix A ⬿). Do the data in the case study support this diagnosis? If so, identify the supportive data.
2. *Pain, acute; tissue perfusion, ineffective;* and *anxiety* are diagnoses in the NANDA taxonomy. Do the data in the case study support these diagnoses? If so, identify the supporting data.
3. Use the data in the case study to develop additional nursing diagnoses. Identify the data to support the PES (problem, etiology, signs or symptoms) statement.

► *Prepare Teaching Plan*

LEARNING NEED: Mr. Tibbs has an increased risk for heart disease because he is African American and has been diagnosed with hypertension and diabetes. His symptoms include those that are typical in MI. He was reluctant to seek medical care, but at his wife's insistence, he received care shortly after the onset of symptoms.

The documentation for Mr. Tibbs indicates that he will be admitted to the CCU for care of his acute cardiovascular problem. The symptoms suggest that Mr. Tibbs suffered an MI.

APPLICATION OF OBJECTIVE 2: Discuss risk factors for MI

Content	Teaching Strategy	Evaluation
Risk factors: 1. Race (African Americans have higher risk.) 2. Gender (Males are at greater risk.) 3. High blood pressure 4. Diabetes 5. Family history 6. Aging 7. High cholesterol 8. Cigarette smoking 9. Stress 10. Obesity 11. Lack of exercise	• Lecture • Discussion • Slides Lecture allows information to be provided to a large group. Discussion encourages learner participation and permits for questions and answers. Audiovisual materials such as pictures and slides provide visual reinforcement of information. Printed material can be used by the learner during and after the session to review materials.	• Written examination

While in the CCU, he will receive information about his condition and requirements for his posthospital healthcare regimen.

The case study provides data that is representative of risks, symptoms, and behaviors of many individuals. Therefore, the following teaching plan is based on the need to provide information to members of any community about MI and the importance of immediate care when symptoms arise.

GOAL: Participants will seek healthcare to promote cardiovascular health.

OBJECTIVES: Upon completion of this learning session, the participants will be able to:

1. Describe MI.
2. Discuss risk factors for MI.
3. Describe symptoms of MI.
4. Identify lifesaving procedures.

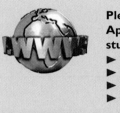

Please refer to the Companion Website at www.prenhall.com/damico and click on Chapter 17, the Application Through Critical Thinking module, to complete the following activities related to this case study:
- ► **Critical Thinking questions**
- ► **Extended Nursing Diagnosis challenge**
- ► **Documentation activity**
- ► **Teaching Plan for Objectives 1, 3, and 4**

EXPLORE MediaLink

Additional resources for this chapter are found on the Student CD-ROM accompanying this textbook and on the Companion Website.

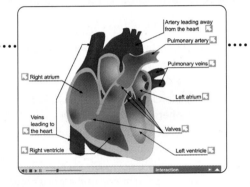

CD-ROM CONTENT

Content for this chapter includes:
Objectives
Key Concepts
NCLEX-RN® Review Questions
Model Documentation Forms
Audio Glossary
Heart Sounds
   Irregular Heart Rate
   S_1 and S_2 Heart Sounds
   S_3 and S_4 Heart Sounds
   S_1 Splitting Sound
   S_2 Splitting Sound
   Mid-Diastolic Murmur
   Mid-Systolic Murmur
   Murmur Grade—Faint
   Murmur Grade—Moderate
   Murmur Grade—Loud
Animations
   Heart and Major Vessels
   Chambers of the Human Heart
   Normal Heart Hemodynamics
Games and Challenges
Clinical Spotlight Videos
   Disease Investigation: Heart Disease
   Coronary Heart Disease
   Dysrhythmia
Head-to-Toe Physical Examination Video

COMPANION WEBSITE CONTENT

www.prenhall.com/damico

Content for this chapter includes:
Objectives
NCLEX-RN® Review Questions
Client Interaction Case Study Challenge
Application Through Critical Thinking
   Case Study Teaching Plan Challenge
MediaLinks
MediaLink Application
Tool Box
   Chapter Documentation Form Example
   Characteristics of Heart Sounds
   Additional Heart Sounds
   Distinguising Heart Murmurs
   Classification of Heart Murmurs
   Electrocardiograph Wave
   Events of the Cardiac Cycle
   Health Promotion
      Healthy People 2010
      Client Education
New York Times

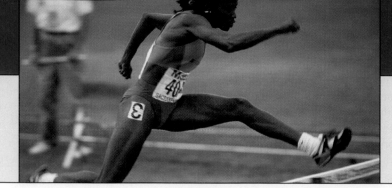

18
Peripheral Vascular System

CHAPTER OBJECTIVES

Upon completion of this chapter, you will be able to:

1. Identify the anatomy and physiology of the peripheral vascular and lymphatic systems.
2. Develop questions that guide the focused interview.
3. Explain client preparation for assessment of the peripheral vascular system.
4. Describe techniques required for assessment of the peripheral vascular system.
5. Differentiate normal from abnormal findings in physical assessment of the peripheral vascular system.
6. Describe developmental, psychosocial, cultural, and environmental variations in assessment techniques and findings of the peripheral vascular system.
7. Discuss the focus areas of *Healthy People 2010* as they relate to issues of the peripheral vascular system.
8. Apply critical thinking in selected simulations related to physical assessment of the peripheral vascular system.

MEDIALINK

www.prenhall.com/damico

The CD-ROM in the back of this textbook and the Media-Link website contain NCLEX-RN® review questions, interactive exercises, case study challenges, animations, videos, documentation and checklist forms, and review materials. For a complete listing of the media content specific to Chapter 18, see the Explore MediaLink at the end of the chapter.

CHAPTER OUTLINE

The **peripheral vascular system** is made up of the blood vessels of the body. Together with the heart and the lymphatic vessels, they make up the body's circulatory system, which transports blood and lymph throughout the body. This chapter discusses assessment of the 60,000-mile network of veins and arteries that make up the peripheral vascular system, as well as the peripheral lymphatic vessels.

The vascular system plays a key role in the development of heart disease, one of the leading causes of death. People with high blood pressure have an increased risk of developing heart disease and stroke. Hypertension, the "silent killer," produces many physiological changes before any symptoms are experienced. This characteristic has tended to undermine efforts at treatment. Hypertension is considered one of the focus areas discussed in *Healthy People 2010*. The objectives and health promotion strategies for hypertension are included in the *Healthy People 2010* feature on page 505.

Therefore, the nurse's efforts must be directed at prevention of problems of the circulatory system and promotion of a healthful way of life. A client's psychosocial health, self-care practices, and factors related to the client's family, culture, and environment all influence vascular health.

ANATOMY AND PHYSIOLOGY REVIEW

The peripheral vascular system is composed of arteries, veins, and lymphatics. Each of these will be described in the following sections.

ARTERIES

The **arteries** of the peripheral vascular system receive oxygen-rich blood from the heart and carry it to the organs and tissues of the body. The pumping heart (ventricular systole) creates a high-pressure wave or **pulse** that causes the arteries to expand and contract. This pulse propels the blood through the vessels and is palpable in arteries near the skin or over a bony surface. The thickness and elasticity of arterial walls help them to withstand these constant waves of pressure and to propel the blood to the body periphery. The thickness or viscosity of blood, the heart rate or cardiac output, and the ability of the vessels to expand and contract influence the arterial pulse. It is described as a smooth wave with a forceful ascending portion that domes and becomes less forceful as it descends. (Review Chapter 17 for more detailed information. ∞)

In the arm, the pulsations of the *brachial artery* can be palpated in the antecubital region. The divisions of the brachial artery, the *radial* and *ulnar arteries,* can be palpated for pulsations over the anterior wrist. The major arteries of the arm are shown in Figure 18.1 ●.

In the leg, the pulsations of the femoral artery can be palpated inferior to the inguinal ligament, about halfway between the anterior superior iliac spine and the symphysis pubis. The *femoral artery* continues down the thigh and becomes the *popliteal artery* as it passes behind the knee. Pulsations of the popliteal artery are palpable over the popliteal region. Below the knee, the popliteal artery divides into the anterior and posterior tibial arteries. The *anterior tibial artery* travels to the dorsum of the foot, and its pulsation can be felt just lateral to the prominent extensor tendon of the big toe close to the ankle. This pulse is known as the dorsalis pedis. Pulsations of the *posterior tibial artery* can be felt where it passes behind the medial malleolus of the ankle. The major arteries of the leg are illustrated in Figure 18.2 ●.

The movement of blood through the systemic arterial system occurs in waves that cause two types of pressure. The blood pressure has two distinct parts, a systolic pressure and a diastolic pressure. The systolic pressure occurs during cardiac systole or ventricular contraction. It is the force of the blood that is exerted on the arterial wall during this cardiac action. The diastolic pressure occurs during cardiac diastole or ventricular relaxation. It is the force of the blood on the arterial wall during ventricular filling. Blood pressure is influenced by age, sympathoadrenal activity, blood volume, and ability of the vessels to contract and dilate. Blood pressure was discussed in greater detail in Chapter 7. ∞

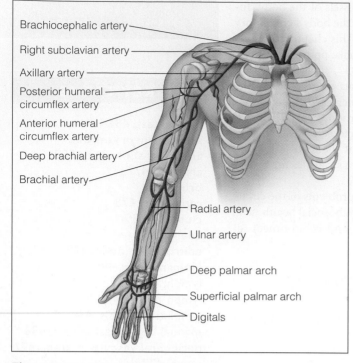

Figure 18.1 ● Main arteries of the arm.

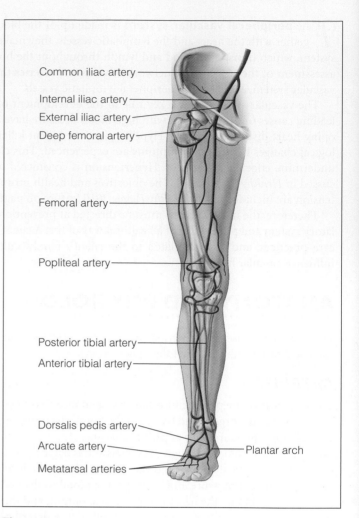

Figure 18.2 ● Main arteries of the leg.

VEINS

The **veins** of the systemic circulation deliver deoxygenated blood from the body periphery back to the heart. Veins have thinner walls and a larger diameter than arteries and are able to stretch and dilate to facilitate venous return. Venous return is assisted by contraction of skeletal muscles during activities such as walking, and by pressure changes related to inspiration and expiration. In addition, veins have one-way intraluminal valves that close tightly when filled to prevent backflow. Thus, venous blood flows only toward the heart. Problems with the lumen or valves of the leg veins can lead to *stasis,* or pooling of blood in the veins of the lower extremities.

The femoral and the popliteal veins are deep veins of the legs and carry about 90% of the venous return from the legs. The great and small saphenous veins are superficial veins that are not as well supported as the deep veins by surrounding tissues and therefore are more susceptible to venous stasis. The major veins of the leg are depicted in Figure 18.3 ●.

CAPILLARIES

Exchanges of gases and nutrients between the arterial and venous systems are conducted within beds of **capillaries,** the smallest vessels of the circulatory system. Blood pressure in the arterial end of the capillary bed forces fluid out across the capillary membrane and into the body tissues.

LYMPHATIC SYSTEM

The lymphatic system consists of the vast network of vessels, fluid, various tissue, and organs throughout the body. These vessels help transport escaped fluid back to the vascular system.

The lymphoid organs have a major role regarding body defenses and the immune system. These structures help fight infection and provide the individual immunocompetence. The spleen, tonsils, and thymus gland are examples of lymphoid organs.

The **lymphatic vessels** form their own circulatory system in which their collected fluid flows to the heart. The vessels extend from the capillaries of their system to the two main lymphatic trunks. The *right lymphatic duct* collects lymph from the right upper extremity, which is the right side of the thorax and head. The *thoracic duct* collects lymph from the remaining part of the body. The thoracic duct responds to the protein and fluid pressure at the capillary end of the vessels that help keep the lymph properly circulated. During circulation, as blood continues through the capillary bed toward the smallest veins, called *venules,* more fluid leaves the capillaries than can be absorbed by the veins. The lymphatic system retrieves this excess fluid, called **lymph,** from the tissue spaces and carries it to the lymph nodes throughout the body. **Lymph nodes** are clumps of tissue located along the lymphatic vessels either deep or superficially in the body. The lymph nodes usually are covered and protected by connective tissue and are therefore not palpable. Some of the more superficial nodes are located in the neck, the axillary region, and the inguinal region. Deeper clusters are located in the ab-

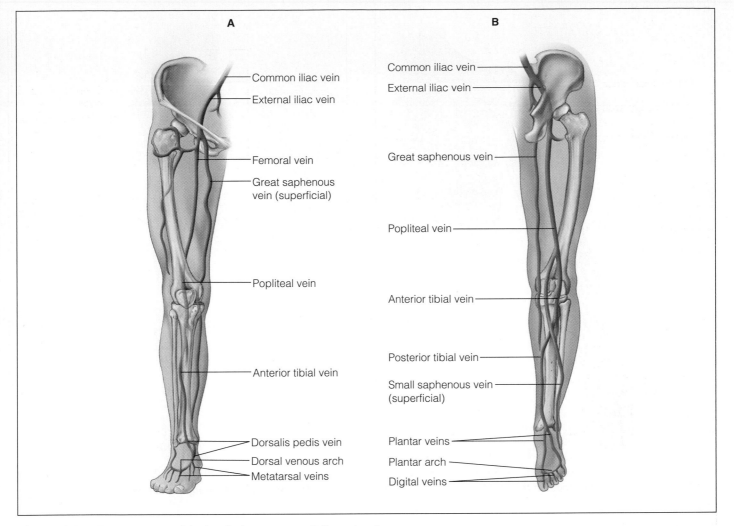

A

Common iliac vein

External iliac vein

Femoral vein

Great saphenous
vein (superficial)

Popliteal vein

Anterior tibial vein

Dorsalis pedis vein

Dorsal venous arch

Metatarsal veins

B

Common iliac vein

External iliac vein

Great saphenous vein

Popliteal vein

Anterior tibial vein

Posterior tibial vein

Small saphenous vein
(superficial)

Plantar veins

Plantar arch

Digital veins

Figure 18.3 ● The main veins of the leg. A. Anterior view. B. Posterior view.

domen and thoracic cavity. The lymph nodes filter lymph
fluid, removing any pathogens before the fluid is returned to
the bloodstream.

The **epitrochlear node** located on the medial surface of
the arm above the elbow drains the ulnar surface of the forearm
and the third, fourth, and fifth digits. The nodes in the axilla of
the arm drain the rest of the arm. The major lymph nodes of
the arm are shown in Figure 18.4 ●.

The legs have two sets of superficial inguinal nodes, a vertical group and a horizontal group. The vertical group is located
close to the saphenous vein and drains that area of the leg. The
horizontal group of nodes is found below the inguinal ligament. These nodes drain the skin of the abdominal wall, the external genitals, the anal canal, and the gluteal area. The major
lymph nodes of the leg are illustrated in Figure 18.5 ●.

The functions of the peripheral vascular system are the following:

● Delivering oxygen and nutrients to tissues of the body
● Transporting carbon dioxide and other waste products from
  the tissues for excretion
● Removing pathogens from the body fluid by filtering lymph

SPECIAL CONSIDERATIONS

The nurse must use critical thinking and the nursing process to
identify factors to consider when conducting a comprehensive
health assessment. Factors that impact the client's health status
include but are not limited to age, developmental level, race,
ethnicity, work history, living conditions, socioeconomics, and
emotional well-being.

DEVELOPMENTAL CONSIDERATIONS

Interpretation of data from health assessment is dependent
upon the ability to differentiate normal from abnormal findings. Normal variations in anatomy and physiology occur with
growth and development. Specific variations associated with
the peripheral vascular system for different age groups are discussed in the following sections.

Infants and Children

Assessing the blood pressure of an infant less than 1 year of age
is difficult without special equipment. It is usually not necessary if the infant is moving well and the skin color is good.

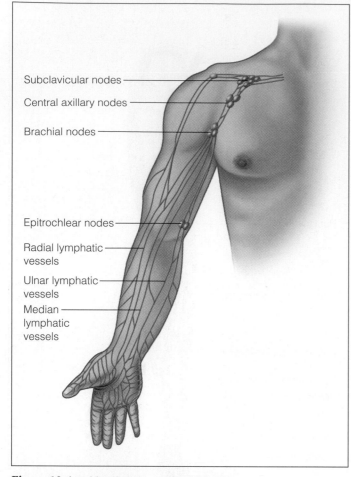

Figure 18.4 ● Main lymph nodes of the arm.

Subclavicular nodes

Central axillary nodes

Brachial nodes

Epitrochlear nodes

Radial lymphatic vessels

Ulnar lymphatic vessels

Median lymphatic vessels

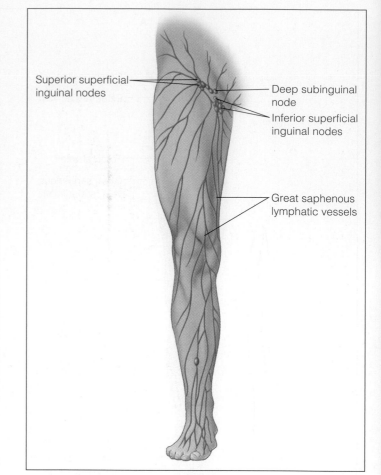

Figure 18.5 ● Main lymph nodes of the leg.

Superior superficial inguinal nodes

Deep subinguinal node

Inferior superficial inguinal nodes

Great saphenous lymphatic vessels

However, if the child is lethargic and tires easily during feeding or the skin becomes cyanotic when the infant cries, the blood pressure should be measured with a Doppler flowmeter. A newborn's blood pressure is much lower than that of an adult and gradually increases with age. The systolic pressure of a newborn is 50 to 80 mm Hg; the diastolic pressure is 25 to 55 mm Hg.

All children 18 months of age and older should have their blood pressure evaluated during their well-child examination. The cuff should be no larger than two thirds of the child's arm or smaller than half of the length of the child's arm between the elbow and the shoulder. Pediatric blood pressure cuffs are available.

In young children, the blood pressure should be measured on the thigh to rule out a significant difference between upper and lower extremity pressure. Such a difference in pressure could indicate a narrowing (coarctation) of the aorta. In a baby less than 1 year of age, the systolic pressure in the thigh should equal that of the arm. A child over 1 year of age will have a systolic pressure in the thigh that is 10 to 40 mm Hg higher than that in the arm. The diastolic pressure in the thigh equals that in the arm.

The pulse increases if the child has a fever. For every degree of fever, the pulse may increase 8 to 10 beats per minute (bpm). The lymphatic system develops rapidly from birth until puberty and then subsides in adulthood. The presence of enlarged lymph nodes in a child may not indicate illness. However, if an infection is present, the nodes may enlarge considerably.

Chapter 25 describes a complete assessment of infants, children, and adolescents. ○○

The Pregnant Female

Blood pressure should be monitored throughout the pregnancy to test for pregnancy-induced hypertension. Blood volume during pregnancy almost doubles. In the second trimester, blood pressure may decrease because of the dilation of the peripheral vessels. However, blood pressure usually returns to the prepregnancy level by the third trimester. If the client has a history of hypertension prior to her pregnancy, the blood pressure may increase dramatically during the third trimester, posing the threat of cerebral hemorrhage. Pressure from the uterus on the lower extremities can obstruct venous return and lead to hypotension when the client is lying on her back, or it can cause edema, varicosities of the leg, and hemorrhoids. Chapter 26 describes a complete assessment of the pregnant female. ○○

The Older Adult

The aging process causes arteriosclerosis or calcification of the walls of the blood vessels. The arterial walls lose elasticity and become more rigid. This increase in peripheral vascular resistance results in increased blood pressure. The enlargement of calf veins can pose the risk of blood clots in leg veins. However, the amount of circulatory inadequacy at any given age is not predictable. The aging process may not cause any symptoms in some older clients.

Most hypertension is asymptomatic, but a severe elevation may produce a headache, epistaxis (nosebleed), shortness of breath, or chest pain. When evaluating the various arterial pulses, the nurse should keep in mind that the heart rate slows with the aging process. Some persons may normally have a rate of 50 bpm; however, the client should be evaluated if the pulse is below 60 bpm. Likewise, it is common for older clients to manifest irregular pulses often with occasional pauses or extra beats. Again, any client with an irregular pulse should be referred for further examination. Chapter 27 describes a complete assessment of the older adult. ◯◯

PSYCHOSOCIAL CONSIDERATIONS

Stress is among the factors that contribute to development of hypertension. Work-related stress has often been associated with hypertension. Stress can result from the rigors of everyday life in a complex and ever changing world. Globalization and resulting economic fluctuations, spread of disease, and terrorist threats have created a stressful environment. An individual's ability to cope can determine the risk of developing hypertension in response to stress.

CULTURAL AND ENVIRONMENTAL CONSIDERATIONS

There is a greater incidence of hypertension in African Americans and Hispanics than in Caucasians. Obesity is a risk factor for hypertension and is increasing in the United States. The incidence of obesity is greatest in Hispanic females and African American children.

Risk factors for varicose veins include Irish and German descent, family history of varicosities, a sedentary lifestyle, obesity, and multiple pregnancies.

Clients whose jobs require them to stand for most of the day, such as hairdressers and cashiers, are at greater risk for developing varicose veins. Desk jobs that require sitting for prolonged periods also contribute to venous stasis and varicose veins.

Cultural Considerations

- Skin color variations across ethnic groups may affect assessment of circulation. The nurse must use skin temperature, capillary refill, and pulse characteristics when pink undertones are not easily detected.
- African Americans have a higher incidence of hypertension than other groups.
- Diabetes increases the risk for peripheral vascular disease and is increasing in prevalence in Native Americans and Hispanics.

- Obesity is a risk factor for hypertension and peripheral vascular disease. Obesity is increasing in all groups at all ages but occurs most frequently in Hispanic females and African American children.
- Smoking increases the risk for hypertension and peripheral vascular disease. Smoking is most prevalent in African American and Hispanic males.

Gathering the Data

*H*ealth assessment of the peripheral vascular system includes gathering subjective and objective data. During the interview the nurse uses a variety of communication techniques to elicit general and specific information about the client's state of health or illness. Health records and the results of laboratory tests are important secondary sources to be reviewed and included in the data-gathering process. In physical assessment of the peripheral vascular system, the techniques of inspection, palpation, and auscultation will be used. Before proceeding, it may be helpful to review the information about each of the data-gathering processes and practice the techniques of health assessment.

FOCUSED INTERVIEW

The focused interview for the peripheral vascular system concerns data related to the structures and functions of that system. Subjective data is gathered during the focused interview. The nurse must be prepared to observe the client and listen for cues related to the functions of the systems. The nurse may use closed or open-ended questions to obtain information. Often a number of follow-up questions or requests for descriptions are required to clarify data or gather missing information.

The focused interview guides the physical assessment of the peripheral vascular system. The information is always considered in relation to normal parameters and expectations. Therefore, the nurse must consider age, gender, race, culture, environment, health practices, past and concurrent problems, and therapies when framing questions and using techniques to elicit information. In order to address all of the factors when conducting a focused interview, categories of questions related to the peripheral vascular system status and function have been developed. These categories include general questions that are asked of all clients; those addressing illness or infection; questions related to symptoms, pain, or behaviors; those related to habits or practices; questions that are specific to clients according to age; those for the pregnant female; and questions that address environmental concerns. The data will be used to help meet the goal of improving peripheral vascular health as indicated in *Healthy People 2010*.

The nurse must consider the client's ability to participate in the focused interview and physical assessment. If a client is experiencing pain or anxiety, attention must focus on relief of symptoms.

FOCUSED INTERVIEW QUESTIONS	RATIONALES

The following section provides sample questions and bulleted follow-up questions in each of the previously mentioned categories. A rationale for each of the questions is provided. The list of questions is not all-inclusive but represents the types of questions required in a comprehensive focused interview related to the peripheral vascular and lymphatic systems.

GENERAL QUESTIONS

1. **Describe your circulation.**
   - Have you felt cold or hot?
   - Have you had numbness anywhere?
   - Has your skin been pale or blue?
   - Has it changed in the last 2 months or 2 years?

▶ This gives clients the opportunity to provide their own perceptions about circulation.

2. **Have you or any member of your family ever had heart problems, respiratory disease, diabetes, varicose veins, or blood clots?**

▶ These problems can damage the peripheral circulation, and they tend to be hereditary.

QUESTIONS RELATED TO ILLNESS

1. **Have you ever been diagnosed with a disease of your circulatory or lymphatic system?**
   - When were you diagnosed with the problem?
   - What treatment was prescribed for the problem?
   - Was the treatment helpful?
   - What kinds of things do you do to help with the problem?
   - Has the problem ever recurred (acute)?
   - How are you managing the disease now (chronic)?

▶ The client has an opportunity to provide information about specific illnesses. If a diagnosed illness is identified, follow-up about the date of diagnosis, treatment, and outcomes is required. Data about each illness identified by the client is essential to an accurate health assessment. Illnesses can be classified as acute or chronic, and follow-up regarding each classification will differ.

2. **An alternative to question 1 is to list possible illnesses, such as hypertension, arteriosclerosis, Raynaud's disease, varicose veins, thrombophlebitis, and aneurysms, and ask the client to respond yes or no as each is stated.**

▶ This is a comprehensive and easy way to elicit information about all diagnoses. Follow-up would be carried out for each identified diagnosis as in question 1.

QUESTIONS RELATED TO SYMPTOMS OR BEHAVIORS

When gathering information about symptoms, many questions are required to elicit details and descriptions that assist in the analysis of the data. Discrimination is made in relation to the significance of a symptom, in relation to specific diseases or problems, and in relation to potential follow-up examination or referral. One rationale may be provided for a group of questions in this category.

The following questions refer to specific symptoms and behaviors associated with the peripheral vascular and lymphatic systems. For each symptom, questions and follow-up are required. The details to be elicited are the characteristics of the symptom; the onset, duration, and frequency of the symptom; the treatment or remedy for the symptom, including over-the-counter and home remedies; the determination if diagnosis has been sought; the effect of treatments; and family history associated with a symptom or illness.

FOCUSED INTERVIEW QUESTIONS	**RATIONALES**

QUESTIONS RELATED TO SYMPTOMS

1. **Have you noticed any skin changes on your arms or legs?**
   - If so, describe the changes.
   - Have you noticed any swelling or shiny skin, particularly on your legs?

2. **If the client reports swelling: Is the swelling in one leg or both legs?**
   - When did this swelling start?
   - Is the swelling worse in the morning or at the end of the day, or is the swelling constant?
   - What relieves the swelling?

3. **Have you noticed any changes in temperature in your arms or legs, such as extreme coolness or heat?**

4. **Have you noticed any skin changes such as sores or ulcers on your legs?**
   - If so, is there any pain associated with the sores?

5. **Have you noticed any changes in the feeling in your legs, such as numbness or tingling?**

6. **Have you noticed a change in the growth of hair on your legs?**

7. **Does your skin look shiny or feel taut?**

8. **Do you have any swollen glands? If so, where are they in your body?**
   - How long have they been swollen?
   - Is there any pain or redness associated with these swollen glands?
   - Have you had any other symptoms such as fever, fatigue, or bleeding?

9. **For male clients: Have you experienced any difficulty in achieving an erection?**

► Shiny skin and swelling is sometimes caused by fluid leaking into tissue spaces because of incompetent valves in the veins.

► Answers to these questions may help the nurse determine the reason for the swelling.

► Extreme coolness may indicate arterial insufficiency.

► Leg ulcers can be an indication of chronic arterial or venous problems.

► Decreased circulation in the lower extremities can cause a loss of sensation, particularly in persons with diabetes.

► Peripheral arterial insufficiency can result in hair loss or skin changes.

► Enlarged lymph glands usually are associated with an infectious process in the body.

► Impotence may occur as a result of a diminished arterial flow to the pelvic arteries. This condition is a common finding in peripheral vascular disease and is not always reported because of client embarrassment.

QUESTIONS RELATED TO PAIN

1. **Do you ever have pains in your legs, or leg cramps?**
   - If so, please describe the pain or cramp, the location, and the time it most often occurs.

► Pain associated with arterial insufficiency is usually described as gnawing, sharp, or stabbing and increases with exercise. Pain is relieved with the cessation of movement and when legs are dangling. The pain is most commonly in the calf of the leg but it may also be in the lower leg or top of the foot. **Venous insufficiency** is described as aching or a feeling of fullness. It intensifies with prolonged standing or sitting in one position. Swelling and varicosities in the legs may also be present. The condition is relieved by elevating the legs or by walking.

QUESTIONS RELATED TO BEHAVIORS

1. **Do you smoke?**
   - If so, how long have you smoked?
   - How many cigarettes, cigars, or pipes of tobacco do you smoke per day?

2. **Do you exercise regularly?**
   - If so, describe your exercise routine.
   - How often do you exercise?
   - For how long?

► Nicotine is a vasoconstrictor and aggravates peripheral vascular disease.

► Exercise not only helps to prevent vascular disease but also improves the survival rate of people who have already suffered a heart attack and reduces the likelihood of their suffering a second attack. Even modest levels of physical activity are beneficial, according to the American Heart Association.

FOCUSED INTERVIEW QUESTIONS	RATIONALES

QUESTIONS RELATED TO AGE

The focused interview must reflect the anatomical and physiological differences that exist along the age span. The following questions are presented as examples of those that would be specific for children, the pregnant female, and older adults.

QUESTIONS REGARDING INFANTS AND CHILDREN

1. **Has the infant become lethargic?**
   - Does the infant tire during feeding or become cyanotic when crying?

   ► These are signs of hypotension or hypoxemia associated with vascular disease.

2. **Has the child had blood pressure screening?**

   ► It is recommended that blood pressure screening begin at age 18 months.

3. **Does the child have any enlarged lymph nodes?**

   ► Enlarged lymph nodes in a child may not indicate illness. However, in infection considerable enlargement is found.

QUESTIONS FOR THE PREGNANT FEMALE

1. **Have you had your blood pressure monitored?**

   ► Monitoring can reduce risks for pregnancy-induced hypertension.

2. **Are you experiencing swelling of the face, hands, or legs?**

   ► Pitting edema in the lower extremities is common in pregnancy, especially at the end of the day and into the third trimester.

QUESTIONS FOR THE OLDER ADULT

No additional questions for the older adult are required.

QUESTIONS RELATED TO THE ENVIRONMENT

Environment refers to both the internal and external environments. Questions related to the internal environment include all of the previous questions and those associated with internal or physiological responses. Questions regarding the external environment include those related to home, work, or social environments.

INTERNAL ENVIRONMENT

1. **Are you now experiencing or have you ever had an experience of intermittent or prolonged anxiety or emotional upset?**
   - Describe the situation.
   - Can you determine precipitating factors?
   - Have you sought care or treatment for the problem?
   - What do you do when the problem arises?

   ► Anxiety and situations of emotion impact the sympathetic nervous system, producing hormonal responses that affect vascular function.

2. **What medications are you taking, either over-the-counter or prescription?**

   ► Contraceptive medications have been associated with blood clots in the peripheral vascular system. Aspirin is an anticoagulant.

EXTERNAL ENVIRONMENT

The following questions deal with the physical environment of the client. That includes the indoor and outdoor environments of the home and the workplace, those encountered for social engagements, and any encountered during travel.

1. **Describe your daily activities.**

   ► Sedentary activities and prolonged periods of sitting and standing at work or in the home can promote peripheral vascular problems, varicosities, or problems associated with venous stasis.

CLIENT INTERACTION

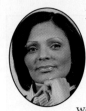

Ms. Mercedes Carlos, age 35, is an accountant at a local firm. She is married and has two children, 6 and 4 years of age. They recently returned from a 10-day vacation in Florida where they visited many of the theme parks. The flight home was delayed 2 hours, and they were seated on the plane for more than 4 hours. Ms. C. reports to the employee health office complaining of right leg pain and edema of the right ankle and foot that seems to be worse when standing or sitting at the desk. Following is an excerpt of the nurse-client interaction.

INTERVIEW

Nurse: Good morning Ms. Carlos. What brings you here?

Ms. Carlos: I've been having some trouble with my leg. I just got back from vacation at a theme park in Florida. Our trip was great. Some of the lines at the parks were long. We did a lot of standing, walking, and sitting.

Nurse: How long was your trip?

Ms. Carlos: We were away for 10 days. We got home Saturday night, and here I am Tuesday morning seeing you.

Nurse: Tell me about the pain and swelling in your right leg.

Ms. Carlos: The pain started in my lower right leg about the fifth day of our trip. When I got back to the hotel, I would rest with my legs up and the pain seemed to go away.

Nurse: Did you have pain every day thereafter?

Ms. Carlos: Yes, and then after our flight home I noticed my foot was swollen. That was the first I noticed any swelling.

Nurse: Have you ever had a problem like this before?

Ms. Carlos: During my last pregnancy I had a problem like this. The doctor told me I could be developing varicose veins. After the delivery I never had a problem until now. I'm too young to have varicose veins.

ANALYSIS

Throughout the interview, the nurse uses closed and open-ended statements to obtain information. The opening question by the nurse was to determine the client's problem or chief complaint. Additional statements by the nurse give direction to the client to provide specific subjective data.

Please refer to the Companion Website at **www.prenhall.com/damico** and click on Chapter 18, the **Client Interaction** module, to answer questions about this case. In addition, see other resources for this chapter including NCLEX review questions and other interactive exercises and materials.

Physical Assessment

ASSESSMENT TECHNIQUES AND FINDINGS

Physical assessment of the peripheral vascular and lymphatic systems requires the use of inspection, palpation, auscultation, and assessment of blood pressure. During each aspect of the assessment, the nurse is gathering objective data about circulation. Inspection includes looking at skin color, appearance of superficial vasculature, and shape and size of the extremities and nails. Palpation of pulses and auscultation of blood pressure and arteries provide information about vascular status. Knowledge of normal parameters and expected findings is essential in determining the meaning of the data as the physical assessment is performed.

The adult has a normal systolic blood pressure of less than 120 and diastolic blood pressure below 80. The carotid pulses are palpable, symmetrical, and synchronous with S_1 of the heart. Auscultation of carotid arteries yields a soft sound, occasionally with transmission of heart sounds, but absence of bruits. The upper extremities should be of equal size and warm, with pink undertones and no edema. Capillary refill should occur in less than 2 seconds. The brachial and radial arteries should be equal in rate and symmetrical in amplitude. The epitrochlear nodes are not palpable. The lower extremities are warm and equal in size, the color is consistent with the rest of the body, hair is evenly distributed, and the extremities have no edema, lesions, or varicosities. The inguinal nodes are nonpalpable. The femoral, popliteal, posterior tibial, and dorsalis pedis pulses are equal and symmetrical in rate and amplitude. The toes have hair and toenails are pink and without clubbing.

Physical assessment of the peripheral vascular and lymphatic systems proceeds in an organized pattern. Blood pressure is assessed in upper and lower extremities. A cephalocaudal pattern for assessment of the vascular and lymphatic system begins with the carotid arteries and follows through inspection of the upper and lower extremities and palpation of pulses and lymph nodes within them. Additional assessment techniques include **Allen's test** to determine patency of the radial and ulnar arteries, the **manual compression test** to determine the length of varicose veins, and Trendelenburg's test to evaluate valve competence when varicosities are present.

HELPFUL HINTS

• The client should don an examination gown, but undergarments may remain in place.
• The client should remove watches and jewelry that may interfere with assessment.
• Socks and stockings should be removed.
• The client will sit, stand, and lie in a supine position during various aspects of the assessment. The nurse should provide assistance and support when required and ensure that the client's respiratory effort will not be affected by moving about or when lying flat.
• Use Standard Precautions.

EQUIPMENT

examination gown	stethoscope
sphygmomanometer	doppler

TECHNIQUES AND NORMAL FINDINGS

**ABNORMAL FINDINGS
SPECIAL CONSIDERATIONS**

BLOOD PRESSURE

1. **Instruct the client.**
   • Explain that you will be assessing blood pressure in the arms and legs. Tell the client you will inflate the cuff twice for each location. The first time you will only touch a pulse area, and the second time you will use the stethoscope. Tell the client to breathe normally and relax the extremity. The only discomfort should occur when the cuff is fully inflated and will be relieved as the cuff deflates. Tell the client to report any other problems.

   • Ask the client to remain still and not to speak during the auscultation, as you will not hear well when the stethoscope is in place for the blood pressure reading.

   • Explain that you will take the blood pressure while the client is sitting and then when lying down. The readings will be compared.

2. **Position the client.**
   • Place the client in a sitting position on the examination table (see Figure 18.6 ●).

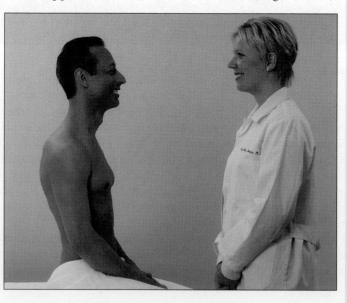

Figure 18.6 ●
The client is positioned for the examination.

TECHNIQUES AND NORMAL FINDINGS	ABNORMAL FINDINGS SPECIAL CONSIDERATIONS

TECHNIQUES AND NORMAL FINDINGS

- Take the blood pressure in both arms. Assess the palpable systolic pressure (see Figure 18.7A ●).
- Auscultate the blood pressure (see Figure 18.7B ●).

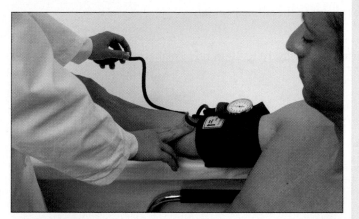

Figure 18.7A ●
Blood pressure measurements. A. Palpable blood pressure.

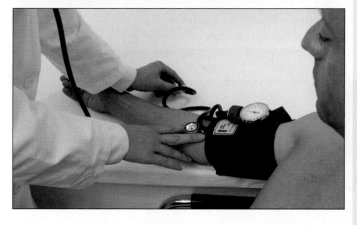

Figure 18.7B ●
Blood pressure measurements. B. Auscultation of blood pressure.

- The blood pressure normally does not vary more than 5 to 10 mm Hg in each arm.

- Table 18.1 includes current guidelines regarding interpretation of blood pressure readings for adults.

Table 18.1	National Institutes of Health (NIH) Blood Pressure Guidelines	
BP CLASSIFICATION	**SYSTOLIC BP MM HG**	**DIASTOLIC BP MM HG**
Normal	<120	and <80
Prehypertension	120–139	or 80–89
Stage 1 Hypertension	140–159	or 90–99
Stage 2 Hypertension	≥160	or ≥100

ABNORMAL FINDINGS SPECIAL CONSIDERATIONS

▶ Assessing the palpable systolic pressure helps to avoid an inaccuracy due to auscultatory gap when auscultating blood pressure.

▶ A difference of 10 mm Hg or more between the arms may indicate an obstruction of arterial flow to one arm.

▶ A systolic reading below 90 or a diastolic reading under 60 may be an early indication of shock, which requires immediate medical attention.

TECHNIQUES AND NORMAL FINDINGS	ABNORMAL FINDINGS SPECIAL CONSIDERATIONS

3. **Assist the client to a supine position.**

4. **Take the blood pressure in both arms.**
   - Pressures are lower when taken in the supine position.
   - Standards for blood pressure are set for clients in the sitting position.

▶ It is important to document the client's position for each assessment of blood pressure.

5. **Take the blood pressure in both legs.**
   - The blood pressure in the popliteal artery is usually 10 to 40 mm Hg higher than that in the brachial artery.

CAROTID ARTERIES

1. **Inspect the neck for carotid pulsations.**
   - With the client in a supine position, inspect the neck from the hyoid bone to the clavicles. Bilateral pulsations will be seen between the trachea and sternocleidomastoid muscle.

▶ The absence of pulsation may indicate internal or external obstruction.

2. **Palpate the carotid pulses.**
   - Place the pads of your first two or three fingers on the client's neck between the trachea and the sternocleidomastoid muscle, just below the angle of the jaw (see Figure 18.8 ●).

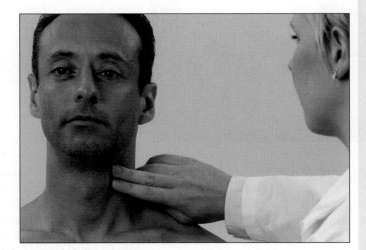

Figure 18.8 ●
Palpating the
carotid artery.

   - Ask the client to turn the head slightly toward your hand to relax the sternocleidomastoid muscle.
   - Palpate firmly, but not so hard that you occlude the artery.

▶ If both carotid arteries are palpated at the same time, the result can be a drop in blood pressure or a reduction in the pulse rate, from the stimulation of baroreceptors.

   - Palpate one side of the neck at a time. If you are having difficulty finding the pulse, try varying the pressure of your fingers, feeling carefully below the angle.

▶ A rate over 90 bpm is considered abnormal unless the client is anxious or has recently been exercising or smoking. A rate below 60 is also considered abnormal.

   - Note the rate, rhythm, amplitude, and symmetry of the carotid pulses. Compare this rate to the apical pulse.

▶ However, some athletes have a resting pulse as low as 50 bpm. An irregular rhythm, or a pulse with extra beats or missed beats is considered abnormal. An exaggerated pulse or a weak, thready pulse is abnormal. A discrepancy between the two carotid pulses is abnormal.

TECHNIQUES AND NORMAL FINDINGS	**ABNORMAL FINDINGS SPECIAL CONSIDERATIONS**

3. Auscultate the carotid pulses.

- Using the diaphragm of the stethoscope, auscultate each carotid artery high in the neck, inferior to the angle of the jaw, and medial to the sternocleidomastoid muscle. Ask the client to hold his or her breath for several seconds to decrease tracheal sounds. You may need to have the client turn the head slightly to the side not being examined.

- Repeat the procedure using the bell of the stethoscope.

ALERT!

It is important not to put pressure on the bell of the stethoscope as this may occlude the sounds in the blood vessel.

- While auscultating, you should hear a very quiet sound. Normal heart sounds could be transmitted to the neck, but there should be no swishing sounds.

▶ A swishing sound indicates the presence of a **bruit,** an obstruction causing turbulence, such as a narrowing of the vessel due to the buildup of cholesterol.

▶ An increased cardiac output such as that seen in hyperthyroidism or anemia also will produce a bruit.

ARMS

1. Assess the hands.

- Take the client's hands in your hands. Note the color of skin and nail beds, the temperature and texture of the skin, and the presence of any lesions or swelling. Look at the fingers and nails from the side and observe the angle of the nail base. The angle should be about 160 degrees.

▶ Flattening of the angle of the nail and enlargement of the tips of the fingers (**clubbing**) is a sign of oxygen deprivation in the extremities. In clients with chronic hypoxia (oxygen deprivation), there may be a rounding of the tip of the finger described as "turkey drumsticks." The nail may feel spongy instead of firm, and there may be a blue discoloration of the nail.

2. Observe for capillary refill in both hands.

- Holding one of the client's hands in your hand, apply pressure to one of the client's fingernails for 5 seconds.

- The area under pressure should turn pale. Release the pressure and note how rapidly the normal color returns.

- In a healthy client, the color should return in less than 1 to 2 seconds.

- Repeat the procedure for the other hand.

▶ A delayed capillary refill could indicate decreased cardiac output or constriction of the peripheral vessels. However, cigarette smoking, anemia, or cold temperatures can also cause delayed capillary refill.

3. Place both arms together and compare their size.

- They should be nearly equal in size.

▶ **Edema** (increased accumulation of fluid) in the arms could indicate an obstruction of the lymphatic system.

4. Palpate the radial pulse.

- The radial pulses are found on the ventral and medial side of each wrist. Ask the client to extend one hand, palm up.

- Palpate with two fingers over the radial bone (see Figure 18.9 ●).

TECHNIQUES AND NORMAL FINDINGS

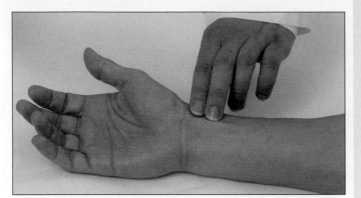

Figure 18.9 ●
Palpating the
radial pulse.

- Repeat the procedure for the other arm. Note the rate, rhythm, amplitude, and symmetry of the pulses.
- Characteristics of peripheral pulse are included in Box 18.1.

▶ It is not necessary to palpate the ulnar pulses, located medial to the ulna on the flexor surface of the wrist. They are deeper than the radial pulses and are difficult to palpate.

Box 18.1   Assessing Peripheral Pulses

Assess peripheral pulses by palpating with gentle pressure over the artery. Use the pads of your first three fingers.

Note the following characteristics:
- Rate—the number of beats per minute
- Rhythm—the regularity of the beats
- Symmetry—pulses on both sides of body should be similar
- Amplitude—the strength of the beat, assessed on a scale of 0 to 4:
    - 4 = Bounding
    - 3 = Increased
    - 2 = Normal
    - 1 = Weak
    - 0 = Absent or nonpalpable

---

5. **Palpate both brachial pulses.**
   - The brachial pulses are found just medial to the biceps tendon.
   - Ask the client to extend the arm.
   - Palpate over the brachial artery just superior to the antecubital region (see Figure 18.10 ●).

▶ If any pulses are difficult to palpate, a Doppler flowmeter should be used. When positioned over a patent artery, this device emits sound waves as the blood moves through the artery.

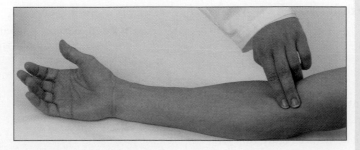

Figure 18.10 ●
Palpating the
brachial pulse.

- Repeat the procedure for the other arm.
- Note the rate, rhythm, amplitude, and symmetry of the pulses.
- Grade the amplitude on the 4-point scale as before.

TECHNIQUES AND NORMAL FINDINGS	ABNORMAL FINDINGS SPECIAL CONSIDERATIONS

6. Perform Allen's test.

- If you suspect an obstruction or insufficiency of an artery in the arm, Allen's test may determine the patency of the radial and ulnar arteries.
- Ask the client to place the hands on the knees with palms up.
- Compress the radial arteries of both wrists with your thumbs.
- Ask the client to open and close his or her fist several times.
- While you are still compressing the radial arteries, ask the client to open his or her hands.
- The palms should become pink immediately, indicating patent ulnar arteries.

▶ If normal color does not return, the ulnar arteries may be occluded.

- Next, occlude the ulnar arteries and repeat the same procedure to test the patency of the radial arteries (see Figure 18.11 ●).

▶ If normal color does not return, the radial arteries may be occluded.

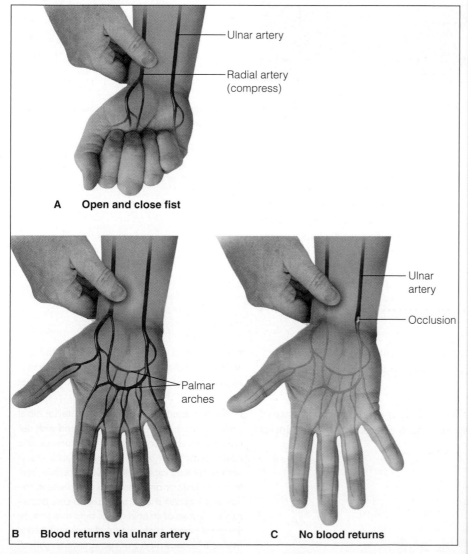

A   **Open and close fist**

Ulnar artery

Radial artery (compress)

Ulnar artery

Occlusion

Palmar arches

B   **Blood returns via ulnar artery**   C   **No blood returns**

Figure 18.11 ● Allen's test.

TECHNIQUES AND NORMAL FINDINGS	ABNORMAL FINDINGS SPECIAL CONSIDERATIONS

7. Palpate the epitrochlear lymph node in each arm.

- The epitrochlear node drains the forearm and the third, fourth, and fifth fingers.
- Hold the client's right hand in your right hand. With your left hand, reach behind the elbow to the groove between the biceps and triceps muscles (see Figure 18.12 ●).

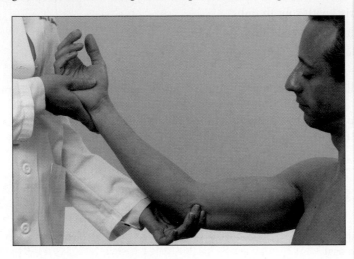

Figure 18.12 ● Palpating the epitrochlear lymph node.

- Note the size and consistency of the node. Normally, it is not palpable or is barely palpable.

  ▶ An enlarged node may indicate an infection in the hand or forearm.

- Repeat the procedure for the left arm.

8. Palpate the axillary lymph nodes.

- With the palmar surface of your fingers, reach deep into the axilla. Gently palpate the anterior border of the axilla (anterior or subpectoral nodes), the central aspect along the rib cage (central nodes), the posterior border (subscapular/posterior nodes), and along the inner aspect of the upper arm (lateral nodes). Refer to Figure 16.20 on page 415 for a depiction of palpating the axillary lymph nodes. ∞

LEGS

1. Inspect both legs.

- Observe skin color, hair distribution, and any skin lesions.
- Skin color should match the skin tone of the rest of the body. Hair is normally present on the legs.
- If the hair has been removed, there is still usually hair on the dorsal surface of the great toes. Hair growth should be symmetrical. The skin should be intact with no lesions.

  ▶ If peripheral vessels are constricted, the skin will be paler than the rest of the body. If the vessels are dilated, the skin will have a reddish tone.

  ▶ A rusty discoloration over the anterior tibial surface with the skin intact is associated with decreased arterial circulation. The characteristic color stems from blood leaking out of a vessel with decreased capacity for it to be reabsorbed.
  ▶ If skin lesions or ulcerations are present, the size and location should be noted. Ulcers occurring as a result of arterial deficit tend to occur on pressure points, such as tips of toes and lateral malleoli. Venous ulcers occur at medial malleoli because of fragile tissue with poor drainage.
  ▶ If any blackened tissue is discovered, the client must be referred to a physician immediately. The presence of blackened tissue can indicate tissue death (necrosis).

TECHNIQUES AND NORMAL FINDINGS	**ABNORMAL FINDINGS** **SPECIAL CONSIDERATIONS**

2. Compare the size of both legs.

- Both legs should be symmetrical in size. If the legs are unequal in size, measure the circumference of each leg at the widest point. It is important to measure each leg at the same point.

▶ A discrepancy in the size of the legs could indicate an accumulation of fluid (edema) resulting from increased pressure in the capillaries or an obstruction of a lymph vessel. Unequal size of the legs could also indicate a blood clot in the deep vessels of the leg.

3. Palpate the legs for temperature.

- Palpate from the feet up the legs, using the dorsal surface of your hands.
- Note any discrepancies.
- The skin should be the same temperature on both legs.

▶ If the peripheral vessels are constricted, the skin will feel cool. If the peripheral vessels are dilated, the skin will feel warm. A difference in the temperature of the feet may be a sign of arterial insufficiency.

4. Assess the legs for the presence of superficial veins.

- With the client in a sitting position and legs dangling from the examination table, inspect the legs.
- Now ask the client to elevate the legs.
- The veins may appear as nodular bulges when the legs are in the dependent position, but any bulges should disappear when the legs are elevated.
- Palpate the veins for tenderness or inflammation (phlebitis).

▶ **Varicosities** (distended veins) frequently occur in the anterolateral aspect of the thigh and lower leg or on the posterolateral aspect of the calf. These bulging veins do not disappear when legs are elevated. Varicose veins are dilated but have a diminished blood flow and an increased intravenous pressure. An incompetent valve, a weakness in the vein wall, or an obstruction in a proximal vein causes varicosities.

5. Perform the manual compression test.

- If varicose veins are present, you can determine the length of the varicose vein and the competency of its valves with the manual compression test.
- Ask the client to stand.
- With the fingers of one hand, palpate the lower part of the varicose vein.
- Keeping that hand on the vein, compress the vein firmly at least 15 to 20 cm higher with the fingers of your other hand (see Figure 18.13 ●).

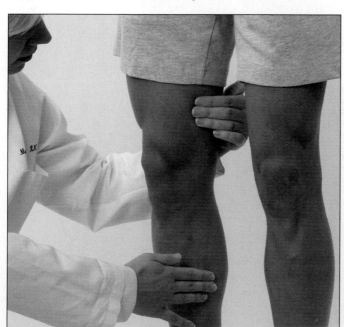

Figure 18.13 ●
Performing the
manual
compression
test.

TECHNIQUES AND NORMAL FINDINGS

- You will not feel any pulsation beneath your lower fingers if the valves of the varicose vein are still competent.

6. **Perform Trendelenburg's test.**
   - A second test to evaluate valve competence in the presence of varicosities is Trendelenburg's test.
   - Assist the client to a supine position.
   - Elevate the leg to 90 degrees until the venous blood has drained from the leg.
   - Place a tourniquet around the upper thigh (see Figure 18.14A ●).
   - Help the client to stand.
   - Watch for filling of the venous system (see Figure 18.14B ●).

▶ If the valves are incompetent, an impulse in the vein will be felt between your two hands.

▶ A rapid filling of the superficial veins from above indicates incompetent valves.

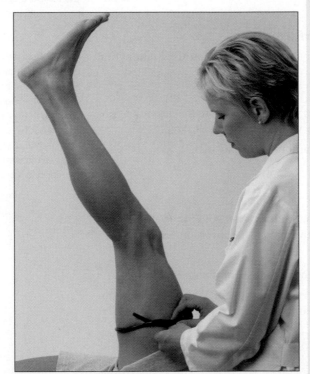

Figure 18.14A ●
Performing the
Trendelenburg's test.
A. Applying tourniquet.

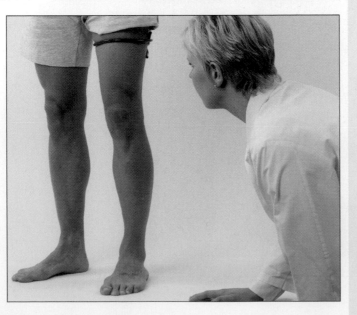

Figure 18.14B ●
Performing the
Trendelenburg
test. B. Watching
for filling.

| **TECHNIQUES AND NORMAL FINDINGS** | **ABNORMAL FINDINGS** **SPECIAL CONSIDERATIONS** |

- The saphenous vein should fill from below in about 30 to 35 seconds.
- After the client has been standing for 20 to 30 seconds, remove the tourniquet and note whether the varicose veins fill from above.

  ▶ A sudden filling of superficial veins after removing the tourniquet indicates backward filling past incompetent valves.

- Competent valves prevent sudden retrograde filling.

7. Test for Homans' sign.

- Assist the client to a supine position.
- Flex the client's knee about 5 degrees.
- Now sharply dorsiflex the client's foot (see Figure 18.15 ●).

  ▶ A positive **Homans' sign** could indicate a blood clot in one of the deep veins of the leg. However, a positive Homans' sign could also indicate an inflammation of one of the superficial leg veins or an inflammation of one of the tendons of the leg. The reliability of Homans' sign in indicating disease has been shown to be inconsistent. Follow-up studies such as a venous Doppler examination may be required to identify the presence of a clot in the deep veins of the leg.

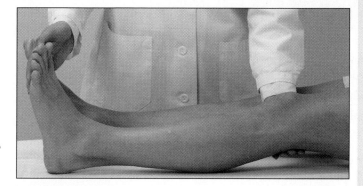

Figure 18.15 ●
Testing for
Homans' sign.

- Ask whether the client feels calf pain.
- This maneuver exerts pressure on the posterior tibial vein and should not cause pain.

8. Palpate the inguinal lymph nodes.

- Move the client's gown aside over the inguinal region. Palpate over the top of the medial thigh (see Figure 18.16 ●).

  ▶ Lymph nodes that are larger than 1 cm or tender may be an indication of an infection in the legs.

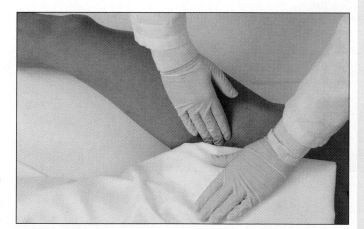

Figure 18.16 ●
Palpating the
inguinal lymph
nodes.

- If the nodes can be palpated, they should be movable and not tender.
- Repeat the procedure for the other leg.

9. Palpate both femoral pulses.

- The femoral pulses are inferior and medial to the inguinal ligament.
- Ask the client to flex the knee and externally rotate the hip. Palpate over the femoral artery (see Figure 18.17 ●).

  ▶ If it is not possible to palpate the femoral pulse, an artery may be occluded.

TECHNIQUES AND NORMAL FINDINGS

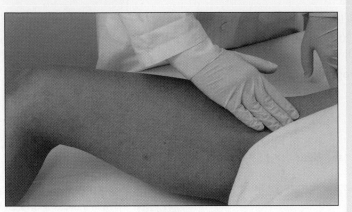

Figure 18.17 ●
Palpating the
femoral artery.

- The femoral artery is deep, and you may need to place one hand on top of the other to locate the pulse. Repeat the procedure for the other leg.
- Note the rate, rhythm, amplitude, and symmetry of the pulses.
- Grade the amplitude on the 4-point scale.

10. Palpate both popliteal pulses.

- The pulsations of the popliteal artery can be palpated deep in the popliteal fossa lateral to the midline.
- Ask the client to flex the knee and relax the leg.

▶ If the popliteal pulse cannot be palpated, an artery may be occluded.

- Palpate the popliteal pulse.
- If you cannot locate the pulse, ask the client to roll onto the abdomen and flex the knee (see Figure 18.18 ●).

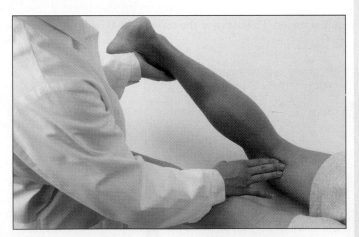

Figure 18.18 ●
Palpating the
popliteal pulse.

- Palpate deeply for the pulse.
- Repeat the procedure for the other leg.
- Note the rate, rhythm, amplitude, and symmetry of the pulses.
- Grade the amplitude on the 4-point scale.

11. Palpate both dorsalis pedis pulses.

- The dorsalis pedis pulses may be felt on the medial side of the dorsum of the foot.

▶ The absence of a dorsalis pedis pulse may not be indicative of occlusion because another artery may be supplying blood to this area of the foot. Edema in the foot will make palpation difficult.

TECHNIQUES AND NORMAL FINDINGS	ABNORMAL FINDINGS SPECIAL CONSIDERATIONS

- Palpate the pulse lateral to the extensor tendon of the great toe (see Figure 18.19 ●).

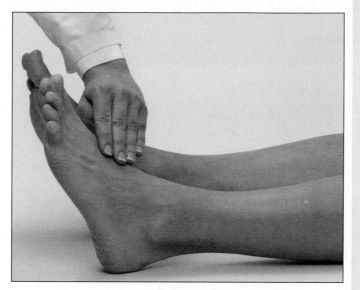

Figure 18.19 ●
Palpating the dorsalis pedis pulse.

- Use light pressure.
- Repeat the procedure for the other foot.
- Note the rate, rhythm, amplitude, and symmetry of the pulses.
- Grade the amplitude on the 4-point scale.

12. Palpate both posterior tibial pulses.

- The posterior tibial pulses may be palpated behind and slightly inferior to the medial malleolus of the ankle, in the groove between the malleolus and the Achilles tendon.
- Palpate the pulse by curving your fingers around the medial malleolus (see Figure 18.20 ●).

▶ If it is not possible to palpate the posterior tibial pulse, an artery may be occluded. If the client has edematous ankles, this pulse may be difficult to palpate.

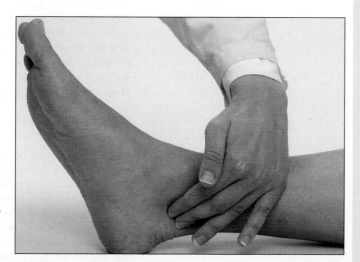

Figure 18.20 ●
Palpating the posterior tibial pulse.

- Repeat the procedure for the other foot. Note the rate, rhythm, amplitude, and symmetry of the pulses.
- Grade the amplitude on the 4-point scale.

TECHNIQUES AND NORMAL FINDINGS	ABNORMAL FINDINGS SPECIAL CONSIDERATIONS

13. Assess for arterial supply to the lower legs and feet.

- If you suspect an arterial deficiency, test for arterial supply to the lower extremities. Ask the client to remain supine.
- Elevate the client's legs 12 inches above the heart.
- Ask the client to move the feet up and down at the ankles for 60 seconds to drain the venous blood (see Figure 18.21 ●).

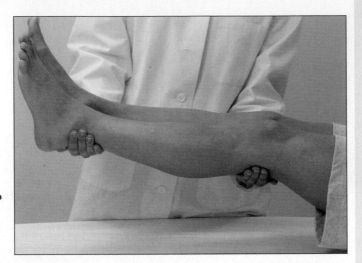

Figure 18.21 ●
Testing the arterial supply to the lower extremities.

- The skin will be blanched in color because only arterial blood is present.
- Now ask the client to sit up and dangle the feet.
- Compare the color of both feet.
- The original color should return in about 10 seconds.
- The superficial veins in the feet should fill in about 15 seconds.

- The feet of a dark-skinned person may be difficult to evaluate, but the soles of the feet should reflect a change in color.

▶ Marked pallor of the elevated extremities may indicate arterial insufficiency.

▶ A marked bluish red color of the dependent feet occurs with severe arterial insufficiency. This color is due to a lack of oxygenated blood to the area, which leads to a loss of vasomotor tone and venous stasis.

▶ Delayed filling of the superficial veins of the feet also could indicate arterial insufficiency. Motor loss may occur with arterial insufficiency.

▶ Sensory loss may occur with arterial insufficiency.

▶ Pitting edema can be related to a failure of the right side of the heart or an obstruction of the lymphatic system. Edema in only one leg may indicate an occlusion of a large vein in the leg. Diminished arterial flow thickens toenails, which often become yellow and loosely attached to the nail bed. Clients with diabetes often acquire fungal and bacterial infections of the nail because of increased glucose collecting in the skin under the nail.

TECHNIQUES AND NORMAL FINDINGS	ABNORMAL FINDINGS SPECIAL CONSIDERATIONS

14. Test the lower legs for muscle strength.

- With the client in a sitting position, instruct the client to extend each knee while you apply opposing force. Instruct the client to flex the knees again. The client should be able to perform the movement against resistance. The strength of the muscles in both legs is equal. Testing of muscle strength is discussed in greater detail in Chapter 23. ⬭

15. Test the lower legs for sensation.

- Use a cotton wisp, lightly applied to symmetrical areas on each lower extremity to assess light touch. The rounded end and the sharp end of a safety pin are used to assess pain sensation. The ends are applied to symmetrical areas of the lower legs in a random pattern of sharp and dull to assess sensation. The client should have eyes closed during the assessment. Ask the client to state "now" when the cotton wisp is felt, and "sharp" or "dull" when the ends of the safety pin are applied.

- The client should sense touch and pain. Testing for sensation is discussed in greater detail in Chapter 24. ⬭

16. Check for edema of the legs.

- Press the skin for at least 5 seconds over the tibia, behind the medial malleolus, and over the dorsum of each foot (see Figure 18.22 ●).

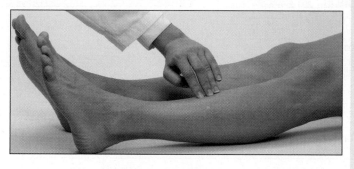

Figure 18.22 ● Palpating for edema over the tibia.

- Look for a depression in the skin (called pitting edema) caused by the pressure of your fingers (see Figure 18.23 ●).

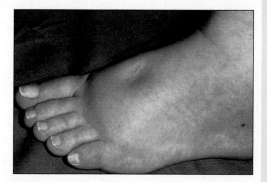

Figure 18.23 ● Pitting edema of the lower extremities.

TECHNIQUES AND NORMAL FINDINGS	ABNORMAL FINDINGS SPECIAL CONSIDERATIONS

- If edema is present, you should grade it on a scale of 1+ (mild) to 4+ (severe) (see Figure 18.24 ●).

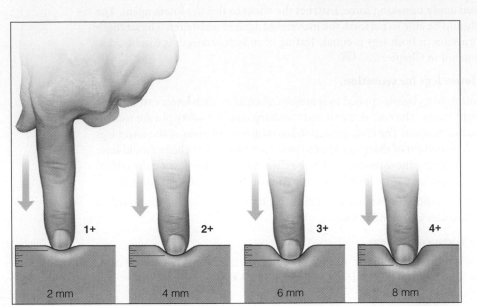

Figure 18.24 ● Grading pitting edema.

17. Inspect the toenails for color and thickness.

- Nails should be pink and not thickened. Clubbing should not be present.

Refer to the Companion Website at **www.prenhall.com/damico** and click on the **Documentation** module for documentation samples and documentation practice exercises.

Findings from physical assessment of the peripheral vascular and lymphatic systems include normal and abnormal pulses (see Table 18.2) and common alterations of the peripheral vascular and lymphatic systems as shown in Figures 18.25 through 18.31.

Table 18.2	Normal and Abnormal Pulses		
NAME OF PULSE	**CHARACTERISTICS**	**ARTERIAL WAVEFORM PATTERN**	**CONTRIBUTING CONDITIONS**
Normal	• Regular, even in intensity		• Normal
Absent	• No palpable pulse, no waveform		• Arterial line disconnected • Cardiac arrest
Weak/thready	• Intensity of pulse is +1 • May wax and wane • May be difficult to find		• Shock • Severe peripheral vascular disease
Bounding	• Intensity of pulse is +4 • Very easy to observe in arterial locations near surface of skin • Very easy to palpate and difficult to obliterate with pressure from fingertips		• Hyperdynamic states such as seen with hyperthyroidism, exercise, anxiety, vasodilation seen in high cardiac output syndromes • May be due to normal aging secondary to arterial wall stiffening • Aortic regurgitation • Anemia
Biferiens	• Has two systolic peaks with a dip in between • Easier to detect in the carotid location • In the case of hypertrophic obstructive cardiomyopathy only one systolic peak palpated, but waveform demonstrates double systolic peak		• Aortic regurgitation • Combination of aortic regurgitation and stenosis • Hypertrophic obstructive cardiomyopathy
Pulsus Alternans	• Alternating strong and weak pulses • Equal interval between each pulse		• Aortic regurgitation • Terminal left ventricular heart failure • Systemic hypertension
Pulsus Bigeminus	• Alternating strong and weak pulses, but the weak pulse comes in *early* after the strong pulse		• Regular bigeminal dysrhythmias such as PVCs and PACs
Pulsus Paradoxus	• Reduced intensity of pulse during inspiration versus expiration	Expiration Inspiration	• Cardiac tamponade • Acute pulmonary embolus • Pericarditis • May be present in clients with chronic lung disease • Hypovolemic shock • Pregnancy
Water-hammer, Corrigan's Pulse	• Rapid systolic upstroke and no dicrotic notch secondary to rapid collapse		• Aortic regurgitation
Unequal	• Difference in intensity or amplitude between right and left pulses	Right femoral Left femoral	• Dissecting aneurysm (location of aneurysm determines where the difference in amplitude is felt)

Arterial Insufficiency

Arterial insufficiency is inadequate circulation in the arterial system, usually due to the buildup of fatty plaque or calcification of the arterial wall resulting in diminished pulses; cool, shiny skin; absence of hair on toes; pallor on elevation, red color when dependent; and deep muscle pain, usually in the calf or lower leg aggravated by activity and elevation of the limb. Pain is quickly relieved by rest. Ulcers due to arterial insufficiency are usually seen on the toes or areas of trauma of the feet or lateral malleolus (see Figure 18.25 ●). The ulcer is pale in color with well-defined edges and no bleeding.

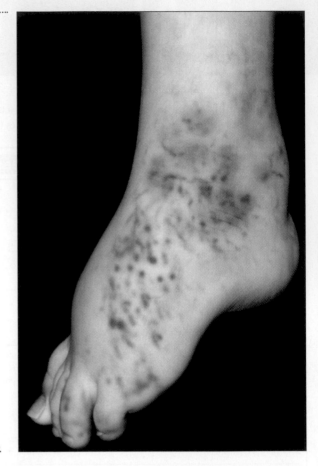

Figure 18.25 ● Arterial insufficiency.

Arterial Aneurysm

Arterial aneurysm is a bulging or dilation caused by a weakness in the wall of an artery (see Figure 18.26 ●). It can occur in the aorta and abdominal, renal, or femoral arteries. Aneurysms can sometimes be detected by a characteristic bruit over the artery; however, if they are located deep in the abdomen, they can be difficult to discover.

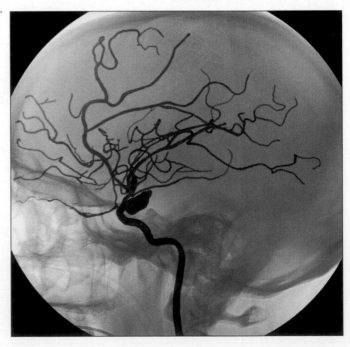

Figure 18.26 ● Arterial aneurysm.

Venous Insufficiency

Venous insufficiency is inadequate circulation in the venous system usually due to incompetent valves in deep veins or a blood clot in the veins. Temperature of skin is normal, but edema is usually present and is accompanied by a feeling of fullness in the legs. Skin around the ankles may be thickened and have a brown discoloration (see Figure 18.27 ●). Discomfort is aggravated by prolonged standing or sitting and is relieved by rest but only after several hours. Ulcers related to venous insufficiency are often found on the medial malleolus and are characterized by bleeding and uneven edges. There is minimal pain associated with the ulcer, and the skin surrounding the ulcer is coarse.

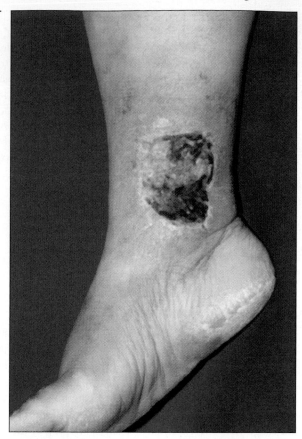

Figure 18.27 ● Venous insufficiency.

Varicose Veins

Varicose veins are veins that have become dilated and have a diminished rate of blood flow and increased intravenous pressure (see Figure 18.28 ●). The condition may be the result of incompetent valves that permit the reflux of blood or an obstruction of a proximal vein.

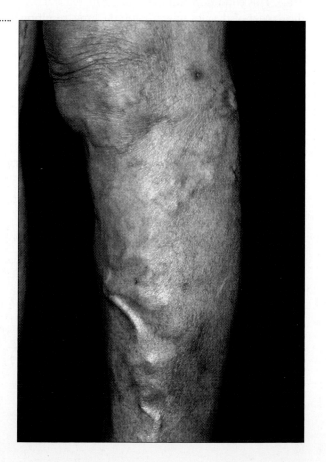

Figure 18.28 ● Varicose veins.

Raynaud's Disease

Raynaud's disease is a condition in which the arterioles in the fingers develop spasms, causing intermittent skin pallor or cyanosis and then rubor (red color). The spasms may last from minutes to hours, occurring bilaterally. The client may describe numbness or pain during the pallor or cyanotic state, and burning or throbbing pain during the rubor. This condition is seen most commonly in young, otherwise healthy females, frequently secondary to connective tissue disease, drug intoxication, pulmonary hypertension, or trauma (see Figure 18.29 ●).

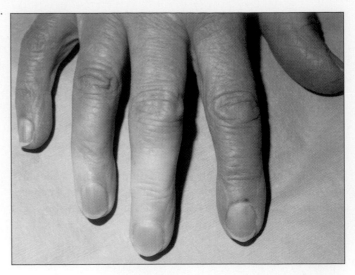

Figure 18.29 ● Raynaud's disease.

Deep Vein Thrombosis

Deep vein thrombosis is the occlusion of a deep vein, such as in the femoral or pelvic circulation, by a blood clot. There may be no symptoms or the client may describe intense, sharp pain along the iliac vessels, in the popliteal space, or in the calf muscles. Pain may increase with sharp dorsiflexion of the foot (Homans' sign), but this maneuver is not absolutely reliable for diagnosis. There may also be slight swelling of the leg, some edema, low-grade fever, and tachycardia (rapid heartbeat). This condition requires immediate referral because of the danger of the clot migrating to the lung, resulting in a pulmonary embolism (see Figure 18.30 ●).

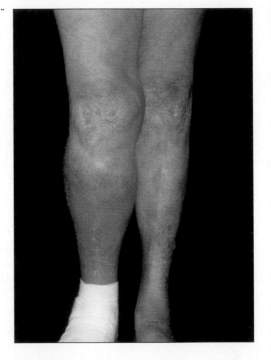

Figure 18.30 ● Deep vein thrombosis.

Lymphedema

Lymphedema is unilateral swelling associated with an obstruction in lymph nodes (see Figure 18.31 ●).

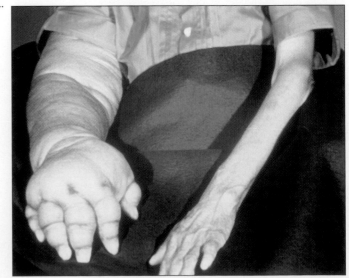

Figure 18.31 ● Lymphedema.

Health Promotion

HEALTHY PEOPLE 2010

FOCUS AREA	PREVALENCE	OBJECTIVES	ACTIONS
High Blood Pressure	• Hypertension occurs most frequently in older adults. • Over 50 million adults have hypertension. • Hypertension is more prevalent in African Americans than whites. • Hypertension is a risk factor for heart, kidney, and cerebrovascular disease. • Obesity increases the risk for development of hypertension.	• Increase blood pressure screening. • Increase the number of adults who know their blood pressure reading. • Increase the number of people with hypertension who have blood pressure under control. • Increase the number of people with hypertension who take actions to reduce blood pressure (weight loss, increase of activity, smoking cessation).	• Blood pressure screening. • Referral to ongoing care. • Education regarding the risks associated with hypertension. • Programs for weight reduction, increase of activity, and smoking cessation.
Stroke	• Approximately 600,000 strokes occur annually in the United States. • Deaths from stroke are 80% higher in African Americans than whites. • Hypertension, cigarette smoking, high blood cholesterol, and obesity increase the risk for stroke.	• Reduce stroke deaths. • Increase awareness of early warning signs of stroke.	• Education regarding warning signs. • Smoking cessation programs. • Education aimed at adolescents regarding risk factors.

CLIENT EDUCATION

The following are physiological, behavioral, and cultural factors that affect the health of the peripheral vascular system across the age span. Several of these factors are cited as trends in *Healthy People 2010*. The nurse provides advice and education to reduce risks associated with these factors and to promote and maintain health of the peripheral vascular and lymphatic systems.

LIFE SPAN CONSIDERATIONS

RISK FACTORS

• Palpable lymph nodes often occur in healthy infants and children.

• The hormonal changes of pregnancy cause vascular changes and increased blood volume, which can result in hypo- or hypertension. As the pregnancy progresses, drainage of the iliac veins and inferior vena cava is obstructed. As a result, venous pressure increases causing edema, varicosities, and hemorrhoids.

• Obesity is increasingly prevalent across the age span. Obesity increases the risk for diabetes, hypertension, and cardiac disease.

• Varicose veins occur in both sexes and are associated with enlargement of calf veins in aging, as well as prolonged standing or sitting in one position and constrictive clothing.

CLIENT EDUCATION

• Advise parents that lymph nodes enlarge during infection but may remain enlarged even when the child is well. Abdominal pain may be a result of enlarged mesenteric lymph nodes that accompany an upper respiratory infection. Parents should be encouraged to seek care when lymph node enlargement is unaccounted for and supported when seeking advice about the discomfort associated with expected lymph involvement.

• Provide prenatal education and care to reduce risk for and associated with hypertension and vascular changes.

• Provide education about healthy eating and exercise to prevent obesity and the associated vascular problems.

• Provide education and encouragement to prevent varicosities with elevation of legs, avoidance of tight clothing such as socks or garters to reduce the risk of hypertension and varicosities.

CULTURAL CONSIDERATIONS

RISK FACTORS

- African Americans are at greater risk for developing hypertension than other groups.
- Guidelines for hypertension include a "prehypertensive" category for those with a systolic blood pressure between 120 and 139 and diastolic between 80 and 89. Those with prehypertension are at risk for progression to hypertension.

CLIENT EDUCATION

- Advise all clients to have blood pressure screening. African Americans and those in the prehypertensive category must receive information about blood pressure monitoring and activities to reduce risks including healthy dietary practices, weight reduction, and exercise.

ENVIRONMENTAL CONSIDERATIONS

RISK FACTORS

- Diabetes increases the risk for vascular diseases including hypertension, arterial or venous insufficiency, and coronary artery disease.
- The use of oral contraceptives increases the risk for development of thrombosis, especially in females who smoke.
- Peripheral vascular disease (PVD) can result in slow-healing ulcers. Risks for PVD include obesity, family history, diabetes, coronary artery disease (CAD), aging, and high cholesterol.
- Medications for hypertension may have side effects including nausea, headache, dizziness, decreased sex drive, and impotence in males. Noncompliance with treatment increases the risks for complications of hypertension.

CLIENT EDUCATION

- Advise those with a family history of diabetes about screening. Early diagnosis can reduce risks for complications.
- Explain the risks of oral contraceptives to female clients, provide information about the signs of thrombosis, and advise them to seek healthcare if symptoms arise.
- Educate clients with diabetes or peripheral vascular disease about skin assessment and care, particularly of the feet.
- Educate clients about the importance of following recommended treatment for hypertension. Advise clients to discuss side effects with their healthcare provider so that effective treatment can be provided.

BEHAVIORAL CONSIDERATIONS

RISK FACTORS

- Hypertension increases the risk for cardiac disease and stroke. Risk factors for hypertension include obesity, lack of exercise, alcohol consumption, smoking, and stress.
- Prolonged immobility is a risk factor for development of deep vein thrombosis (DVT), which can occur in those who are severely ill, postsurgery, involved in prolonged sitting at work, or in travel.
- Smoking is associated with increased risk for peripheral vascular diseases and hypertension.

CLIENT EDUCATION

- Advise all clients to have blood pressure screening. African Americans and those in the prehypertensive category must receive information about blood pressure monitoring and activities to reduce risks including healthy dietary practices, weight reduction, and exercise.
- Provide general education about immobility as a risk for DVT, especially to older clients and those who are involved in air or other travel. Include advice to get up and walk and to increase intake of water when traveling.
- Educate clients about the risks of smoking and encourage them to join a cessation program.

Application Through Critical Thinking

CASE STUDY

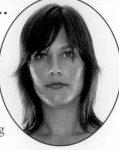

Jenny Battaglia, a 26-year-old female, is seen in the emergency department for pain in her lower legs. The client states that she has had pain in her calves for about 48 hours, starting when she got home from vacation. She does not recall any injury. She says it started like cramping but has not improved with rest or taking Tylenol. She thinks there is little swelling and some tenderness.

The nurse knows that an organized approach to data collection is essential. Further, every effort must be made to get a comprehensive picture of the situation and to avoid missing pieces of information that will guide decision making for the client.

The approach to care of the client will be determined by the client's condition. When a client is in acute distress—for example, with dyspnea, with a bleeding injury, in shock, or in severe pain—data gathering focuses on the immediate problem and its resolution.

Ms. Battaglia is uncomfortable but does not appear to be in acute distress and denies severe discomfort. She states, "I'm a little nervous. I've never really been sick and have only been in the emergency department once before for a couple of stitches when I was 10." The nurse tells Ms. Battaglia that they will begin an examination to determine the cause of her problem.

The assessment reveals the following: A thin female. The client is suntanned, and without pink undertone to her skin. B/P 116/64 (R) arm, sitting, pulse 88, 3+. Upper extremities symmetrical in size, no edema, radial and brachial pulses equal, regular, lower extremities, edema, rubor (redness) bilateral posterior lower legs, warm and tender to touch. Pulses present, equal, 3+. Positive Homans' sign.

The nurse considers the data and determines that Ms. Battaglia is not in acute distress. However, pallor, edema in lower extremities, and the positive Homans' sign suggest a vascular problem. The nurse decides to continue the health assessment by further interview for missing subjective information.

The interview reveals that Ms. Battaglia has no personal or family history of vascular problems, cardiovascular disease, or diabetes. She is not married and lives with her boyfriend. She takes aspirin or Tylenol occasionally for headaches or menstrual cramps. She has no allergies. She is para 0 gravida 0, LMP 2 weeks prior to ED visit, regular menses, has taken birth control pills for 3 years.

The nurse asks Ms. Battaglia several questions about the leg pain. The client states it is 5 to 7 on a scale of 1 to 10 and continuous. Nothing she has done has relieved the pain. It started 48 hours ago "at the end of my vacation" and wakes her at night.

The nurse asks if travel was involved in the vacation. Ms. Battaglia says, "Yes, we flew to Aruba for 6 days. That's how I got a tan. We had a great time and I was feeling rested, ready to go back to work, and looked forward to seeing family and friends." Further questions reveal that the flight was 6 hours and Ms. Battaglia "slept almost all the way back, I never really moved."

The data suggest to the nurse that Ms. Battaglia has deep vein thrombosis. Ms. Battaglia is admitted to a medical unit. She will be on bed rest and receive anticoagulation.

► Complete Documentation

The following is a sample narrative complete documentation for Jenny Battaglia.

SUBJECTIVE DATA: Pain in lower legs for about 48 hr. Started when she got home from vacation. No recall of injury. Started as cramping, no improvement with rest or Tylenol. She thinks there is some swelling and tenderness. "A little nervous." No personal or family history of vascular problems, cardiac disease, or diabetes. Single, lives with boyfriend. Tylenol or aspirin

occasionally for headache or menstrual cramps. No allergies. Gravida 0, Para 0, LMP 2 weeks prior to ED visit, regular menses. Oral contraceptives for 3 years. Air travel—flight of 6 hr—Jenny slept almost all the time.

OBJECTIVE DATA: Suntanned, without pink undertone. Vital signs: B/P 116/64 right, sitting. Radial pulse 88, 3 + T 99.20°. Pain: 5 to 7 on a scale of 1 to 10, continuous, wakes at night. Upper extremities symmetrical in size, no edema, warm brachial and radial pulses = regular. Cap refill <2 sec L & R. Extremities—below knees, posterior bilateral rubor, edema 1+, warm, tender to touch. Pulses present, 3+. Positive Homans' sign. No lesions, no visible superficial vessels. Feet warm, no edema. Toenails—polish—unable to assess.

► Critical Thinking Questions

1. Identify the data that suggest the presence of DVT.
2. How would the data be clustered?
3. Describe the areas for client education derived from this case study.

► Applying Nursing Diagnoses

1. *Tissue perfusion, ineffective* is a nursing diagnosis in the NANDA taxonomy (see Appendix A ⚭).Does the case study for Ms. Battaglia provide data to support this diagnosis? If so, identify the data.
2. Explain your analysis of the data in the case study to formulate additional diagnoses.
3. Provide PES (problem, etiology, signs or symptoms) statements for additional diagnoses for Ms. Battaglia.

► Prepare Teaching Plan

LEARNING NEED: The data in the case study reveals that Ms. Battaglia is at risk for development of DVT because she is using oral contraceptives and has experienced recent air travel. Her symptoms are typical for DVT. She will be admitted for treatment of DVT and will receive education regarding her treatment regimen and follow-up care.

The case study provides data that is representative of risks, symptoms, and behaviors of many individuals. Therefore, the following teaching plan is based on the need to provide information to members of any community about DVT.

GOAL: The participants in this learning program will have increased awareness of risk factors and strategies to prevent DVT.

OBJECTIVES: At the completion of this learning session, the participants will be able to:

1. Describe DVT.
2. Identify risk factors associated with DVT.
3. List the symptoms of DVT.
4. Discuss strategies to prevent DVT.

ASSESSMENT FORM

EXAM	FINDINGS

Peripheral Vascular System

Blood Pressure

	Sitting	Standing	Supine
Left	_____	_____	_____
Right	116/64	_____	_____

Upper Extremity

Skin
- Left: Color _suntanned no pink undertone_ Temperature _warm_
- Right: Color _suntanned no pink undertone_ Temperature _warm_

Capillary Refill   Left __<2 sec__   Right __<2 sec__

Arm Size   Left = Right ✓

Edema
- Left   0 ✓   1+ _____   2+ _____   3+ _____   4+ _____
- Right   0 ✓   1+ _____   2+ _____   3+ _____   4+ _____

Pulses

Radial	Rate 88	Rhythm Regular	Amplitude 3+
Ulnar	Rate 88	Rhythm Regular	Amplitude 3+
Brachial	Rate 88	Rhythm Regular	Amplitude 3+

Lower Extremity

Skin
- Legs
  - Left: Color _posterior knee rubor_   Temperature _Warm_
  - Right: Color _posterior knee rubor_   Temperature _Warm_
- Feet
  - Left: Color _Pink_   Temperature _Warm_
  - Right: Color _Pink_   Temperature _Warm_

Leg Size   Left = Right   ✓ yes _____ no _____

Edema
- Legs
  - Left   0 _____   1+ ✓   2+ _____   3+ _____   4+ _____
  - Right   0 _____   1+ ✓   2+ _____   3+ _____   4+ _____
- Feet
  - Left   0 ✓   1+ _____   2+ _____   3+ _____   4+ _____
  - Right   0 ✓   1+ _____   2+ _____   3+ _____   4+ _____

Superficial Veins
- Left   0
- Right   0

Lesions
- Left   0
- Right   0

Homans' Sign   Left _____ ✓ _____ + _____ -   Right _____ ✓ _____ + _____ -

Toenails   Left _unable to assess_   Right _unable to assess_

Pulses

Femoral	Rate present	Rhythm Regular	Amplitude 3+
Popliteal	Rate present	Rhythm Regular	Amplitude 3+
Posterior Tibial	Rate present	Rhythm Regular	Amplitude 3+
Dorsalis Pedis	Rate present	Rhythm Regular	Amplitude 3+

APPLICATION OF OBJECTIVE 2: Identify risk factors associated with DVT

Content	Teaching Strategy	Evaluation

• Age—over 40 years of age
• Family history of clotting disorder or DVT
• Circulation problems
• Obesity
• Cancer treatment
• Pregnancy or recent birth
• Oral contraception or hormonal therapy
• Immobility:
  1. Sitting for long periods during auto or air travel
  2. Surgery or illness
  3. Recent surgery
  4. Trauma
• Smoking
• Dehydration
	• Lecture
	• Discussion
	• Audiovisual materials
	• Printed materials
	
	Lecture is appropriate when disseminating information to large groups.
	
	Discussion allows participants to bring up concerns and to raise questions.
	
	Audiovisual materials reinforce verbal presentation.
	
	Printed material, especially to be taken away with learners, allows review, reinforcement, and repeated reading at the learner's pace.
		• Written examination.
		
		May use short answer, fill-in, or multiple-choice items or a combination of items.
		
		If these are short and easy to evaluate, the learner receives immediate feedback.

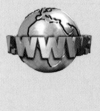

Please refer to the Companion Website at www.prenhall.com/damico and click on Chapter 18, the Application Through Critical Thinking module, to complete the following activities related to this case study:
- ▶ **Critical Thinking questions**
- ▶ **Extended Nursing Diagnosis challenge**
- ▶ **Documentation activity**
- ▶ **Teaching Plan for Objectives 1, 3, and 4**

EXPLORE MediaLink

Additional resources for this chapter are found on the Student CD-ROM accompanying this textbook and on the Companion Website.

CD-ROM CONTENT

Content for this chapter includes:
Objectives
Key Concepts
NCLEX-RN® Review Questions
Model Documentation Forms
Audio Glossary
Animations
  Blood Pressure: Systole and Diastole
  Lymphatics
  Capillary Pressure
Games and Challenges
Head-to-Toe Physical Examination Video

COMPANION WEBSITE CONTENT

www.prenhall.com/damico

Content for this chapter includes:
Objectives
NCLEX-RN® Review Questions

Client Interaction Case Study Challenge
Application Through Critical Thinking
  Case Study Teaching Plan Challenge
MediaLinks
MediaLink Application
Tool Box
  Chapter Documentation Form Example
  Assessing Peripheral Pulses
  National Institutes of Health (NIH) Blood Pressure Guidelines
  Grading Pitting Edema
  Normal and Abnormal Pulses
  Health Promotion
    Healthy People 2010
    Client Education
New York Times

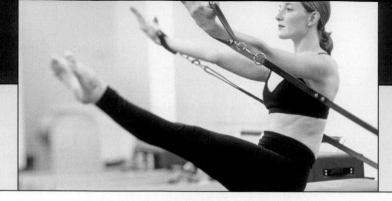

19
Abdomen

MEDIALINK

www.prenhall.com/damico

The CD-ROM in the back of this textbook and the Media-Link website contain NCLEX-RN® review questions, interactive exercises, case study challenges, animations, videos, documentation and checklist forms, and review materials. For a complete listing of the media content specific to Chapter 19, see the Explore MediaLink at the end of the chapter.

The **abdomen** is not a system unto itself. It is the largest cavity of the body and contains many organs and structures that belong to various systems of the body. For example, the liver, gallbladder, and stomach belong to the digestive system. The kidneys, ureters, and bladder belong to the urinary system. These structures and many other structures are assessed when performing an abdominal assessment. The primary focus of this chapter is the assessment of the structures of the digestive system.

The primary responsibility of the digestive system is to take in, break down, and absorb nutrients to be used by all cells of the body. The ability to perform these functions is influenced by the health of many other body systems. The parasympathetic fibers of the nervous system increase digestion while the sympathetic fibers inhibit the process. The respiratory system provides oxygen needed for the metabolic processes and removes the carbon dioxide created by metabolism. The hormones of the endocrine system help regulate digestion and the metabolic processes.

Abnormalities of the gastrointestinal system include colorectal cancer, hepatitis, and foodborne illnesses, all of which are focus areas in *Healthy People 2010*. Health-related goals in these focus areas are to reduce deaths from colorectal cancer, to decrease the number of foodborne infections, to decrease anaphylaxis from foods, and to reduce the number of cases of hepatitis A, B, and C as illustrated in the *Healthy People 2010* feature on page 549.

ANATOMY AND PHYSIOLOGY REVIEW

The abdomen is composed of the alimentary canal, the intestines, accessory digestive organs, the urinary system, the spleen, and reproductive organs. Each of these structures or systems will be discussed in the following sections.

ABDOMEN

The abdomen is situated in the anterior region of the body. It is inferior to the diaphragm of the respiratory system and superior to the pelvic floor. The abdominal muscles, the intercostal margins, and the pelvis form the anterior borders of the abdomen. The vertebral column and the lumbar muscles form the posterior borders of the abdomen.

The anatomy and physiology review of the abdomen has a two-point focus. The primary focus is the gastrointestinal system, and the secondary focus is the abdominal structures of other systems. The gastrointestinal system consists of the alimentary canal and the accessory organs of the digestive system. The **alimentary canal**, a continuous, hollow, muscular tube, begins at the mouth and terminates at the anus. The accessory organs include the teeth, salivary glands, liver, gallbladder, and pancreas (see Figure 19.1 ●).

The anatomy, physiology, and assessment of the mouth, teeth, tongue, salivary glands, and pharynx are discussed in Chapter 14 of this text. ⚭ Before proceeding with the assessment of the abdomen, it may be helpful to review the information in that chapter.

ALIMENTARY CANAL

The alimentary canal is the continuous hollow tube extending from the mouth to the anus. The boundaries include the mouth, pharynx, esophagus, stomach, small and large intestines, rectum, and anus.

Esophagus

The esophagus, a collapsible tube, connects the pharynx to the stomach. Approximately 25 cm (10 in.) in length, it passes through the mediastinum and diaphragm to meet the stomach at the cardiac sphincter. The primary function of the esophagus is to propel food and fluid from the mouth to the stomach.

Stomach

The stomach extends from the esophagus at the cardiac sphincter to the duodenum at the pyloric sphincter. Located in the left side of the upper abdomen, the stomach is

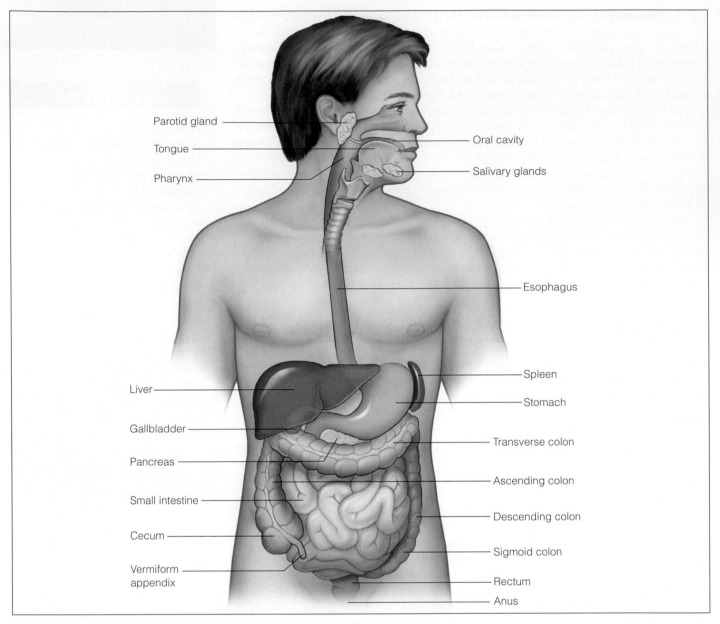

Figure 19.1 ● Organs of the alimentary canal and related accessory organs.

directly inferior to the diaphragm. The diameter and volume of the stomach are directly related to the food it contains. Food mixes with digestive juices in the stomach and becomes chyme before entering the small intestine. The primary function of the stomach is the chemical and mechanical breakdown of food.

Small Intestine

The small intestine is the body's primary digestive and absorptive organ. Approximately 6 m (18 to 21 ft) in length, it has three subdivisions. The first segment, the duodenum, meets the stomach at the pyloric sphincter and extends to the middle region, called the jejunum. The ileum extends from the jejunum to the ileocecal valve at the cecum of the large intestine. Intestinal juices, bile from the liver and gallbladder and pancreatic enzymes, mix with the chyme to promote digestion and facilitate the absorption of nutrients. The primary functions of the small intestine are the continuing chemical breakdown of food and the absorption of digested foods.

Large Intestine

The last portion of the alimentary canal is the large intestine, which extends from the ileocecal valve to the anus. The large intestine is approximately 1.5 m (5 to 5.5 ft) in length. It consists of the cecum, ascending colon, transverse colon, descending colon, sigmoid colon, rectum, and anus. The vermiform appendix is attached to the large intestines at the cecum. The appendix contains masses of lymphoid tissue that make only a minor contribution to immunity; however, when inflamed, the appendix causes significant health problems. The large intestine is wider and shorter than the small intestine. It is on the periphery of the abdominal cavity, surrounding the small intestine and other structures. The main functions of the large intestine are absorbing water from indigestible food residue and eliminating the residue in the form of feces.

ACCESSORY DIGESTIVE ORGANS

The **accessory digestive organs**—the liver, gallbladder, and pancreas—contribute to the digestive process of foods. These structures connect to the alimentary canal by ducts.

Liver

The largest gland of the body, the liver is located in the right upper portion of the abdominal cavity directly inferior to the diaphragm and extends into the left side of the abdomen. The lower portion of the rib cage, which makes only the lower border of the liver palpable, protects the liver. The only digestive function of the liver is the production and secretion of bile for fat emulsification. It has a major role in the metabolism of proteins, fats, and carbohydrates. The liver has the ability to store some vitamins, produce substances for coagulation of blood, produce antibodies, and detoxify harmful substances.

Gallbladder

Chiefly a storage organ for bile, the gallbladder, a thin-walled sac, is nestled in a shallow depression on the ventral surface of the liver. The gallbladder releases stored bile into the duodenum when stimulated and thus promotes the emulsification of fats. The main functions of the gallbladder are storing of bile and assisting in the digestion of fats.

Pancreas

An accessory digestive organ, the pancreas is a triangular-shaped gland located in the left upper portion of the abdomen. The head of the pancreas is nestled in the C curve of the duodenum, and the body and tail of the pancreas lie deep to the left of the stomach and extend toward the spleen at the lateral aspect of the abdomen. The pancreas is an endocrine and exocrine gland. As an endocrine gland, it secretes insulin, an important factor in carbohydrate metabolism. As an exocrine gland, it releases pancreatic juice, which contains a broad spectrum of enzymes that mixes with bile in the duodenum. The main function of the pancreas is assisting with the digestion of proteins, fats, and carbohydrates.

OTHER RELATED STRUCTURES

Some structures located in the abdomen have no connection to the digestive process. They are part of other systems and are considered with the general assessment of the abdomen.

Peritoneum

The **peritoneum** is a thin, double layer of serous membrane in the abdominal cavity. The visceral peritoneum covers the external surface of most digestive organs. The parietal peritoneum lines the walls of the abdominal cavity. The serous fluid secreted by the membranes helps lubricate the surface of the organs, allowing motion of structures without friction.

Muscles of the Abdominal Wall

Having no bony reinforcements, the anterior and lateral abdominal walls depend upon the musculature for support and protection. The four pairs of abdominal muscles, when well toned, support and protect the abdominal viscera most effectively (see Figure 19.2 ●). The muscle groups include the rectus

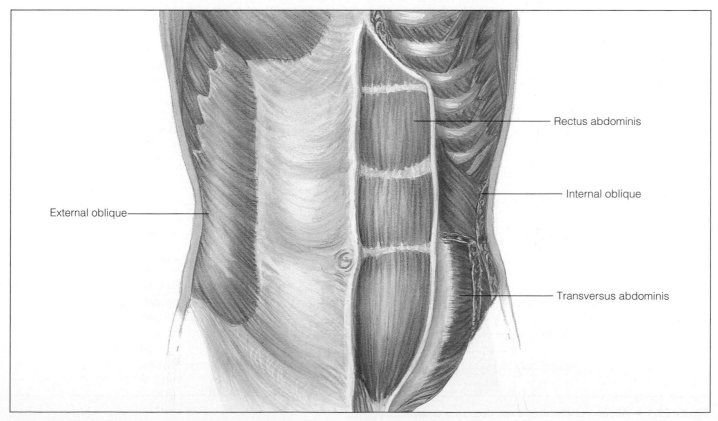

External oblique

Rectus abdominis

Internal oblique

Transversus abdominis

Figure 19.2 ● Muscles of the abdominal wall.

abdominis, external oblique, internal oblique, and transverse abdominis. Secondary functions of these muscle groups include lateral flexion, rotation, and anterior flexion of the trunk. Simultaneous contraction of the muscle groups increases intra-abdominal pressure by compressing the abdominal wall. Weakness in the muscular structure will produce herniation of structures.

Aorta

As the descending aorta passes through the diaphragm and enters the abdominal cavity, it becomes the abdominal aorta. This penetration occurs at the T_{12} level of the vertebral column slightly to the left of the midline of the body. The abdominal aorta continues to the L_4 level of the vertebral column where it bifurcates to form the right and left common iliac arteries. The many branches of the abdominal aorta serve all the parietal and visceral structures (see Figure 19.3 ●).

Kidneys, Ureters, and Bladder

The kidneys lie within the abdomen behind the peritoneum. Responsible for the filtration of nitrogenous wastes and the production of urine, the kidneys are protected by the lower ribs. The slender tubelike structures that carry the urine from the kidneys to the bladder are the ureters. The urinary bladder, a smooth, collapsible muscular sac, is located in the pelvis of the abdominal cavity. The primary function of the bladder is to store urine until it can be released. As the bladder fills with urine, it may rise above the symphysis pubis into the abdominal cavity. Assessment of the kidneys, ureters, and bladder is discussed in Chapter 20 of this text. ⏺

Spleen

The spleen, the largest of the lymphoid organs, is located in the left upper portion of the abdomen directly inferior to the diaphragm. Surrounded by a fibrous capsule, the spleen provides a site for lymphocyte proliferation and immune surveillance and response. It filters and cleanses blood, destroying worn-out red blood cells and returning their breakdown products to the liver.

Reproductive Organs

In the female, the uterus, fallopian tubes, and ovaries are in the pelvic portion of the abdominal cavity. In the male, the prostate gland surrounds the urethra just below the bladder. The assessment of these structures is discussed in Chapters 21 and 22 of this text. ⏺

LANDMARKS

Reference points and anatomical structures need to be identified when assessing the abdomen. Defined landmarks help to

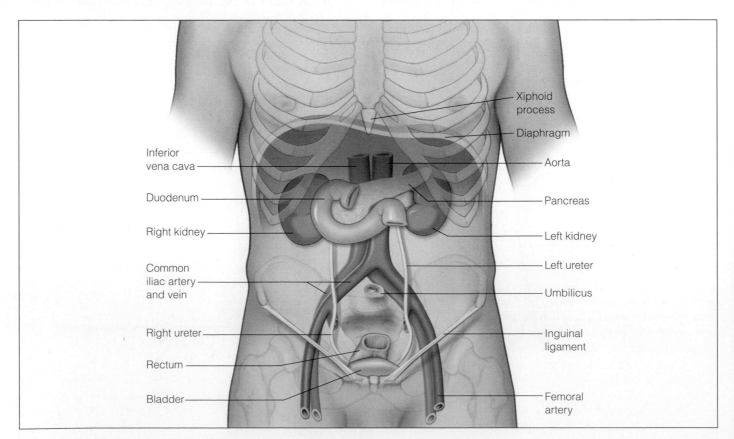

Figure 19.3 ● Abdominal vasculature and deep structures.

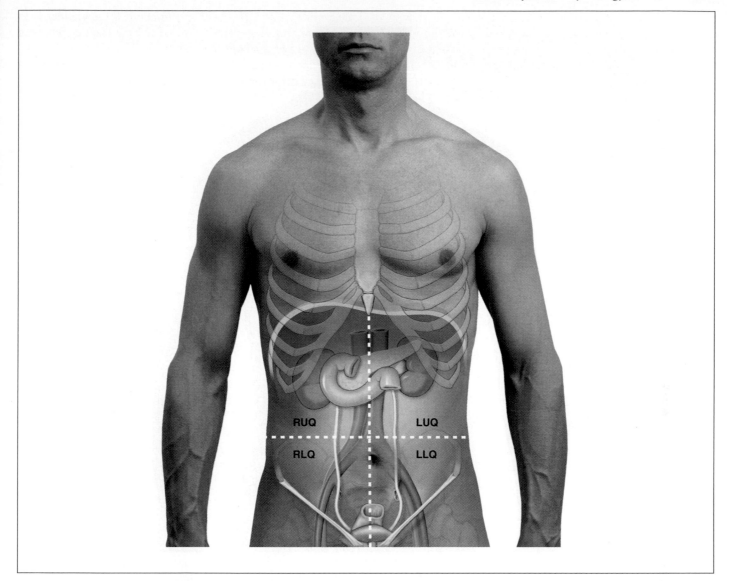

Figure 19.4 ● Mapping of the abdomen into four quadrants.

identify specific underlying structures and provide a source for description and recording of findings. Landmarks for the abdomen include the xiphoid process, umbilicus, costal margin, iliac crests, and pubic bone.

Mapping is the process of dividing the abdomen into quadrants or regions for the purpose of examination. To obtain the four quadrants, the nurse extends the midsternal line from the xiphoid process through the umbilicus to the pubic bone and then draws a horizontal line perpendicular to the first line, through the umbilicus. These two perpendicular lines form four equal quadrants of the abdomen as illustrated in Figure 19.4 ●. The quadrants are simply named right upper quadrant (RUQ), right lower quadrant (RLQ), left upper quadrant (LUQ), and left lower quadrant (LLQ).

The second mapping method divides the abdomen into nine regions. To obtain these abdominal regions, one extends the right and left midclavicular lines to the groin and then draws a horizontal line across the lowest edge of the costal margin. The final step is to draw another horizontal line at the level of the iliac crests. The abdomen has now been divided into nine regions as shown in Figure 19.5 ●. The names of the regions are right hypochondriac, epigastric, left hypochondriac, right lumbar, umbilical, left lumbar, right inguinal, hypogastric or pubic, and left inguinal.

Of the two methods described, the quadrant method is more commonly used. When using the quadrant method, it is important to pay attention to structures that are in the midline of the abdomen and do not belong to any specific quadrant. These structures include the abdominal aorta, urinary bladder, and uterus.

The nurse should select one mapping method and use it consistently. Once a method has been selected, the nurse visualizes the underlying structures before proceeding (see Figure 19.6 ●). The gallbladder sits in the upper right quadrant of the abdomen inferior to the liver and lateral to the right midclavicular line (MCL). The kidneys are posterior to the abdominal contents and situated in the retroperitoneal space, protected by the eleventh

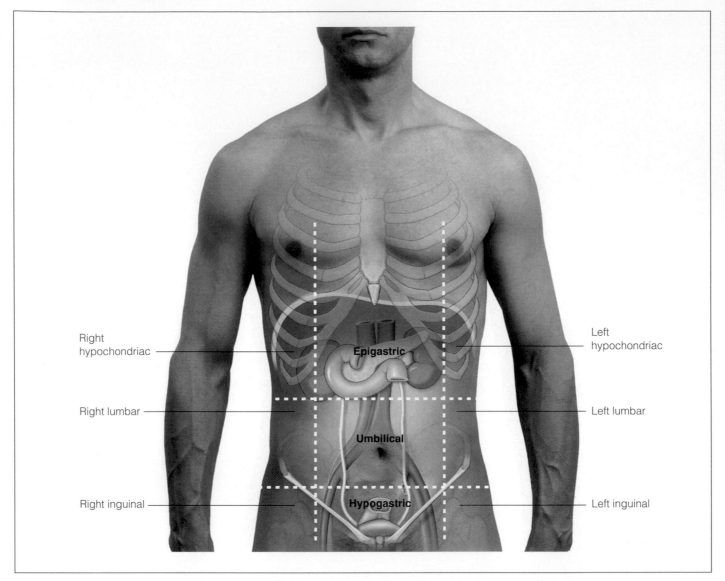

Right hypochondriac

Epigastric

Left hypochondriac

Right lumbar

Umbilical

Left lumbar

Right inguinal

Hypogastric

Left inguinal

Figure 19.5 ● Mapping of the abdomen into nine regions.

and twelfth pairs of ribs. The costovertebral angle is formed as the ribs articulate with the vertebra. The liver displaces the right kidney, thus making the lower pole palpable. The spleen, part of the lymphatic system, is at the level of the tenth rib lateral to the left midaxillary line. The lower pole moves into the abdomen toward the midline when enlarged.

SPECIAL CONSIDERATIONS

Subjective and objective data inform the nurse about the client's health status. A variety of factors may influence health and include age, developmental level, race, ethnicity, work history, living conditions, socioeconomics, and emotional well-being. These factors will be discussed in the following sections.

DEVELOPMENTAL CONSIDERATIONS

Data collection and interpretation of findings in relation to changes that accompany growth and development are impor-

tant. Expected variations in the abdomen for different age groups are discussed in the following sections.

Infants and Children

The abdomen of the newborn and infant is round. The umbilical cord, containing two arteries and one vein, is ligated at the time of delivery. The stump dries and ultimately forms the umbilicus. The toddler has a characteristic "potbelly" appearance as depicted in Figure 19.7 ●. Respirations are abdominal; therefore, movement of the abdomen is seen with breathing. This breathing pattern is evident until about the sixth year, at which age respirations become thoracic.

Peristaltic waves are usually more visible in infants and children than in adults because the muscle wall of the abdomen is thinner. Children have the tendency to swallow more air than adults when eating, thus creating a greater sound of tympany when percussion is performed. The area of tympany on the right side of the abdomen is smaller because the liver is larger in children.

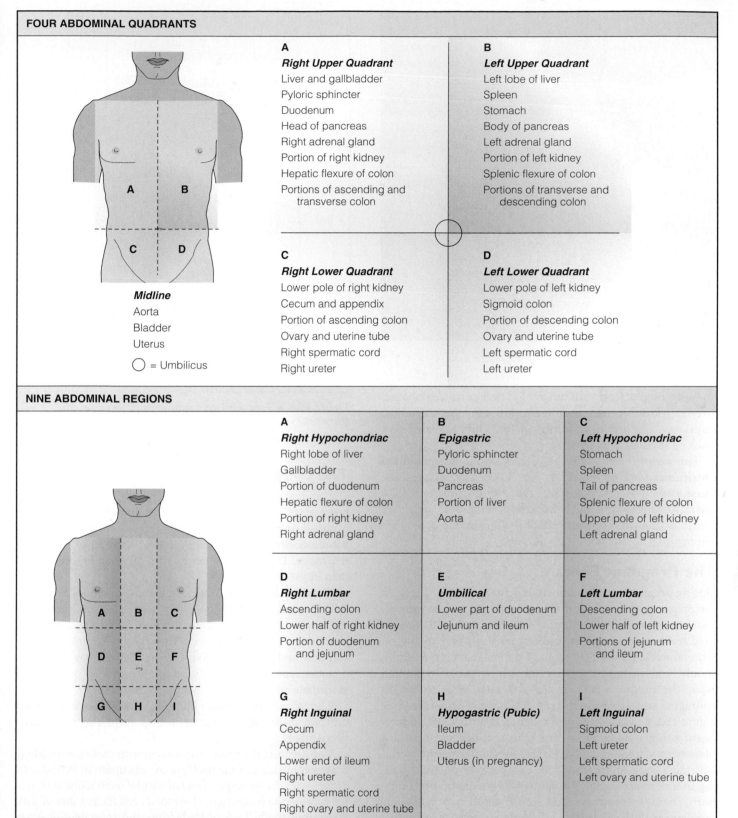

FOUR ABDOMINAL QUADRANTS

A
Right Upper Quadrant
Liver and gallbladder
Pyloric sphincter
Duodenum
Head of pancreas
Right adrenal gland
Portion of right kidney
Hepatic flexure of colon
Portions of ascending and
   transverse colon

B
Left Upper Quadrant
Left lobe of liver
Spleen
Stomach
Body of pancreas
Left adrenal gland
Portion of left kidney
Splenic flexure of colon
Portions of transverse and
   descending colon

C
Right Lower Quadrant
Lower pole of right kidney
Cecum and appendix
Portion of ascending colon
Ovary and uterine tube
Right spermatic cord
Right ureter

D
Left Lower Quadrant
Lower pole of left kidney
Sigmoid colon
Portion of descending colon
Ovary and uterine tube
Left spermatic cord
Left ureter

Midline
Aorta
Bladder
Uterus
◯ = Umbilicus

NINE ABDOMINAL REGIONS

A
Right Hypochondriac
Right lobe of liver
Gallbladder
Portion of duodenum
Hepatic flexure of colon
Portion of right kidney
Right adrenal gland

B
Epigastric
Pyloric sphincter
Duodenum
Pancreas
Portion of liver
Aorta

C
Left Hypochondriac
Stomach
Spleen
Tail of pancreas
Splenic flexure of colon
Upper pole of left kidney
Left adrenal gland

D
Right Lumbar
Ascending colon
Lower half of right kidney
Portion of duodenum
   and jejunum

E
Umbilical
Lower part of duodenum
Jejunum and ileum

F
Left Lumbar
Descending colon
Lower half of left kidney
Portions of jejunum
   and ileum

G
Right Inguinal
Cecum
Appendix
Lower end of ileum
Right ureter
Right spermatic cord
Right ovary and uterine tube

H
Hypogastric (Pubic)
Ileum
Bladder
Uterus (in pregnancy)

I
Left Inguinal
Sigmoid colon
Left ureter
Left spermatic cord
Left ovary and uterine tube

Figure 19.6 ● Upper torso: Organs of the four abdominal quadrants. Lower torso: Organs of the nine abdominal regions.

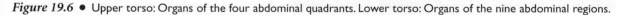

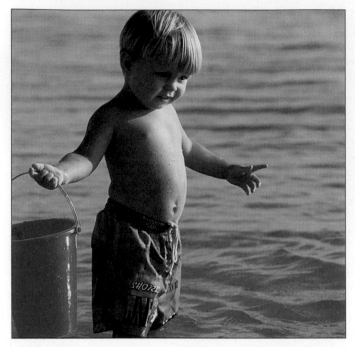

Figure 19.7 • Potbelly stance of toddler.

Congenital defects such as cleft lip, cleft palate, esophageal atresia, pyloric stenosis, and hernias influence the nutritional status, growth, and development of the child and therefore must be assessed with care.

The size of the abdomen at all ages is an indication of the nutritional state of the child. For children of all ages, the nurse should ascertain feeding and eating habits and food tolerance. Symptoms such as nausea, vomiting, and skin rashes of the child and the actions taken by the parent are important.

The Pregnant Female

During pregnancy, the abdomen undergoes many changes. As the pregnancy progresses, the uterus enlarges and moves into the abdominal cavity. The height of the fundus should be measured and compared against predictable levels based on the gestational week. By the 14th week of the pregnancy, the fundus should be above the pubic bone and easily palpable. By the 36th week, the fundus is high in the abdomen, close to the diaphragm, and compresses many abdominal structures (see Figure 19.8 ●). Constipation, flatulence, hemorrhoids, and frequent voiding are common problems resulting from the displacement of abdominal organs and pressure from the uterus. Changing levels of hormones decrease peristaltic activity leading to a decrease in bowel sounds. Acid indigestion or heartburn, nausea, vomiting, and constipation are additional problems with the gastrointestinal system during pregnancy.

The skin of the abdomen undergoes some characteristic changes. Striae gravidarum (stretch marks) become most visible during the second half of the pregnancy (see Chapter 26 ⊙). Linea nigra, a dark line, extends from the umbilicus to the pubic bone along the midline of the abdomen (see Figure 11.7 on page 187 ⊙). The muscles of the abdominal wall are stretched and may lose tone.

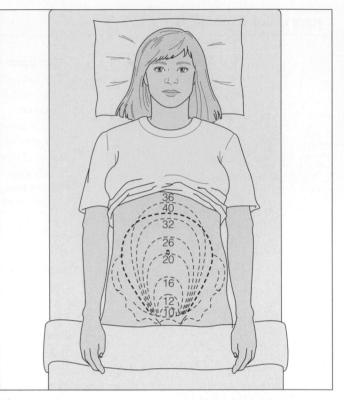

Figure 19.8 • Fundal height measurements during specific gestational weeks.

The Older Adult

The appearance of the abdomen changes with the aging process. In the older adult, the abdomen may be more rounded or protuberant due to increased adipose tissue distribution, decreased muscle tone, and reduced fibroconnective tissue. The abdomen tends to be softer and more relaxed than in the younger adult.

The digestive system of the older adult undergoes characteristic changes; however, these may not be as pronounced as changes in other body systems. There is a gradual decrease in secretion of saliva, digestive enzymes, peristalsis, intestinal absorption, and intestinal activity. These changes may lead to indigestion, constipation, and gastroesophageal reflux and could exacerbate any preexisting changes or disease.

The loss of teeth makes chewing and swallowing of food difficult. Ill-fitting, broken, or lost dentures also alter nutritional status.

Constipation is a common problem with older adults. Many factors contribute to the problem of constipation. Periodontal disease with the subsequent loss of natural teeth is one such factor because the inability to chew foods results in a diet of soft, nonfibrous foods. Lack of fresh fruits and vegetables or other sources of bulk or fiber contributes to the pattern of constipation. The older adult may self-limit the daily fluid intake, especially water, to decrease frequency of urination with the increased potential for constipation. Other changes the nurse should anticipate with this age group are dry mouth, delayed esophageal and gastric emptying, decreased gastric acid production, and decreased liver size.

PSYCHOSOCIAL CONSIDERATIONS

High stress levels may cause or aggravate abdominal problems. Gastritis, gastric or duodenal ulcers, and ulcerative colitis are several examples of stress-related problems.

Self-perception may have a subtle influence on the client's weight. Clients who perceive themselves as naturally thin may show greater dedication to restricting their caloric intake and exercising to maintain that self-image. Conversely, clients who perceive themselves as naturally fat may overeat and avoid exercise, feeling that there is nothing they can do to alter their weight.

Surgical scars may alter an individual's body image. Gastrointestinal surgery may require a colostomy, which might be a temporary or permanent change. Many adults consider "wearing a bag" a significant limitation, causing embarrassment and anxiety. This often leads to depression and withdrawal.

CULTURAL AND ENVIRONMENTAL CONSIDERATIONS

Culture, customs, family, and religious practices influence the foods clients choose to eat. Certain foods may be prescribed in certain cultures or religions; however, a healthy diet usually can be achieved even with significant food restrictions. Clients used to a diet of meat and potatoes may not fully appreciate the value of fresh fruits and vegetables.

The financial security of the client also has an impact on eating habits. In some areas, certain foods may not be available year-round or may be much more costly than in other areas. For example, fresh fruits and vegetables typically increase in price in many regions in winter months. Unfortunately, highly processed foods are often lower in fiber than their fresh counterparts.

Cultural Considerations

- Chronic hepatitis C occurs more commonly in African Americans and Hispanics.
- Alcoholic and drug abuse liver disease occurs more frequently in Native Americans and African Americans.
- Gallstones and gallbladder cancer occur more frequently in Mexican Americans and Native Americans.
- African Americans have a greater incidence of colorectal cancer than Caucasians.
- *Helicobacter pylori,* a major cause of peptic ulcer disease, occurs more frequently in African Americans and Hispanics.
- Obesity is a risk factor for gastrointestinal diseases and is on the rise in the United States. Currently, 54% of adults and 25% of children in the United States are overweight. Adult obesity is seen more frequently in African American and Hispanic females.
- Japanese individuals are at greater risk of gastric cancer.
- Lactose intolerance occurs with greatest frequency in non-Caucasian Americans and Jewish Americans.
- Linguistic and cultural factors must be considered to avoid miscommunication and misinterpretation of information about diagnoses when caring for many immigrant populations.
- The nurse must be sensitive to cultural issues about disrobing for an abdominal assessment.
- Females may require the presence of another female during physical assessment of the abdomen, especially when the examiner is not of the same sex.

Gathering the Data

*H*ealth assessment of the abdomen includes the gathering of subjective and objective data. Subjective data collection occurs during the client interview, before the actual physical assessment. During the interview the nurse uses a variety of communication techniques to elicit general and specific information about the client's state of abdominal health or illness. Health records, the results of laboratory tests, and radiologic studies are important secondary sources to be reviewed and included in the data-gathering process.

During physical assessment of the abdomen, four techniques of physical assessment will be used. However, the order of the techniques changes to inspection, auscultation, percussion, and palpation. Auscultation is performed after inspection. This order prevents augmentation or disturbance of abdominal sounds that could occur from percussion and palpation. Percussion and palpation could influence peristaltic activity, therefore changing the findings upon auscultation. The diaphragm of the stethoscope should be used when auscultating for bowel sounds. The nurse should not apply heavy pressure to the diaphragm since this could influence peristaltic activity and ultimately the natural sounds of the intestinal activity. The bell is used when auscultating the aorta and other arteries.

FOCUSED INTERVIEW

The focused interview for assessment of the abdomen concerns data related to the structures and functions of organs within the abdomen. Subjective data related to the status and function of the structures within the abdomen is gathered during the focused interview. The nurse must be prepared to observe the client and listen for cues related to the function of the organs and systems within the abdomen. The nurse may use open-ended or closed questions to obtain information. Often a number of follow-up questions or requests for descriptions are required to clarify data or gather missing information.

The focused interview guides the physical assessment of the abdomen. The information is always considered in relation to norms and expectations about the function of organs and systems within the abdomen. Therefore, the nurse must consider age, gender, race, culture, environment, health practices, past and concurrent problems, and therapies when framing questions and using techniques to elicit information. In order to address all of the factors when conducting a focused interview,

categories of questions related to status and function of organs and systems within the abdomen have been developed. These categories include general questions that are asked of all clients, those addressing illness or infection, questions related to symptoms or behaviors, those related to habits or practices, questions that are specific to clients according to age, those for the pregnant female, and questions that address environmental concerns.

The nurse must consider the client's ability to participate in the focused interview and physical assessment of the abdomen. If a client is experiencing pain, cramping, problems with elimination (including frequency or urgency), difficulty swallowing, nausea and vomiting, or the anxiety that accompanies any of these problems, attention must focus on identification of immediate problems and relief of symptoms.

FOCUSED INTERVIEW QUESTIONS	RATIONALES

The following section provides sample questions and bulleted follow-up questions in each of the previously mentioned categories. A rationale for each of the questions is provided. The list of questions is not all-inclusive, but represents the types of questions required in a comprehensive focused interview related to the abdomen. Subjective data collected and questions asked during the health history and focused interview provide information to help meet the goals for gastrointestinal health described in Healthy People 2010.

GENERAL QUESTIONS

1. **Describe your appetite. Has it changed in the last 24 hours? In the last month? In the last year?**
   - What do you believe has caused the change in your appetite?
   - Have you done anything to address the change?
   - Have you spoken to a healthcare professional about the change?
   - Has anything else occurred with the change in appetite?

▶ These questions elicit basic information about the client's eating. In addition, appetite change can be indicative of underlying physical and emotional problems. If a change has occurred, it is important to elicit the client's perception of the change and to identify factors that may have contributed to the change.

2. **What is your weight? Has your weight changed?**
   - Over what period of time did the weight change occur?
   - What do you believe has contributed to your weight change?
   - Have any problems or symptoms accompanied the weight change?
   - Have you discussed this with a healthcare professional?

▶ Weight loss or gain can accompany physical and emotional problems. Dietary consumption is one of the leading factors in weight control. The nurse should determine if weight gain is associated with decrease in activity, changes in metabolic rates, hormonal factors, or fluid retention. Emotional problems may cause an individual to over- or underconsume foods. Weight loss may be an appropriate or desired outcome for some individuals. The nurse must determine if the weight loss was purposeful. Weight loss can accompany problems associated with diabetes, hyperthyroidism, and some cancers.

   - Questions about dietary intake can be included in the follow-up about weight or may be included in questions about behaviors. These questions would include the following: Tell me what you have had to eat and drink in the last 24 hours. Be sure to include snacks. How much of each item did you consume? Is this a typical eating pattern for you?

▶ In addition to obtaining data about weight, the nurse is building on the nutritional data already collected. The nurse is establishing the client's dietary patterns, paying special attention to overconsumption and underconsumption.

FOCUSED INTERVIEW QUESTIONS	**RATIONALES**

3. **Describe your bowel habits. Describe the color and consistency of your stool.**
   - Have you experienced any changes in your elimination pattern or in your stool?
   - What kind of change has occurred in your elimination pattern or stool?
   - When did the change begin?
   - Can you identify anything you believe may have caused the change?
   - What have you done about the problem?
   - Have you discussed the changes with a healthcare professional?
   - Questions about the use of medications such as laxatives or antidiarrheals may be included as follow-up questions here. However, this information may have been obtained in the health history or can be included in questions about behaviors.

▶ These questions provide initial information about bowel functioning. The nurse determines if the client has an established pattern for bowel elimination. If the client indicates that there has been a change in the pattern of elimination or in the characteristics of the stool, follow-up questions are indicated. Tarry stool indicates bleeding in the upper part of the gastrointestinal tract. A clay color indicates lack of bile in the stool.

4. **Do you have feelings of bloating or increased gas?**
   - What do you think causes this? Have any changes been made in your diet or medications?
   - What do you do to decrease these feelings?
   - What do you do to relieve the symptoms?
   - Do you use antacids?
   - Do you increase water intake?
   - Do you exercise?

▶ Some foods (broccoli, cauliflower, figs) and intolerance to lactose will cause this feeling. Some medications are constipating. Severe bloating and gas can be indicative of abdominal pathology.

5. **Do you have any physical problems that affect your appetite, affect your bowel functioning, or contribute to abdominal problems?**
   - Describe the way your abdominal function is affected.
   - How long has this been occurring?
   - Have you sought relief for the problem?
   - What have you done to relieve the problem?
   - Did the remedy help?
   - Have you sought advice from a healthcare professional?

▶ This question is used to elicit information about abdominal or other problems that may impact the structures and functions within the abdomen. For example, pain from any source may diminish appetite, and intake of medications for nonabdominal problems may affect digestion and abdominal comfort. If the client identifies any problems that affect abdominal functions, follow-up is required for clear descriptions and details about what, when, and how problems occur, how abdominal function is impacted, and the duration of the problem.

6. **Is there anyone in your family who has had an abdominal disease or problem?**
   - What is the disease or problem?
   - Who in the family now has or has had the disease?
   - When was it diagnosed?
   - Describe the treatment.
   - How effective was the treatment?

▶ This may reveal information about abdominal diseases associated with familial or genetic predisposition.

▶ Follow-up is required to obtain details about specific problems, as well as their occurrence, treatment, and outcomes.

QUESTIONS RELATED TO ILLNESS OR INFECTION

1. **Have you ever been diagnosed with an abdominal disease?**
   - When were you diagnosed with the problem?
   - What treatment was prescribed for the problem?
   - Was the treatment helpful?
   - What kinds of things do you do to help with the problem?
   - Has the problem ever recurred (acute)?
   - How are you managing the disease now (chronic)?

▶ The client has an opportunity to provide information about specific abdominal diseases. If a diagnosed illness is identified, follow-up about the date of diagnosis, treatment, and outcomes is required. Data about each illness identified by the client is essential to an accurate health assessment. Illness can be classified as acute or chronic, and follow-up regarding each classification will differ.

2. **An alternative to question 1 is to list possible abdominal illnesses, such as cholecystitis, cholelithiasis, ulcers, diverticulosis, and cirrhosis, and ask the client to respond yes or no as each is stated.**
   - Follow-up would be carried out for each identified diagnosis as in question 1.

▶ This is a comprehensive and easy way to elicit information about all abdominal diagnoses.

FOCUSED INTERVIEW QUESTIONS	RATIONALES

3. **Do you now have or have you ever had an infection within the abdomen?**
   - When were you diagnosed with the infection?
   - What treatment was prescribed for the problem?
   - Was the treatment helpful?
   - What kinds of things do you do to help with the problem?
   - Has the problem ever recurred (acute)?
   - How are you managing the infection now (chronic)?

▶ If an infection is identified, follow-up about the date of the infection, treatment, and outcomes is required. Data about each infection identified by the client is essential to an accurate health assessment. Infections can be classified as acute or chronic, and follow-up regarding each classification will differ.

4. **An alternative to question 3 is to list possible abdominal infections, such as hepatitis, cholecystitis, and diverticulitis, and ask the client to respond yes or no as each is stated.**

▶ This is a comprehensive and easy way to elicit information about all abdominal diagnoses. Follow-up would be carried out for each identified diagnosis as in question 3.

QUESTIONS RELATED TO SYMPTOMS OR BEHAVIORS

When gathering information about symptoms, many questions are required to elicit details and descriptions that assist in the analysis of the data. Discrimination is made in relation to the significance of a symptom, in relation to specific diseases or problems, and in relation to potential follow-up examination or referral. One rationale may be provided for a group of questions in this category.

The following questions refer to specific symptoms and behaviors associated with the organs and structures within the abdomen. For each symptom, questions and follow-up are required. The details to be elicited are the characteristics of the symptom; the onset, duration, and frequency of the symptom; the treatment or remedy for the symptom, including over-the-counter (OTC) and home remedies; the determination if a diagnosis has been sought; the effect of treatments; and family history associated with a symptom or illness.

QUESTIONS RELATED TO SYMPTOMS

Questions 1 through 20 refer to nausea as a symptom associated with abdominal problems and are comprehensive enough to provide an example of the number and types of questions required in a focused interview when a symptom exists. The remaining questions refer to other symptoms associated with abdominal problems. The number and types of questions are limited to identification of the symptom. Follow-up is included only when required for clarification.

1. **Do you have nausea?**

2. **How long have you had the nausea?**

▶ Determining the duration of symptoms is helpful in determining the significance of symptoms in relation to specific diseases and problems.

3. **How often are you nauseated?**

4. **Do you know what is causing the nausea?**

5. **Is there a difference in the nausea at different times of the day?**

▶ Question 1 identifies the existence of a symptom, and questions 2 through 5 add knowledge about the symptom.

6. **Describe your nausea.**

7. **Is the nausea accompanied by burning, indigestion, or bloating?**

▶ The description of the nausea may indicate a symptom associated with a specific disease or problem.

FOCUSED INTERVIEW QUESTIONS	**RATIONALES**

8. Do you vomit when you experience the nausea?

9. What does the vomitus look like?

10. Does the vomitus have any odor?

▶ The color and odor of vomitus may be associated with specific diseases or problems. For example, brown vomitus with a fecal odor can indicate an intestinal obstruction.

11. What was the cause, in your opinion?

12. How frequently do you have this experience?

13. What do you do to relieve the symptoms?

14. When you vomit, describe what comes up and the amount.

▶ Vomiting can be related to a variety of pathologic conditions, such as food poisoning, ulcers, varices of the esophagus, hepatitis, and beginning of an intestinal obstruction. Medications, prescribed and OTC, may contribute to or cause vomiting.

15. Do you have pain with the nausea?
   - Describe the type, severity, and location of the pain.
   - What do you do for the pain?
   - Is the remedy effective?

▶ Pain may occur because of associated muscle pain when vomiting or may be indicative of an underlying abdominal disease. Follow-up elicits details that assist in the data analysis.

16. Have you sought treatment for the nausea?

17. When was the treatment sought?

18. What occurred when you sought that treatment?

19. Was something prescribed or recommended for the nausea?

20. What was the effect of the remedy?

▶ These questions provide information about the need for diagnosis, referral, or continued evaluation of the symptom. They also provide information about the client's knowledge of a current diagnosis or problem, and his or her response to intervention.

21. Do you use OTC or home remedies for the nausea?

22. What are the OTC or home remedies that you use?

23. How often do you use them?

24. How much of them do you use?

▶ Questions 21 through 24 provide information about drugs and substances that may relieve symptoms or provide comfort. Some substances may mask symptoms, interfere with the effect of prescribed medications, or harm the client.

25. Do you have any difficulty chewing or swallowing your food?

26. Do you wear dentures?

27. Do you have any crowns?

28. Do your gums bleed easily?

▶ Ill-fitting dentures, failure to wear them, and missing or diseased teeth make chewing and swallowing difficult. Disorders of the throat and esophagus can also make swallowing difficult.

29. Do you have indigestion?
   - Questions would include onset, frequency, and duration as well as knowledge about causative factors including food intolerance and discomfort associated with medication or treatments for other problems. For example, when did the indigestion start?

30. Do you suffer from diarrhea or constipation?

FOCUSED INTERVIEW QUESTIONS	RATIONALES

31. What do you think is the cause?

32. What have you done to correct the situation?

33. Have these measures helped the situation?

34. Do you experience any rectal itching or bleeding?

► Dark, tarry stool indicates bleeding, usually in the upper or middle part of the intestinal tract. Bright red (frank) blood usually indicates lower tract bleeding.

QUESTIONS RELATED TO PAIN

1. Are you having any abdominal pain at this time?

2. Where is the pain?

► Questions 2 through 6 are standard questions associated with pain to determine the location, frequency, duration, and intensity of the pain.

3. How often do you experience the pain?

4. How long does the pain last?

5. How long have you had the pain?

6. How would you rate the pain on a scale of 1 to 10, with 10 being the worst pain?

7. Does the pain radiate?

8. Where does the pain radiate?

9. Is there a trigger for the pain?

10. Does the pain affect your breathing or any other functions?

11. What do you think is causing the pain?

12. What do you do to relieve the pain?

► Pain could indicate cardiac disease, ulcers, cholecystitis, renal calculi, diverticulitis, urinary cystitis, or ectopic pregnancy.

QUESTIONS RELATED TO BEHAVIORS

1. What have you had to eat and drink in the last 24 hours?

2. What snacks do you have in a 24-hour period?

3. What size portions do you eat?

4. Is the 24-hour pattern you described typical for the way you eat?

► This provides input about diet and nutrition, which may contribute to obesity or problems with weight loss. This provides information about meeting nutritional requirements.

5. How much coffee, tea, cola, alcoholic beverages, or chocolate do you consume in a 24-hour period?

► Caffeine and alcohol irritate the gastrointestinal system and can contribute to ulcers and irritable bowel syndrome.

QUESTIONS RELATED TO AGE

The focused interview must reflect the anatomical and physiological differences that exist along the age span. The following questions are examples of those that would be specific for infants and children, the pregnant female, and the older adult.

FOCUSED INTERVIEW QUESTIONS

RATIONALES

QUESTIONS REGARDING INFANTS AND CHILDREN

1. Is the baby breast-fed or bottle-fed?

2. Does the baby tolerate the feeding?

3. How frequently does the baby eat?

4. Have you recently started the baby on any new foods?

5. Is the baby colicky? What do you do to relieve the colic?

6. How much water does the baby drink?

▶ These questions assist in evaluation of gastrointestinal function by the baby's ability to take in nutrients, digest them, and eliminate waste products. The types of formula and food consumed influence color, consistency, amount, and frequency of the stool.

7. Does the toddler eat at regular times?

8. What and how much does the toddler eat?

9. Is the toddler able to feed himself or herself?

10. What type of snacks does the toddler eat?

▶ Eating habits, patterns, and preferences established in the early years of life are likely to have a lasting effect.

11. Is the child toilet trained?

12. Describe how toilet training is taught to the child.

13. Have there been any lapses in toilet training?

14. If so, how frequently? How recently?

15. How do you typically respond to this?

▶ As the nervous system matures, the child gradually achieves control of the anal sphincter. The nurse should explore the developmental level and readiness of the child.

16. What does the child eat?

17. Does the child bring a lunch and snack to school or buy it at school?

18. When at home, how often does the child snack, and what are the snacks?

19. Does the family have one meal a day together?

20. What kind of food do you eat at this meal?

21. Describe the atmosphere at this meal.

▶ The quality of the food is more important than the quantity of food. Mealtime should be enjoyable. Often this is the only time the family is together.

FOCUSED INTERVIEW QUESTIONS	RATIONALES

QUESTIONS FOR THE PREGNANT FEMALE

1. Are you experiencing any nausea or vomiting?

2. Are you experiencing any elimination problems such as constipation?

3. Are you experiencing heartburn or flatulence?

▶ Nausea is common during early pregnancy and may be due to changing hormone levels and changes in carbohydrate metabolism. Fatigue is also a factor. Vomiting is less common. If it occurs more than once a day or for a prolonged period, the client should be referred to a physician.

▶ A number of factors increase the likelihood of constipation during pregnancy. Among these are displacement of the intestines by the growing uterus, bowel sluggishness caused by increased progesterone and steroid metabolism, and the use of oral iron supplements, which are prescribed for many clients during pregnancy.

▶ Heartburn (regurgitation of gastric contents into the esophagus) is primarily caused by displacement of the stomach by the enlarging uterus. Flatulence results from the decreased gastrointestinal motility, common during pregnancy, and pressure on the large intestine from the growing uterus.

QUESTIONS FOR THE OLDER ADULT

1. Are you ever incontinent of feces?

2. How often are you constipated?

3. Do you take laxatives?

4. How often?

5. Which laxative do you take?

6. How many foods containing fiber or roughage do you eat during a typical day?

7. Are you able to get to the store for groceries?

8. Do you eat alone? With someone?

▶ Muscle tone decreases with age, and the older adult may lose sphincter control.

▶ Constipation is a common problem with older adults. Influencing factors include decreased peristaltic activity, decreased desire to eat, and self-limited fluid intake. To help relieve the problem, some older clients take over-the-counter laxatives. With prolonged use, laxatives can become habit forming.

▶ Older adults tend to have diets low in fiber or roughage. Loss of natural teeth and ill-fitting dentures make chewing difficult.

▶ Responses to questions 7 and 8 help determine mobility patterns, availability of food, and social isolation at mealtimes.

QUESTIONS RELATED TO THE ENVIRONMENT

Environment refers to both the internal and external environments. Questions related to the internal environment include all of the previous questions and those associated with internal or physiological responses. Questions regarding the external environment include those related to home, work, or social environments.

FOCUSED INTERVIEW QUESTIONS

RATIONALES

INTERNAL ENVIRONMENT

1. How would you describe your stress level?

2. Do you think you are coping well?

3. Could your coping skills be better?

▶ Prolonged stress is linked to gastrointestinal disease.

EXTERNAL ENVIRONMENT

1. Do you work with any chemical irritants?

▶ Exposure to benzol, lead, or nickel may lead to gastric irritation. Excessive exposure to chemical hepatotoxins such as carbon tetrachloride may lead to postnecrotic cirrhosis.

2. Have you recently done any traveling?

3. Where did you travel?

▶ Water purification and food storage methods vary in different regions and different countries. Exposure to food- or waterborne microorganisms can lead to gastroenteritis, hepatitis, diarrhea, or parasite infestation.
   Follow-up questions would include all of the questions mentioned that address symptoms and problems.

CLIENT INTERACTION

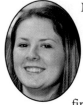

Ms. Emily Zabriski is a 20-year-old college student living on campus. She has purchased the 7-day meal plan and has lunch and dinner in the student dining room. Breakfast is usually one cup of coffee and one glass of orange juice "to go." This is determined by the time of her first class and how late she gets up.

Not having slept last night, Ms. Zabriski reports to the health center on campus early in the morning with complaints of nausea, vomiting, diarrhea, abdominal pain, and cramping in the right and left lower quadrants. She has experienced these symptoms for approximately 18 hours. The following is an excerpt of the focused interview.

INTERVIEW

Nurse: Good morning, Ms. Zabriski. I see by your report you have had nausea, vomiting, diarrhea, lower abdominal pain, and cramping for about 18 hours.

Ms. Zabriski: Yes, that is correct.

Nurse: First, I want you to rate and describe your pain. On a scale of 1 to 10 with 10 being the most severe pain ever, select a number.

Ms. Zabriski: Oh, it is a 2 to 3 right now. When I vomit or have diarrhea it goes up, maybe to 8, then comes down. I have a lot of cramps.

Nurse: With your pain at a 2 to 3 level do you think you could answer a few questions?

Ms. Zabriski: Oh, that won't be a problem. It is only a problem when I'm going to vomit or have diarrhea. Right now I'm OK.

Nurse: These symptoms could occur for any number of reasons. What do you think is causing your problem?

Ms. Zabriski: I don't understand what you mean.

Nurse: These symptoms could be caused by stress, food allergies, an intestinal disease such as Crohn's disease, or pregnancy, just to mention a few.

Ms. Zabriski: It could be something I ate, or maybe it is a stomach virus. Five dorm mates on my floor have the same thing.

Nurse: Let us talk about you. Since you indicated maybe it was something you ate, tell me about your eating prior to getting sick.

Ms. Zabriski: I had lunch in the student dining room. I had a glass of ice tea, cottage cheese with fruit salad, and a small bag of chips.

Nurse: What have you had to eat since lunch yesterday?

Ms. Zabriski: Well, I started to vomit and have cramps about 1½ hours after I ate. Now even crackers won't stay down.

Nurse: When was the last time you drank something?

Ms. Zabriski: I tried some diet cola after I vomited the first time and that came up.

Nurse: What have you taken to try to stop the nausea, vomiting, and diarrhea?

Ms. Zabriski: Nothing, I thought it would stop and go away, but it hasn't. That's why I'm here.

ANALYSIS

The nurse used several communication strategies to obtain information from Ms. Zabriski. First, the nurse determined Ms. Zabriski's level of pain and discomfort, and ability to participate in the interview. When asked what could be causing the symptoms, Ms. Zabriski responded with uncertainty. The nurse provided clarity with some diagnoses that could contribute to the symptoms. Following the response by Ms. Zabriski, the nurse brought the focus to Ms. Zabriski and not the dorm mates. The interview continued with the nurse obtaining specific subjective data using open-ended questions.

 Please refer to the Companion Website at **www.prenhall.com/damico** and click on Chapter 19, the **Client Interaction** module, to answer questions about this case. In addition, see other resources for this chapter including NCLEX review questions and other interactive exercises and materials.

Physical Assessment

ASSESSMENT TECHNIQUES AND FINDINGS

Physical assessment of the abdomen requires the use of inspection, auscultation, percussion, and palpation. This order differs from that of physical assessment of other systems. The nurse should remember to auscultate after inspection. Delaying percussion and palpation prevents disturbance of the normal bowel sounds. During each of the procedures the nurse is gathering data related to problems with underlying abdominal organs and structures. Inspection includes looking at skin color, structures of the abdomen, abdominal contour, pulsations, and abdominal movements. Knowledge of normative values or expected findings is essential in determining the meaning of the data as the physical assessment is performed.

The skin of the abdomen should be consistent with the skin of the rest of the body. The umbilicus should be midline in an abdomen that may be round, flat, convex, or protuberant. The abdomen should be symmetrical and free of bulges. Pulsations

and wavelike movements below the xiphoid process are normal in thin adults.

Physical assessment of the abdomen follows an organized pattern. It begins with a client survey followed by inspection, auscultation, percussion, and palpation of the abdomen. The lateral aspects of the abdomen are included when conducting each of the assessments.

HELPFUL HINTS
- Provide an environment that is warm and comfortable.
- Encourage the client to void prior to the examination.
- Provide instructions about what is expected of the client. For example, taking several deep breaths to relax abdominal muscles.
- Pay attention to nonverbal cues that may indicate discomfort. Facial gestures, legs flexed at the knees, and abdominal guarding with the hands are all indices of discomfort.
- When a client is experiencing abdominal pain, examine that area last.
- Stand on the right side of the client, unless otherwise indicated, because the liver and right kidney are in the right side of the abdomen.
- Maintain the dignity of the client through appropriate draping techniques.
- Use Standard Precautions.

EQUIPMENT

examination gown and drape	skin marker
clean, nonsterile examination gloves	metric ruler
examination light	tissues
stethoscope	tape measure

| **TECHNIQUES AND NORMAL FINDINGS** | **ABNORMAL FINDINGS SPECIAL CONSIDERATIONS** |

SURVEY

A quick survey of the client enables the nurse to identify any immediate problems as well as the client's ability to participate in the assessment.

Inspect the overall appearance, posture, and position of the client. Observe for signs of pain or discomfort and signs of anxiety or distress.

▶ Clients experiencing anxiety may demonstrate pallor and shallow breathing. They may be diaphoretic and use their hands to guard their abdomen.
▶ Acknowledgment of the problem and a discussion of the procedures often provides some relief. If the client is experiencing severe pain or discomfort, the problem must be addressed and a complete abdominal assessment may need to be delayed.

INSPECTION OF THE ABDOMEN

1. **Position the client.**
   - The client should be in a supine position with a small pillow placed beneath the head and knees. Drape the examination gown over the chest, exposing the abdomen. Place the drape at the symphysis pubis, covering the client's pubic area and legs (see Figure 19.9 ●).

▶ These measures relax the abdominal musculature and prevent unnecessary exposure of the client.

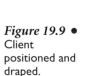

Figure 19.9 ● Client positioned and draped.

   - Stand at the right side of the client. Lighting must be adequate to detect color differences, lesions, and movements of the abdomen.

2. **Instruct the client.**
   - Explain that you will be looking at the client's abdomen. Tell the client to breathe normally.

▶ If the client is guarding the abdomen, demonstrated by posture or breathing, the client should be asked to take several deep breaths. This assists in relaxation of abdominal musculature.

3. **Map the abdomen.**
   - Visualize the imaginary horizontal and vertical lines delineating the abdominal quadrants and regions as identified in Figures 19.4 and 19.5.
   - Visualize the underlying structures as identified in Figure 19.6A and B.

4. **Determine the contour of the abdomen.**
   - Observe the profile of the abdomen between the costal margins and the symphysis pubis.
   - The abdominal profile should be viewed at eye level. You may need to sit or kneel to observe the abdominal profile.
   - Normal findings include flat, rounded, or scaphoid contours (see Figure 19.10 ●).

▶ A protuberant abdomen is normal in pregnancy. It may indicate obesity or ascites in a nonpregnant client.

TECHNIQUES AND NORMAL FINDINGS	ABNORMAL FINDINGS SPECIAL CONSIDERATIONS

Flat. A straight horizontal line is observed from the costal margin to the symphysis pubis. This contour is common in a thin person.

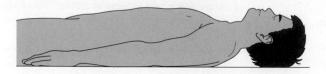

Rounded. Sometimes called a convex abdomen. The horizontal line now curves outward, indicating an increase in abdominal fat or a decrease in muscle tone. This contour is considered a normal variation in the toddler and the pregnant female.

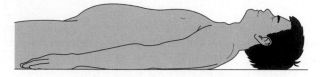

Scaphoid. Sometimes called a concave abdomen. The horizontal line now curves inward toward the vertebral column, giving the abdomen a sunken appearance. In the adult, this contour is seen in the very thin person.

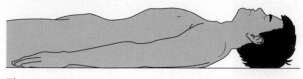

Figure 19.10 ● Contour of the abdomen.

Protuberant. Similar to the rounded abdomen, only greater. This contour is anticipated in pregnancy. It is also seen in the adult with obesity, ascites, and other conditions.

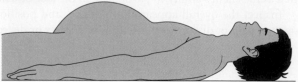

5. **Observe the position of the umbilicus.**

   ● The umbilicus is normally in the center of the abdomen. It may be inverted or protruding. The umbilicus should be clean and free of inflammation or drainage.

   ALERT!

   A client with drainage from the umbilicus following laparoscopic surgery should be referred to the physician immediately.

   ▶ A protruding or displaced umbilicus is a normal variation in pregnant females. In the non-pregnant adult, it could indicate an abdominal mass or distended urinary bladder. Inflammation or drainage may indicate an infection or complication from recent laparoscopic surgery. A displaced or protruding umbilicus may be a sign of a hernia in a child.

6. **Observe skin color.**

   ● The abdominal skin should be consistent in color and luster with the skin of the rest of the body. The skin is smooth, moist, and free of lesions.

   ▶ Taut, glistening skin could indicate ascites.

TECHNIQUES AND NORMAL FINDINGS	ABNORMAL FINDINGS SPECIAL CONSIDERATIONS

7. Observe the location and characteristics of lesions, scars, and abdominal markings.

- Lesions such as macules, moles, and freckles are considered normal findings.

▶ **Striae,** commonly called stretch marks, are silvery, shiny, irregular markings on the skin. These are seen in obesity, pregnancy, and ascites (refer to Figure 19-29 on page 546).
▶ Scars indicate previous surgery or trauma and the possibility of underlying adhesions. The location of all lesions must be documented as baseline data and for determination of change in future assessment.

8. Observe the abdomen for symmetry, bulging, or masses.

- First observe the abdomen while standing at the client's side. Second, observe the abdomen while standing at the foot of the examination table. Compare the right and left sides. The sides should appear symmetrical in shape, size, and contour.

▶ Asymmetry may indicate masses, adhesions, or strictures of underlying structures.

- Third, return to the client's side and use a tangential light across the abdomen. No shadows should appear.

▶ Shadows may indicate bulges or masses.

- Observe the abdomen from eye level, by sitting or kneeling, and shine the light across the abdomen. The abdomen should appear symmetrical without bulges or masses.

▶ Bulges could indicate tumors, cysts, or hernias.

- You may repeat all of the assessments above while asking the client to take a deep breath and raise the head off the pillow.

▶ Deep breathing and head raising accentuate masses.

9. Observe the abdominal wall for movement.

- Movements can include pulsations or peristaltic waves. In thin clients it is normal to observe a pulsation of the abdominal aorta below the xiphoid process. The observation of peristaltic waves in thin clients is normal.

▶ Marked pulsations could indicate aortic aneurysm or increased pulse pressure. Increased peristaltic activity could indicate gastroenteritis or an obstructive process.

AUSCULTATION OF THE ABDOMEN

Auscultation of the abdomen refers to listening to bowel sounds, vascular sounds, and friction rubs through the stethoscope.

> **ALERT!**
>
> *It is important to auscultate before percussing and palpating, because the latter techniques could alter peristaltic action.*

The pattern for auscultation of bowel sounds is to begin in the RLQ and then proceed through each of the remaining quadrants. The diaphragm of the stethoscope is used to auscultate bowel sounds. The pattern for auscultation of vascular sounds is to begin at the midline below the xiphoid process for the aorta and to proceed from side to side over renal, iliac, and femoral arteries. The bell of the stethoscope is used to auscultate vascular sounds.

The pattern for auscultation for friction rubs is to begin in the RLQ and proceed through each of the remaining quadrants and to listen over the liver and spleen.

The normal bowel sounds heard upon auscultation of the abdomen are irregular, high-pitched, gurgling sounds.

▶ Hyperactive bowel sounds are loud, high-pitched, and rushing. They may occur more frequently with gastroenteritis or diarrhea.

TECHNIQUES AND NORMAL FINDINGS

ABNORMAL FINDINGS SPECIAL CONSIDERATIONS

Normal bowel sounds occur from 5 to 30 times per minute. Borborygmi (stomach growling) refers to more frequent sounds heard in clients who have not eaten in a few hours.

Auscultation of the normal abdomen will not produce vascular sounds or friction rubs.

▶ Hypoactive sounds that are slow and sluggish are common following abdominal surgery or bowel obstruction.
▶ Absent bowel sounds may be indicative of paralytic ileus.
▶ Vascular sounds include bruits and venous hum. A **bruit** is pulsatile and blowing. A venous hum is soft, continuous, and low-pitched. **Friction rub** refers to a rough, grating sound caused by the rubbing together of organs or an organ rubbing on the peritoneum.

1. **Instruct the client.**
   • Explain that you will be listening to the client's abdomen with the stethoscope. The client will be in the supine position. Tell the client to breathe normally. Explain that you will be moving the stethoscope around the client's abdomen and stopping to listen when the stethoscope is placed down. Inform the client that this will cause no discomfort.

2. **Auscultate for bowel sounds.**
   • Use the diaphragm of the stethoscope. Start in the RLQ and move through the other quadrants. Note the character and frequency of the sounds. Count the sounds for at least 60 seconds (see Figure 19.11 ●).

▶ Hyperactive sounds are common in gastroenteritis and diarrhea. Hypoactive sounds are common following abdominal surgery and occur in end-stage intestinal obstruction. Absence of bowel sounds may indicate paralytic ileus.

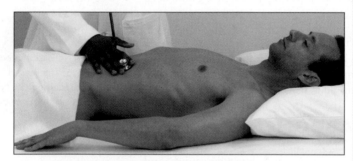

Figure 19.11 ●
Auscultating the abdomen for bowel sounds.

   • Normal bowel sounds are irregular, gurgling, and high-pitched. They occur from 5 to 30 times per minute. Borborygmi is a normal finding.

▶ Clients with paralytic ileus or intestinal obstruction require immediate attention.

ALERT

It may be difficult for the novice nurse to hear bowel sounds in some clients. All four quadrants are auscultated for a total of at least 5 minutes before documenting absent bowel sounds.

3. **Auscultate for vascular sounds.**
   • Use the bell of the stethoscope. Listen at the midline below the xiphoid process for aortic sounds. Move the stethoscope from side to side as you listen over the renal, iliac, and femoral arteries (see Figure 19.12 ●).

▶ Bruits heard during systole and diastole may indicate arterial occlusion.
   A venous hum usually indicates increased portal tension.

| TECHNIQUES AND NORMAL FINDINGS | ABNORMAL FINDINGS SPECIAL CONSIDERATIONS |

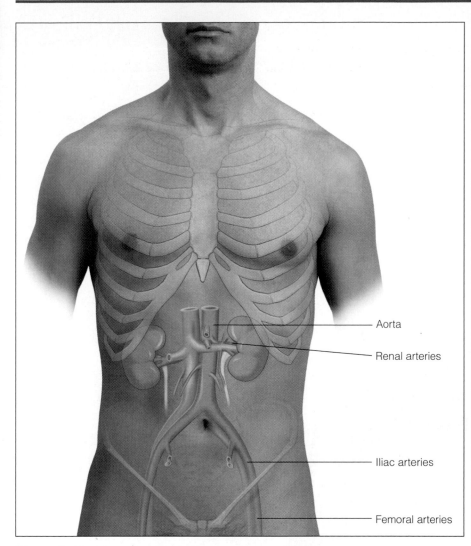

Figure 19.12 • Auscultatory areas for vascular sounds.

Labels on figure: Aorta, Renal arteries, Iliac arteries, Femoral arteries

4. Auscultate for friction rubs.

- Auscultate the abdomen, listening for a coarse, grating sound. Listen carefully over the liver and spleen. Friction rubs are not normally heard.

PERCUSSION OF THE ABDOMEN

1. Visualize the landmarks.

- Observe the abdomen and visualize the horizontal and vertical lines. Visualize the organs and underlying structures of the abdomen.

2. Recall the expected findings.

- Percussion allows you to assess underlying structures. The normal sounds heard over the abdomen are tympany, a loud hollow sound; and dullness, a short high-pitched sound heard over solid organs and the distended bladder.

▶ Hyperresonance is louder than tympany and is heard over air-filled or distended intestines. Flat sounds are short and abrupt and heard over bone. Correct placement of the fingers is important.

TECHNIQUES AND NORMAL FINDINGS	ABNORMAL FINDINGS SPECIAL CONSIDERATIONS

3. **Instruct the client.**

- Explain that you will be tapping on the client's abdomen in a variety of areas.
- Tell the client to breathe normally through this examination. If muscle tension is detected, ask the client to take several deep breaths.

4. **Percuss the abdomen.**

- Place your pleximeter finger on the abdomen during the examination. Review the technique of percussion in Chapter 6. ⊙⊃ Start in the RLQ and percuss through all of the remaining quadrants (see Figure 19.13 ●).

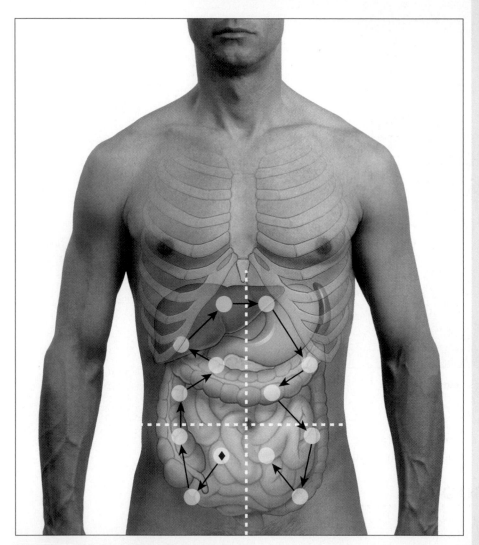

Figure 19.13 ● Percussion pattern for abdomen.

- Percussion over the abdomen produces tympany. Tympany is more pronounced over the gastric bubble. Dullness is heard over the liver and spleen.

▶ Dullness may indicate an enlarged uterus, distended urinary bladder, or ascites. Dullness in the LLQ may indicate the presence of stool in the colon. It is important to ask when the client last had a bowel movement.

| TECHNIQUES AND NORMAL FINDINGS | ABNORMAL FINDINGS SPECIAL CONSIDERATIONS |

PERCUSSION OF THE LIVER

Percuss the liver to determine the upper and lower borders at the anterior axillary line, midclavicular line, and midsternal line. Measure the distance between marks drawn to identify the borders.

1. **Instruct the client.**
   - Explain that you will be tapping the client's abdomen and chest on the right side. Explain that you will be making marks on the abdomen and using a ruler to measure the marks in order to evaluate the size of the liver. Tell the client to remain relaxed and that there should be no discomfort during this assessment.

2. **Percuss the liver.**
   - Begin percussion at the level of the umbilicus and move toward the rib cage along the extended right MCL (see Figure 19.14 ●).

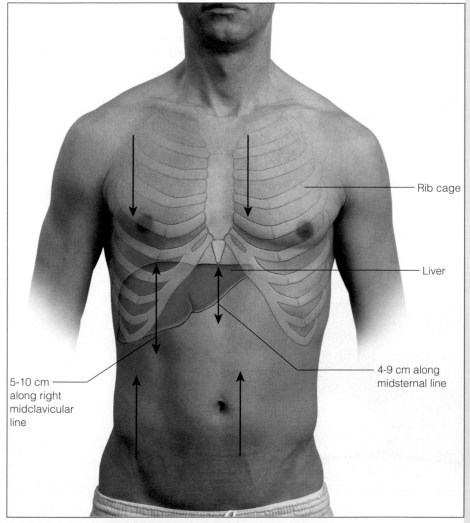

Rib cage

Liver

4-9 cm along midsternal line

5-10 cm along right midclavicular line

Figure 19.14 ● Percussion pattern for liver.

TECHNIQUES AND NORMAL FINDINGS	ABNORMAL FINDINGS SPECIAL CONSIDERATIONS

- The first sound you should hear is tympany. When the sound changes to dullness, you have identified the lower border of the liver. Mark the point with a skin-marking pen. The lower border is normally at the costal margin.

▶ Dullness below the costal margin suggests liver enlargement or downward displacement due to respiratory disease. Dullness above the fifth or sixth intercostal space could indicate an enlarged liver (hepatomegaly) or displacement upward due to ascites or a mass.

- Percuss downward from the fourth intercostal space along the right MCL. The first sound you should hear is resonance because you are over the lung. Percuss downward until the sound changes to dullness. This is the upper border of the liver. Mark the point with a pen. The upper border should be at the level of the sixth intercostal space.

- Measure the distance between the two points. The distance should be approximately 5 to 10 cm (2 to 4 in.). This distance is called the *liver span*.

- Percuss along the midsternal line, using the same technique as before. The liver size at the midsternal line should be approximately 4 to 9 cm (1.5 to 3 in.).

- To determine the movement of the liver with breathing, ask the client to take a deep breath and hold it. Percuss upward along the extended MCL.

- The lower liver border should descend about 1 inch. Remember, liver size is influenced by age, gender, height, and disease process.

▶ Movement of the liver is diminished when atelectasis or pneumothorax of the right lung exists.

PERCUSSION OF THE SPLEEN

The spleen is located in the left side of the abdomen. Percussion is conducted to identify enlargement of the organ.

1. **Instruct the client.**
   - Explain that you will be tapping on the left side of the client's abdomen to examine the spleen. Tell the client to continue to relax, taking deep breaths if required.

2. **Percuss the spleen.**
   - Percuss the abdomen on the left side posterior to the midaxillary line (see Figure 19.15 ●).

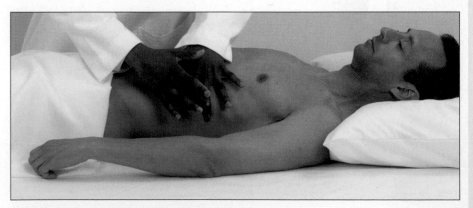

Figure 19.15 ● Percussing the spleen.

TECHNIQUES AND NORMAL FINDINGS	ABNORMAL FINDINGS SPECIAL CONSIDERATIONS

- A small area of splenic dullness will usually be heard from the sixth to tenth intercostal spaces.

► Splenic dullness at the left anterior axillary line indicates splenomegaly, an enlarged spleen. The dull percussion sound is identifiable before an enlarged spleen is palpable. The spleen enlarges anteriorly and inferiorly (see Figure 19.16 ●).

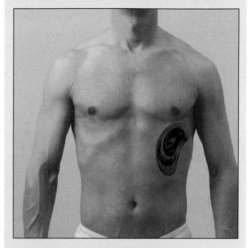

Figure 19.16 ● Splenic enlargement.

PERCUSSION OF THE GASTRIC BUBBLE

Percussion of the gastric bubble is conducted to determine the area occupied by the stomach.

1. **Instruct the client.**
   - Explain that you will be tapping on the client's abdomen over the stomach area. Repeat the explanation about relaxation if required.

2. **Percuss the gastric bubble.**
   - Percuss the abdomen in the area between the left costal margin and the midsternal line extended below the xiphoid process.
   - The percussion sound will be tympany.
   - The sound is influenced by the stomach contents.

► A dull percussion sound suggests a stomach mass. Dull percussion sounds may occur after a meal.
► A very loud sound and an increased area suggest gastric dilation.

PALPATION OF THE ABDOMEN

Palpation of the abdomen is conducted to determine organ size and placement, muscle tightness or guarding, masses, tenderness, and the presence of fluid. This is performed after auscultation to avoid changing the natural sounds and movements of the abdomen. Identify painful areas and palpate these areas last.

You will use both light and deep palpation.

► Muscle tightness or guarding may indicate abdominal pain. Guarding is involuntary contraction of abdominal muscles associated with peritonitis.
► Abdominal pain from an organ is often experienced as referred pain—that is, felt on the surface of the abdomen or back.

TECHNIQUES AND NORMAL FINDINGS	ABNORMAL FINDINGS SPECIAL CONSIDERATIONS

1. **Instruct the client.**
   - Explain that you will be touching the client's abdomen with your hands. Explain that you are going to use light touch and then slight pressure to explore the abdomen. Instruct the client to inform you of any discomfort. Observe the client's facial expression for signs of pain. Also watch for the tendency to guard the abdomen with the hands, or to flex the knees.
   - Instruct the client to take several deep breaths to relax the muscles of the abdomen.

2. **Lightly palpate the abdomen.**
   - Place the palmar surface of your hand on the abdomen and extend your fingers. Lightly press into the abdomen with your fingers (see Figure 19.17 ●).

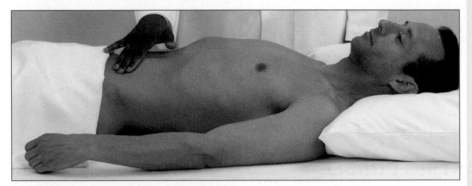

Figure 19.17 ● Light palpation of abdomen.

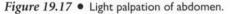

   - Move your hand over the four quadrants by lifting your hand and then placing it in another area. Do not drag or slide your hand over the surface of the skin.
   - The abdomen should be soft, smooth, nontender, and pain-free.

3. **Deeply palpate the abdomen.**
   - Proceed as for light palpation, described in the previous step. Exert pressure with your hand to depress the abdomen about 2 inches.
   - Palpate all four quadrants in an organized sequence.

   - In an obese client or a client with an enlarged abdomen, use a bimanual technique. Place the fingers of your nondominant hand over your dominant hand (see Figure 19.18 ●).

▶ Masses, tumors, or obstructions may be palpated.

▶ In the pregnant female the uterus is palpable. The height of the fundus varies according to the week of gestation.

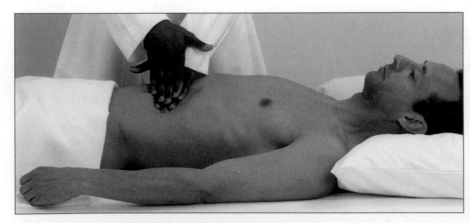

Figure 19.18 ● Deep palpation of abdomen.

TECHNIQUES AND NORMAL FINDINGS	ABNORMAL FINDINGS SPECIAL CONSIDERATIONS

- Identify the size of the underlying organs and any masses for tenderness. The pancreas is nonpalpable because of its size and location.

▶ A mass in the LLQ may be stool in the colon.
▶ A vaguely palpable sensation of fullness in the epigastric region may be pancreatic in origin.

PALPATION OF THE LIVER

The liver is palpated to detect enlargement, pain, and consistency.

1. **Instruct the client.**
   - Explain that you will be using your hands to palpate the client's liver. Explain that you will place one hand under the ribs in the back and ask the client to take a deep breath while you apply slight pressure in an upward motion under the ribs on the client's right side. Instruct the client to tell you of any pain and observe the client for cues of discomfort.

2. **Palpate the liver.**
   - Stand on the right side of the client. Place your left hand under the lower portion of the ribs (ribs 11 and 12). Tell the client to relax into your left hand. Lift the rib cage with your left hand.
   - Place your right hand into the abdomen using an inward and upward thrust at the costal margin (see Figure 19.19 ●). Ask the client to take a deep breath. The descent of the diaphragm will cause the liver to descend, and the lower border will meet your right hand.

▶ Pain on palpation indicates gallbladder disease, hepatitis, or enlargement of the liver (hepatomegaly) associated with congestive heart failure.

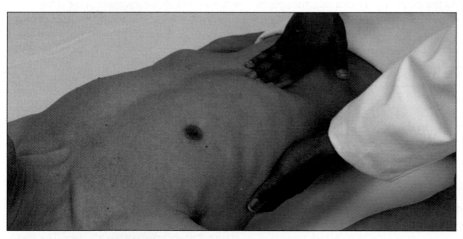

Figure 19.19 ● Palpating the liver.

- Normally, the liver is nonpalpable, except in thin clients. If you feel the lower border of the liver it will be smooth, firm, and nontender.

▶ Nodules occur with cirrhosis or metastatic carcinoma.

PALPATION OF THE SPLEEN

The spleen is palpated to detect enlargement. Careful palpation is required because the spleen is fragile and sensitive.

1. **Instruct the client.**
   - Explain that you will be touching the client with both hands to palpate the spleen. Explain that you will be lifting the client slightly with your left hand while applying slight pressure with fingers under the ribs on the left side. Instruct the client to inform you of any pain or discomfort.

TECHNIQUES AND NORMAL FINDINGS	ABNORMAL FINDINGS SPECIAL CONSIDERATIONS

TECHNIQUES AND NORMAL FINDINGS

ABNORMAL FINDINGS
SPECIAL CONSIDERATIONS

2. **Palpate the spleen.**

- Stand on the client's right side. Place your left hand under the lower border of the rib cage on the left side and elevate the rib cage. This moves the spleen anteriorly. Press the fingers of your right hand into the left costal margin area of the client (see Figure 19.20 ●).

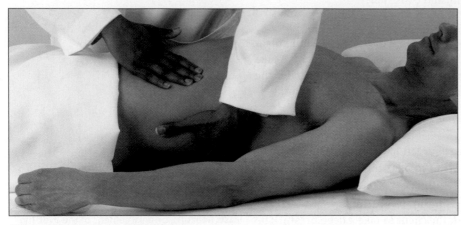

Figure 19.20 ● Palpating the spleen.

- Ask the client to take a slow deep breath. As the diaphragm descends, the spleen moves forward to the fingertips of your right hand. The spleen is normally not palpable.

▶ Splenomegaly, enlargement of the spleen, occurs in acute infections such as mononucleosis. The enlarged spleen is palpable.

ADDITIONAL PROCEDURES

1. **Palpate the aorta for pulsations.**

- Using your fingertips, press deeply and firmly in the upper abdomen to the left of midline below the xiphoid process.
- The average adult aorta is 3 cm wide.

▶ Obesity and masses make palpation of the aorta difficult.

▶ The widened aorta may indicate aneurysm.

2. **Palpate for rebound tenderness.**

- With the client in a supine position, hold your hand at a 90-degree angle to the abdominal wall in an area of no pain or discomfort. Press deeply into the abdomen, using a slow steady movement.
- Rapidly remove your fingers from the client's abdomen (see Figure 19.21 ●).
- Ask if the client feels any pain. Normally, the client feels the pressure but no pain.

▶ The experience of sharp stabbing pain as the compressed area returns to a noncompressed state is known as **Blumberg's sign.** This finding occurs in peritoneal irritation and requires immediate medical attention. Pain referred to McBurney's point (1 to 2 in., 2.5 to 5.1 cm, above the anterosuperior iliac spine, on a line between the ileum and the umbilicus) on palpation of the left lower abdomen is Rovsing's sign, suggestive of peritoneal irritation in appendicitis.

| TECHNIQUES AND NORMAL FINDINGS | ABNORMAL FINDINGS SPECIAL CONSIDERATIONS |

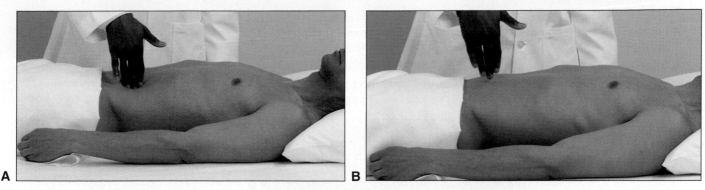

Figure 19.21 ● Palpating for rebound tenderness. A. Applying pressure. B. Rapid release of pressure.

3. Percuss the abdomen for ascites.

● **Ascites** is an abnormal collection of fluid in the peritoneal cavity. With the client in a supine position, percuss at the midline to elicit tympany. Continue to percuss in lateral directions away from the midline and listen for dullness (see Figure 19.22 ●).

▶ Ascites is found in congestive heart failure, cirrhosis, and renal failure, and in many types of cancer.

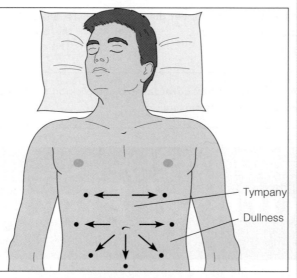

Figure 19.22 ●
Percussion pattern for ascites.

● Mark the skin, identifying possible levels of fluid.

● An alternative method, called *shifting dullness,* is to position the client on the right or left side. Percuss the abdomen. Because fluid settles, anticipate tympany at a superior level and dullness at lower levels (see Figure 19.23 ●).

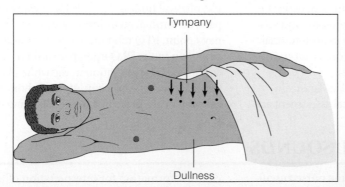

Figure 19.23 ●
Percussion pattern for ascites.

● If ascites is suspected, measure the abdominal girth with a tape measure.

TECHNIQUES AND NORMAL FINDINGS	ABNORMAL FINDINGS SPECIAL CONSIDERATIONS

4. Test for psoas sign.

- Perform this test when lower abdominal pain is present and you suspect appendicitis.

- With the client in a supine position, place your left hand just above the level of the client's right knee. Ask the client to raise the leg to meet your hand. Flexion of the hip causes contraction of the psoas muscle (see Figure 19.24 ●).

▶ Pain during this maneuver is indicative of irritation of the psoas muscle associated with the peritoneal inflammation or appendicitis.

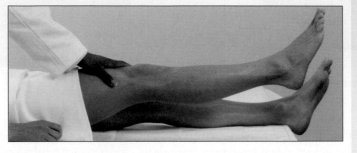

Figure 19.24 ●
Psoas sign.

- Normally there is no abdominal pain associated with this maneuver.

5. Test for Murphy's sign.

- While palpating the liver, ask the client to take a deep breath. The diaphragm descends, pushing the liver and gallbladder toward your hand.
    In a healthy client, liver palpation is painless.

▶ Sharp abdominal pain and the need to halt the examination is a positive Murphy's sign. This occurs in clients with cholecystitis.

 Refer to the Companion Website at **www.prenhall.com/damico** and click on the **Documentation** module for documentation samples and documentation practice exercises.

Abnormal Findings

*A*bnormal findings in the abdomen occur in association with general health and in illness. For example, protrusion of the abdomen is seen in obese individuals and in pregnancy. Abdominal hernias are often seen in otherwise healthy adults and children. Untreated hernias, however, can lead to obstructive intestinal complications that give rise to acute symptoms and serious health problems. Further, alterations of the gastrointestinal tract include nutritional problems, eating disorders, cancers, ulcers, and inflammatory and infectious processes.

For accurate diagnosis in many abdominal and gastrointestinal problems, the health history and physical assessment are accompanied by observations of products of elimination and require diagnostic testing. Diagnostic testing includes laboratory studies of blood, urine, and feces, as well as radiographic and magnetic resonance imaging (MRI). In appendicitis, for example, physical findings include facial expressions demonstrating pain, abdominal guarding, tenderness to palpation at McBurney's point, RLQ rebound tenderness, and a positive *Rovsing's sign* (pain in the RLQ upon palpation of the LLQ). Diagnosis is confirmed by an elevation in the white blood cell count and a flat-plate abdominal x-ray. Abnormal findings from abdominal assessment are presented in the following sections.

ABNORMAL ABDOMINAL SOUNDS

When conducting an abdominal assessment, the nurse auscultates for bowel sounds and for vascular sounds. Table 19.1 includes information for interpretation of abnormal abdominal sounds.

Table 19.1	Abnormal Abdominal Sounds		
SOUND	**LOCATION**	**CAUSATIVE FACTORS**	
Bowel Sounds			
Hyperactive sounds	Any quadrant	Gastroenteritis, diarrhea	
Hyperactive sounds followed by absence of sound	Any quadrant	Paralytic ileus	
High-pitched sounds with cramping	Any quadrant	Intestinal obstruction	
Vascular Sounds			
Systolic bruit (blowing)	Midline below xiphoid	Aortic arterial obstruction	
	Left and right lower costal borders at clavicular line	Stenosis of renal arteries	
	Left and right abdomen at clavicular line between umbilicus and anterior iliac spine	Stenosis of iliac arteries	
Venous hum (continuous tone)	Epigastrium and around umbilicus	Portal hypertension	
Rubbing			
Friction rub (harsh, grating)	Left and right upper quadrants, over liver and spleen	Tumor or inflammation of organ	

ABDOMINAL PAIN

Pain is associated with acute and chronic conditions that affect the digestive organs and abdominal structures. Table 19.2 provides information about several disorders that cause abdominal pain. Disruption of function of the abdominal

Table 19.2	Pain in Common Abdominal Disorders		
DISORDER	**DEFINITION**	**PAIN CHARACTERISTICS**	**PRECIPITATING FACTORS**
Appendicitis	Acute inflammation of vermiform appendix	Epigastric and periumbilical Localizes to RLQ Sudden onset	Obstruction (fecal stone, adhesions)
Cholecystitis	Acute or chronic inflammation of wall of gallbladder	RUQ, radiates to right scapula Sudden onset	Fatty meals, obstruction of duct in cholelithiasis
Diverticulitis	Inflammation of diverticula (outpouches of mucosa through intestinal wall)	Cramping LLQ Radiates to back	Ingestion of fiber-rich diet, stress
Duodenal Ulcer	Breaks in mucosa of duodenum	Aching, gnawing, epigastric	Stress, use of NSAIDs
Ectopic Pregnancy	Implantation of blastocyte outside of the uterus, generally in the fallopian tube	Fullness in the rectal area Abdominal cramping, unilateral pain	Tubal damage, pelvic infection, hormonal disorders, lifting, bowel movements
Gastritis	Inflammation of mucosal lining of the stomach (acute and chronic)	Epigastric pain	Acute: NSAIDs, alcohol abuse, stress, infection Chronic: *H. pylori* Autoimmune responses
Gastroesophageal Reflux Disorder (GERD)	Backflow of gastric acid to the esophagus	Heartburn, chest pain	Food intake, lying down after meals
Intestinal Obstruction	Blockage of normal movement of bowel contents	Small intestine: aching Large intestine: spasmodic pain Neurogenic: diffuse abdominal discomfort Mechanical: colicky pain associated with distention	Mechanical: physical block from impaction, hernia, volvulus Neurogenic: manipulation of bowel during surgery, peritoneal irritation
Irritable Bowel Syndrome (Spastic Colon)	Problems with GI motility	LLQ accompanied by diarrhea and/or constipation Pain increases after eating and decreases after bowel movement	Stress, intolerated foods, caffeine, lactose intolerance, alcohol, familial linkage
Pancreatitis	Inflammation of the pancreas	Upper abdominal, knifelike, deep epigastric or umbilical area pain	Ductal obstruction, alcohol abuse, use of acetaminophen, infection

structures may result in referred pain. **Referred pain** is located where the development of structures occurred in the fetus. Figure 19.25 ● includes referred cutaneous pain areas in the female.

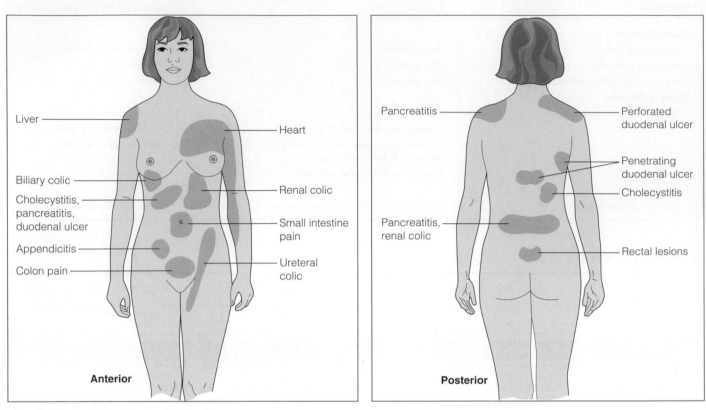

Liver
Heart
Biliary colic
Cholecystitis, pancreatitis, duodenal ulcer
Renal colic
Small intestine pain
Appendicitis
Ureteral colic
Colon pain

Anterior

Pancreatitis
Perforated duodenal ulcer
Penetrating duodenal ulcer
Cholecystitis
Pancreatitis, renal colic
Rectal lesions

Posterior

Figure 19.25 ● Referred cutaneous pain areas.

ABDOMINAL DISTENTION

Abdominal distention occurs for a variety of reasons including obesity, gaseous distention, and ascites. Each of these is described in the following sections.

Obesity

Distention or protuberance of the abdomen occurs in obesity. (see Figure 19.26 ●) The increase in the size of the abdomen is caused by a thickened abdominal wall and fat deposited in the mesentery and omentum. Percussion produces normal tympanic sounds.

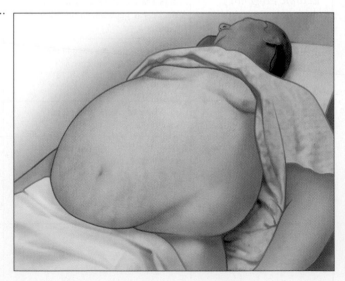

Figure 19.26 ● Obesity.

Gaseous Distention

Gaseous distention of the abdomen is a result of increased production of gas in the intestines, which occurs with the ingestion of some foods (see Figure 19.27 ●). Gaseous distention is also associated with altered peristalsis in which gas cannot move through the intestines. This type of distention is seen in paralytic ileus and intestinal obstruction. Gaseous distention can be localized or generalized. Percussion produces tympany over a large area.

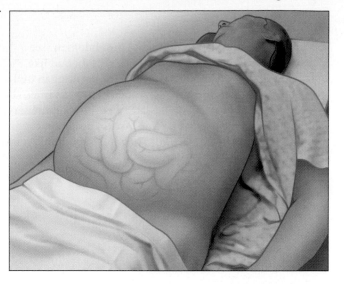

Figure 19.27 ● Distended abdomen.

Tumor

The presence of an abdominal tumor produces abdominal distention (see Figure 19.28 ●). The abdomen is firm to palpation and dull to percussion. This type of distention is common in ovarian and uterine tumors.

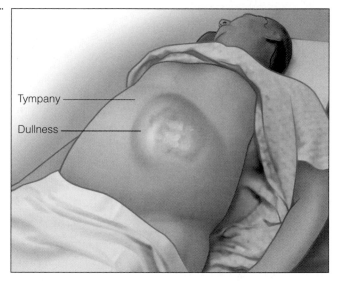

Tympany

Dullness

Figure 19.28 ● Abdominal tumor.

Ascites

Ascites is the accumulation of fluid in the abdomen (see Figure 19.29 ●). The abdomen becomes protuberant like bulging flasks. Fluid descends with gravity, resulting in dullness to percussion in the lower abdomen. Ascites may also be assessed by placing the client in a lateral position and observing fluid shift to the dependent side. Ascites occurs in cirrhosis, congestive heart failure (CHF), nephrosis, peritonitis, and neoplastic diseases.

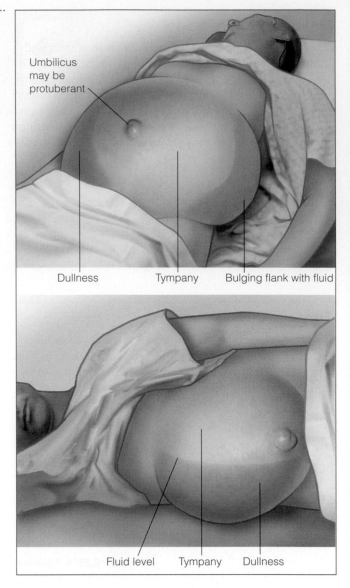

Umbilicus may be protuberant

Dullness　　　Tympany　　　Bulging flank with fluid

Fluid level　　Tympany　　Dullness

Figure 19.29 ● Ascites.

ABDOMINAL HERNIAS

A **hernia,** commonly called a rupture, is a protrusion of an organ or structure through an abnormal opening or weakened area in a body wall. The abdominal wall is the most common site of hernias. This weakening could be congenital or acquired. If the protruding or displaced abdominal contents return to their normal position when the client relaxes, the hernia is said to be reducible or reduced. When the displaced or protruding structures do not return to their normal position, the hernia is said to be incarcerated or nonreducible. An incarcerated hernia can become strangulated. In strangulated hernias, the blood supply to the displaced abdominal contents is compromised. The strangulated visceral contents can become gangrenous. Overstretched rectus muscles with weakened fascia cause an umbilical hernia.

Umbilical Hernia

An *umbilical hernia* occurs at the umbilicus (see Figure 19.30 ●). The abdominal rectus muscle separates or weakens, allowing abdominal structures, usually the intestines, to push through and come closer to the skin. Umbilical hernias are more common in children than in adults.

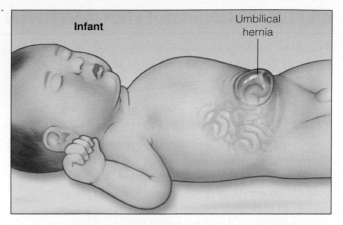

Figure 19.30 ● Umbilical hernia.

Ventral (Incisional) Hernias

A *ventral hernia* is also known as an incisional hernia because it occurs at the site of an incision (see Figure 19.31 ●). The incision weakens the muscle, and the abdominal structures move closer to the skin. Causes include obesity, repeated surgeries, infection during the postoperative period, impaired wound healing, and poor nutrition.

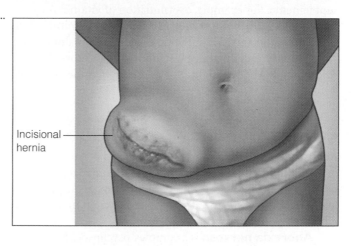

Figure 19.31 ● Ventral hernia.

Hiatal Hernia

A *hiatal hernia* is due to a weakening in the diaphragm that allows a portion of the stomach and the esophagus to move into the thoracic cavity. This hernia is classified as sliding or rolling and is more common in adults than children. Abdominal hernias are illustrated in Figure 19.32 ●.

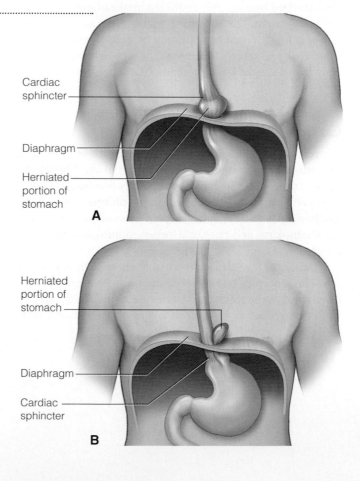

Figure 19.32 ● Abdominal hernias. A. Sliding hiatal hernia. B. Rolling hiatal hernia.

ALTERATIONS OF THE GASTROINTESTINAL TRACT

Alterations of the gastrointestinal tract include nutritional problems, eating disorders, cancers, and inflammatory diseases. These alterations are described in the following sections.

Nutritional Problems

Nutritional problems include malnutrition, obesity, and overweight. **Malnutrition** is an imbalance, whether a deficit or excess, of the required nutrients of a balanced diet. *Undernutrition* denotes inadequate intake of the nutrients needed to maintain optimal body functioning. *Overnutrition* is an excessive intake of nutrients, either as food or as food supplements. For example, overnutrition of vitamin A can lead to toxicity symptoms such as nausea and vomiting. Both undernutrition and overnutrition are forms of malnutrition.

Obesity is defined as a weight of 20% or more above recommended body weight. Severe obesity signifies an excess of 100% or 100 lb above recommended body weight. Obesity has been linked to an increased risk for a number of gastrointestinal problems, such as cancers of the gallbladder and colon. In addition, research suggests that obese people experience a variety of psychosocial problems, such as job discrimination and social isolation.

Overweight is defined as a weight of 10 to 20% in excess of recommended body weight. The likelihood of developing significant health problems is lower in those who are overweight than in those who are obese.

Eating Disorders

An eating disorder is a condition in which a person's current intake of food differs significantly from that person's normal intake. Eating disorders typically result from an attempt to lose weight; however, the attempt to lose weight may be a misguided response to psychosocial problems.

Anorexia nervosa is a complex psychosocial problem characterized by a severely restricted intake of nutrients and a low body weight. The anorexic typically experiences intense fear of gaining weight or becoming fat, feels fat even when emaciated, and refuses to maintain body weight over a minimal normal weight for age and height. Many anorexics experience constipation, gastrointestinal bloating or distention, nausea, and abdominal pain.

Bulimia nervosa is an eating disorder characterized by binge eating and purging or another compensatory mechanism to prevent weight gain. Typically, the bulimic consumes large portions of high-calorie food, typically about 4,000 calories at one time. The individual then tries to force the food out of the body by vomiting or using laxatives, enemas, diuretics, or diet pills. Many bulimics experience tooth decay, dehydration, laxative dependence, and rectal bleeding.

Cancers

Cancer of the esophagus is a malignant growth of the esophagus, most common in males over 50 years of age. The lower third of the esophagus is most commonly involved. Clients commonly complain of weight loss, **dysphagia** (difficulty swallowing), and odynophagia (pain on swallowing). Alcohol abuse, smoking, and poor oral hygiene appear to be predisposing factors.

Cancer of the stomach is a malignant growth of the stomach. The cancerous lesions are found most frequently in the distal third of the stomach. The disease is often in the advanced stages before a diagnosis is made. Dietary habits seem to be an influencing factor. Weight loss, nausea, vomiting, abdominal pain, abdominal distention, and some bleeding are the common complaints of the client.

Colorectal cancer is a malignant lesion involving any part of the large intestine, sigmoid colon, or rectum. Predisposing factors include poor dietary habits and chronic constipation. Signs and symptoms vary according to the location of the growth. A change in bowel habits or patterns is a characteristic with any location. In many cases, when an intestinal obstruction occurs, surgery is required and the client may need a permanent colostomy.

Inflammatory Processes

Ulcerative colitis is a recurrent inflammatory process causing ulcer formation in the lower portions of the large intestine and rectum. This condition is common in adolescents and young adults. The distribution of the inflammatory process is diffuse. The ulcerative areas abscess and later become necrotic. Diarrhea, abdominal pain, and cramping with weight loss are common symptoms of the disease process.

Esophagitis is an inflammatory process of the esophagus. It is caused by a variety of irritants. The more common causes include smoking, alcohol abuse, reflux of gastric contents, and ingestion of extremely hot or cold foods and liquids.

Peritonitis is a local or generalized inflammatory process of the peritoneal membrane of the abdomen. The precipitant can be an infectious process (pelvic inflammatory disease), perforation of an organ (ruptured duodenal ulcer), internal bleeding (ruptured ectopic pregnancy), or trauma (stab wound to abdomen).

Hepatitis is an inflammatory process of the liver. Its causes include viruses, bacteria, chemicals, and drugs. Types of hepatitis include the following.

Hepatitis A virus (HAV) infectious hepatitis is transmitted via enteric routes (feces or oral routes).

Hepatitis B virus (HBV) is transmitted parenterally, sexually, or perinatally.

Hepatitis C virus (HCV) is transmitted via blood and blood products, parenterally, and through unknown factors.

Hepatitis D virus (HDV) is the same as HBV and requires HBV to replicate.

Hepatitis E virus (HEV) is a non-A, non-B type transmitted enterically. HEV is most common in those who travel to India, Africa, Asia, and Central America.

Crohn's disease is a chronic inflammatory process of the ileum. It is sometimes called regional ileitis, which is a misnomer because it can involve any part of the lower intestinal tract. Crohn's disease is characterized by "skipped" sections of involvement. It is most common in young adults and usually has an insidious onset. The inflammation involves all layers of the intestinal mucosa. Transverse fissures develop in the bowel, producing a characteristic cobblestone appearance.

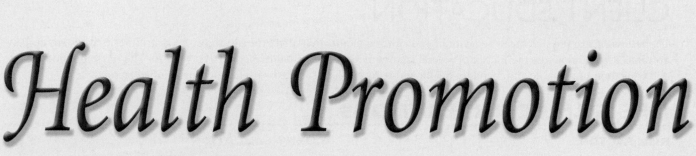

Health Promotion

HEALTHY PEOPLE 2010

FOCUS AREA	PREVALENCE	OBJECTIVES	ACTIONS
Colorectal Cancer	• Colorectal cancer is the second leading cause of cancer deaths in the United States.	• Reduce death rate from colorectal cancer.	• Education about risks and screening.
Foodborne Illness	• Very young, elderly, and immunocompromised individuals experience serious foodborne illnesses. • Risks of foodborne illnesses increase as a result of emerging pathogenic organisms, improper food storage or preparation, increasing global supply of foods, inadequate training of food handlers, and an aging population. • Food allergies are present in almost 4% of children under age 6 and 1 to 2% of the adult population.	• Reduce infections by foodborne pathogens. • Reduce anaphylaxis deaths from food allergies.	• Education about food handling in retail areas and in the home. • Education about food labeling and preparation.

(continued)

Health Promotion

HEALTHY PEOPLE 2010—continued

FOCUS AREA	PREVALENCE	OBJECTIVES	ACTIONS
Hepatitis	• Hepatitis C virus (HCV) is the most common bloodborne viral infection in the United States. • Hepatitis B virus (HBV) occurs in more than 15,000 children born of mothers infected with HBV. • Hepatitis A virus (HAV) occurs most frequently in children, and children are a source for new community infections.	• Reduce hepatitis C, B, and A.	• Screening. • Education about hepatitis. • Immunization programs.

CLIENT EDUCATION

The following are physiological, behavioral, and cultural factors that affect the health of the gastrointestinal system and abdominal structures across the life span. Several factors reflect trends cited in *Healthy People 2010*. The nurse provides advice and education to promote and maintain health and reduce risks associated with the aforementioned factors.

LIFE SPAN CONSIDERATIONS

RISK FACTORS

- Congenital defects such as cleft lip, cleft palate, esophageal atresia, pyloric stenosis, and hernias affect the nutritional status as well as the growth and development of infants and children.
- Pregnant females experience hormonal shifts that result in nausea, vomiting, and constipation.

- A decrease in digestive enzymes and decreased peristalsis occur in older adults.

- Obesity has become increasingly prevalent across the age span in the United States.

- Dental diseases occur at all ages and impact nutrition by affecting the desire for food and the ability to chew foods.
- Foodborne illness occurs in all age groups; however, children, older adults, and those with immunosuppression are at greatest risk.
- Hepatitis infections can be acute or chronic and occur in all ages. Hepatitis A occurs most frequently in children and young adults. Hepatitis can be an acute self-limiting illness or a chronic debilitating disease. It can result in liver necrosis and death. Individuals who travel to India, Asia, Africa, and Central America are at risk for hepatitis E.

CLIENT EDUCATION

- Educate parents of children with congenital defects about alterations in foods and feeding patterns.

- Tell pregnant clients that dietary changes including small, frequent meals of dry foods are helpful in relieving the nausea and vomiting in early pregnancy.
- Inform clients that increased fluid intake, fruits, and high-fiber foods increase regularity in bowel elimination in pregnant females and in older adults.
- Tell clients that regular exercise promotes and maintains the efficiency of gastrointestinal function.
- Provide information about healthy eating from infancy to old age to prevent obesity and contribute to improved gastrointestinal function.
- Advise clients about regular dental hygiene and care to reduce risks for malnutrition.
- Provide information about safe food preparation, handling, and storage as it is important in reducing the incidence of foodborne illnesses and hepatitis.
- Tell clients that immunization for hepatitis is important across the age span. Recommended schedules should be followed.

CULTURAL CONSIDERATIONS

RISK FACTOR

- The types of foods one eats and the ways in which foods are prepared are influenced by culture. Frequent ingestion of fried foods can result in obesity and health problems associated with high cholesterol.

CLIENT EDUCATION

- Discuss alternative methods of food preparation and seasoning to decrease the incidence of obesity and gastrointestinal disorders that occur with greater frequency in cultural groups who prepare spicy and fried foods.

ENVIRONMENTAL CONSIDERATIONS

RISK FACTORS

- Medications can impact the function and integrity of the gastrointestinal system. For example, aspirin and NSAIDs can irritate the mucosa of the gastrointestinal tract. Pain medications often slow the peristaltic process.
- Stress is associated with increased frequency, duration, and acuity of gastrointestinal and abdominal problems including ulcerative diseases and eating disorders.

CLIENT EDUCATION

- Provide instruction about prescribed and OTC medications to reduce the risks of side effects that impact gastrointestinal health and other physiological functions or systems.
- Provide information about stress reduction techniques, support groups, and resources in the community to assist with crisis management and ongoing stressful situations.

BEHAVIORAL CONSIDERATIONS

RISK FACTOR

- Alcohol abuse is associated with gastritis and liver disease. The number of adolescents who abuse alcohol is on the rise. Alcohol use is greater in Caucasians and Hispanics than in African Americans.

CLIENT EDUCATION

- Advise adolescents, parents, and adults about alcohol abuse in relation to gastrointestinal and liver diseases. Teach clients how to recognize behaviors associated with alcohol abuse, and about prevention programs and addiction services to reduce the incidence of physical and emotional problems associated with alcohol abuse.

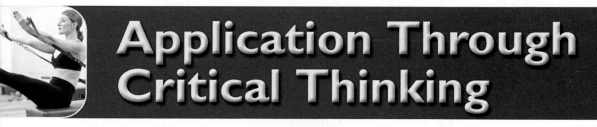

Application Through Critical Thinking

CASE STUDY

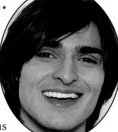

*L*uiz Hernandez, a 28-year-old Hispanic male, is seeking care for abdominal pain and weight loss in the neighborhood clinic. He has been seen here for employment physicals, which revealed no acute or chronic health problems.

During the interview the nurse learns that the client has had abdominal pain, on and off, for a couple of months and that the pain is getting worse. The pain is in the middle of his stomach and is like an ache. Mr. Hernandez says he has also had no interest in food, feels gassy, and has lost about 10 lb.

When asked about factors that precipitate or affect the pain, the client reveals that the pain occurs most frequently late in the morning and afternoon and that he wakes up at night with the pain. When asked if he has tried any remedy for the pain, Mr. Hernandez states that he uses an antacid once in a while and it helps, and that he takes mint because that is what

his mother gave to the family members when they had stomach troubles.

In response to questions about weight loss, Mr. Hernandez says that he thinks he has been losing weight because he just hasn't been feeling hungry and many of the foods he is used to eating do not appeal to him. He also states that he is starting to get nervous about the pain, and when he is nervous he never feels like eating. The nurse asks if he is nervous about this clinic visit. The client replies that he was really nervous when he arrived but is feeling a little better now that he is talking about what is going on. He further states, "I am still scared about what might be causing this."

The nurse continues the interview with questions about the client's past and family history. No acute or chronic problems are revealed. The nurse asks the client about use of medications and his habits. Mr. Hernandez states that he uses Tylenol occasionally for a headache. He does not smoke and uses alcohol socially, mostly on weekends.

The physical examination reveals vital signs of B/P 132/84—P 88—RR 22. The skin is cool, dry, and pale. The abdomen is soft and not distended, bowel sounds are present in all quadrants, and there is no tenderness on palpation.

The plan for this client is to begin antacids three times a day, after meals, and at bedtime, schedule an endoscopy, obtain cultures for *H. pylori*, and arrange for a follow-up visit in 1 week.

▶ Complete Documentation

The following is sample documentation for Luis Hernandez.

SUBJECTIVE DATA: Aching midabdominal pain for several months, getting worse. Feels "gassy." No interest in food. Weight loss 10 lb. Pain occurs late in a.m. and p.m., wakes at night. Antacid used infrequently with relief. Uses mint for symptoms. Nervous about pain and what it might mean.

OBJECTIVE DATA: Skin pale, cool, dry. Abdomen soft, nontender. BS + 4Qs. VS: B/P 132/84—P 88—RR 22.

S—Aching, midabdominal pain for several months, getting
worse
Feels "gassy"
No interest in food
Loss of 10 lb
Pain occurs late in a.m. & p.m., wakes at night
Antacid used infrequently with relief
Uses mint for symptoms
Nervous about pain and what it might mean
O—Pallor
Skin cool, dry
VS: B/P 132/84—P 88—RR 22
Abdomen soft, nontender, BS + 4 Qs
A—Increasing late a.m. and p.m. mid-abdominal pain over
several months. Relief with antacids, nervous, and H.
pylori gastric ulcer
P—Begin antacid tid pc and HS
Endoscopy
Follow + findings with cultures for H. pylori
Schedule follow-up appointment

▶ Critical Thinking Questions

1. What data suggests the need for *H. pylori* cultures?
2. How would data be clustered to formulate nursing diagnoses?
3. What would be included in an educational plan for this client?

▶ Applying Nursing Diagnoses

1. *Nausea* is a nursing diagnosis in the NANDA taxonomy (see Appendix A). Do the data in the case study support this diagnosis? If so, identify the data.
2. *Pain, acute* is a diagnosis in the NANDA taxonomy. Do the data for Luis Hernandez support this diagnosis?
3. Refer to the NANDA taxonomy in Appendix A to formulate additional nursing diagnoses for Mr. Hernandez.

▶ Prepare Teaching Plan

LEARNING NEED: Mr. Hernandez sought healthcare for abdominal pain and weight loss. The data reveal that he experiences pain late in the morning and afternoon and that he often wakes at night with pain. He uses antacids with some relief. He admits to being nervous about the problem. Following the interview and physical examination, the plan of care includes antacids and a scheduled diagnostic test for *H. pylori*.

The case study provides data that is representative of symptoms and behaviors associated with *H. pylori* and peptic ulcer disease. Individuals and community groups could benefit from education about *H. pylori*. The following teaching plan is intended for a group of learners and focuses on *H. pylori* and ulcers.

GOAL: The participant will have increased awareness of ulcers and *H. pylori* infection.

OBJECTIVES: Upon completion of this educational session, the participants will be able to:

1. Define peptic ulcer.
2. Discuss causes of peptic ulcer disease.
3. Describe symptoms of peptic ulcer.
4. Identify diagnostic tests for peptic ulcer.
5. List treatments for peptic ulcer.

See teaching plan on next page.

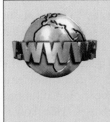

Please refer to the Companion Website at www.prenhall.com/damico and click on Chapter 19, the Application Through Critical Thinking module, to complete the following activities related to this case study:
▶ Critical Thinking questions
▶ Extended Nursing Diagnosis challenge
▶ Documentation activity
▶ Teaching Plan for Objectives 1, 3, 4, and 5

APPLICATION OF OBJECTIVE 2: Discuss causes of peptic ulcer disease

Content	Teaching Strategy	Evaluation
• In the past it was believed that ulcers were caused by stress or eating too much acidic food. Now it is known that this is not true.	• Lecture	• Written examination. May use short answer, fill-in, or multiple-choice items or a combination of items.
• Most stomach ulcers are caused by infection.	• Discussion	If these are short and easy to evaluate, the learner receives immediate feedback.
• The infection is caused by a bacteria named *Helicobacter pylori* or *H. pylori*.	• Audiovisual materials such as illustrations of the gastrointestinal system	• Question-and-answer period. With small groups, can prompt discussion. Provides immediate feedback.
• *H. pylori* causes more than 90% of peptic ulcers.	These reinforce verbal presentation.	
• *H. pylori* infects almost two thirds of the world's population.	Printed materials allow review and reinforcement at the learner's own pace.	
• In the United States, *H. pylori* is more prevalent in the older adults, African Americans, Hispanics, and those in lower socioeconomic groups.		
• Most people with *H. pylori* never have symptoms.		
• *H. pylori* can be transmitted from person to person. Always wash hands after using bathroom and before eating.		
• Peptic ulcers are also caused by long-term use of nonsteroidal anti-inflammatory drugs (NSAIDs) such as ibuprofen and aspirin.		
• Peptic ulcers can be caused by tumors in the stomach or pancreas.		

EXPLORE MediaLink

Additional resources for this chapter are found on the Student CD-ROM accompanying this textbook and on the Companion Website.

CD-ROM CONTENT

Content for this chapter includes:
Objectives
Key Concepts
NCLEX-RN® Review Questions
Model Documentation Forms
Audio Glossary
Animations
Digestive System Anatomy
Games and Challenges
Clinical Spotlight Videos
Gastro-Esophageal Reflux Disease
Ulcers
Head-to-Toe Physical Examination Video

COMPANION WEBSITE CONTENT

www.prenhall.com/damico

Content for this chapter includes:
Objectives
NCLEX-RN® Review Questions

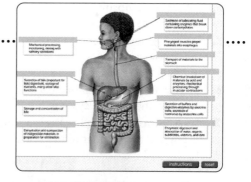

Client Interaction Case Study Challenge
Application Through Critical Thinking
　　Case Study Teaching Plan Challenge
MediaLinks
MediaLink Application
Tool Box
Chapter Documentation Form Example
Abnormal Abdominal Sounds
Pain in Common Abdominal Disorders
Referred Cutaneous Pain Areas
Health Promotion
　　Healthy People 2010
　　Client Education
New York Times

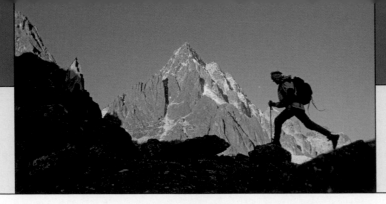

20
Urinary System

MEDIALINK

www.prenhall.com/damico

The CD-ROM in the back of this textbook and the Media-Link website contain NCLEX-RN® review questions, interactive exercises, case study challenges, animations, videos, documentation and checklist forms, and review materials. For a complete listing of the media content specific to Chapter 20, see the Explore MediaLink at the end of the chapter.

The urinary system is composed of the kidneys, ureters, bladder, and urethra. The **glomeruli** (tufts of capillaries) of the kidneys filter more than one liter (1 L) of fluid each minute. As a result, wastes, toxins, and foreign matter are removed from the blood. The urinary system acts through the kidneys to prevent the accumulation of nitrogenous wastes, promotes fluid and electrolyte balance, assists in maintenance of blood pressure, and contributes to *erythropoiesis* (development of mature red blood cells).

The organs of the urinary system are distributed among the retroperitoneal space, abdomen, and genitals. Assessment of the urinary system is incorporated into assessment of the abdomen and reproductive systems. Urinary function is interdependent with other body systems. In addition, psychosocial and developmental factors impact the function of the urinary system.

Chronic kidney disease is one of the focus areas as stated in *Healthy People 2010*. A goal is to reduce the number of new cases, the many complications, disabilities, deaths, and ultimately the cost for treatment as described in the *Healthy People 2010* feature on page 578.

ANATOMY AND PHYSIOLOGY REVIEW

The structures of the urinary system include the kidneys, ureters, urinary bladder, urethra, and renal vasculature (blood vessels). Each of the structures will be described in the following sections.

KIDNEYS

The **kidneys** are bean-shaped organs located in the retroperitoneal space on either side of the vertebral column. Extending from the level of the twelfth thoracic vertebra to the third lumbar vertebra, the upper portion of the kidneys is protected by the lower rib cage. The right kidney is displaced downward by the liver and sits slightly lower than the left kidney. A layer of fat cushions each kidney, and the kidney itself is surrounded by tissue called the renal capsule (see Figure 20.1 ●). The renal fascia connects the kidney and fatty layer to the posterior wall of the abdomen. Each adult kidney weighs approximately 150 g (5 oz) and is 11 to 13 cm (4 to 5 in.) long, 5 to 7 cm (2 to 3 in.) wide, and 2.5 to 3 cm (1 in.) thick. The lateral surface of the kidney is convex. The medial surface is concave and contains the hilus, a vertical cleft that opens into a space within the kidney referred to as the renal sinus. The ureters, renal blood vessels, nerves, and lymphatic vessels pass through the hilus into the renal sinus. The superior part of the kidney is referred to as the upper pole, whereas the inferior surface is called the lower pole.

The inner portion of the kidney is called the *renal medulla.* The renal **medulla** is composed of structures called pyramids and calyces. The pyramids are wedgelike structures made up of bundles of urine-collecting tubules. At their apex, the pyramids have papillae that are enclosed by cuplike structures called calyces. The calyces collect urine and transport it into the renal pelvis, which is the funnel-shaped superior end of the ureter (see Figure 20.2 ●).

The outer portion of each kidney is called the renal **cortex.** It is composed of over 1 million nephrons, which form urine. The first part of each nephron is the renal corpuscle, which consists of a tuft of capillaries called a glomerulus. These glomeruli begin the filtration of the blood. Larger blood components, such as red blood cells and larger proteins, are separated from most of the fluid, which passes into the glomerular capsule (or Bowman's capsule). The filtrate then moves into a proximal convoluted tubule, then into the loop of Henle, and finally into a distal convoluted tubule, from which it is collected as urine by a collecting tubule. Along the way, some of the filtrate is resorbed along with electrolytes and chemicals such as glucose, potassium, phosphate, and sodium. Each collecting tubule guides the urine from several nephrons out into the renal pyramids and calyces, and from there through the renal pelvis and into the ureters.

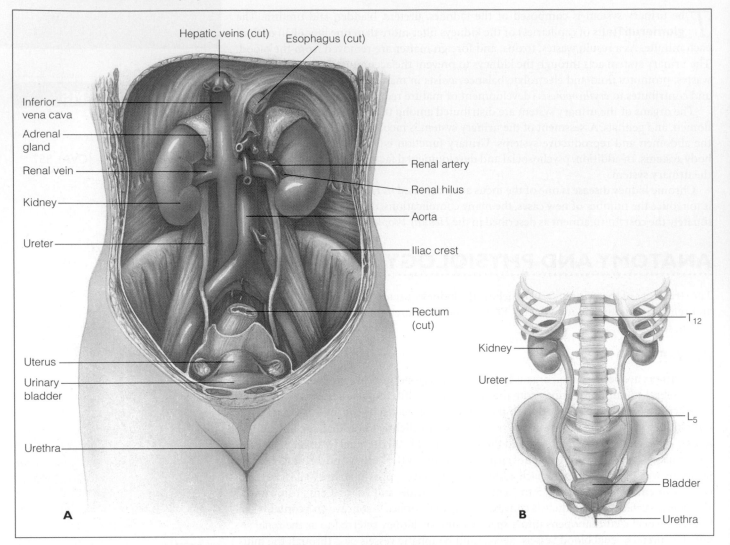

Hepatic veins (cut)
Esophagus (cut)
Inferior vena cava
Adrenal gland
Renal vein
Kidney
Ureter
Uterus
Urinary bladder
Urethra
Renal artery
Renal hilus
Aorta
Iliac crest
Rectum (cut)

A

T₁₂
Kidney
Ureter
L₅
Bladder
Urethra

B

Figure 20.1 ● The urinary system. A. Anterior view of the urinary organs of a female. B. Relationship of the kidneys to the vertebrae.

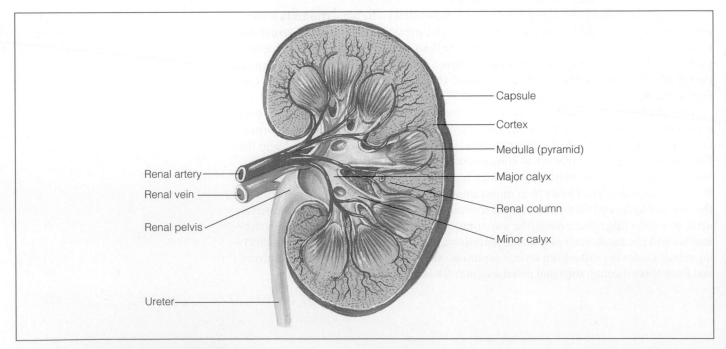

Renal artery
Renal vein
Renal pelvis
Ureter
Capsule
Cortex
Medulla (pyramid)
Major calyx
Renal column
Minor calyx

Figure 20.2 ● Internal anatomy of the kidney.

The major functions of the kidneys are the following:

- Eliminating nitrogenous waste products, toxins, excess ions, and drugs through urine
- Regulating volume and chemical makeup of the blood
- Maintaining balance between water and salts, and acids and bases
- Producing renin, an enzyme that assists in the regulation of blood pressure
- Producing the hormone erythropoietin, which stimulates production of red blood cells in the bone marrow
- Assisting in the metabolism of vitamin D

RENAL ARTERIES

The kidneys require a tremendous amount of oxygen and nutrients and receive about 25% of the cardiac output. Although not part of the urinary system, an extensive network of arteries intertwines within the renal network. These arteries include renal arteries, arcuate arteries, interlobular arteries, afferent arteries, and efferent arterioles. The vasa recta are looping capillaries that connect with the juxtamedullary nephrons and continue into the medulla alongside the loop of Henle. The vasa recta help to concentrate urine. The major function of the renal arteries is providing a rich supply of blood (approximately 1,200 ml per minute when an individual is at rest) to the kidneys.

URETERS

The **ureters** are mucous-lined narrow tubes approximately 25 to 30 cm (10 to 12 in.) in length and 6 to 12 mm (0.25 to 0.5 in.) in diameter. As the ureter leaves the kidney, it travels downward behind the peritoneum to the posterior wall of the urinary bladder. The middle layer of the ureters contains smooth muscle that is stimulated by transmission of electric impulses from the autonomic nervous system. Their peristaltic action propels urine downward to the urinary bladder. The major function of the ureters is transporting urine from the kidney to the urinary bladder.

URINARY BLADDER

The urinary bladder is a hollow, muscular, collapsible pouch that acts as a reservoir for urine. It lies on the pelvic floor in the retroperitoneal space. The bladder is composed of two parts: the rounded muscular sac made up of the detrusor muscle, and the portion between the body of the bladder and the urethra known as the neck. In males, the bladder lies anterior to the rectum, and the neck of the bladder is encircled by the prostate gland of the male reproductive system. In females, the bladder lies anterior to the vagina and uterus. The detrusor muscle allows the bladder to expand as it fills with urine, and to contract to release urine to the outside of the body during micturition (voiding). When empty, the bladder collapses upon itself forming a thick-walled, pyramidal organ that lies low in the pelvis behind the symphysis pubis. As urine accumulates, the fundus, the superior wall of the bladder, ascends in the abdominal cavity and assumes a rounded shape that is palpable. When moderately filled (500 ml), the bladder is approximately 12.5 cm

(5 in.) long. When larger amounts of urine are present, the bladder becomes distended and rises above the symphysis pubis.

The major functions of the urinary bladder are the following:

- Storing urine temporarily
- Contracting to release urine during micturition

URETHRA

The **urethra** is a mucous-lined tube that transports urine from the urinary bladder to the exterior. In females, the urethra is approximately 3 to 4 cm (1.5 in.) long and lies along the anterior wall of the vagina. The female urethra terminates in the external urethral orifice or meatus, which lies between the clitoris and the vagina. The male urethra is approximately 20 cm (8 in.) long and runs the length of the penis. It terminates in the external urethral orifice in the glans penis. In addition to providing a passageway for urine, the male urethra also carries semen outside of the body. Because the female urethra is short and its meatus lies close to the anus, it can become contaminated with bacteria more readily than the male urethra. A more detailed review of the penis, prostate gland, and male and female external genitalia is presented in Chapters 21 and 22. The major function of the urethra is providing a passage for the elimination of urine.

LANDMARKS

During assessment of the urinary system, the nurse uses three landmarks to locate and palpate the kidneys and urinary bladder. These landmarks are the costovertebral angle, the rectus abdominis muscle, and the symphysis pubis. The **costovertebral angle (CVA)** is the area on the lower back formed by the vertebral column and the downward curve of the last posterior rib as depicted in Figure 20.3A ●. It is an important anatomical landmark because the lower poles of the kidney and ureter lie below this surface. The rectus abdominis muscles are a longitudinal pair of muscles that extend from the pubis to the rib cage on either side of the midline as illustrated in Figure 20.3B ●. These muscles are used as guidelines for positioning the hands when palpating the kidneys through the abdominal wall. The symphysis pubis is the joint formed by the union of the two pubic bones by cartilage at the midline of the body (Figure 20.3B). The bladder is cradled under the symphysis pubis. When the bladder is full, the nurse is able to palpate it as it rises above the symphysis pubis.

SPECIAL CONSIDERATIONS

The client's health status is influenced by a number of factors, including age, developmental level, race, ethnicity, work history, living conditions, socioeconomics, and emotional health. During a comprehensive health assessment, effective communication and critical thinking enable the nurse to identify the ways in which one or more factors influence the client's health, beliefs, and practices.

DEVELOPMENTAL CONSIDERATIONS

Changes in anatomical structures and functions occur as a normal part of growth and development. Knowledge of normal, age-related variations in findings from health assessment is

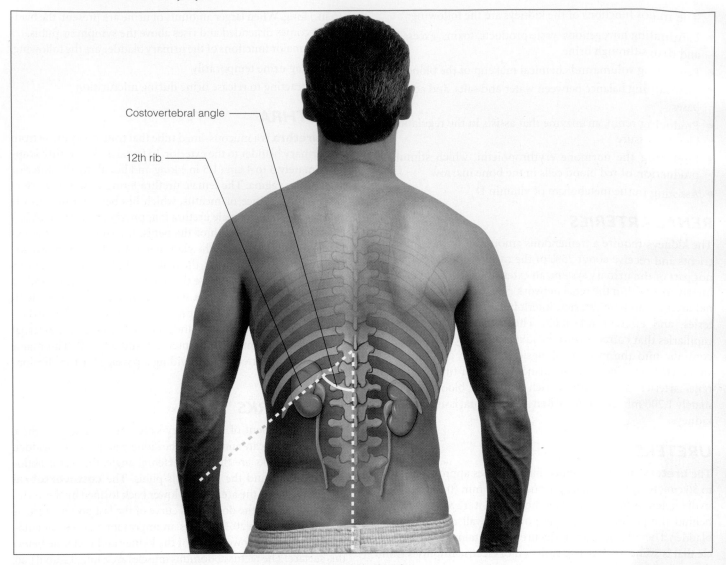

Costovertebral angle

12th rib

Figure 20.3A ● Landmarks for urinary assessment. A. The costovertebral angle.

essential in interpretating data and planning care for clients. Specific variations in the urinary system for different age groups are presented in the following sections.

Infants and Children

Renal blood flow increases with a significant allotment to the renal medulla at birth. The glomerular filtration rate also increases at birth compared to the fetal filtration rate and continues to increase until the first or second year of life. The fluid and electrolyte balance in an infant or child is fragile. Illnesses that cause dehydration, loss of fluids, or lack of fluid intake may rapidly lead to metabolic acidosis and fluid imbalance. Serious, chronic dysfunction of this system may impair the child's growth and development.

It is important to consider the health practices of the family when the genital areas are unclean in infants or children of any age. Presence of a diaper rash is a clue that the nurse should explore the family's hygiene practices; however, diaper rash is often difficult to control, and supportive teaching is indicated.

The nurse examines infants for anomalies such as scrotal edema, undescended testes, and noncentral placement of the urinary meatus. Bed-wetting is a difficult problem for both the child and the family and may influence the child's relationship with the family. The child's confidence and social development may also be affected by bed-wetting. Bed-wetting is not generally considered problematic unless the child has no daytime dryness after 4 years of age or nighttime dryness after 6 years of age.

The Pregnant Female

During the first trimester, the enlarging uterus presses against the bladder, increasing the frequency of urination. Frequency decreases during the second trimester and then recurs during the third trimester as the presenting part of the fetus descends into the pelvis and again presses on the bladder.

During pregnancy, the amount of urine produced increases, causing the client to feel the need to urinate more frequently. There is also a tendency for the urine to test positive for sugar. In the postpartum period, edema and hyperemia of the bladder mucosa cause decreased sensation and contribute to overdistention of the bladder. Incomplete emptying of the bladder often accompanies this condition, increasing the client's susceptibility to urinary tract infection (UTI).

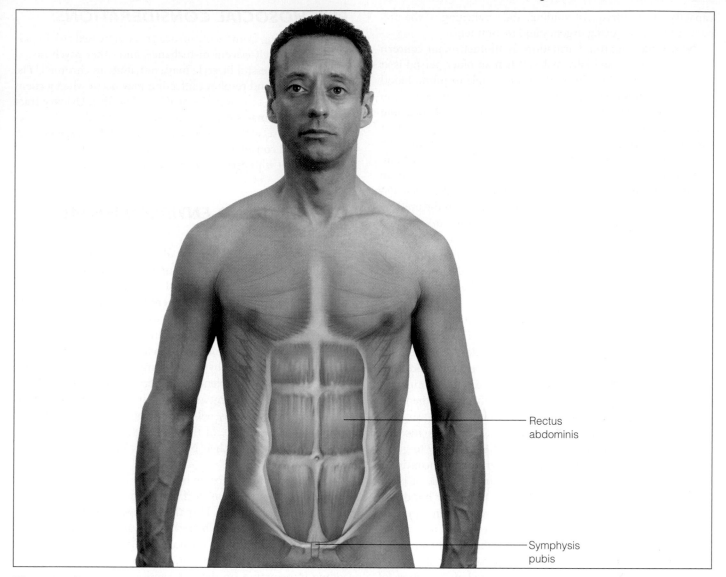

Rectus
abdominis

Symphysis
pubis

Figure 20.3B ● Landmarks for urinary assessment. B. The rectus abdominis muscles and the symphysis pubis.

The Older Adult

The effects of aging take their toll on the kidneys. The weight of the kidneys may drop by as much as 30%, particularly in the renal cortex. Renal blood flow and perfusion gradually decrease. The capillary system in the glomeruli atrophies. Although the vasculature in the renal medulla remains relatively well preserved, the arcuate and interlobular arteries may become distorted, resulting in a tortuous configuration. All structures of the renal cortex and the renal medulla experience some degree of decline, especially the nephrons. About 30 to 50% of the glomeruli degenerate because of fibrosis, hyalinization, and fat deposition. All of these factors contribute to the loss of filtration surface area in the glomerular capillary tufts by the age of 75. Creatinine clearance decreases slowly after 40 years of age, as does the ability to concentrate and dilute urine.

The older client's decreased sensation of thirst and resultant decreased intake of water relates directly to the body's compen-

satory response of concentrating urine. However, antidiuretic hormone is not as effective as in a younger client; thus, concentrations and activity of renin and aldosterone are reduced with advanced age by as much as 30 to 50%. This combination of circumstances places the older client at risk for hyperkalemia.

The older adult also has a reduced capacity to produce ammonia, which interacts with acids. Reduced ability to clear medications and acids, along with reduced ability to resorb bicarbonate and glucose, makes the older client more susceptible to toxicity related to medications, the effects of respiratory or metabolic acidosis, increased concentrations of glucose in the urine, and the loss of fluids.

Urinary elimination becomes a major concern as an individual advances in age and significant changes in urinary and bladder function begin to occur. Major changes in both males and females include urinary retention leading to increased urinary infections; involuntary bladder contractions resulting in urgency, frequency, and incontinence; decreased bladder capacity causing frequent voiding; and weakening of the urinary sphincters causing urgency and incontinence.

Nocturia (nighttime urination) is another major concern of older persons, especially males. When an older person is at rest in a horizontal position, the heart is able to pump blood through the kidneys more efficiently, facilitating the excretion of urine. This factor, combined with weakened bladder and urethral muscles, contributes to nocturnal micturition. Other causes of nocturia, such as urinary infection, hyperglycemia, medication use, and stool impactions, should not be ruled out.

Benign prostatic hypertrophy (hyperplasia) is a common cause of urinary retention and obstruction in males. As males age, the prostate gland enlarges, encroaching upon the urethra. Unrecognized urinary tract obstruction from an enlarged prostate results in damage to the upper urinary tract.

Postmenopausal females experience a decrease in estrogen that affects the strength of the pubic muscles and may lead to urine leakage, reduced acidity in the lower urinary tract, and UTI.

The nurse should allow older clients with urinary tract problems extra time to explain their concerns. Quite often, older adults have difficulty talking about bladder or bowel concerns because they consider the subject too personal. Additionally, some clients may find it distasteful to discuss elimination with anyone of the opposite sex. It is helpful to use the terms with which the client is comfortable and familiar.

When assessing an individual who experiences incontinence, the nurse should ask about the client's ability to get to the bathroom. Many clients who are diagnosed as incontinent simply cannot get to the bathroom on time because of other age-related conditions such as arthritis, strokes, or blindness. Whenever possible, the nurse should observe clients in their own settings to determine what disabilities or environmental barriers (e.g., stairs, distance) hinder the ability to function.

The physical assessment of the older person is similar to that of any other adult. Because the abdominal musculature of older persons tends to be more flaccid than that of younger adults, less pressure is used during deep palpation. The kidneys of the older client are more difficult to palpate abdominally because the mass of the adrenal cortex decreases with age. The nurse should omit blunt percussion in a frail older person. Palpation of the costovertebral angles and flanks can be used instead to reveal any pain or tenderness. A digital examination of the prostate gland is generally included as part of the urinary assessment in older males. Palpation of the urethra through the anterior vaginal wall is recommended for all older females.

PSYCHOSOCIAL CONSIDERATIONS

Clients suffering from incontinence are at increased risk for social isolation, self-esteem disturbance, and other psychosocial problems. A stressful lifestyle may contribute to chronic UTIs. Stasis of urine and resultant infection may occur when a client feels "too busy" to empty the bladder as needed. Urinary tract infections in females may also result from sexual trauma, sexual intercourse with a new partner, or coital frequency. The nurse should consider the possibility of sexual abuse in a child or adolescent who presents with a UTI.

CULTURAL AND ENVIRONMENTAL CONSIDERATIONS

When considering the influence of culture on a client's healthcare practices, the nurse must be open-minded and sensitive to the specific values and beliefs of the client without passing judgment. Not all individuals adhere to the norms, values, and practices of their culture. Consideration for the client's privacy and modesty is essential when obtaining subjective and objective data regarding urinary elimination. Though not every client is embarrassed by these components of assessment, many individuals experience considerable uneasiness. It is essential to afford the client as much privacy and dignity as possible. Some individuals will not disrobe or allow a physical examination by anyone of the opposite sex. Other clients will not allow a sample of their body fluids to be taken and examined by strangers.

Clients with hypertension or diabetes mellitus are especially vulnerable to kidney damage if they do not follow a strict medication and diet regimen. Hispanics and African Americans experience higher rates of hypertension and diabetes mellitus; however, these conditions are not limited to these populations. The nurse can help all clients maintain optimal health by providing information on diet, prevention of hypertension, and the importance of compliance with medication regimens.

Renal **calculi** (stones) occur with greater frequency in Caucasians than in African American or Asian American populations. Also, people who live in the southwestern United States or other areas where the mineral content of water is high are more susceptible to renal calculi.

Information obtained during the focused interview may identify whether the client is taking herbs prescribed by a healer. The nurse should obtain as complete information about the herb remedies as possible.

 Cultural Considerations

- African Americans have a higher incidence of hypertension, which is a risk factor for chronic renal disease.
- The incidence of diabetes is increasing with highest rates in Hispanic females. Diabetes is a risk factor for urinary tract infection and chronic renal disease.
- Hygiene practices differ across cultures. Hygiene can influence the development of urinary tract infections.
- The functions of the urinary system are considered private in many cultures.

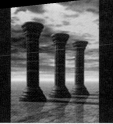

Assessment of the health of the urinary system includes gathering subjective and objective data. Subjective data collection occurs during the client interview, before the actual physical assessment. During the interview the nurse uses a variety of communication techniques to elicit general and specific information about the client's state of health or illness. Health records and the results of laboratory tests are important secondary sources to be reviewed and included in the data-gathering process. During physical assessment of the urinary system, the techniques of inspection, palpation, percussion, and auscultation will be used to collect objective data. Before proceeding, it may be helpful to review the information about each of the data-gathering processes and practice the techniques of health assessment.

FOCUSED INTERVIEW

The focused interview for the urinary system concerns data related to the structures and functions of that system. Subjective data is gathered during the focused interview. The nurse must be prepared to observe the client and listen for cues related to the functions of the urinary system. The nurse may use open-ended or closed questions to obtain information. Often a number of follow-up questions or requests for descriptions are required to clarify data or gather missing information. Follow-up questions are aimed at identifying the source of problems, duration of difficulties, measures to alleviate problems, and clues about the client's knowledge of his or her own health.

Discussion of urinary examination may be difficult for some clients because it is considered a private matter. The nurse should try to determine and use the terms used by the client in referring to parts of the body and urination.

The focused interview guides the physical assessment of the urinary system. The information is always considered in relation to norms and expectations about the function of the urinary system. Therefore, the nurse must consider age, gender, race, culture, environment, health practices, past and concurrent problems, and therapies when framing questions and using techniques to elicit information. In order to address all of the factors when conducting a focused interview, categories of questions have been developed. These categories include general questions that are asked of all clients; those addressing illness or infection; questions related to symptoms, pain, or behaviors; those related to habits or practices; questions that are specific to clients according to age; those for the pregnant female; and questions that address internal and external environmental concerns.

The nurse must consider the client's ability to participate in the focused interview and physical assessment of the urinary system. If a client is experiencing pain, urgency, incontinence, or the anxiety that accompanies any of these problems, attention must focus on relief of symptoms.

FOCUSED INTERVIEW QUESTIONS	RATIONALES

The following section provides sample questions and follow-up questions in each of the categories previously mentioned. A rationale for questions is provided. The list of questions is not all-inclusive but rather represents the types of questions required in a comprehensive focused interview related to the urinary system. The follow-up bulleted questions are asked to seek clarification with additional information from the client to enhance the subjective database. The subjective data collected and the questions asked during the health history and focused interview will provide data to help meet the goal of decreasing new cases of chronic kidney disease and promoting health as stated in Healthy People 2010.

GENERAL QUESTIONS

1. **What are your normal patterns when you urinate?**
   - How often do you urinate each day?
   - How much do you pass each time you urinate? (Note: The nurse may use terms familiar to the client such as "pass water" when asking about urination.)

   ▶ Many factors influence the number of times and amount that a client voids. Among these are size of the bladder, amount of fluid intake, type of fluid or solid intake, medications, amount of perspiration, and the client's temperature. The adult may void five or six times per day in amounts averaging 100 to 400 ml. Adults may urinate as much as 2 L of fluid. The child may void more frequently in smaller amounts. The key point is to determine the client's normal patterns.

FOCUSED INTERVIEW QUESTIONS	RATIONALES
2. Have you noticed any change from your normal urination patterns? • Have you noticed any changes in your pattern recently? • Have you had any of these changes: urinating more often, urinating less often, urinating more fluid, or urinating less fluid?	▶ Changes in urinary elimination patterns signal fluid retention, which may indicate heart failure, kidney failure, or improper nutritional intake. Other considerations include obstructions, infections, and endocrine alterations.
3. When you urinate, do you feel you are able to empty your bladder completely? • If not, describe your feeling.	▶ The feeling of being unable to empty the bladder may indicate the client is retaining urine or developing increased residual urine, which may contribute to the development of infection.
4. Are you always able to control when you are going to urinate? • If not, do you have to hurry to the bathroom as soon as you feel the urge to urinate? • When you feel the urge to urinate, are you able to get to the toilet? • Have you ever had an "accident" and wet yourself? • Have you ever urinated by accident when you have coughed, sneezed, or lifted a heavy object?	▶ Urgency and stress incontinence may be caused by an infection, an inflammatory process, or the loss of muscle control over urination, for example, after the vaginal delivery of a child or vaginal hysterectomy.
5. Do you ever have to get up at night to urinate? • If so, can you describe why? • Is there any predictable pattern? • How many times per night? • Describe your fluid intake for a day.	▶ Nocturia may indicate the presence of aging changes in the older adult, cardiovascular changes, diuretic therapy, or habit. Nocturia can be influenced by the amount and timing of fluid intake.
6. Do you have difficulty starting the flow of the stream? • Does the stream flow continuously, or does it start and stop? • Do you need to strain or push during urination to empty your bladder completely?	▶ Difficulties of this sort may signify the presence of prostate disease in the male.
7. If you have urinary problems, have they caused you embarrassment or anxiety? • Have your urinary problems affected your social, personal, or sexual relationships?	▶ These are important considerations, because they may affect clients' ability to function in other parts of their lives.
8. Has anyone in your family had a kidney disease or urinary problem? • If so, when did they have it? • How was it treated? • Do they still have it?	▶ A family history of kidney disease may signify a genetic predisposition to the development of renal disorders in some individuals.
9. Have you had a recent urine analysis or blood work evaluating your kidneys? • If so, do you know the results?	▶ It is valuable for clients to know the results of their lab work and to provide the healthcare professional with their impression of the results.

QUESTIONS RELATED TO ILLNESS OR INFECTION

1. Have you ever been diagnosed with a disease of the kidney or bladder? • When were you diagnosed with the problem? • What treatment was prescribed for the problem? • Was the treatment helpful? • What kinds of things do you do to help with the problem? • Has the problem ever recurred (acute)? • How are you managing the disease now (chronic)?	▶ The client has an opportunity to provide information about specific urinary illnesses. If a diagnosed illness is identified, follow-up about the date of diagnosis, treatment, and outcomes is required. Data about each illness identified by the client is essential to an accurate health assessment. Illnesses can be classified as acute or chronic, and follow-up regarding each classification will differ. ▶ An alternative to question 1 is to list possible illnesses of the urinary system, such as renal calculi, nephrosis, and renal failure, and ask the client to respond yes or no as each is stated. This is a comprehensive and easy way to elicit information about all diagnoses. Follow-up would be carried out for each identified diagnosis as in question 1.

FOCUSED INTERVIEW QUESTIONS	RATIONALES

2. Do you now have or have you had an infection in the urinary system?
- When were you diagnosed with the infection?
- What treatment was prescribed for the problem?
- Was the treatment helpful?
- What kinds of things do you do to help with the problem?
- Has the problem ever recurred (acute)?
- How are you managing the infection now (chronic)?

► If an infection is identified, follow-up about the date of infection, treatment, and outcomes is required. Data about each infection identified by the client is essential to an accurate health assessment. Infections can be classified as acute or chronic, and follow-up regarding each classification will differ.

3. An alternative to question 2 is to list possible urinary system infections, such as cystitis, pyelonephritis, and prostatitis, and ask the client to respond yes or no as each is stated.

► This is a comprehensive and easy way to elicit information about all urinary system infections. Follow-up would be carried out for each identified infection as in question 2.

4. Have you ever had surgery on the urinary system?
- If so, describe the procedure. How long ago did you have it done? Is the problem corrected?
- If not, describe it.
- Has anyone in your family ever had surgery on the urinary system?
- If so, please describe the procedures.
- How long ago was the surgery?
- Is the problem corrected?
- If not, describe it.

5. Do you have any of these problems: high blood pressure, diabetes, frequent bladder infections, kidney stones?
- If so, how has the problem been treated?
- Describe any associated symptoms.
- Do you still have problems with this condition?
- Do you have any idea what causes this problem?

► High blood pressure may contribute to the development of renal disease. Diabetes may significantly contribute to the development of renal disease. Infections may be caused by inadequate fluid intake, inadequate hygiene, and structural anomalies. In some clients this is an infrequent situation; in others it is a common malady. Kidney stones may be an isolated event or a recurring condition. Parathyroid disorders and any condition that causes an increase in calcium may contribute to the formation of kidney stones.

6. Do you have any of these neurologic diseases: multiple sclerosis, Parkinson's disease, spinal cord injury, stroke?
- If so, which one?
- When was it diagnosed? How are you being treated?

► These conditions contribute to the retention and stasis of urine, thus placing the client at risk for chronic urinary infections.

7. Do you have any cardiovascular disease?
- If so, what was the diagnosis?
- When was it diagnosed?
- How are you being treated?

► Hypertension in particular may significantly contribute to the development of renal failure.

8. Have you had influenza, a skin infection, a respiratory tract infection, or other infection recently?
- If so, what was it?
- What medication did the physician prescribe?
- Did you take all of the medication?
- Is this a recurrent problem?

► If the infection was untreated, the client may be at risk for developing a renal infection.

QUESTIONS RELATED TO SYMPTOMS OR BEHAVIORS

When gathering information about symptoms, many questions are required to elicit details and descriptions that assist in the analysis of the data. Discrimination is made in relation to the significance of a symptom, in relation to specific diseases or problems, and in relation to potential follow-up examination or referral. One rationale may be provided for a group of questions in this category.

FOCUSED INTERVIEW QUESTIONS	RATIONALES

The following questions refer to specific symptoms and behaviors associated with the urinary system. For each symptom, questions and follow-up are required. The details to be elicited are the characteristics of the symptom; the onset, duration, and frequency of the symptom; the treatment or remedy for the symptom, including over-the-counter (OTC) and home remedies; the determination if diagnosis has been sought; the effect of treatments; and family history associated with a symptom or illness.

1. **Have you noticed any changes in the quality of the urine?**
   - If so, describe the change.
   - Has your urine been cloudy?
   - Does it have an odor?
   - Has the color changed?
   - If there has been a color change, what is it?
   - Is the color change happening each time you urinate?
   - Is there a pattern?
   - Can you predict the color change?

   ▶ Color changes offer clues to the presence of infection, kidney stones, or neoplasm. The quantity of urine may indicate the presence of renal failure or may reflect hydration status.

2. **If the urine is bloody (hematuria), the nurse should ask these questions:**
   - Have you fallen recently?
   - Do you experience burning when the blood is present? Have you seen clots in the urine?
   - Have you noticed any stones or other material in the urine?
   - Have you noticed any granular material on the toilet paper after you wipe?

   ▶ The client may offer valuable information about the source and characteristics of bleeding, because this symptom is present in a wide variety of conditions. Hematuria is a serious finding and warrants additional follow-up.

3. **Is your urine foamy and amber in color?**

   ▶ This finding may indicate the presence of hepatic illness.

4. **Have you had any weight gain recently?**
   - If so, describe it.
   - Are you retaining fluid?
   - Are your rings, clothing, or shoes becoming tighter?
   - Has this change been gradual or did it come on suddenly?

   ▶ This may alert the nurse to the presence of hypertension, associated heart failure, or endocrine problems. These ultimately affect the renal circulation and function of the kidneys.

5. **Have you noticed any discharge from the urethra?**
   - If so, describe the color, odor, amount, and frequency.
   - When did it start?
   - Is this a recurrent problem? If so, what was the diagnosis?
   - How was it treated?
   - Did you follow the treatment as prescribed by the physician?

   ▶ Discharge signals the potential presence of an infective process.

6. **Have you noticed any redness or other discoloration in the urethral area or penis? If so, describe the characteristics.**

   ▶ Redness may indicate the presence of inflammation, irritation, or infection.

7. **For male clients:** Do you have prostate problems?
   - If so, describe the symptoms and treatment.
   - When was your last prostate exam?

   ▶ Enlargement of the prostate gland contributes to problems in urination, including frequency, difficulty starting a stream, or incomplete emptying of the bladder.

8. **Has your skin changed recently?**
   - Describe the change.
   - Has the color changed?
   - Is it itchy all the time?

   ▶ Clients with chronic renal failure have itchy skin (pruritus), and a uremic frost may develop on the skin as an adaptive response to renal failure.

9. **Have you recently had nausea, vomiting, diarrhea, or chills?**
   - If so, which one? Describe it.
   - How was it treated?
   - Has it recurred?

   ▶ These conditions may indicate the presence of infection or recurring infection.

10. **Have you had any shortness of breath or difficulty breathing lately? If so, describe it.**

    ▶ This may alert the nurse to the presence of hypertension and associated heart failure. These ultimately affect the renal circulation and function of the kidneys.

11. **Do you have difficulty concentrating, reading, or remembering things?**

    ▶ Difficulty remembering may be associated with renal dysfunction. There are many conditions that contribute to memory disturbances.

FOCUSED INTERVIEW QUESTIONS	**RATIONALES**

QUESTIONS RELATED TO PAIN

When assessing pain the nurse needs to gather information about the characteristics of the pain, which include quality, severity, location, duration, predictability, onset, relief, and radiation.

1. **Do you ever have pain, burning, or other discomfort before, during, or after urination?**
   - If so, describe the discomfort, location, and timing.
   - Do you have symptoms all of the time or some of the time?
   - Is the discomfort predictable? For instance, is it related to time of the day, or certain foods or beverages?
   - Do you feel it after sexual intercourse?

▶ Painful urination may indicate the presence of an infective process.

2. **Do you have any pain or discomfort in your back, sides, or abdomen?**
   - If so, show me where the pain or discomfort is located.
   - Describe the pain.
   - What aggravates or alleviates the symptoms?

▶ Back or abdominal pain often accompanies renal disease.

3. **Have you noticed any pain or discomfort when your urine is bloody?**
   - If so, describe the type, location, and timing of the discomfort.

▶ Hematuria without pain is often associated with cancer.

QUESTIONS RELATED TO BEHAVIORS

1. **Describe your diet.**
   - Describe what you have eaten and drunk over the last week.
   - How is your appetite?
   - On a typical day, how much do you eat and drink?
   - Do you drink alcoholic beverages?
   - How many glasses of water do you drink a day?
   - Are there any foods or beverages that bother you?
   - Do any foods or beverages cause you discomfort either before or upon urination?
   - Do any foods or beverages cause you to feel bloated or gassy?
   - Do any foods or beverages affect the color, clarity, or smell of your urine?
   - How much salt do you use?
   - Do you retain fluid after consuming certain foods or beverages?

▶ Questions such as these may provide information regarding the client's hydration status, potential allergic reaction to foods, and retention of fluid.

2. **Do you smoke or are you exposed to passive smoke?**
   - If so, what type of smoking (cigarette, cigar, pipe)?
   - For how long?
   - How many packs per day?

▶ Smoking has been linked to hypertension, which over time may contribute to the development of renal failure.

3. **Do you use any recreational drugs?**
   - If so, describe the type, amount, and frequency.
   - How long have you been using these drugs?

▶ Substance abuse over time may lead to kidney failure, potential for inadequate nutrition and hydration, and susceptibility to infection.

4. **How often do you have intercourse?**
   - Do you urinate after intercourse?
   - Are you aware of any sexual partners who may have sexually transmitted diseases?

▶ Some clients may have a tendency to develop UTIs if they do not urinate after intercourse.

5. ***For female clients:* How do you cleanse yourself after urination or bowel movement?**
   - Do you use bubble bath?
   - Do you use sprays, powders, or feminine hygiene products?

▶ Cleansing materials such as bubble bath, sprays, and powders may increase the incidence of UTIs. Improper cleansing methods after elimination may also lead to infection.

FOCUSED INTERVIEW QUESTIONS	RATIONALES

QUESTIONS RELATED TO AGE

The focused interview must reflect the anatomical and physiological differences that exist along the age span. The following questions are examples of those that would be specific for infants and children, the pregnant female, and the older adult.

QUESTIONS REGARDING INFANTS AND CHILDREN

1. **Have you ever been told that the child has a kidney that has failed to grow?**

   ▶ Renal agenesis may involve one or both kidneys. A genetic factor may be associated with the development of this condition in some cases. Bilateral renal agenesis is invariably fatal. Unilateral renal agenesis may be asymptomatic and is often incidentally diagnosed by abdominal ultrasound or computed tomography (CT) scan secondary to another condition. In infants with unilateral renal agenesis, the remaining kidney may be enlarged, and there is increased risk of problems with the remaining kidney (Bianchi, Crombleholme, & D'Alton, 2000).

2. **Has the child ever been diagnosed with a kidney disorder?**
   - If so, what is it called, what were the symptoms, and how was it treated?
   - Is it still being treated?

   ▶ Some disorders, such as infections, are easily treated and do not recur; others, such as glomerulonephritis, may be chronic.

3. **Has the child had hearing problems?**

   ▶ The ears and kidneys develop at the same time in utero. Congenital deafness is associated with renal disease.

4. **Have you ever observed any unusual shape or structure in the child's genital anatomy?**

   ▶ Parents may report abnormally shaped external genitals, as seen in hypospadias and epispadias. In children with exstrophy of the bladder, the lower urinary tract is visible.

5. **Has the child ever had problems with involuntary urination?**
   - If so, what are the characteristics?
   - What was the diagnosis?
   - How was it treated?
   - Is it still occurring?

   ▶ **Enuresis** is the medical term for involuntary urination after age 4. If it occurs at night, it is termed nocturnal enuresis after age 6. This condition may have extensive impact on the social, mental, and physical well-being of the family and child.

6. **Have you started toilet training with the child?**
   - If yes, how successful has it been?
   - Are there any current problems with toilet training?
   - What method are you using for toilet training?

   ▶ These questions elicit information about maturity of the neurologic and urinary systems.

7. **Has the child decreased play activity?**

   ▶ Loss of interest in play may signal fatigue, which may be associated with renal failure.

8. **Are you changing the baby's diaper more or less than you were?**

   ▶ There are a variety of contributors to changes in elimination patterns, but renal failure, dehydration, overhydration, diet changes, obstruction, and stress may contribute to a change in normal pattern.

THE PREGNANT FEMALE

1. **Have you noticed any changes in your urinary pattern?**

   ▶ Often, the developing fetus places increasing pressure on the mother's bladder, causing urinary urgency. As a result, the client voids more often, in smaller amounts.

2. **Have you noticed unusual swelling in your ankles, feet, fingers, or wrists?**
   - Have you noticed any headaches?

   ▶ These signs may be associated with pregnancy-induced hypertension and preeclampsia.

FOCUSED INTERVIEW QUESTIONS	RATIONALES

QUESTIONS FOR THE OLDER ADULT

1. **Have you noticed any unusual swelling in your ankles, feet, fingers, or wrists?**

▶ Swelling may be indicative of congestive heart failure. Associated with the swelling can be weight gain, fatigue, activity intolerance, and shortness of breath.

2. *For male clients:* **Have you noticed difficulty initiating the stream of urine, voiding in small amounts, and feeling the need to void more frequently than in the past?**

▶ These symptoms may be due to an enlarged prostate.

QUESTIONS RELATED TO THE ENVIRONMENT

Environment refers to both the internal and external environments. Questions related to the internal environment include all of the previous questions and those associated with internal or physiological responses. Questions regarding the external environment include those related to home, work, or social environments.

INTERNAL ENVIRONMENT

1. **What medications do you currently take?**
   - What medications have you been taking in the last several months?
   - Describe the type, the dose, and the reason why you are taking the medication.
   - How often do you take it?
   - Every day, as needed, or only when you remember?

▶ It is important to know the client's compliance with the medication regimen. If the client has not completed a regimen of antibiotic therapy to clear a urinary tract infection, kidney infection, or sexually transmitted disease, the infection may persist.

2. **Do you take any vitamins, protein powders, or dietary supplements?**
   - If so, which ones?
   - How much do you take?
   - How many days a week do you take it?
   - How many times a day?
   - Why do you take it?

▶ Excessive ingestion may contribute to the development of renal disorders.

EXTERNAL ENVIRONMENT

The following questions deal with substances and irritants found in the physical environment of the client. The physical environment includes the indoor and outdoor environments of the home and workplace, those encountered for social engagements, and any encountered during travel.

1. **Do you live in an environment or work in an industry that exposes you to toxic chemicals?**

▶ These may contribute to the development of cancer of the urinary system.

2. **Have you traveled recently to a foreign country or any unfamiliar place?**

▶ The client may have been exposed to bacterial, viral, or fungal agents that affect renal function.

CLIENT INTERACTION

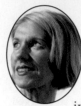

Ms. Angela Carbone, age 55, comes to the Medi-Center at 10:30 A.M. with the chief complaint of left back pain. She has some nausea and no vomiting. She complains of dysuria and gross hematuria and indicates she had a kidney stone on the right side several years ago. The following is an excerpt from the focused interview with Ms. Carbone.

INTERVIEW

Nurse: Good morning. Ms. Carbone. Are you having pain now?

Ms. Carbone: Yes I am.

Nurse: On a scale of 1 to 10 with 10 being the highest, how do you rate your pain?

Ms. Carbone: Now it is about 4 but I'm afraid it will become 10 or 12 like the last time.

Nurse: I need to ask you some questions to get information from you. Will you be able to talk to me for a few minutes?

Ms. Carbone: I think so! I'll try. I'll let you know if I can't sit any more.

Nurse: Tell me about the pain.

Ms. Carbone: I have back pain on my left side, right here (pointing to the left costovertebral area). It feels like it moves down my back but not all the time. It really hurts and is getting worse each day.

Nurse: When did the pain start?

Ms. Carbone: It started about 5 days ago. That's when I noticed my urine was darker than usual.

Nurse: Did you do anything to help reduce the pain?

Ms. Carbone: Not really. At first I thought I slept funny. Then my urine got darker. I tried to drink three glasses of water a day, but I became nauseated and had to stop drinking.

Nurse: Earlier you commented that you are afraid the pain will become 10 or 12 like the last time. Tell me more.

Ms. Carbone: I had a kidney stone about 3 years ago on my right side. Now the pain is similar on the left side.

ANALYSIS

The nurse immediately asked Ms. Carbone about her current pain status to determine her ability to participate in the interview. Throughout the interview, the nurse used open-ended and leading statements. These statements encouraged verbalization by the client to explore and describe actions and feelings in detail. The open and leading statements permitted the client to provide detail, thereby eliminating the need for multiple closed questions.

Please refer to the Companion Website at **www.prenhall.com/damico** and click on Chapter 20, the **Client Interaction** module, to answer questions about this case. In addition, see other resources for this chapter including NCLEX review questions and other interactive exercises and materials.

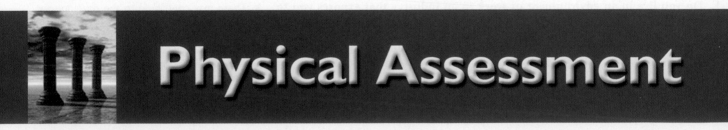

Physical Assessment

ASSESSMENT TECHNIQUES AND FINDINGS

Physical assessment of the urinary system includes the use of inspection, palpation, percussion, and auscultation. The skills are used to gather information about the function of the urinary system. Knowledge of normal parameters and expected findings is essential in determining the meaning of the data as the nurse performs the physical assessment.

Adult skin is moist and supple with pink undertones. The abdomen is symmetrical and free of lesions, bruises, and swelling. The renal arteries are without bruits. The costovertebral angle and flanks are symmetrical, even in color, and nontender to palpation and percussion. The kidneys are not enlarged; they are rounded, smooth, firm, and nontender. The bladder is nonpalpable, and percussion reveals tympany above the symphysis pubis.

Physical assessment of the urinary system follows an organized pattern. It begins with a survey of the client's general appearance followed by inspection of the abdomen. The renal arteries are auscultated and then the costovertebral angles and flank areas are inspected, palpated, and percussed. The kidneys are palpated. Bladder size is determined by palpation and percussion of the lower abdomen.

EQUIPMENT

examination gown and drape	stethoscope
clean, nonsterile examination gloves	specimen container

TECHNIQUES AND NORMAL FINDINGS	**ABNORMAL FINDINGS SPECIAL CONSIDERATIONS**

GENERAL SURVEY

A quick survey of the client enables the nurse to identify any immediate problem as well as the client's ability to participate in the assessment.

1. **Instruct the client.**
   - Explain that you will be looking, listening, touching, and tapping on parts of the abdomen. Tell the client you will explain each procedure as it occurs. Tell the client to report any discomfort and that you will stop the examination if the procedure is uncomfortable.

2. **Position the client.**
   - Begin the examination with the client in a supine position with the abdomen exposed from the nipple line to the pubis (see Figure 20.4 ●).

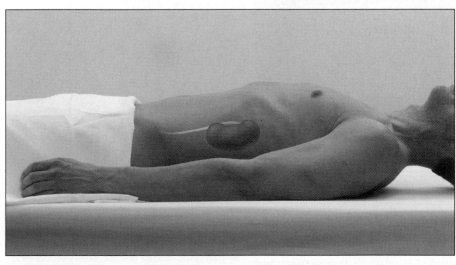

Figure 20.4 ● Position the client.

3. **Assess the general appearance.**
   - Assess general appearance and inspect the client's skin for color, hydration status, scales, masses, indentations, or scars.

TECHNIQUES AND NORMAL FINDINGS

ABNORMAL FINDINGS
SPECIAL CONSIDERATIONS

- The client should not show signs of acute distress and should be mentally alert and oriented.

► Clients with kidney disorders frequently look tired and complain of fatigue. If a kidney disorder is suspected, it is important to look for signs of circulatory overload (pulmonary edema) or peripheral edema (puffy face or fingers), or indications of pruritus (scratch marks on the skin).

► Elevated nitrogenous wastes (azotemia) in the blood contribute to mental confusion.

4. **Inspect the abdomen for color, contour, symmetry, and distention.**

- It may be helpful to stand at the foot of the exam table and inspect the abdomen from there (see Figure 20.5 ●).

► A distended bladder may be visible in the suprapubic area, indicating the need to void and perhaps the inability to do so.

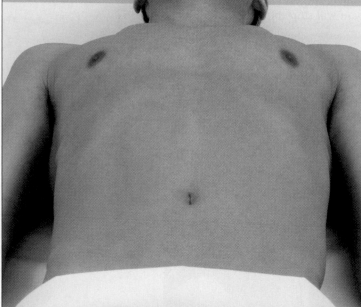

Figure 20.5 ●
Inspecting the abdomen from the foot of the bed.

- Note that visual inspection of the suprapubic area may confirm the presence or absence of a distended bladder.

- Normally, the client's abdomen is not distended, is relatively symmetrical, and is free of bruises, masses, and swellings. (A complete discussion of abdominal assessment is provided in Chapter 19. ⬭)

► Many diseases may contribute to abdominal distention. These include renal conditions such as polycystic kidney disease; enlarged kidneys, as seen in acute pyelonephritis; ascites (accumulation of fluid) due to hepatic disease; and displacement of abdominal organs. Pressure from the abdominal contents on the diaphragm may alter the client's breathing pattern.

5. **Auscultate the right and left renal arteries to assess circulatory sounds.**

- Gently place the bell of the stethoscope over the extended midclavicular line (MCL) on either side of the abdominal aorta, which is located above the level of the umbilicus (see Figure 20.6 ●).

TECHNIQUES AND NORMAL FINDINGS	ABNORMAL FINDINGS SPECIAL CONSIDERATIONS

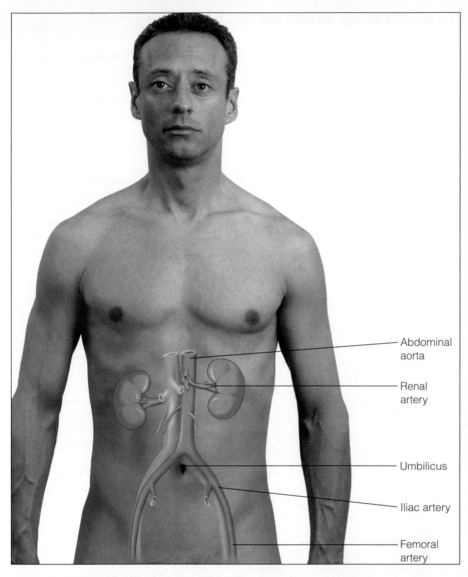

Figure 20.6 ● Auscultating the renal arteries.

- Be sure to auscultate both the right and left sides, and over the epigastric and umbilical areas.

- In most cases, no sounds are heard; however, an upper abdominal bruit is occasionally heard in young adults and is considered normal. On a thin adult, renal artery pulsation may be auscultated.

THE KIDNEYS AND FLANKS

1. **Position the client.**
   - Place the client in a sitting position facing away from you with the client's back exposed.

2. **Inspect the left and right costovertebral angles for color and symmetry.**
   - The color should be consistent with the rest of the back.

▶ A protrusion or elevation over a costovertebral angle occurs when the kidney is grossly enlarged or when a mass is present.

TECHNIQUES AND NORMAL FINDINGS

ABNORMAL FINDINGS SPECIAL CONSIDERATIONS

3. **Inspect the flanks (the side areas between the hips and the ribs) for color and symmetry.**

   • The costovertebral angles and flanks should be symmetrical and even in color.

ALERT!

Do not percuss or palpate the client who reports pain or discomfort in the pelvic region. Do not percuss or palpate the kidney if a tumor of the kidney is suspected, such as a neuroblastoma or Wilms' tumor. Palpation increases intra-abdominal pressure, which may contribute to intraperitoneal spreading of this neuroblastoma. Deep palpation should be performed only by experienced practitioners.

---

4. **Gently palpate the area over the left costovertebral angle (see Figure 20.7 ●).**

   • Watch the reaction and ask the client to describe any sensation the palpation causes. Normally, the client expresses no discomfort.

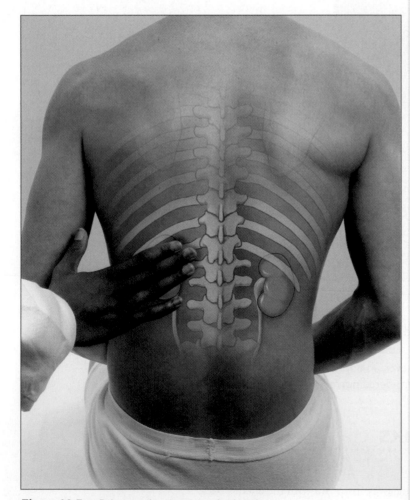

Figure 20.7 ● Palpating the costovertebral angle.

▶ This finding must be carefully correlated to other diagnostic cues as the assessment proceeds. If ecchymosis is present (Grey Turner's sign), there may be other signs of trauma such as blunt, penetrating wounds or lacerations.

▶ Pain, discomfort, or tenderness from an enlarged or diseased kidney may occur over the costovertebral angle, flank, and abdomen. When questioned, the client complains of a dull, steady ache. This type of pain is associated with polycystic formation, pyelonephritis, and other disorders that cause kidney enlargement. In the client with polycystic kidney disease, a sharp, sudden, intermittent pain may mean that a cyst in the kidney has ruptured. If the costovertebral angle is tender, red, and warm, and the client is experiencing chills, fever, nausea, and vomiting, the underlying kidney could be inflamed or infected.

▶ The pain caused by calculi (stones) in the kidney or upper ureter is unique and different in character, severity, and duration than that caused by kidney enlargement. This pain occurs as calculi travel from the kidney to the ureters and the urinary bladder.

▶ Some clients experience no pain, and others feel excruciating pain. A stationary stone causes a dull, aching pain. As stones travel down the urinary tract, spasms occur. These spasms produce sharp, intermittent, colicky pain (often accompanied by chills, fever, nausea, and vomiting) that radiates from the flanks to the lower quadrants of the abdomen, and in some cases, the upper thigh and scrotum or labium.

▶ If the client reports severe pain, **hematuria** (blood in the urine) or **oliguria** (diminished volume of urine), and nausea and vomiting, it is important to be alert for hydroureter, a frequent complication that occurs when a renal calculus moves into the ureter. The calculus blocks and dilates the ureter, causing spasms and severe pain. Hydroureter can lead to shock, infection, and impaired renal function. If the nurse suspects hydroureter or obstruction at any point in the urinary tract, medical collaboration must be sought immediately.

TECHNIQUES AND NORMAL FINDINGS	**ABNORMAL FINDINGS SPECIAL CONSIDERATIONS**

5. Use blunt or indirect percussion to further assess the kidneys.

- Place your left palm flat over the left costovertebral angle.
- Thump the back of your left hand with the ulnar surface of your right fist, causing a gentle thud over the costovertebral angle (see Figure 20.8 ●).

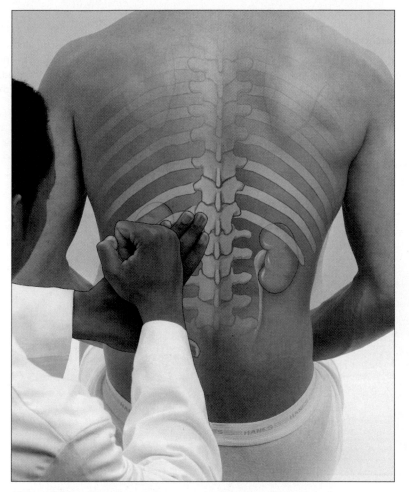

Figure 20.8 ● Blunt percussion over the left costovertebral angle.

- Repeat the procedure on the right side. Ask the client to describe the sensation as you examine each side.
- The client should feel no pain or tenderness with pressure or percussion.

► Pain or discomfort during and after blunt percussion suggests kidney disease. This finding is correlated with other assessment findings.

THE LEFT KIDNEY

1. Attempt to palpate the lower pole of the left kidney.

- Although it is not usually palpable, attempt to palpate the lower pole of the kidney for size, contour, consistency, and sensation. Note that the rib cage obscures the upper poles.

► When enlargement occurs in the presence of conditions such as neoplasms and polycystic disease, the kidneys may be palpable. Otherwise, they are rarely palpable.

TECHNIQUES AND NORMAL FINDINGS

ALERT!

Because deep kidney palpation can cause tissue trauma, novice nurses should not attempt either deep palpation or capture of the kidney unless supervised by an experienced nurse or nurse practitioner. Deep kidney palpation should not be done in clients who have had a recent kidney transplant or an abdominal aortic aneurysm.

- Position the client in a supine position. All palpation should be performed from the client's right side.

- While standing on the client's right side, reach over the client and place your left hand between the posterior rib cage and the iliac crest (the left flank).

- Place your right hand on the left upper quadrant of the abdomen lateral and parallel to the left rectus muscle just below the costal margin.

- Instruct the client to take a deep breath. As the client inhales, lift the client's left flank with your left hand and press deeply with your right hand (approximately 4 cm) to attempt to palpate the lower pole of the kidney (see Figure 20.9 ●).

▶ Care must be taken not to mistake an enlarged spleen for an enlarged left kidney. An enlarged kidney feels smooth and rounded, whereas an enlarged spleen feels sharper, with a more delineated edge.

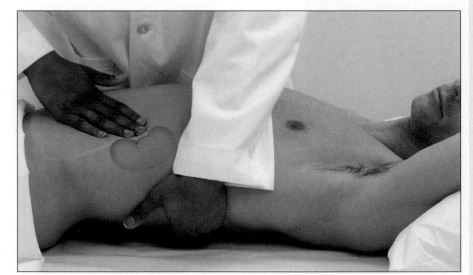

Figure 20.9 ● Palpating the left kidney.

2. **Attempt to capture the left kidney.**

- Because of its position deep in the retroperitoneal space, the left kidney is not normally palpable. The capture maneuver may enable you to palpate it. This maneuver is possible because the kidneys descend during inspiration and slide back into their normal position during exhalation.

- Standing on the client's right side, place your left hand under the client's back to elevate the flank as before. Place your right hand on the left upper quadrant of the abdomen lateral and parallel to the left rectus muscle with the fingertips just below the left costal margin. Instruct the client to take a deep breath and hold it. As the client inhales, attempt to capture the kidney between your two hands. Ask the client to exhale slowly and then to briefly hold the breath. At the same time, slowly release the pressure of your fingers.

- As the client exhales, you will feel the captured kidney move back into its previous position. The kidney surface should be rounded, smooth, firm, and nontender.

▶ An enlarged palpable kidney could be painful for the client. This suggests tumor, cyst, or hydronephrosis.

| **TECHNIQUES AND NORMAL FINDINGS** | **ABNORMAL FINDINGS SPECIAL CONSIDERATIONS** |

THE RIGHT KIDNEY

1. **Attempt to palpate the lower pole of the right kidney.**
   - Standing on the client's right side, place your left hand under the back parallel to the right twelfth rib (about halfway between the costal margin and iliac crest) with your fingertips reaching for the costovertebral angle. Place your right hand on the right upper quadrant of the abdomen lateral to the right rectus muscle and just below the right costal margin.
   - Instruct the client to take a deep breath. As the client inhales, lift the flank with your left hand and use deep palpation to feel for the lower pole of the kidney.

2. **Attempt to capture the right kidney.**
   - Place your left hand under the client's right flank.
   - Place your right hand on the right upper quadrant of the abdomen with the fingertips lateral and parallel to the right rectus muscle just below the right costal margin.
   - Instruct the client to take a deep breath and hold it. As the client inhales, attempt to capture the kidney between your two hands.
   - Ask the client to exhale slowly and then to briefly hold the breath. At the same time, slowly release the pressure of your fingers.
   - As the client exhales you will feel the captured kidney move back into its previous position. The kidney surface should be rounded, smooth, firm, and nontender.
   - The lower pole of the right kidney is palpable in some individuals, especially in thin, relaxed females. If palpable, the lower pole of the kidney has a smooth, firm, uninterrupted surface.
   - During the capture maneuver, some clients describe a nonpainful sensation as the kidney slides between the nurse's fingers back into its normal position.

▶ It is important not to mistake an enlarged liver for an enlarged right kidney. An enlarged kidney feels smooth and rounded, whereas an enlarged liver is closer to the midline and has a more distinct border. Polycystic kidney disease or carcinoma should be suspected when there is gross enlargement of the kidney. The kidneys may be two or three times their normal size in clients with polycystic disease.

THE URINARY BLADDER

1. **Palpate the bladder to determine symmetry, location, size, and sensation.**
   - Use light palpation over the lower portion of the abdomen. The abdomen should be soft.
   - Use deep palpation to locate the fundus (base) of the bladder, approximately 5 to 7 cm (2 to 2.5 in.) below the umbilicus in the lower abdomen. Once you have located the fundus of the bladder, continue to palpate, outlining the shape and contour (see Figure 20.10 ●).

▶ A distended bladder feels smooth, round, and taut. An asymmetrical contour or nodular surface suggests abnormal growth that should be correlated with other findings. In males with urethral obstruction due to hypertrophy or hyperplasia of the prostate, the bladder is enlarged.

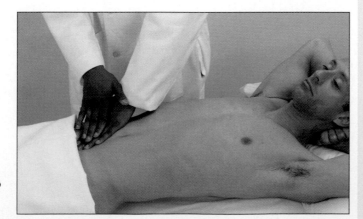

Figure 20.10 ●
Palpating the bladder.

TECHNIQUES AND NORMAL FINDINGS	ABNORMAL FINDINGS SPECIAL CONSIDERATIONS

- Slide your fingers over the surface of the bladder and continue palpating to determine smoothness and continuity.
- The surface of the bladder should feel smooth and uninterrupted. An empty bladder is usually not palpable. When the bladder is moderately full, it should be firm, smooth, symmetrical, and nontender. As the bladder fills, the fundus can reach the level of the umbilicus. A full bladder is firm and buoyant.

2. **Percuss the bladder to determine its location and degree of fullness.**

ALERT!

If the bladder is distended with urine and the client is unable to void, obtain an order to catheterize the client. Reduce the contents of a distended bladder slowly to prevent atony of the bladder wall.

- Begin with direct percussion of the bladder over the suprapubic area.
- Move your fingers upward toward the umbilicus as you continue to percuss. A full bladder produces a dull tone upon percussion. Continue percussing upward toward the umbilicus until no more dull tones are heard. The point at which dull tones cease is the upper margin of the bladder.
- Some practitioners conclude the assessment of the urinary system with the inspection and palpation of the penis and urethral meatus in the male client or the inspection of the urethral meatus in the female client. Other practitioners consider these structures with the assessment of the genitalia. These techniques are discussed in Chapters 21 and 22. ⬭

 Refer to the Companion Website at **www.prenhall.com/damico** and click on the **Documentation** module for documentation samples and documentation practice exercises.

Common alterations of the urinary system include bladder cancer, kidney and urinary tract infections, calculi, tumors, renal failure, and changes in urinary elimination. Each of these alterations will be discussed in the following sections.

Bladder Cancer

Seen later in life, bladder cancer occurs more frequently in males than in females. Smoking has been linked to this disease. The client may be totally asymptomatic or have hematuria, flank pain, and frequent urination.

Glomerulonephritis

This entity is an inflammation of the glomerulus. The key clinical manifestations are hematuria with red blood cell casts and proteinuria.

Renal Calculi

Calculi are stones that block the urinary tract. They are usually composed of calcium, struvite, or a combination of magnesium, ammonium, phosphate, and uric acid. Pain is the primary symptom. The pain may radiate and is variable in location and severity. Other symptoms include spasms, nausea, vomiting, pain on urination, frequency and urgency of urination, and gross hematuria.

Renal Tumor

Renal tumors may be either benign or malignant, with malignant being more common. Research has shown that there is an association with renal tumors and smoking. The key manifestations of renal tumors are hematuria, flank pain, weight loss, and palpable mass in the flank.

Renal Failure

Renal failure may be acute or it may progress to a chronic state. Acute renal failure that does not progress to a chronic state includes three stages: oliguria, diuresis, and recovery. Other symptoms include fluid retention, hyperkalemia, hyperphosphatemia, nausea, and vomiting. Uremia is the classic hallmark of chronic renal failure. Anorexia, nausea, vomiting, mentation changes, uremic frost, pruritus, weight loss, fatigue, and edema are common symptoms of uremia.

Urinary Tract Infection

Bacteria cause urinary tract infections. The bladder is the most common site of the infection, which results in inflammation of the bladder called cystitis; however, infection may include the kidneys. Clients may be asymptomatic, but the classic symptoms include urgency, frequency, dribbling, pain upon urination, and suprapubic or lower back pain. Hematuria, as well as cloudy and foul-smelling urine, may accompany the other signs.

Changes in Urinary Elimination

The following are examples of alterations in urinary elimination:

Dysreflexia affects clients with spinal cord injuries at level T_7 or higher. Bladder distention causes a sympathetic response that can trigger a potentially life-threatening hypertensive crisis.

Incontinence is the inability to retain urine. If this is the client's problem, the nurse must determine which of the five types of incontinence is present.

- *Functional incontinence* occurs when the client is unable to reach the toilet in time because of environmental, psychosocial, or physical factors.
- *Reflex incontinence* occurs in clients with spinal cord damage when urine is involuntarily lost.
- *Stress incontinence,* involuntary urination, occurs when intra-abdominal pressure is increased during coughing, sneezing, or straining. Aging changes may also contribute to stress incontinence.
- *Urge incontinence* may be caused by consuming a significant volume of fluids over a relatively short period of time. Urge incontinence may also be due to diminished bladder capacity.
- *Total incontinence* is related to a neurologic condition.

Urinary retention is a chronic state in which the client cannot empty the bladder. In most cases, the client voids small amounts of overflow urine when the bladder reaches its greatest capacity.

Health Promotion

HEALTHY PEOPLE 2010

FOCUS AREA	PREVALENCE	OBJECTIVES	ACTIONS
Chronic and End-Stage Renal Disease (ESRD)	• Almost 10 to 12 million people over the age of 12 have chronic renal disease. • End-stage renal disease results from chronic damage to the kidneys for over a decade or more. • Diabetes and hypertension increase the risk for ESRD. • The number of new cases of ESRD is increasing and correlates to an increase in cases of type 2 diabetes. • African Americans are at the highest risk for renal disease. • American Indians, Native Alaskans, Asians, and Pacific Islanders have higher rates of renal disease than whites. • Mexicans have a high risk for renal disease related to higher incidence of type 2 diabetes.	• Decrease the rate of new cases of ESRD. • Increase the number of dialysis patients on waiting lists for transplant. • Decrease kidney failure due to diabetes.	• Early identification of people at risk. • Control of diabetes and hypertension. • Education related to diet and exercise.
Diabetes	• The incidence of diabetes, especially type 2, is increasing. • Diabetes is the seventh leading cause of death in the United States. • Diabetes occurs most often after 60 years of age. • Hispanics, African Americans, and Asians are at greater risk for development of diabetes than whites. • Rising obesity and physical inactivity are expected to contribute to increasing incidence of diabetes. • Diabetes increases the risk for development of acute and chronic diseases of the urinary system.	• Prevent diabetes. • Increase the number of diabetics who receive formal education. • Increase the number of diabetics with annual testing for urinary microalbumin. • Reduce death rates associated with diabetes.	• Education related to diet and exercise. • Establishment of programs to promote physical activity. • Obesity prevention and treatment. • Diabetic education including risks, diagnosis, treatment, and long-term management. • Education regarding the significance of symptoms, especially urinary.

CLIENT EDUCATION

The following are physiological, behavioral, and cultural factors that affect the health of the urinary system across the age span. Several factors reflect trends cited in *Healthy People 2010*. The nurse provides advice and education to reduce risks associated with these factors and to promote and maintain urinary health.

LIFE SPAN CONSIDERATIONS

RISK FACTORS

- Tissues of the urinary system in infants are stretchy. As a result of this and other conditions, hydronephrosis and reflux diseases may develop.

- Bed-wetting (enuresis) is common in children, especially males.

- Prostate enlargement occurs in aging and can lead to problems with urinary elimination.

CLIENT EDUCATION

- Tell parents that hydronephrosis can be diagnosed antenatally by ultrasound. Parents then need support and counseling about treatment. Further UTI in infants is usually the first sign of reflux disorders. Parents need guidance regarding healthcare of infants when symptoms arise. Reflux disorders generally resolve without treatment. Parents need support and guidance regarding prevention of further infection, and long-term care recommendations when problems do not resolve or result in chronic renal disorders.

- Inform parents that most bed-wetting ceases by the age of 4 or 5. Parents should be encouraged to seek healthcare if the problem persists at ages 6 and 7. Limiting fluid intake before bedtime or waking the child to void are some methods to address the problem.

- Encourage males over 40 years of age to have regular prostate examinations.

CULTURAL CONSIDERATIONS

RISK FACTOR

- Hypertension is a risk factor for chronic kidney disease. African Americans have increased incidence of hypertension.

CLIENT EDUCATION

- Advise clients to discuss all medications—including OTC, herbal, and folk medications—with their healthcare provider.

ENVIRONMENTAL CONSIDERATIONS

RISK FACTORS

- UTIs can occur at any age. Females are more susceptible because of the short urethra.

- Renal calculi occur more frequently in individuals with a family history of calculi. Calculi can develop following UTI, in clients with parathyroid disorders and hypercalcemia.

- Clients with diabetes are at increased risk for problems in the urinary system.

CLIENT EDUCATION

- Inform clients that UTIs are generally caused by bacteria and treated with antibiotics. Inform clients of the importance of taking all of the medication, even when symptoms subside.

- Provide information, especially to females, about methods to prevent UTI.

- Tell clients that renal calculi are caused by a variety of problems. Guidance for reducing the risk for development of stones in those with a family history includes drinking enough fluid in a 24-hour period to produce 2 quarts of urine. Dietary changes and medications may be prescribed for clients with renal calculi. Support and encouragement to follow guidelines is an important role of the nurse.

- Advise clients with diabetes to follow their prescribed regimen and to schedule urinary and renal function screenings with their healthcare provider.

BEHAVIORAL CONSIDERATIONS

RISK FACTORS

- The use of analgesics has been linked with renal disease.

- Cigarette smoking has been linked with bladder cancer and renal tumors.

CLIENT EDUCATION

- Instruct about the use of analgesics, especially OTC medications to prevent renal disease. Clients should be advised to follow the instructions on the label, avoid prolonged use of combination ingredients (those with aspirin, acetaminophen, and caffeine in one pill), and drink six to eight glasses of water a day when using analgesics.

- Advise clients to discuss all medications—including OTC, herbal, and folk medications—with their healthcare provider.

- Educate clients to prevent the start of smoking and provide advice and support to foster smoking cessation.

Application Through Critical Thinking

CASE STUDY

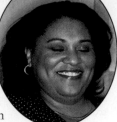

Ms. Sadie Basset is a 52-year-old African American female who arrives at the Metropolitan Women's Clinic complaining of itching, burning, and frequency of urination. She tells Louise Lo, RN, "I feel like I have to go to the bathroom every 10 minutes. I'm just miserable. I'm burning all the time, and I have tenderness here." (She points to her lower abdominal area.) Ms. Basset states that sometimes she feels a sharp abdominal pain and a sudden urge to urinate. On a few of these occasions, she has had difficulty getting to the bathroom on time and has even had a few "accidents." Ms. Lo asks if Ms. Basset has any illnesses. Ms. Basset reports that she was diagnosed with diabetes mellitus a few weeks ago.

After the interview, Ms. Lo performs a physical examination. Blood pressure is 106/82, pulse 68, respirations 20, and temperature 101.2°F. Abdomen is flat and soft. Bowel sounds are active and present in all four quadrants. The client complains of tenderness over the suprapubic area on palpation. The urinary meatus is red and edematous with no apparent discharge. Induration of the urinary meatus is noted on palpation of the anterior vaginal wall. The urinary stream is strong and steady. The urine is dark yellow with a hint of blood. It is cloudy and has a strong, foul odor.

Ms. Lo determines that there are four targets of concern for Ms. Basset: urge incontinence, pain, elevated temperature, and lack of knowledge.

▶ Complete Documentation

The following is sample documentation for Sadie Basset.
SUBJECTIVE DATA: Complains of itching, burning, and frequency of urination. "I feel like I'm going to the bathroom every 10 minutes. I'm just miserable. I'm burning all the time and I have tenderness here" (points to lower abdomen). Sometimes feels a sharp abdominal pain and sudden urge to urinate. Occasional difficulty getting to bathroom and few "accidents." Diagnosed with diabetes 2 weeks ago.
OBJECTIVE DATA: VS: B/P 106/82—P 68—RR 20. Temperature 101.2°F. Abdomen flat, soft. Bowel sounds present all quadrants. Tenderness over suprapubic area on palpation. Urinary meatus red, edematous, no discharge. Induration of meatus. Urinary stream strong, steady. Urine dark yellow, cloudy, strong, foul odor, Hematest positive.

▶ Critical Thinking Questions

1. Identify the data that support Ms. Lo's targets of concern.

ASSESSMENT FORM

Chief Complaint: *Frequent urination—urinary, urgency.*
Pain lower abdomen.

History: *Diabetes—diagnosed 2 weeks ago.*

Vital Signs: *B/P 106/82—P 68—RR 20—T 101.2°F*

Abdomen: *Soft, flat BS + X 4. Tender over suprapubic area.*

External Genitalia: *Meatus red, no edema, no discharge,*
indurated.

Urine: *Stream strong and steady. Dark, cloudy, strong,*
foul odor, Hematest positive.

---

2. What additional missing data is required to determine treatment for this client?
3. Describe a plan of nursing care for Ms. Basset.

▶ Applying Nursing Diagnoses

1. *Impaired urinary elimination* is a nursing diagnosis in the NANDA taxonomy (see Appendix A ∞). Do the data from the case study for Sadie Basset support this diagnosis? If so, identify the data to support the diagnosis.
2. *Knowledge, deficiency* is a diagnosis in the NANDA taxonomy. Do the data in the case study support this diagnosis? If so, identify the data to support the diagnosis.
3. Refer to the NANDA taxonomy to formulate additional nursing diagnoses for Sadie Basset.

▶ Prepare Teaching Plan

LEARNING NEED: Sadie Basset is a newly diagnosed diabetic with frequent, painful urination and lower abdominal pain. Her urine is dark, cloudy, and foul smelling with a hint of blood. The data indicate that she has a UTI. Diabetes increases the risk for development of UTI. Therefore, the nurse has a twofold responsibility. First, the nurse must ascertain Ms. Basset's ability to adhere to the prescribed regimen for diabetes. Second, in the presence of this acute problem, the nurse must address this client's need to learn about UTI.

GOAL: Sadie Basset will reduce her risk for further episodes of UTI.

OBJECTIVES: Upon completion of this learning experience, Sadie Basset will be able to:

1. Describe UTI.
2. Identify factors that contribute to the development of UTI.
3. Describe measures to prevent UTI.

APPLICATION OF OBJECTIVE 3: Describe measures to prevent UTI

Content	Teaching Strategy	Evaluation
• Follow the prescribed diabetic regimen. • Report changes in blood glucose readings. • Drink six to eight glasses of water daily. • Urinate as soon as you feel the urge. Do not wait. • Cleanse the genital area from front to back to prevent organisms from the rectal area from entering the vagina or urethra. • Shower rather than bathe in a tub. • Avoid irritation of the urethra that can occur with douching, vaginal sprays, perfumed soaps, and bubble bath. Avoid wet clothing. • Avoid tight clothing and pantyhose without cotton linings. • Cleanse the genital area before and after intercourse. • Urinate after intercourse.	One-on-one discussion. Permits repetition and introduction of sensitive information.	Verbal questioning in which Ms. Basset describes the eight measures to prevent UTI.

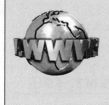

Please refer to the Companion Website at www.prenhall.com/damico and click on Chapter 20, the Application Through Critical Thinking module, to complete the following activities related to this case study:
▶ **Critical Thinking questions**
▶ **Extended Nursing Diagnosis challenge**
▶ **Documentation activity**
▶ **Teaching Plan for Objectives 1 and 2**

EXPLORE MediaLink

Additional resources for this chapter are found on the Student CD-ROM accompanying this textbook and on the Companion Website.

CD-ROM CONTENT

Content for this chapter includes:
Objectives
Key Concepts
NCLEX-RN® Review Questions
Model Documentation Forms
Audio Glossary
Games and Challenges
Clinical Spotlight Videos
Kidney Stones
Renal Failure
Head-to-Toe Physical Examination Video

COMPANION WEBSITE CONTENT

www.prenhall.com/damico

Content for this chapter includes:
Objectives
NCLEX-RN® Review Questions

Client Interaction Case Study Challenge
Application Through Critical Thinking Case Study
   Teaching Plan Challenge
MediaLinks
MediaLink Application
Tool Box
Chapter Documentation Form Example
Health Promotion
   Healthy People 2010
   Client Education
New York Times

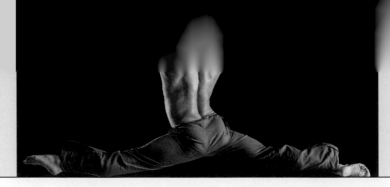

21

Male Reproductive System

MEDIALINK

www.prenhall.com/damico

The CD-ROM in the back of this textbook and the Media-Link website contain NCLEX-RN® review questions, interactive exercises, case study challenges, animations, videos, documentation and checklist forms, and review materials. For a complete listing of the media content specific to Chapter 21, see the Explore MediaLink at the end of the chapter.

The male reproductive system produces hormones, which impact physical development and sexual behavior. The reproductive organs in males provide for sexual pleasure and producing offspring. The structures of the male reproductive system produce and transport sperm (the male reproductive cells) and protective fluid (semen) for the deposition of sperm within the female reproductive tract and produce the male sex hormones. Many factors including psychosocial health, self-care habits, family, culture, and environment impact reproductive health. Therefore, the nurse must consider these factors while conducting the interview and physical assessment. The nurse must have a thorough understanding of the constituents of a healthy reproductive system and consider the relationship of other body systems to the reproductive system.

During the physical assessment, the nurse will assess and evaluate the occasional ambiguous cues of actual and potential reproductive disease and the variety of contributors to the development of pathology. The nurse documents and communicates the findings to the other members of the healthcare team. Additionally, the nurse has a key role in teaching the client how to establish and maintain reproductive wellness. The goal of client education is the promotion of optimum health according to the client's individual needs. Reproductive health is reflected in the focus areas of *Healthy People 2010*. Goals related to sexually transmitted diseases and prostate cancer are included in the Healthy People 2010 feature, on page 619.

ANATOMY AND PHYSIOLOGY REVIEW

The male reproductive system includes the penis, scrotum, testes, spermatic cord, duct system, accessory glands, and inguinal and perianal areas. These will be described in the following sections.

MALE REPRODUCTIVE SYSTEM

The male reproductive system is divided anatomically into external and internal genital organs. The penis and scrotum, the two external organs, are easily inspected and palpated. Only some of the internal structures are palpable. A basic understanding of anatomical structure and function is fundamental to performing assessment techniques correctly and safely. Figure 21.1 ● illustrates the gross anatomy of the male reproductive system.

Some of the male reproductive organs serve dual roles as part of the reproductive system and the urinary system. As part of the urinary system, the male genitals serve as a passageway for expelling urine. The functions of the male reproductive system are manufacturing and protecting sperm for fertilization, transporting sperm to the female vagina, regulating hormonal production of and secretion of male sex hormones, and providing sexual pleasure.

Scrotum

The **scrotum** is a loosely hanging, pliable, pear-shaped pouch of darkly pigmented skin that is located behind the penis. It houses the testes, which produce sperm. Spermatogenesis (sperm production) requires an environment in which the temperature is slightly lower than core body temperature; thus, the scrotum hangs outside of the abdominopelvic cavity and is usually about 37.4°F (3°C) cooler than core body temperature. A vertical septum within the scrotum divides it into two sections, each containing a testis, epididymis, vas deferens, and spermatic cord, as well as other functional structures (see Figures 21.2 ● and 21.3 ●).

Pubic hair scantily covers the scrotum. It is visibly asymmetrical, with the left side extending lower than the right, because the left spermatic cord is longer.

Below the scrotal surface lie two muscles, the cremaster muscle and the dartos muscle, which play a protective role in sperm production and viability. In cold temperatures, the dartos muscle wrinkles the scrotal skin, whereas the cremaster muscle contracts, causing the testes to elevate toward the body. Warmer temperatures cause the reverse reaction. The testes also become more wrinkled and contract toward the body during sexual arousal.

The major functions of the scrotum are protecting the testes, epididymides, and part of the spermatic cord, and protecting sperm production and viability through the maintenance of an appropriate surface temperature.

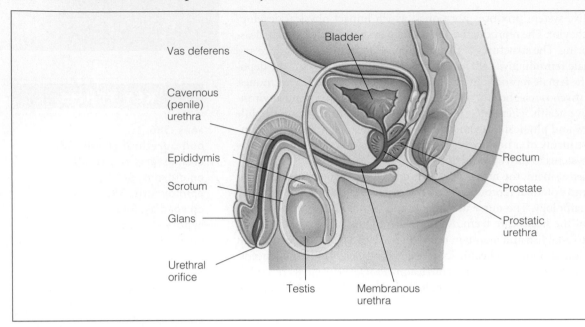

Figure 21.1 ● Gross anatomy of the male reproductive organs.

Testes

The **testes** are two firm, rubbery, olive-shaped structures that measure 4 to 5 cm long and 2 to 2.5 cm wide. They manufacture sperm and are thus the primary male sex organs. Each testis has two coats, the outer tunica vaginalis and the inner tunica albuginea, that separate it from the scrotal wall. Within each testis are the seminiferous tubules that produce sperm, and Leydig's cells that produce testosterone. Testosterone plays

a significant role in sperm production and the development of male sexual characteristics. The testes receive their blood supply from the testicular arteries. The testicular veins not only remove deoxygenated blood from the testes, but also form a network called the pampiniform plexus (Figure 21.2). This plays a crucial supportive role in regulating the temperature in the testes by cooling arterial blood before it passes into the testes. The major functions of the testes are producing spermatozoa and secreting testosterone.

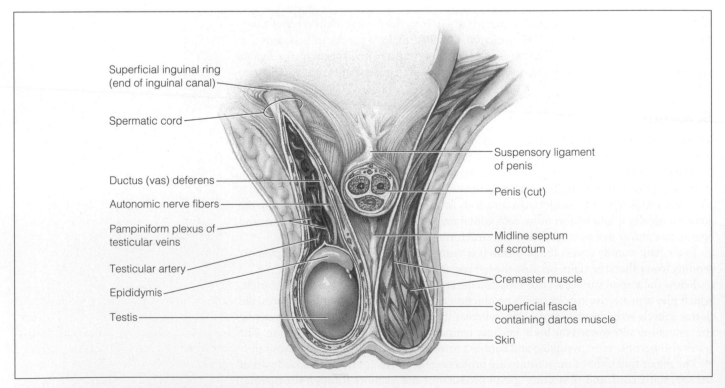

Figure 21.2 ● Contents of the scrotum, anterior view.

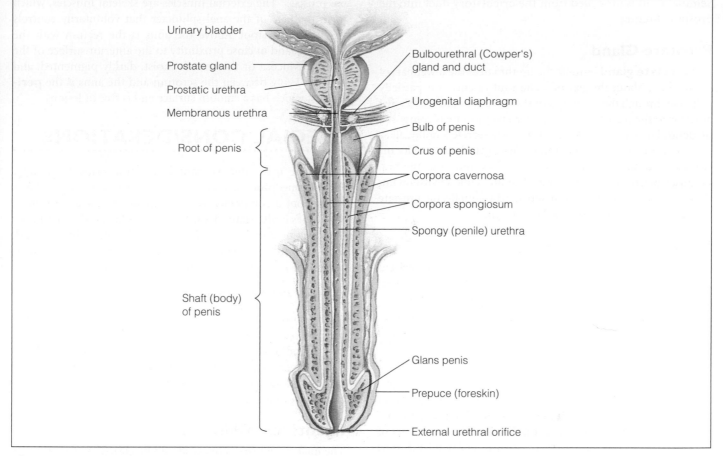

Figure 21.3 • Structure of the penis.

Spermatic Cord

The **spermatic cord** is composed of fibrous connective tissue. Its purpose is to form a protective sheath around the nerves, blood vessels, lymphatic structures, and muscle fibers associated with the scrotum (Figure 21.2).

DUCT SYSTEM

The duct system plays a crucial role in the transportation of sperm. The three structures comprising the duct system are the epididymis, the ductus deferens, and the urethra (Figures 21.2 and 21.3).

Epididymis

Positioned on top of and just posterior to each testicle is a commal- or crescent-shaped **epididymis**, which is palpable upon physical examination. It is actually a long, coiled tube, about 18 to 20 ft in length, which forms the beginning of the male duct system. Once the immature sperm have been produced in the testes, they are transported into the epididymis where they mature and become mobile. During orgasm, forceful contraction of muscles in this structure propels the sperm into the ductus deferens. The major functions of the epididymis are storing sperm as they mature and transporting sperm to the ductus deferens.

Ductus Deferens

Also known as the vas deferens, this tubular structure stretches from the end of the epididymis to the ejaculatory duct. Extending

about 46.15 cm (18 in.) long, the tube runs through the inguinal canal, on the backside of the bladder, and to the ejaculatory duct as it enters into the prostate gland. Mature sperm remain in the ductus deferens until ready for transport. The major functions of the ductus deferens are serving as an excretory duct in the transport of sperm and serving as a reservoir for mature sperm.

Urethra

The **urethra** serves as a conduit for the transportation of both urine and semen to the outside of the body. It is composed of three sections: the prostatic urethra, the membranous urethra, and the spongy (penile) urethra (Figure 21.3).

ACCESSORY GLANDS

The accessory glands play a crucial role in the formation of semen. These glands include the seminal vesicles, the prostate gland, and the bulbourethral gland.

Seminal Vesicles

The **seminal vesicles** are a pair of saclike glands, 7.5 cm long, located between the bladder and rectum. These vesicles are the source of 60% of the semen produced. Semen, a thick yellow fluid, is composed of a high concentration of fructose, amino acids, prostaglandins, ascorbic acid, and fibrinogen. It is secreted into the ejaculatory duct, where it mixes with sperm, which has been propelled from the ductus deferens. Semen nourishes and dilutes the sperm, enhancing its motility.

Seminal fluid is propelled from the ejaculatory duct into the prostatic urethra.

Prostate Gland

The **prostate gland** borders the urethra near the lower part of the bladder. About the size of a chestnut (2 cm), it is partially palpable through the front wall of the rectum because it lies just anterior to the rectum (Figure 21.1). The prostate is composed of glandular structures that continuously secrete a milky, alkaline solution. During sexual intercourse, glandular activity increases, and the alkaline secretions flow into the urethra. Because sperm motility is reduced in an acidic environment, these secretions aid sperm transport. Additionally, the prostate gland produces about one third of all semen.

Bulbourethral Glands

Also referred to as Cowper's glands, the **bulbourethral glands** are located below the prostate within the urethral sphincter (Figure 21.3). These glands are small (4.5 to 5 mm) and round. Just before ejaculation, the bulbourethral glands secrete a clear mucus into the urethra that lubricates the urethra and increases its alkaline environment.

PENIS

The **penis** is centrally located between the left and right groin areas and lies directly in front of the scrotum. Internally, the penile shaft consists of the penile urethra and three columns of highly vascular, erectile tissue: the two dorsolateral columns (corpora cavernosa) and the midventral column surrounding or encasing the urethra (Figure 21.3). The penis contracts and elongates during sexual arousal when its vasculature dilates as it fills with blood. This process allows the penis to become firm and erect so that it can deposit sperm into the female vagina. The distal end of the urethra (the external meatus) appears as a small opening centrally located on the glans of the penis, the cone-shaped distal end of the organ. In uncircumcised males, the glans is covered by a layer of skin called the foreskin. The major functions of the penis are serving as an exit for urine and as a passageway for sperm to exit and be deposited into the vagina during sexual intercourse.

INGUINAL AREAS

The inguinal areas are located laterally to the pubic region over the iliac region or the upper part of the hip bone. Within this area are the inguinal ligaments and the inguinal canals, which lie above the inguinal ligaments. The inguinal canals are associated with the abdominal muscles and actually represent a potential weak link in the abdominopelvic wall. When a separation of the abdominal muscle exists, the weak points of these canals afford an area for the protrusion of the intestine into the groin region. This is called an **inguinal hernia.** Table 21.1 describes types, characteristics, and signs and symptoms of inguinal hernias.

PERIANAL AREA

The **anus** is the terminal end of the gastrointestinal system. The anal canal is between 2 and 4 cm long, opens onto the perineum at the midpoint of the gluteal folds, and has internal and external muscles. The external muscles are skeletal muscles, which form the part of the anal sphincter that voluntarily controls evacuation of stool. Above the anus is the rectum with the prostate gland in close proximity to the anterior surface of the rectum. Mucosa of the anus is moist, darkly pigmented, and hairless. Lying between the scrotum and the anus is the **perineum,** which has a smooth surface and is free of lesions.

SPECIAL CONSIDERATIONS

The nurse uses effective communication, critical thinking, the nursing process, and appropriate assessment techniques throughout a comprehensive assessment process to determine the client's health status. Health status is influenced by a number of factors including age, developmental level, race, ethnicity, work history, living conditions, socioeconomics, and emotional well-being. These factors will be described in the following sections.

DEVELOPMENTAL CONSIDERATIONS

Changes in anatomy and physiological function occur as normal parts of growth and development. The accurate interpretation of findings from assessment is dependent upon knowledge of the expected variations across the age span. The following sections address specific age-related variations in the male reproductive system.

Infants and Children

The male newborn's genitals should be clearly evident and not ambiguous. If there is ambiguity, referral for genetic counseling is indicated. The penis may vary in size but averages about 2.5 cm in length and is slender. The urethral meatus should be in the center of the glans. If the opening is located on the underside of the glans, **hypospadias** is present. If the opening is on the superior aspect of the glans, **epispadias** exists. *Chordee,* a tight band of skin, causes bowing of the penis. The penis appears to have a C shape. This is associated with epispadias and hypospadias. The foreskin may be somewhat tight and not retractable until 2 or 3 years of age. If it is still tight after this time, **phimosis** exists. Cultural values and religious beliefs determine whether the family or caregiver circumcises the child. The family requires teaching about either maintaining the cleanliness of the uncircumcised penis or caring for the penis in the days following a circumcision.

The male infant's scrotum should be consistent in color with other body parts. It should seem oversized in comparison with the penis. This proportion changes as the infant grows. If the scrotum is enlarged and filled with fluid, a hydrocele may be present. The testes should be palpable and are about 2 cm in diameter at birth. Undescended testes, called cryptorchidism, is a common finding, especially if the infant is preterm. The testes should descend spontaneously within the first year of life. If both testes do not descend, the male will be infertile and will be at a greater risk for the development of testicular cancer. Enlargement of the testes in adolescence indicates the presence of a tumor. Testes smaller than 1.5 to 2.0 cm may indicate adrenal hyperplasia.

The onset of puberty in the male child occurs between 10 and 15 years of age. At this time, under the influence of elevat-

Table 21.1	Inguinal Hernias	
TYPE OF HERNIA	**CHARACTERISTICS**	**SIGNS AND SYMPTOMS**
Direct Hernia 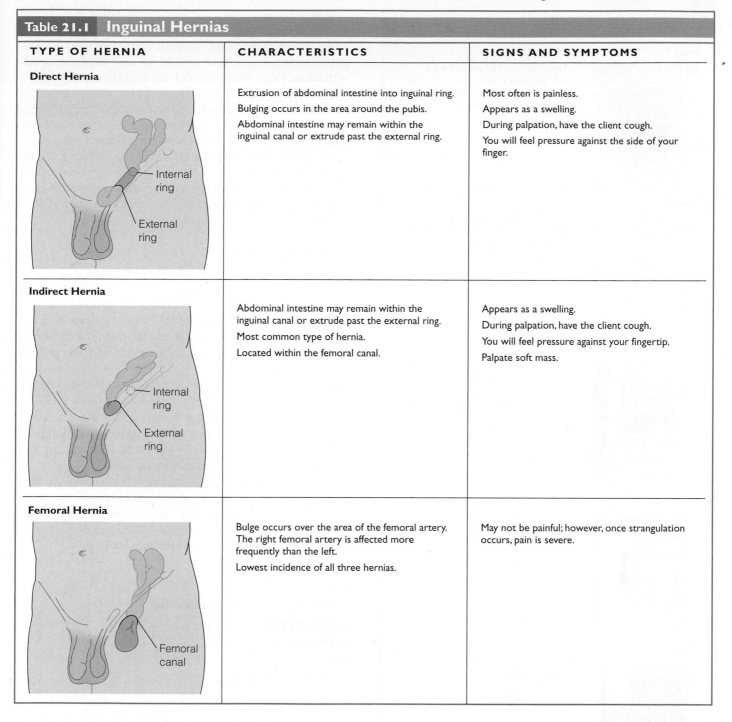	Extrusion of abdominal intestine into inguinal ring. Bulging occurs in the area around the pubis. Abdominal intestine may remain within the inguinal canal or extrude past the external ring.	Most often is painless. Appears as a swelling. During palpation, have the client cough. You will feel pressure against the side of your finger.
Indirect Hernia	Abdominal intestine may remain within the inguinal canal or extrude past the external ring. Most common type of hernia. Located within the femoral canal.	Appears as a swelling. During palpation, have the client cough. You will feel pressure against your fingertip. Palpate soft mass.
Femoral Hernia	Bulge occurs over the area of the femoral artery. The right femoral artery is affected more frequently than the left. Lowest incidence of all three hernias.	May not be painful; however, once strangulation occurs, pain is severe.

ing levels of testosterone, the male child begins to develop adult sexual characteristics. The testes and scrotum enlarge. Pubic, facial, and axillary hair develops. The penis begins to elongate, and the testes begin to produce mature sperm. The male child will experience unexpected erections and nocturnal emissions (wet dreams). Open, supportive communication is essential at this time. The nurse can show male children pictures of the sexual maturation of genitals to demonstrate that their development is normal. Table 21.2 includes Tanner's staging for evaluating sexual maturity. The male child often displays a fascination with his genitals. Masturbation and exploration of the genitals are usual practices in infants, toddlers, and preschoolers. Males may express curiosity in comparing

their genitals with those of other children, both male and female, in preschool and school ages.

Precocious puberty is an endocrine disorder characterized by the development of adult male characteristics in males under age 10. It includes dense pubic hair, penile enlargement, and enlargement of the testes. Precocious puberty may be idiopathic or caused by a genetic trait, lesions in the pituitary gland or hypothalamus, or testicular tumors. Referral to an endocrinologist may be required for definitive diagnosis.

It is important to assess not only the physical development of the male child's sexual organs but also the presence of abnormalities such as infection, tumors, and hernias. Assessment is completed using the same methods as described for the adult male.

Table 21.2 Maturation Stages in the Male

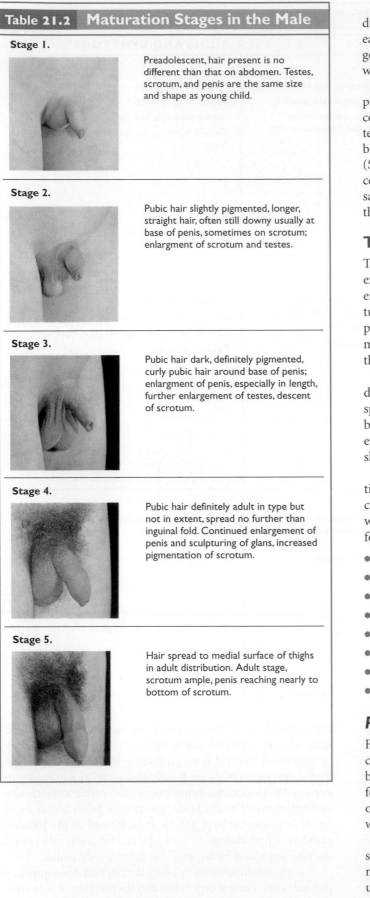

Stage 1. Preadolescent, hair present is no different than that on abdomen. Testes, scrotum, and penis are the same size and shape as young child.

Stage 2. Pubic hair slightly pigmented, longer, straight hair, often still downy usually at base of penis, sometimes on scrotum; enlargment of scrotum and testes.

Stage 3. Pubic hair dark, definitely pigmented, curly pubic hair around base of penis; enlargment of penis, especially in length, further enlargement of testes, descent of scrotum.

Stage 4. Pubic hair definitely adult in type but not in extent, spread no further than inguinal fold. Continued enlargement of penis and sculpturing of glans, increased pigmentation of scrotum.

Stage 5. Hair spread to medial surface of thighs in adult distribution. Adult stage, scrotum ample, penis reaching nearly to bottom of scrotum.

It is essential to assess for sexual molestation in male children. Some signs of sexual molestation are trauma, depression, eating disorders, bruising, swelling, and inflammation in the genital and anal areas. Additionally, the male child may appear withdrawn. Often the male child will deny the experience.

Adolescents often express interest in the changes related to puberty. The desire to explore sexual relationships and sexual contact, from kissing and fondling to intercourse, may be intense. Thus, adolescents need counseling on relationship issues, birth control, protection against sexually transmitted diseases (STDs), and delaying sexual activity. An adolescent may be concerned about or confused by an attraction to individuals of the same sex. It is important to provide open communication so that the adolescent may express concerns.

The Older Adult

The older male client experiences the following changes to the external genitals. Pubic hair thins and grays, the prostate gland enlarges, the size of the penis and testes may diminish, the scrotum hangs lower, and the testes are softer to palpation. Sperm production decreases in middle age; however, the older male may remain able to contribute viable sperm and father children throughout his life span.

Sexual function and ability change as well. Testosterone production decreases, resulting in diminished libido. Sexual response is often slower and not as intense. The older male may be slower to achieve erection, yet may be able to maintain the erection longer. Ejaculation can be less forceful and last for a shorter time, and less semen may be ejaculated.

Even though older male adults can achieve sexual gratification and participate in a satisfying sexual relationship, a decrease in sexual drive may contribute to the client's withdrawing from sexual experiences and relationships. The following factors are known to influence sexual drive.

- Chronic or acute diseases
- Certain medications
- Loss of spouse or significant other
- Loss of privacy
- Depression
- Fatigue
- Any stressful situation
- Use of alcohol or illicit drugs

PSYCHOSOCIAL CONSIDERATIONS

Fatigue, depression, and stress can decrease sexual desire in a client of any age. Grief over the loss of a relationship, whether because of separation, divorce, or death, can have long-term effects on a client's willingness to seek new relationships. Feelings of betrayal—for example, when a partner becomes intimate with another person—can have the same effect.

Past or recent trauma, as from childhood abuse, physical assault, and sexual assault, whether or not penetration occurred, may have a significant impact on a client's ability to enjoy a sexual relationship. This may be true even if the trauma is completely repressed.

A male's body image may be affected by his perception of his penis size in relation to that of other males. Some males fear that they are "too small" to satisfy a female sexually. Caring and sensitive teaching is needed to help the client understand that variations in penis size are normal and that there is little correlation between penis size and a partner's sexual satisfaction.

Males who have had a surgical sterilization procedure may feel suddenly freed from the worry of unwanted pregnancy and experience an increase in sexual desire, or they may suddenly feel less masculine than before the surgery and withdraw from sexual relationships.

CULTURAL AND ENVIRONMENTAL CONSIDERATIONS

Some cultures and religions have specific beliefs or encourage specific behaviors related to circumcision and sexual practices. For example, the Jewish religion requires the child to be circumcised by the seventh day of life by the clergy. Muslims practice circumcision, but not on the seventh day of life. In addition, many religions forbid premarital sex. When assessing clients, the nurse must never assume that they share all the beliefs or follow all the practices of their religious or cultural group or of the nurse.

Testicular cancer is the most common type of cancer in males between the ages of 20 and 35; thus, even adolescent males should perform a monthly testicular self-examination (see Box 21.1). Prostate cancer is the second leading cause of cancer-related deaths in males. Screening for prostate-specific antigen (PSA) and an annual prostate exam after the age of 50 is essential. Prostate cancer is more common in males of African ancestry. The signs of the condition are not usually noticeable until the prostatic cancer is advanced. The signs are usually confounding because benign prostatic disease presents with similar symptoms. These signs are dribbling, retention of urine, difficulty initiating the urinary stream, and cystitis. Risk factors include a family history of prostatic cancer and smoking.

Adults living in overcrowded conditions may feel that their lack of privacy inhibits their ability to experience sexual gratification. Today, one or more grandparents or older relatives may live with their adult child, and sexual expression and gratification may be compromised for all of the adults in the family.

Sexual, physical, or verbal abuse among family members may cause significant sexual dysfunction. Some family members may

---

Box 21.1 Testicular Self-Examination

Testicular cancer has no early warning signs. Thus, males should perform a testicular self-exam monthly, beginning in adolescence. Describe to the client how to perform the exam:

- The best time to perform the exam is in the shower or bath, since the heat and steam will warm your hands and the water will help your hands to glide over the skin surface. If your hands are cold, a reflex response will occur, causing your testicles to move up against your body. They will then be more difficult for you to feel.
- Feel each testicle by applying gentle pressure with your thumb, index, and middle fingers. If your testicle hurts while you feel it, you are pressing too hard.
- The contour of the testicle should be smooth, rounded, and firm.
- You will feel the epididymis on top of and behind each testicle.
- You should not feel any distinct lumps or areas of hardness, nor should your testicle be enlarged. If any of these signs are present, make an appointment with your physician immediately.

---

be aware of the experience but be unwilling or unable to stop the perpetrators or help the victims.

Negative family reactions to an individual's sexual orientation and lifestyle choices can constrain a person's ability and willingness to find a sexual partner and maintain a satisfying sexual relationship. The family's influence may be so strong that individuals choose partners acceptable to the family who do not meet their own needs or desires. This can have a negative emotional and physical impact on the individuals. Homosexual experimentation is common in adolescence and may not signify homosexuality or bisexuality.

Males who work in the microelectronics industry—in which the design and production of semiconductors, circuit boards, and other components of high-speed electronic equipment occur—may be exposed to arsenic, glycol ethers, lead, and radiation. These substances have been linked to birth defects. Lead is also still present in some homes, especially those built before 1979. Males who have been exposed to lead may experience decreased libido, diminished sperm count, and abnormal sperm morphology. Exposure to vinyl chloride, a gas used in the manufacture of building and construction materials, wire and cable insulation, glass, paper, household goods, and medical supplies, may increase the risk for chromosomal changes in the male germ cells. Federal regulations regarding exposure to vinyl chloride have been adopted to prevent known health risks.

Cultural Considerations

- Penile cancer is rare in the United States; however, it accounts for almost 10% of male cancers in Africa and South America.
- Prostate cancer occurs more frequently in African Americans than in Caucasians.
- Testicular cancer occurs more frequently in Caucasians than in any other ethnic group.
- Bladder cancer occurs twice as frequently in Caucasians as in African Americans.

- The rates for STDs are higher in African American and Hispanic populations than in Caucasians.
- Circumcision of the male is required in some religions (Judaism, Islam) and preferred in many cultures to promote hygiene. It is seen with the least frequency in Hispanics.
- In many cultures, physical assessment is limited to same-sex examiners.

*H*ealth assessment of the male reproductive system includes gathering subjective and objective data. Subjective data collection occurs during the client interview, before the actual physical assessment. During the interview the nurse uses a variety of communication techniques to elicit general and specific information about the client's state of health or illness. Health records, the results of laboratory tests, and x-rays are important secondary sources to be reviewed and included in the data-gathering process. During physical assessment of the male reproductive system, the techniques of inspection and palpation will be used.

FOCUSED INTERVIEW

The focused interview for the male reproductive system concerns data related to the structures and functions of this body system. Subjective data related to the status of the reproductive system is gathered during the focused interview. The nurse must be prepared to observe the client and listen for cues related to the function of this body system. The nurse may use open-ended or closed questions to obtain information. Often a number of follow-up questions or requests for descriptions are required to clarify data or gather missing information. Follow-up questions are aimed at identifying the source of problems, duration of difficulties, measures to alleviate problems, and clues about the client's knowledge of his own health.

Because of the dual functions of some of the male reproductive structures, some of the data gathered during the focused interview will relate to the status of the urinary system as well as the reproductive system. Some commonly reported problems are those related to altered patterns of voiding, the presence of masses or lesions, unusual discharge, pain and tenderness, changes in sexual functioning, suspected contact with a sexual partner who may have an STD, and infertility. Examination of the anus and rectum is included in examination of the male reproductive system. Related problems include hemorrhoids, fissures, and infectious processes.

Nurses need to understand their own feelings and comfort about various aspects of sexuality to be efficient in gathering data. It is essential for the nurse to put aside personal beliefs and values about sexual practices and focus in a culturally competent and nonjudgmental manner on gathering data to determine the health status of the male client.

During the focused interview, the nurse will need to create an atmosphere that facilitates open communication and comfort for the client. Male clients commonly experience anxiety, fear, and embarrassment when the nurse requests information about a topic that, in most clients' minds, is very personal. These emotions may be expressed either verbally or nonverbally. With this in mind, the nurse should approach the client in as nonthreatening a manner as possible and assure the male client that the information provided and the results of the physical examination will remain confidential. Furthermore, the nurse should be aware of personal behaviors that may serve as a hindrance to effective communication. The nurse should sit down with the male client to convey that it is important to spend time discussing the client's concerns. The nurse's verbal and nonverbal communication should convey a nonjudgmental attitude while requesting only the information needed to assess the client's health status. It is a good idea to begin with questions that are the least threatening and have the least sexual connotation because the information the nurse gathers may reveal some abnormality that may threaten sexual activity and health. A conversational approach with the use of open-ended statements may be helpful, especially with male adolescents. As the client provides information, the male client's choice of terminology can serve as a guide in deciding which terms would be most appropriate to use. When discussing any sensitive or controversial topic, it is always best to start with a general statement that opens the door for male clients to express their thoughts.

The focused interview guides the physical assessment of the male reproductive system. The information is always considered in relation to normal parameters and expectations about the function of the system. Therefore, the nurse must consider age, gender, race, culture, environment, health practices, past and concurrent problems, and therapies when framing questions and using techniques to elicit information. In order to address all of the factors when conducting a focused interview, categories of questions related to reproductive status and function have been developed. These categories include general questions that are asked of all clients, those addressing illness or infection, questions related to symptoms or behaviors, those related to habits or practices, questions that are specific to clients according to age, and questions that address environmental concerns.

The nurse must consider the client's ability to participate in the focused interview and physical assessment of the male reproductive system. If a client is experiencing discomfort or anxiety, the nurse should focus on relief of symptoms.

FOCUSED INTERVIEW QUESTIONS

RATIONALES

The following section provides sample questions and bulleted follow-up questions in each of the categories previously mentioned. A rationale for each of the questions is provided. The list of questions is not all-inclusive but does represent the types of questions required in a comprehensive focused interview related to the male reproductive system. The subjective data collected and questions asked during the health history and focused interview will provide information to help meet the goal of promoting reproductive health and preventing STDs as described in the Healthy People 2010 *feature on page 619.*

GENERAL QUESTIONS

1. **Do you have any concerns about your sexual health?**
   - Have you had concerns in the past? If so, please tell me about those concerns.

   ▶ These questions may prompt the male client to discuss any concerns about reproductive health.

2. **Are you sexually active? If so, how would you describe your sexual relationship(s)?**

   ▶ The male client may feel pressured to be in a sexual relationship. These pressures may be external (expectations of family, friends, or work associates) or internal (fear of being viewed by others as less than desirable or not of an accepted sexual orientation, fear of being alone, or fear of not being loved and accepted).

3. **Are there any obstacles to your ability to achieve sexual satisfaction?**

   ▶ Causes of inability to achieve sexual satisfaction include fear of acquiring an STD, fear of being unable to satisfy the partner, fear of pregnancy, confusion regarding sexual preference, unwillingness to participate in sexual activities enjoyed by the partner, job stress, financial considerations, crowded living conditions, loss of partner, attraction to or sexual involvement with individuals that the partner does not know about, criticism of sexual performance by the partner, or history of sexual trauma.

4. **Have you noticed a change in your sex drive recently?**

   ▶ This may be indicative of some physical or psychological problems that need follow-up. If the client answers yes, the nurse should ask the following question.

5. **Can you associate the change with anything in particular?**

   ▶ Often clients can relate a decrease in sex drive with stress, illness, drug therapy, or some other factor.

6. *For clients who are sexually active:*
   - What type of contraception do you use?
   - What kind of sexual activities do you engage in?

   ▶ Questions about types of sexual activities provide information related to risk for STDs.

7. **Do your family and friends support your relationship with your sexual partner?**

   ▶ The client's family and friends can influence the client's sexual relationship in a variety of ways. The client may feel tension if the partner is not accepted.

8. **Are you able to talk to your partner about your sexual needs?**
   - Does your partner accept your needs and help you fulfill them?
   - Are you able to do the same for your partner?

   ▶ Communication with a sexual partner helps in establishing a fulfilling relationship.

9. **Some clients come to a healthcare provider to discuss sexual abuse.**
   - Have you ever been forced to have sexual intercourse or other sexual contact against your will?
   - Have you ever been molested or raped?

   ▶ The opening statement lets the client know that sexual abuse is a topic that can be addressed in this encounter. The questions allow the client to describe abusive encounters in some detail.

FOCUSED INTERVIEW QUESTIONS	RATIONALES

10. *If the client answers yes, the nurse should ask the following questions.*
    - When did the abuse occur?
    - Who abused you?
    - What was the experience?
    - How often did this happen?
    - What was done about the situation and for you?

11. *For clients who are sexually active:*
    - Are you in a relationship with one partner?
    - If not, how many sexual partners have you or your partner had over the last year?

▶ Sexual activity with many different partners increases the risk of acquiring STDs. Sexual activity with more than four partners in a lifetime increases risk for certain gynecologic cancers in the female.

12. **Do you have children?**
    - If so, how many?
    - *If the client answers no:* Have you tried to have children?
    - *If the client answers yes:* How long have you been trying to have a child?

▶ The couple is not considered potentially infertile unless they have been unable to conceive for a year.

13. *If the client indicates that his partner has shown inability to conceive after 1 year:* **How often do you and your partner have intercourse?**

▶ For couples attempting to have a child, it is important to engage in intercourse routinely, two to three times a week. Although nurses do not treat infertility, they may be involved in teaching the client about certain measures that may be helpful, such as temperature tracking in the female partner, to determine the optimal time for intercourse. Concerns about infertility can produce great anxiety for many couples.

14. **Have you ever had mumps?**

▶ Mumps occurring after puberty has been linked to sterility in males.

15. **Have you ever sought professional help for fertility problems? If so, describe this experience.**

▶ This provides the opportunity to identify diagnostic testing and procedures for infertility. In addition, the client can describe psychosocial or emotional issues surrounding the fertility problem.

16. **Has an inability for your partner to conceive placed a strain on your relationship?**
    - How has this problem affected your relationship?
    - How are you feeling about this?

▶ The client has the opportunity to express emotional or psychosocial concerns surrounding a partner's infertility.

17. **Are you able to be sexually aroused?**
    - Has this ability changed over time or recently?

▶ A variety of factors may influence an individual's ability to become sexually aroused. These include use of prescribed or illicit drugs, disorders of the nervous system, diabetes, stress, and fear (e.g., of intimacy, inability to satisfy a partner, or acquiring an STD).

18. **Are you able to achieve and maintain an erection?**
    - Have any aspects in your ability to achieve an erection changed?
    - Are you satisfied with the length of time it takes to achieve and maintain an erection?

▶ The ability to achieve an erection depends on both physiological factors and state of mind.

19. **When you have an erection, is the shaft of the penis straight or crooked?**

▶ **Peyronie's disease** causes the shaft of the penis to be crooked during an erection.

20. **Are you able to achieve orgasm?**
    - Are you satisfied with your ability to control the timing of your orgasms?

▶ Premature ejaculation is defined by some researchers as orgasm immediately after, or even before, penetration. It may also be defined as ejaculation before the male's sexual partner reaches orgasm in more than half of the male's sexual experiences. It is often a devastating disorder that may severely compromise sexual relationships. The client can learn techniques to delay ejaculation.

FOCUSED INTERVIEW QUESTIONS	**RATIONALES**

QUESTIONS RELATED TO ILLNESS OR INFECTION

1. **Have you ever been diagnosed with an illness or disease of the reproductive organs?**
   - When were you diagnosed with the problem?
   - What treatment was prescribed for the problem?
   - Was the treatment helpful?
   - What kinds of things do you do to help with the problem?
   - Has the problem ever recurred (acute)?
   - How are you managing the disease now (chronic)?

► The client has an opportunity to provide information about specific illnesses. If a diagnosed illness is identified, follow-up about the date of diagnosis, treatment, and outcomes is required. Data about each illness identified by the client is essential to an accurate health assessment. Illnesses can be classified as acute or chronic, and follow-up regarding each classification will differ.

2. **An alternative to question 1 is to list possible disorders of the male reproductive system, such as benign prostatic disease, erectile dysfunction, and cancer of the penis, prostate, or testicles, and ask the client to respond yes or no as each is stated.**

► This is a comprehensive and easy way to elicit information about illnesses of the reproductive system. Follow-up would be required for each diagnosis as in question 1.

3. **Have you ever had a sexually transmitted disease (such as herpes, gonorrhea, syphilis, or chlamydia)?**
   - *If the client answers yes:* Was it treated?
   - Did you inform your partner?
   - Did you have sexual relations with your partner while you were infected?
   - *If the client answers yes:* Did you use condoms?
   - What treatment did you receive?

► Serious, sometimes fatal, complications can develop if treatment is delayed. For example, untreated syphilis can eventually involve the cardiovascular and central nervous systems, and genital herpes is contagious and infects partners with every sexual encounter.

   The nurse should talk about herpes and how contagious it is and that the male can infect every partner he has intercourse with.

4. **Are you aware of having had any exposure to HIV?**
   - *If the client answers yes:* Describe the situation and how you feel you were exposed.

► This question helps to determine at-risk practices and knowledge of the transmission of HIV.

5. **What are your views on sexual relations and the potential for acquiring HIV?**
   - Have you ever been tested for HIV?
   - What were the results?

► Further information about at-risk sexual activity and the determination of HIV status or transmissibility is obtained.

6. **Do you have sexual intercourse without condoms?**
   - *If the client answers yes:* On one occasion or routinely?

► The incidence of HIV is still on the rise. HIV has reached epidemic proportions in India and South Africa. Despite the wide availability of information on the risk and methods of protection for sexually active individuals, many people continue to have unprotected sex.

7. **Have you had surgery on any of your reproductive organs?**
   - If so, what was the surgery?

► Some surgeries, such as penile implants, require periodic follow-up for problems, including possible infection. Surgeries such as prostatectomy (removal of the prostate) or surgeries that alter body image, such as colostomy, may have bearing on sexual function as well as attitude about oneself in relation to sexuality.

QUESTIONS RELATED TO SYMPTOMS OR BEHAVIORS

When gathering information about symptoms, many questions are required to elicit details and descriptions that assist in the analysis of the data. Discrimination is made in relation to the significance of a symptom, in relation to specific diseases or problems, and in relation to potential follow-up examination or referral. One rationale is provided for a group of questions in this category.

FOCUSED INTERVIEW QUESTIONS	RATIONALES

The following questions refer to specific symptoms and behaviors associated with the male reproductive system. For each symptom, questions and follow-up are required. The details to be elicited are the characteristics of the symptom; the onset, duration, and frequency of the symptom; the treatment or remedy for the symptom, including over-the-counter (OTC) and home remedies; the determination if diagnosis has been sought; the effect of treatments; and family history associated with a symptom or illness.

QUESTIONS RELATED TO SYMPTOMS

1. **Have you felt any lumps or masses on your penis, scrotum, or surrounding areas? If so, describe the mass.**
   - Exactly where is it?
   - Describe the size.
   - Is it soft or hard?
   - Is it movable?
   - When did you first notice the mass?
   - Is it painful?
   - Has there been any pattern to the swelling: an increase, decrease, or unchanged pattern?
   - What treatments have you tried?

   ▶ This information helps the nurse to understand the nature of the mass or lump.

2. **Have you noticed any swelling of your scrotum, penis, or surrounding areas?**
   - If so, when did it start?
   - Is it painful?
   - Has there been any pattern to the swelling: an increase, decrease, or unchanged pattern?
   - What treatments have you tried?

   ▶ This information could help identify problems of rapid onset, which sometimes have the potential to be more detrimental. Swelling in the inguinal area may signal the presence of a hernia. Sources of swelling in the scrotal area include an acute or chronic inflammatory process, a hydrocele, scrotal edema, or scrotal hernia.

3. **Have you noticed any unusual discharge from your penis?**
   - If so, of what color?
   - Is there any odor to the discharge?
   - Is it a small, moderate, or large amount?
   - When did you first notice the discharge?
   - Is there any burning or pain with the discharge?

   ▶ Discharge characteristics may indicate whether an infectious process is occurring.

4. **Have you noticed any change in color of your penis or scrotum?**
   - If so, describe the change and the location.

   ▶ Inflammatory processes may cause redness in the affected area.

5. **Have you had any unusual itching in your genital area?**
   - If so, where? Have you noticed any rash, scaling, or lumps?

   ▶ Causes may include environmental allergens, soaps, lotions, and the presence of pubic lice (crabs).

6. **Have you had any problems with your rectal area such as pain, itching, bruising, burning, or bleeding?**
   - When did the problem begin?
   - Do you know the cause of the problem?
   - Have you sought healthcare for the problem?
   - Was a diagnosis made?
   - What treatment was prescribed?
   - What do you do to help with the problem?
   - Has the treatment helped?

   ▶ Pain, itching, bleeding, or burning may indicate the presence of infection, irritation, or injury to the anus or rectum. Bleeding, pain, and irritation may result from passing hard stools, from hemorrhoids, from injuries, or from trauma including anal sex. Fungal infection may result in chronic pruritus or irritation of the perianal area.

   ▶ When symptoms with the anorectal area are associated with hemorrhoids or hard stool, follow-up would include information about diet and bowel habits.

   Irritation or injury to the perianal area can occur as a result of sexual practices or sexual abuse. Sensitive questioning about these topics is required when sexual activity is described or when abuse is suspected or disclosed.

FOCUSED INTERVIEW QUESTIONS

RATIONALES

QUESTIONS RELATED TO PAIN

1. **Have you noticed any pain, tenderness, or soreness in the areas of your penis or scrotum?**
   - If so, describe the pain.
   - Is it dull? Sharp? Radiating? Intermittent? Continuous?
   - Does anything make the pain better or worse?

2. **Are you having any pain in the area now?**

▶ Testicular torsion may cause excruciating acute pain in the testicular area. Often, the affected testicle will be higher in the scrotal sac than the nonaffected testicle. A dull, aching pain is a common symptom of **epididymitis**, a common infection in males.

▶ This question helps the nurse determine if the problem is current, experienced in the past only, or chronic.

QUESTIONS RELATED TO BEHAVIORS

1. **Do you check your genitals on a routine basis?**
   - Do you know how to perform testicular self-exam?
   - How often do you perform this exam?
   - What technique do you use?

2. **How often do you get physical examinations?**

3. **Are you circumcised? If so, have you had any difficulty keeping this area clean?**

4. **Are you and your partner using contraception?**
   - If so, what kind?
   - Are you using it consistently?

5. **Would you like to know more about the use of birth control?**

6. **How do you protect yourself from sexually transmitted diseases, including HIV?**

7. **Do you drink alcohol? If so, how many drinks per week do you consume?**

8. **Do you use recreational drugs? If so, what type and how much?**

▶ Self-examination of the genitals should be performed at least monthly for early detection of changes that need follow-up. Teaching may be indicated if the client is not performing self-examination. Refer to Box 21.1.

▶ Screening for problems such as prostate or testicular cancer usually is performed during a routine physical.

▶ If the client is having problems with maintaining hygiene of the area, client teaching may be necessary.

▶ This helps to determine knowledge of the product being used and practice of contraception.

▶ This is a very important question to ask adolescents who shy away from talking about sexual practices but have verbalized that they are sexually active.

▶ Abstinence is the only 100% effective protection against STDs. Latex condoms offer significant protection, especially when treated with spermicide; however, they are not 100% effective.

▶ Chronic alcoholism has been linked to impotence. Additionally, intake of alcoholic beverages can contribute to an individual "taking chances," such as failing to use condoms, and can impact fertility.

▶ Taken in sufficient amounts, some drugs, such as marijuana and opiates, may decrease libido and lead to impotence. Drug use may also contribute to failure to use protection against STDs.

FOCUSED INTERVIEW QUESTIONS	**RATIONALES**

QUESTIONS RELATED TO AGE

The focused interview must reflect the anatomical and physiological differences that exist along the age span. The following questions are examples of those that would be specific for children and older adults.

QUESTIONS REGARDING INFANTS AND CHILDREN

1. **Have you noticed any redness, swelling, or discharge that is discolored or foul smelling in the child's genital areas?**

   ▶ These may indicate inflammatory processes or infection.

2. **Have you noticed any asymmetry, lumps, or masses in the infant's genitals?** *If the parent or caregiver answers yes:*
   - Where are they?
   - Are they movable?
   - Hard or soft?
   - Does touching the mass elicit a pain response from the child?

   ▶ These symptoms may indicate the development of an obstructive process, hydrocele, or inguinal hernia.

3. **Has the child complained of itching, burning, or swelling in the genital area?**

   ▶ These symptoms may indicate the presence of pinworms or infections such as yeast infections.

The nurse should ask the preschool child, school-age child, or adolescent the following questions:

1. **Has anyone ever touched you when you didn't want him or her to? Where? (The nurse may want to have the child point to a picture.)**

   ▶ The nurse must try to determine exactly what the person did to the child. Has there been more than touching? Has any other form of sexual contact occurred? The child may feel responsible for the situation and not wish to discuss it. The abuser is most often a parent or relative. The nurse should assure the child that he has not been bad and that it helps to talk to an adult about it. Referral should be made to a specialist immediately for sexual abuse examination. Careful documentation is required. Information may be considered forensic evidence.

2. **Has anyone ever asked you to touch him or her when you didn't want to? (If the child answers yes, the child may be sexually abused. The nurse should try to obtain additional information by asking the following questions but remember to be sensitive:)**

3. **Where did he or she ask you to touch him or her?**

4. **Who touched you? How many times did this happen? Who knows about this?**

Many of the questions the nurse asks adolescents are similar to those the nurse would ask male adults. It is important to explore adolescents' feelings and concerns regarding their sexual development—for instance, concerns about wet dreams. The male adolescent should be reassured that these changes are normal. Some adolescents may be confused about their feelings of sexual attraction to the opposite or same sex. The nurse should ask open-ended questions and assure the male adolescent that such feelings are normal.

Whether or not a male adolescent admits to being sexually active, the nurse should offer information on teenage pregnancy, birth control, and protection against STDs. Some teenagers may be fearful that the nurse will relay this information to their parents. The nurse should reinforce that all information is confidential except in situations of sexual abuse.

Use of gender-neutral terms prevents value judgments about sexual orientation. This question allows clients to define what they think sex is. Many teens consider anything not involving vaginal penetration as not being sex.

FOCUSED INTERVIEW QUESTIONS	RATIONALES

QUESTIONS FOR THE OLDER ADULT

The questions for older male adults are the same as those for younger male adults. In addition, the nurse should explore whether older clients perceive any changes in their sexuality related to advancing age. For example, an older male may find he needs more time to achieve erection. The older adult can be reassured that these changes are normal and do not necessarily indicate disease.

QUESTIONS RELATED TO ENVIRONMENT

Environment refers to both the internal and external environments. Questions related to the internal environment include all of the previous questions and those associated with internal or physiological responses. Questions regarding the external environment include those related to home, work, or social environments.

INTERNAL ENVIRONMENT

1. Do you know if your mother received (diethylstilbestrol DES) treatment during pregnancy?

▶ Some reports indicate that sons of DES mothers have higher than average rates of genitourinary problems such as hypospadias, infertility, and undescended or enlarged testicles. They may be at risk for testicular cancer and have low sperm counts. Physician referral is indicated if the client's response is yes.

2. Do you take any prescribed or over-the-counter medications, home remedies, herbal or cultural medicines, or dietary supplements?

▶ Medications, herbs, dietary supplements, and home remedies can alter, enhance, or interfere with one another in terms of therapeutics and can result in side effects affecting reproductive functioning. For example, saw palmetto is used to improve prostate health. Herbal testosterone products such as nettle root are also available.

EXTERNAL ENVIRONMENT

The following questions deal with substances and irritants found in the physical environment of the client. The physical environment includes the indoor and outdoor environments of the home and workplace, those encountered for social engagements, and any encountered during travel.

1. Have you been exposed to lead, chemicals, or toxins in the environment?

▶ Lead exposure may result in decreased libido and sperm abnormalities.

2. Do you use protective equipment when engaged in work or athletic activities?

▶ The use of protective equipment including athletic supports and cups reduces the incidence of testicular damage.

CLIENT INTERACTION

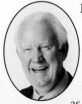

Mr. Edward O'Reilly, age 71, comes to the Urgi-Medi Center at 8:00 P.M. accompanied by his son. He tells the clerk at the reception desk that he needs to see Nurse Jack, stating, "I haven't passed my water since yesterday afternoon." His son tells the clerk his father called him about 5:00 P.M. just as he was leaving work, screaming, "I can't go! I'm going to burst. I have a lot of pressure down there." Mr. O'Reilly is observed pacing in the reception area waiting for the nurse. His chart indicates he came to the center 2 weeks ago with a similar complaint. At that time a diagnosis of benign prostatic hypertrophy was made, along with a recommendation for a transurethral resection of the prostate (TURP). The following is an excerpt from the focused interview.

INTERVIEW

Nurse: Good evening, Mr. O'Reilly. I see by the report you are having trouble voiding again.

Mr. O'Reilly: Oh, I'm glad you are here tonight. I can't talk to Ms. Pat about my problem.

Nurse: Tell me about the problem.

Mr. O'Reilly: I have not passed any water since yesterday afternoon, not even a few drops. I have to go really bad. The pressure down there really hurts. I need the tube again.

Nurse: The last time you were able to pass your water, did you have trouble starting the stream?

Mr. O'Reilly: Oh, yes. That's been getting worse. I need to push very hard to start and then I leak when I'm finished.

Nurse: You leak?

Mr. O'Reilly: Yes, I'm like my grandson; I always have wet briefs. I leak and it never stops. I'm so embarrassed.

Nurse: When was the last time you tried to pass your water?

Mr. O'Reilly: I didn't sleep much last night. I'm always trying. I tried before I left the house, nothing, and then when I was waiting for you, and nothing. Nothing, don't you understand me?

ANALYSIS

Several strategies were used by the nurse in this clinical example. First, the client's request to see a male nurse was honored. The nurse used open-ended statements and reflection, and sought clarification as needed. The use of client terminology was employed to put the client at ease.

Please refer to the Companion Website at **www.prenhall.com/damico** and click on Chapter 21, the **Client Interaction** module, to answer questions about this case. In addition, see other resources for this chapter including NCLEX review questions and other interactive exercises and materials.

Physical Assessment

ASSESSMENT TECHNIQUES AND FINDINGS

The adult male has clean, evenly distributed pubic hair in a diamond pattern thinning as it extends toward the umbilicus. The penis is free of hair and of a size appropriate to the stage of development. The skin is of darker pigment than the rest of the body and loose over a flaccid penis. The dorsal vein is midline on the shaft of the penis. The glans penis is smooth and free of lesions or discharge. The urinary meatus is in the center of the tip of the penis. The scrotum is pear shaped with wrinkled, loose skin, and is lower on the left side. The inguinal areas are flat. The penis and scrotum are nontender to palpation. The testes are mobile, smooth, elastic, and solid. The spermatic cord is palpable, smooth, and resilient. The inguinal canal is free of masses or lumps. The anus is darkly pigmented and the perianal area is smooth. The bulbourethral gland is smooth and lesion-free, and the prostate gland is nontender, smooth, and firm.

Physical assessment of the male reproductive system follows an organized pattern. It begins with inspection and palpation of the external genitalia. This is followed by inspection of the perianal area, palpation of the bulbourethral and prostate glands via rectal examination, and examination of stool for occult blood.

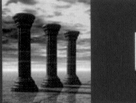

EQUIPMENT

examination gown and drape	flashlight
clean, nonsterile examination gloves	lubricant
examination light	slides and swabs to obtain a specimen of abnormal discharge

HELPFUL HINTS

- Provide an environment that is warm and private.
- Explain each step in the procedure and provide specific instructions about what is expected of the client. For example, the nurse should state whether the client will be expected to sit, stand or bear down during an assessment.
- Males from puberty through adulthood respond in a variety of ways when the genitals are exposed for examination. It is imperative to maintain the client's dignity throughout the assessment.
- Explore cultural issues and seek remedies for concerns at the onset of the interaction.
- Use Standard Precautions.

TECHNIQUES AND NORMAL FINDINGS	**ABNORMAL FINDINGS SPECIAL CONSIDERATIONS**

INSPECTION

1. **Instruct the client.**

   - Have the male client empty his bladder and bowel before the examination.

   - Explain to the client that you will be looking at and touching his genitals and pubic area. Tell him that the assessment should not cause physical discomfort. However, he must tell you of pain or discomfort at any point during the examination.

   - Reassure the client that anxiety and embarrassment are normal. Explain that relaxation and focus on instructions will make the assessment easier. If the client experiences an erection during the examination, explain that this is normal and has no sexual connotation.

2. **Position the client.**

   - The client stands in front of the examiner for the first part of the assessment.

3. **Position yourself on a stool sitting in front of the client.**

4. **Inspect the pubic hair.**

   - Observe the pubic hair for normal distribution, amount, texture, and cleanliness (see Figure 21.4 ●).

► The amount, distribution, and texture of pubic hair vary according to the client's age and race. Absent or extremely sparse hair in the pubic area may be indicative of sexual underdevelopment. The pubic hair of elderly males may be gray and thinning (see Table 21.2).

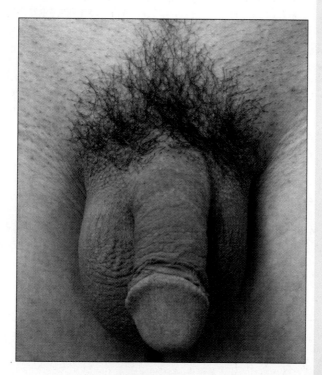

Figure 21.4 ●
Inspecting the pubic hair.

   - Confirm that pubic hair is distributed heavily at the symphysis pubis in a diamond- or triangular-shaped pattern, thinning out as it extends toward the umbilicus. The hair will thin as it reaches the inner thigh area and over the scrotum. Hair should be absent on the penis.

   - If the client has complained of itching in his pubic area, comb through the pubic hair with two or three fingers.

TECHNIQUES AND NORMAL FINDINGS	ABNORMAL FINDINGS SPECIAL CONSIDERATIONS

- Confirm the absence of small bluish gray spots, or nits (eggs), at the base of the pubic hairs.

▶ These signs indicate the presence of crab or pubic lice. Marks may be visible from persistent scratching to relieve the intense itching crabs cause.

5. **Inspect the penis.**

- Inspect the penis size, pigmentation, glans, location of the dorsal vein, and the urethral meatus.

- Start by confirming that the penis size is appropriate for the stage of development of the client. In adult males, penis size varies.

▶ Penis size varies according to the developmental stage of the client (see Table 21.2).

- Note the pigmentation of the penis.

- Pigmentation should be evenly distributed over the penis. The color depends on the client's race but will be slightly darker than the color of the skin over the rest of his body.

▶ Pigmentation of the penis of males with lighter complexions ranges from pink to light brown. In dark-skinned clients, the penis is light to dark brown.

- Assess the looseness of the skin over the shaft of the penis. The skin should be loose over the flaccid penis.

- Confirm that the dorsal vein is midline on the shaft.

- Inspect the glans penis. It should be smooth and free of lesions or discharge. No redness or inflammation should be present. **Smegma**, a white, cheesy substance, may be present. This finding is considered normal.

▶ Discharge or lesions may indicate the presence of infective diseases such as *herpes, genital warts, or syphilis,* or may indicate cancer. If discharge is present, the substance should be cultured. Consistency, color, and odor are noted.

- If the client is uncircumcised, either ask the client to pull the foreskin back or do so yourself. To retract the foreskin, gently pull the skin down over the penile shaft from the side of the glans using the thumb and first two fingers or forefinger (see Figure 21.5 ●).

▶ Phimosis is a condition in which the foreskin is so tight that it cannot be retracted.
▶ Paraphimosis describes a condition in which the foreskin, once retracted, becomes so tight that it cannot be moved back over the glans.

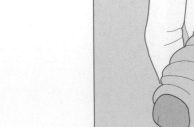

Figure 21.5 ●
Retracting the foreskin.

| **TECHNIQUES AND NORMAL FINDINGS** | **ABNORMAL FINDINGS SPECIAL CONSIDERATIONS** |

- Gently move the foreskin back into place over the glans. The foreskin should move smoothly.

6. **Assess the position of the urinary meatus.**
   - The meatus should be located in the center of the tip of the penis (see Figure 21.6 ●).

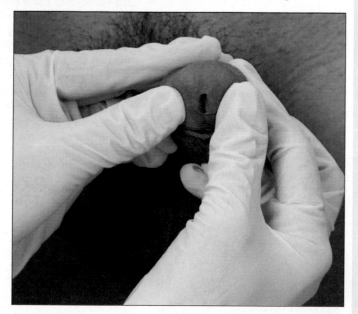

Figure 21.6 ●
Assessing the position of the urinary meatus.

7. **Inspect the scrotum.**
   - Ask the client to hold his penis up so that the scrotum is fully exposed (see Figure 21.7 ●). Optionally, you may hold the penis up by letting it rest on the back of your nondominant hand.

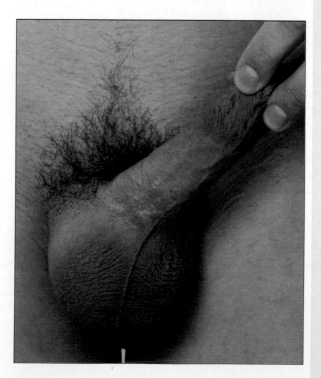

Figure 21.7 ●
Inspecting the scrotum.

▶ Immediate assistance must be sought if the foreskin cannot be retracted. Prolonged constriction of the vessels can obstruct blood flow and lead to tissue damage or necrosis.

▶ In rare cases, the urinary meatus is located on the upper side of the glans (*epispadias*) or the under side of the glans (*hypospadias*). These conditions are usually corrected surgically shortly after birth.

▶ A pinpoint appearance of the urinary meatus is indicative of **urethral stricture.**

TECHNIQUES AND NORMAL FINDINGS

- Observe the shape of the scrotum and how it hangs. It should be pear shaped, with the left side hanging lower than the right.

- Inspect the front and back of the scrotum. The skin should be wrinkled, loosely fitting over its internal structures. Note any swelling, redness, distended veins, and lesions. If swelling is present, note if it is unilateral or bilateral.

- If you detect a mass, you may want to perform transillumination.

- In a darkened room, place a lighted flashlight behind the area in which the abnormal mass was palpated (see Figure 21.8 ●).

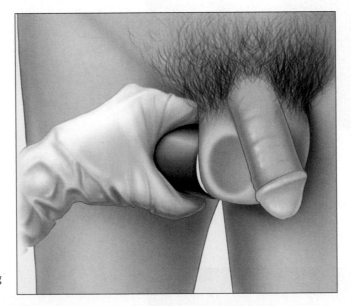

Figure 21.8 ●
Transilluminating
the scrotum.

- Note that the light shines through the scrotum with a red glow. The testicle shows up as a nontransparent oval structure.

- Repeat these steps on the other side and compare the results.

8. **Inspect the inguinal area.**
   - The inguinal area should be flat. This may be difficult to confirm if the client is overweight. Even in the presence of adipose tissue, the contour of the inguinal area should be consistent with the rest of the body. Lymph nodes are present in this location, but not normally visible.
   - Inspect both the right and left inguinal areas with the client breathing normally.
   - Have the client hold his breath and bear down as if having a bowel movement.
   - Observe for any evidence of lumps or masses. The contour of the inguinal areas should remain even.

▶ An appearance of flatness could suggest testicular abnormality. Elderly males may have a pendulous, sagging scrotal sac.

▶ Scrotal swelling and inflammation could suggest problems such as **orchitis** (inflammation of the testicles), *epididymitis* (inflammation of the epididymis), *scrotal edema* (an accumulation of fluid in the scrotum), *scrotal hernia,* or *testicular torsion* (twisting of the testicle onto the spermatic cord). Swelling and inflammation may also be seen in renal, cardiovascular, and other systemic disorders.

▶ Note any area where the light does not transilluminate. Light will not penetrate a mass. Masses may indicate *testicular tumor,* **spermatocele** (a cyst located in the epididymis), or other conditions.

▶ Masses or lumps may be related to the presence of an inguinal hernia or cancer within the reproductive, abdominal, urinary, lymphatic, and other systems.

| **TECHNIQUES AND NORMAL FINDINGS** | **ABNORMAL FINDINGS SPECIAL CONSIDERATIONS** |

PALPATION

1. **Palpate the penis.**
   - Place the glans between your thumb and forefinger.
   - Gently compress the glans, allowing the meatus to gape open (see Figure 21.9 ●). The meatus should be pink, patent, and free of discharge.

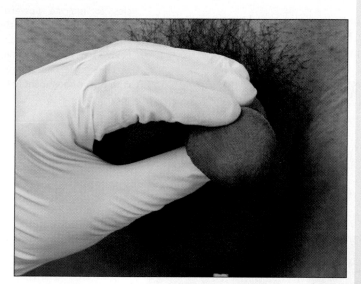

Figure 21.9 ●
Palpating the penis.

   - Note any discharge or tenderness.

   - Continue gentle palpation and compression up the entire shaft of the penis.

2. **Palpate the scrotum.**
   - Ask the client to hold his penis up to expose the scrotum.
   - Gently palpate the left and then the right scrotal sacs (see Figure 21.10 ●). Each scrotal sac should be nontender, soft, and boggy. The structures within the sacs should move easily with your palpation.

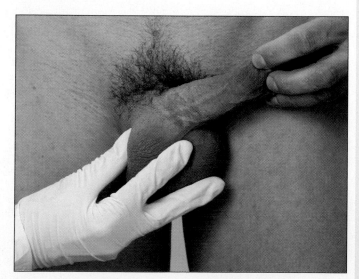

Figure 21.10 ●
Palpating the scrotum.

   - Note any tenderness, swelling, masses, lesions, or nodules.

▶ The client may be hesitant to verbalize pain when palpation is performed. It is important to watch for nonverbal facial and body gestures.

▶ A *urethral stricture* is suspected if the meatus is only about the size of a pinpoint.

▶ Signs of *urethritis* include redness and edema around the glans and foreskin, eversion of urethral mucosa, and drainage. If urethritis is suspected, the client should be asked if he experiences itching and tenderness around the meatus and painful urination. If drainage is present, observe for color, consistency, odor, and amount. Obtain a specimen if indicated. Suspect a gonococcal infection (gonorrhea) if the drainage is profuse and thick, purulent, and greenish yellow.

▶ Consider inflammation or infection higher up in the urinary tract if redness, edema, and discharge are visible around the urethral opening, because the mucous membrane in the urethra is continuous with the mucous membrane in the rest of the tract.

▶ Be alert for any lesions, masses, swelling, or nodules.

▶ Note characteristics of any abnormal findings. Culture any discharge.

▶ Assess shape, size, consistency, location, and mobility of any masses. If the client expresses pain, lift the scrotum. If the pain is relieved, the client may have epididymitis, inflammation of the epididymis.

TECHNIQUES AND NORMAL FINDINGS	ABNORMAL FINDINGS SPECIAL CONSIDERATIONS

ALERT!

If you cannot insert your finger with gentle pressure, do not force your finger into the opening.

3. **Palpate the testes.**

    - Be sure that your hands are warm.

    - Approach each testis from the bottom of the scrotal sac and gently rotate it between your thumb and fingertips (see Figure 21.11 ●). Each testis should be nontender, oval shaped, walnut-sized, smooth, elastic, and solid.

    ▶ The cremasteric reflex may cause the testicles to migrate upward temporarily. Cold hands, a cold room, or the stimulus of touch could cause this response. To prevent this reflexive action when examining a child, have him sit tailor style. Gentle pressure over the canal with the nondominant hand can reduce this response.

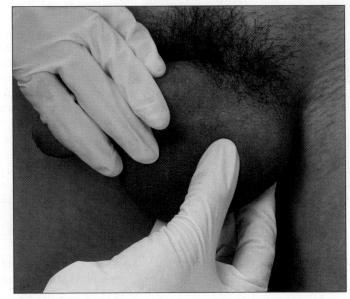

Figure 21.11 ●
Palpating the testes.

4. **Palpate the epididymis.**

    - Slide your fingertips around to the posterior side of each testicle to find the epididymis, a small, crescent-shaped structure.

    ▶ In some clients, the epididymis may be palpated on the front surface of each testis.

5. **Palpate the spermatic cord.**

    - Slide your fingers up just above the testicle, feeling for a vertical, ropelike structure about 3 mm wide.

    ▶ A cord that is hard, beaded, or nodular could indicate the presence of a varicosity or varicocele. A **varicocele** is a distended cord and is a common cause of male infertility. Upon palpation, it may feel like a "bag of worms."

| **TECHNIQUES AND NORMAL FINDINGS** | **ABNORMAL FINDINGS SPECIAL CONSIDERATIONS** |

- Gently grasp the cord between your thumb and index finger (see Figure 21.12 ●).

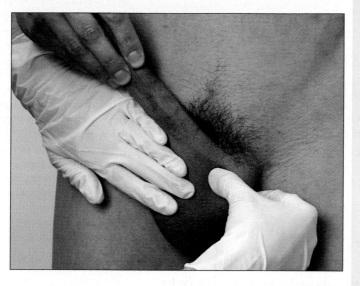

Figure 21.12 ●
Palpating the
spermatic cord.

- Do not squeeze or pinch. Trace the cord up to the external inguinal ring using a gentle rotating motion.
- The cord should feel thin, smooth, nontender to palpation, and resilient.

6. **Palpate the inguinal region.**
   - Start by preparing the client for palpation in the right inguinal area.
   - Ask the client to shift his balance so that his weight is on his left leg.
   - Place your right index finger in the upper corner of the right scrotum.
   - Slowly palpate the spermatic cord up and slightly to the client's left.
   - Allow the client's scrotal skin to fold over your index finger as you palpate.
   - Proceed until you feel an opening that feels like a triangular slit. This is the external ring of the inguinal canal. Attempt to gently glide your finger into this opening (see Figure 21.13 ●).

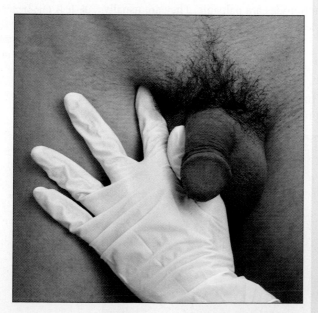

Figure 21.13 ●
Palpating the inguinal
canal.

TECHNIQUES AND NORMAL FINDINGS

- If the opening has admitted your finger, ask the client to either cough or bear down.
- Palpate for masses or lumps.

ALERT!

Do not pinch or squeeze any mass, lesion, or other structure.

- Repeat this procedure by palpating the client's left inguinal area. Use your left index finger when performing the palpation.

7. **Palpate the inguinal lymph chain.**
   - Using the pads of your first three fingers, palpate the inguinal lymph nodes.
   - Confirm that nodes are nonpalpable and the area is nontender (see Figure 21.14 ●).

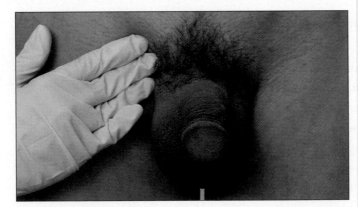

Figure 21.14 ●
Palpating the inguinal lymph nodes.

- Occasionally some of the inguinal lymph nodes are palpable. They are usually less than 0.5 cm in size, spongy, movable, and nontender.

8. **Inspect the perianal area.**
   - Reposition the client. Ask the client to turn and face the table and bend over at the waist. The client can rest his arms on the table (see Figure 21.15 ●).

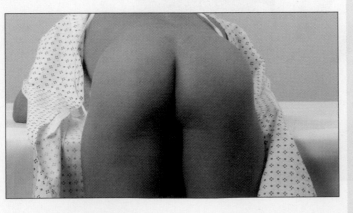

Figure 21.15 ●
Positioning for assessment of internal structures.

▶ An *inguinal hernia* feels like a bulge or mass.

▶ A *direct inguinal hernia* can be palpated in the area of the external ring of the inguinal ligament. It will be felt either right at the external ring opening or just behind it.

▶ An *indirect inguinal hernia* is more common, especially in younger males. It is located deeper in the inguinal canal than the direct inguinal hernia. It can pass into the scrotum, whereas a direct inguinal hernia rarely protrudes into the scrotum.

▶ It is also possible that a *femoral hernia* may be present. It is more commonly found in the right inguinal area and near the inguinal ligament. Table 21.1 illustrates these three types of hernias. If the client displays an acute bulge with tenderness, pain, nausea, or vomiting, he may have a strangulated hernia. Help him to lie down and request immediate medical assistance.

▶ It is important to assess if a node is larger than 0.5 cm or if multiple nodes are present. Tenderness in this area suggests infection of the scrotum, penis, or groin area.

TECHNIQUES AND NORMAL FINDINGS	ABNORMAL FINDINGS SPECIAL CONSIDERATIONS

- If the client is unable to tolerate this position, he may lie on his left side on the examination table with both knees flexed.
- Inspect the sacrococcygeal and perianal areas. The skin should be smooth and without lesions.

▶ Tufts of hair or dimpling at the sacrococcygeal area are associated with pilonidal cysts. Rashes, redness, excoriation, or inflammation in the perianal area can signal infection or parasitic infestation.

9. Palpate the sacrococcygeal and perianal areas.

- The areas should be nontender and without palpable masses.

▶ Tenderness, mass, or inflammation may indicate pilonidal cyst, anal abscess, fissure, or pruritus.

10. Inspect the anus.

- Spread the buttocks apart. Visualize the anus. The skin is darker and coarse. The area should be free of lesions.
- Ask the client to bear down. The tissue stretches, but there are no bulges or discharge.

▶ Lesions may include skin tags, warts, hemorrhoids, or fissures.

▶ Fistulas, fissures, internal hemorrhoids, or rectal prolapse are more easily detected when the client bears down.

11. Palpate the bulbourethral gland and the prostate gland.

- Lubricate your right index finger with lubricating gel.
- Tell the client that you are going to insert your finger into his rectum in order to palpate his prostate gland. Explain that the insertion may cause him to feel as if he needs to have a bowel movement. Tell him that this technique should not cause pain but to inform you immediately if it does.
- Place the index finger of your dominant hand against the anal opening (see Figure 21.16 ●). Be sure that your finger is slightly bent and not forming a right angle to the buttocks. If you insert your index finger at a right angle to the buttocks, the client may experience pain.

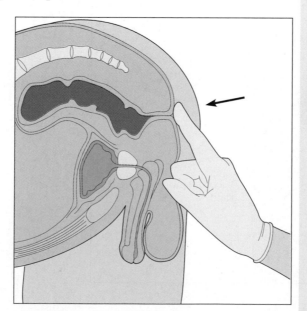

Figure 21.16 ●
Placing the finger against the anal opening

TECHNIQUES AND NORMAL FINDINGS	ABNORMAL FINDINGS SPECIAL CONSIDERATIONS

- Apply gentle pressure as you insert your bent finger into the anus (see Figure 21.17 ●).

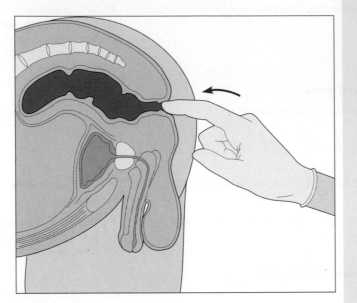

Figure 21.17 ●
Inserting the finger into the anus.

- As the sphincter muscle tightens, stop inserting your finger.
- Resume as the sphincter muscle relaxes.
- Press your right thumb gently against the perianal area.
- Palpate the bulbourethral gland by pressing your index finger gently toward your thumb (see Figure 21.18 ●). This should not cause the client to feel pain or tenderness. No swelling or masses should be felt.

▶ If the bulbourethral gland is inflamed, the client may feel pain upon palpation. Referral for further examination is warranted.

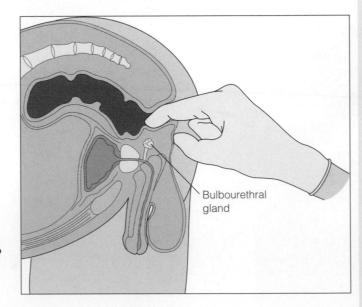

Bulbourethral gland

Figure 21.18 ●
Palpating the bulbourethral gland.

| **TECHNIQUES AND NORMAL FINDINGS** | **ABNORMAL FINDINGS SPECIAL CONSIDERATIONS** |

- Release the pressure between your index finger and thumb. Continue to insert your index finger gently (see Figure 21.19 ●).

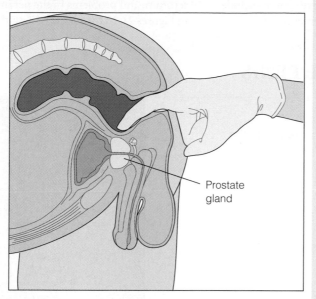

Prostate gland

Figure 21.19 ●
Palpating the prostate gland.

- Palpate the posterior surface of the prostate gland.
- Confirm that it is smooth, firm, even somewhat rubbery, nontender, and extends out no more than 1 cm into the rectal area.

▶ Note tenderness, masses, nodules, hardness, or softness. Nodules are characteristic of *prostate cancer*. Tenderness indicates inflammation.

- Remove your finger slowly and gently.
- Remove your gloves.
- Help the client to a standing position.
- Wash your hands.
- Give the client tissues to wipe the perianal area.

12. Stool Examination

- Inspect feces remaining on the gloved finger. Feces are normally brown and soft.

▶ Rectal bleeding is suspected when bright red blood is on the surface of the stool. Feces mixed with bright red blood is associated with bleeding above the rectum. Black, tarry stool is associated with upper gastrointestinal tract bleeding.

- Test feces for occult blood. Normally, the test is negative. A positive test may signal the presence of occult blood but may occur if red meat was eaten within 3 days of the test.

 Refer to the Companion Website at **www.prenhall.com/damico** and click on the **Documentation** module for documentation samples and documentation practice exercises.

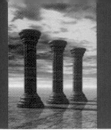
Abnormal findings of the male reproductive system include inguinal hernias, disorders of the penis, abnormalities of the scrotum, and problems in the perianal area. These are depicted in Figures 21.20 through 21.37 on the following pages.

ABNORMALITIES OF THE PENIS

Hypospadias

Hypospadias is congenital displacement of the meatus to the inferior surface of the penis (see Figure 21.20 ●)

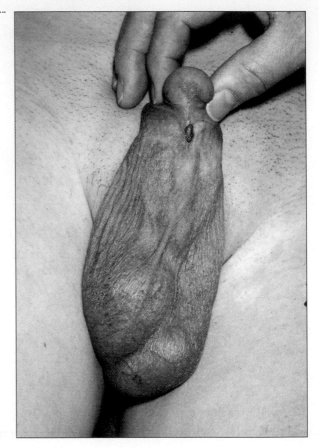

Figure 21.20 ● Hypospadias

Peyronie's Disease

In Peyronie's disease, hard plaques are found along the dorsum and are palpable under the skin. These plaques result in pain and bending of the penis during erection.

Carcinoma

Carcinoma of the penis usually occurs in the glans. It appears as a reddened nodule growth, or ulcerlike lesion (see Figure 21.21 ●).

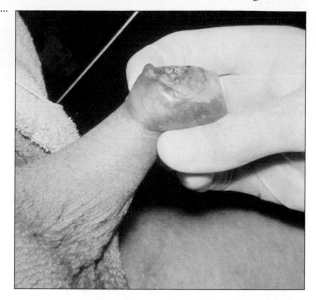

Figure 21.21 ● Carcinoma.

Genital Warts

Caused by human papillomavirus, genital warts are rapidly growing, papillar lesions (see Figure 21.22 ●).

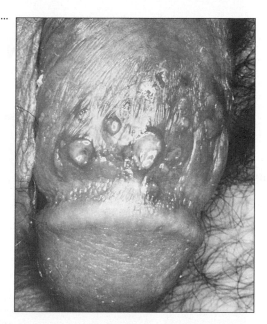

Figure 21.22 ● Genital warts.

Syphilitic Chancre

These nontender lesions appear as round or oval reddened ulcers (see Figure 21.23 ●). Lymphadenopathy is present.

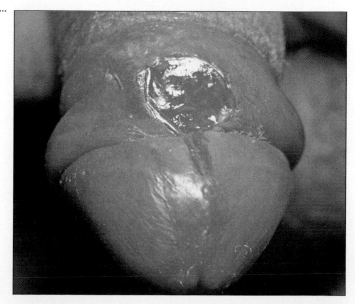

Figure 21.23 ● Syphilitic chancre.

Genital Herpes

Small vesicles appear in clusters on any part of the surface of the penis (see Figure 21.24 ●). These are painful, and the area around the vesicles is erythematous.

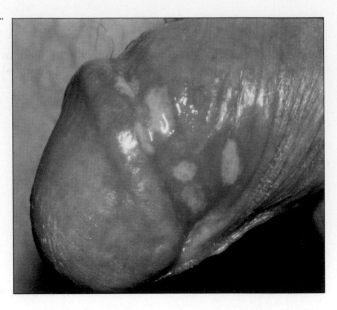

Figure 21.24 ● Genital herpes.

ABNORMAL FINDINGS IN THE SCROTUM

Hydrocele

Hydrocele is a fluid-filled mass that is nontender (see Figure 21.25 ●). The mass occurs within the tunica vaginalis.

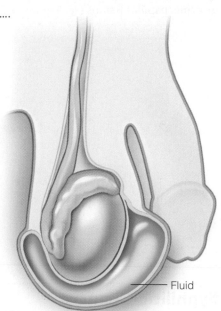

Fluid

Figure 21.25 ● Hydrocele.

Scrotal Hernia

Scrotal hernia is commonly an indirect inguinal hernia located within the scrotum (see Figure 21.26 ●).

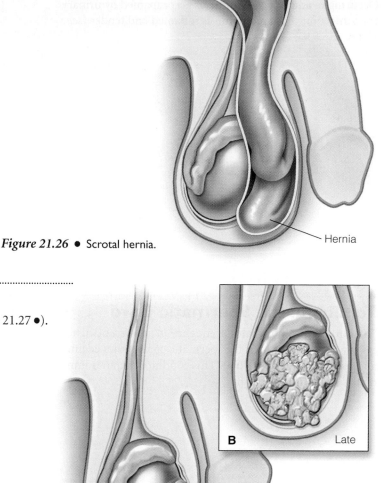

Figure 21.26 ● Scrotal hernia.

Testicular Tumor

Testicular tumor is a painless nodule on the testes (see Figure 21.27 ●). As it grows, the entire testicle seems to be overtaken.

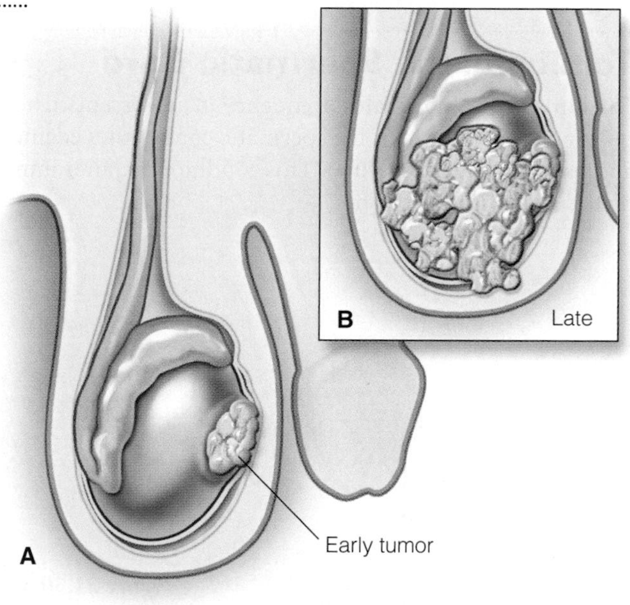

Figure 21.27 ● Testicular tumor. A. Early. B. Late.

Orchitis

This inflammatory process results in painful, tender, and swollen testes (see Figure 21. 28 ●).

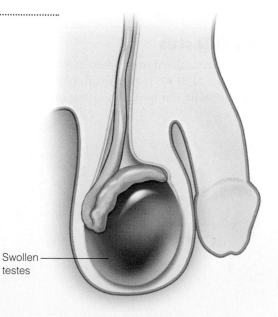

Figure 21.28 ● Orchitis.

Epididymitis

Occuring in adults, epididymitis is accompanied by urinary tract infection. The epididymis is inflamed and tender (see Figure 21.29 ●).

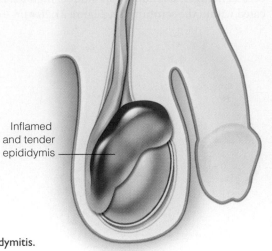

Inflamed and tender epididymis —

Figure 21.29 ● Epididymitis.

Torsion of the Spermatic Cord

Torsion occurs with greatest frequency in adolescents. The twisting of the testicle or the spermatic cord creates edema and pain (see Figure 21.30 ●). This condition requires immediate surgical intervention.

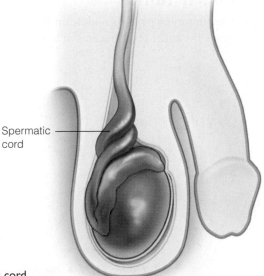

Spermatic cord —

Figure 21.30 ● Torsion of the spermatic cord.

Small Testes

Testes are considered small when they are less than 2 cm long (see Figure 21.31 ●). Testes can atrophy in liver disease, in orchitis, and with estrogen administration.

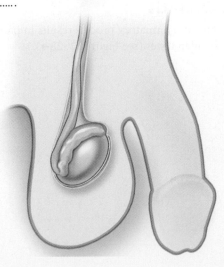

Figure 21.31 ● Small testes.

Cryptorchidism

Cryptorchidicm is absence of a testicle in the scrotal sac (see Figure 21.32 ●). This condition may result from undescended testicles.

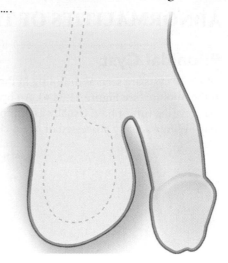

Figure 21.32 ● Cryptorchidism

Scrotal Edema

Edema of the scrotum is seen in conditions causing edema of the lower body including renal disease and heart failure (see Figure 21.33 ●).

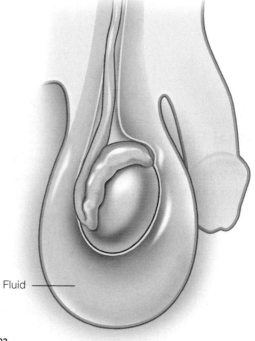

Fluid ———

Figure 21.33 ● Scrotal edema.

ABNORMALITIES OF THE PERIANAL AREA

Pilonidal Cyst

Pilonidal cysts are seen as dimpling in the sacrococcygeal area at the midline (see Figure 21.34 ●). An opening is visible and may reveal a tuft of hair. Usually asymptomatic, these cysts may become acutely abscessed or drain chronically.

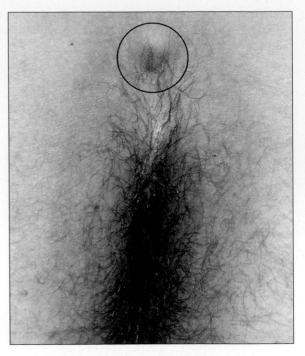

Figure 21.34 ● Pilonidal cyst.

Anal Fissure

Tears in the anal mucosa are known as fissures. These are usually seen in the posterior anal area. They are most frequently associated with passage of hard stools.

Hemorrhoids

Varicosities of the hemorrhoidal veins are called hemorrhoids or piles. These are considered normal findings in adults when they are asymptomatic.

Internal hemorrhoids occur in the venous plexus superior to the mucocutaneous junction of the anus (see Figure 21.35A ●). Internal hemorrhoids are rarely painful. They are identified by bright red bleeding unmixed with stool.

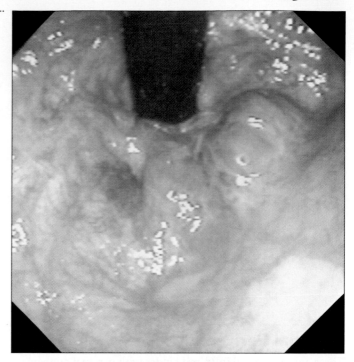

Figure 21.35A ● Hemorrhoids, internal.

External hemorrhoids occur in the inferior venous plexus inferior to the mucocutaneous junction (see Figure 21.35B ●). External hemorrhoids rarely bleed. External hemorrhoids cause anal irritation and create difficulty with cleansing the area.

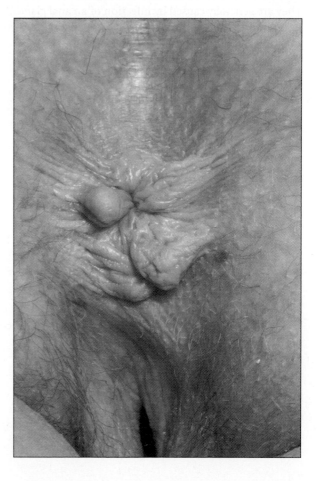

Figure 21.35B ● Hemorrhoids, external.

Prolapse of the Rectum

A prolapse occurs when the rectal mucosa, with or without the muscle, protrudes through the anus (see Figure 21.36 ●). In mucosal prolapse, a round or oval pink protrusion is seen outside the anus. When the muscular wall is involved, a large red protrusion is visible.

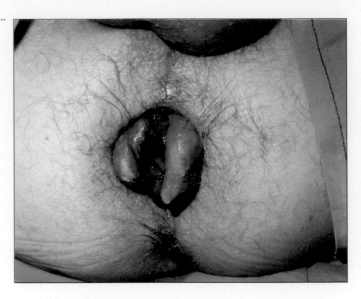

Figure 21.36 ● Prolapse of the rectum.

Perianal Perirectal Abscess

These abscesses are painful and tender with perianal erythema. They are generally caused by infection of an anal gland. Anal abscesses can lead to fistulas, which are openings between the anal canal and the outside skin (see Figure 21.37 ●).

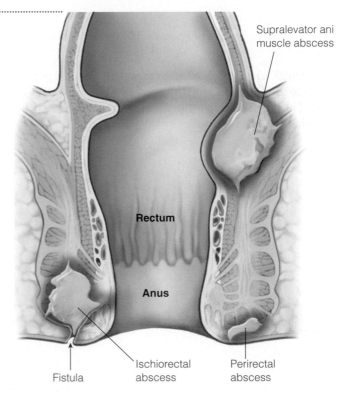

Figure 21.37 ● Perianal perirectal abscess.

Health Promotion

HEALTHY PEOPLE 2010

FOCUS AREA	PREVALENCE	OBJECTIVES	ACTIONS
Sexually Transmitted Diseases (STDs)	• Higher rates of STDs occur in African American and Hispanic populations than in whites. • HIV infection is highest in African American males between 25 and 44 years of age. • Substance abuse increases irresponsible sexual behavior. As a result there can be an increase in STD. • The use of alcohol and illicit drugs is higher in white males than in other groups.	• Reduce the numbers of individuals with STD. • Increase the use of condoms. • Reduce HIV infections.	• Individual, school, and community programs to promote responsible sexual behavior. • Education about risks associated with substance abuse.
Prostate Cancer	• Prostate cancer is second as a cause of cancer deaths in males in the United States. • Almost 80% of prostate cancer occurs in males over 65 years of age.	• Reduce the prostate cancer death rate.	• Screening for prostate cancer. • The benefits of early screening and detection are uncertain. Clinical trials of screening measures are in progress.

CLIENT EDUCATION

The following are physiological, behavioral, and cultural factors that affect the health of the male reproductive system across the age span. Several factors reflect trends cited in *Healthy People 2010*. The nurse provides advice and education to reduce risks associated with the aforementioned factors and to promote and maintain the health of the male reproductive system.

LIFE SPAN CONSIDERATIONS

RISK FACTORS

- Infants may be born with ambiguous external genital organs.

- Approximately 3% of males are born with cryptorchidism (undescended testicles). Cryptorchidism is a risk factor for testicular cancer.
- Adolescents are interested in exploring their sexuality, and the number of sexually active teenagers is increasing.
- The occurrence of an STD in infants and children often indicates sexual abuse.

- Changes in reproductive organs and sexual drive occur with aging.

CLIENT EDUCATION

- Counsel and support parents when making decisions about intervention for ambiguous external genitalia.
- Advise parents that surgery to correct cryptorchidism should occur before age 1 to decrease the risk of testicular cancer.
- Inform males from adolescence through the middle adult years about testicular self-examination (see Box 21.1).
- Instruct parents and guardians to observe and seek treatment for problems with external genitalia that may signal the presence of an STD (drainage, itching, painful urination).
- Advise parents to observe for changes in behavior, appetite, activity in school, and friends that can signal problems associated with sexual activity, concern about sexual identity, or abuse.
- Advise older males that changes in external genitalia are a normal part of aging.

CULTURAL CONSIDERATIONS

RISK FACTOR

- Prostate cancer occurs more frequently in African American males than in other ethnic groups.

CLIENT EDUCATION

- Advise males to follow recommendations for screening for prostate cancer, which include laboratory testing for prostate-specific antigen (PSA) and digital rectal exam (DRE) annually after 50 years of age. African American males, especially those with a family history of prostate cancer, should begin screening at age 45. Males should be informed of symptoms of prostate enlargement, which requires follow-up. These include frequent urination, dysuria, difficulty initiating or stopping urination, a change in the urine stream, and pain in the back, hips, or upper thighs.

ENVIRONMENTAL CONSIDERATIONS

RISK FACTOR

- Uncircumcised males are at greater risk of irritation to the penis and possibly penile cancer.

CLIENT EDUCATION

- Instruct clients and parents of uncircumcised infant males regarding retraction of the foreskin when cleaning the penis.

BEHAVIORAL CONSIDERATIONS

RISK FACTORS

- Human papillomavirus (HPV) increases the risk for penile cancer. HPV occurs in males who begin sexual relations at an early age, have multiple partners, have sexual relations with a female who has had multiple partners, and have unprotected sexual activity.
- Smoking and eating foods with high fat amounts are associated with increased risk of cancers of the male reproductive system.
- Psychosocial factors including anxiety, stress, and grief can affect sexual behavior across the age span.

CLIENT EDUCATION

- Provide information about safe sex practices to all males to reduce risk of all STDs.

- Inform clients about smoking cessation programs and reduction of fat in their diet as methods to reduce the risk of cancers of the male reproductive system.
- Provide counseling when clients experience a decrease in sexual desire or ability to perform. Explore the reason for the problems. Physiological changes may be involved and include the effects of some medications and treatments. Psychosocial problems including stress, anxiety, or grief may contribute to the problem and warrant counseling.

Application Through Critical Thinking

CASE STUDY

James Lewis is a 24-year-old male who is seen in the clinic for "pain in the groin." During the interview the client states, "I have a soreness in my groin area on both sides." Mr. Lewis denies any trauma to the area, states he has not done any heavy lifting, nor has he been involved in athletic activities or "working out." He reports that he is in good health. He does not take any medications ex-

cept vitamins and occasionally some nonaspirin product for a headache. He denies nausea, vomiting, diarrhea, or fever. He has no pain in his legs or back. He tells the nurse his appetite is okay but he is tired. He thinks his fatigue is because he's been "a little worried about this problem and really having a hard time deciding to come in for help."

When asked about the onset of the problem, Mr. Lewis explains that he "started feeling some achiness about a week ago." When asked if he has ever experienced these feelings before, he replies, "No." He is then asked to describe or discuss any other symptoms. He looks away, shifts in his chair, and then says, "Well, I have had some burning when I pass urine and it's kind of cloudy."

When asked if he has ever had a problem like this before, he replies, "Yes, about 2 months ago." With further questioning, the nurse learns that Mr. Lewis was diagnosed with gonorrhea and treated with an injection and pills he was supposed to take for a week. He says he was not supposed to have sex until he finished the pills. When asked if he followed the prescribed treatment, he reluctantly responds that he finished all but a couple of pills and he did have sex with one of his girlfriends about 4 or 5 days after he got the injection.

Mr. Lewis tells the nurse he did not inform his girlfriends of his problem and he generally avoids condoms because "I've known these girls for a long time."

The physical examination yields the following information: B/P 128/86—P 96—RR 20—T 98.6. His color is pale, and the skin is moist and warm. External genitalia are intact, without lesions or erythema. There is lymphadenopathy in bilateral groin areas. Compression of the glans yields milky discharge. A smear of urethral discharge is obtained.

The nurse knows that Mr. Lewis's original gonococcal infection was treated with an injection, most likely ceftriaxone. The nurse also knows that chlamydia is present in almost half of the clients with gonorrhea and is treated with a 7-day regimen of oral antibiotics. Between 40 and 60% of clients with gonorrhea have lymphadenopathy.

Based on the data, the nurse suspects that Mr. Lewis has a reinfection with gonorrhea and may have a concomitant chlamydial infection.

The nurse recommends single-injection treatment for gonorrhea and a new oral regimen for chlamydia. A urine specimen will be obtained and submitted with the urethral discharge smear. The client will be scheduled for a follow-up phone conference about the laboratory results in 48 hours and a return visit in 7 days. The nurse conducts an information, education, and advice session prior to discharge from the clinic.

► Complete Documentation

The following is sample documentation for James Lewis.
SUBJECTIVE DATA: Seeking care for "pain in groin." Pain in groin bilateral. Denies trauma, heavy lifting, athletic activity, or "working out." Reports he is in "good health." Takes no medications except vitamins and nonaspirin product for a headache. Denies nausea, vomiting, diarrhea, or fever. No pain in back or legs. Reports "okay" appetite. Reports fatigue. "Became a little worried about this problem and decided to come in for help." Achiness 1 week ago. Burning on urination, cloudy urine. Gonorrhea diagnosis 2 months ago, treated with injection and oral meds. Did not complete prescription and had intercourse "4 or 5 days after injection." Did not inform partners of diagnosis, generally avoids condoms.
OBJECTIVE DATA: VS: B/P 120/86—P 96—RR 20—T 98.6°F. Color pale, skin moist and warm. External genitalia intact, no lesions or erythema. Lymphadenopathy bilateral groin. Milky discharge on compression of glans. Culture to lab.

► Critical Thinking Questions

1. Describe the critical thinking process as applied by the nurse to direct the care of this client.
2. What additional data should the nurse seek when conducting the health assessment for this client?

ASSESSMENT FORM	
Reason for Visit: *"Pain in groin"*	
History:	
Reproductive Disease:	*Gonorrhea 2 mos. ago (did not finish oral meds)*
Medications:	*Vitamins, nonaspirin product for headache*
Sexual History:	*Multiple partners*
Condom Use:	*None*
HIV Testing:	*Unknown*
Erectile Function:	*Unknown*
Safety:	*Not inform partners of diagnosis*
Other:	*Burning on urination, cloudy urine, fatigue, okay appetite*
Physical Findings:	
External Genitalia:	*No lesions, no erythema*
Meatus:	*Milky discharge on compression of glans (specimen to labs)*
Inguinal Area:	*Lymphadenopathy (bilateral)*

3. What data informed the nurse of a need to provide education for the client?

4. What data will the nurse seek upon the return visit with Mr. Lewis?

▶ Applying Nursing Diagnoses

1. *Ineffective sexuality patterns* is a nursing diagnosis in the NANDA taxonomy (see Appendix A ⬤). Do the data for James Lewis support this diagnosis? If so, identify the data that support the diagnosis.

2. Identify additional diagnoses suggested in the data. Develop PES statements.

▶ Prepare Teaching Plan

LEARNING NEED: The data from the case study reveal that James Lewis has an ongoing problem with sexually transmitted diseases, particularly gonorrhea. The data reveal that Mr. Lewis has not followed recommendations for a previous infection. Education and counseling will be provided for this client.

The case study provides data that is representative of concerns about sexually transmitted disease, especially gonorrhea, of many individuals. Therefore, the following teaching plan is based on the need to provide information to members of any community about gonorrhea.

GOAL: The participants in this learning program will have the knowledge to prevent contraction and transmission of gonorrhea.

OBJECTIVES: At the completion of this learning session the participants will be able to:

1. Describe gonorrhea.

2. Identify symptoms of gonorrhea.

3. Discuss treatment strategies.

4. Describe methods to prevent contraction and transmission of gonorrhea.

APPLICATION OF OBJECTIVE 4: Describe methods to prevent contraction and transmission of gonorrhea

Content	Teaching Strategy	Evaluation
• Avoid sexual partners whose health status is unclear. • Use condoms correctly and consistently during sexual intercourse. • When infected, notify all sexual contacts so they can be treated. Refrain from sexual contact for 1 week after treatment is completed. Take all prescribed medications exactly as ordered until they are gone.	• Lecture • Discussion • Audiovisual materials • Printed materials Lecture is appropriate when disseminating information to large groups. Discussion allows participants to bring up concerns and to raise questions. Audiovisual materials such as illustrations of the genitals and reproductive structures reinforce verbal presentation. Printed material allows review, reinforcement, and reading at the learner's pace.	• Written examination. May use short answer, fill-in-the-blank, multiple-choice items, or a combination of items. If these are short and easy to evaluate, the learner receives immediate feedback.

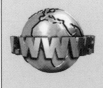

Please refer to the Companion Website at www.prenhall.com/damico and click on Chapter 21, the Application Through Critical Thinking module, to complete the following activities related to this case study:

▶ **Critical Thinking questions**
▶ **Extended Nursing Diagnosis challenge**
▶ **Documentation activity**
▶ **Teaching Plan for Objectives 1, 2, and 3**

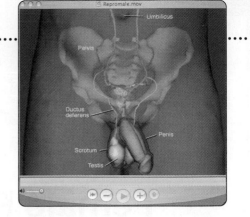

EXPLORE MediaLink

Additional resources for this chapter are found on the Student CD-ROM accompanying this textbook and on the Companion Website.

CD-ROM CONTENT

Content for this chapter includes:

Objectives
Key Concepts
NCLEX-RN® Review Questions
Model Documentation Forms
Audio Glossary
Animations
   Male Genitalia Anatomy
   Male Urinary Tract Anatomy
Games and Challenges
Clinical Spotlight Videos
   Testicular Self-Examination
   Identifying Child Abuse
   Circumcision
Head-to-Toe Physical Examination Video

COMPANION WEBSITE CONTENT

www.prenhall.com/damico

Content for this chapter includes:

Objectives
NCLEX-RN® Review Questions

Client Interaction Case Study Challenge
Application Through Critical Thinking
   Case Study Teaching Plan Challenge
MediaLinks
MediaLink Application
Tool Box
   Chapter Documentation Form Example
   Maturation Stages in the Male
   Health Promotion
      Healthy People 2010
      Client Education
New York Times

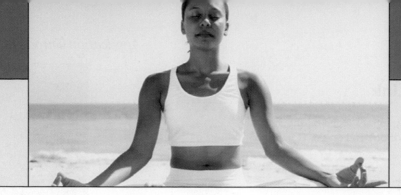

22

Female Reproductive System

MEDIALINK

www.prenhall.com/damico

The CD-ROM in the back of this textbook and the Media-Link website contain NCLEX-RN® review questions, interactive exercises, case study challenges, animations, videos, documentation and checklist forms, and review materials. For a complete listing of the media content specific to Chapter 22, see the Explore MediaLink at the end of the chapter.

*T*he female reproductive system provides for both human reproduction and sexual gratification. Many factors influence the female client's reproductive health on both physiological and psychological levels. Assessment of the client's psychosocial health, self-care habits, family, culture, and environment is an important part of the focused interview. The nurse must keep these findings in mind when conducting the physical assessment. The nurse also must have a thorough understanding of the constituents of a healthy reproductive system and be able to consider the relationship of other body systems to the reproductive system.

Throughout assessment of the female reproductive system, the nurse considers not only the function of the reproductive system but also the client's sexual fulfillment on both a physical and psychological basis. Reproductive health is reflected in the focus areas of *Healthy People 2010*. Goals concerning unintended pregnancy, maternal deaths, and STDs are included in the *Healthy People 2010* feature on page 661.

Nurses need to understand their own feelings and comfort about various aspects of sexuality to be efficient in gathering data. They must put aside personal beliefs and values about sexual practices and focus in a nonjudgmental manner on gathering data to determine the health status of the client.

It is essential to create an atmosphere that facilitates open communication and comfort for the client. Clients commonly experience anxiety, fear, and embarrassment when requested for information about a topic that, in most clients' minds, is very personal. These emotions may be expressed either verbally or nonverbally. The nurse should approach the client in as nonthreatening a manner as possible and assure the client that the information provided and the results of the physical examination will remain confidential.

ANATOMY AND PHYSIOLOGY REVIEW

The female reproductive system is unique in that it experiences cyclic changes in direct response to hormonal levels of estrogen and progesterone during the childbearing years. The uterus changes throughout the ovarian cycle during which the ova (eggs) are prepared for fertilization with sperm. During the menstrual cycle, the uterine lining is prepared for the development of a fetus. The onset of menopause represents the end of the childbearing years.

Unlike the male reproductive system, the female reproductive tract is completely separate from the urinary tract. However, structures of the two tracts lie within close proximity.

The functions of the female reproductive system are the following:

- Manufacturing and protecting ova for fertilization
- Transporting the fertilized ovum for implantation and embryonic/fetal development
- Regulating hormonal production and secretion of several sex hormones
- Providing sexual stimulation and pleasure

EXTERNAL GENITALIA

Female external genitalia include the mons pubis, labia, glands, clitoris, and perianal area. These will be described in the following sections.

Mons Pubis

The mons pubis is the mound of adipose tissue overlying the symphysis pubis (see Figure 22.1 ●). In the mature female, it is thickly covered with hair and provides protection to the underlying reproductive structures.

Labia Majora and Labia Minora

The **labia** are a dual set of liplike structures lying on either side of the vagina (Figure 22.1). The exterior labia majora are two thick, elongated pads of tissue that become more full toward the center. An extension of the external skin surface, the labia majora are covered with coarse hair extending from the mons pubis. The enclosed labia minora are

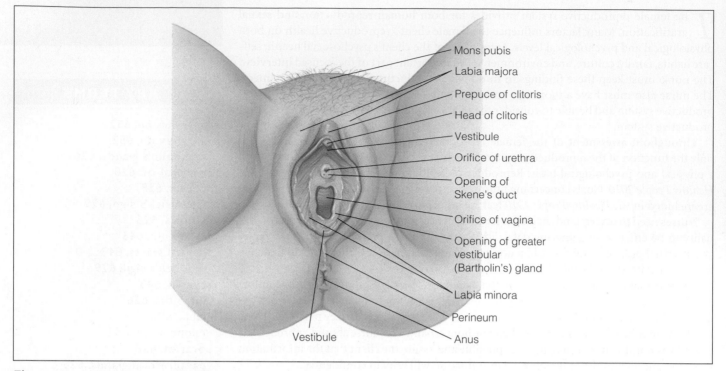

Figure 22.1 ● External female genitalia.

two thin, elongated pads of tissue that overlie the vaginal and urethral openings, as well as several glandular openings. Anteriorly, the labia minora join to form the prepuce, which covers the clitoris. Posteriorly, the labia join to form the *fourchette* (small fold of membrane). The labia minora border an almond-shaped area of tissue known as the *vestibule.* It extends from the clitoris to the fourchette. The urethral meatus, vaginal opening (**introitus**), Skene's glands, and Bartholin's glands lie within the vestibule. The major function of the labia is providing protection from infection and physical injury to the urethra and vagina, and ultimately other urinary and reproductive structures.

Skene's and Bartholin's Glands

The Skene's glands, also called **paraurethral glands,** are located just posterior to the urethra (Figure 22.1). They open into the urethra and secrete a fluid that lubricates the vaginal vestibule during sexual intercourse. The **Bartholin's glands,** or greater vestibular glands, are located posteriorly at the base of the vestibule and produce mucus, which is released into the vestibule (Figure 22.1). This mucus actively promotes sperm motility and viability.

Clitoris

Located at the anterior of the vestibule is the **clitoris,** a small, elongated mound of erectile tissue (Figure 22.1). As the labia minora merge together anteriorly, a small hoodlike covering is formed that lies over the top of the clitoris. The clitoris is homologous with the penis. It is permeated with numerous nerve fibers responsive to touch. When stimulated, the clitoris becomes erect as its underlying corpus cavernosa become vaso-

congested. The major function of the clitoris is serving as the primary organ of sexual stimulation.

Perianal Area

The perianal area is bordered anteriorly by the top of the labial folds, laterally by the ischial tuberosities, and posteriorly by the anus (Figure 22.1). The anus is the terminal end of the gastrointestinal system. The anal canal opens onto the perineum at the midpoint of the gluteal folds. The external muscles of the anal canal are skeletal muscles, which form the part of the anal sphincter that voluntarily controls stool evacuation. The anal mucosa is smooth, moist, hairless, and darkly pigmented.

INTERNAL REPRODUCTIVE ORGANS

The internal female reproductive organs are the vagina, uterus, cervix, fallopian tubes, and ovaries. These organs will be described in the following paragraphs.

Vagina

The **vagina** is a long, tubular, muscular canal (approximately 9 to 15 cm in length) that extends from the vestibule to the cervix at the inferior end of the uterus (see Figure 22.2A ●). The muscularity of the vaginal wall and its thick, transverse rugae (ridges) allow it to dilate widely to accommodate the erect penis and, during childbirth, the head of the fetus. At the point of juncture with the cervix, a continuous circular cleft called the *fornix* is formed. The major functions of the vagina are serving as the female organ of copulation, the birth canal, and the channel for the exit of menstrual flow.

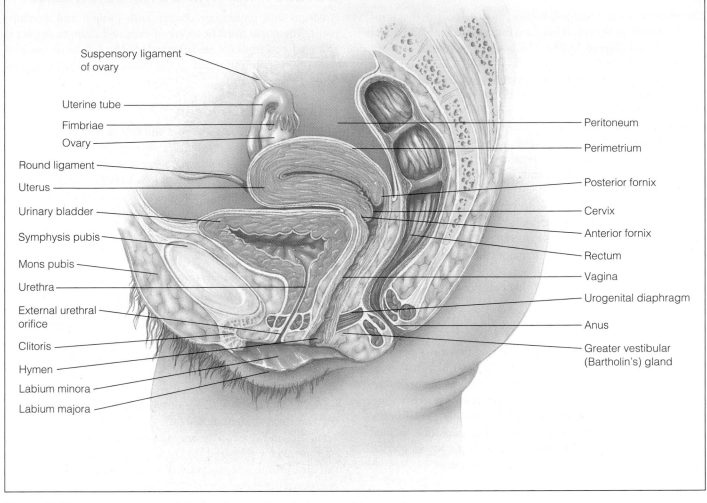

Figure 22.2A ● Internal organs of the female reproductive system within the pelvis.

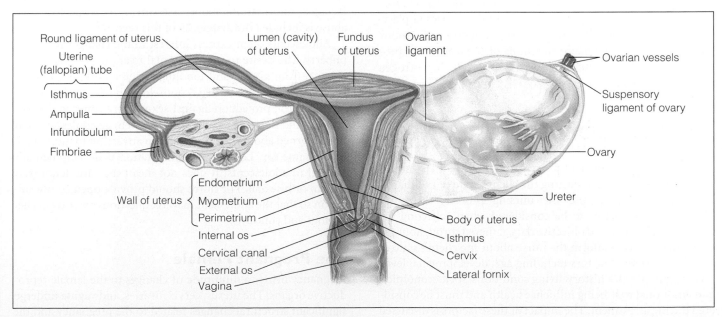

Figure 22.2B ● Cross-section of the anterior view of the female pelvis.

Uterus

The **uterus** is a pear-shaped, hollow, muscular organ that is located centrally in the pelvis between the neck of the bladder and the rectal wall (Figure 22.2A). The body of the uterus is about 4 cm wide and 6 to 8 cm in length. Its walls are 2 to 2.5 cm thick and are composed of serosal, muscular, and mucosal layers. Anatomically, the uterus is divided into three segments. These segments are the fundus, the corpus, and the cervix. The **cervix** projects into the vagina about 2.5 cm and is about 2.5 cm round. A small central canal connects the vagina to the inside of the uterus. The external **cervical os** is the inferior opening (the vaginal end of the canal), and the *internal cervical os* opens directly into the uterine chamber.

The uterus is easily moved within the pelvic cavity, but its basic position is secured with several ligaments that attach it to the pelvic floor. The ligaments also prevent the uterus from dropping into the vaginal canal. The major functions of the uterus are serving as the site of implantation of the fertilized ovum and as a protective sac for the developing embryo and fetus.

Uterine Tubes

The **uterine tubes** (or fallopian tubes) are two ducts on either side of the fundus of the uterus (Figure 22.2B ●). They are about 7 to 10 cm in length and extend from the uterus almost to the ovaries. An ovum released by an ovary travels to the uterus within the uterine tubes. Normally fertilization takes places within the uterine tubes. The major functions of the fallopian tubes include serving as the site of fertilization and providing a passageway for unfertilized and fertilized ova to travel to the uterus.

Ovaries

Lying close to the distal end of either side of the uterine tubes are the **ovaries** (Figure 22.2B). These almond-shaped glandular structures produce ova, as well as estrogen and progesterone. They are about 3 cm long and 2 cm wide. The ovarian ligaments and suspensory ligaments hold the ovaries in place. The ovaries become fully developed after puberty and atrophy after menopause. The major functions of the ovaries are producing ova for fertilization by sperm and producing estrogen and progesterone.

SPECIAL CONSIDERATIONS

Throughout the assessment process, the nurse gathers subjective and objective data reflecting the client's state of health. Using critical thinking and the nursing process, the nurse identifies many factors to be considered when collecting the data. The subjective and objective data gathered throughout the assessment process inform the nurse about the client's state of health. A variety of factors including age, developmental level, race, ethnicity, work history, living conditions, socioeconomics, and emotional well-being influence health and must be considered during assessment. The impact of these factors is discussed in the following sections.

DEVELOPMENTAL CONSIDERATIONS

Anatomy and physiology change with growth and development. The nurse must be aware of expected changes as data is gathered and findings are interpreted. The following sections describe specific variations in the female reproductive system across the age span.

Infants and Children

The female infant's labia majora will be enlarged at birth in response to maternal hormones. The labia majora should cover the labia minora. The urinary meatus and vaginal orifice should be visible. No inflammation should be present. Bloody and mucoid discharge (false menses) is commonly seen in newborns due to exposure to maternal hormones in utero.

The female child reaches puberty a few years before the male. Changes begin to occur at any time from 8 to 13 years of age; most commonly, breast changes begin at age 9 and menstruation at age 12. Release of estrogen initiates the changes, which are first demonstrated in the development of breast buds and growth of pubic hair, followed several years later by menstruation. Table 22.1 describes Tanner's stages of maturation in girls.

The female child may experience a precocious puberty. These children develop the adult female sex characteristics of dense pubic and axillary hair, breasts, and menstrual bleeding before 8 years of age. Early maturation may be caused by hypothalamic tumor. Further, the early development of sexual characteristics allows for pregnancy before the child is intellectually or emotionally prepared for the experience. Early maturation can also lead to anemia related to menstrual bleeding and to emotional difficulties.

It is essential to assess for sexual molestation with female children. Some signs of sexual molestation are trauma, depression, eating disorders, bruising, swelling, and inflammation in the vaginal, perineal, and anal areas. Additionally, the child may appear withdrawn. Often the child will deny the experience. Detailed information about assessment in suspected child abuse is included in Chapter 25 of this text. ∞

Adolescents often express interest in the changes related to puberty. The desire to explore sexual relationships and sexual contact, from kissing and fondling to intercourse, may be intense. Thus, adolescents need counseling on relationship issues, birth control, protection against sexually transmitted diseases (STDs), and delaying sexual activity. A female adolescent may be concerned about or confused by an attraction to individuals of the same sex. Lesbian experimentation is developmentally normal in adolescents. It does not mean they are definitively lesbian or bisexual. The nurse should provide open communication so that the adolescent may ask questions and express her feelings and concerns.

The Pregnant Female

Pregnancy brings a multitude of changes to the female reproductive organs. The uterus, cervix, ovaries, and vagina undergo significant structural changes related to the pregnancy and the influence of hormones.

Table 22.1 Maturation Stages in the Female

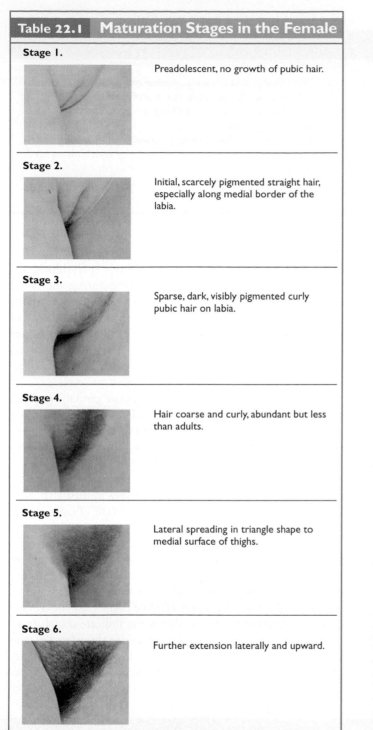

Stage 1.
Preadolescent, no growth of pubic hair.

Stage 2.
Initial, scarcely pigmented straight hair, especially along medial border of the labia.

Stage 3.
Sparse, dark, visibly pigmented curly pubic hair on labia.

Stage 4.
Hair coarse and curly, abundant but less than adults.

Stage 5.
Lateral spreading in triangle shape to medial surface of thighs.

Stage 6.
Further extension laterally and upward.

The uterus becomes hypertrophied and weighs about 1 kg (2.2 lb) by the end of pregnancy. Its capacity increases to about 5 L. The growth of the uterus during pregnancy causes it to push up into the abdominal cavity and displace the liver and intestines from their normal positions. Contractions of the uterus occur. Throughout the pregnancy, the female may have irregular Braxton Hicks contractions, which are usually not painful. However, by the end of the pregnancy, these contractions may become more intense and cause pain.

During pregnancy, the vascularity of the cervix increases and contributes to the softening of the cervix. This softening is called **Goodell's sign.** The vascular congestion creates a blue-purple blemish or change in cervical coloration. This change is considered normal and is referred to as **Chadwick's sign.** Estrogen causes the glandular cervical tissue to produce thick mucus, which builds up and forms a mucous plug at the endocervical canal. The mucous plug prevents the introduction of any foreign matter into the uterus. At the initiation of labor, this plug is expelled. This expulsion is called the "bloody show."

The vagina undergoes changes similar to those of the uterus during pregnancy. Hypertrophy of the vaginal epithelium occurs. The vaginal wall softens and relaxes to accommodate the movement of the infant during birth. The vagina also displays Chadwick's sign. A thorough discussion of the pregnant female is found in Chapter 26. ∞

The Older Adult

Reproductive ability in the female usually peaks in her late 20s. Over time, estrogen levels begin to decline. Between the ages of 46 and 55, menstrual periods become shorter and less frequent until they stop entirely. Menopause is said to have occurred when the female has not experienced a menstrual period in over a year. Other symptoms of menopause include mood changes and unpredictable episodes of sweating or hot flashes.

As the female progresses into older age, her sexual organs atrophy. Vaginal secretions are not as plentiful, and she may experience pain during intercourse. Intercourse may produce vaginal infections. The clitoris becomes smaller.

Even though older adults can achieve sexual gratification and participate in a satisfying sexual relationship, a decrease in sexual drive may contribute to the client's withdrawing from sexual experiences and relationships. Chronic or acute disease, medications, loss of a spouse or significant other, loss of privacy, depression, fatigue, stress, and use of alcohol and illicit drugs are factors known to influence sexual drive.

PSYCHOSOCIAL CONSIDERATIONS

Fatigue, depression, and stress can decrease sexual desire in a female client of any age. Grief over the loss of a relationship, whether because of separation, divorce, or death, can have long-term effects on a client's willingness to seek new relationships. Feelings of betrayal—for example, when a partner becomes intimate with another person—can have the same effect.

Past or recent trauma, as from childhood abuse, physical assault, and sexual assault, whether or not penetration occurred, may have a significant impact on a female client's ability to enjoy a sexual relationship. This may be true even if the trauma is unremembered.

Some females may fear sexual intimacy because of an altered body image related to their weight, body type, breast size, or other factors. Reproductive surgeries can affect a female client's self-image and sexual expression. For example, clients who have had a hysterectomy may feel free from the worry of unwanted pregnancy and experience an increase in sexual desire, or they may feel less feminine than before the surgery and withdraw from sexual relationships.

Cultural Considerations

- Female circumcision or female genital mutilation (FGM) is a traditional or cultural practice in Africa, Asia, and Middle Eastern countries.
- FGM is increasingly found in the United States and Canada among immigrants from Africa, Asia, and the Middle East.
- The death rate from cervical cancer is higher than average in African Americans, Hispanics, and Native Americans.
- Leiomyosarcoma, one form of uterine cancer, occurs with greater frequency in African Americans than in other groups.

- In many cultures and religions, physical examination by a health-care provider of the opposite sex is prohibited.
- Discussion of sexual activity and reproductive function is unacceptable in many cultures.
- Language barriers often prevent females from seeking or obtaining information or actual care associated with female reproductive issues.

CULTURAL AND ENVIRONMENTAL CONSIDERATIONS

Some cultures and religions have specific beliefs or encourage specific behaviors related to menstruation, female circumcision, and sexual practices. For example, many religions such as Roman Catholicism forbid premarital sex. When assessing clients, the nurse must never assume that they share all of the beliefs or follow all the practices of their religious or cultural group.

Lack of privacy can inhibit the ability to engage in experiences that promote sexual gratification. Many adults today live with older parents or grandparents. As a result, the sexual experiences for all may be affected.

Sexual dysfunction can result from sexual, physical, or verbal abuse among family members. Negative family reactions to an individual's sexual orientation and lifestyle choices may impact the individual's ability to find a sexual partner and maintain a satisfying sexual relationship. Females may choose partners who do not meet their own needs or desires because of family pressures. This can have a negative emotional and physical impact, especially among female adolescents.

Females who work in the microelectronics (high-speed electronics, such as circuit boards) industry may be exposed to arsenic, glycol ethers, lead, and radiation. These substances have been linked to birth defects and spontaneous abortions. Lead is also still present in some homes. Exposure to vinyl chloride (used in construction and building materials) may increase the

risk for stillbirths and premature births. Exposure to high concentrations of halogenated hydrocarbons polychlorinated biphenyls (PCBs), found in plastics manufacturing and in the electrical industries, is associated with low birth weight, spontaneous abortion, hyperpigmentation of infants, and microcephaly (abnormally small head size). Oncology nurses exposed to antineoplastic drugs may have spontaneous abortions, fetal anomalies, change in the regularity of their menstrual cycle, or even cessation of their menstrual cycle.

Maintaining the cleanliness of the female genitalia requires daily washing, and changing of underclothes. Douching is not only unnecessary but may even be harmful. Douching has been shown to promote irritation, rashes, and infection in some females. The likelihood of rashes or infections can be reduced by keeping the genitals dry by changing sweaty underclothes after physical exercise, changing into dry clothes immediately after bathing or swimming, and changing an infant's diaper immediately after it is wet.

Although research has shown that infections can be transmitted sexually even when the partners are using a latex condom, its use significantly lowers the incidence of transmission. A history of human papillomavirus (HPV) and more than four sexual partners in a lifetime increases a female client's risk for cervical cancer. A history of STDs in children may indicate sexual abuse.

The risk for cervical cancer is increased in those females who participate in early (before age 18) and frequent sexual activity and have a history of many sexual partners. Obesity is a risk factor for uterine cancer.

Gathering the Data

*H*ealth assessment of the female reproductive system includes gathering subjective and objective data. Collection of subjective data occurs during the client interview, before the physical assessment. The nurse uses a variety of communication techniques to elicit general and specific information about

the health of the reproductive system. Health records and the results of laboratory and clinical examinations are important secondary sources to be reviewed and included in the data-gathering process. Physical assessment of the female reproductive system includes the techniques of inspection and palpation as well as the use of equipment and techniques specific to the assessment of the female reproductive system.

FOCUSED INTERVIEW

The focused interview of the female concerns data related to the structures and functions of the reproductive system. Subjective data related to that system is gathered during the focused interview. The nurse should be prepared to observe the client and listen for cues related to the function of this body system. Open-ended or closed questions are used to obtain information. Often a number of follow-up questions or requests for descriptions are required to clarify data or gather missing information. Follow-up questions are aimed at identifying the source of problems, duration of difficulties, measures to alleviate problems, and clues about the client's knowledge of her own health.

Information about the genital areas, reproduction, and sexual activity is generally considered very private. The nurse must be sensitive to the client's need for privacy and carefully explain that all information is confidential. A conversational approach with the use of open-ended statements is often helpful in a situation that promotes anxiety and embarrassment. The client's terminology about body parts and functions should guide the nurse's questions.

The focused interview guides the physical assessment of the female reproductive system. The information is always considered in relation to normal parameters and expectations about the health of the system. Therefore, the nurse must consider age, gender, race, culture, environment, health practices, past and concurrent problems, and therapies when framing questions and using techniques to elicit information. In order to address all of the factors when conducting a focused interview, categories of questions related to status and function of the reproductive system have been developed. These categories include general questions that are asked of all clients; those addressing illness or infection; questions related to symptoms, pain, or behaviors; those related to habits or practices; questions that are specific to clients according to age; and questions that address environmental concerns.

The nurse must consider the client's ability to participate in the focused interview and physical assessment of the reproductive system. If a client is experiencing pain or anxiety, attention must focus on relief of these symptoms. Because of the close proximity of some of the female reproductive structures to the urethra, data gathered during the focused interview will relate to the status of the urinary system as well. Questions related to the health and function of the female urinary system are discussed in Chapter 20. ⟳

Abnormal vaginal discharge, pelvic pain, inflammation, infection, and suspicion of contracting an STD are some of the more frequent problems that the female reports. Examination of the perianal area is included in assessment of the female reproductive system. Related problems include hemorrhoids, fissures, and infectious processes.

FOCUSED INTERVIEW QUESTIONS

RATIONALES

The following section provides sample questions and bulleted follow-up questions in each of the previously mentioned categories. A rationale for the questions is provided. The list of questions is not all-inclusive but represents the types of questions required in a comprehensive focused interview related to the female reproductive system. The subjective data from questions asked during the health history and focused interview will provide information to meet the goal of promoting reproductive health and preventing STD as described in the Healthy People 2010 *feature on page 661.*

GENERAL QUESTIONS

1. **Do you have any concerns about your reproductive health? Have you had concerns in the past? If so, please tell me about those concerns.**

▶ This question may prompt the client to discuss any concerns about reproductive health.

2. **How old were you when you had your first menstrual period?**

▶ Onset of menses is influenced by a variety of factors including percent of body fat. Menarche (onset of menstruation) between the ages of 11 and 14 indicates normal development. Late onset is associated with endocrine problems.

3. **What was the first day of your last menstrual period?**

▶ This establishes a pattern for the client and has significance for physical assessment in relation to physical changes that occur at points throughout the cycle.

4. **How many days does your cycle usually last?**
   - Is this consistent with each period?
   - How many days does bleeding occur?

▶ A cycle is defined as the first day of one period to the first day of the next. These questions establish the pattern for the client.

FOCUSED INTERVIEW QUESTIONS	RATIONALES

FOCUSED INTERVIEW QUESTIONS

5. **Describe your menstrual flow.**
   - Is this consistent each period?
   - How many tampons or pads do you use each day?
   - For how many days?

6. **How do you usually feel during your period? Is this a pattern for you?**

7. **How do you usually feel just before your period?**
   - Has this gotten worse or better?
   - Do you use any self-care remedies?

8. **Do you take any medications for cramps?**
   - If so, what do you take and how much?
   - If not, how do you relieve your cramps?

9. **Have you ever been pregnant? If so, how many times?**

10. **Did you have any problems during pregnancy, the delivery, or postpartum?** *If the client answers yes:* **Describe the problem(s).**

11. **Was delivery vaginal or by cesarean section?**

12. **Have you ever had a miscarriage?**
   - What were you told was the cause?
   - Was surgery required?
   - Have you ever had an abortion?
   - At how many weeks, and by what method?
   - How has it been emotionally since the abortion or miscarriage?

13. **Do you have children?**
   - If so, how many?
   - *If the client answers no:* Have you tried to have children?
   - *If the client answers yes:* How long have you been trying to have a child?

14. ***If the client indicates inability to conceive after 1 year:*** **How often do you and your partner have intercourse?**

15. **Have you ever sought professional help for fertility problems? If so, describe this experience.**

16. **Has an inability to conceive placed a strain on your relationship with your partner?**
   - How has this problem affected your relationship?
   - How are you feeling about this?

RATIONALES

▶ Clotting and excessive bleeding warrant additional follow-up. Any uterine bleeding that the client views as unusual warrants additional follow-up. The client's assessment of her menstrual flow is subjective. Generally, an excessively heavy flow is characterized by use of more than one pad or tampon per hour.

▶ This may provide clues as to whether discomfort is occurring. Dysmenorrhea (painful or difficult menstruation) is the most common gynecologic disorder.

▶ Premenstrual syndrome (PMS) presents with a variety of signs and symptoms including irritability, headache, cramping, and breast engorgement. PMS usually occurs a few days before menstruation. Typically, sudden relief occurs with the onset of full menstrual flow.

▶ This helps to determine if the female is able to continue with her daily routine.

▶ Questions 9 through 11 provide information about significant obstetric history, which impacts current status and anticipated physical findings.

▶ Strong emotions often accompany the issue of termination of a pregnancy by either spontaneous or surgical abortion. The nurse may want to follow up.

▶ The couple is not considered potentially infertile unless they have been unable to conceive for a year.

▶ For couples attempting to have a child, it is important to engage in intercourse routinely, two to three times a week. Although nurses do not treat infertility, they may be involved in teaching the client about certain measures that may be helpful, such as temperature tracking to determine the optimal time for intercourse. Concerns about infertility can produce great anxiety and depression for many females.

▶ The client can explain and describe specific diagnostic procedures and treatments for infertility as well as the emotional response to the processes and procedures.

▶ Specific questions enable the client to affirm or deny relationship problems, to discuss changes in the relationship, and to discuss feelings about the partnership.

FOCUSED INTERVIEW QUESTIONS	**RATIONALES**
17. Are you sexually active?	▶ The client may feel pressured to be in a sexual relationship. These pressures may be external (expectations of family, friends, or work associates) or internal (fear of being viewed by others as less than desirable or not of an accepted sexual orientation, fear of being alone, or fear of not being loved and accepted).
18. Are there any obstacles to your ability to achieve sexual satisfaction?	▶ Causes of inability to achieve sexual satisfaction include fear of acquiring an STD, fear of being unable to satisfy the partner, fear of pregnancy, confusion regarding sexual preference, unwillingness to participate in sexual activities enjoyed by the partner, job stress, financial considerations, crowded living conditions, loss of partner, attraction to or sexual involvement with individuals that the partner does not know about, criticism of sexual performance by the partner, or history of sexual trauma.
19. Have you noticed a change in your sex drive recently?	▶ This may be indicative of some physical or psychological problems that need follow-up.
20. *If the client answers yes to question 19:* Can you associate the change with anything in particular?	▶ Often clients can relate a decrease in sex drive with stress, illness, drug therapy, or some other factor.
21. *If the client is sexually active:* Do you use contraceptives? Which type?	▶ This question provides information about the client's knowledge about contraception, at-risk behaviors, and specific contraceptive devices or medications.

QUESTIONS RELATED TO ILLNESS OR INFECTION

1. Do you now have or have you ever had an illness associated with the female reproductive system1? • When were you diagnosed with the problem? • What was the treatment for the illness? • Was the treatment helpful? • What kinds of things do you do to help with the problem? • Has the problem ever recurred? • How are you managing the problem now?	▶ This allows the client to provide her own perceptions about problems with her reproductive system.
2. An alternative to question 1 is to list common problems with the reproductive system, such as dysmenorrhea, uterine fibroids, and uterine, ovarian, or vulvar cancer, and ask the client to respond yes or no as each is stated.	▶ This is a comprehensive and easy way to elicit information about illnesses associated with the female reproductive system. Follow-up would be carried out for each identified diagnosis as in question 1.
3. Do you now have or have you ever had an infection of the reproductive system? • When were you diagnosed with the infection? • What treatment was prescribed for the problem? • Was the treatment helpful? • What kinds of things do you do to help with the problem? • Has the problem ever recurred (acute)? • How are you managing the infection now (chronic)?	▶ If an infection is identified, follow-up about the date of infection, treatment, and outcomes is required. Data about each infection identified by the client is essential to an accurate health assessment. Infections can be classified as acute or chronic, and follow-up regarding each classification will differ.
4. An alternative to question 3 is to list possible infections, such as vaginitis, cystitis, and pelvic inflammatory disease (PID), and ask the client to respond yes or no as each is stated.	▶ This is a comprehensive and easy way to elicit information about all reproductive system infections. Follow-up would be carried out for each identified infection as in question 3.

FOCUSED INTERVIEW QUESTIONS	RATIONALES

5. **Have you ever had any surgery of the reproductive system?**
   - If so, what was it? When? Where?
   - What was the outcome?

6. **Have you ever had an abnormal Pap smear?**
   - If so, how long ago was this?
   - What treatment, if any, did you receive?
   - Have you had follow-up Pap smears? When? What were the results?

▶ Questions 5 and 6 provide information about client knowledge in regard to pathologies and treatments. This establishes variations in expected findings in physical examination.

7. **Have you ever had a sexually transmitted disease such as herpes, gonorrhea, syphilis, HPV, or chlamydia?**
   - *If the client answers yes:* Was it treated?
   - Did you inform your partner?
   - Was your partner treated?
   - Did you have sexual relations with your partner while you were infected?
   - *If the client answers yes:* Did you use condoms?
   - What treatment did you receive?

▶ Serious, sometimes fatal, complications can develop if treatment is delayed. STDs can be detected only by testing. If untreated, STDs can cause sterility and problems with the reproductive and other body systems.

8. **Are you aware of having had any exposure to HIV?**
   - *If the client answers yes:* Describe the situation and how you believe you were exposed.
   - What are your views on sexual relations and the potential for acquiring HIV?

9. **Have you ever been tested for HIV?**
   - *If the client answers yes:* On one occasion or routinely?
   - What were the results of the test?

▶ The incidence of HIV is still greatly on the rise. Despite the wide availability of information on the risk and methods of protection for sexually active individuals, many females continue to have unprotected sex.

QUESTIONS RELATED TO SYMPTOMS OR BEHAVIORS

When gathering information about symptoms, many questions are required to elicit details and descriptions that assist in the analysis of the data. Discrimination is made in relation to the significance of a symptom, in relation to specific diseases or problems, and in relation to potential follow-up examination or referral. One rationale may be provided for a group of questions in this category.

The following questions refer to specific symptoms and behaviors associated with the female reproductive system. For each symptom, questions and follow-up are required. The details to be elicited are the characteristics of the symptom; the onset, duration, and frequency of the symptom; the treatment or remedy for the symptom, including over-the-counter and home remedies; the determination if diagnosis has been sought; the effect of treatments; and family history associated with a symptom or illness.

QUESTIONS RELATED TO SYMPTOMS

1. **Have you noticed any rashes, blisters, ulcers, sores, or warts on your genital area or surrounding areas?**

▶ Rashes may occur with yeast infections, which are the most common female genital infection. Yeast infections generally produce redness, pruritus (itching), and cheeselike discharge. Herpes infection causes small painful ulcerations, whereas syphilitic chancres are not painful. In the older client, a raised, reddened lesion may indicate carcinoma of the vulva. Reddened lesions that eventually weep and form crusts characterize contact dermatitis. Venereal warts are cauliflower shaped.

FOCUSED INTERVIEW QUESTIONS	RATIONALES

2. **Have you felt any lumps or masses in any of these areas?**
   - If so, describe the mass. Exactly where is it?
   - About what size?
   - Is it soft or hard?
   - Is it movable?
   - When did you first notice the mass?
   - Is it painful?
   - Have you noticed any change in it since it developed?
   - Have you used any remedies such as ice, heat, or creams?

▶ Sebaceous cysts can be noted in the labial area. A lump created by an abscess of the Bartholin's gland causes localized pain. An abscess of the Bartholin's gland may indicate the presence of gonorrhea.

3. **Have you noticed any swelling or redness of your genitals?**

▶ Vulvovaginitis may cause edema in the area, including the vulva. Redness and swelling may indicate an alteration in health such as an abscess of the Bartholin's gland, which may be caused by gonorrhea. Bruising may indicate sexual trauma.

4. **Do you have any structures extruding from your vagina?**
   - Have you felt any pressure from your vagina?
   - Have you felt bulging or masses from within your vagina?

▶ Uterine prolapse may be so severe that the uterus protrudes into and at times out of the vagina. Surgery may be indicated.

5. **Have you experienced any itching in your labia or vaginal area?**
   - If so, when did it start?
   - Has it been treated and, if so, how?
   - Have there been any associated urinary symptoms?

▶ Crab lice, atrophic vaginitis, candidiasis, and contact dermatitis may cause intense itching.

6. **Have you noticed any discharge from your vagina?**
   - If so, what color is it?
   - Is there any odor to it?
   - Is it a small, moderate, or large amount?
   - When did you first notice the discharge?

▶ Vaginal discharge is a typical complaint of clients with vaginitis. The most common presenting symptom in females with STDs is vaginal discharge; however, the client may have no symptoms.

7. **Have you had any vaginal bleeding outside the time of your normal menstrual period?**

▶ Abnormal bleeding may be related to hormonal influences and be easily corrected. Conditions such as uterine fibroids and several forms of cancer can also cause abnormal bleeding patterns.

8. *If the client answers yes to question 7:* **When did it occur? How much bleeding was there?**

▶ The nurse should obtain quantitative data by asking whether panties were saturated or how many pads or tampons were saturated in 24 hours. A calendar should be used to determine the number of days since the client's last menstrual period.

9. **Have you had any problems in and around your rectal area, such as pain, itching, burning, or bleeding?**
   - When did the problem begin?
   - Do you know the cause of the problem?
   - Have you sought healthcare for the problem?
   - Was a diagnosis made?
   - What treatment was prescribed?
   - What do you do to help with the problem?
   - Has the treatment helped?

▶ Pain, itching, bleeding, or burning may indicate the presence of abuse, infection, irritation, or injury to the anus, rectum, or perineum. Rectal bleeding, pain, and irritation may result from passing hard stools, from hemorrhoids, or from injuries. Fungal infection may result in pruritus or irritation of the perianal area.

▶ When symptoms in the perianal area are associated with hemorrhoids or hard stool, follow-up would include questions about diet, exercise, and bowel habits.

Irritation or injury to the perianal area can occur as a result of sexual practices or sexual abuse. Sensitive questioning about these topics is required when sexual activity is described or when sexual abuse is suspected or disclosed.

FOCUSED INTERVIEW QUESTIONS	RATIONALES

QUESTIONS RELATED TO PAIN

1. **Do you have any pain, tenderness, or soreness in your pelvic area?**
   - If so, describe the pain.
   - Is it dull? Sharp? Radiating? Intermittent? Continuous?
   - When did it start?
   - Are you having any pain in the area now?
   - What makes the pain better or worse?
   - Do you have associated symptoms of headache, vomiting, or diarrhea?

▶ Common causes of gynecologic pain include infection, menstrual difficulties, endometriosis (abnormal condition involving the endometrial lining of the uterus), ectopic pregnancy (fetus implanted in abnormal location), threatened abortion, pelvic masses, uterine fibroids, and ovarian cancer.

QUESTIONS RELATED TO BEHAVIORS

1. **Do you check your genitals on a routine basis?** *If the client answers yes:* **How often?**

▶ Self-examination of the genitals should be performed at least monthly for early detection of changes that need follow-up. Teaching may be indicated if the client is not performing self-examination.

2. **How often do you get physical examinations?**

▶ Screening for problems such as cervical or endometrial cancer is typically performed during routine physical or gynecologic examinations.

3. **Do you use tampons?**
   - If so, how frequently do you change the tampons?
   - Are you aware of the risk for toxic shock syndrome with the use of tampons?
   - Are you aware of the signs of toxic shock?

▶ Tampons, when not used cautiously (for example, lack of frequent changes), have been linked with toxic shock syndrome.

4. **What kinds of products do you use for hygiene in the genital area?**

▶ Use of soap, sprays, powders, and douche products can irritate the tissues of the reproductive system. Some studies suggest that females who have used talc in the genital area for many years may be at increased risk of developing ovarian cancer.

5. *If the client is sexually active:* **Are you in a mutually monogamous relationship? If not, how many sexual partners have you or your partner had over the last year?**

▶ Sexual activity with many different partners increases the risk of acquiring STDs and possibly certain gynecologic cancers.

6. **Are you able to be sexually aroused?**
   - Has this ability changed over time or recently?

▶ A variety of factors may interfere with a female's ability to be sexually aroused. These factors include prescribed or illicit drug use, disorders of the nervous or endocrine systems, stress, and fear (e.g., of intimacy, inability to satisfy a partner, acquiring an STD, or becoming pregnant).

7. **Are you satisfied with your sexual experiences?**
   - *If the client expresses dissatisfaction:* Are you able to achieve orgasm?
   - Have you noticed a change in your ability to have an orgasm?

▶ A variety of factors may interfere with a female's ability to experience orgasm.

8. **Are you using contraception?**
   - If so, what kind?
   - Are you using it consistently?

▶ This provides information about knowledge of contraception in general and regarding the products indicated by the client.

9. **Would you like to know more about the use of birth control?**

▶ This is a very important question to ask adolescents who shy away from talking about sexual practices but have verbalized that they are sexually active.

10. **How do you protect yourself from sexually transmitted diseases, including HIV?**

▶ Abstinence is the only 100% effective protection against STDs. Latex condoms offer significant protection, especially when treated with spermicide; however, they are not 100% effective.

FOCUSED INTERVIEW QUESTIONS	RATIONALES

QUESTIONS RELATED TO AGE

The focused interview must reflect the anatomical and physiological differences that exist along the life span. The following questions are examples of those that would be specific for infants and children, adolescents, the pregnant female, and the older adult.

QUESTIONS REGARDING INFANTS AND CHILDREN

1. **Have you noticed any redness, swelling, or discharge that is discolored or foul smelling in the child's genital areas?**

2. **Has the child complained of itching, burning, or swelling in the genital area?**

▶ These may indicate inflammatory processes or infection.

▶ These symptoms may indicate the presence of pinworms, yeast infections and other infections, trauma, or sexual abuse.

The nurse should ask the preschool or school-age child the following questions:

1. **Has anyone ever touched you when you didn't want him or her to?**
   - Where? (*The nurse may want to have the child point to a picture or doll.*)
   - Has anyone ever asked you to touch him or her when you didn't want to?
   - Where did he or she ask you to touch him or her?
   - *If the child answers yes, the child may be experiencing sexual abuse. The nurse should try to obtain additional information by asking the following questions but remember to be sensitive:*
   - Who touched you?
   - How many times did this happen?
   - Who knows about this?

▶ The nurse must try to determine exactly what the person did to the child. Has there been more than touching? Has any other form of sexual contact occurred? The child may feel responsible for the situation and not wish to discuss it. The abuser may be a parent or relative. The nurse should assure the child that she has not been bad and that it helps to talk to an adult about it. Referral should be made to a specialist immediately for sexual abuse assessment.

QUESTIONS REGARDING ADOLESCENTS

Many of the questions nurses ask adolescents are similar to questions they ask adults. It is important to explore adolescents' feelings and concerns regarding their sexual development. The nurse can reassure the adolescent that these changes are normal. Some adolescents may be confused about their feelings of sexual attraction to the opposite or same sex. The nurse should ask open-ended questions and assure the adolescent that such feelings are normal.

Whether or not an adolescent admits to being sexually active, it is important to offer information on teenage pregnancy, birth control, and protection against STDs. Some teenagers may be fearful that the nurse will relay this information to their parents. The nurse should reinforce that all information is confidential unless sexual abuse is reported.

1. **Are you having sex with anyone now?**

▶ Use of gender-neutral terms prevents value judgments about sexual orientation. This question allows clients to define what they think sex is. Many teens consider anything not involving vaginal penetration as not being sex. The nurse must stress that oral sex is indeed sexual activity.

QUESTIONS FOR THE PREGNANT FEMALE

Questions for the pregnant female would include menstrual, obstetric, gynecologic, family, and partner histories.

This information would provide data about the client and her partner and identify risk factors. Specific questions for the pregnant female are included in Chapter 26 of this text. ∞

FOCUSED INTERVIEW QUESTIONS	RATIONALES

The questions for aging female adults are the same as those for younger adults. In addition, the nurse should explore whether older clients perceive any changes in their sexuality related to advancing age. For example, an older female may notice a decrease in vaginal lubrication even when she is fully aroused. The female older adult can be reassured that these changes are normal and do not indicate disease.

QUESTIONS FOR THE OLDER ADULT

1. **When did menopause begin for you?**

   ▶ This information establishes a reference for the onset of physiological changes that accompany menopause.

2. **Tell me about physical changes you have noticed since menopause.**

   ▶ It is common for aging females to experience a variety of symptoms, including mood changes and "hot flashes." Vaginal dryness causes dyspareunia.

3. **Have you had any vaginal bleeding since starting menopause?**

   ▶ Some females assume that postmenopausal bleeding is normal and tend to ignore it. Postmenopausal bleeding may be suggestive of inadequate estrogen therapy and endometrial cancer. It could also be indicative of serious problems such as genital tract cancer.

QUESTIONS RELATED TO ENVIRONMENT

Environment refers to both the internal and external environments. Questions related to the internal environment include all of the previous questions and those associated with internal or physiological responses. Questions regarding the external environment include those related to home, work, or social environments.

INTERNAL ENVIRONMENT

1. **Do you know if your mother received diethylstilbestrol (DES) treatment during pregnancy with you?**

   ▶ Studies indicate that daughters of mothers who received DES during pregnancy have a significantly higher number of reproductive tract problems, including cervical cancer, infertility, and ectopic pregnancy. This may have some bearing on the current problem. If the client answers yes to this question, the nurse should refer her to a physician.

2. **Do you drink alcohol? How many drinks per week?**

   ▶ Intake of alcoholic beverages can contribute to an individual "taking chances" such as failing to ask the partner to use condoms.

3. **Do you use illicit drugs? If so, what type and how much?**

   ▶ Taken in sufficient amounts, some drugs, such as marijuana and opiates, may decrease libido. Drug use may also contribute to failure to use protection against STDs.

EXTERNAL ENVIRONMENT

The following questions deal with substances and irritants found in the physical environment of the client. The physical environment includes the indoor and outdoor environments of the home and the workplace, those encountered for social engagements, and any encountered during travel.

1. **Do your family and friends support your relationship with your sexual partner?**

   ▶ The client's family and friends can influence the client's sexual relationship in a variety of ways. The client may feel tension if the partner is not accepted.

FOCUSED INTERVIEW QUESTIONS

2. **Are you able to talk to your partner about your sexual needs?**
   - Does your partner accept your needs and help you fulfill them?
   - Are you able to do the same for your partner?

3. **Some clients come to a healthcare provider to discuss sexual abuse.**
   - Have you ever been forced to have sexual intercourse or other sexual contact against your will?
   - Have you ever been molested or raped?
   - *If the client answers yes:* When was this?
   - Who abused you?
   - What was the experience?
   - What was done about the situation and for you?

For more information about assessment of abuse, contact the Nursing Network on Violence Against Women International. Link to their Website through the Companion Website.

RATIONALES

▶ The ability to openly discuss sexual needs and preferences fosters strong and lasting relationships.

CLIENT INTERACTION

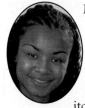

Ms. Tanya Jacobs comes to the clinic and tells the admission clerk she needs help and needs to see a female nurse. She further indicates she would like to see Mary Bart, RN, again today if she is working. When asked why she is seeking healthcare, Ms. Jacobs responds, "I have a bad itch down there." About 5 minutes later Mary Bart greets Ms. Jacobs Part of the focused interview follows.

INTERVIEW

Nurse: Tell me about the problem.

Ms. Jacobs: I don't know where or how to begin. I'm so embarrassed.

Nurse: First, we need to address your feelings of embarrassment, and then it might be easier for you to talk about your problem. I understand that discussion of problems with your genitals is embarrassing. These are difficult issues to discuss. I will keep all that is said here confidential. I will let you take your time as you tell me about the problem. Your discussion will help to determine the cause of the problem and the best way to take care of it.

Ms. Jacobs: I just don't know how this could happen. I haven't seen my boyfriend in 2 weeks. He is away, and I get this itch. What did I do wrong?

Nurse: Perhaps you have done nothing wrong. As you give me more information, I will help you. Where would you like to begin?

Ms. Jacobs: Just ask me some questions.

Nurse: Let's first talk about the itch. Try to be as specific as possible. Where is it?

Ms. Jacobs: You know, in my private area.

Nurse: On the outside or inside?

Ms. Jacobs: The outside.

Nurse: When did you first notice the itch?

Ms. Jacobs: Two days ago.

Nurse: Do you have a rash?

Ms. Jacobs: No.

Nurse: Is your private area red?

Ms. Jacobs: Yes.

Nurse: What have you done to relieve the itch and redness?

Ms. Jacobs: I try not to scratch, but that is why I'm here. I can't stand it. It seems to be getting worse.

ANALYSIS

The nurse realized that discussing matters related to the reproductive system and genitalia might be very difficult for the client. Ms. Jacobs' stated embarrassment and her verbal burst of information were verbal and nonverbal cues interpreted by the nurse to set the tone for the interview. The interview began with an open-ended statement. This allowed the client to respond within the area of greatest comfort. The nurse recognized the emotional aspect of this situation and addressed this before seeking more information. Closed statements were used to obtain specific subjective data. The nurse listened to the client and did not impose judgment.

Please refer to the Companion Website at **www.prenhall.com/damico** and click on Chapter 22, the **Client Interaction** module, to answer questions about this case. In addition, see other resources for this chapter including NCLEX review questions and other interactive exercises and materials.

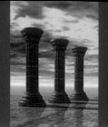

Physical Assessment

ASSESSMENT TECHNIQUES AND FINDINGS

Physical assessment of the female reproductive system includes the techniques of inspection and palpation. In addition, the speculum is used to visualize the vagina and cervix. During each of the procedures, the nurse is gathering data related to the health and function of the reproductive system. Knowledge of normal or expected findings is essential in determining the meaning of the data as the nurse conducts the physical assessment.

The adult female has pubic hair that is distributed in an even, inverted triangular pattern over the mons pubis. Hair distribution is less dense over the labia, perineum, and inner thighs. The labia majora are symmetrical, smooth, and without lesions. The labia minora are smooth, pink, and moist. The clitoris is smooth, midline, and about 1 cm in length. The urethra is slitlike, midline, smooth, pink, and patent. The vaginal opening is pink and round. On bearing down, there should be no urine leakage at the meatus or protrusions from the vagina. The perineum is smooth and firm. The anus is intact, moist, darkly pigmented, and without lesions. Upon palpation the vaginal wall is rugated and soft; the Skene's glands and Bartholin's glands are nontender and without discharge. The examination with the speculum reveals a pink, moist, round, and centrally positioned cervix. The cervix is free of lesions with clear, odorless secretions present. Palpation of the cervix reveals it as firm, smooth, and mobile like the tip of the nose. The fornices are smooth and nontender. The uterus is palpated and found tilted upward above the bladder with the cervix tilted forward. Variations in uterine position may be anteverted, midline, or retroverted. When ovaries are palpable, they are smooth, firm, mobile, and almond shaped. They may be slightly tender. The uterine tubes are nonpalpable. The rectovaginal system is thin, smooth, and nontender.

Physical assessment of the female reproductive system follows an organized pattern. It begins with inspection of the external genitalia and perianal area, palpation of the vagina and glands, and speculum examination and specimen collection. This is followed by palpation of the cervix, fornices, uterus, uterine tubes, and ovaries. The assessment ends with the rectovaginal examination.

EQUIPMENT

examination gown and examination drape
clean, nonsterile examination gloves
lubricant
Pap smear equipment
speculum
handheld mirror

HELPFUL HINTS

- Provide a warm, private environment.
- Have the client void and empty bowels before the examination.
- Use appropriate draping to maintain the client's dignity.
- Determine if the client has had this kind of assessment before. If not, booklets with diagrams are helpful before proceeding.
- It is helpful to show the client pictures of equipment, slides, and the bimanual examination.
- Use an unhurried, deliberate manner and ask the client how she is doing as the examination proceeds.
- Explore and remedy cultural or language issues at the onset of the interaction.
- Use Standard Precautions.

TECHNIQUES AND NORMAL FINDINGS	ABNORMAL FINDINGS SPECIAL CONSIDERATIONS

INSPECTION

1. Instruct the client.

- Explain to the client that you will be looking at and touching her external genital area. Tell her that it should not cause discomfort, but if pain occurs she should tell you and you will stop. Explain that deep breathing is a good way to relax during the examination.
- Tell the client you will provide instructions and explanations at each point in the assessment.

TECHNIQUES AND NORMAL FINDINGS	ABNORMAL FINDINGS SPECIAL CONSIDERATIONS

2. Position the client.

- Ask the client to lie down on the examination table.
- Assist her into the lithotomy position (supine with knees and hips flexed so that feet rest flat on the examination table), and then have her slide her hips as close to the end of the table as possible.
- Place her feet in the stirrups (see Figure 22.3 ●).

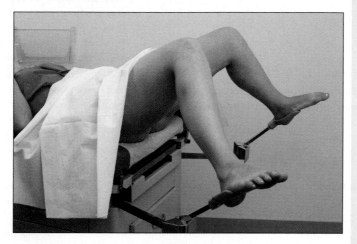

Figure 22.3 ●
Positioning the client.

3. Inspect the pubic hair.

- Confirm that the hair grows in an inverted triangle and is scattered heavily over the mons pubis. It should become sparse over the labia majora, perineum, and inner thighs (see Figure 22.4 ●).

▶ A sparse hair pattern may be indicative of delayed puberty. It is also a common and normal finding in females of Asian ancestry. The elderly client's pubic hair will become sparse, scattered, and gray. Table 22.1 depicts Tanner's stages of female development.

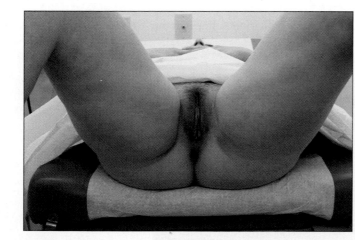

Figure 22.4 ●
Inspecting the pubic hair.

- If the client has complained of itching in the pubic area, comb through the pubic hair with two or three fingers.
  Confirm the absence of small, bluish gray spots, or nits (eggs), at the base of the pubic hairs.

▶ These signs indicate pubic lice (crabs). Marks may be visible from persistent scratching to relieve the intense itching caused by the lice.

TECHNIQUES AND NORMAL FINDINGS

4. Inspect the labia majora.

- Confirm that the labia majora are fuller and rounder in the center of the structure and that the skin is smooth and intact.
- Compare the right and left labia majora for symmetry.
- Observe for any lesions, warts, vesicles, rashes, or ulcerations. If you notice drainage, note the color, distribution, location, and characteristics.

- Remember to change gloves as needed during the exam to prevent cross-contamination. Also remember to culture any abnormal discharge.
  Confirm the absence of any swelling or inflammation in the area of the labia majora.

▶ The labia majora of older females may be thinner and wrinkled.

▶ These findings may signal a variety of conditions. *Contact dermatitis* appears as a red rash with associated lesions that are weepy and crusty. There often are scratches due to intense itching.
▶ **Genital warts** are raised, moist, cauliflower-shaped papules.
▶ Red, painful vesicles accompanied by localized swelling are seen in *herpes infection*.
▶ Swelling over red, inflamed skin that is tender and warm to palpation may indicate an abscess in the Bartholin's gland. The abscess may be caused by gonorrhea.

5. Inspect the labia minora.

- Confirm that the labia minora are smooth, pink, and moist.

- Observe for any redness or swelling. Note any bruising or tearing of the skin.

▶ The older female may have drier, thinner labia minora.
▶ Redness and swelling indicate the presence of an infective or inflammatory process. Bruising or tearing of the skin may suggest forceful intercourse or sexual abuse, especially in the case of adolescents and children.

6. Inspect the clitoris.

- Place your right or left hand over the labia majora and separate these structures with your thumb and index finger.
- The clitoris should be midline, about 1 cm in length, with more fullness in the center. It should be smooth. (Figure 22.5 ●)
- Observe for any redness, lesions, or tears in the tissue.

▶ An elongated clitoris may signal elevated levels of testosterone and warrants further investigation and referral to a physician.

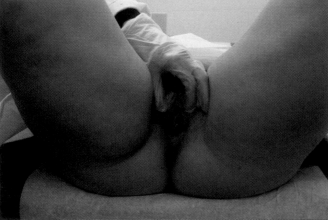

Figure 22.5 ●
Inspection of
the clitoris.

7. Inspect the urethral orifice.

- Confirm that the urethral opening is midline, pink, smooth, slitlike, and patent.

- Ask the client to cough. No urine should leak from the urethral opening.
- Inspect for any redness, inflammation, or discharge.

▶ Urine leakage indicates stress incontinence and weakening of the pelvic musculature.

▶ These symptoms indicate urinary tract infection.

TECHNIQUES AND NORMAL FINDINGS	ABNORMAL FINDINGS SPECIAL CONSIDERATIONS

TECHNIQUES AND NORMAL FINDINGS

8. **Inspect the vaginal opening, perineum, and anal area.**
   - Confirm that the vaginal opening or introitus is pink and round. It may be either smooth or irregular.
   - Locate the **hymen,** which is a thin layer of skin within the vagina. It may be present in females who have never had sexual intercourse.
   - Inspect for tears, bruising, or lacerations.

   - The **perineum,** the space between the vaginal opening and anal area, should be smooth and firm.
   - Scars from episiotomy procedures may be observed in parous females. These are normal.
   - The anus should be intact, moist, and darkly pigmented. There should be no lesions.
   - Have the client bear down.

   - Inspect for any protrusions from the vagina.

ABNORMAL FINDINGS SPECIAL CONSIDERATIONS

▶ Tears, bruising, or lacerations could be due to forceful, consensual sex or rape. Additional follow-up is needed after examination. It is important not to ask any questions that the client may interpret as probing or threatening during the physical assessment.

▶ Thin, fragile perineal tissues indicate atrophy. Tears and fissures may indicate trauma.

▶ A **prolapsed uterus** may protrude right at the vaginal wall with straining, or it may hang outside of the vaginal wall without any straining (see Figure 22.6 ●).

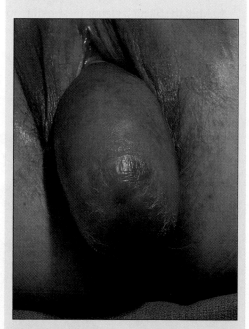

Figure 22.6 ● Prolapsed uterus.

▶ A **cystocele** is a hernia that is formed when the urinary bladder is pushed into the anterior vaginal wall.

▶ A **rectocele** is a hernia that is formed when the rectum pushes into the posterior vaginal wall.

TECHNIQUES AND NORMAL FINDINGS	ABNORMAL FINDINGS SPECIAL CONSIDERATIONS

PALPATION

1. **Palpate the vaginal walls.**

   • Explain to the client that you are going to palpate the vaginal walls. Tell her that she will feel you insert a finger into the vagina.

   • Place your left hand above the labia majora and spread the labia minora apart with your thumb and index finger.

   • With your right palm facing toward the ceiling, gently place your right index finger at the vaginal opening.

   • Insert your right index finger gently into the vagina.

   • Gently rotate the right index finger counterclockwise. The vaginal wall should feel rugated, consistent in texture, and soft.

   • Ask the client to bear down or cough.

   • Note any bulging in this area.

   ▶ Bulging may occur with uterine prolapse, cystocele, or rectocele.

2. **Palpate the urethra and Skene's glands.**

   • Explain to the client that you are going to palpate her urethra. Tell her that she will again feel pressure against her vaginal wall.

   • Your left hand should still be above the labia majora and you should still be spreading the labia minora apart with your thumb and index finger.

   • Your right index finger should still be inserted in the client's vagina.

   • With your right index finger, apply very gentle pressure upward against the vaginal wall.

   • Milk the Skene's glands by stroking outward (see Figure 22.7 ●).

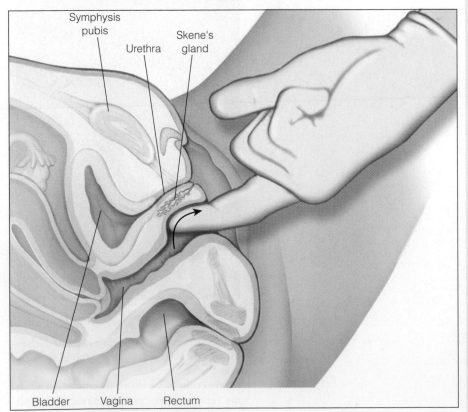

Symphysis pubis
Urethra
Skene's gland
Bladder Vagina Rectum

Figure 22.7 ● Palpating Skene's glands.

TECHNIQUES AND NORMAL FINDINGS	ABNORMAL FINDINGS SPECIAL CONSIDERATIONS

- Now apply the same upward and outward pressure on both sides of the urethra.
- No pain or discharge should be elicited.

▶ Discharge from the urethra or Skene's glands may indicate an infection such as gonorrhea. A culture must be obtained.

3. Palpate the Bartholin's glands.

- With your right index finger still inserted in the client's vagina, gently squeeze the posterior region of the labia majora between your right index finger and right thumb (see Figure 22.8 ●).

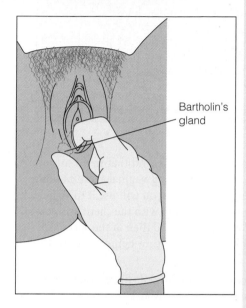

Bartholin's gland

Figure 22.8 ● Palpating Bartholin's glands.

- Perform this maneuver bilaterally, palpating both Bartholin's glands.
- No lump or hardness should be felt. No pain response should be elicited. No discharge should be produced.

▶ Lumps, hardness, pain, or discharge suggest the presence of an abscess and infective process. Often the source is a gonorrheal infection. A culture should be obtained of any discharge.

INSPECTION WITH A SPECULUM

Be sure that the client has not douched within 24 hours before obtaining cervical and vaginal specimens. Otherwise, the results of the test may be inaccurate.

1. Select the speculum.

- The speculum should be the proper size for the client.
- Use a speculum that has been prewarmed with a heating pad. Do not prewarm a speculum with warm water, because it is not desirable to introduce water into the vagina. Do not use gel lubricant, as it may distort the cells in your specimens.

2. Hold the speculum in your dominant hand.

- Place the index finger on top of the blades, the third finger on the bottom of the blades, and be sure to move the thumb just underneath the thumbscrew before inserting (see Figure 22.9 ●).

▶ If the client has vaginitis, the speculum examination should be delayed until the problem has been treated unless this is the client's chief complaint and the reason for her visit.

TECHNIQUES AND NORMAL FINDINGS	ABNORMAL FINDINGS SPECIAL CONSIDERATIONS

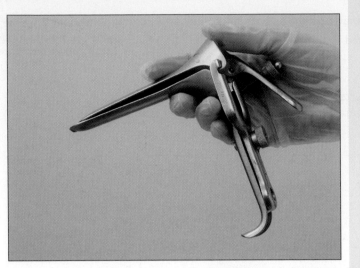

Figure 22.9 ● Holding the speculum.

3. **Insert the speculum.**

   - Tell the client that you are going to examine her cervix, and that to do so, you are going to insert a speculum. If this is the client's first vaginal examination, show her the speculum, and briefly demonstrate how you will use it to visualize her cervix. Have a mirror available to share findings with the client. Also explain that she will feel pressure, first of your fingers, and then of the speculum. You may also want to show her a booklet with a picture demonstrating the technique.

   - With your nondominant hand, place your index and middle fingers on the posterior vaginal opening and apply pressure gently downward.

   - Turn the speculum blades obliquely.

   - Place the blades over your fingers at the vaginal opening and slowly insert the closed speculum at a 45-degree downward angle (see Figure 22.10 ●). This angle matches the downward slope of the vagina when the client is in the lithotomy position.

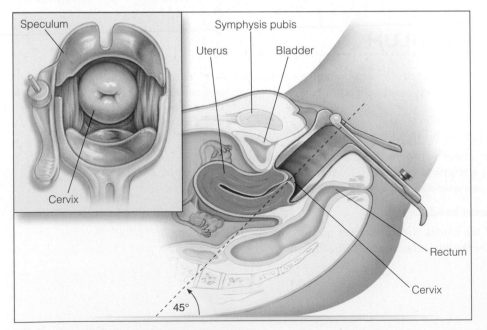

Figure 22.10 ● Speculum inserted into vagina.

TECHNIQUES AND NORMAL FINDINGS	ABNORMAL FINDINGS SPECIAL CONSIDERATIONS

- Ask the client to bear down as you insert the speculum. It is normal for the client to tense as the speculum is inserted, and bearing down helps to relax the muscles.
- Once the speculum is inserted, withdraw your fingers and turn the speculum clockwise until the blades are in a horizontal plane.
- Advance the blades at a downward 45-degree angle until they are completely inserted.
- This maneuver should not cause the client pain.
- Avoid pinching the labia or pulling on the client's pubic hair. If insertion of the speculum causes the client pain, stop immediately and reevaluate your technique.
- To open the speculum blades, squeeze the speculum handle.
- Sweep the speculum blades upward until the cervix comes into view.
- Adjust the speculum blades as needed until the cervix is fully exposed between them.
- Tighten the thumbscrew to stabilize the spread of the blades.

4. **Visualize the cervix.**
   - Confirm that the cervix is pink, moist, round, and centrally positioned, and that it has a small opening in the center called the os.
   - Note any bluish coloring.

     ▶ A bluish coloring is seen during the second month of pregnancy and is called *Chadwick's sign.* Otherwise, a bluish color is indicative of cyanosis.

   - Confirm that any secretions are clear or white and without odor.

     ▶ Green discharge that has a foul smell is associated with gonorrhea. Thick discharge is seen in *candidiasis.* Frothy, yellow-green discharge is seen in *trichomoniasis.* A yellow discharge can also be visualized in chlamydial infection. *Bacterial vaginitis* presents with a creamy-gray to white discharge that has a fishy odor.

   - Confirm that the cervix is free from erosions, ulcerations, lacerations, and polyps.

     ▶ Erosions are associated with carcinoma or infections. Ulcerations can be due to carcinoma, syphilis, and tuberculosis. Yellow cysts or nodules are *nabothian cysts,* benign cysts that may appear after childbirth.

OBTAINING THE PAP SMEAR AND GONORRHEA CULTURE

The Pap (Papanicolaou) smear consists of three specimens: an endocervical swab, a cervical scrape, and a vaginal pool sample.

Have ready prelabeled slides for specimens, either (a) one labeled *endocervical,* one labeled *vaginal,* and one labeled *cervical* or (b) one slide that has sections for each sample.

1. **Perform an endocervical swab.**
   - Carefully insert a saline-moistened, cotton-tipped applicator or Cytobrush®GT into the vagina and into the cervical os.

     ▶ Moistening the applicator with saline prevents the cells from being absorbed into the cotton.

     The cytobrush is recommended over the cotton-tipped applicator because more endocervical cells adhere to it, thus yielding more accurate results.

TECHNIQUES AND NORMAL FINDINGS	ABNORMAL FINDINGS SPECIAL CONSIDERATIONS

- Do not force insertion of the applicator.

- Rotate the applicator in a complete circle (see Figure 22.11 ●).

- Roll a thin coat across the slide labeled *endocervical.*

▶ If the applicator cannot be slipped into the cervical os, a tumor may be blocking the opening.

▶ A thin coat is preferred because a thick coat may be difficult to assess under the microscope.

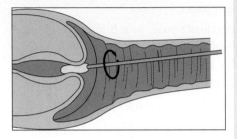

Figure 22.11 ● The endocervical swab.

- Spray fixative on the slide immediately or place it in a container filled with fixative.

2. **Obtain a cervical scrape.**
   - Insert the longer end of a bifid spatula into the client's vagina.
   - Advance the fingerlike projection of the bifid end gently into the cervical os.
   - Allow the shorter end to rest on the outer ridge of the cervix.
   - Rotate the applicator one full 360-degree turn clockwise to scrape cells from the cervix (see Figure 22.12 ●).

▶ If the client has had a hysterectomy, obtain the scrape from the surgical stump.

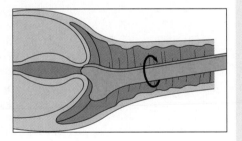

Figure 22.12 ● The cervical scrape.

- Do not rotate the applicator more than once or turn it in a counterclockwise manner.
- Spread a thin smear across the slide labeled *cervical* from each side of the applicator.
- Spray fixative on the slide immediately or place in a container filled with fixative.

3. **Obtain a vaginal pool sample.**
   - Insert the paddle end of the spatula into the vaginal recess area (fornix). Alternatively, you may use a saline-moistened cotton applicator.

TECHNIQUES AND NORMAL FINDINGS	ABNORMAL FINDINGS SPECIAL CONSIDERATIONS

TECHNIQUES AND NORMAL FINDINGS

- Gently rotate the spatula back and forth to obtain a sample (see Figure 22.13 ●).

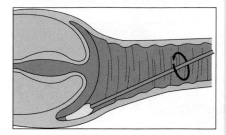

Figure 22.13 ● The vaginal pool sample.

- Apply the specimen to the slide labeled *vaginal*.
- Spray fixative on the slide immediately.

4. Obtain a gonorrhea culture.

- Obtain a gonorrhea culture if the assessment findings indicate.

▶ Nurses must be sure to check with the laboratory in their institution because techniques and protocols may differ.

- Insert a saline-moistened cotton applicator into the cervical os.
- Leave the applicator in place for 20 seconds to allow full saturation of the cotton.
- Using a Z-shaped pattern, roll a thin coat of the secretions onto the Thayer-Martin culture plate labeled *cervical*.

5. Remove the speculum.

- Gently loosen the thumbscrew on the speculum while holding the handles securely.

▶ The infections that contribute to the development of discolored or foul-smelling vaginal discharge are the same as those listed in the previous section on identifying cervical discharge.

- Slant the speculum from side to side as you slide it from the vaginal canal.
- While you withdraw the speculum, note that the vaginal mucosa is pink, consistent in texture, rugated, and nontender. Discharge is thin or stringy, and clear or opaque.
- Close the speculum blades before complete removal.

BIMANUAL PALPATION

Stand at the end of the examination table. The client remains in the lithotomy position.

1. Palpate the cervix.

- Lubricate the index and middle fingers of your gloved dominant hand.
- Inform the client that you are going to palpate her cervix.
- Place your nondominant hand against the client's thigh, then insert your lubricated index and middle fingers into her vaginal opening.
- Proceed downward at a 45-degree angle until you reach the cervix.

<table>
<tr><td>

TECHNIQUES AND NORMAL FINDINGS

</td><td>

</td></tr>
</table>

- Keep the other fingers of that hand rounded inward toward the palm and put the thumb against the mons pubis away from the clitoris (see Figure 22.14 ●).

▶ Pressure on the clitoris may be painful for the client.

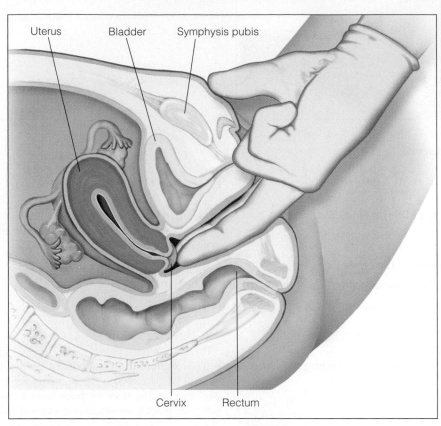

Figure 22.14 ● Palpating the cervix.

- Palpate the cervix. It should feel firm and smooth, somewhat like the tip of a nose.
- Gently try to move it. It should move easily about 1 to 2 cm in either direction.

▶ Nodules, hardness, or lack of mobility suggest a tumor.

▶ If the woman is pregnant, the cervix will be soft. This is a normal finding and is called Goodell's sign.

2. **Palpate the fornices.**
   - Slip your fingers into the vaginal recess areas, called the fornices.
   - Palpate around the grooves.
   - Confirm that the mucosa of the vagina and cervix in these areas is smooth and nontender.
   - Leave your fingers in the anterior fornix when you have checked all sides.

3. **Palpate the uterus.**
   - Place the fingers of your nondominant hand on the client's abdomen.

▶ Note any tenderness, which could be indicative of inflammation.

TECHNIQUES AND NORMAL FINDINGS	ABNORMAL FINDINGS SPECIAL CONSIDERATIONS

- Invaginate the abdomen midway between the umbilicus and the symphysis pubis by pushing with your fingertips downward toward the cervix (see Figure 22.15 ●).

▶ Note tenderness, masses, nodules, or bulging. These findings may indicate inflammation, infection, cysts, tumors, or wall prolapse. Note size, shape, consistency, and mobility of nodules and masses.

▶ In the obese female, it may be difficult to clearly differentiate the uterine structures, and an ultrasound study may be needed.

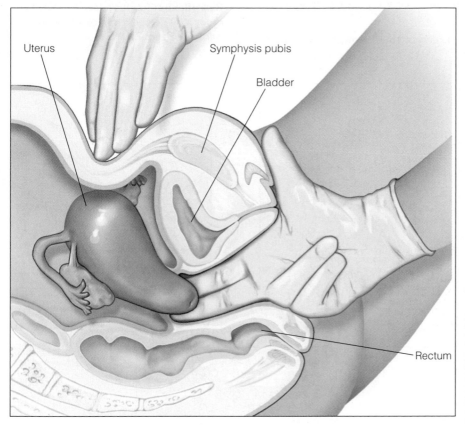

Uterus

Symphysis pubis

Bladder

Rectum

Figure 22.15 ● Palpating the uterus.

- Palpate the front wall of the uterus with the hand that is inside the vagina.
- As you palpate, note the position of the uterine body to determine that the uterus is in a normal position. When in a normal position, the uterus is tilted slightly upward above the bladder, and the cervix is tilted slightly forward.

TECHNIQUES AND NORMAL FINDINGS	ABNORMAL FINDINGS SPECIAL CONSIDERATIONS

- Normal variations of uterine position are:
  - **Anteversion** (uterus tilted forward, cervix tilted downward; see Figure 22.16A ●)
  - **Midposition** (uterus lies parallel to tailbone, cervix pointed straight; see Figure 22.16B ●)
  - **Retroversion** (uterus tilted backward, cervix tilted upward; see Figure 22.16C ●)

▶ Abnormal variations of uterine position are:
- **Anteflexion** (uterus folded forward at about a 90-degree angle, and cervix tilted downward; see Figure 22.16D ●)
- **Retroflexion** (uterus folded backward at about a 90-degree angle, cervix tilted upward; see Figure 22.16E ●)

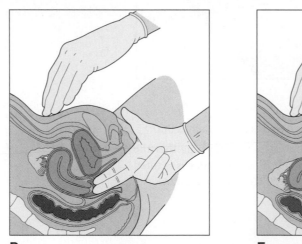

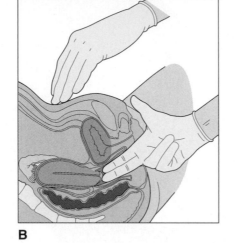
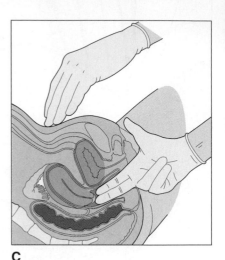
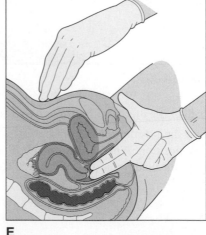

A B C

D E

Figure 22.16 ● Variations in uterine position. A. Anteversion. B. Midposition. C. Retroversion. D. Anteflexion. E. Retroflexion.

- Move the inner fingers to the posterior fornix, and gently raise the cervix up toward your outer hand.
- Palpate the front and back walls of the uterus as it is sandwiched between the two hands.

▶ Masses, tenderness, nodules, or bulging require further evaluation.

4. **Palpate the ovaries.**
   - While positioning the outer hand on the left lower abdominal quadrant, slip the vaginal fingers into the left lateral fornix.

▶ Extreme tenderness, nodularity, and masses are suggestive of inflammation, infection, cysts, malignancies, or tubal pregnancy.

TECHNIQUES AND NORMAL FINDINGS	ABNORMAL FINDINGS SPECIAL CONSIDERATIONS

- Push the opposing fingers and hand toward one another, and then use small circular motions to palpate the left ovary with your intravaginal fingers (see Figure 22.17 ●).

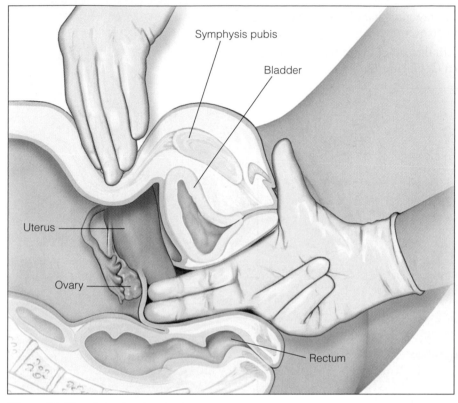

Figure 22.17 ● Palpating the ovaries.

- If you are able to palpate the ovary, it will feel mobile, almond shaped, smooth, firm, and nontender to slightly tender. Often you will be unable to palpate the ovaries, especially the right ovary.

▶ In obese females, it may not be possible to palpate the ovaries. In the female client who has been postmenopausal for more than 2½ years, palpable ovaries are considered abnormal because the ovaries usually atrophy with the postmenopausal decrease in estrogen.

- Slide your vaginal fingers around to the right lateral fornix and your outer hand to the lower right quadrant to palpate the right ovary.
- Confirm that the uterine tubes are not palpable.

▶ If the uterine tubes are palpable, an inflammation or some other disease process such as salpingitis or ectopic pregnancy may be present.

- Remove your hand from the vagina and put on new gloves.

▶ This prevents cross-contamination from the vagina to the rectum.

5. **Perform the rectovaginal exam.**
   - Tell the client that you are going to insert one finger into her vagina and one finger into her rectum in order to perform a rectovaginal exam. Tell her that this maneuver may make her feel as though she needs to have a bowel movement.
   - Lubricate the gloved index and middle fingers of the dominant hand.
   - Ask the client to bear down.
   - Touch the client's thigh with your nondominant hand to prepare her for the insertion.
   - Insert the index finger into the vagina (at a 45-degree downward slope) and the middle finger into the rectum.

▶ Note tenderness, masses, nodules, bulging, and thickened areas.

TECHNIQUES AND NORMAL FINDINGS

- Compress the rectovaginal septum between your index and middle fingers.
- Confirm that it is thin, smooth, and nontender.
- Place your nondominant hand on the client's abdomen.
- While maintaining the position of your intravaginal hand, press your outer hand inward and downward on the abdomen over the symphysis pubis.
- Palpate the posterior side of the uterus with the pad of the rectal finger while continuing to press down on the abdomen (see Figure 22.18 ●).

Figure 22.18 ●
Rectovaginal palpation.

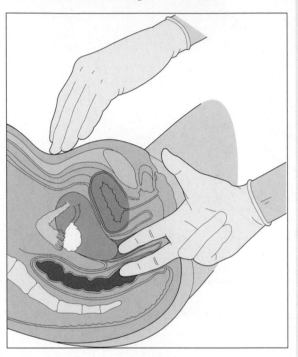

- Confirm that the uterine wall is smooth and nontender.

▶ Tenderness, masses, nodules, bulging, or thickened areas require further evaluation.

- If the ovaries are palpable, note that they are normal in size and contour.
- Remove your fingers from the vagina and rectum slowly and gently.

6. **Examine the stool.**

- Remove your gloves.

▶ Rectal bleeding is suspected when bright red blood is on the surface of the stool. Feces mixed with blood signals bleeding above the rectum.

- Assist the client into a comfortable position.
- Inspect feces remaining on the glove. Feces is normally brown and soft. Test feces for occult blood. Normally the test is negative.
- Wash your hands.
- Give the client tissues to wipe the perineal area. Some clients may need a perineal pad.
- Inform the client that she may have a small amount of spotting for a few hours after the speculum examination.

▶ Black, tarry stool indicates upper gastrointestinal tract bleeding.

 Refer to the Companion Website at **www.prenhall.com/damico** and click on the **Documentation** module for documentation samples and documentation practice exercises.

$\mathcal{A}$bnormal findings from assessment of the female reproductive system include but are not limited to problems with the external genitalia, perianal area, cervix, internal reproductive organs, and inflammatory processes. Problems in the perianal area are described in this chapter. Abnormal findings in the external genitalia are depicted and described in Figures 22.19 through 22.22. Abnormal findings of the cervix are illustrated and described in Figure 22.23. Abnormal findings of the internal reproductive organs such as myomas/fibroids, ovarian cancer, and ovarian cysts are illustrated and explained in Figures 22.24 through 22.26. Common inflammatory processes in the female reproductive system are depicted and described in Figures 22.27 through 22.30.

EXTERNAL GENITALIA

Pediculosis Pubis

Nits are on and around roots of pubic hair and cause itching. The area is reddened and excoriated (see Figure 22.19 ●).

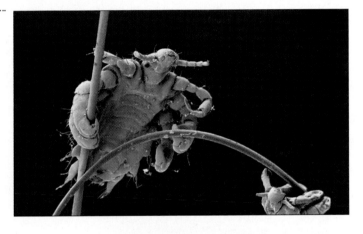

Figure 22.19 ● Pediculosis pubis (crab lice).

Herpes Simplex

Small vesicles appear on genitalia and may spread to the inner thigh (see Figure 22.20 ●). Ulcers are painful and erupt upon rupture of vesicles. The virus may be dormant for long periods.

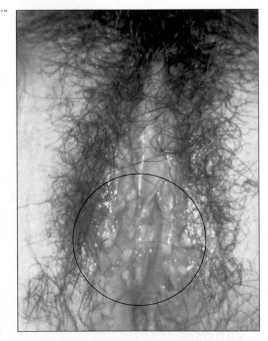

Figure 22.20 ● Herpes simplex.

Syphilitic Lesion

A syphilitic lesion is a nontender solitary papule that gradually changes to a draining ulcer (see Figure 22.21 ●).

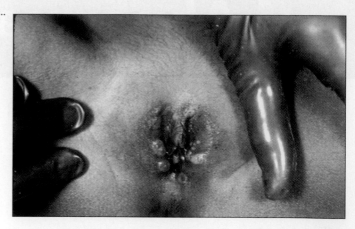

Figure 22.21 ● Syphilitic lesion.

Human Papillomavirus (HPV)

Wartlike, painless growths appear in clusters (see Figure 22.22 ●). These are seen on the vulva, inner vagina, cervix, or anal area.

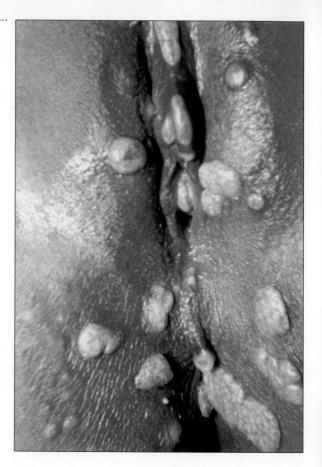

Figure 22.22 ● Human papillomavirus (genital warts).

Abscess of Bartholin's Gland

An abscess of Bartholin's gland includes labial edema and erythema with a palpable mass. There is purulent drainage from the duct.

CERVIX

Cyanosis

Cyanosis associated with hypoxic conditions such as congestive heart failure (CHF) can cause this. Blue coloring of the cervix is normal in pregnancy.

Carcinoma

Ulcerations with vaginal discharge, postmenopausal bleeding or spotting, or bleeding between menstrual periods are characteristics of cervical carcinoma. Diagnosis is confirmed by Pap smear.

Erosion

Inflammation and erosion are visible on the surface of the cervix (see Figure 22.23 ●). It is difficult to distinguish this from carcinoma without a biopsy.

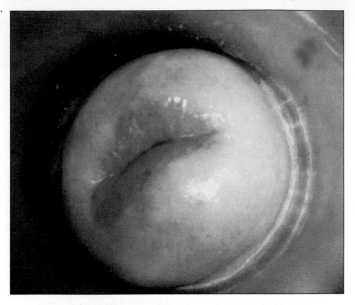

Figure 22.23 ● Erosion of the cervix.

Polyp

A soft growth extends from the os. A polyp is usually bright red and may bleed.

Diethylstilbestrol (DES) Syndrome

Abnormalities of the cervix arise in females who had prenatal exposure to DES. Epithelial abnormalities occur as granular patchiness extending from the cervix to the vaginal walls.

INTERNAL REPRODUCTIVE ORGANS

Myomas/Fibroids

Characteristics

- May be influenced by estrogen.

Signs and Symptoms

- May be asymptomatic.
- May cause excessive bleeding during menses.
- Uterus may become enlarged.
- May cause abdominal distention, pain, intestinal obstruction, frequent urination, and constipation.

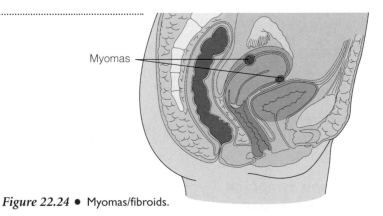

Figure 22.24 ● Myomas/fibroids.

Treatment

- Depends upon symptoms, and whether the client is currently pregnant or wishes to become pregnant.
- Surgery.

Ovarian Cancer

Ovarian cancer (see Figure 22.25 ●) is a type of cancer that begins in the cells of the ovaries and includes the epitheleal, germ, and includes the epithelial and germ cells.

Characteristics

- Occurs in 1 of 57 adult females in the United States. Known as the silent killer of women.
- Incidence higher in females with a family history (first-degree relative), younger women (but mostly female, over 50, with highest risk over age 60), those who have not had children, those who have had breast or colon cancer, and those who have used fertility drugs, talc in the genital area, and hormone replacement therapy (HRT).

Signs and Symptoms

- In early stages, may be symptomatic. Some clients experience gastrointestinal disturbances (pressure, bloating, cramps, indigestion), pain in the calves of the legs, lower back pain, loss of appetite, weight gain or loss with no known reason, nausea, diarrhea, constipation, and frequent urination.
- Progression of tumor leads to severe abdominal pressure and bloating, ascites, constipation, urinary frequency, abnormal bleeding from the vagina, and severe pain.

Treatment

- Depending upon the stage and general health of the female, may include surgery, chemotherapy, and radiation therapy.

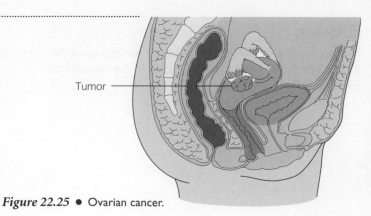

Figure 22.25 ● Ovarian cancer.

Ovarian Cysts

Ovarian cysts are fluid-filled sacs within the ovary or on the surface of the ovary (see Figure 22.26 ●).

Characteristics

- Nonmalignant cysts that may develop during puberty through menopause.

Signs and Symptoms

- Can be asymptomatic.
- Some clients experience pelvic pain, abdominal distention, and lower back pain.

Treatment

- May be spontaneously resorbed within several months.
- Medications may include clomiphene citrate, progesterone, or hydrocortisone.
- Surgery may be indicated.

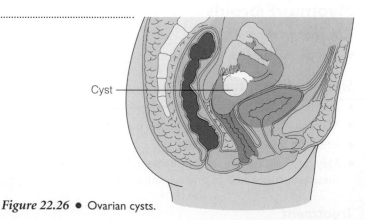

Figure 22.26 ● Ovarian cysts.

INFLAMMATORY PROCESSES

Atrophic Vaginitis

Estrogen deficiency in postmenopausal females results in dryness, itching, and burning sensations in the vagina. The vaginal mucosa may appear pale with mucousy discharge (see Figure 22.27 ●).

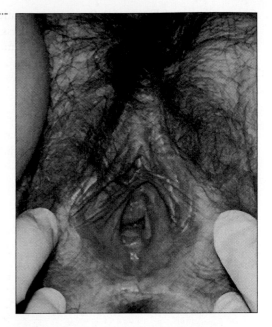

Figure 22.27 ● Atrophic vaginitis.

Candidiasis

Alteration of the pH of the vagina or antibiotic use predispose the female to this condition. The vulva and vagina are erythematous. Thick, cheesy white discharge is seen (see Figure 22.28 ●).

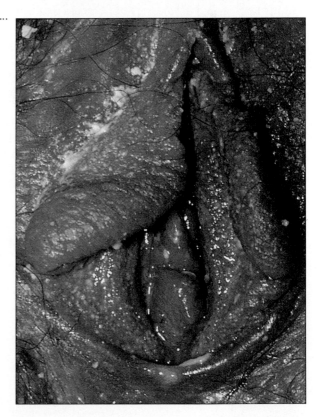

Figure 22.28 ● Candidiasis (yeast infection).

Chlamydia

Chlamydia is an STD that is often asymptomatic. This is characterized by purulent discharge with tenderness to movement of the cervix. Chlamydia can cause sterility if untreated.

Gonorrhea

Gonorrhea is generally asymptomatic. One may see vaginal discharge or bleeding and abscesses in Bartholin's or Skene's glands (see Figure 22.29 ●).

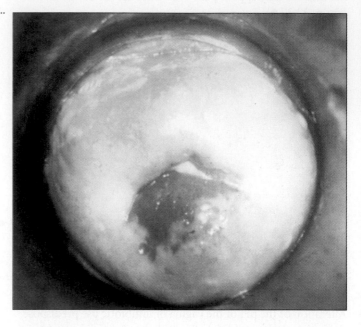

Figure 22.29 ● Gonorrhea.

Trichomoniasis

The female experiences painful urination, vulvular itching, and purulent vaginal discharge in this STD. The vagina and vulva are reddened and the discharge is yellow and foul smelling (see Figure 22.30 ●).

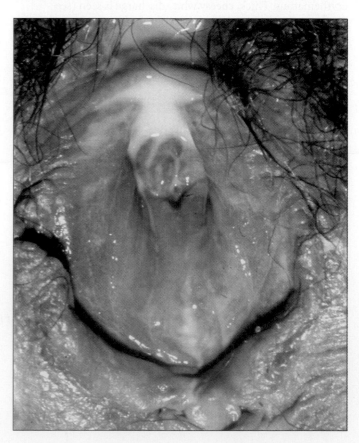

Figure 22.30 ● Trichomoniasis.

Health Promotion

HEALTHY PEOPLE 2010

FOCUS AREA	PREVALENCE	OBJECTIVES	ACTIONS
Unintended Pregnancy	• Fifty percent of all pregnancies in the United States are unintended. • Unintended pregnancy occurs most frequently in teenagers, women over 40 years of age, and low-income African American women.	• Increase the proportion of intended pregnancies. • Increase contraceptive use. • Reduce pregnancies in adolescents.	• Education about family planning. • Education about contraception. • Educational programs in schools and communities regarding sexual activity, pregnancy, and contraception.
Maternal Deaths	• Maternal mortality in African Americans is four times the rate of white women. • Maternal mortality is associated with ectopic pregnancy, induced abortions, and eclampsia.	• Reduce maternal deaths.	• Promotion of prenatal care to identify and mitigate risks.
Sexually Transmitted Disease (STD)	• Women have a higher risk for STD than males. • STD complications include pelvic inflammatory disease (PID), ectopic pregnancy, and chronic pelvic pain. • STDs affect adolescents and young adults more than older women. • HIV infection and the development of AIDS is increasing in the young heterosexual female population.	• Reduce the incidence of STD. • Reduce the proportion of females who require treatment for PID. • Reduce HIV infections. • Increase the number of adolescents who abstain from or delay sexual activity.	• Education about the transmission of STD. • Educational programs for individuals, groups, schools, and communities about responsible sexual behavior. • Information and education about condom use. • Education about the need for treatment and intervention in STD. • Screening for STD.
Cervical Cancer	• Cervical cancer is responsible for almost 2% of female cancer deaths in the United States. • New cases of cervical cancer are higher in African American and Hispanic women than in whites. • Sexually transmitted human papillomavirus is a causative factor in most cervical cancer.	• Reduce the death rate from cervical cancer.	• Education to promote screening for cervical cancer. • Education about sexual behavior and STD.

CLIENT EDUCATION

The following are physiological, behavioral, and cultural risk factors that affect female reproductive health across the age span. Several factors are cited as trends in *Healthy People 2010*. The nurse provides advice and education to reduce risks associated with these factors and to promote and maintain reproductive health.

LIFE SPAN CONSIDERATIONS

RISK FACTORS

- Infants may be born with ambiguous external genitalia.

- Young females experience changes associated with puberty between the ages of 8 and 13 years.

- Adolescents are interested in exploring their sexual identity and sexual contact.

- Changes in the reproductive system occur with aging and include physiological changes as well as changes in sexual activity.

CLIENT EDUCATION

- Counsel and advise parents about decisions regarding ambiguous genitalia, including genetic testing.
- Provide information to young females and parents regarding the changes that accompany the onset of puberty, including menstruation.
- Advise and counsel adolescents regarding sexual activity. Information should include the risks associated with sexual activity including STDs.
- Provide aging females with information about changes that accompany menopause. Aging females should be advised that atrophy of the reproductive organs occurs, vaginal lubrication diminishes, and sexual intercourse may be painful. Lubricants are available to decrease discomfort.

CULTURAL CONSIDERATIONS

RISK FACTOR

- Culture and language influence knowledge and practices related to the reproductive system.

CLIENT EDUCATION

- Be sensitive to cultural differences regarding discussion of reproductive function. In addition, information regarding hygiene, risk, and treatments should be provided in the native language of the client. Obtain a translator if needed.

ENVIRONMENTAL CONSIDERATIONS

RISK FACTORS

- The proximity of the urinary tract to genitalia and the perianal area requires the need for careful hygiene.

- Psychological and physical problems may be a result of sexual trauma or abuse.

- Females with a family history of reproductive cancer are at greater risk for the disease.

CLIENT EDUCATION

- Inform females of all ages about cleansing of the genitoperineal area to decrease risk of urinary tract infections. The use of bubble baths, perfumed soaps, antiseptics, and douche solutions may promote local irritation to the genitalia. Advise about avoidance of those hygiene products.
- Provide information about the safe use of tampons to all females to reduce risks of infection and toxic shock syndrome.
- Tell parents or caregivers that behavioral and physical changes may signal abuse. Withdrawal, changes in grades or participation in activities, changes in physical appearance, sleeplessness, or appetite change are among the behaviors that warrant follow-up. Encourage all females to report inappropriate sexual advances or abuse.
- Inform adult females of recommendations for Pap smears for cervical cancer screening. These recommendations include having the first Pap smear by age 21 or within 3 years of initiating vaginal intercourse. Annual Pap tests are recommended. At age 30, Pap testing may occur every 2 to 3 years in females who have had three normal tests. At 70 years, females with three or more normal tests may discontinue Pap tests. Advise clients to reduce their risk for cervical cancer by delaying initial sexual encounters until adulthood, limiting the number of partners (thereby reducing exposure to HPV), and not smoking. Inform clients with a first-degree relative with ovarian cancer that the cancer antigen (CA) 125 assay is used to measure the level of CA 125, which is a tumor marker.

- Psychosocial factors influence sexual desire and enjoyment.

- Provide clients with information about the actions and interactions of medications in relation to health and function of the reproductive and other systems and sexual activity. For example, antibodies can alter the vaginal flora and lead to vaginal yeast infections. Eating active culture yogurt while on antibiotics can reduce this risk. Some medications for cardiovascular problems diminish sexual desire. The use of oral contraceptives increases the risk for thrombosis, especially in smokers. Therefore, smoking cessation and precautions regarding periods of prolonged immobility, such as air flights, are important aspects of education about medications.

BEHAVIORAL CONSIDERATIONS

RISK FACTOR

- Risks for problems with the female reproductive system correlate to the numbers and types of sexual contacts.

CLIENT EDUCATION

- Discuss the risks associated with multiple sexual partners, including HPV, HIV, other STDs, and hepatitis C. Discuss safe sex practices.

Application Through Critical Thinking

CASE STUDY

Jessica Johnson, a 24-year-old, Caucasian female arrives in the clinic with lower abdominal pain and nausea. She states, "I've had this throbbing pain for 3 days and it kept getting worse." She further states, "I haven't been able to eat. I feel awful. You have to do something for the pain."

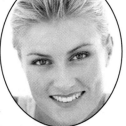

The nurse explains that more information is needed so that the proper treatment can be initiated. In further interview the following information is obtained. Ms. Johnson's last menstrual period was 1 week ago and she had more crampiness than usual. She has had brownish, thick vaginal discharge on and off since then. She has had some itchiness in the vaginal area and burning when she voids. She states she has to go to the bathroom all the time: "All I did was pee little bits, until this pain got to me. I have hardly gone since last night."

When asked about the pain, Ms. Johnson says it is mostly 8 on a scale of 1 to 10 and getting pretty constant. "Nothing I do helps, except a little if I curl up and hold still."

Physical examination reveals a thin, pale female.

VS: B/P 108/64—P 92—RR 20—T 101.4°F. Skin is hot, dry, poor turgor.

Mucous membranes dry. Posture—abdominal guarding.

Abdomen BS × 4 tender in R & LLQ to palpation. Vulvar pruritus, thick purulent vaginal drainage, pain upon cervical and uterine movement.

Cultures from vaginal secretions obtained	To lab
Blood drawn for CBC	To lab
Urine specimen obtained—clear, yellow	To lab

The client's clinic record reveals that she has been sexually active since age 16. She has had multiple partners and one abortion. She has been treated for sexually transmitted disease three times, most recently 2 months prior to this visit. The client is on birth control pills. She has no allergies to medications, and no family history of cardiovascular, abdominal, neurologic, urologic, endocrine, or reproductive disease.

Interpretation of the data suggests a diagnosis of pelvic inflammatory disease (PID). The options are outpatient treatment with antibiotics and education about limitations in activity and sexual practices, or inpatient treatment with intravenous fluids, antibiotics, analgesia, and bed rest.

Because Ms. Johnson is acutely ill, with pain and dehydration, she is admitted to the acute care facility with a diagnosis of PID.

► Complete Documentation

The following is sample documentation for Jessica Johnson.
SUBJECTIVE DATA: Throbbing abdominal pain for 3 days and getting worse. Rated 8 on scale of 1 to 10 with slight relief when "curled up and still." Nausea, unable to eat. LMP 1 week ago with increased crampiness. Brownish thick vaginal discharge. Vaginal itchiness. Urgent, burning urination of small amounts until past 12 hours. Sexually active with history of multiple partners, recent STD. No family history of disease, no allergies to medication.

OBJECTIVE DATA: Thin, pale female. Dry mucous membranes, skin hot, dry, poor turgor. Abdominal guarding, BS present X 4, tender RLQ, LLQ to light palpation. Vulvar pruritus, purulent vaginal discharge, adnexal tenderness with vaginal and bimanual examination.

ASSESSMENT FORM

Vital Signs

B/P: *108/64*

P: *92*

T: *101.4°F*

Pain: Location: *R & L LQ*

Rating: *8*

Duration: *constant*

Relief: *curling up and being still*

Onset: *3 days*

Quality: *throbbing*

Skin

Color: *pink*

Temperature: *hot*

Moisture: *dry*

Turgor: *poor*

Lesions: *none*

Respiratory

Respiratory rhythm: *regular*

Rate: *20*

Lung sounds: *clear all fields*

Abdomen

Contour: *round*

BS: *+ all Q*

Pain: *tender (R) (L) LQ*

Stool: *none*

Appetite: *poor—nausea*

Urinary

Frequency: *increased until past 12 hours*

Amount: *"a little at a time"*

Color: *yellow*

Effort: *burning*

Endocrine

LMP: *1 week ago*

Blood sugar: *unknown*

Genitalia

Vulvar pruritus, purulent vaginal discharge

Adnexal tenderness with vaginal and bimanual examination

► Critical Thinking Questions

1. What clusters of information suggest the diagnosis of PID?
2. What additional information is required to develop a plan of care for Jessica Johnson?
3. What would discharge planning for Ms. Johnson include?

► Applying Nursing Diagnoses

1. *Ineffective sexuality patterns* is a diagnosis in the NANDA taxonomy (see Appendix A ⃝⃝). Do the data in the case study support this diagnosis? Explain your response.
2. Use the data from the case study and the NANDA taxonomy (see Appendix A ⃝⃝) to develop nursing diagnoses for Jessica Johnson.
3. Identify the data to support each diagnosis identified in the NANDA taxonomy.

► Prepare Teaching Plan

LEARNING NEED: Jessica Johnson initiated sexual activity at 16 years of age. She has had multiple partners and frequent episodes of STD. These data indicate a need to learn about PID and to discuss this infection with her partner.

GOAL: Jessica Johnson will decrease her risk for repeated episodes of PID.

OBJECTIVES: Jessica Johnson will be able to:

1. Describe PID.
2. Relate personal practices to the occurrence of PID.
3. Describe treatment modalities for PID.

APPLICATION OF OBJECTIVE 2: Relate personal practices to the occurrence of PID (Cognitive)

Content	Teaching Strategy	Evaluation
• Frequent douching will mask symptoms or push organisms internally. • Sexual activity before age 25. • Multiple partners. • Partner with multiple partners. • Use of IUD. • Not practicing safe sex—use of condoms will help decrease risk. • Untreated STD.	One-on-one discussion encourages learner participation, permits reinforcement of content, and is appropriate for sensitive subject matter.	Jessica relates her personal practices to the occurrence of PID.

Please refer to the Companion Website at www.prenhall.com/damico and click on Chapter 22, the Application Through Critical Thinking module, to complete the following activities related to this case study:
► Critical Thinking questions
► Extended Nursing Diagnosis challenge
► Documentation activity
► Teaching Plan for Objectives I and 3

EXPLORE MediaLink

Additional resources for this chapter are found on the Student CD-ROM accompanying this textbook and on the Companion Website.

CD-ROM CONTENT

Content for this chapter includes:
Objectives
Key Concepts
NCLEX-RN® Review Questions
Model Documentation Forms
Audio Glossary
Animations
Female Reproductive Anatomy
Contraception
Games and Challenges
Clinical Spotlight Videos
Premenstrual Syndrome
Disease Investigation: Gonorrhea
Child Abuse
Head-to-Toe Physical Examination Video

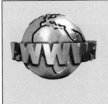

Client Interaction Case Study Challenge
Application Through Critical Thinking Case Study
Teaching Plan Challenge
MediaLinks
MediaLink Application
Tool Box
Chapter Documentation Form Example
Health Promotion
    Healthy People 2010
    Client Education
New York Times

COMPANION WEBSITE CONTENT

www.prenhall.com/damico

Content for this chapter includes:
Objectives
NCLEX-RN® Review Questions

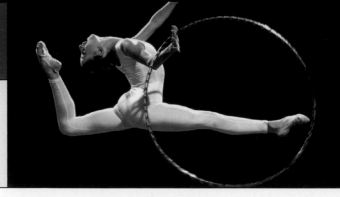

23

Musculoskeletal System

MEDIALINK

www.prenhall.com/damico

The CD-ROM in the back of this textbook and the Media-Link website contain NCLEX-RN® review questions, interactive exercises, case study challenges, animations, videos, documentation and checklist forms, and review materials. For a complete listing of the media content specific to Chapter 23, see the Explore MediaLink at the end of the chapter.

The primary function of the musculoskeletal system is to provide structure and movement for the human body. The 206 bones of the musculoskeletal system and accompanying skeletal muscles allow the body to stand erect and move, and they support and protect body organs. This system produces red blood cells, stores fat and minerals, and generates body heat.

A thorough assessment of the musculoskeletal system provides data relevant to activity, exercise, nutrition, and metabolism. The physical assessment of the musculoskeletal system is extensive, requiring a head-to-toe approach because it extends throughout the body. Musculoskeletal assessment could be combined with assessment of other body systems to obtain data reflecting the client's total health status, because every other body system is affected by or affects this body system. For example, the nervous system innervates bone and joint capsules and helps stimulate and regulate muscle activity. Should the client have difficulty moving a specific part of the body, the nurse will need to determine the origin of the problem as being neurologic or musculoskeletal. Red blood cells are formed in the bone marrow; therefore, if the cell count is low, the nurse will need to determine the source of the problem.

Bone density and curvatures vary widely among people of different cultural groups. Working conditions requiring heavy lifting, repetitive motions, or substantial physical activity present potential risks to this system. Participation in hobbies and athletic activities can contribute to "wear and tear" damage to joints and create risks for trauma to bones, muscles, and joints. Changes in bone density and injury to bone and muscle are factors in the goals for health promotion as discussed in *Healthy People 2010*. Actions to achieve the goals are included in the *Healthy People 2010* feature on page 724.

ANATOMY AND PHYSIOLOGY REVIEW

The musculoskeletal system consists of the body's bones, skeletal muscles, and joints. A thorough discussion of these anatomical structures is included in the following section.

BONES

The bones support and provide a framework for the soft tissues and organs of the body. They are classified according to shape and composition. Bone shapes include *long bones* (femur, humerus), *short bones* (carpals, tarsals), *flat bones* (the parietal bone of the skull, the sternum, ribs), and *irregular bones* (vertebrae, hip bones) as shown in Figure 23.1 ●. Bones are composed of osseous tissue that is arranged in either a dense, smooth, compact structure, or a cancellous, spongy structure with many small open spaces (see Figure 23.2 ●). The bones of the human skeleton are illustrated in Figure 23.3 (see page 669) ●.

The major functions of the bones include providing a framework for the body, protecting structures, acting as levers for movement, storing fat and minerals, and producing blood cells.

SKELETAL MUSCLES

A skeletal muscle is composed of hundreds of thousands of elongated muscle cells or fibers arranged in striated bands that attach to skeletal bones (see Figure 23.4 on page 670 ●). Although some skeletal muscles react by reflex, most skeletal muscles are voluntary and are under an individual's conscious control. Figure 23.5 (see pages 671–672) ● illustrates the muscles of the human body. The major functions of the skeletal muscles include providing for movement, maintaining posture, and generating body heat.

JOINTS

A **joint** (or *articulation*) is the point where two or more bones in the body meet. Joints may be classified structurally as fibrous, cartilaginous, or synovial. Bones joined by fibrous tissue, such as the sutures joining the bones of the skull, are called **fibrous joints.**

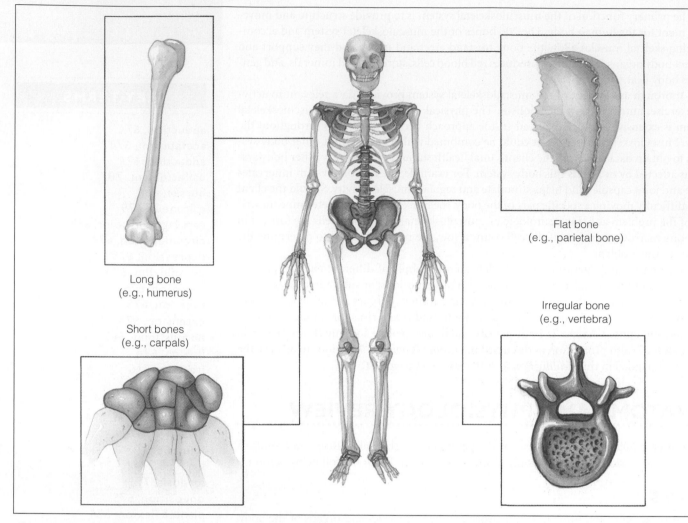

Figure 23.1 ● Classification of bones according to shape.

Bones joined by cartilage, such as the vertebrae, are called **cartilaginous joints.** Bones separated by a fluid-filled joint cavity are called **synovial joints.** The structure of synovial joints allows tremendous freedom of movement, and all joints of the limbs are synovial joints. Most synovial joints are reinforced and strengthened by a system of *ligaments,* which are bands of flexible tissue that attach bone to bone. Some ligaments are protected from friction by small, synovial-fluid-filled sacs called **bursae. Tendons** are tough fibrous bands that attach muscle to bone, or muscle to muscle. Tendons, subjected to continuous friction, develop fluid-filled bursae called *tendon sheaths* to protect the joint from damage.

During the assessment of the musculoskeletal system, the nurse assesses the joint, its range of motion, and its surrounding structures of muscles, ligaments, tendons, and bursae. Table 23.1 (see pages 673–674) describes the classification of synovial joints, and Table 23.2 (see pages 674–675) describes the movements of the joints. A description of selected joints to be examined during the physical assessment of the musculoskeletal system follows.

Temporomandibular Joint

The temporomandibular joint (TMJ) permits articulation between the mandible and the temporal bone of the skull

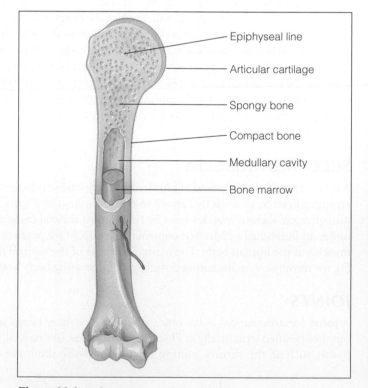

Figure 23.2 ● Composition of a long bone.

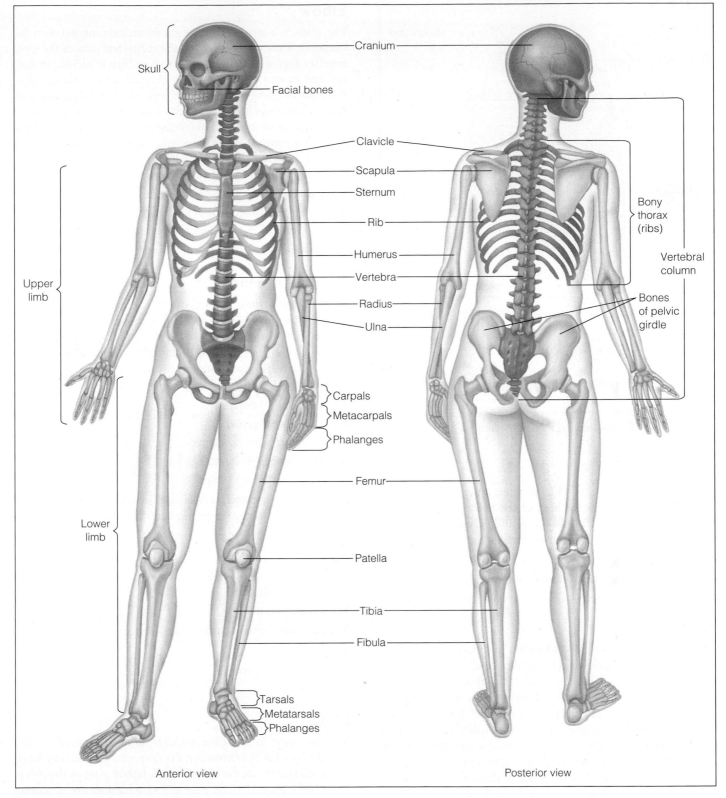

Anterior view

Posterior view

Figure 23.3 ● Bones of the human skeleton.

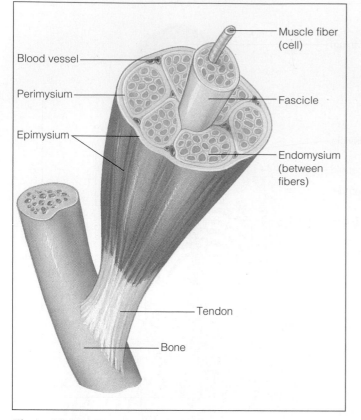

Blood vessel
Perimysium
Epimysium
Muscle fiber (cell)
Fascicle
Endomysium (between fibers)
Tendon
Bone

Figure 23.4 • Composition of a skeletal muscle.

(see Figure 23.6 on page 676 •). Lying just anterior to the external auditory meatus, at the level of the tragus of the ear, the temporomandibular joint allows an individual to speak and chew. Temporomandibular movements include the following:

- Opening and closing of the lower jaw
- Protraction and retraction of the lower jaw
- Side-to-side movement of the lower jaw

Shoulder

The shoulder joint is a ball-and-socket joint in which the head of the humerus articulates in the shallow glenoid cavity of the scapula (see Table 23.1). The shoulder is supported by the rotator cuff, a sturdy network of tendons and muscles, as well as a series of ligaments (see Figure 23.7 on page 676 •). The major landmarks of the shoulder include the scapula, the acromion process, the greater tubercle of the humerus, and the coracoid process. The subacromial bursa, which allows the arm to abduct smoothly and with ease, lies just below the acromion process. Movements of the shoulder include the following:

- Abduction (180 degrees)
- Adduction (50 degrees)
- Horizontal forward flexion (180 degrees)
- Horizontal backward extension (50 degrees)
- Circumduction (360 degrees)
- External rotation (90 degrees)
- Internal rotation (90 degrees)

Elbow

The elbow is a hinge joint that allows articulation between the humerus of the upper arm, and the radius and ulna of the forearm (see Figure 23.8 on page 676 •). Landmarks include the lateral and medial epicondyles on either side of the distal end of the humerus, and the olecranon process of the ulna. The olecranon bursa sits between the olecranon process and the skin. The ulnar nerve travels between the medial epicondyle and the olecranon process. When inflamed, the synovial membrane is palpable between the epicondyles and the olecranon process. Elbow movements include the following:

- Flexion of the forearm (160 degrees)
- Extension of the forearm (160 degrees)
- Supination of the forearm and hand (90 degrees)
- Pronation of the forearm and hand (90 degrees)

Wrist and Hand

The wrist (or *carpus*) consists of two rows of eight short carpal bones connected by ligaments as illustrated in Figure 23.9 (see page 677) •. The distal row articulates with the metacarpals of the hand. The proximal row includes the scaphoid and lunate bones, which articulate with the distal end of the radius to form the wrist joint. Wrist movements include the following:

- Extension (70 degrees)
- Flexion (90 degrees)
- Hyperextension (30 degrees)
- Radial deviation (20 degrees)
- Ulnar deviation (55 degrees)

Each hand has metacarpophalangeal joints, and each finger has interphalangeal joints. Finger movements include the following:

- Abduction (20 degrees)
- Extension
- Hyperextension (30 degrees)
- Flexion (90 degrees)
- Circumduction

Thumb movements include the following:

- Extension
- Flexion (80 degrees)
- Opposition

Hip

The hip joint is a ball-and-socket joint composed of the rounded head of the femur as it fits deep into the **acetabulum,** a rounded cavity on the right and left lateral sides of the pelvic bone (see Figure 23.10 on page 677 •). Although not as mobile as the shoulder, the hip is surrounded by a system of cartilage, ligaments, tendons, and muscles that contribute to its strength and stability. Landmarks include the iliac crest (not shown), the greater trochanter of the femur, and the anterior inferior iliac spine. Hip movements include the following:

- Extension (90 degrees)
- Hyperextension (15 degrees)
- Flexion with knee flexed (120 degrees)

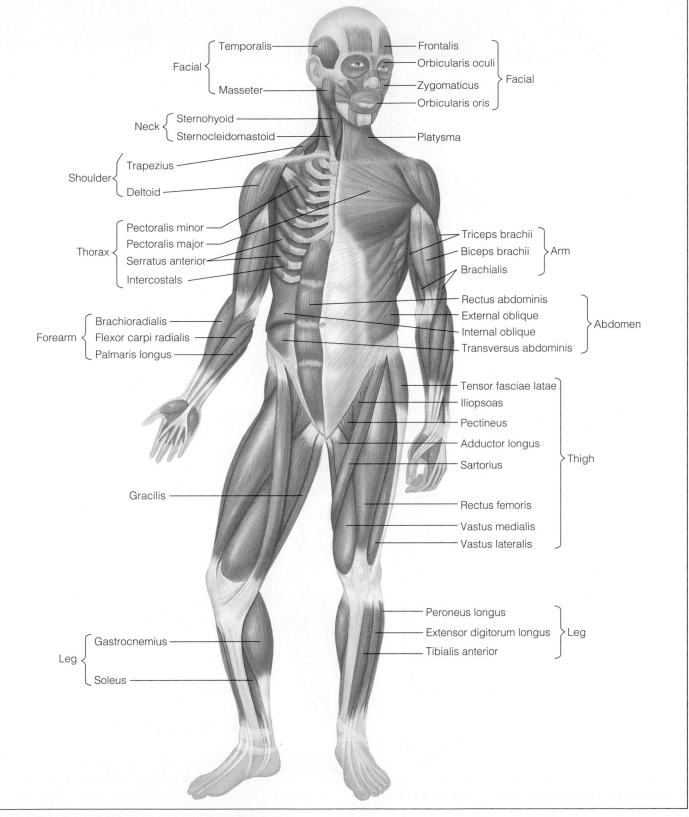

Facial
- Temporalis
- Masseter

Facial
- Frontalis
- Orbicularis oculi
- Zygomaticus
- Orbicularis oris

Neck
- Sternohyoid
- Sternocleidomastoid

Platysma

Shoulder
- Trapezius
- Deltoid

Thorax
- Pectoralis minor
- Pectoralis major
- Serratus anterior
- Intercostals

Arm
- Triceps brachii
- Biceps brachii
- Brachialis

Forearm
- Brachioradialis
- Flexor carpi radialis
- Palmaris longus

Abdomen
- Rectus abdominis
- External oblique
- Internal oblique
- Transversus abdominis

Thigh
- Tensor fasciae latae
- Iliopsoas
- Pectineus
- Adductor longus
- Sartorius
- Rectus femoris
- Vastus medialis
- Vastus lateralis

Gracilis

Leg
- Gastrocnemius
- Soleus

Leg
- Peroneus longus
- Extensor digitorum longus
- Tibialis anterior

Figure 23.5A ● Anterior view of muscles of the human body.

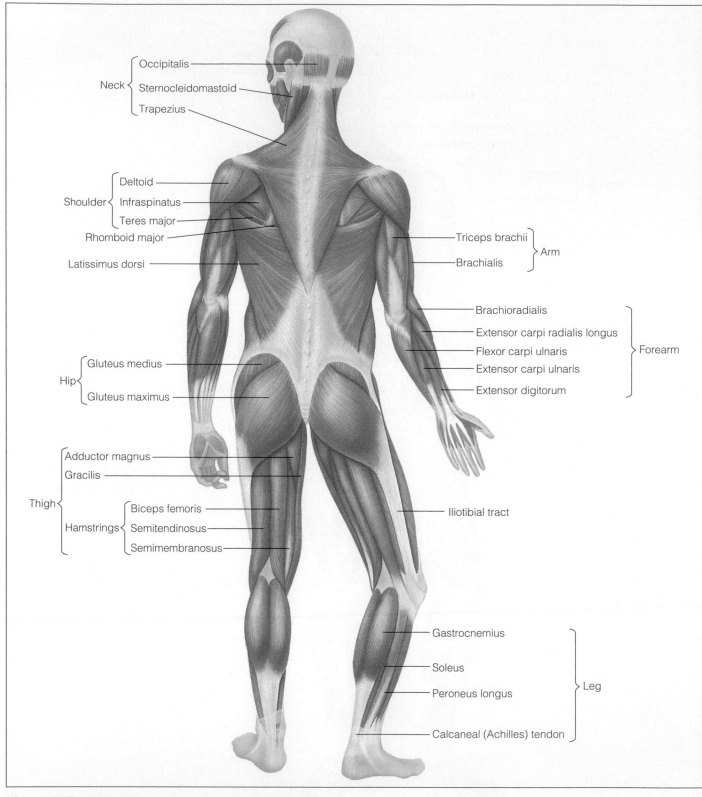

Figure 23.5B ● Posterior view of muscles of the human body.

Table 23.1 **Classification of Synovial Joints**

TYPE OF JOINT

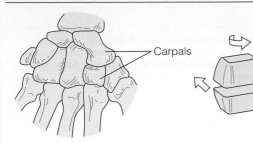

A Plane joint

In *plane joints,* the articular surfaces are flat, allowing only slipping or gliding movements. Examples include the intercarpal and intertarsal joints, and the joints between the articular processes of the ribs.

Carpals

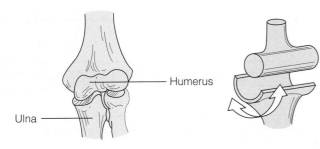

B Hinge joint

In *hinge joints,* a convex projection of one bone fits into a concave depression in another. Motion is similar to that of a mechanical hinge. These joints permit flexion and extension only. Examples include the elbow and knee joints.

Humerus

Ulna

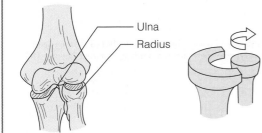

C Pivot joint

In *pivot joints,* the rounded end of one bone protrudes into a ring of bone (and possibly ligaments). The only movement allowed is rotation of the bone around its own long axis or against the other bone. An example is the joint between the atlas and axis of the neck.

Ulna
Radius

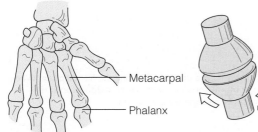

D Condyloid joint

In *condyloid joints,* the oval surfaces of two bones fit together. Movements allowed are flexion and extension, abduction, adduction, and circumduction. An example is the radiocarpal (wrist) joints.

Metacarpal

Phalanx

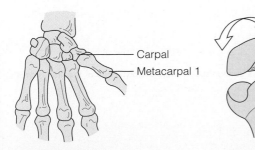

E Saddle joint

In *saddle joints,* each articulating bone has both concave and convex areas (resembling a saddle). The opposing surfaces fit together. The movements allowed are the same as for condyloid joints, but the freedom of motion is greater. The carpometacarpal joints of the thumbs are an example.

Carpal
Metacarpal 1

(continued)

Table 23.1	Classification of Synovial Joints *(continued)*

TYPE OF JOINT

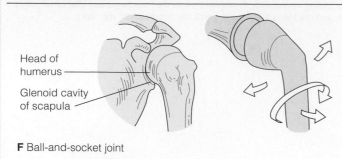

F Ball-and-socket joint

In *ball-and-socket joints,* the ball-shaped head of one bone fits into the concave socket of another. This joints allow movement in all axes and planes, including rotation. The shoulder and hip joints are the only examples in the body.

Head of humerus

Glenoid cavity of scapula

Table 23.2	Joint Movement

TYPE OF MOVEMENT

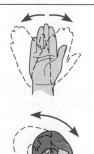

Gliding movements are the simplest type of joint movements. One flat bone surface glides or slips over another similar surface. The bones are merely displaced in relation to one another.

Flexion is a bending movement that decreases the angle of the joint and brings the articulating bones closer together. **Extension** increases the angle between the articulating bones. (**Hyperextension** is a bending of a joint beyond 180 degrees.)

Flexion of the ankle so that the superior aspect of the foot approaches the shin is called **dorsiflexion.** Extension of the ankle (pointing the toes) is called **plantar flexion.**

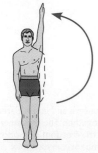

Abduction is movement of a limb away from the midline or median plane of the body, along the frontal plane. When the term is used to describe movement of the fingers or toes, it means spreading them apart. **Adduction** is the movement of a limb toward the body midline. Bringing the fingers close together is adduction.

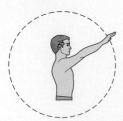

Circumduction is the movement in which the limb describes a cone in space: while the distal end of the limb moves in a circle, the joint itself moves only slightly in the joint cavity.

Table 23.2	Joint Movement *(continued)*

TYPE OF MOVEMENT

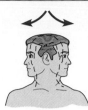

Rotation is the turning movement of a bone around its own long axis. Rotation may occur toward the body midline or away from it.

The terms **supination** and **pronation** refer only to the movements of the radius around the ulna. Movement of the forearm so that the palm faces anteriorly or superiorly is called *supination*. In *pronation*, the palm moves to face posteriorly or inferiorly.

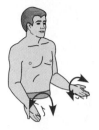

The terms **inversion** and **eversion** refer to movements of the foot. In *inversion*, the sole of the foot is turned medially. In *eversion*, the sole faces laterally.

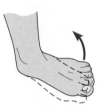

Protraction is a nonangular anterior movement in a transverse plane.
Retraction is a nonangular posterior movement in a transverse plane.

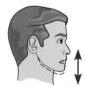

Elevation is a lifting or moving superiorly along a frontal plane. When the elevated part is moved downward to its original position, the movement is called **depression.** Shrugging the shoulders and chewing are examples of alternating elevation and depression.

Opposition *of the thumb* is only allowed at the saddle joint between metacarpal I and the carpals. It is the movement of touching the thumb to the tips of the other fingers of the same hand.

- Flexion with knee extended (90 degrees)
- Internal rotation (40 degrees)
- External rotation (45 degrees)
- Abduction (45 degrees)
- Adduction (30 degrees)

Knee

The knee is a complex joint consisting of the patella (knee cap), femur, and tibia (see Figure 23.11 on page 678 ●). It is supported and stabilized by the cruciate and collateral ligaments, which have a sta-

bilizing effect on the knee and prevent dislocation. The landmarks of the knee include the tibial tuberosity and the medial and lateral condyles of the tibia. Knee movements include the following:

- Extension (0 degree)
- Flexion (130 degrees)
- Hyperextension (15 degrees)

Ankle and Foot

The ankle is a hinge joint that accommodates articulation between the tibia, fibula, and *talus*, a large, posterior tarsal of the foot

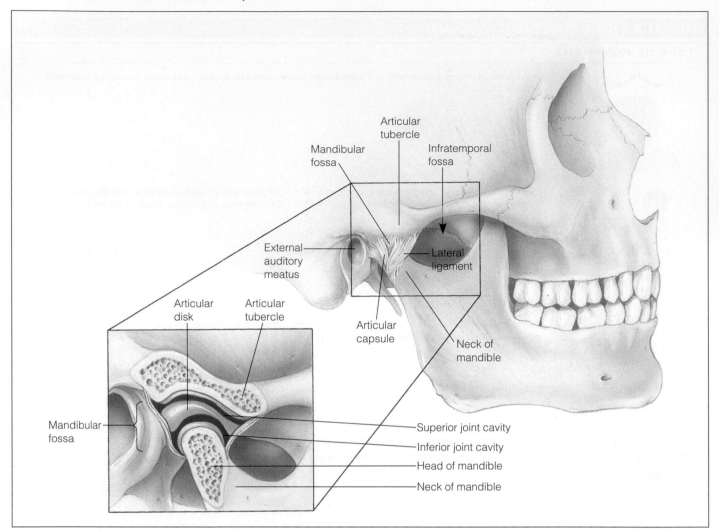

Figure 23.6 ● Temporomandibular joint. The enlargement shows a sagittal section through the joint.

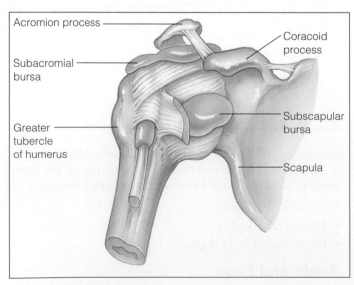

Figure 23.7 ● Shoulder joint.

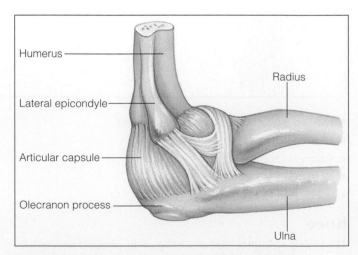

Figure 23.8 ● Elbow joint. Lateral view of the right elbow.

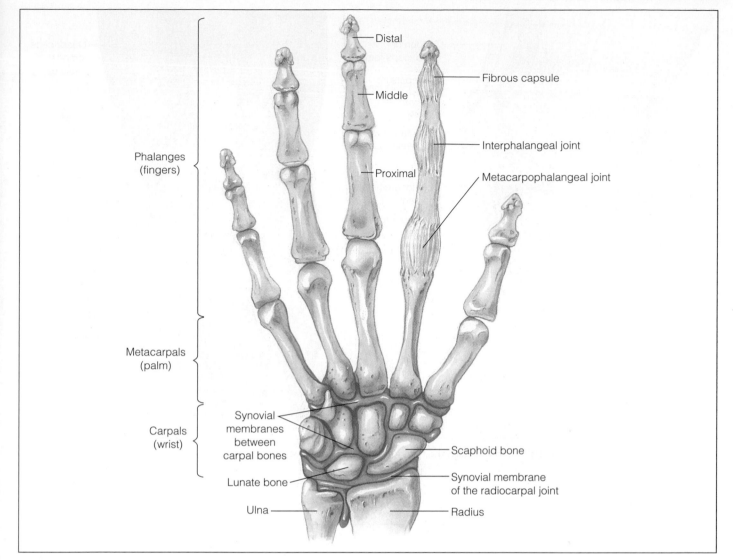

Figure 23.9 ● Bones of the wrist, hand, and phalanges.

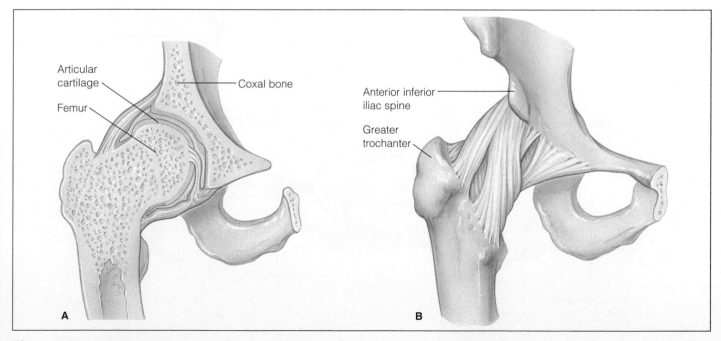

Figure 23.10 ● Hip joint. A. Cross section. B. Anterior view.

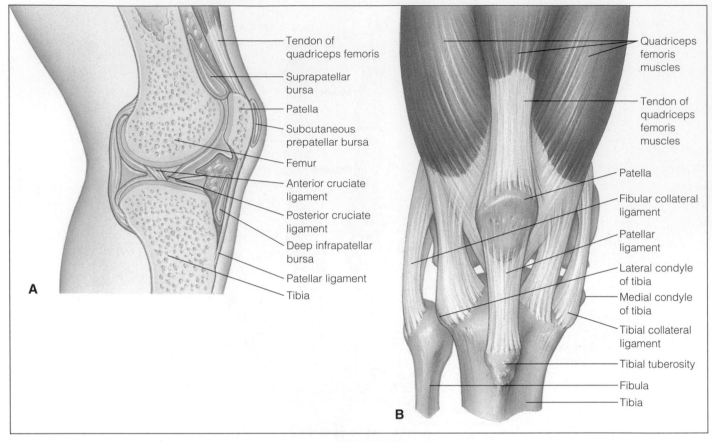

Figure 23.11 ● Knee joint. A. Sagittal section through the right knee. B. Anterior view.

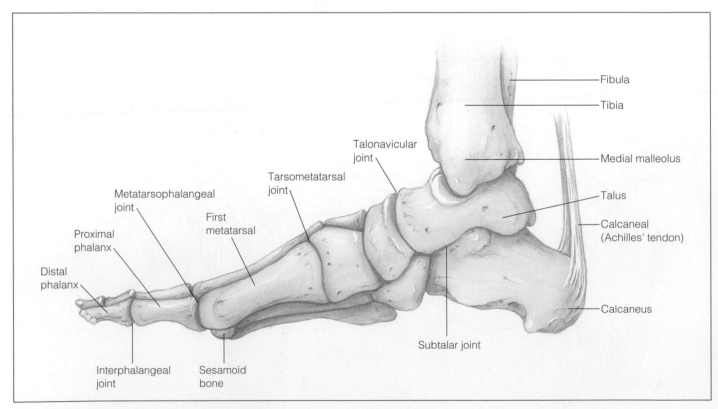

Figure 23.12 ● Medial view of joints of right ankle and foot.

(see Figure 23.12 ●). The **calcaneus** (or heel bone) is just inferior to the talus. It is stabilized by a set of taut ligaments that are anchored from bony prominences at the distal ends of the tibia and fibula (the lateral and medial malleoli), and then extend and attach to the foot. Movements of the ankle and foot include the following:

- Dorsiflexion of ankle (20 degrees)
- Plantar flexion of ankle (45 degrees)
- Inversion of foot (30 degrees)
- Eversion of foot (20 degrees)

Movements of the toes include the following:

- Extension
- Flexion
- Abduction (10 degrees)
- Adduction (20 degrees)

Spine

The spine is composed of 26 irregular bones called vertebrae (see Figure 23.13 ●). There are 7 *cervical vertebrae,* which sup-port the base of the skull and the neck. All 12 of the *thoracic vertebrae* articulate with the ribs. The 5 *lumbar vertebrae* support the lower back. They are heavier and denser than the other vertebrae, reflecting their weight-bearing function. The *sacrum* shapes the posterior wall of the pelvis, offering strength and stability. The *coccyx* is a small, triangular tailbone at the base of the spine.

Viewed laterally, the spine has cervical and lumbar concavities and a thoracic convexity. As a person bends forward, the normal concavity should flatten, and there should be a single convex C-shaped curve. Figure 23.5B shows the main muscles of the neck and the spine. Movements of the neck include the following:

- Flexion (45 degrees)
- Extension (55 degrees)
- Hyperextension (10 degrees)
- Lateral flexion (bending) (40 degrees)
- Rotation (70 degrees)

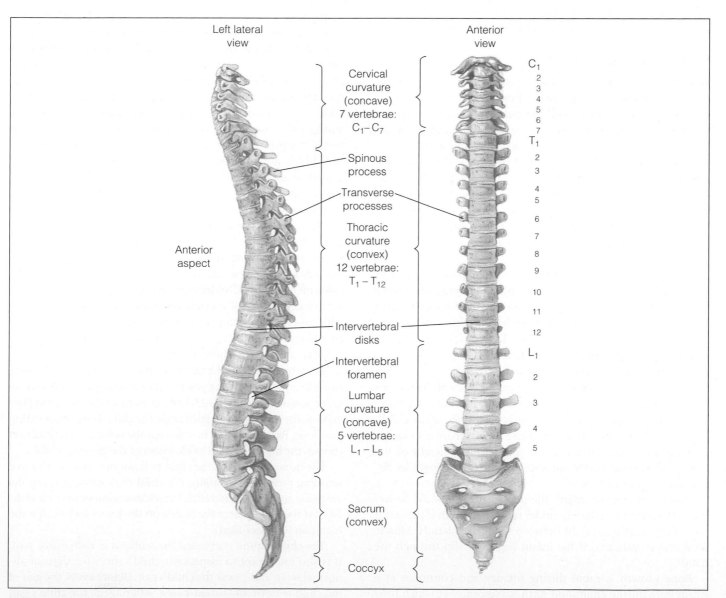

Figure 23.13 ● The spine.

Movements of the spine include the following:

- Lateral flexion (35 degrees)
- Extension (30 degrees)
- Flexion (90 degrees)
- Rotation (30 degrees)

SPECIAL CONSIDERATIONS

There are a variety of factors or special considerations that contribute to health status. Among these are age, developmental level, race, ethnicity, work history, living conditions, socioeconomics, and emotional well-being. The following sections describe special considerations to include when gathering subjective and objective data.

DEVELOPMENTAL CONSIDERATIONS

Accurate interpretation of findings requires knowledge of the variations in anatomy and physiology that occur with growth and development. Specific variations in the musculoskeletal system across the age span are described in the following sections.

Infants and Children

Fetal positioning and the delivery process may cause musculoskeletal anomalies in the infant. These include *tibial torsion,* a curving apart of the tibias, and *metatarsus adductus,* a tendency of the forefoot to turn inward. Many such anomalies correct themselves spontaneously as the child grows and walks.

Newborns normally have flat feet; arches develop gradually during the preschool years. Before learning to walk, infants tend to exhibit genu varum (bowlegs). Then, as the child begins to walk, this tendency gradually reverses. By the age of 4, most children tend to exhibit genu valgum (knock knees). This condition also resolves spontaneously, usually by late childhood or early adolescence.

The nurse should inspect the newborn's spine. Any tuft of hair, cyst, or mass may indicate spina bifida and requires further evaluation. The nurse also palpates the length of the clavicles at each office visit, noting any lumps or irregularities and observing the range of motion of the arms. The clavicle is frequently fractured during birth, and the fracture often goes unnoticed until a callus forms at the fracture site.

The infant is assessed for congenital hip dislocation at every office visit until 1 year of age. Additionally, *Allis' sign* is used to detect unequal leg length. The nurse is positioned at the child's feet. With the infant supine, the nurse flexes the infant's knees, keeping the femurs aligned, and compares the height of the knees. An uneven height indicates unequal leg length as depicted in Figure 23.14 ●.

While holding the infant, the nurse's hands should be beneath the infant's axillae. Shoulder muscle strength is present if the infant remains upright between the nurse's hands. Muscle weakness is indicated if the infant begins to slip through the hands.

Bone growth is rapid during infancy and continues at a steady rate during childhood until adolescence, at which time

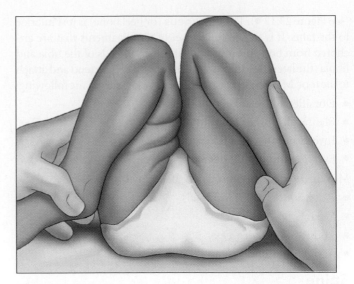

Figure 23.14 ● Allis' sign—demonstration of unequal knee height.

both girls and boys experience a growth spurt. Long bones increase in width because of the deposition of new bony tissue around the diaphysis (shaft). Long bones also increase in length because of a proliferation of cartilage at the growth plates at the epiphyses (ends) of the long bones. Longitudinal growth ends at about 21 years of age, when the epiphyses fuse with the diaphysis. Throughout childhood, ligaments are stronger than bones. Therefore, childhood injuries to the long bones and joints tend to result in fractures instead of sprains. Individual muscle fibers grow throughout childhood, but growth is especially increased during the adolescent growth spurt. Muscles vary in size and strength due to genetics, exercise, and diet.

Much of the examination of the child and adolescent includes the same techniques of inspection, palpation, and assessment of range of motion and muscle strength used in the examination of the adult. However, children also have unique assessment needs. Children present wonderful opportunities for assessing range of motion and muscle strength as they play with toys in the waiting area or examination room. The nurse should encourage children to jump, hop, skip, and climb. Most children are eager to show off their abilities.

At each office visit, the nurse should ask children to demonstrate their favorite sitting position. If a child assumes the reverse tailor position (see Figure 23.15 ●), common when watching television, the nurse should encourage the child to try other sitting positions. Parents should be told that the reverse tailor position stresses the hip, knee, and ankle joints of the growing child.

The nurse should ask the child to lie supine, then to rise to a standing position. Normally, the child rises without using the arms for support. Generalized muscle weakness may be indicated if the child places the hands on the knees and pushes the trunk up (Gowers' sign).

The child's spine is assessed for scoliosis at each office visit. It is also important to inspect the child's shoes for signs of abnormal wear, and assess the child's gait. Before age 3, the gait of the child is normally broad-based. After age 3, the child's gait

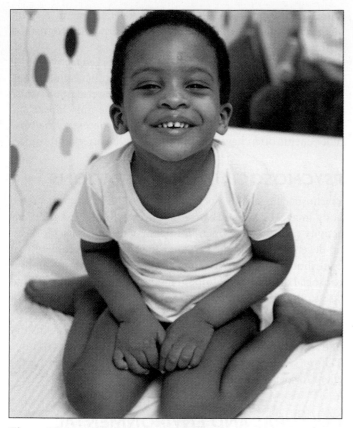

Figure 23.15 ● Reverse tailor position.

narrows. At each visit, the nurse assesses the range of motion of each arm. **Subluxation** of the head of the radius occurs commonly when adults dangle children from their hands or remove their clothing forcibly.

The nurse must obtain complete information on any sports activity the child or adolescent engages in, because par-

ticipation in these can indicate the need for special assessments or preventive teaching such as the use of helmets and other safety equipment.

The Pregnant Female

Estrogen and other hormones soften the cartilage in the pelvis and increase the mobility of the joints, especially the sacroiliac, sacrococcygeal, and symphysis pubis joints. As the pregnancy progresses, lordosis (exaggeration of the lumbar spinal curve) compensates for the enlarging fetus. The female's center of gravity shifts forward, and she shifts her weight farther back on her lower extremities. This shift strains the lower spine, causing the lower back pain that is so common during late pregnancy (see Figure 23.16 ●). As the pregnancy progresses, she may develop a waddling gait because of her enlarged abdomen and the relaxed mobility in her joints. Typically, a female resumes her normal posture and gait shortly after the pregnancy.

The Older Adult

As individuals age, physiological changes take place in the bones, muscles, connective tissue, and joints. These changes may affect the older client's mobility and endurance. Bone changes include decreased calcium absorption and reduced osteoblast production. If the older adult has a chronic illness, such as chronic obstructive lung disease or hyperthyroidism, or takes medications containing glucocorticoids, thyroid hormone preparation, or anticonvulsants, bone strength may be greatly compromised because of decrease in the bone density. Elderly persons who are housebound and immobile or whose dietary intake of calcium and vitamin D is low may also experience reduced bone mass and strength. During aging, bone resorption occurs more rapidly than new bone growth, resulting in the loss of bone density typical of osteoporosis. The entire skeleton is affected, but the vertebrae and long bones are especially

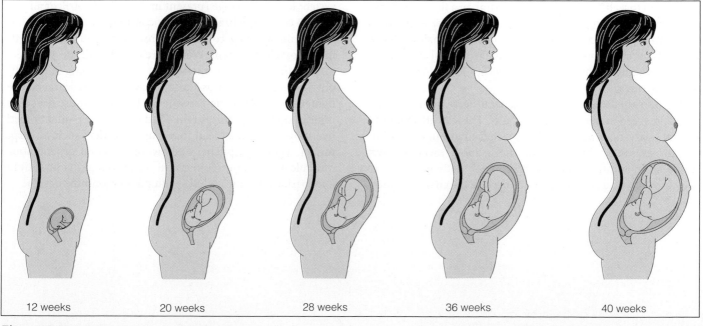

| 12 weeks | 20 weeks | 28 weeks | 36 weeks | 40 weeks |

Figure 23.16 ● Postural changes with pregnancy.

vulnerable. Most aging adults develop some degree of osteoporosis, but it is more marked in Caucasian females, especially those of Scandinavian ancestry.

The decreased height of the aging adult occurs because of a shortening of the vertebral column. Thinning of the intervertebral disks during middle age and an erosion of individual vertebrae due to osteoporosis contribute to this shortening. There is an average decrease in height of 1 to 2 inches from the 20s through the 70s, and a further decrease in the 80s and 90s because of additional collapse of the vertebrae. Kyphosis, an exaggerated convexity of the thoracic region of the spine, is common. When the older adult is standing, the nurse may notice a slight flexion of the hips and knees. These changes in the vertebral column may cause a shift in the individual's center of gravity, which in turn may put the older adult at an increased risk for falls.

The size and quantity of muscle fibers tend to decrease by as much as 30% by the 80th year of life. The amount of connective tissue in the muscles increases, and they become fibrous or stringy. Tendons become less elastic. As a result, the older client experiences a progressive decrease in reaction time, speed of movements, agility, and endurance.

Degeneration of the joints causes thickening and decreased viscosity of the synovial fluid, fragmentation of connective tissue, and scarring and calcification in the joint capsules. In addition, the cartilage becomes frayed, thin, and cracked, allowing the underlying bone to become eroded. Because of these changes, the joints of older people are less shock absorbent and have decreased range of motion and flexibility. These normal degenerative joint changes that occur from aging and use are referred to as *osteoarthrosis*. In some individuals, *Heberden's nodes*—hard, typically painless, bony enlargements associated with osteoarthritis—may occur in the distal interphalangeal joints.

The gait of an older client alters as the bones, muscles, and joints change with advancing age. Both males and females tend to walk slower, supporting themselves as they move. Elderly males tend to walk with the head and trunk in a flexed position, using short, high steps, a wide gait, and a smaller arm swing. The bowlegged stance that is observed in older females is due to reduced muscular control, thus altering the normal angle of the hip and leading to increased susceptibility to falls and subsequent fractures.

As individuals age, there is a general decrease in reaction time and speed of performance of tasks. This can affect mobility and safety, especially with unexpected environmental stimuli (for example, objects on the floor, loose carpeting, wet surfaces). In addition, any health problem that contributes to decreased physical activity tends to increase the chance of alterations in the health of the musculoskeletal system. A well-balanced diet and regular exercise help to slow the progression of these musculoskeletal changes.

The physical assessment of the musculoskeletal system of the elderly person is similar to that of any other adult. When testing range of motion, the nurse must be careful not to cause pain, discomfort, or damage to the joint. The musculoskeletal exam is conducted at a slower pace when necessary because older clients often have health problems that affect endurance.

PSYCHOSOCIAL CONSIDERATIONS

Psychosocial problems such as anxiety, depression, fear, altered body image, or a disturbance in self-esteem may promote inactivity or isolation, which in turn may lead to musculoskeletal degeneration. By the same token, any health problem that contributes to inactivity may trigger or contribute to psychosocial disturbances. Impaired physical mobility may lead to stress, hopelessness, ineffective coping, social isolation, or other problems.

Physical abuse should be considered if a client has a history of frequent fractures, sprains, or other musculoskeletal trauma. The nurse must follow the state's guidelines for referring the client to social or protective services.

CULTURAL AND ENVIRONMENTAL CONSIDERATIONS

The bone density of people of African ancestry is significantly higher than that of people of European heritage. Asians typically have lower bone density than people of European descent. The curvature of long bones varies widely among cultural groups and seems to be related to genetics and body weight. Thin people have less curvature than people of average weight; obese people display an increased curvature.

The number and distribution of vertebrae vary. While 24 vertebrae is the average (present in about 85 to 90% of all people), 23 or 25 vertebrae are not uncommon.

Certain working conditions present potential risks to the musculoskeletal system. Workers required to lift heavy objects may strain and injure their back. Jobs requiring substantial physical activity, such as those of construction workers, firefighters, or athletes, increase the likelihood of musculoskeletal injuries such as sprains, strains, and fractures. Frequent repetitive movements may lead to misuse disorders such as carpal tunnel syndrome, pitcher's elbow, or vertebral degeneration. Musculoskeletal injuries may also arise when individuals sit for long periods of time at desks with poor ergonomic design.

Cultural Considerations

- Asians and Caucasians have a higher incidence of osteoporosis than African Americans.
- African Americans have greater bone density compared to Caucasians or Asians.
- Ankylosing spondylitis occurs more frequently in males than in females, and in individuals who are of Native American or European descent.
- Systemic lupus erythematosus occurs more frequently in females, and with greater frequency and severity in African Americans than in Hispanics or Caucasians.

- Sickle cell anemia, which can result in joint disruption, occurs in descendants of individuals from sub-Saharan Africa, South America, Cuba, Central America, Saudi Arabia, India, and Mediterranean countries such as Turkey, Greece, and Italy. In the United States, it occurs most frequently in African Americans.
- Osteoarthritis occurs more frequently in African American males than in Caucasian males and develops twice as frequently in African American females as in Caucasian females.
- Paget's disease occurs more frequently in Caucasians than in other cultural groups.

Gathering the Data

$\mathcal{H}$ealth assessment of the musculoskeletal system includes gathering subjective and objective data. Subjective data collection occurs during the client interview, before the physical assessment. During the interview, various communication techniques are used to elicit general and specific information about the status of the client's musculoskeletal system and ability to function. Health records, the results of laboratory tests, x-rays, and imaging reports are important secondary sources to be included in the data-gathering process. During physical assessment of the musculoskeletal system, the techniques of inspection and palpation will be used to gather objective data.

FOCUSED INTERVIEW

The focused interview for the musculoskeletal system concerns data related to the structures and functions of that system. Subjective data is gathered during the focused interview. The nurse must be prepared to observe the client and to listen for cues related to the function of the musculoskeletal system. The nurse may use open-ended or closed questions to obtain information. A number of follow-up questions or requests for descriptions may be required to clarify data or gather missing information. Follow-up questions are intended to identify the sources of problems, duration of difficulties, and measures used to alleviate or manage problems. They also provide clues about the client's knowledge of his or her own health.

The focused interview guides the physical assessment of the musculoskeletal system. The information is always considered in relation to norms and expectations about musculoskeletal function. Therefore, the nurse must consider age, gender, race, culture, environment, health practices, past and concurrent problems, and therapies when framing questions and using techniques to elicit information. In order to address all of the factors when conducting a focused interview, categories of questions related to the status and function of the musculoskeletal system have been developed. These categories include general questions that are asked of all clients; those addressing illness or infection; questions related to symptoms, pain, or behaviors; those related to habits or practices; questions that are specific to clients according to age; those for the pregnant female; and questions that address environmental concerns.

The nurse must consider the client's ability to participate in the focused interview and physical assessment of the musculoskeletal system. Illness, discomfort, and disease may affect the ability to participate in the interview. Participation in the focused interview may be influenced by the ability to communicate in the same language. Language barriers interfere with the accuracy of data collection and cause anxiety in the client and examiner. A nurse may have to use a translator in conducting interviews and during the physical assessment. If the client is experiencing acute pain, recent injury, or anxiety, attention must be focused on relief of discomfort and relief of symptoms before proceeding with the in-depth interview.

FOCUSED INTERVIEW QUESTIONS	RATIONALES

The following section provides sample questions and bulleted follow-up questions in each of the categories previously mentioned. A rationale for each of the questions is provided. The list of questions is not all-inclusive but represents the types of questions required in a comprehensive focused interview related to the musculoskeletal system. As these questions are asked, the subjective data obtained helps to identify strengths or risks associated with the musculoskeletal system as described in Healthy People 2010.

GENERAL QUESTIONS

1. **Describe your mobility today, 2 months ago, and 2 years ago.**

2. **Are you able to carry out all of your regular activities?**
   - Describe the change in your activity.
   - Do you know what is causing the problem?
   - What do you do about the problem?
   - How long has this been happening?
   - Have you discussed this with a healthcare professional?

3. **Do you have any chronic diseases such as diabetes mellitus, hypothyroidism, sickle cell anemia, lupus, or rheumatoid arthritis?**
   - If so, describe the disease and its progression, treatment, and effects on daily activities.

4. **Please describe any musculoskeletal problems of any family member.**
   - What is the disease or problem?
   - Who in the family has had the problem?
   - When was it diagnosed?
   - Describe the treatment.
   - How effective has the treatment been?

▶ This gives clients the opportunity to provide their own perceptions about mobility.

▶ Musculoskeletal problems affect activities of daily living (ADLs) because of pain or decreased mobility.

▶ These conditions can predispose the client to musculoskeletal problems such as osteomyelitis.

▶ Some conditions such as rheumatoid arthritis are genetic or familial and recur in a family.

QUESTIONS RELATED TO ILLNESS, INFECTION, OR INJURY

1. **Have you ever been diagnosed with a musculoskeletal illness?**
   - When were you diagnosed with the problem?
   - What treatment was prescribed for the problem?
   - Was the treatment helpful?
   - What kinds of things do you do to help with the problem?
   - Has the problem ever recurred (acute)?
   - How are you managing the disease now (chronic)?

2. **An alternative to question 1 is to list possible musculoskeletal illnesses, such as arthritis myalgia and lupus, and ask the client to respond yes or no as each is stated.**

3. **Have you ever had an infection in your bones, muscles, or joints?**
   - When were you diagnosed with the infection?
   - When did the problem begin?
   - What treatment was prescribed?
   - Was the treatment helpful?
   - What do you do to help the problem?
   - Has the problem ever recurred (acute)?
   - How are you managing the problem now (chronic)?

▶ The client has an opportunity to provide information about a specific illness. If a diagnosed illness is identified, follow-up about the date of diagnosis, treatment, and outcomes is required. Data about each illness identified by the client is essential to an accurate health assessment. Illnesses can be classified as acute or chronic, and follow-up regarding each classification will differ.

▶ This is a comprehensive and easy way to elicit information about all musculoskeletal diagnoses. Follow-up would be carried out for each identified diagnosis as in question 1.

▶ Osteomyelitis, an infection of the bone, frequently recurs in clients with a history of previous infections.

FOCUSED INTERVIEW QUESTIONS	RATIONALES

4. **Have you had any fractures? If so, tell me about the frequency, cause, injuries, treatment, and present problems with daily activities.**

▶ Older adults who have osteoporosis and osteomalacia (adult vitamin D deficiency) are prone to develop multiple fractures of the bone. Physical abuse should be considered when an individual has a history of frequent fractures; however, disease or hereditary illness can predispose fractures.

5. **Have you ever experienced any penetrating wounds (punctures from a nail or sharp object, stabbing, or gunshot)? If so, please describe them.**

▶ Penetrating wounds may be a causative factor for osteomyelitis. Follow-up for questions 4 and 5 would follow the format for questions 1 and 3.

QUESTIONS RELATED TO SYMPTOMS OR BEHAVIORS

When gathering information about symptoms, many questions are required to elicit details and descriptions that assist in the analysis of the data. Discrimination is made in relation to the significance of a symptom, in relation to specific diseases or problems, and in relation to potential follow-up examination or referral. One rationale may be provided for a group of questions in this category.

The following questions refer to specific symptoms and behaviors associated with the musculoskeletal system. For each symptom, questions and follow-up are required. The details to be elicited are the characteristics of the symptom; the onset, duration, and frequency of the symptom; the treatment or remedy for the symptom, including over-the-counter and home remedies; the determination if diagnosis has been sought; the effect of treatments; and family history associated with a symptom or illness.

1. **Tell me about any swelling, heat, redness, or stiffness you have had in your muscles or joints.**

▶ Swelling, heat, redness, and stiffness are associated with disorders of the musculoskeletal system such as arthritis or sprains.

2. **How long have you had the symptom?**

▶ Determining the duration of symptoms is helpful in identifying the significance of the symptoms in relation to specific diseases and problems.

3. **Do you know what causes the symptom?**

4. **Does the symptom differ at different times of day?**

5. **Have you sought treatment?**

6. **When was the treatment sought?**

7. **What happened when you sought treatment?**

8. **Was something prescribed or recommended?**

9. **What was the effect of the remedy?**

▶ Questions 3 through 9 elicit information about the need for diagnosis, referral, or continued evaluation of the symptom; information about the client's knowledge about a current diagnosis or underlying problems; and the client's response to intervention.

10. **Do you now use, or have you ever used, over-the-counter (OTC) or home remedies for the symptom?**

11. **What are the OTC or home remedies that you use?**

12. **How often do you use them?**

13. **How much of them do you use?**

▶ Questions 10 through 13 elicit information about drugs and substances that may relieve symptoms or provide comfort. Some substances may mask symptoms, interfere with the effect of prescribed medication, or harm the client.

14. **Do you experience constipation or abdominal distention?**

▶ These diagnostic cues commonly occur in clients who have decreased mobility, atrophy of the abdominal muscles, or spinal deformity.

15. **Do you have difficulty breathing? If so, describe.**

▶ Spinal deformities, osteoporosis, and any other condition that restricts trunk movement may interfere with normal breathing movements.

FOCUSED INTERVIEW QUESTIONS	RATIONALES

QUESTIONS RELATED TO PAIN

1. **Please describe any pain you experience in your bones, muscles, or joints.**
   - How would you rate the pain on a scale of 0 to 10, with 10 being the worst?
   - When did the pain begin?
   - What were you doing when the pain began?
   - What activities increase the pain?
   - What activities seem to decrease or eliminate the pain?
   - Does this pain radiate from one place to another?
   - Do you experience any unusual sensations along with the pain?

▶ These questions help determine if the pain has a sudden or gradual onset. Also, certain activities such as lifting heavy objects can strain ligaments and vertebrae in the back, causing acute pain. Weight-bearing activities may increase the pain if the client has degenerative disease of hip, knee, and vertebrae. The pain from hiatal hernia and from cardiac, gallbladder, and pleural conditions may be referred to the shoulder. Lumbosacral nerve root irritation may cause pain to be felt in the leg. Sensations of burning, tingling, or prickling (paresthesia) may accompany compression of nerves or blood vessels in that body region.

2. **What do you do to relieve the pain?**

3. **Is that treatment effective?**

▶ Questions 2 and 3 are intended to determine if the client has selected a treatment based on past experience, knowledge of musculoskeletal illness, or use of complementary and alternative medicine and its effectiveness.

QUESTIONS RELATED TO BEHAVIORS

1. **Do you smoke?**
   - If so, how much?
   - How much caffeine do you consume each day?
   - How many cups of coffee, tea, or cola?
   - How much alcohol do you drink?

▶ Smoking, caffeine consumption, and alcohol consumption increase the client's risk for osteoporosis.

2. **Tell me about your exercise program.**

▶ A sedentary lifestyle leads to muscle weakness, contributes to poor coordination skills, and predisposes postmenopausal females to osteoporosis.

QUESTIONS RELATED TO AGE

The focused interview must reflect the anatomical and physiological differences that exist along the life span. The following questions are examples of those that would be specific for infants and children, the pregnant female, and the older adult.

QUESTIONS REGARDING INFANTS AND CHILDREN

1. **Were you told about any trauma to the infant during labor and delivery?**
   - If so, describe the trauma.

▶ Traumatic births increase the risk for fractures, especially of the clavicle.

2. **Did the baby require resuscitation after delivery?**

▶ Periods of anoxia can result in increased muscle tone.

3. **Have you noticed any deformity of the child's spine or limbs, or any unusual shape of the child's feet and toes?**
   - If yes, please describe these deformities and any treatment the child has had.

▶ Some deformities correct themselves as the child grows. Others may require physical therapy or surgery.

4. **Please describe any dislocations or broken bones the child has had, including any treatment.**

▶ Dislocations or broken bones are more common in children with certain developmental disabilities or sensory or motor disorders such as cerebral palsy or Down syndrome. They may also signal physical abuse. The latter will require further investigation.

FOCUSED INTERVIEW QUESTIONS	RATIONALES

5. *For the school-age child:* Do you play any sports at school or after school?
   - If so, describe the sports activities.

▶ Sports activities can cause musculoskeletal injuries, especially if played without adequate adult supervision or the use of protective equipment.

QUESTIONS FOR THE PREGNANT FEMALE

1. Please describe any back pain you are experiencing.
   - Tell me about the effects of the pain on your daily activities.

▶ Lordosis may occur in the last months of pregnancy along with complaints of back pain.

QUESTIONS FOR THE OLDER ADULT

1. Have you noticed any muscle weakness over the past few months?
   - If so, explain what effect this muscle weakness has on your daily activities.

▶ Muscle weakness is common as a person ages, especially in people with sedentary lifestyles.

2. Have you fallen in the past 6 months?
   - If so, how many times?
   - What prompted the fall(s)?
   - Describe your injuries.
   - What treatment did you receive?
   - What effect did your injuries have on your daily activities?

▶ Older adults have an increased rate of falls because of a change in posture that can affect their balance. Loss of balance may also be caused by sensory or motor disorders, inner ear infections, the side effects of certain medications, and other factors.

3. Do you use any walking aids such as a cane or walker to help you get around?
   - If so, please describe the aid or show it to me.

▶ These aids help the older adult ambulate, but they can also cause falls, especially if the client does not use the device properly.

4. *For postmenopausal females:* Do you take calcium supplements?

▶ Calcium supplementation may slow the development of some of the musculoskeletal changes associated with age, such as osteoporosis.

QUESTIONS RELATED TO THE ENVIRONMENT

Environment refers to both the internal and external environments. Questions related to the internal environment include all of the previous questions and those associated with internal or physiological responses. Questions regarding the external environment include those related to home, work, or social environments.

INTERNAL ENVIRONMENT

1. Describe your typical daily diet.
   - Do you have problems eating or drinking dairy products?
   - If so, describe the problems you experience.

▶ Protein deficiency interferes with bone growth and muscle tone; calcium deficiency predisposes an individual to low bone density, resulting in osteoporosis; and vitamin C deficiency inhibits bone and tissue healing. Clients with intolerance to milk products frequently ingest low amounts of calcium, leading to musculoskeletal problems such as osteoporosis.

2. Have you had any recent weight gain?
   - If so, how much weight?

▶ Increased weight puts added stress on the musculoskeletal system.

3. Are you currently taking any medications such as steroids, estrogen, muscle relaxants, or any other drugs?

▶ These drugs may cause a variety of symptoms such as weakness, swelling, and increased muscle size that could affect the musculoskeletal system.

EXTERNAL ENVIRONMENT

1. How much sunlight do you get each day?

▶ Twenty minutes of sunshine each day helps the body manufacture vitamin D. Vitamin D deficiency can lead to osteomalacia.

FOCUSED INTERVIEW QUESTIONS	RATIONALES

2. What kind of work do you do?
  ● Do you work on a computer?

▶ Frequent repetitive movements may lead to misuse syndromes such as carpal tunnel syndrome, an inflammation of the tissues of the wrist that causes pressure on the median nerve. Work that requires heavy lifting or twisting may lead to lower back problems.

3. Describe your hobbies or athletic activities.

▶ Participation in athletic or sports activities can predispose the individual to trauma or "wear and tear" injuries. Sitting for long periods of time and repetitive motion such as in sewing, crocheting, and woodworking can cause musculoskeletal damage.

CLIENT INTERACTION

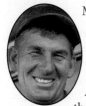

Mr. Alexander French, a 49-year-old truck driver, returns to the pain clinic at 10:30 A.M. accompanied by his wife. His health history includes having been diagnosed with a herniated intervertebral disk at L$_{4-5}$ about 10 months ago. At that time, he declined surgery and selected the alternative method of treatment, which included wearing a back brace, and home exercises to help strengthen his back muscles. Now his chief complaint is back pain radiating to his left leg. The following is an excerpt from the focused interview.

INTERVIEW

Nurse: Good morning, Mr. French. I see by your report you are having back pain again. Your last visit was about 3 months ago for a routine follow-up with no pain.

Mr. French: Yes, that is correct. Yes, to both of your thoughts.

Nurse: First we need to determine your pain level right now and find a comfortable position for you.

Mr. French: Right now my pain is about 4 on a scale of 0 to 10 and it sometimes shoots down my left leg. It was higher at home but I took my pills before coming here. That's why my wife drove and is here with me. I will be able to sit for awhile. When I can't sit any longer, I will tell you.

Nurse: I need more information about the cause, actions you have taken to decrease the pain, and activities since your last visit. Where shall we begin?

Mr. French: I'll start with the cause. I was outside Saturday after it stopped snowing, and I shoveled our front walk. Then I helped the children build a big snowman. I was tired and had a backache that evening but I tried to ignore it.

Nurse: You ignored it?

Mr. French: I should have taken the medicine right away. I should have had my brace on when I was shoveling and building the snowman with the children.

Nurse: You weren't wearing your back brace?

Mr. French: That's right. I wear it every day to work. I never forget since I move heavy boxes from the truck. I had been feeling so good, no problems, and the snow was not heavy. I guess when I lifted the second snowball for the snowman, that did me in though.

ANALYSIS

Several techniques were used to obtain subjective data from the client. The nurse first clarified the reason for the visit and then determined the client's pain level and position for comfort. Using open-ended statements and listening to the client, the nurse encouraged the client to focus on details of the topics being discussed. The nurse introduced several thoughts and questions at one time. This could have hindered the communication process during the interview.

Please refer to the Companion Website at **www.prenhall.com/damico** and click on Chapter 23, the **Client Interaction** module, to answer questions about this case. In addition, see other resources for this chapter including NCLEX review questions and other interactive exercises and materials.

ASSESSMENT TECHNIQUES AND FINDINGS

Physical assessment of the musculoskeletal system requires the use of inspection and palpation. During each of the procedures the nurse is gathering data related to the client's skeleton, joints, musculature, strength, and mobility. Knowledge of normal or expected findings is essential in determining the meaning of the data as the nurse conducts the physical assessment.

Adults have erect posture, an even gait, and symmetry in size and shape of muscles. A healthy adult is capable of active and complete range of motion in all joints. Joints are nonswollen and nontender. Muscle strength is equal bilaterally, and the movements against resistance are smooth and symmetrical. The spine is midline and cervical; thoracic and lumbar curves are present. The extremities are of equal length. The arm span is equal to height, and the distance from head to pubis is equal to the distance from pubis to toes.

Physical assessment of the musculoskeletal system follows an organized pattern. It begins with a client survey and proceeds in a cephalocaudal direction to include inspection, palpation, assessment of range of motion of each joint, and assessment of muscle size, symmetry, and strength.

EQUIPMENT

examination gown	skin marking pen
clean, nonsterile examination gloves	goniometer
examination light	tape measure

HELPFUL HINTS

- Age and agility influence the client's ability to participate in the assessment.
- It is often more helpful to demonstrate the movements you expect of the client during this assessment than to use easily misunderstood verbal instructions. A "Simon Says" approach works well, especially with children.
- When assessing range of motion, do not push the joint beyond its normal range.
- Stop when the client expresses discomfort.
- Measure the joint angle with a goniometer when range of motion appears limited.
- Use an orderly approach: head to toe, proximal to distal, compare the sides of the body for symmetry.
- The musculoskeletal assessment may be exhausting for some clients. Provide rest periods or schedule two sessions.
- Use Standard Precautions.

TECHNIQUES AND NORMAL FINDINGS	ABNORMAL FINDINGS SPECIAL CONSIDERATIONS

SURVEY

A quick survey of the client enables the nurse to identify any immediate problems and to determine the client's ability to participate in the assessment.

Inspect the overall appearance, posture, and position of the client. Observe for deformities, inflammation, and immobility (see Figure 23.17 ●).

▶ If a client is experiencing pain or inflammation, these issues must be addressed first. The complete assessment of the musculoskeletal system may have to be delayed until acute problems are attended to. Limited strength and mobility must be considered throughout the assessment.

TECHNIQUES AND NORMAL FINDINGS	ABNORMAL FINDINGS SPECIAL CONSIDERATIONS

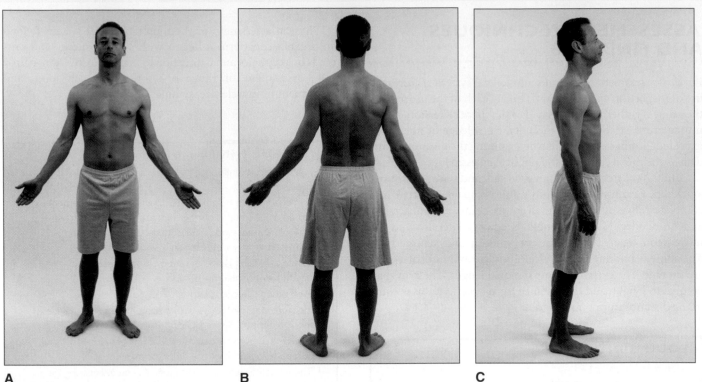

A   B   C

Figure 23.17 ● Survey and posture of client. A. Anterior view. B. Posterior view. C. Lateral view.

ASSESSMENT OF THE JOINTS

1. **Position the client.**
   - The client should be in a sitting position with an examination gown on.

2. **Instruct the client.**
   - Explain that you will be looking at all of the client's joints and muscles. Tell the client you will be touching bones, muscles, and joints and you will ask the client to move different parts of the body to determine the mobility of the joints. Explain that part of the exam will require the client to move against the resistance you provide. It is helpful to demonstrate or describe the movements expected of the client for one joint and to apply resistance as the client repeats the expected movement. Then explain that each joint will be assessed in a similar manner with the same amount of resistance and that you will provide direction with each examination. Explain that the assessment should not cause discomfort and tell the client to inform you of pain, discomfort, or difficulty with any assessment. Explain that you will provide assistance or support when necessary and can provide rest periods throughout the examination.

3. **Inspect the temporomandibular joint on both sides.**
   - The joints should be symmetrical and not swollen or painful.

4. **Palpate the temporomandibular joints.**
   - Place the finger pads of your index and middle fingers in front of the tragus of each ear. Ask the client to open and close the mouth while you palpate the temporomandibular joints (see Figure 23.18 ●).

▶ An enlarged or swollen joint shows as a rounded protuberance.

▶ Discomfort, swelling, crackling sounds, and limited movement of the jaw are unexpected findings that require further evaluation for dental or neurologic problems or TMJ syndrome.

TECHNIQUES AND NORMAL FINDINGS	ABNORMAL FINDINGS SPECIAL CONSIDERATIONS

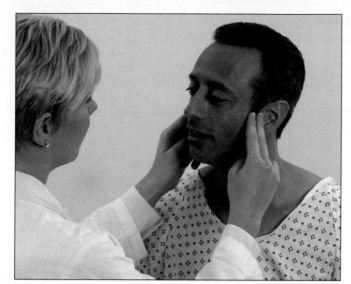

Figure 23.18 •
Palpating the
temporomandi-
bular joints.

- As the client's mouth opens, your fingers should glide into a shallow depression of the joints. Confirm the smooth motion of the mandible.
- The joint may audibly and palpably click as the mouth opens. This is normal.

5. Palpate the muscles of the jaw.

- Instruct the client to clench the teeth as you palpate the masseter and temporalis muscles. Confirm that the muscles are symmetrical, firm, and nontender.

▶ Swelling and tenderness suggest arthritis and myofascial pain syndrome.

6. Test for range of motion of the temporomandibular joints.

- Ask the client to open the mouth as wide as possible. Confirm that the mouth opens with ease to as much as 3 to 6 cm between the upper and lower incisors.
- With the mouth slightly open, ask the client to push out the lower jaw, and return the lower jaw to a neutral position. The jaw should protrude and retract with ease.
- Ask the client to move the lower jaw from side to side. Confirm that the jaw moves laterally from 1 to 2 cm without deviation or dislocation.
- Ask the client to close the mouth. The mouth should close completely without pain or discomfort.

▶ Temporomandibular joint dysfunction should be suspected if facial pain and limited jaw movement accompany clicking sounds as the jaw opens and closes.

7. Test for muscle strength and motor function of cranial nerve V.

- Instruct the client to repeat the movements in step 6 as you provide opposing force. The client should be able to perform the movements against your resistance. The strength of the muscles on both sides of the jaw should be equal.
- For more detailed testing of cranial nerve V, including sensory function, see Chapter 24. ⬤⬤

THE SHOULDERS

1. With the client facing you, inspect both shoulders.

- Compare the shape and size of the shoulders, clavicles, and scapula. Confirm that they are symmetrical and similar in size both anteriorly and posteriorly.

▶ Swelling, deformity, atrophy, and misalignment, combined with limited motion, pain, and crepitus (a grating sound caused by bone fragments in joints), suggest degenerative joint disease, traumatized joints (strains, sprains), or inflammatory conditions (rheumatoid arthritis, bursitis, or tendinitis).

TECHNIQUES AND NORMAL FINDINGS	ABNORMAL FINDINGS SPECIAL CONSIDERATIONS

2. **Palpate the shoulders and surrounding structures.**

- Begin palpating at the sternoclavicular joint; then move laterally along the clavicle to the acromioclavicular joint.
- Palpate downward into the subacromial area and the greater tubercle of the humerus.
- Confirm that these areas are firm and nontender, the shoulders symmetrical, and the scapulae level and symmetrical.

3. **Test the range of motion of the shoulders.**

- Instruct the client to use both arms for the following maneuvers:
  - Shrug the shoulders by flexing them forward and upward.
  - With the elbows extended, raise the arms forward and upward in an arc. (The client should demonstrate a forward flexion of 180 degrees.)
  - Return the arms to the sides. Keeping the elbows extended, move the arms backward as far as possible (see Figure 23.19 ●). (The client should demonstrate an extension of as much as 50 degrees.)

▶ Shoulder pain without palpation or movement may result from insufficient circulation to the myocardium. This cue, known as *referred pain*, can be a precursor to a myocardial infarction (heart attack). If the client exhibits other symptoms such as chest pain, indigestion, and cardiovascular changes, medical assistance must be obtained immediately.

▶ If the client expresses discomfort, it is important to determine if the pain is referred. Conditions that increase intra-abdominal pressure, such as hiatal hernia and gastrointestinal disease, may cause pain in the shoulder area. When limitation or increase in range of motion (ROM) is assessed, the goniometer should be used to precisely measure the angle.

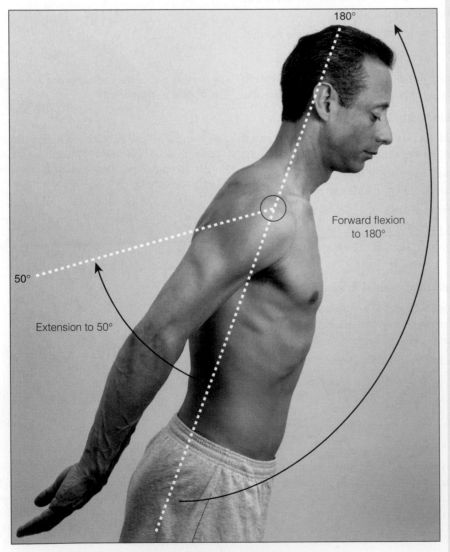

Figure 23.19 ● Flexion and extension of the shoulders.

TECHNIQUES AND NORMAL FINDINGS	ABNORMAL FINDINGS SPECIAL CONSIDERATIONS

- Place the back of the client's hands as close as possible to scapulae (internal rotation; see Figure 23.20 ●).
- Ask the client to clasp his or her hands behind the head (external rotation; see Figure 23.21 ●).

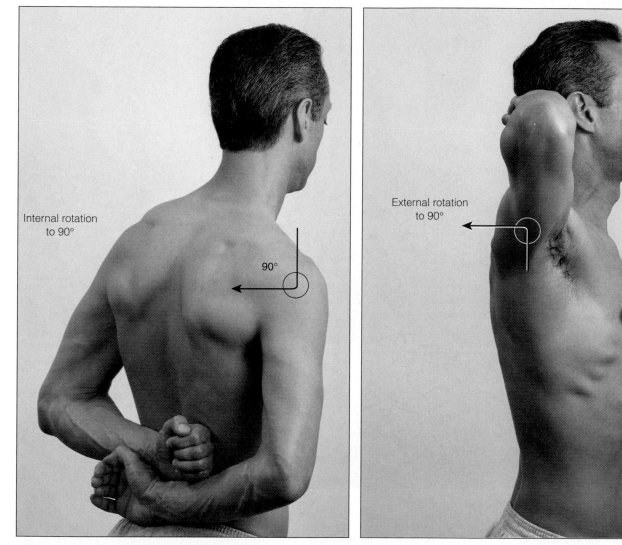

Internal rotation to 90°

90°

External rotation to 90°

Figure 23.20 ● Internal rotation of the shoulders.

Figure 23.21 ● External rotation of the shoulders.

- With elbows extended, ask the client to swing the arms out to the sides in arcs, touching the palms together above the head. The client should demonstrate abduction of 180 degrees.

► In rotator cuff tears, the client is unable to perform abduction without lifting or shrugging the shoulder. This sign is accompanied by pain, tenderness, and muscle atrophy.

TECHNIQUES AND NORMAL FINDINGS	ABNORMAL FINDINGS SPECIAL CONSIDERATIONS

- With the elbows extended, ask the client to swing each arm toward the midline of the body (see Figure 23.22 ●).

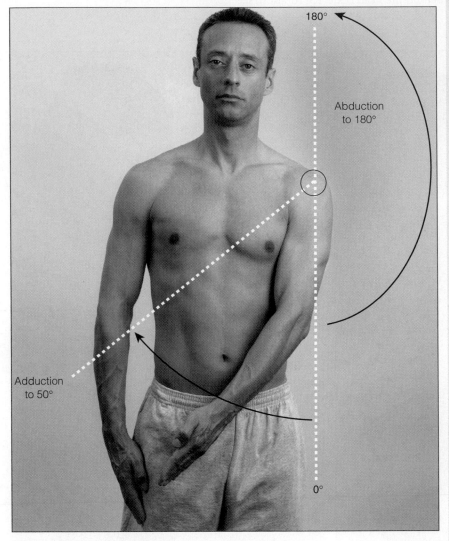

Figure 23.22 ● Abduction and adduction of the shoulder.

- The client should demonstrate adduction of as much as 50 degrees.

4. **Test for strength of the shoulder muscles.**

- Instruct the client to repeat the movements in step 3 as you provide opposing force. The client should be able to perform the movements against your resistance. The strength of the shoulder muscles on both sides should be equal.

- Muscle strength is rated on a scale of 0 to 5 with 0 representing absence of strength and 5 indicating maximum or normal strengths. Table 23.3 includes information about rating muscle strength.

▶ Full resistance during the shoulder shrug indicates adequate cranial nerve XI (spinal accessory) function. See Chapter 24 for more detail. ⬭

| TECHNIQUES AND NORMAL FINDINGS | ABNORMAL FINDINGS SPECIAL CONSIDERATIONS |

Table 23.3	Rating Muscle Strength	
RATING	**DESCRIPTION OF FUNCTION**	**CLASSIFICATION**
5	Full range of motion against gravity with full resistance	Normal
4	Full range of motion against gravity with moderate resistance	Good
3	Full range of motion with gravity	Fair
2	Full range of motion without gravity (passive motion)	Poor
1	Palpable muscle contraction but no movement	Trace
0	No muscle contraction	Zero

ELBOWS

1. **Support the client's arm and inspect the lateral and medial aspects of the elbow.**
   - The elbows should be symmetrical.

   ▶ Swelling, deformity, or malalignment requires further evaluation. If there is a subluxation (partial dislocation), the elbow looks deformed, and the forearm is misaligned.

2. **Palpate the lateral and medial aspects of the olecranon process.**
   - Use your thumb and middle fingers to palpate the grooves on either side of the olecranon process.

   ▶ In the presence of inflammation, the grooves feel soft and spongy, and the surrounding tissue may be red, hot, and painful.

   - The joint should be free of pain, thickening, swelling, or tenderness.

   ▶ Inflammatory conditions of the elbow include arthritis, bursitis, and epicondylitis. *Rheumatoid arthritis* may result in nodules in the olecranon bursa or along the extensor surface of the ulna. Nodules are firm, nontender, and not attached to the overlying skin. *Lateral epicondylitis* (tennis elbow) results from constant, repetitive movements of the wrist or forearm. Pain occurs when the client attempts to extend the wrist against resistance. *Medial epicondylitis* (pitcher's or golfer's elbow) results from constant, repetitive flexion of the wrist. Pain occurs when the client attempts to flex the wrist against resistance.

3. **Test the range of motion of each elbow.**
   - Instruct the client to perform the following movements:
     - Bend the elbow by bringing the forearm forward and touching the fingers to the shoulder (see Figure 23.23 ●). The elbow should flex to 160 degrees.

TECHNIQUES AND NORMAL FINDINGS

- Straighten the elbow. The lower arm should form a straight line with the upper arm. The elbow in a neutral position is at 0 degree extension. The elbow should extend to 0 degree.

- Holding the arm straight out, turn the palm upward facing the ceiling, then downward facing the floor (see Figure 23.25 ●). The elbow should supinate and pronate to 90 degrees.

▶ To use the goniometer, begin with the joint in a neutral position and then flex the joint as far as possible. Measure the angle with the goniometer. Fully extend the joint and measure the angle with the goniometer. Compare the goniometer measurements to the expected degree of flexion and extension. See Figure 23.24 ● for an example.

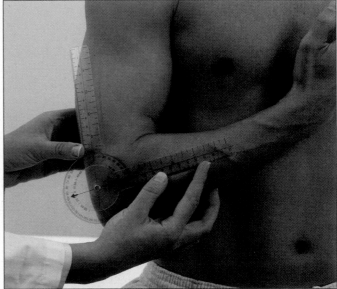

Figure 23.24 ● Goniometer measure of joint range of motion.

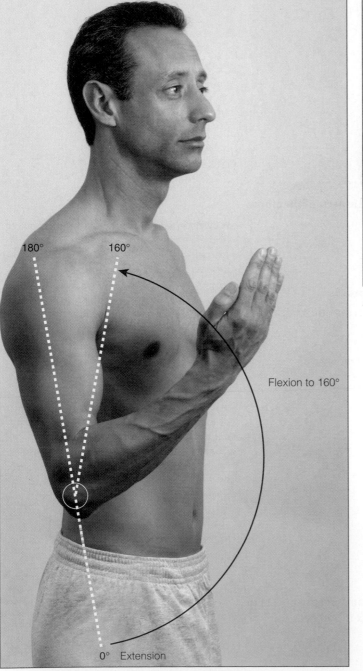

Figure 23.23 ● Flexion and extension of the elbow.

TECHNIQUES AND NORMAL FINDINGS	ABNORMAL FINDINGS SPECIAL CONSIDERATIONS

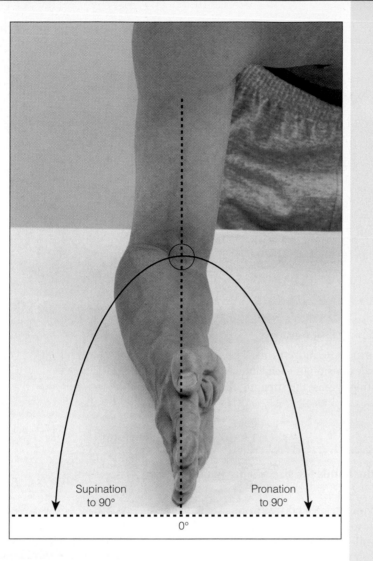

Figure 23.25 ● Supination and pronation of the elbow.

Supination to 90°   Pronation to 90°

0°

- The client should be able to put each elbow through the normal range of motion without difficulty or discomfort.

4. Test for muscle strength.

- Stabilize the client's elbow with your nondominant hand while holding the wrist with your dominant hand.
- Instruct the client to flex the elbow while you apply opposing resistance (see Figure 23.26 ●).

TECHNIQUES AND NORMAL FINDINGS	ABNORMAL FINDINGS SPECIAL CONSIDERATIONS

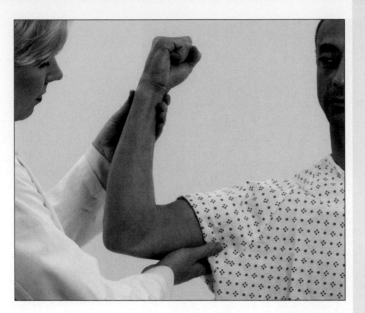

Figure 23.26 ● Testing muscle strength using opposing force.

- Instruct the client to extend the elbow against resistance.
- The client should be able to perform these movements. The strength of the muscles associated with flexion and extension of each elbow should be equal. Muscle strength is measured by testing against the strength of the examiner as resistance is applied.

WRISTS AND HANDS

1. **Inspect the wrists and dorsum of the hands for size, shape, symmetry, and color.**
   - The wrists and hands should be symmetrical and free from swelling and deformity. The color should be similar to that of the rest of the body. The ends of either the ulna or radius may protrude further in some individuals.

   ▶ Redness, swelling, or deformity in the joints requires further evaluation. It is important to note any nodules on the hands or wrists, or atrophy of the surrounding muscles. In acute rheumatoid arthritis, the wrist, proximal interphalangeal, and metacarpophalangeal joints are likely to be swollen, tender, and stiff. As the disease progresses, the proximal interphalangeal joints deviate toward the ulnar side of the hand; the interosseous muscles atrophy, and rheumatoid nodules form, giving the rheumatic hand its characteristic appearance.

2. **Inspect the palms of the hands.**
   - There is a rounded protuberance over the thenar eminence (the area proximal to the thumb).

   ▶ Carpal tunnel syndrome is a nerve disorder in which an inflammation of tissues in the wrist causes pressure on the median nerve (which innervates the hand). Thenar atrophy is a common finding associated with carpal tunnel syndrome; however, some atrophy of the thenar eminence occurs with aging.

3. **Palpate the wrists and hands for temperature and texture.**
   - The temperature of the wrists and hands should be warm and similar to the rest of the body. The skin should be smooth and free of cuts. The skin around the interphalangeal joints may have a rougher texture.

TECHNIQUES AND NORMAL FINDINGS	ABNORMAL FINDINGS SPECIAL CONSIDERATIONS

4. Palpate each joint of the wrists and hands.

- Move your thumbs from side to side gently but firmly over the dorsum, with your fingers resting beneath the area you are palpating (see Figures 23.27A ● and B ●). As you palpate, make sure you keep the client's wrist straight.

- To palpate the interphalangeal joints, pinch them gently between your thumb and index finger (see Figure 23.27C ●). All joints should be firm and nontender, with no swelling.

- As you palpate, note the temperature of the client's hand.

▶ A ganglion is a typically painless, round, fluid-filled mass that arises from the tendon sheaths on the dorsum of the wrist and hand. It may require surgery. Ganglia that are more prevalent when the wrist is flexed do not interfere with range of motion or function.

▶ A cool temperature in the extremities may indicate compromised vascular function, which may in turn influence muscle strength.

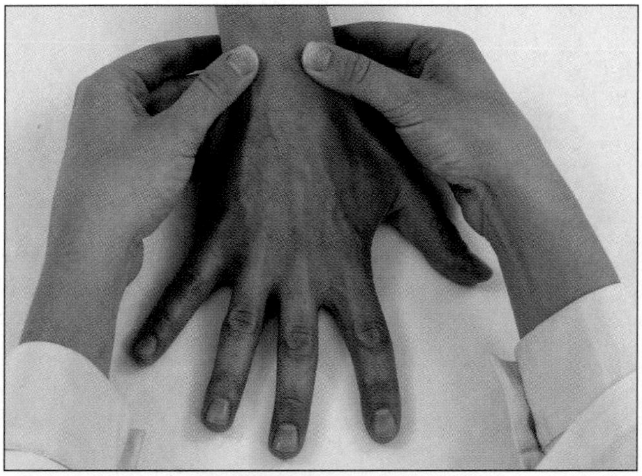

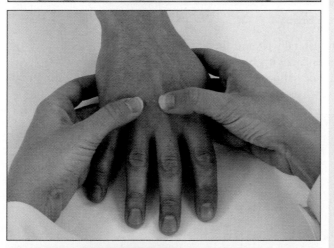

Figure 23.27A ●
Palpating the wrist.

Figure 23.27B ●
Palpating the hand.

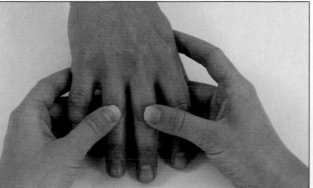

Figure 23.27C ●
Palpating the fingers.

TECHNIQUES AND NORMAL FINDINGS

5. **Test the range of motion of the wrist.**

   • Instruct the client to perform the following movements:

   • Straighten the hand (extension).

   • Using the wrist as a pivot point, bring the fingers backward as far as possible, and then bend the wrist downward (see Figure 23.28 ●). The wrist should hyperextend to 70 degrees and flex to 90 degrees.

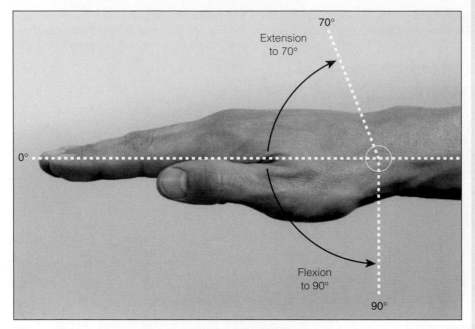

Figure 23.28 ● Hyperextension and flexion of the wrist.

   • Turn the palms down; move the hand laterally toward the fifth finger, then medially toward the thumb (see Figure 23.29 ●). Be sure the movement is from the wrist and not the elbow. Ulnar deviation should reach as much as 55 degrees, and radial deviation should reach as much as 20 degrees.

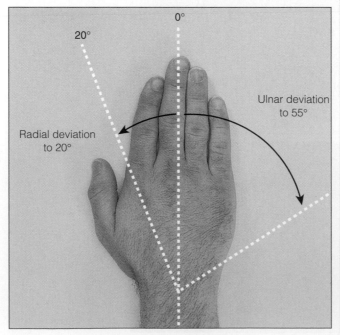

Figure 23.29 ●
Ulnar and radial deviation of the wrist.

| **TECHNIQUES AND NORMAL FINDINGS** | **ABNORMAL FINDINGS SPECIAL CONSIDERATIONS** |

- Bend the wrists downward and press the backs of both hands together (*Phalen's test;* see Figure 23.30 ●). This causes flexion of the wrists to 90 degrees. Normally clients experience no symptoms with this maneuver.

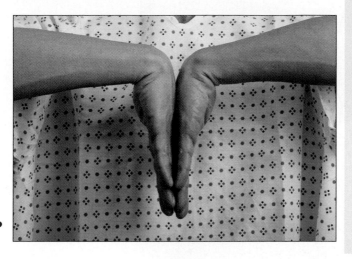

Figure 23.30 ●
Phalen's test.

▶ When a Phalen's test is performed on individuals with carpal tunnel syndrome, 80% experience pain, tingling, and numbness that radiates to the arm, shoulder, neck, or chest within 60 seconds. If carpal tunnel syndrome is suspected, it is important to check for Tinel's sign by percussing lightly over the median nerve in each wrist. If carpal tunnel syndrome is present, the client feels numbness, tingling, and pain along the median nerve (Figure 23.31 ●).

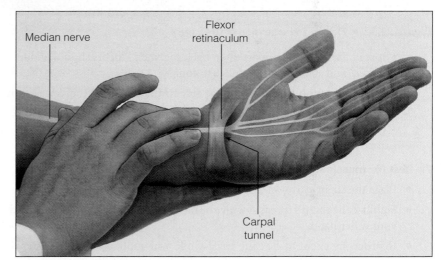

Median nerve

Flexor retinaculum

Carpal tunnel

Figure 23.31 ● Tinel's sign.

6. Test the range of motion of the hands and fingers.

- Instruct the client to perform the following movements:
  - Make a tight fist with each hand with the fingers folded into the palm and the thumb across the knuckles (thumb flexion).
  - Open the fist and stretch the fingers (extension).
  - Point the fingers downward toward the forearm, and then back as far as possible (see Figure 23.32 ●). Fingers should flex to 90 degrees and hyperextend to as much as 30 degrees.

▶ In *Dupuytren's contracture,* the client is unable to extend the fourth and fifth fingers. This is a progressive, painless, inherited disorder that causes severe flexion in the affected fingers, is usually bilateral, and is more common in middle-aged and older males.

TECHNIQUES AND NORMAL FINDINGS	ABNORMAL FINDINGS SPECIAL CONSIDERATIONS

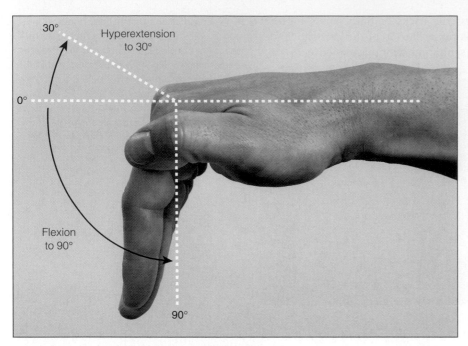

Figure 23.32 ● Flexion and extension of the fingers.

- Spread the fingers far apart, then back together. Fingers should abduct to 20 degrees and should adduct fully (to touch).
- Move the thumb toward the ulnar side of the hand and then away from the hand as far as possible.
- Touch the thumb to the tip of each of the fingers and to the base of the little finger.

7. Test for muscle strength of the wrist.

- Place the client's arm on a table with his or her palm facing up.
- Stabilize the client's forearm with one hand while holding the client's hand with your other hand.
- Instruct the client to flex the wrist while you apply opposing resistance (see Figure 23.33 ●). The client should be able to provide full resistance.

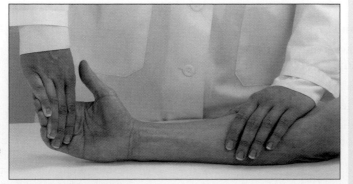

Figure 23.33 ● Testing the muscle strength of the wrist.

8. Test for muscle strength of the fingers.

- Ask the client to spread his or her fingers, and then try to force the fingers together.
- Ask the client to touch his or her little finger with the thumb while you place resistance on the thumb in order to prevent the movement.

▶ Clients with carpal tunnel syndrome manifest weakness when attempting opposition of the thumb.

TECHNIQUES AND NORMAL FINDINGS	ABNORMAL FINDINGS SPECIAL CONSIDERATIONS

HIPS

1. **Inspect the position of each hip and leg with the client in a supine position.**
   - The legs should be slightly apart and the toes should point toward the ceiling.

   ▶ External rotation of the lower leg and foot is a classic sign of a fractured femur.

2. **Palpate each hip joint and the upper thighs.**
   - The hip joints are firm, stable, and nontender.

   ▶ Pain, tenderness, swelling, deformity, limited motion (especially limited internal rotation), and crepitus are diagnostic cues that signal inflammatory or degenerative joint diseases in the hip. A fractured femur should be suspected if the joint is unstable and deformed.

3. **Test the range of motion of the hips.**

   ### ALERT!
   Do not ask clients who have undergone hip replacement to perform these movements without the permission of the physician, because these motions can dislocate the prosthesis.

   - Instruct the client to perform the following movements:
     - Raise each leg straight off the bed or table (see Figure 23.34 ●). The other leg should remain flat on the bed. Hip flexion with straight knee should reach 90 degrees. Return the leg to its original position.

   ▶ This maneuver produces back and leg pain along the course of the sciatic nerve in the client with a herniated disk.

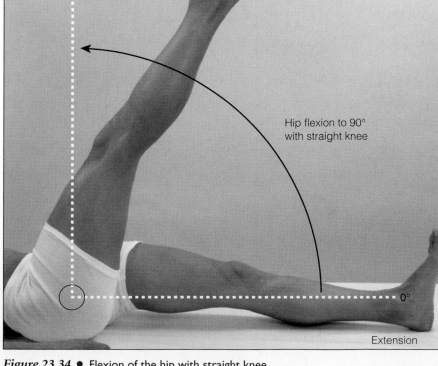

90°

Hip flexion to 90°
with straight knee

0°

Extension

Figure 23.34 ● Flexion of the hip with straight knee.

TECHNIQUES AND NORMAL FINDINGS

- Raise the leg with the knee flexed toward the chest as far as it will go (see Figure 23.35 ●). Hip flexion with flexed knee should reach 120 degrees. Return the leg to its original position.

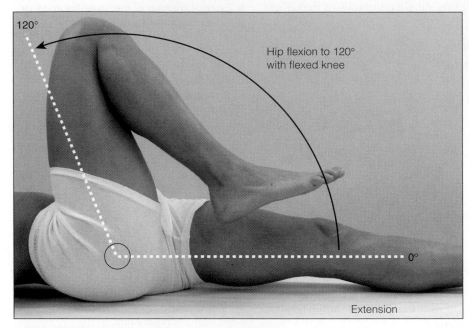

Figure 23.35 ● Flexion of the hip with flexed knee.

- Move the foot away from the midline as the knee moves toward the midline (see Figure 23.36 ●). Internal hip rotation should reach 40 degrees.

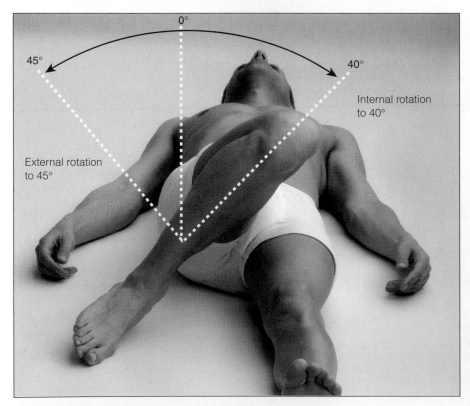

Figure 23.36 ● Internal and external hip rotation.

TECHNIQUES AND NORMAL FINDINGS	**ABNORMAL FINDINGS SPECIAL CONSIDERATIONS**

- Move the foot toward the midline as the knee moves away from the midline. External hip rotation should reach 45 degrees.
- Move the leg away from the midline (see Figure 23.37 ●), then as far as possible toward the midline. Abduction should reach 45 degrees. Adduction should reach 30 degrees.

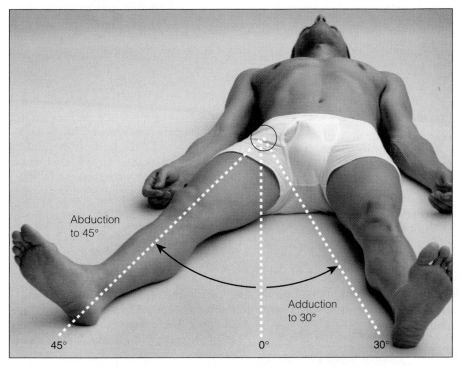

Figure 23.37 ● Abduction and adduction of the hip.

- Assist the client to turn onto his or her abdomen. An alternative position could be side lying. With the client's knee extended, ask the client to raise each leg backward and up as far as possible (see Figure 23.38 ●). Hips should hyperextend to 15 degrees. (You may also perform this test later, during assessment of the spine, with the client standing.)

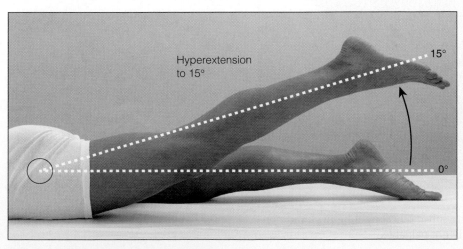

Figure 23.38 ● Hyperextension of the hip.

TECHNIQUES AND NORMAL FINDINGS	ABNORMAL FINDINGS SPECIAL CONSIDERATIONS

4. Test for muscle strength of the hips.

- Assist the client in returning to the supine position.
- Press your hands on the client's thighs and ask the client to raise his or her hip.
- Place your hands outside the client's knees and ask the client to spread both legs against your resistance.
- Place your hands between the client's knees, and ask the client to bring the legs together against your resistance.

KNEES

1. Inspect the knees.

- With the client in the sitting position, inspect the knees.
- The patella should be centrally located in each knee. The normal depressions along each side of the patella should be sharp and distinct. The skin color should be similar to that of the surrounding areas.

▶ Swelling and signs of fluid in the knee and its surrounding structures require further evaluation. Fluid accumulates in the suprapatellar bursa, the prepatellar bursa, and other areas adjacent to the patella when there is inflammation, trauma, or degenerative joint disease.

2. Inspect the quadriceps muscle in the anterior thigh.

- The muscles should be symmetrical.

▶ Atrophy in the quadriceps muscles occurs with disuse or chronic disorders.

3. Palpate the knee.

- Using your thumb, index, and middle fingers begin palpating approximately 10 cm above the patella with your thumb, index, and middle fingers (see Figure 23.39 ●). Palpate downward, evaluating each area.

▶ Any pain, swelling, thickening, or heat should be noted while palpating the knee. These diagnostic cues occur when the synovium is inflamed. Painless swelling frequently occurs in degenerative joint disease. A painful, localized area of swelling, heat, and redness in the knee is caused by the inflammation of the bursa (bursitis), for example, *prepatellar bursitis* (housemaid's knee).

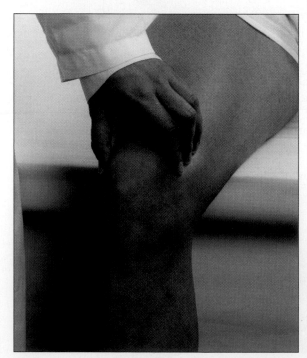

Figure 23.39 ● Palpating the knee.

- The quadriceps muscle and surrounding soft tissue should be firm and non-tender. The suprapatellar bursa is usually not palpable.

TECHNIQUES AND NORMAL FINDINGS	ABNORMAL FINDINGS SPECIAL CONSIDERATIONS

4. Palpate the tibiofemoral joint.

- With the client's knee still in the flexed position, use your thumbs to palpate deeply along each side of the tibia toward the outer aspects of the knee.

► Signs of inflammation, including pain and tenderness, occur when the joint is inflamed or damaged and may indicate degenerative joint disease, synovitis, or a torn meniscus. Bony ridges or prominences in the outer aspects of the joint occur with osteoarthritis.

- Then palpate along the lateral collateral ligament.
- The joint should be firm and nontender.

5. Test for the bulge sign.

- This procedure detects the presence of small amounts of fluid (4 to 8 ml) in the suprapatellar bursa.
- With the client in the supine position, use firm pressure to stroke the medial aspect of the knee upward several times, displacing any fluid (see Figure 23.40 ●).
- Apply pressure to the lateral side of the knee while observing the medial side.
- Normally no fluid is present.

► The medial side of the knee bulges if fluid is in the joint.

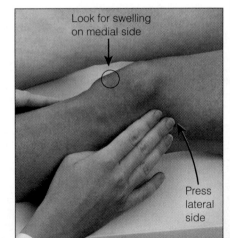

Figure 23.40 ● Testing for the bulge sign.

6. Perform ballottement.

- **Ballottement** is a technique used to detect fluid, or to examine or detect floating body structures. The nurse displaces body fluid and then palpates the return impact of the body structure.

► When there are abnormal fluid levels, fluid forced between the patella and femur causes the patella to "float" over the femur. A palpable click is felt when the patella is snapped back against the femur when fluid is present.

- To detect large amounts of fluid in the suprapatellar bursa, with your thumb and fingers, firmly grasp the thigh just above the knee. This action causes any fluid in the suprapatellar bursa to move between the patella and the femur.
- With the fingers of your left hand, quickly push the patella downward upon the femur (see Figure 23.41 ●).

TECHNIQUES AND NORMAL FINDINGS	ABNORMAL FINDINGS SPECIAL CONSIDERATIONS

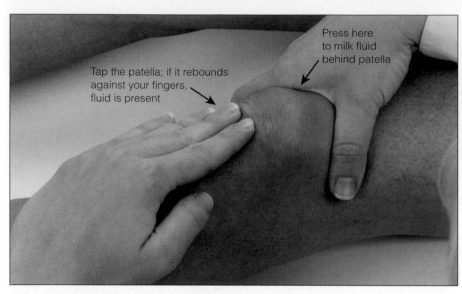

Tap the patella; if it rebounds against your fingers, fluid is present

Press here to milk fluid behind patella

Figure 23.41 ● Testing for ballottement.

- Normally the patella sits firmly over the femur, allowing little or no movement when pressure is exerted over the patella.

7. **Test the range of motion of each knee.**
   - Instruct the client to bend each knee against the chest as far as possible (flexion; see Figure 23.42 ●), and then return the knee to its extended position.

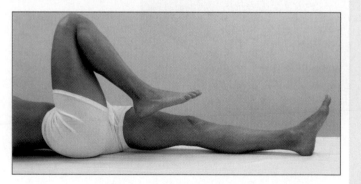

Figure 23.42 ● Flexion of the knee.

8. **Test for muscle strength.**
   - Instruct the client to flex each knee while you apply opposing force.
   - Now instruct the client to extend the knee again.
   - The client should be able to perform the movement against resistance.
   - The strength of the muscles in both knees is equal.

9. **Inspect the knee while the client is standing.**
   - Ask the client to stand erect. If the client is unsteady, allow the client to hold onto the back of a chair.

   ▶ Look for *genu varum* (bowlegs), *genu valgum* (knock knees), or *genu recurvatum* (excessive hyperextension of the knee with weight bearing due to weakness of quadriceps muscles).

   - The knees should be in alignment with the thighs and ankles.
   - Ask the client to walk at a comfortable pace with a relaxed gait.

TECHNIQUES AND NORMAL FINDINGS	ABNORMAL FINDINGS SPECIAL CONSIDERATIONS

ANKLES AND FEET

1. **Inspect the ankles and feet with the client sitting, standing, and walking.**
   - The color of the ankles and feet should be similar to that of the rest of the body. They should be symmetrical, and the skin should be unbroken. The feet and toes should be in alignment with the long axis of the lower leg. No swelling should be present, and the client's weight should fall on the middle of the foot.

▶ The following abnormalities require further evaluation:

Gouty arthritis: The metatarsophalangeal joint of the great toe is swollen, hot, red, and extremely painful.

Hallux valgus (bunion): The great toe deviates laterally from the midline, crowding the other toes. The metatarsophalangeal joint and bursa become enlarged and inflamed, causing a bunion.

Hammertoe: There is flexion of the proximal interphalangeal joint of a toe, while the distal metatarsophalangeal joint hyperextends. A callus or corn frequently occurs on the surface of the flexed joint from external pressure.

Pes planus (flatfoot): The arch of the foot is flattened, sometimes coming in contact with the floor. The deformity may be noticeable only when an individual is standing and bearing weight on the foot.

2. **Palpate the ankles.**
   - Grasp the heel of the foot with the fingers of both hands while palpating the anterior and lateral aspects of the ankle with your thumbs (see Figure 23.43 ●).

▶ Pain or discomfort on palpation and movement frequently indicate degenerative joint disease.

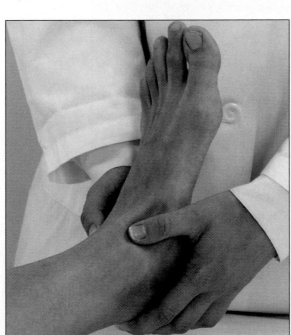

Figure 23.43 ●
Palpating the ankle.

   - The ankle joints should be firm, stable, and nontender.

3. **Palpate the length of the calcaneal (Achilles) tendon at the posterior ankle.**
   - The calcaneal tendon should be free of pain, tenderness, and nodules.

▶ Pain and tenderness along the tendon may indicate tendinitis or bursitis. Small nodules sometimes occur in clients with rheumatoid arthritis.

TECHNIQUES AND NORMAL FINDINGS	ABNORMAL FINDINGS SPECIAL CONSIDERATIONS

4. Palpate the metatarsophalangeal joints just below the ball of the foot.

- The metatarsophalangeal joints should be nontender.

▶ Pain and discomfort with this maneuver suggest early involvement of rheumatoid arthritis. Acute inflammation of the first metatarsophalangeal joint suggests gout.

5. Deeply palpate each metatarsophalangeal joint.

- The joints should be firm and nontender.

▶ Pain, swelling, or tenderness may be associated with inflammation or degenerative joint disease.

6. Test the range of motion of the ankles and feet.

- Instruct the client to perform the following movements:
  - Point the foot toward the nose. Dorsiflexion should reach 20 degrees.
  - Point the foot toward the floor. Plantar flexion should reach 45 degrees.
  - Point the sole of the foot outward, then inward. The ankle should evert to 20 degrees and invert to 30 degrees (see Figure 23.44 ●).

▶ Limited range of motion and painful movement of the foot and ankle without signs of inflammation suggest degenerative joint disease.

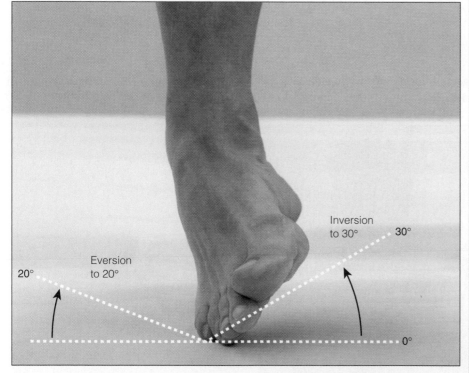

Figure 23.44 ● Eversion and inversion of the ankles.

  - Curl the toes downward (flexion).
  - Spread the toes as far as possible (abduction), and then bring the toes together (adduction).

7. Test muscle strength of the ankle.

- Ask the client to perform dorsiflexion and plantar flexion against your resistance.

8. Test muscle strength of the foot.

- Ask the client to flex and extend the toes against your resistance.

| TECHNIQUES AND NORMAL FINDINGS | ABNORMAL FINDINGS SPECIAL CONSIDERATIONS |

9. Palpate each interphalangeal joint.

- As you did for the hand, note the temperature of the extremity. Confirm that it is similar to the temperature of the rest of the client's body.

▶ Pain, swelling, or tenderness may be associated with inflammation or degenerative joint disease.

A temperature in the lower extremities that is significantly cooler than the rest of the body may indicate vascular insufficiency, which in turn may lead to musculoskeletal abnormalities.

SPINE

1. Inspect the spine.

- With the client in a standing position, move around the client's body to check the position and alignment of the spine from all sides. Confirm that the cervical and lumbar curves are concave, and that the thoracic curve is convex (see Figure 23.45A ●).

▶ Lack of symmetry of the scapulae may indicate thoracic surgery. A scapula may appear higher if a lung has been removed on that side. In addition, the following abnormalities require further evaluation:

▶ **Kyphosis:** An exaggerated thoracic dorsal curve that causes asymmetry between the sides of the posterior thorax (see Figure 23.50 ● on page 717).

▶ **Lordosis:** An exaggerated lumbar curve that compensates for pregnancy, obesity, or other skeletal changes (see Figure 23.52 ● on page 718).

▶ **Flattened lumbar curve:** A reduced lumbar concavity frequently occurs when spasms affect the lumbar muscles.

▶ **List:** The spine leans to the left or right. A plumb line drawn from T_1 does not fall between the gluteal cleft. This condition may occur with spasms in the paravertebral muscles or a herniated disk.

▶ **Scoliosis:** The spine curves to the right or left, causing an exaggerated thoracic convexity on that side (see Figure 23.51 on page 717). The body compensates, and a plumb line dropped from T_1 falls between the gluteal cleft. Unequal leg length may contribute to scoliosis; therefore, if scoliosis is suspected, it is necessary to measure the client's leg length. With the client supine, measure the distance from the anterior superior iliac spine to the medial malleolus, crossing the tape measure at the medial side of the knee (see Figure 23.46 ●).

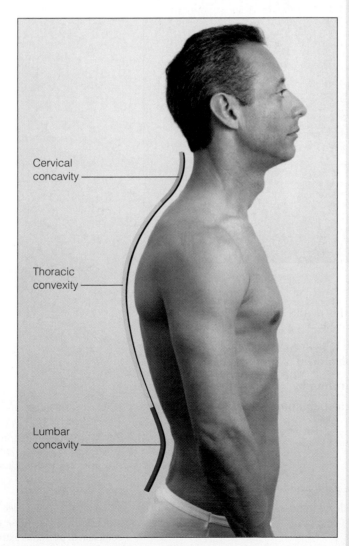

Cervical concavity

Thoracic convexity

Lumbar concavity

Figure 23.45A ●
Lateral view of spine.

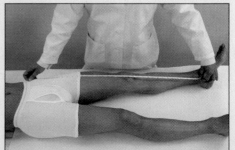

Figure 23.46 ● Measuring leg length.

- Imagine a vertical line falling from the level of T_1 to the gluteal cleft. Confirm that the spine is straight (see Figure 23.45B ●).

TECHNIQUES AND NORMAL FINDINGS

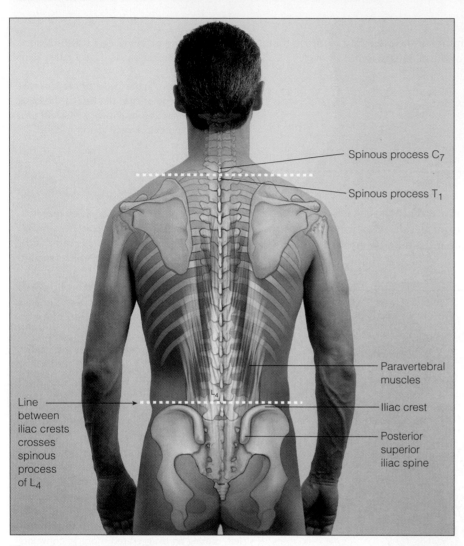

Spinous process C₇

Spinous process T₁

Paravertebral muscles

Iliac crest

Posterior superior iliac spine

Line between iliac crests crosses spinous process of L₄

L₄

Figure 23.45B ● Posterior view of spine.

- Imagine a horizontal line across the top of the scapulae. Confirm that the scapulae are level and symmetrical (see Figure 23.45B). Similarly, check that the heights of the iliac crests and the gluteal folds are level (Figure 23.45B). Ask the client to bend forward, and assess the alignment of the vertebrae.

2. **Palpate each vertebral process with your thumb.**
   - The vertebral processes should be aligned, uniform in size, firm, stable, and nontender.

3. **Palpate the muscles on both sides of the neck and back.**
   - The neck muscles should be fully developed and symmetrical, firm, smooth, and nontender.

▶ A *compression fracture* should be considered if the client is elderly, complains of pain and tenderness in the back, and has restricted back movement. T₈ and L₃ are the most common sites for compression fractures.

▶ *Muscle spasms* feel like hardened or knotlike formations. When they occur, the client may complain of pain and restricted movement. Muscle spasms may be associated with temporomandibular joint dysfunction or with *spasmodic torticollis*, a disorder in which the spasms cause the head to be pulled to one side.

TECHNIQUES AND NORMAL FINDINGS	ABNORMAL FINDINGS SPECIAL CONSIDERATIONS

TECHNIQUES AND NORMAL FINDINGS

4. **Test the range of motion of the cervical spine.**
   - Instruct the client to perform the following movements.
     - Touch the chest with the chin (flexion).
     - Look up toward the ceiling (hyperextension).
     - Attempt to touch each shoulder with the ear on that side, keeping the shoulder level (lateral bending or flexion).
     - Turn the head to face each shoulder as far as possible (rotation).

5. **Test the range of motion of the thoracic and lumbar spine.**
   - Sit or stand behind the standing client. Stabilize the pelvis with your hands and ask the client to bend sideways to the right and to the left. Right and left lateral flexion should reach 35 degrees (see Figure 23.47 ●).

ABNORMAL FINDINGS SPECIAL CONSIDERATIONS

▶ Limited range of motion, crepitation, or pain with movement in the joint requires further evaluation. If the client complains of sharp pain that begins in the lower back and radiates down the leg, perform the straight-leg-raising test: Keeping the knee extended, raise the client's leg until pain occurs, then dorsiflex the client's foot. Record the distribution and severity of the pain and the degree of leg elevation at the time the pain occurs. Also record whether dorsiflexion increases the pain. Pain with straight-leg raising may indicate a herniated disk.

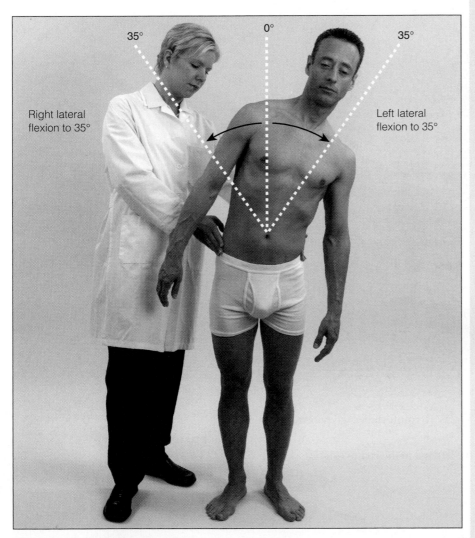

Figure 23.47 ● Lateral flexion of the spine.

TECHNIQUES AND NORMAL FINDINGS

- Ask the client to bend forward and touch the toes (flexion). Confirm that the lumbar concavity disappears with this movement and that the back assumes a single C-shaped convexity (see Figure 23.48 ●).

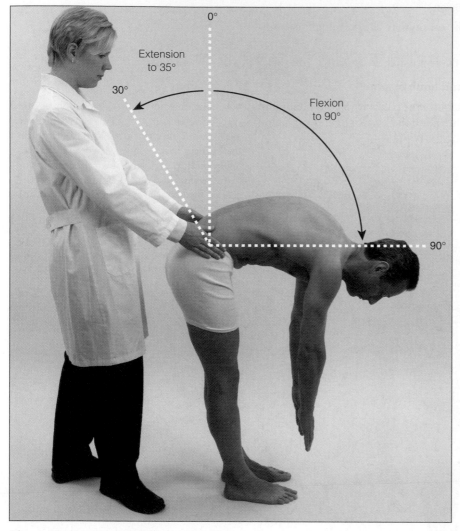

Figure 23.48 ● Forward flexion of the spine.

- Ask the client to bend backward as far as is comfortable. Hyperextension should reach 30 degrees.
- Ask the client to twist the shoulders to the left and to the right. Rotation should reach 30 degrees (see Figure 23.49 ●).

TECHNIQUES AND NORMAL FINDINGS	ABNORMAL FINDINGS SPECIAL CONSIDERATIONS

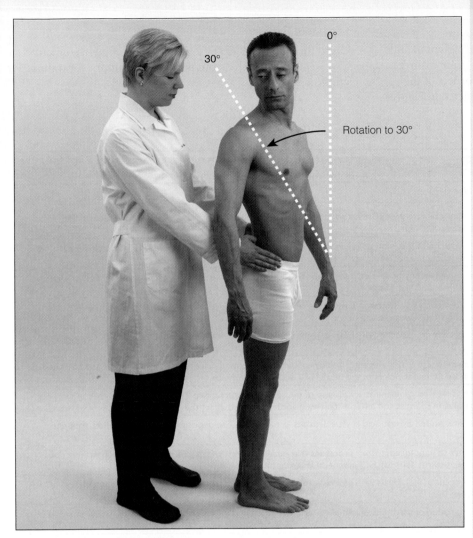

30°   0°

Rotation to 30°

Figure 23.49 ● Rotation of the spine.

Refer to the Companion Website at **www.prenhall.com/damico** and click on the **Documentation** module for documentation samples and documentation practice exercises.

Abnormal Findings

*A*bnormal findings of the musculoskeletal system include rheumatic disease, abnormalities of the spine, joint disorders, and trauma-induced disorders. Common disorders of the musculoskeletal system are described and depicted in Figures 23.50 through 23.67. Table 23.4 lists and defines rheumatic diseases. Table 23.5 lists and provides definitions for trauma-induced disorders.

Table 23.4 Rheumatic Diseases

DISEASE	DESCRIPTION
Osteoarthritis	In osteoarthritis the joint cartilage erodes, resulting in pain and stiffness. Disability is associated with osteoarthritic changes in the spine, knees, and hips.
Rheumatoid Arthritis	Inflammation of the synovium of the joint occurs in rheumatoid arthritis. The inflammation leads to pain, swelling, damage to the joint, and loss of function. Rheumatoid arthritis affects the hands and feet symmetrically.
Juvenile Rheumatoid Arthritis	This form of arthritis can affect any body part. Inflammation causes pain, swelling, stiffness, and loss of function of joints. Symptoms may include fever and skin rash.
Systemic Lupus Erythematosus (SLE)	SLE is an autoimmune disease. The autoimmune response results in inflammation and damage to joints and other organs including the kidneys, lungs, blood vessels, and heart.
Scleroderma	In scleroderma there is an overproduction of collagen in the skin or organs, which results in damage to skin, blood vessels, and joints.
Fibromyalgia	Fibromyalgia is a chronic disease that is characterized by pain in the muscles and soft tissues that support and surround joints. Pain is experienced in tender points of the head, neck, shoulders, and hips.
Ankylosing Spondylitis	Ankylosing spondylitis is a chronic inflammatory disease of the spine. It occurs more frequently in males than in females. Fusion of the spine results in stiffness and inflexibility. This disorder may also affect the hips.
Gout	Gout is a type of arthritis caused by uric acid crystal deposits in the joints. The deposits cause inflammation, pain, and swelling in the joint.
Infectious Arthritis	Infectious arthritis refers to joint inflammatory processes that occur as a result of bacterial or viral infection. Infectious arthritis can occur as parvovirus arthritis, as gonococcal arthritis, or in Lyme disease.
Psoriatic Arthritis	Psoriatic arthritis may occur in individuals with psoriasis. Joint inflammation occurs in the fingers and toes and occasionally in the spine.
Bursitis	Bursitis refers to inflammation of the bursae (fluid-filled sacs) that surround joints. The pain of bursitis may limit range of motion of the affected area.
Tendinitis	Overuse or inflammatory processes can result in tendinitis. The inflammation of the tendon results in pain and limitation in movement.
Polymyositis	Polymyositis refers to inflammation and weakness in skeletal muscles. This disease can affect the entire body and result in disability.

Table 23.5 Trauma-Induced Disorders

DISORDER	DESCRIPTION
Dislocation	A displacement of the bone from its usual anatomical location in the joint.
Joint Sprain	A stretching or tearing of the capsule or ligament of a joint due to forced movement beyond the joint's normal range.
Fracture	A partial or complete break in the continuity of the bone from trauma.
Muscle Strain	A partial muscle tear resulting from overstretching or overuse of the muscle.

ABNORMALITIES OF THE SPINE

Kyphosis

Kyphosis is an exaggeration of the normal convex curve of the thoracic spine (see Figure 23.50 ●). It may result from congenital abnormality, rheumatic conditions, compression fractures, or other disease processes including syphilis, tuberculosis, and rickets.

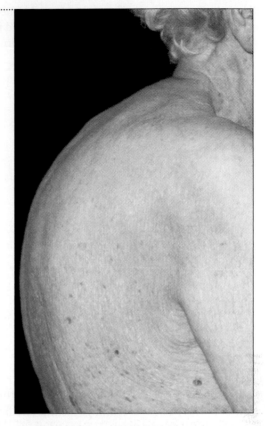

Figure 23.50 ● Kyphosis (hunchback).

Scoliosis

Scoliosis is a lateral curvature of the spine (see Figure 23.51 ●). Scoliosis may occur congenitally or as a result of disease or injury. In addition, scoliosis can occur from habitual improper posture, unequal leg length, weakening of musculature, and chronic head tilting in visual disorders. Functional scoliosis is flexible. It is visible when standing.

Structural scoliosis is irreversible and visible when standing and bending.

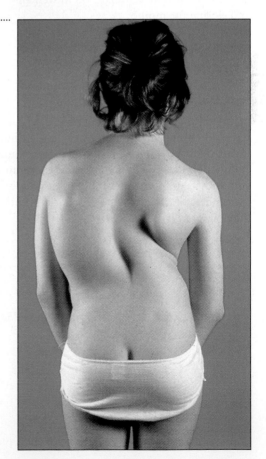

Figure 23.51 ● Scoliosis.

Lordosis

Lordosis is an exaggeration of the normal lumbar curve (see Figure 23.52 ●). This occurs in pregnancy and in obesity to compensate for the protuberance of the abdomen.

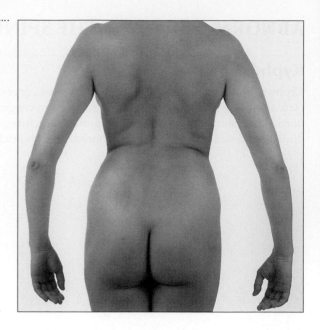

Figure 23.52 ● Lumbar lordosis.

JOINT DISORDERS

Head and Neck

TMJ Syndrome

Inflammation or trauma can result in temporomandibular joint (TMJ) syndrome. Findings include swelling and crepitus or pain in the joint, especially on movement such as opening and closing the mouth.

Shoulder

Rotator Cuff Tear

More common after the age of 40, rotator cuff tears arise from repeated impingement, injury, or falls. Findings include muscle atrophy of the infraspinatus and supraspinatus, tenderness and pain. Impaired abduction of the glenohumeral joint occurs with a complete tear of the supraspinatus tendon. The appearance of shoulder shrugging occurs with attempts at abduction (see Figure 23.53 ●).

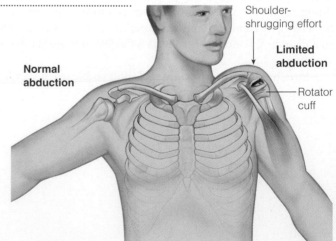

Figure 23.53 ● Rotator cuff tear.

Elbow

Olecranon Bursitis

Trauma or inflammation from rheumatoid or gouty arthritis results in swelling of the olecranon bursa (see Figure 23.54 ●).

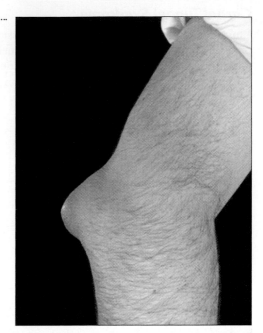

Figure 23.54 ● Olecranon bursitis.

Wrist and Hand

Joint Effusion

Inflammatory joint disease results in fluid in the joint capsule (see Figure 23.55 ●). The result is distention of the tissue seen.

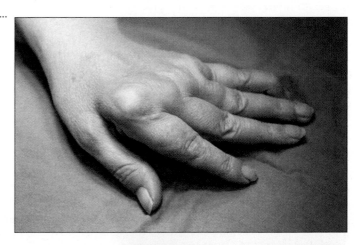

Figure 23.55 ● Joint effusion of the hand.

Rheumatoid Nodules

Firm, nontender subcutaneous nodules occur along the extensor surface of the ulna (see Figure 23.56 ●). They often are seen distal to the olecranon bursa in the hands and fingers.

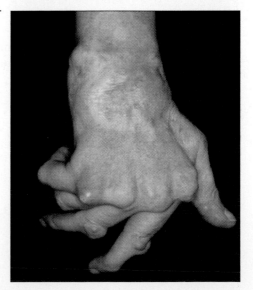

Figure 23.56 ● Rheumatoid nodules.

Carpal Tunnel Syndrome

Chronic repetitive motion results in compression of the medial nerve which lies inside the carpal tunnel. Decreased motor function leads to atrophy of the thenar eminence (see Figure 23.57 ●). Findings include pain, numbness, and positive Phalen's test.

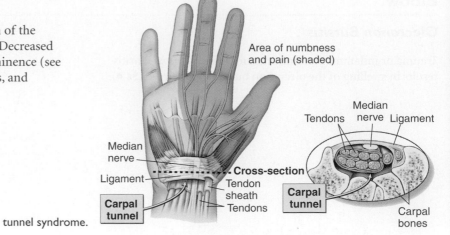

Figure 23.57 ● Carpal tunnel syndrome.

Dupuytren's Contracture

Flexion contracture of the fingers is a result of hyperplasia of the fascia of the palmar surface of the hand (see Figure 23.58 ●). Range of motion is impaired. This contracture may be inherited or occur with diabetes or alcoholic cirrhosis.

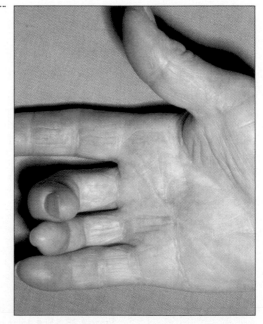

Figure 23.58 ● Dupuytren's contracture.

Ulnar Deviation

In rheumatoid arthritis the chronic inflammation of the metacarpophalangeal and interphalangeal joints leads to ulnar deviation (see Figure 23.59 ●).

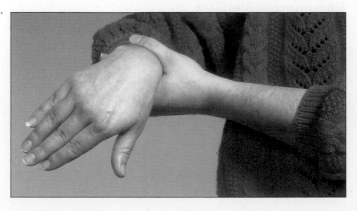

Figure 23.59 ● Ulnar deviation.

Swan-Neck and Boutonnière Deformities

Flexion contractures associated with rheumatoid arthritis include (1) swan-neck contractures, in which the proximal interphalangeal joints are hyperextended while the distal interphalangeal joints are fixed in flexion; and (2) boutonnière deformities, in which the proximal interphalangeal joint is flexed in conjunction with distal interphalangeal joint hyperextension (see Figure 23.60 ●).

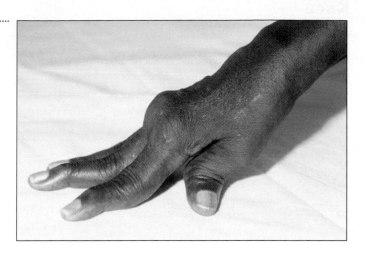

Figure 23.60 ● Swan-neck and boutonnière deformities.

Osteoarthritis

Bouchard's and Heberden's nodes occur in osteoarthritis (see Figure 23.61 ●). These nodes are hard nodules over the proximal and distal interphalangeal joints.

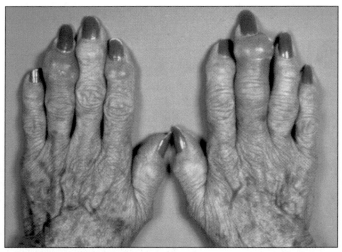

Figure 23.61 ● Osteoarthritis.

© 1972–2004 American College of Rheumatology Clinical Slide Collection. Used with permission.

Rheumatoid Arthritis

Rheumatoid arthritis results in symmetrical fusiform swelling in the soft tissue around the proximal interphalangeal joints (see Figure 23.62 ●).

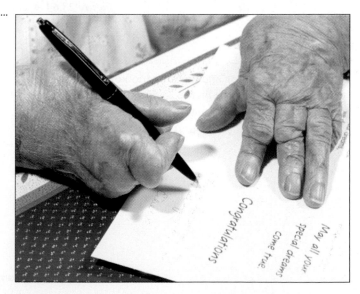

Figure 23.62 ● Rheumatoid arthritis.

Knee

Synovitis

Effusion within the synovinum results in distention of the suprapatellar area and the lateral aspects of the knee (see Figure 23.63 ●).

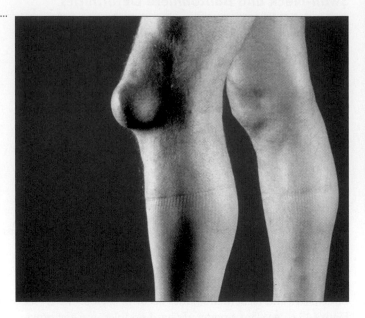

Figure 23.63 ● Synovitis.

Foot

Gout

Altered purine metabolism results in inflammation of the joints. Gout is usually seen in the metatarsophalangeal joint of the first toe (see Figure 23.64 ●). Hard nodules known as **tophi** may appear over the joint. Gout is manifested in erythema, pain, and edema.

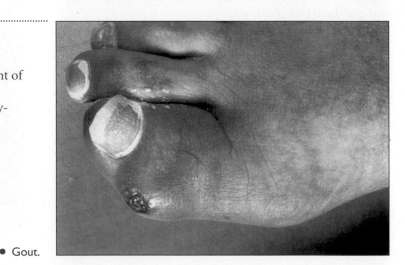

Figure 23.64 ● Gout.

Bunion

Bunions are thickening and inflammation of the bursa of the joint of the great toe (see Figure 23.65 ●). There is lateral displacement of the toe with marked enlargement of the joint.

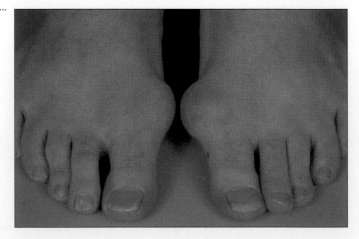

Figure 23.65 ● Bunion.

Hallux Valgus

In **hallux valgus** the great toe is abnormally adducted at the metatarsophalangeal joint (see Figure 23.66 ●).

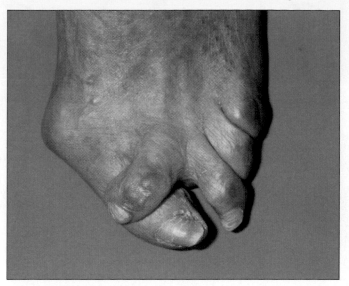

Figure 23.66 ● Hallux valgus.

Hammertoe

In hammertoe the metatarsophalangeal joint of the toe hyper-extends with flexion of the interphalangeal joint of the toe (see Figure 23.67 ●).

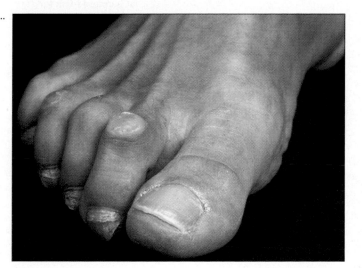

Figure 23.67 ● Hammertoe.

Health Promotion

HEALTHY PEOPLE 2010

FOCUS AREA	PREVALENCE	OBJECTIVES	ACTIONS
Physical Activity	• Regular physical activity reduces the risks for many diseases, enhances wellness, and maintains independence in older adults. • People with low physical activity and other risk factors including obesity and high blood pressure are at increased risk for coronary heart disease (CHD). • Persons with low income and education participate in less leisure physical activity than those with higher income or education. • Women participate in less leisure physical activity than men. • African Americans and Hispanics have less leisure physical activity than whites. • Participation in physical activity decreases with age and grade in school.	• Increase the numbers of adults and children who participate in moderate and vigorous physical activity. • Increase the numbers of those who perform activities to improve and maintain strength, flexibility, and endurance.	• Education about the benefits of physical activity. • Individual, community, and school programs to increase physical activity.
Arthritis	• Arthritis affects more than 20% of the adult population. • Arthritis is a common chronic illness in children. • Activity limitation because of arthritis occurs with the greatest frequency in African Americans. • Lower education and income levels produce higher rates of arthritis and disability. • African Americans have fewer joint replacements, which relieve the pain and disability in arthritis.	• Reduce the number of adults who have activity limitation due to arthritis. • Increase the number of individuals with arthritis who maintain independence. • Increase the numbers of people who seek healthcare for chronic joint pain. • Reduce disparities in joint replacement.	• Education about healthcare for chronic joint disease. • Encouragement and education about arthritis self-help groups and exercise programs. • Weight reduction programs. • Education to dispel myths about arthritis as "a part of getting old."

FOCUS AREA	PREVALENCE	OBJECTIVES	ACTIONS
Osteoporosis	• Osteoporosis occurs in about 18% of females and 5% of males over age 50. • Almost 1.5 million fractures per year are associated with osteoporosis. • White postmenopausal women have the highest risk for development of osteoporosis.	• Reduce the proportion of adults with osteoporosis.	• Programs to promote exercise, better nutrition (especially calcium and Vitamin D), smoking cessation, and reduced alcohol consumption to prevent development of osteoporosis. • Counseling for menopausal women regarding prevention of bone loss.
Chronic Back Conditions	• Limitation of activity is caused by back pain in people under 45 years of age. • Work-related factors such as heavy lifting, heavy physical work, and forceful movements are associated with almost 50% of chronic back conditions. • Back pain increases with age. • Women experience more impairment from back pain than men. • Obesity increases the risk for back pain.	• Reduce activity limitations.	• Education about ergonomics in the workplace and home activities. • Weight reduction programs. • Programs to promote physical activity, flexibility, and strength in older adults.

CLIENT EDUCATION

The following are physiological, behavioral, and cultural risk factors that affect the health of the musculoskeletal system across the life span. Several factors are cited as trends in *Healthy People 2010*. The nurse provides advice and education to reduce risks associated with the aforementioned factors and to promote and maintain musculoskeletal health.

LIFE SPAN CONSIDERATIONS

RISK FACTORS

• Diet impacts musculoskeletal health across the age span.

• Decreased bone density, muscle strength, and flexibility occur with aging.

CLIENT EDUCATION

• Instruct about healthy diet. Include recommendations for daily calcium intake and to eat a balance of protein, fats, and carbohydrates. Calcium-rich foods include dairy products, green leafy vegetables, and sardines. Vitamins C and D are important for tissue strength, healing, and promoting absorption of calcium. Laying down of bone occurs predominantly in adolescence. Nutrition discussion is critical. Image-conscious females may abstain from dairy and other calcium-rich foods to avoid the fat content in these foods.

• Recommend regular exercise according to age and ability to maintain or improve musculoskeletal function.

CULTURAL CONSIDERATIONS

RISK FACTORS

- Osteoporosis occurs with the greatest frequency in Caucasian females.
- African Americans have higher bone density than do Caucasians or Asians.
- Systemic lupus erythematosus occurs more frequently in females and those of African descent than in males and Caucasians or Hispanics.
- Sickle cell anemia, an inherited blood disorder, can result in delayed growth and bone damage. Sickle cell anemia occurs in descendants of individuals from Africa, South and Central America, Saudi Arabia, the Mediterranean, and India. Link to the Cell Anemia Association through the Companion Website.
- Accidents and trauma affect musculoskeletal health and function.

CLIENT EDUCATION

- Caucasian and Asian females need to have information about the increased risk of osteoporosis and preventive measures including changes in diet and exercise programs.
- Advise at-risk clients to seek information and screening for connective and hematologic diseases that affect joint and musculoskeletal health and function.
- Advise at-risk clients to seek information and screening for connective and hematologic diseases that affect joint and musculoskeletal health and function.
- Teach clients safety measures to avoid injury and trauma to the body. Safety measures include seat belt use when driving or as a passenger in a vehicle. Helmets and protective gear should be used when playing recreational or team sports.

ENVIRONMENTAL CONSIDERATIONS

RISK FACTORS

- Obesity increases the risks of disorders of the bones, muscles, and joints.

- Medication can impact the function and integrity of the musculoskeletal system.

CLIENT EDUCATION

- Advise that maintenance of healthy or ideal weight or weight reduction is important in reducing risks of joint disease and injury.
- Obesity can create problems with self-esteem and contribute to immobility and isolation. Weight reduction increases body image and mobility.
- Advise clients to provide information about alternative, complementary, or prescribed medicine in order to avoid potential harmful interactions or reactions with prescribed therapies.

BEHAVIORAL CONSIDERATIONS

RISK FACTORS

- Smoking and alcohol use contribute to the development of osteoporosis.
- Sedentary lifestyles increase the risk for musculoskeletal problems.
- Accidents and trauma affect musculoskeletal health and function.

CLIENT EDUCATION

- Educate and advise about smoking cessation programs to reduce the incidence of osteoporosis.
- Recommend regular exercise according to age and ability to maintain or improve musculoskeletal function.
- Educate about safety in the home, at work, and when participating in sports or athletic activities as important to reduce traumatic and other musculoskeletal injuries.

Application Through Critical Thinking

CASE STUDY

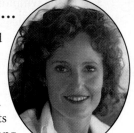

Mrs. Rhonda Barber is a 43-year-old teacher. She visits the clinic for assessment of swelling and stiffness all over, but especially in her hands.

The health history reveals that Mrs. Barber has had some stiffness in her joints when awakening from sleep and after long periods of physical activity "like housework" for several months. She became "alarmed" when her hands were "hot, red, and swollen" and that she "could hardly move them." She has had no recent illness but has "felt weak and tired" and has not had much of an appetite lately. She reports no family history of musculoskeletal disease. She reports that she has had regular physical examinations including blood work, and that nothing has been abnormal. Her last exam was 6 months ago. She takes no prescribed medications but has been using Advil and Aleve for the stiffness with moderate relief. She states that she is concerned about her hands because she must write on the board and correct papers. She also fears that "if something is really wrong and I don't get relief, I won't be able to care for my family or myself for that matter."

Physical assessment reveals a well-developed female 5'3" tall, weighing 120 lb. Her skin is pale and warm. Her gait is steady. She has normal ROM in the upper and lower extremities. ROM of her wrists, hands, and fingers is limited. The joints of her fingers are erythematous, hot, and edematous bilaterally. Her joints are tender to touch and painful upon movement. Pain is 6 to 7 on a scale of 1 to 10.

The nurse suspects that Mrs. Barber may have rheumatoid arthritis. The nurse will obtain laboratory tests and x-rays.

▶ Complete Documentation

The following is a sample documentation from assessment of Rhonda Barber.

SUBJECTIVE DATA: Stiffness in joints when waking and after long periods of physical activity for several months. "Alarmed" when hands were hot, red, swollen, and could hardly move them. No recent illness. Weak, tired, and loss of appetite lately. No family history of musculoskeletal disease. Regular physical examinations with normal results and normal "blood work." Last examination 6 months ago. No prescribed medications. Advil and Aleve for stiffness—moderate relief. Concerned about ability to work as teacher and "if something is really wrong," about ability to care for family.

OBJECTIVE DATA: Well-developed 43-year-old female. 5'3", 120 lb. Skin pale, warm. Gait steady. Full ROM all extremities except hands and fingers. Joints of fingers erythematious, hot,

---

ASSESSMENT FORM

REASON FOR VISIT

Joint stiffness, heat, redness, swelling of hands for several months. Concerned about ability to work and care for family.

HISTORY

No history of recent illness. No family history of musculoskeletal disease. No prescribed medications. Advil and Aleve for stiffness—moderate relief. Regular physical examinations—no abnormalities. Last = 6 months.

FINDINGS

Skin pale, warm

5'3" 120 lb.

Gait steady

Joints—all WNL except hands and fingers

Bilateral hands/fingers—erythematous, hot, swollen, tender to touch, pain on movement

Pain 6 to 7 on scale of 1 to 10

---

edematous bilaterally, tender to touch and painful on movement. Pain 6 to 7 on scale of 1 to 10.

▶ Critical Thinking Questions

1. Describe the thoughts and actions of the nurse that led to the suspicion of rheumatoid arthritis.
2. What information would help in developing a plan of care for Mrs. Barber?
3. How would the nurse discriminate between findings for rheumatoid arthritis and osteoarthritis?

▶ Applying Nursing Diagnoses

1. The NANDA taxonomy (see Appendix A ⌾) includes the nursing diagnosis of *impaired physical mobility.* Do the data for Mrs. Barber support this diagnosis? If so, identify the data required for the PES statement.
2. The NANDA taxonomy includes a diagnosis of *role conflict.* Do the data in the case study support this diagnosis? If so, identify the data.
3. Refer to the NANDA taxonomy to identify additional nursing diagnoses for Mrs. Barber.

▶ *Prepare Teaching Plan*

LEARNING NEED: The data in the case study revealed that Mrs. Barber may have rheumatoid arthritis. Her symptoms are typical for rheumatoid arthritis. She will undergo laboratory tests and x-rays to confirm the diagnosis.

The case study provides data that is representative of risks, symptoms, and behaviors of many individuals. Therefore, the following teaching plan is based on the need to provide information to members of any community about arthritis.

GOAL: The participants in this learning program will have increased awareness of risk factors and symptoms associated with arthritis.

OBJECTIVES: At the completion of this learning session, the participants will be able to:

1. Describe arthritis.
2. Identify risk factors associated with arthritis.
3. List the symptoms of arthritis.
4. Discuss strategies in diagnosis and treatment of arthritis.

APPLICATION OF OBJECTIVE 2: Identify risk factors associated with arthritis

Content	Teaching Strategy	Evaluation
• Age. Osteoarthritis risk increases after age 45. • Gender. Females have a higher incidence of arthritis. • Hereditary factors. Family history and genetic factors increase risk for arthritis. • Obesity. Obesity increases risk for arthritis in weight-bearing joints. • Joint injury through sports or repeated stress in some occupations can increase the risk of osteoarthritis. • Joint misalignment or deformity can increase the risk for arthritis.	• Lecture • Discussion • Audiovisual materials • Printed materials Lecture is appropriate when disseminating information to large groups. Discussion allows participants to bring up concerns and to raise questions. Audiovisual materials such as illustrations reinforce verbal presentation. Printed material, especially to be taken away with learners, allows review, reinforcement, and reading at the learner's pace.	• Written examination. May use short answer, fill-in, or multiple-choice items or a combination of items. If these are short and easy to evaluate, the learner received immediate feedback.

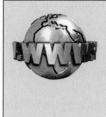

Please refer to the Companion Website at www.prenhall.com/damico and click on Chapter 23, the Application Through Critical Thinking module, to complete the following activities related to this case study:
▶ **Critical Thinking questions**
▶ **Extended Nursing Diagnosis challenge**
▶ **Documentation activity**
▶ **Teaching Plan for Objectives 1, 3, and 4**

EXPLORE MediaLink

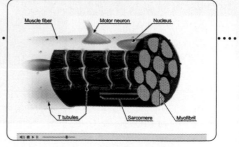

Additional resources for this chapter are found on the Student CD-ROM accompanying this textbook and on the Companion Website.

CD-ROM CONTENT

Content for this chapter includes:
Objectives
Key Concepts
NCLEX-RN® Review Questions
Model Documentation Forms
Audio Glossary
Animations
Muscle Contractions
Muscles
Joint Movements
Games and Challenges
Clinical Spotlight Videos
Arthritis
Carpal Tunnel
Muscle Atrophy
Muscular Dystrophy
Head-to-Toe Physical Examination Video

COMPANION WEBSITE CONTENT

www.prenhall.com/damico

Content for this chapter includes:
Objectives
NCLEX-RN® Review Questions
Client Interaction Case Study Challenge
Application Through Critical Thinking Case Study
  Teaching Plan Challenge
MediaLinks
MediaLink Application
Tool Box
Joint Movements
Rating Muscle Strength
Chapter Documentation Form Example
Health Promotion
  Healthy People 2010
  Client Education
New York Times

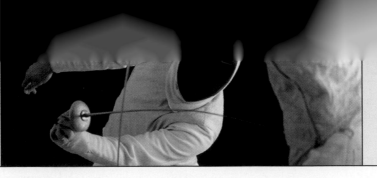

24

Neurologic System

MediaLink

www.prenhall.com/damico

The CD-ROM in the back of this textbook and the Media-Link website contain NCLEX-RN® review questions, interactive exercises, case study challenges, animations, videos, documentation and checklist forms, and review materials. For a complete listing of the media content specific to Chapter 24, see the Explore MediaLink at the end of the chapter.

The complex integration, coordination, and regulation of body systems, and ultimately all body functions, are achieved through the mechanics of the nervous system. The intricate nature of the nervous system permits the individual to perform all physiological functions, perform all activities of daily living, function in society, and maintain a degree of independence. A threat to any aspect of neurologic function is a threat to the whole person. A neurologic deficit could alter self-concept, produce anxiety related to decreased function and loss of self-control, and restrict the client's mobility. Thus, it is essential to assess the psychosocial health status of a client experiencing a neurologic deficit. Because factors such as diet, alcohol intake, smoking, and other healthcare practices can influence neurologic health, the nurse must consider the client's self-care practices when assessing the client's neurologic system. Factors relating to the client's occupation, environment, and genetic background also contribute to neurologic health. These are among the considerations regarding neurologic health as described in *Healthy People 2010*. Actions to promote neurologic health are discussed in the *Healthy People 2010* feature on page 777.

The nervous system is immature at birth. Many reflexes that are present in the newborn begin to disappear as the system matures. The older adult experiences a decrease in neurologic function; the senses diminish, as do the reactions to stimuli. Degeneration of the nervous system may lead to a variety of psychosocial problems such as social isolation, lowered self-esteem, stress, anxiety, and ineffective coping.

A healthy diet, exercise, and rest help ensure optimum neurologic functions. Alcohol causes neurologic impairments ranging from mild sedation to severe motor deficits. Caffeine is a mild stimulant that may cause restlessness, tremors, and insomnia.

A variety of home, work, and environmental factors may cause neurologic impairments. For example, lead-based paint in older homes may cause lead poisoning and encephalopathy in children.

A thorough neurologic assessment gives the nurse detailed data regarding the client's health status and self-care practices. It is imperative to develop and refine assessment skills regarding the wellness and normal parameters of the neurologic functions in the body. The nurse needs to foster a keen discriminatory skill concerning the subtle changes that could be occurring in the client. Neurologic assessment is an integral aspect of the client's health and must be carefully considered when conducting a thorough health assessment.

ANATOMY AND PHYSIOLOGY REVIEW

The neurologic system, a highly integrated and complex system, is divided into two principal parts: the central nervous system (CNS) and the peripheral nervous system (PNS). The **central nervous system** consists of the brain and the spinal cord, whereas the cranial nerves and the spinal nerves make up the **peripheral nervous system.** The two systems work together to receive an impulse, interpret it, and initiate a response, enabling the individual to maintain a high level of adaptation and homeostasis. The nervous system is responsible for control of cognitive function and both voluntary and involuntary activities.

The basic cell of the nervous system is the *neuron.* This highly specialized cell sends impulses throughout the body. Many of the nerve fibers that have a large diameter or are long in length are covered with a *myelin sheath.* This white, fatty coverage helps to protect the neuron while increasing the delivery of a nerve impulse, hence the term *white matter of the nervous system.*

CENTRAL NERVOUS SYSTEM

The central nervous system includes the brain and spinal cord. These structures will be described in the following sections.

Brain

The brain is the largest portion of the central nervous system. It is covered and protected by the meninges, the cerebrospinal fluid, and the bony structure of the skull. The **meninges** are three connective tissue membranes that cover, protect, and nourish the

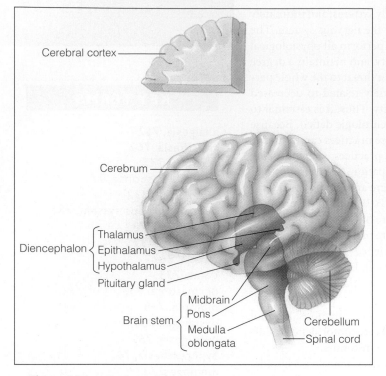

Figure 24.1 ● Regions of the brain.

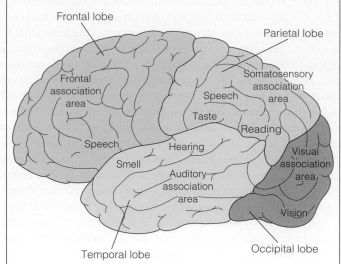

Figure 24.2 ● Lobes of the cerebrum.

central nervous system. The cerebrospinal fluid also helps to nourish the central nervous system; however, its primary function is to cushion the brain and prevent injury to the brain tissue. The brain is made up of the cerebrum, diencephalon, cerebellum, and brain stem (see Figure 24.1 ●).

CEREBRUM. The **cerebrum** is the largest portion of the brain. The outermost layer of the cerebrum, the *cerebral cortex,* is composed of gray matter. Responsible for all conscious behavior, the cerebral cortex enables the individual to perceive, remember, communicate, and initiate voluntary movements. The cerebrum consists of the frontal, parietal, and temporal lobes. The lobes of the cerebrum are illustrated in Figure 24.2 ●.

The frontal lobe of the cerebrum helps control voluntary skeletal movement, speech, emotions, and intellectual activities. The prefrontal cortex of the frontal lobe controls intellect, complex learning abilities, judgment, reasoning, concern for others, and creation of abstract ideas.

The parietal lobe of the cerebrum is responsible for conscious awareness of sensation and somatosensory stimuli, including temperature, pain, shapes, and two-point discrimination—for example, the ability to sense a round versus square object placed in the hand or hot versus cold materials against the skin.

The visual cortex, located in the occipital lobe, receives stimuli from the retina and interprets the visual stimuli in relation to past experiences.

The temporal lobe of the cerebrum is responsible for interpreting auditory stimuli. Impulses from the cochlea are transmitted to the temporal lobe and are interpreted regarding pitch, rhythm, loudness, and perception of what the individual hears. The olfactory cortex is also in the temporal lobe and transmits impulses related to smell.

DIENCEPHALON. The diencephalon is composed of the thalamus, hypothalamus, and epithalamus. The **thalamus** is

the gateway to the cerebral cortex. All input channeled to the cerebral cortex is processed by the thalamus.

The hypothalamus, an autonomic control center, influences activities such as blood pressure, heart rate, force of heart contraction, digestive motility, respiratory rate and depth, and perception of pain, pleasure, and fear. Regulation of body temperature, food intake, water balance, and sleep cycles are also regulated by the hypothalamus.

The epithalamus helps control moods and sleep cycles. It contains the choroid plexus, where the cerebrospinal fluid is formed.

CEREBELLUM. The **cerebellum** is located below the cerebrum and behind the brain stem. It coordinates stimuli from the cerebral cortex to provide precise timing for skeletal muscle coordination and smooth movements. The cerebellum also assists with maintaining equilibrium and muscle tone.

BRAIN STEM. The **brain stem** contains the midbrain, pons, and medulla oblongata. Located between the cerebrum and spinal cord, the brain stem connects pathways between the higher and lower structures. Ten of the 12 pairs of cranial nerves originate in the brain stem. As an autonomic control center, the brain stem influences blood pressure by controlling vasoconstriction. It also regulates respiratory rate, depth, and rhythm as well as vomiting, hiccuping, swallowing, coughing, and sneezing.

Spinal Cord

The **spinal cord** is a continuation of the medulla oblongata. About 42 cm (17 in.) in length, it passes through the skull at the foramen magnum and continues through the vertebral column to the first lumbar vertebra. The meninges, cerebrospinal fluid, and bony vertebrae protect the spinal cord. The spinal cord has the ability to transmit impulses to and from the brain via the ascending and descending pathways. Some reflex activity takes place within the spinal cord; however, for this activity to be useful, the brain must interpret it.

REFLEXES

Reflexes are stimulus-response activities of the body. They are fast, predictable, unlearned, innate, and involuntary reactions to stimuli. The individual is aware of the results of the reflex activity and not the activity itself. The reflex activity may be simple and take place at the level of the spinal cord, with interpretation at the cerebral level. For example, if the tendon of the knee is sharply stimulated with a reflex hammer, the impulse follows the afferent nerve fibers. A synapse occurs in the spinal cord, and the impulse is transmitted to the efferent nerve fibers, leading to an additional synapse and stimulation of muscle fibers. As the muscle fibers contract, the lower leg moves, causing the knee-jerk reaction. The individual is aware of the reflex after the lower leg moves and the brain has interpreted the activity. Figure 24.3 ● illustrates two simple reflex arcs.

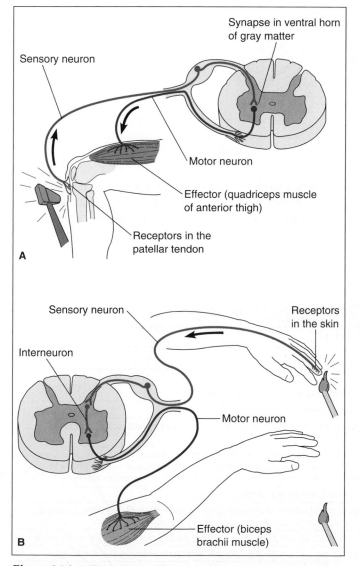

Figure 24.3 ● Two simple reflex arcs. A. In the two-neuron reflex arc, the stimulus is transferred from the sensory neuron directly to the motor neuron at the point of synapse in the spinal cord. B. In the three-neuron reflex arc, the stimulus travels from the sensory neuron to an interneuron in the spinal cord, and then to the motor neuron. (Sensory nerves are shown in blue; motor nerves, in red.)

PERIPHERAL NERVOUS SYSTEM

The peripheral nervous system includes the 12 pairs of cranial nerves and the paired spinal nerves. They will be described in the following paragraphs.

Cranial Nerves

The 12 pairs of cranial nerves originate in the brain and serve various parts of the head and neck (see Figure 24.4 ●). The first 2 pairs originate in the anterior brain, and the remaining 10 pairs originate in the brain stem. The vagus nerve is the only cranial nerve to serve a muscle and body region below the neck. The cranial nerves are numbered using roman numerals and many times are discussed by number rather than name. Composition of the cranial nerve fibers varies, producing sensory nerves, motor nerves, and mixed nerves. A summary of the name, number, function, and activity of the cranial nerves is presented in Table 24.1.

Spinal Nerves

The spinal cord supplies the body with 31 pairs of spinal nerves that are named according to the vertebral level of origin as shown in Figure 24.5 ●.

There are 8 pairs of cervical nerves, 12 pairs of thoracic nerves, 5 pairs of lumbar nerves, 5 pairs of sacral nerves, and 1 pair of coccygeal nerves. At the cervical level, the nerves exit superior to the vertebra except for the eighth cervical nerve. This nerve exits inferior to the seventh cervical vertebra. All remaining descending nerves exit the spinal cord and vertebral column inferior to the same-numbered vertebrae. Spinal nerves are all classified as mixed nerves because they contain motor and sensory pathways that produce motor and sensory activities. Each pair of nerves is responsible for a particular area of the body. The nerves provide some overlap of body segments they serve. This overlap is more complete on the trunk than on the extremities.

A **dermatome** is an area of skin innervated by the cutaneous branch of one spinal nerve. All spinal nerves except the first cervical (C_1) serve a cutaneous region. The anterior and posterior views of the dermatomes of the body are shown in Figure 24.6 ●.

SPECIAL CONSIDERATIONS

Throughout the assessment process, the nurse gathers subjective and objective data reflecting the client's state of health. Using critical thinking and the nursing process, the nurse identifies many factors to be considered when collecting the data. Some of these factors include but are not limited to age, developmental level, race, ethnicity, work history, living conditions, and socioeconomics. Physical and emotional wellness are also among the many factors or special considerations that impact a client's health status. The following sections describe the ways in which neurologic health is affected by these special considerations.

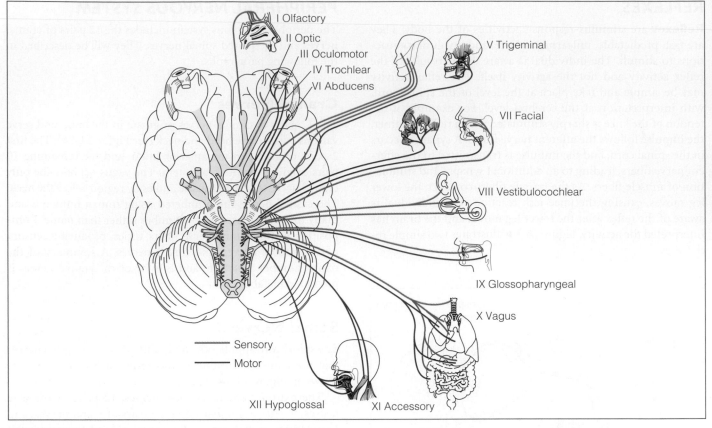

Figure 24.4 • Cranial nerves and their target regions. (Sensory nerves are shown in blue; motor nerves, in red.)

DEVELOPMENTAL CONSIDERATIONS

Growth and development are dynamic processes that describe change over time. The following discussion presents specific variations for different age groups across the life span. The structures and functions of the neurologic system undergo change as a result of normal growth and development. Accurate interpretation of subjective and objective data from assessment of the neurologic system is dependent upon knowledge of expected variations. The discussion of age-related variations is presented in the following sections.

Table 24.1	Cranial Nerves		
NAME	**NUMBER**	**FUNCTION**	**ACTIVITY**
Olfactory	I	Sensory	Sense of smell.
Optic	II	Sensory	Vision.
Oculomotor	III	Motor	Pupillary reflex, extrinsic muscle movement of eye.
Trochlear	IV	Motor	Eye-muscle movement.
Trigeminal	V	Mixed	*Ophthalmic branch:* Sensory impulses from scalp, upper eyelid, nose, cornea, and lacrimal gland.
			Maxillary branch: Sensory impulses from lower eyelid, nasal cavity, upper teeth, upper lip, alate. *Mandibular branch:* Sensory impulses from tongue, lower teeth, skin of chin, and lower lip. Motor action includes teeth clenching, movement of mandible.
Abducens	VI	Mixed	Extrinsic muscle movement of eye.
Facial	VII	Mixed	Taste (anterior two thirds of tongue). Facial movements such as smiling, closing of eyes, frowning. Production of tears and salivary stimulation.
Vestibulocochlear	VIII	Sensory	*Vestibular branch:* Sense of balance or equilibrium. *Cochlear branch:* Sense of hearing.
Glossopharyngeal	IX	Mixed	Produces the gag and swallowing reflexes. Taste (posterior third of the tongue).
Vagus	X	Mixed	Innervates muscles of throat and mouth for swallowing and talking. Other branches responsible for pressoreceptors and chemoreceptor activity.
Accessory	XI	Motor	Movement of the trapezius and sternocleidomastoid muscles. Some movement of larynx, pharynx, and soft palate.
Hypoglossal	XII	Motor	Movement of tongue for swallowing, movement of food during chewing, and speech.

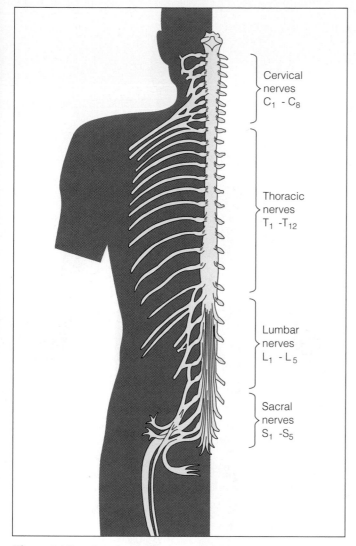

Figure 24.5 ● Spinal nerves.

Infants and Children

The growth of the nervous system is very rapid during the fetal period. This rate of growth does not continue during infancy. Some research indicates that no neurons are formed after the third trimester of fetal life. It is believed that during infancy the neurons mature, allowing for more complete actions to take place. The cerebral cortex thickens, brain size increases, and myelinization occurs. The maturational advances in the nervous system are responsible for the cephalocaudal and proximal-to-distal refinement of development, control, and movement.

The neonate has several primitive reflexes at birth. These include but are not limited to sucking, stepping, startle (Moro), and the Babinski reflex in which stimulation of the sole of the foot from the heel toward the toes results in dorsiflexion of the great toe and fanning of other toes. The Babinski reflex and the tonic neck reflex are normal until around 2 years of age. (See Table 25.4, Primitive Reflexes of Early Childhood, on page 793. ⬭) By about 1 month of age, the reflexes begin to disappear, and the child takes on more controlled and complex activity.

The cry of the newborn helps place the infant on the health-illness continuum. *Strong* and *lusty* are terms used to describe the cry of a healthy newborn. An absent, weak, or "catlike" or shrill cry usually indicates cerebral disease.

Throughout infancy and the early childhood years, it is important to assess the fine and gross motor skills, language, and personal-social skills of the child. The nurse identifies benchmarks or mileposts related to age and level of functioning of the child and compares the child's actual functioning to an anticipated level of functioning. Developmental delays or learning disabilities may be related to neurologic conditions such as fetal alcohol syndrome, autism, and attention deficit disorder.

The Pregnant Female

As the uterus grows to accommodate the fetus, pressure may be placed on nerves in the pelvic cavity, thus producing neurologic changes in the legs. As the pressure is relieved in the pelvis, the changes in the lower extremities are resolved. As the fetus grows, the center of gravity of the female shifts, and the lumbar curvature of the spine is accentuated. This change in posture can place pressure on roots of nerves, causing sensory changes in the lower extremities. These sensory changes are reversible following relief of pressure and postural changes. Hyperactive reflexes may indicate pregnancy-induced hypertension (PIH).

The Older Adult

As the individual ages, many neurologic changes occur. Some of these changes are readily visible, whereas others are internal and are not easily detected. The internal changes could be primary in nature, or secondary to other changes, and contribute to the aging process. In general, the aging process causes a subtle, slow, but steady decrease in neurologic function. These changes can be more pronounced and more troublesome for the individual when they are accompanied by a chronic illness such as heart disease, diabetes, or arthritis. Impulse transmission decreases, as does reaction to stimuli. Reflexes are diminished or disappear, and coordination is not as strong as it once was. Deep tendon reflexes are not as brisk. Coordination and movement may be slower and not as smooth as they were at one time.

The senses—hearing, vision, smell, taste, and touch—are not as acute as they once were. Taste is not as strong; therefore, the older adult tends to use more seasonings on food. Visual acuity and hearing also begin to diminish as the individual ages.

As muscle mass decreases, the older individual moves and reacts more slowly than during youth. The client's gait may now include short, shuffling, uncertain, and perhaps unsteady steps. The posture of the older adult demonstrates more flexion than in earlier years.

Assessment techniques used with the older adult are the same as those used for the younger or middle-aged adult. However, because the older adult tires more easily, the nurse may need to do the total assessment in more than one visit. The nurse should allow more time than usual when performing the neurologic assessment of the older adult. It is also imperative to obtain a detailed history, because chronic health problems can influence the findings.

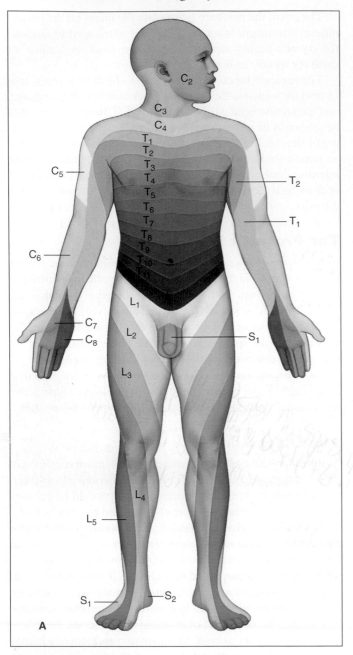

Figure 24.6A ● Dermatomes of body, anterior view.

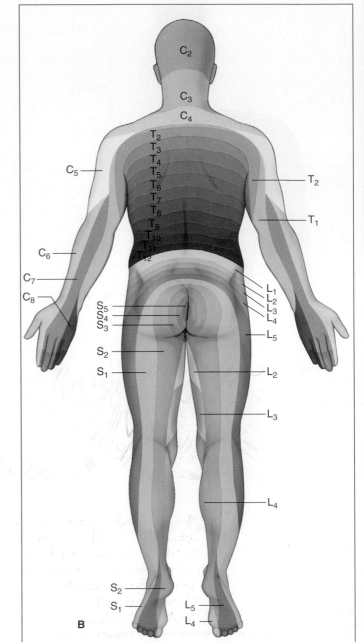

Figure 24.6B ● Dermatomes of body, posterior view.

PSYCHOSOCIAL CONSIDERATIONS

Changes in nervous system functioning may alter an individual's ability to control body movements, speech, elimination patterns, and to engage in activities of daily living. Inevitably, these changes will affect the individual's psychosocial health. Clients' self-esteem may suffer as they suddenly or progressively become unable to carry out the roles they previously assumed in their family and society. Another common psychosocial problem associated with neurologic disorders is social isolation. For example, an individual in the first stage of Alzheimer's disease will decline invitations to social functions because the individual feels anxious and confused in unfamiliar surroundings. Such problems indicate a need for improved coping strategies and increased support systems.

As stresses accumulate, an individual becomes increasingly susceptible to neurologic problems, such as forgetfulness, confusion, inability to concentrate, sleeplessness, and tremors. For example, a college senior who is studying for examinations, writing applications for graduate school, and who has just broken up with his or her significant other, might experience one or all of these symptoms. Chronic stress may also contribute to clinical depression in some clients.

CULTURAL AND ENVIRONMENTAL CONSIDERATIONS

Huntington's disease is a genetically transferred neurologic disorder. However, the genetic link to most other degenerative

Cultural Considerations

- African Americans are more likely than Caucasians to have very low birth weight babies. Very low birth weight babies are at risk for neurologic problems including intraventricular hemorrhage.
- African Americans have higher rates of Alzheimer's disease compared to Caucasians in the United States.

- There is an increased familial risk for development of Alzheimer's in African Americans.
- High blood pressure increases the risk of brain attack (stroke).
- African Americans have a higher incidence of high blood pressure.

neurologic disorders, such as Alzheimer's disease, multiple sclerosis, myasthenia gravis, and others, is unclear.

Research is also inconclusive on the effects of environmental toxins on the development of degenerative neurologic disorders; however, some studies suggest that Alzheimer's disease in some clients may be due to aluminum intoxication. Other research indicates that toxins such as carbon monoxide, manganese, and mercury may cause some cases of Parkinson's disease. Peripheral neuropathy, damage to the peripheral nerves, occurs more often among farm workers exposed to the organophosphates in many insecticides.

Lead poisoning also causes peripheral neuropathy and encephalopathy. Although not as common as in the past, the risk for lead poisoning still remains high among preschool children who live in old apartments or houses in which walls are painted with lead-based paints. Lead poisoning is not limited to those who live in low-cost, inner-city dwellings, but may also occur in wealthy families living in restored older homes.

Gathering the Data

$\mathcal{H}$ealth assessment of the neurologic system includes gathering subjective and objective data. Subjective data is collected during the client interview, prior to the physical assessment. During the interview, various communication techniques are used to elicit general and specific information about the status of the client's neurologic system and ability to function. Health records, results of laboratory tests, x-rays, and imaging reports are important secondary sources to be included in the data-gathering process. During the physical assessment, the techniques of inspection and palpation, as well as techniques and methods specific to neurologic function, will be used.

FOCUSED INTERVIEW

The focused interview for the neurologic system concerns data related to the functions of this body system. Subjective data is collected during the focused interview. The nurse must be prepared to observe the client and to listen for cues related to the function of the neurologic system. The nurse may use openended or closed questions to obtain information. A number of follow-up questions or requests for descriptions may be required to clarify data or gather missing information. Follow-up questions are intended to identify the sources of problems, duration of difficulties, measures to alleviate or manage problems, and clues about the client's knowledge of his or her own health.

The focused interview guides the physical assessment of the neurologic system. The information is always considered in relation to norms and expectations of neurologic function. Therefore, the nurse must consider age, gender, race, culture, environment, health practices, past and concurrent problems, and therapies when framing questions and using techniques to elicit information. In order to address all of the factors when conducting a focused interview, categories of questions related to the status and function of the neurologic system have been developed. These categories include general questions that are asked of all clients; those addressing illness or infection; questions related to symptoms, pain, or behaviors; those related to habits or practices; questions that are specific for clients according to age; those for the pregnant female; and questions that address environmental concerns.

The nurse must consider the client's ability to participate in the focused interview and physical assessment of the neurologic system. Participation in the focused interview is influenced by the ability to communicate in the same language. Language barriers interfere with the accuracy of the data and cause anxiety in the client. The nurse may have to use a translator in conducting an interview and in the physical assessment. If the client is experiencing pain, recent injury, or anxiety, attention must focus on relief of symptoms or discomfort before proceeding with an in-depth interview.

FOCUSED INTERVIEW QUESTIONS

RATIONALES

The following section provides sample questions and bulleted follow-up questions in each of the previously mentioned categories. A rationale for each question is provided. The list of questions is not all-inclusive, but rather represents the types of questions required in a comprehensive focused interview related to the neurologic system. As these questions are asked, the subjective data obtained helps to identify client strengths or risks associated with the neurologic system described in Healthy People 2010.

GENERAL QUESTIONS

1. **Please complete this sentence: "After I get out of bed in the morning, a typical day in my life includes____."**

   ▶ The nurse is asking the client to describe activities of daily living (ADLs). If this data has been obtained in another area of the assessment, the nurse should alter the lead statement accordingly. The client usually perceives this opening as nonthreatening. It places a focus on activities, self-care practices, and the client's level of wellness. The nurse can then employ therapeutic communication skills to seek clarification and encourage the client to relate all of the activities of the day.

2. **Explain what brings you here today.**

   ▶ This open-ended statement allows the client to state what is important. It increases the client's control in what may be a stressful situation, thereby producing a less threatening environment. Based on the client's response, the nurse should adjust the sequence of questions to explore the client's concern.

3. **Have you had a change in your ability to carry out your daily activities?**
   - Describe the change.
   - Do you know what is causing the change?
   - What do you do about the problem?
   - How long has this been happening?
   - Have you discussed this with your healthcare provider?

   ▶ Neurologic problems can interfere with the ability to carry out ADLs.

4. **Do you have any chronic disease such as diabetes or hypertension?**

   ▶ Chronic diseases such as diabetes and hypertension can predispose clients to neurologic problems.

5. **Do any members of your family now have, or have they ever had, a neurologic problem or disease?**
   - What is the disease or problem?
   - Who in the family has the problem?
   - When was it diagnosed?
   - How has it been treated?
   - How effective has the treatment been?

   ▶ Some conditions are familial and recur in families.

QUESTIONS RELATED TO ILLNESS, INFECTION, OR INJURY

1. **Have you ever been diagnosed with a neurologic illness?**
   - When were you diagnosed with the problem?
   - What treatment was prescribed for the problem?
   - What kinds of things do you do to help with the problem?
   - Has the problem ever recurred (acute)?
   - How are you managing the disease now (chronic)?

   ▶ The client has the opportunity to provide information about a specific illness. If a diagnosed illness is identified, follow-up about the date of diagnosis, treatment, and outcomes is required. Data about each illness identified by the client is essential to an accurate health assessment. Illnesses can be classified as acute or chronic, and follow-up regarding each classification will differ.

FOCUSED INTERVIEW QUESTIONS	**RATIONALES**

2. An alternative to question 1 is to list possible neurologic illnesses such as stroke, paresis, epilepsy, multiple sclerosis, and myasthenia gravis and ask the client to respond yes or no as each is stated.

▶ This is a comprehensive and easy way to elicit information about all neurologic diagnoses.

3. Have you ever had an infection of the neurologic system? Follow-up would be the same as in question 1.

4. An alternative to question 3 is to list neurologic infections such as poliomyelitis, meningitis, and encephalitis and ask the client to state yes or no as each is stated. The rationale is the same as in question 2.

5. Have you ever had an injury to your head or back?
   - If so, please explain what happened.
   - When did this happen?
   - What treatments did you receive?
   - As a result of this injury, what problems do you have today? Follow-up would be the same as in question 1.

▶ The database being developed relates to past incidents and residual deficits.

QUESTIONS RELATED TO SYMPTOMS OR BEHAVIORS

When gathering information about symptoms, many questions are required to elicit details and descriptions that assist in analysis of the data. Discrimination is made in relation to the significance of a symptom, in relation to specific diseases or problems, and in relation to the potential need for follow-up examination or referral.

The following questions refer to specific symptoms associated with the neurologic system. For each symptom, questions and follow-up are required. The details to be elicited are the characteristics of the symptom, the treatment or remedy for the symptom including over-the-counter (OTC) and home remedies, the determination if diagnosis has been sought, the effects of treatments, and family history associated with a symptom.

1. **Do you have fainting spells? Do you have a history of seizures or convulsions?**
   - If so, when did you have your first episode?
   - What happens to you immediately before the seizure?
   - What have you been told about what your body does during the seizure?
   - How do you feel after the seizure?
   - What medications do you take?
   - Do you take your medications regularly?
   - When was the last time you had a seizure?

▶ The client should be encouraged to identify the type of seizures: partial, complex, or mixed. The questions focus on an aura, muscular activity, postictal period, and use of medications. Lifestyle changes are important, because these individuals need to be cautioned regarding driving and the use of dangerous equipment. (Epilepsy is described later in this chapter.)

2. **Has your vision changed in any way?**
   - Do you ever see two objects when you know there is just one?
   - Are you able to see off to the sides without turning your head?
   - When you go from a bright room to a darker room, do your eyes adjust to the change rapidly?

▶ Changes in vision may indicate problems with the cranial nerves, a brain tumor, increased intracranial pressure, or ocular disease.

3. **What changes, if any, have you noticed in your hearing?**
   - Have you noticed any ringing in the ears?

▶ Changes in hearing and ringing in the ears may indicate a problem with cranial nerve or auditory functions.

4. **Have you noticed any change with your ability to smell or taste?**

▶ A change in the ability to smell or taste may also indicate a problem with cranial nerve function.

5. **Describe your balance.**
   - Are you steady on your feet?
   - Are you able to function without difficulty?
   - Is one leg stronger than the other?
   - Do you notice any tremors?

▶ All of these questions relate to activities of the cerebellum.

FOCUSED INTERVIEW QUESTIONS	RATIONALES

- Could you bend down to pick up a straight pin and stand up again?
- Do you drop things easily?
- Do you find yourself being very clumsy—tripping, spilling things, and knocking things over?
- If so, how long have the symptoms been present?
- Are the symptoms continuous?
- Are they getting worse? What do you do to control or limit the symptoms?

6. **Do you have numbness or tingling in any part of your body?**
   - How long have you had this?
   - Do you know what causes it?
   - Have you sought treatment?
   - What do you do to relieve the problem?

▶ Numbness or tingling may result from neurologic changes alone or as a result of systemic or circulatory disease.

QUESTIONS RELATED TO PAIN

1. **Are you having any pain?**
   - If so, where is it?
   - When did the pain begin?
   - Is the pain constant or intermittent?
   - What relieves or decreases the pain?
   - What increases the pain?
   - Does the pain interfere with your daily activities?
   - How would you describe the pain—sharp, dull, acute, burning, stabbing, or stinging?
   - On a scale of 1 to 10 with 10 being highest, how would you rate the pain?

▶ Pain, a completely subjective experience, can be acute or chronic. This database provides information regarding cultural variations, self-care practices, and placement on the health-illness continuum.

2. **Do you get headaches?**
   - If so, describe them.
   - Where are they located?
   - Are they always in the same area?
   - How often do they occur?
   - Are you able to function with these headaches?
   - What do you think causes your headaches?
   - What do you do to help relieve the pain?
   - Does this remedy work?
   - On a scale of 1 to 10, rate the severity of your headaches.

▶ The nurse is developing the database to determine if headaches are migraines, tension, cluster, unilateral, bilateral, or associated with other disease. (Refer to the section on the types of headaches in Chapter 12 on pages 253–254 ⚭.)

QUESTIONS RELATED TO BEHAVIORS

1. **Do you now use or have you ever used recreational drugs or alcohol?**
   - What was the drug or substance?
   - When did you use it?
   - How long have you used it?
   - Have you experienced problems as a result of this drug?
   - How much alcohol do you consume?
   - For how long?

▶ *Recreational drugs* is a common term used to imply illegal substances. This category could include heroin, cocaine, marijuana, ketamine, oxycodone, and other substances. Use of social drugs and alcohol can create risk for neurologic symptoms or disorders that may be temporary or have long-term consequences.

2. **Describe your memory.**
   - Do you need to make a list or write things down so you won't forget?
   - Do you lose things easily?
   - What did you do today before you came here?

▶ Memory loss is indicative of the aging process and neurologic or psychiatric disease such as Alzheimer's, depression, or stroke. The nurse is developing a baseline regarding the client's memory and the ability to recall recent and distant events.

QUESTIONS RELATED TO AGE

The focused interview must reflect the anatomical and physiological differences that exist along the life span. The following questions are examples of those that would be specific for infants and children, the pregnant female, and the older adult.

FOCUSED INTERVIEW QUESTIONS	RATIONALES

QUESTIONS REGARDING INFANTS AND CHILDREN

1. Describe if you can the pregnancy with this child, including any health problems, medications taken, or alcohol or drugs used.
   - Was the child premature, at term, or late?
   - Describe the birth of the child, including any complications during or shortly after the birth.

▶ Problems during the antepartal period, including the use of medications, alcohol, or drugs, may affect the neurologic health of the child. Similarly, complications during or shortly after birth may have residual effects. For example, research indicates that some cases of epilepsy, a seizure disorder, may be due to prenatal or birth trauma.

2. Has the child ever had a seizure?
   - If so, how often has this happened?
   - Describe what happens when the child has a seizure.
   - Has the child had a high fever when the seizures occurred?

▶ Seizures in feverish infants and toddlers are not uncommon. Seizures without accompanying fever may indicate a seizure disorder such as epilepsy.

3. Have you noticed any clumsiness in the child's activities? For example, does the child frequently drop things, have difficulty manipulating toys, bump into things, have problems walking or climbing stairs, or fall frequently?

▶ These signs may indicate neurologic disease.

4. Are you aware of any surfaces in the home that are painted with lead-based paint?
   - Have you ever seen the child eating paint chips?

▶ Lead poisoning may lead to developmental delays, peripheral nerve damage, or brain damage.

5. How is the child doing in school?
   - Does the child seem to be able to concentrate on homework assignments and complete them on time?
   - Have you ever been told that the child has a learning disability?
   - That the child is hyperactive?
   - Do you agree with this assessment?
   - Why or why not?
   - Have any medications or therapies been prescribed for the hyperactivity?
   - If so, please provide details.

QUESTIONS FOR THE PREGNANT FEMALE

1. Do you have a history of seizures?
   - Have you had any seizures during this pregnancy or previous pregnancies?
   - If so, how often?
   - Please describe the seizures.

2. Are you taking any vitamins or other nutritional supplements?
   - Please describe these.

▶ Prenatal supplements are important to provide for the neurologic health of the growing fetus. For example, vitamin A is required for nerve myelinization, and folic acid has been shown to reduce the incidence of neural tube defects.

QUESTIONS FOR THE OLDER ADULT

1. Do you require more time to perform tasks today than perhaps 2 years ago? Five years ago? Explain.

▶ Endurance decreases with aging; therefore, more time is required for all activities.

2. When you stand up, do you have trouble starting to walk?

▶ Trouble initiating movement may indicate Parkinson's disease, which is more common in older adults.

3. Do you notice any tremors?

▶ Tremors may indicate motor nerve disease, or they may be attributable to certain medications or excessive consumption of caffeine.

4. What safety features have you added to your home?

▶ Safety precautions are essential to prevent neurologic trauma from falls and other accidents.

FOCUSED INTERVIEW QUESTIONS	RATIONALES

QUESTIONS RELATED TO THE ENVIRONMENT

Environment refers to both the internal and external environments. Questions related to the internal environment include all of the previous questions and those associated with internal or physiological responses. Questions related to the external environment include those related to home, work, or social environments.

INTERNAL ENVIRONMENT

1. **Describe your daily diet.**
   - Do you have problems eating or drinking certain products?

▶ The diet provides nutrients and electrolytes responsible for neuromuscular activity and electrical activity in the nervous system.

2. **Are you currently taking any medications?**
   - What are the medications?
   - Do you use prescribed, over-the-counter, herbal, or culturally derived medications?
   - Do you use home remedies?

▶ Medications alone can cause neurologic problems. The interaction of medications, herbs, or other products may alter or affect the absorption or effects of prescribed medications.

EXTERNAL ENVIRONMENT

1. **Are you now or have you ever been exposed to environmental hazards such as insecticides, organic solvents, lead, toxic wastes, or other pollutants?**
   - If so, which one, when, and for what period of time were you exposed?
   - What treatment did you seek?
   - Are you left with any problems because of the exposure?

▶ Such exposure could contribute to neurologic deficits and neoplastic activity in the body.

CLIENT INTERACTION

Mrs. Roberta Andoli, age 59, reports to her primary care provider with the chief complaint of weakness of the right side of her face. Her right eye is tearing and she has noticed some drooling. All of the symptoms have developed within the last 2½ days. A tentative diagnosis of Bell's palsy is made. The following is an excerpt taken from the focused interview.

INTERVIEW

Nurse: Good afternoon, Mrs. Andoli. I would like to talk with you about your reason for coming today.

Mrs. Andoli: My face didn't feel right when I got up today. I can't explain it.

Nurse: Did you notice anything else about your face?

Mrs. Andoli: When I washed my face this morning, I noticed the crease by my nose was gone. When I brushed my teeth the water and toothpaste were dripping out the right side of my mouth. I could not keep the water in on that side.

Nurse: Did you have breakfast this morning?

Mrs. Andoli: Oh yes, I had one cup of tea and cereal with milk, my usual breakfast.

Nurse: Did the tea or cereal milk drip out of your mouth?

Mrs. Andoli: Oh yes, I could have used a bib. I had trouble swallowing and my cereal didn't taste right. I don't know why. My milk was not sour or anything.

Nurse: What other changes have you noticed?

Mrs. Andoli: When I went to put on eye makeup today, I noticed my right eye was funny.

Nurse: I'm not sure I know what funny means.

Mrs. Andoli: My right eye seemed to be opened wider than my left eye this morning. I usually line my eyelids but I didn't this morning. My bottom lid is turned. I don't know what I did. Gee, I'm really a mess.

ANALYSIS

During the interview, the nurse used several strategies to obtain specific subjective data from the client. The nurse built on the first statement made by the client describing feelings of the face. Clarification was sought. Open-ended statements were used to elicit greater information.

Please refer to the Companion Website at **www.prenhall.com/damico** and click on Chapter 24, the **Client Interaction** module, to answer questions about this case. In addition, see other resources for this chapter including NCLEX review questions and other interactive exercises and materials.

ASSESSMENT TECHNIQUES AND FINDINGS

Physical assessment of the neurologic system requires the use of inspection, palpation, auscultation, and special equipment and procedures to test the functions of the system. During each part of the assessment, the nurse is gathering objective data related to the functioning of the client's central and peripheral nervous systems. The examination begins with assessment of the client's mental status and includes cranial nerves, motor and sensory function, balance, and reflexes. Knowledge of normal or expected findings is essential in interpretation of the data.

Adults have erect posture and a smooth gait. Facial expressions correspond to the content and topic of discussion. The speech is clear and vocabulary and word choice are appropriate to age and experience. Adults are well groomed, clean, and attired appropriately for the season and setting. The adult is oriented to person, place, and time and can respond to questions and directions. The adult demonstrates intact short- and long-term memory, is capable of abstract thinking, and can perform calculations. The cranial nerves are intact. Motor function is in-tact, and movements are coordinated and smooth. Sensory function is demonstrated in the ability to identify touch, pain, heat, and cold; to sense vibrations; to identify objects; and to discriminate between place and points of touch on the body. The response to testing of reflexes is 2+ on a scale of 0 to 4+. Carotid arteries are without bruits.

Physical assessment of the neurologic system follows an organized pattern. It begins with assessment of the client's mental status and proceeds to assessment of cranial nerves, motor and sensory function, reflexes, and auscultation of carotid arteries. Assessment proceeds in a cephalocaudal manner. The nurse tests distal to proximal and moves from gross function to fine function, always comparing corresponding body parts. More than one technique can be used to assess one function. For more information about neurologic assessment, link through the Companion Website.

EQUIPMENT

examination gown	applicator
clean, nonsterile examination gloves	hot and cold water in test tubes
percussion hammer	objects to touch such as coins, paper clips, or safety pins
tuning fork	
sterile cotton balls	
penlight	substances to smell, for example, vanilla, mint, and coffee
ophthalmoscope	
stethoscope	
sterile needle	substances to taste such as sugar, salt, lemon, and grape
tongue blade	

HELPFUL HINTS

- Data gathering begins with the initial nurse-client interaction. As nurses meet clients, they make assessments regarding their general appearance, personal hygiene, and ability to walk and sit down. These activities are related to cerebral function.
- Physical assessment of the neurologic system proceeds in a cepahalocaudal and distal to proximal pattern, and includes comparison of corresponding body parts.
- Several assessments may occur at one time. For example, asking the client to smile tests cranial nerve VII, hearing and the functions of the cerebral cortex, indicated by the ability to follow directions and initiate voluntary movements.
- Provide specific information about what is expected of the client. Demonstrate movements.
- Explain and demonstrate the purposes and uses of the equipment.
- Use Standard Precautions.

| TECHNIQUES AND NORMAL FINDINGS | ABNORMAL FINDINGS SPECIAL CONSIDERATIONS |

MENTAL STATUS

The nurse assesses the mental status of the client when meeting the client for the first time. This process begins with taking the health history and continues with each client contact.

▶ A variety of tools are available to conduct mental status assessment. These tools are described in Table 24.2.

Table 24.2	Tools for Assessment of Mental Status	
TOOL	**ASSESSMENT**
Mini-Mental State Examination (MMSE)	Cognitive status—conducted via interview
Addenbrooke's Cognitive Examination	Detects early dementia
Confusion Assessment Method (CAM)	Tests for delirium
Telephone Interview for Cognitive Status (TICS)	Similar to MMSE, cognitive function assessed via telephone interview
Cornell Scale for Depression in Dementia	Assessment of behavioral problems
Dementia Symptoms Scale	Assessment of behavioral problems
Psychogeriatric Dependency Rating Scale	Assessment of behavioral problems
Hopkins Competency Assessment Test	Assessment of ability to make decisions about healthcare
General Health Questionnaire	Assessment of emotional disturbance in those with normal cognitive ability
Hamilton Depression Rating Scale	Assessment of depression in clients with impaired cognition
Short Portable Mental Status Questionnaire (SPMSQ)	Assessment of organic brain deficit

1. **Instruct the client.**
   - Explain to the client that you will be conducting a variety of tests. Tell the client that you will provide instructions before beginning each examination. Explain that moving about and changing position during the examination will be required. Provide reassurance that the tests will not cause discomfort; however, the client must inform you of problems if they arise during any part of the assessment. Identify the types of equipment you will use and describe the purpose in relation to neurologic function. Tell the client that you will begin the assessment with some general questions about the present and past. Then you will ask the client to respond to number and word questions.

2. **Position the client.**
   - The client should be sitting on the examination table wearing an examination gown (see Figure 24.7 ●).

| **TECHNIQUES AND NORMAL FINDINGS** | **ABNORMAL FINDINGS SPECIAL CONSIDERATIONS** |

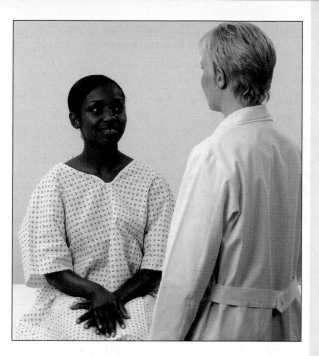

Figure 24.7 •
Positioning the client.

3. **Observe the client.**

   • Look at the client and note hygiene, grooming, posture, body language, facial expressions, speech, and ability to follow directions.

   ▶ Changes could be indicative of depression, schizophrenia, organic brain syndrome, or obsessive-compulsive disorder.

4. **Note the client's speech and language abilities.**

   • Throughout the assessment, note the client's rate of speech, ability to pronounce words, tone of voice, loudness or softness (volume) of voice, and ability to speak smoothly and clearly.

   ▶ Changes in speech could reflect anxiety, Parkinson's disease, depression, or various forms of aphasia.

   • Assess the client's choice of words, ability to respond to questions, and ease with which a response is made.

5. **Assess the client's sensorium.**

   • Determine the client's orientation to date, time, place, and reason for being here. Grade the level of alertness on a scale from full alertness to coma.

   ▶ Neurologic disease can produce a sliding or changing degree of alertness. Change in the level of consciousness may be related to cortical or brain stem disease. A stroke, seizure, or hypoglycemia could also contribute to a change in the level of consciousness.

6. **Assess the client's memory.**

   • Ask for the client's date of birth, Social Security number, names and ages of any children or grandchildren, educational history with dates and events, work history with dates, and job descriptions. Ask questions for which the response can be verified.

   ▶ Loss of long-term memory may indicate cerebral cortex damage, which occurs in Alzheimer's disease.

7. **Assess the client's ability to calculate problems.**

   • Start with a simple problem, such as $4 + 3$, $8 \div 2$, and $15 - 4$.

   ▶ Inability to calculate simple problems may indicate the presence of organic brain disease, or it may simply indicate lack of exposure to mathematical concepts, nervousness, or an incomplete understanding of the examiner's language. In an otherwise unremarkable assessment, a poor response to calculations should not be considered an abnormal finding.

TECHNIQUES AND NORMAL FINDINGS	ABNORMAL FINDINGS SPECIAL CONSIDERATIONS

- Progress to more difficult problems, such as $(10 \times 4) - 8$, or ask the client to start with 100 and subtract 7 ($100 - 7 = 93, 93 - 7 = 86, 86 - 7 = 79$, and so on).
- Remember to use problems that are appropriate for the developmental, educational, and intellectual level of the client.
- Asking the client to calculate change from one dollar for the purchase of items costing 25, 39, and 89 cents is a quick test of calculation.

8. **Assess the client's ability to think abstractly.**

- Ask the client to identify similarities and differences between two objects or topics, such as wood and coal, king and president, orange and apple, and pear and celery. Quote a proverb and ask the client to explain its meaning. For example:
  - "A stitch in time saves nine."
  - "The empty barrel makes the most noise."
  - "Don't put all your eggs in one basket."
- Be aware that age and culture influence the ability to explain American proverbs and slang terms.

▶ Responses made by the client may reflect lack of education, mental retardation, or dementia. Clients with personality disorders such as schizophrenia or depression may make bizarre responses.

9. **Assess the client's mood and emotional state.**

- Observe the client's body language, facial expressions, and communication technique. The facial expression and tone of voice should be congruent with the content and context of the communication.

▶ Lack of congruence of facial expression and tone of voice with the content and context of communication may occur with neurologic problems, emotional disturbance, or a psychogenic disorder such as schizophrenia or depression.

- Ask if the client generally feels this way or if he or she has experienced a change and if so over what period of time.
- Ask the client if it is possible to identify an event or incident that fostered the change in mood or emotional state.
- The client's mood and emotions should reflect the current situation or response to events that trigger mood change or call for an emotional response (e.g., a change in health status, a loss, or a stressful event).

▶ Lack of emotional response, lack of change in facial expression, and flat voice tones can indicate problems with mood or emotional responses. Other abnormal findings in relation to mood and emotional state include anxiety, depression, fear, anger, overconfidence, ambivalence, euphoria, impatience, and irritability. Mood disorders are associated with bipolar disorder, anxiety disorders, and major depression.

10. **Assess perceptions and thought processes.**

- Listen to the client's statements. Statements should be logical and relevant. The client should complete his or her thoughts.

▶ Disturbed thought processes can indicate neurologic dysfunction or mental disorder.

- Determining the client's awareness of reality assesses perception.

▶ Disturbances in sense of reality can include hallucination and illusion. These are associated with mental disturbances as seen in schizophrenia.

11. **Assess the client's ability to make judgments.**

- Determine if the client is able to evaluate situations and to decide upon a realistic course of action. For example, ask the client about future plans related to employment.

| TECHNIQUES AND NORMAL FINDINGS | ABNORMAL FINDINGS SPECIAL CONSIDERATIONS |

TECHNIQUES AND NORMAL FINDINGS

- The plans should reflect the reality of the client's health, psychological stability, and family situation and obligations. The client's responses should reflect an ability to think abstractly.

CRANIAL NERVES

1. **Instruct the client.**
   - Tell the client you will be testing special nerves and the senses of smell, vision, taste, and hearing. Explain that several of the tests will require the client to close both eyes. You will be asking the client to make changes in facial expression. Occasionally, you will touch the client with your hands while using different types of equipment during each test.

2. **Test the olfactory nerve (cranial nerve I).**
   - If you suspect the client's nares are obstructed with mucus, ask the client to blow the nose.
   - Ask the client to close both eyes and to close one naris. Place a familiar odor under the open naris (see Figure 24.8 ●).

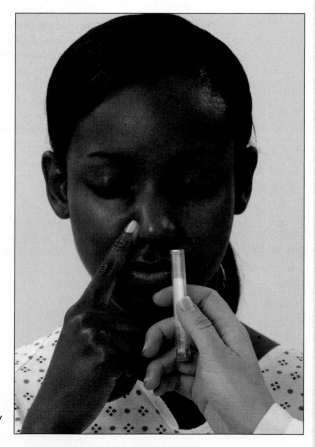

Figure 24.8 ● Olfactory nerve assessment.

   - Ask the client to sniff and identify the odor. Use coffee, vanilla, perfume, cloves, and so on. Repeat with the other naris.

ABNORMAL FINDINGS / SPECIAL CONSIDERATIONS

► Impaired judgment can occur in emotional disturbances, schizophrenia, and neurologic dysfunction.

► **Anosmia,** the absence of the sense of smell, may be due to cranial nerve dysfunction, colds, rhinitis, or zinc deficiency, or it may be genetic. A unilateral change in this sense may be indicative of a brain tumor.

TECHNIQUES AND NORMAL FINDINGS

3. **Test the optic nerve (cranial nerve II).**
   - Test near vision by asking the client to read from a magazine, newspaper, or prepared card. Observe closeness or distance of page to face. Also note the position of the head.
   - Use the Snellen chart to test distant vision and color (see Figure 13.7 on page 277 ⚭).
   - Use the ophthalmoscope to inspect the fundus of the eye. Locate the optic disc and describe the color and shape.
   - See Chapter 13 for a detailed description of the technique for all of these activities. ⚭

▶ Pathologic conditions of the optic nerve include retrobulbar neuritis, papilledema, and optic atrophy. **Retrobulbar neuritis** is an inflammatory process of the optic nerve behind the eyeball. Multiple sclerosis is the most common cause.

▶ **Papilledema** (or *choked disc*) is a swelling of the optic nerve as it enters the retina. A symptom of increased intracranial pressure, papilledema can be indicative of brain tumors or intracranial hemorrhage.

▶ Immediate medical attention is required if intracranial hemorrhage is suspected.

▶ **Optic atrophy** produces a change in the color of the optic disc and decreased visual acuity. It can be a symptom of multiple sclerosis or brain tumor.

4. **Test the oculomotor, trochlear, and abducens nerves (cranial nerves III, IV, and VI).**
   - Test the six cardinal points of gaze.

▶ Pathologic conditions include nystagmus, strabismus, diplopia, or ptosis of the upper lid. **Nystagmus** is the constant involuntary movement of the eyeball. A lack of muscular coordination, *strabismus,* causes deviation of one or both eyes. **Diplopia** is double vision. A dropped lid, or *ptosis* of the lid, is usually related to weakness of the muscles.

   - Test direct and consensual pupillary reaction to light (cranial nerve III).
   - Test convergence and accommodation of the eyes.
   - These three tests are described in detail in Chapter 13. ⚭

5. **Explain the procedure.**
   - Show the client the cotton wisp. Touch the arm with the wisp and explain that the wisp will feel like that when a body part is touched. Ask the client to close both eyes.
   - Touch the arm with the wisp. Ask the client to say "now" when the wisp is felt. Explain that further tests with the wisp will be carried out with the eyes closed, and "now" is to be stated when the wisp is felt.
   - Show the client the opened sterile safety pin. Explain while you touch the arm with the rounded end that the sensation is dull and with the point the sensation is sharp.
   - Tell the client that both eyes must be closed during several tests with the pin.
   - The client is expected to identify each touch or sensation as sharp or dull.
   - Discard the safety pin at the completion of the examination.

6. **Test the trigeminal nerve (cranial nerve V).**
   - Test the sensory function.
   - Ask the client to close both eyes.
   - Touch the face with a wisp of cotton (see Figure 24.9 ●).

| **TECHNIQUES AND NORMAL FINDINGS** | **ABNORMAL FINDINGS SPECIAL CONSIDERATIONS** |

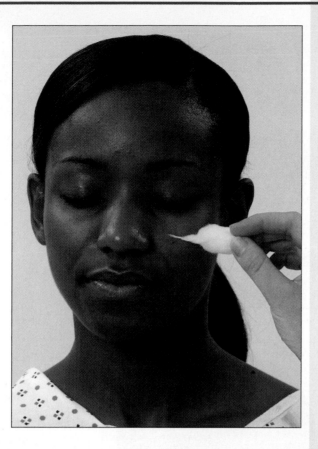

Figure 24.9 ● Testing sensory function of the trigeminal nerve.

- Direct the client to say "now" every time the cotton is felt. Repeat the test using sharp and dull stimuli.

- Be random with the stimulation. Do *not* establish a pattern when testing. Be sure all three branches of the nerve are assessed.

- Test the corneal reflex.
  - Ask the client to look straight ahead.
  - Use a wisp of cotton to touch the cornea from the side.
  - Anticipate a blink.
  - Details for this procedure are presented in Chapter 13. ⟳

- Test the motor function of the nerve. Ask the client to clench the teeth tightly. Bilaterally palpate the masseter and temporalis muscles, noting muscle strength (see Figure 24.10 ●).

- Ask the client to open and close the mouth several times. Observe for symmetry of movement of the mandible without deviation from midline.

▶ Document any loss of sensation, pain, or noted fasciculations (fine rapid muscle movements).

▶ Clients who use contact lenses need to remove them before testing. Most likely these clients will have a decreased or absent reflex because the corneal reflex has diminished in response to long-term contact lens use.

▶ Muscle pain, spasms, and deviation of the mandible with movement can indicate myofascial pain dysfunction.

TECHNIQUES AND NORMAL FINDINGS	ABNORMAL FINDINGS SPECIAL CONSIDERATIONS

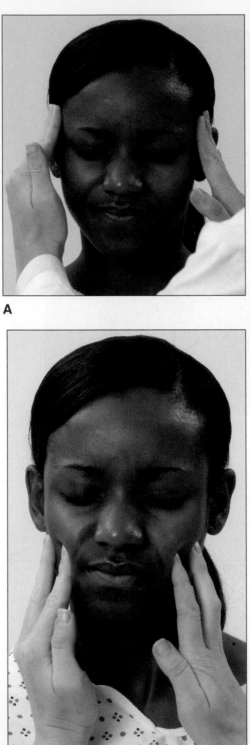

Figure 24.10 • Testing muscle strength. A. Temporalis muscles. B. Masseter muscles.

7. **Test the facial nerve (cranial nerve VII).**

- Test the motor activity of the nerve.
- Ask the client to perform several functions such as the following: smile, show your teeth, close both eyes, puff your cheeks, frown, and raise your eyebrows (see Figure 24.11 •).

▶ Asymmetry or muscle weakness may indicate nerve damage. Muscle weakness includes drooping of the eyelid and changes in the nasolabial folds.

| **TECHNIQUES AND NORMAL FINDINGS** | **ABNORMAL FINDINGS SPECIAL CONSIDERATIONS** |

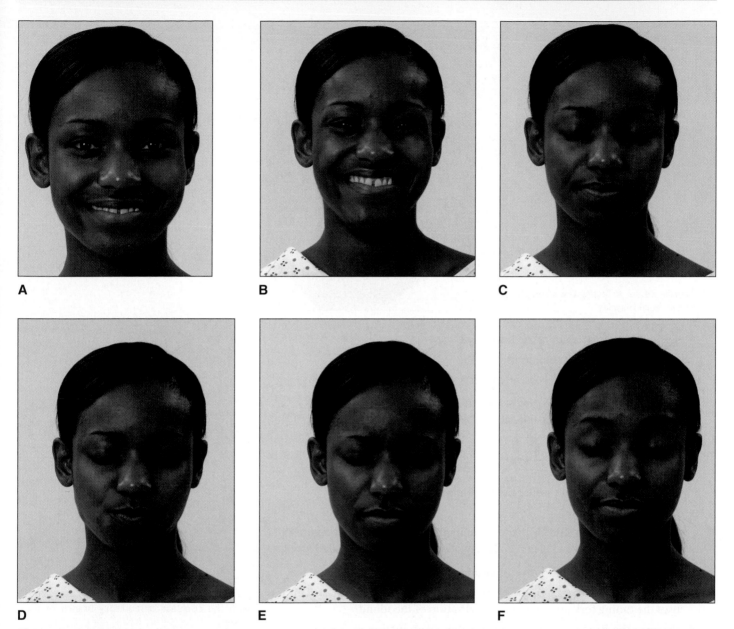

Figure 24.11 ● Testing motor function of cranial nerve VII. A. Smile. B. Show teeth. C. Close both eyes. D. Puff cheeks. E. Frown. F. Raise eyebrows.

- Look for symmetry of facial movements.
- Test the muscle strength of the upper face.
- Ask the client to close both eyes tightly and keep them closed.
- Try to open the eyes by retracting the upper and lower lids simultaneously and bilaterally (see Figure 24.12 ●).

▶ Inability to perform motor tasks could be the results of a lower or upper motor neuron disease.

TECHNIQUES AND NORMAL FINDINGS

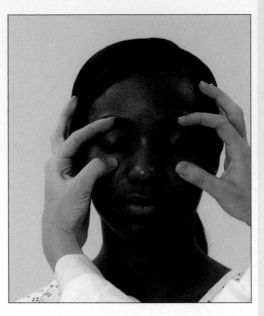

Figure 24.12 • Testing the strength of the facial muscles.

- Test the muscle strength of the lower face.
  - Ask the client to puff the cheeks.
  - Apply pressure to the cheeks, attempting to force the air out of the lips.
- Test the sense of taste.
  - Moisten three applicators and dab one in each of the samples of sugar, salt, and lemon.
  - Touch the client's tongue with one applicator at a time and ask the client to identify the taste.
  - Water may be needed to rinse the mouth between tests.
- Test the corneal reflex.
  - This may have been tested with the trigeminal nerve assessment (see Figure 13.14 on page 282 ⊂⊃). Cranial nerve VII regulates the motor response of this reflex.

8. Test the vestibulocochlear nerve (cranial nerve VIII).

- Test the auditory branch of the nerve by performing the Weber test. This test uses the tuning fork and provides lateralization of the sound.

▶ Tinnitus and deafness are deficits associated with the cochlear or auditory branch of the nerve.

- Perform the Rinne test. This compares bone conduction of sound with air conduction. Both the Weber and Rinne tests are described in detail in Chapter 14. ⊂⊃
- The caloric test, or ice water test as it is sometimes called, tests the vestibular portion of the nerve.
  - This test is usually conducted only when the client is experiencing dizziness or vertigo. (Consult a neurology text for description of this technique.)

▶ Vertigo is associated with the vestibular portion.

- Romberg's test assesses coordination and equilibrium. It is discussed later in this chapter.

9. Test the glossopharyngeal and vagus nerves (cranial nerves IX and X).

- Test motor activity.
  - Ask the client to open the mouth.
  - Depress the client's tongue with the tongue blade.
  - Ask the client to say "ah."

TECHNIQUES AND NORMAL FINDINGS	ABNORMAL FINDINGS SPECIAL CONSIDERATIONS

- Observe the movement of the soft palate and uvula (see Figure 24.13 ●).
- Normally, the soft palate rises and the uvula remains in the midline. *accessory*

▶ Unilateral palate and uvula movement indicate disease of the nerve on the opposite side.

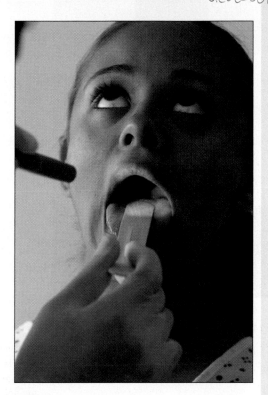

Figure 24.13 ● Testing cranial nerves IX and X.

- Test the gag reflex. This tests the sensory aspect of cranial nerve IX and the motor activity of cranial nerve X.
- Inform the client that you are going to place an applicator in the mouth and lightly touch the throat.
- Touch the posterior wall of the pharynx with the applicator.
- Observe pharyngeal movement.
- Test the motor activity of the pharynx.
  - Ask the client to drink a small amount of water and note the ease or difficulty of swallowing.
  - Note the quality of the voice or hoarseness when speaking.

▶ Clients with a diminished or absent gag reflex have an increased potential for aspiration and need medical evaluation.

▶ **Dysphagia,** difficulty with swallowing, could be related to cranial nerve disease.

▶ Vocal changes could be indicative of lesions, paralysis, or other conditions.

10. Test the accessory nerve (cranial nerve XI).
- Test the trapezius muscle.
- Ask the client to shrug the shoulders.
- Observe the equality of the shoulders, symmetry of action, and lack of fasciculations (see Figure 24.14 ●).

TECHNIQUES AND NORMAL FINDINGS

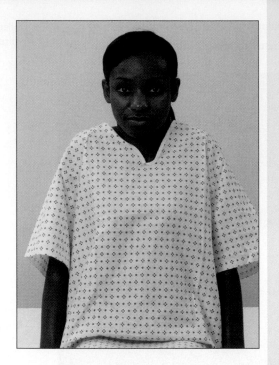

Figure 24.14 • Trapezius muscle movement.

• Test the sternocleidomastoid muscle. neck ROM
  • Ask the client to turn the head to the right and then to the left.
  • Ask the client to try to touch the right ear to the right shoulder without raising the shoulder (see Figure 24.15 •).

▶ Abnormal findings include muscle weakness, muscle atrophy, fasciculations, uneven shoulders, and the inability to raise the chin following flexion.

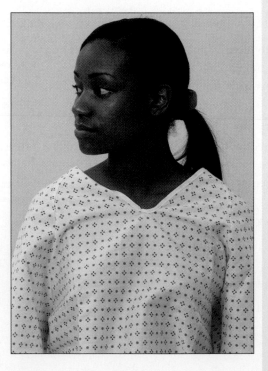

Figure 24.15 •
Sternocleidomastoid muscle movement.

  • Repeat with the left shoulder.
  • Observe ease of movement and degree of range of motion.

| TECHNIQUES AND NORMAL FINDINGS | ABNORMAL FINDINGS SPECIAL CONSIDERATIONS |

- Test trapezius muscle strength.
  - Have the client shrug the shoulders while you resist with your hands (see Figure 24.16 ●).

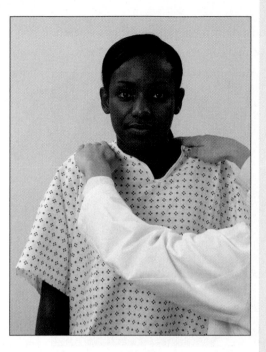

Figure 24.16 ● Testing the strength of the trapezius muscle against resistance.

- Test sternocleidomastoid muscle strength.
  - Ask the client to turn the head to the left to meet your hand.
  - Attempt to return the client's head to midline position (see Figure 24.17 ●).
  - Repeat the preceding steps with the client turning to the right side.

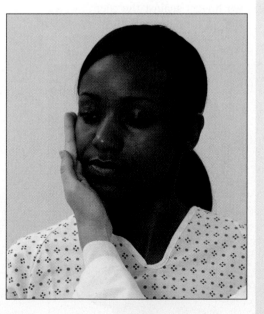

Figure 24.17 ● Testing the strength of the sternocleidomastoid muscle against resistance.

TECHNIQUES AND NORMAL FINDINGS	ABNORMAL FINDINGS SPECIAL CONSIDERATIONS

11. Test the hypoglossal nerve (cranial nerve XII).

- Test the movement of the tongue.
  - Ask the client to protrude the tongue.
  - Ask the client to retract the tongue.
  - Ask the client to protrude the tongue and move it to the right and then to the left.
  - Note ease of movement and equality of movement (see Figure 24.18 ●).

▶ Note atrophy, tremors, and paralysis. An ipsilateral paralysis will demonstrate deviation and atrophy of the involved side.

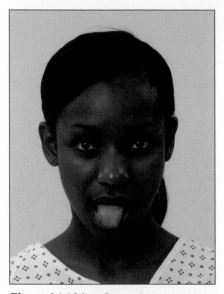

Figure 24.18A ● Protruding movement of tongue.

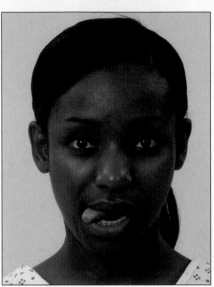

Figure 24.18B ● Lateralization of tongue.

- Test the strength of the tongue.
  - Ask the client to push against the inside of the cheek with the tip of the tongue.
  - Provide resistance by pressing one or two fingers against the client's outer cheek (see Figure 24.19 ●).
  - Repeat on the other side.

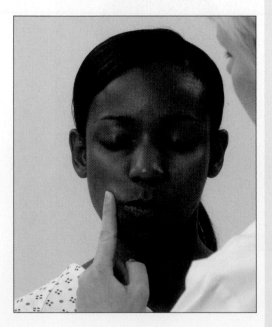

Figure 24.19 ● Testing the strength of the tongue.

| **TECHNIQUES AND NORMAL FINDINGS** | **ABNORMAL FINDINGS SPECIAL CONSIDERATIONS** |

MOTOR FUNCTION

Motor function requires the integrated efforts of the musculoskeletal and the neurologic systems. Assessment of the musculoskeletal system is discussed in detail in Chapter 23. ◯◯ The neurologic aspect of motor function is directly related to activities of the cerebellum, which is responsible for coordination and smoothness of movement, and equilibrium. All of the following tests focus on activities of the cerebellum.

ALERT!

Be ready to support and protect the client to prevent an accident, injury, or fall.

1. **Assess the client's gait and balance.**
   - Ask the client to walk across the room and return (see Figure 24.20 ●).

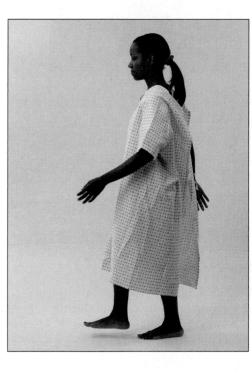

Figure 24.20 ● Evaluation of gait.

   - Ask the client to walk heel to toe (or tandem), by placing the heel of the left foot in front of the toes of the right foot, then the heel of the right foot in front of the toes of the left foot. Be sure the client is looking straight ahead and not at the floor. Continue this pattern for several yards (see Figure 24.21 ●).

▶ A change in gait could be indicative of drug or alcohol intoxication, motor neuron weakness, or muscle weakness.

TECHNIQUES AND NORMAL FINDINGS	ABNORMAL FINDINGS SPECIAL CONSIDERATIONS

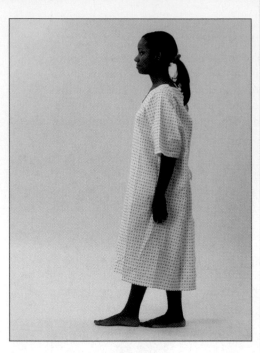

Figure 24.21 ● Heel-to-toe walk.

- Ask the client to walk on his or her toes.
- Ask the client to walk on the heels. Observe the client's posture. Does the posture demonstrate stiffness or relaxation? Note the equality of steps taken, the pace of walking, the position and coordination of arms when walking, and the ability to maintain balance during all of these activities.

2. **Perform Romberg's test.**
   - **Romberg's test** assesses coordination and equilibrium (cranial nerve VIII).
   - Ask the client to stand with feet together and arms at the sides. The client's eyes are open.
   - Stand next to the client to prevent falls. Observe for swaying.
   - Ask the client to close both eyes without changing position.
   - Observe for swaying with the eyes closed. Swaying normally increases slightly when the eyes are closed (see Figure 24.22 ●).

▶ If swaying greatly increases or the client falls, suspect disease of the posterior columns of the spinal cord.

| **TECHNIQUES AND NORMAL FINDINGS** | **ABNORMAL FINDINGS SPECIAL CONSIDERATIONS** |

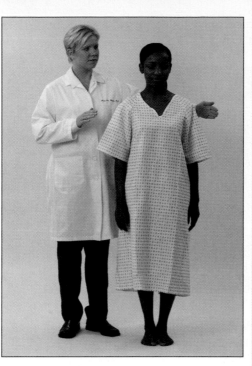

Figure 24.22 ● Romberg's test for balance.

3. **Perform the finger-to-nose test.**

   ● The finger-to-nose test also assesses coordination and equilibrium. It is sometimes called the pass-point test.

   ● Ask the client to resume a sitting position.

   ● Ask the client to extend both arms from the sides of the body.

   ● Ask the client to keep both eyes open.

   ● Ask the client to touch the tip of the nose with the right index finger, and then return the right arm to an extended position.

   ● Ask the client to touch the tip of the nose with the left index finger, and then return the left arm to an extended position.

   ● Repeat the procedure several times.

   ● Ask the client to close both eyes and repeat the alternating movements (see Figure 24.23 ●).

   ● Observe the movement of the arms, the smoothness of the movement, and the point of contact of finger. Does the finger touch the nose, or is another part of the face touched?

▶ With the eyes closed, the client with cerebellar disease will reach beyond the tip of the nose, because the sense of position is affected.

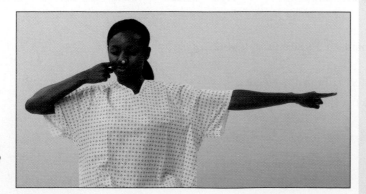

Figure 24.23 ●
Finger-to-nose
test.

TECHNIQUES AND NORMAL FINDINGS

- An alternative technique is to have the client touch the nose with the index finger and then the finger of the nurse (see Figure 24.24 ●).

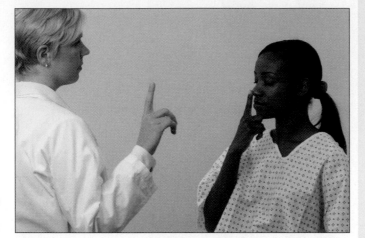

Figure 24.24 ●
Alternative for
pass-point test

4. **Assess the client's ability to perform a rapid alternating action.**

- Ask the client to sit with the hands placed palms down on the thighs (see Figure 24.25A ●).
- Ask the client to turn the hands palms up (see Figure 24.25B ●).
- Ask the client to return the hands to a palms-down position.

▶ Inability to perform this task could indicate upper motor neuron weakness.

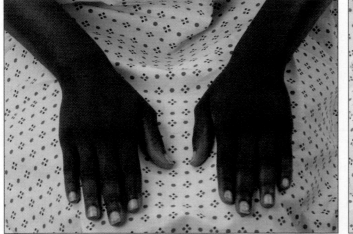

Figure 24.25A ● Testing rapid alternating movement, palms down.

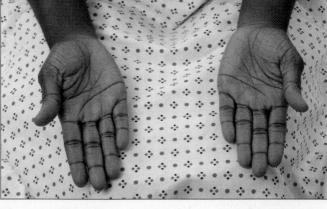

Figure 24.25B ● Testing rapid alternating movement, palms up.

- Ask the client to alternate the movements at a faster pace. If you suspect any deficit, test one side at a time.
- Observe the rhythm, rate, and smoothness of the movements.
- Figure 24.26 ● demonstrates the finger-to-finger test, which is an alternative method to assess coordination.
- Ask the client to touch the thumb to each finger in sequence with increasing pace.

| **TECHNIQUES AND NORMAL FINDINGS** | **ABNORMAL FINDINGS**
SPECIAL CONSIDERATIONS |

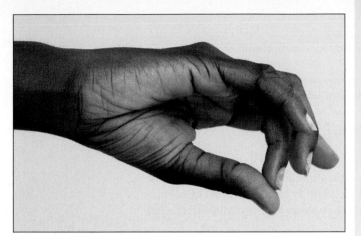

Figure 24.26 ●
Testing co-
ordination using
the finger-to-
finger test.

5. Ask the client to perform the heel-to-shin test.

- Assist the client to a supine position.
- Ask the client to place the heel of the right foot below the left knee.
- Ask the client to slide the right heel along the shin bone to the ankle (see Figure 24.27 ●).

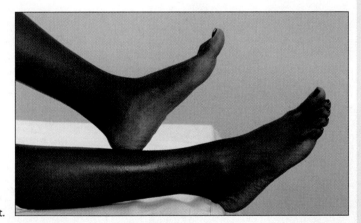

Figure 24.27 ●
Heel-to-shin test.

- Ask the client to repeat the procedure, reversing the legs.
- Observe the smoothness of the action. The client should be able to move the heel in a straight line so that it does not fall off the lower leg.

▶ Inability to perform this test could indicate disease of the posterior spinal tract.

SENSORY FUNCTION

This part of the physical assessment evaluates the client's response to a variety of stimuli. This assessment tests the peripheral nerves, the sensory tracts, and the cortical level of discrimination. A variety of stimuli are used, including light touch, hot/cold, sharp/dull, and vibration. Stereognosis, graphesthesia, and two-point discrimination are also assessed. Each of these assessments is described in the following sections.

TECHNIQUES AND NORMAL FINDINGS	ABNORMAL FINDINGS SPECIAL CONSIDERATIONS

ALERT!

The client may tire during these procedures. If this happens, stop the assessment and continue at a later time. Be sure to test corresponding body parts. Take a distal-to-proximal approach along the extremities. When the client describes sensations accurately at a distal point, it is usually not necessary to proceed to a more proximal point. If a deficit is detected at a distal point, then it becomes imperative to proceed to proximal points while attempting to map that specific area of the deficit. Repeat testing to determine accuracy in areas of deficits.

Remember, always ask the client to describe the stimulus and the location. Do not suggest the type of stimulus or location. Tell the client to keep both eyes closed during testing. To promote full client understanding, you may have to demonstrate what you will do.

1. **Assess the client's ability to identify light touch.**
   - Using a wisp of cotton, touch various parts of the body, including feet, hands, arms, legs, abdomen, and face (see Figure 24.28 ●).

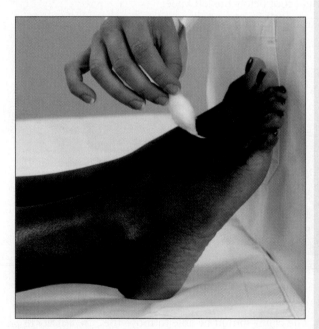

Figure 24.28 ●
Evaluation of light touch.

   - Touch at random locations and use random time intervals.
   - Ask the client to say "yes" or "now" when the stimulus is perceived. Be sure to test corresponding dermatomes.

2. **Assess the client's ability to distinguish the difference between sharp and dull.**
   - Ask the client to say "sharp" or "dull" when something sharp or dull is felt on the skin.
   - Touch the client with the tip of a sterile safety pin (see Figure 24.29A ●).
   - Now touch the client with the blunt end of the pin (see Figure 24.29B ●).

▶ **Anesthesia** is the inability to perceive the sense of touch. **Hyperesthesia** is an increased sensation, whereas *hypoesthesia* is a decreased but not absent sensation.

▶ The absence of pain sensation is called **analgesia.** Decreased pain sensation is called **hypalgesia.** These conditions may result from neurologic disease or circulatory problems such as peripheral vascular disease.

| **TECHNIQUES AND NORMAL FINDINGS** | **ABNORMAL FINDINGS**
SPECIAL CONSIDERATIONS |

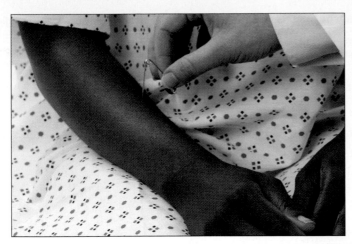

Figure 24.29A ● Testing client's ability to identify sharp sensations.

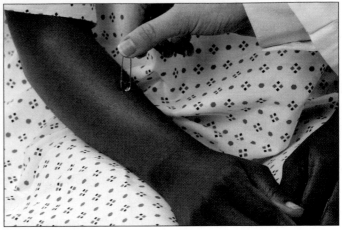

Figure 24.29B ● Testing client's ability to identify dull sensations.

- Alternate between sharp and dull stimulation.
- Touch the client using random locations, random time intervals, and alternating patterns.
- Be sure to test corresponding body parts.
- Discard the pin.

3. **Assess the client's ability to distinguish temperature.**

- Perform this test only if the client demonstrates an absence or decrease in pain sensation.
- Randomly touch the client with test tubes containing warm and cold water.
- Ask the client to describe the temperature.
- Be sure to test corresponding body parts.

4. **Assess the client's ability to feel vibrations.**

- Set a tuning fork in motion and place it on bony parts of the body, such as the toes, ankle, knee, iliac crest, spinal process, fingers, sternum, wrists, or elbows (see Figure 24.30 ●).

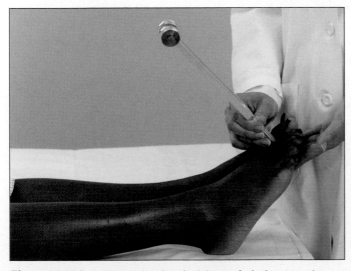

Figure 24.30A ● Testing the client's ability to feel vibrations, the toe.

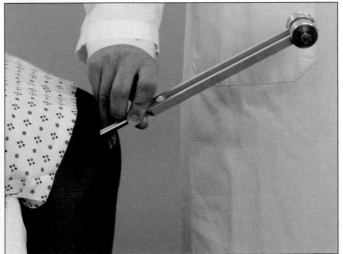

Figure 24.30B ● Testing the client's ability to feel vibrations, the knee.

TECHNIQUES AND NORMAL FINDINGS

- Ask the client to say "now" when the vibration is perceived and "stop" when it is no longer felt.
- If the client's perception is accurate when you test the most distal aspects (toes, ankles, fingers, and wrist), end the test at this time.
- Proceed to proximal points if distal perception is diminished.

5. **Test stereognosis, the ability to identify an object without seeing it.**
   - Direct the client to close both eyes. Place a safety pin in the client's right hand and ask the client to identify it.
   - Place a different object in the left hand and ask the client to identify it.
   - Place a coin in the right hand and ask the client to identify it (see Figure 24.31 ●).

▶ The inability to perceive vibration may indicate neuropathy. This may be associated with aging, diabetes, intoxication, or posterior column disease.

▶ Inability to identify a familiar object could indicate cortical disease.

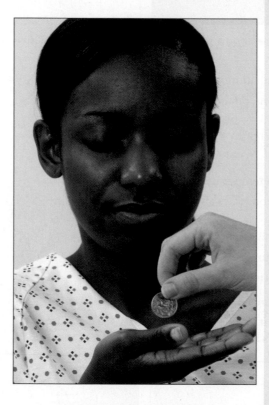

Figure 24.31 ● Testing stereognosis using a coin.

- Place a different coin in the left hand and ask the client to identify it.
- The objects you use must be familiar and safe to hold (no sharp objects).
- Test each object independently.

6. **Test graphesthesia, the ability to perceive writing on the skin.**
   - Direct the client to keep both eyes closed.
   - Using the noncotton end of an applicator or the base of a pen, scribe a number such as 3 into the palm of the client's right hand (see Figure 24.32 ●).

TECHNIQUES AND NORMAL FINDINGS	**ABNORMAL FINDINGS SPECIAL CONSIDERATIONS**

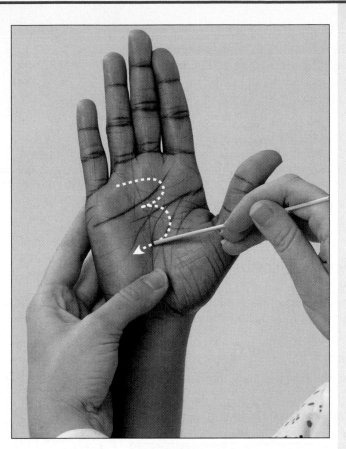

Figure 24.32 ●
Testing
graphesthesia.

- Be sure the number faces the client.
- Ask the client to identify the number.
- Repeat in the left hand using a different number such as 5 or 2.
- Ask the client to identify the number.

7. **Assess the client's ability to discriminate between two points.**

- Simultaneously touch the client with two stimuli over a given area (see Figure 24.33 ●).

▶ Inability to perceive a number on the skin may indicate cortical disease.

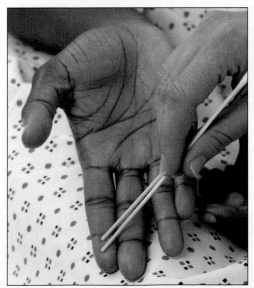

Figure 24.33 ● Two-point
discrimination.

TECHNIQUES AND NORMAL FINDINGS

- Use the unpadded end of two applicators.
- Vary the distance between the two points according to the body region being stimulated. The more distal the location, the more sensitive the discrimination.
- Normally, the client is able to perceive two discrete points at the following distances and locations:

Fingertips	0.3 to 0.6 cm
Hands and feet	1.5 to 2 cm
Lower leg	4 cm

- Ask the client to say "now" when the two discrete points of stimulus are first perceived.

▶ An inability to perceive two separate points within normal distances may indicate cortical disease.

- Note the smallest distance between the points at which the client can perceive two distinct stimuli.
- Discard the applicators.

8. **Assess topognosis, the ability of the client to identify an area of the body that has been touched.**
    - This need not be a separate test. Include it in any of the previous steps by asking the client to identify what part of the body was involved. Also ask the client to point to the area you touched.

▶ Inability of the client to identify a touched area demonstrates sensory or cortical disease.

9. **Assess position sense of joint movement.**
    - Ask the client to close both eyes. Grasp the great toe. Move the joint into dorsiflexion, plantar flexion, and abduction.
    - Ask the client to identify the movement (see Figure 24.34 ●).

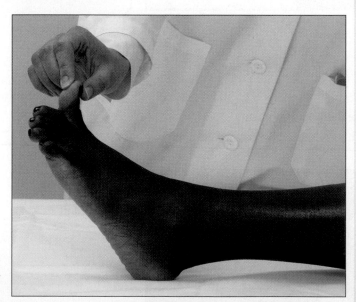

Figure 24.34 ●
Position sense of joint movement.

REFLEXES

Reflex testing is usually the last part of the neurologic assessment. The client is usually in a sitting position; however, you can use a supine position if the client's physical condition so requires. Position the client's limbs properly to stretch the muscle partially.

Proper use of the reflex hammer requires practice. Hold the handle of the reflex hammer in your dominant hand between your thumb and index finger. Use your

TECHNIQUES AND NORMAL FINDINGS	ABNORMAL FINDINGS SPECIAL CONSIDERATIONS

wrist, not your hand or arm, to generate the striking motion. Proper wrist action will provide a brisk, direct, smooth arc for stimulation with the flat or pointed end of the hammer. Stimulate the reflex arc with a brisk tap to the tendon, not the muscle. Through continued practice and experience, you will learn the amount of force to use. Strong force will cause pain, and too little force will not stimulate the arc. After striking the tendon, remove the reflex hammer immediately.

Evaluate the response on a scale from 0 to 4+:

0	no response
1+	diminished
2+	normal
3+	brisk, above normal
4+	hyperactive

Before concluding that a reflex is absent or diminished, repeat the test. Encourage the client to relax. It may be necessary to distract the client to achieve relaxation of the muscle before striking the tendon. Distraction techniques include but are not limited to clenching the teeth, counting ceiling blocks, or humming.

1. **Assess the biceps reflex (C_5, C_6).**

   - Support the client's lower arm with your nondominant hand and arm. The arm needs to be slightly flexed at the elbow with palm up.

   - Place the thumb of your nondominant hand over the biceps tendon.

   - Using the pointed side of a reflex hammer, briskly tap your thumb (see Figure 24.35 ●).

   - Look for contraction of the biceps muscle and slight flexion of the forearm.

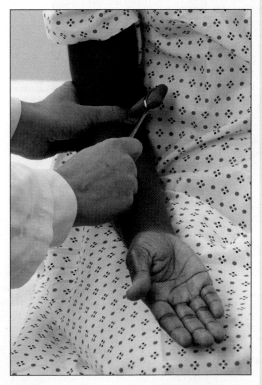

Figure 24.35 ● Testing the biceps reflex.

2. **Assess the triceps reflex (C_6, C_7).**

   - Support the client's elbow with your nondominant hand.

   - Sharply percuss the tendon just above the olecranon process with the flat end of the reflex hammer (see Figure 24.36 ●).

▶ Neuromuscular disease, spinal cord injury, or lower motor neuron disease may cause absent or diminished (hypoactive) reflexes. Hyperactive reflexes may indicate upper motor neuron disease. **Clonus,** rhythmically alternating flexion and extension, confirms upper motor neuron disease.

TECHNIQUES AND NORMAL FINDINGS	ABNORMAL FINDINGS SPECIAL CONSIDERATIONS

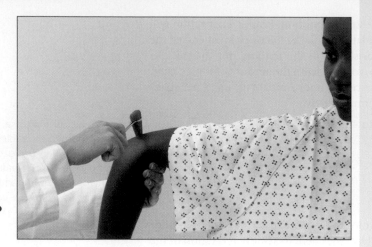

Figure 24.36 ●
Testing the
triceps reflex.

- Observe contraction of the triceps muscle with extension of the lower arm.

3. **Assess the brachioradialis reflex (C₅, C₆).**
   - Position the client's arm so the elbow is flexed and the hand is resting on the client's lap with the palm down (pronation).
   - Using the flat end of the reflex hammer, briskly strike the tendon toward the radius about 2 or 3 inches above the wrist (see Figure 24.37 ●).
   - Observe flexion of the lower arm and supination of the hand.

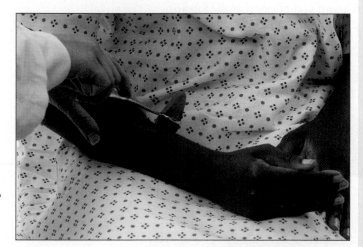

Figure 24.37 ●
Testing the
brachioradialis
reflex.

4. **Assess the patellar (knee) reflex (L₂, L₃, L₄).**
   - Palpate the patella to locate the patellar tendon inferior to the patella.
   - Briskly strike the tendon with the flat end of the reflex hammer (see Figure 24.38 ●).
   - Note extension of lower leg and contraction of the quadriceps muscle.

▶ Flex the leg at the knee. Occasionally, the response is not obtained. Distraction such as that depicted in Figure 24.39 ● may be required.

TECHNIQUES AND NORMAL FINDINGS	ABNORMAL FINDINGS SPECIAL CONSIDERATIONS

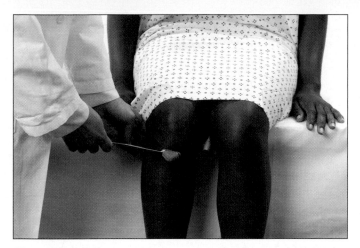

Figure 24.38A • Testing patellar reflex, client in a sitting position.

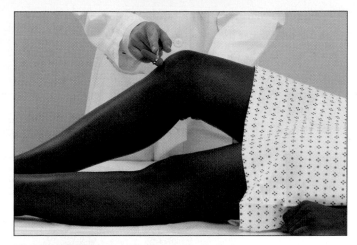

Figure 24.38B • Testing patellar reflex, client in a supine position.

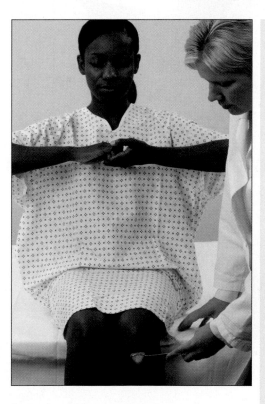

Figure 24.39 • Testing patellar reflex with distraction.

TECHNIQUES AND NORMAL FINDINGS	ABNORMAL FINDINGS SPECIAL CONSIDERATIONS

5. **Assess the Achilles tendon (ankle) reflex (S$_1$).**

- Flex the leg at the knee.
- Dorsiflex the foot of the leg being examined.
- Hold the foot lightly in the nondominant hand.
- Strike the Achilles tendon with the flat end of the reflex hammer (see Figure 24.40 ●).
- Observe plantar flexion of the foot; the heel will "jump" from your hand.

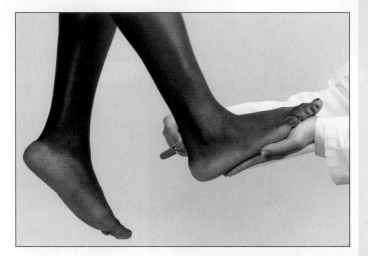

Figure 24.40A ●
Testing the Achilles tendon reflex with client in a sitting position.

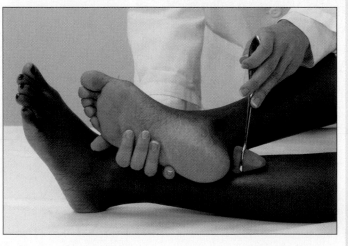

Figure 24.40B ●
Testing the Achilles tendon reflex with client in a supine position.

6. **Assess the plantar reflex (L$_5$, S$_1$).**

- Position the leg with a slight degree of external rotation at the hip.
- Stimulate the sole of the foot from the heel to the ball of the foot on the lateral aspect. Continue the stimulation across the ball of the foot to the big toe.

TECHNIQUES AND NORMAL FINDINGS	ABNORMAL FINDINGS SPECIAL CONSIDERATIONS

- Observe for plantar flexion, in which the toes curl toward the sole of the foot (see Figure 24.41 •). It may be necessary to hold the client's ankle to prevent movement.

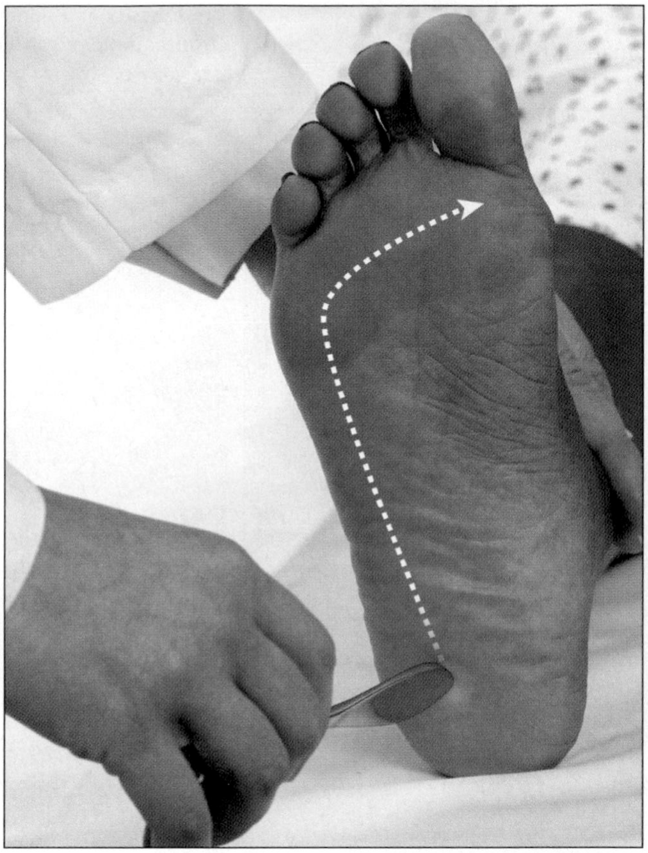

▶ A **Babinski response** is the fanning of the toes with the great toe pointing toward the dorsum of the foot (see Figure 24.42 •). This is called dorsiflexion of the toe and is considered an abnormal response in the adult. It may indicate upper motor neuron disease.

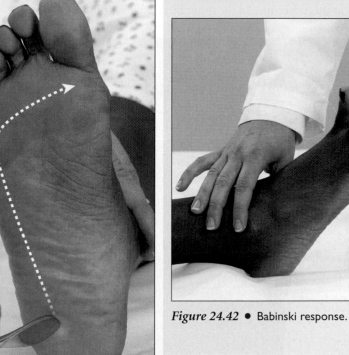

Figure 24.42 • Babinski response.

Figure 24.41 •
Testing the plantar reflex.

▶ A positive Babinski response is considered a normal response in the child until about 2 years of age.

TECHNIQUES AND NORMAL FINDINGS	ABNORMAL FINDINGS SPECIAL CONSIDERATIONS

7. **Assess the abdominal reflexes (T_8, T_9, T_{10} for upper and T_{10}, T_{11}, T_{12} for lower).**

- Using an applicator or tongue blade, briskly stroke the abdomen from the lateral aspect toward the umbilicus (see Figure 24.43 ●).
- Observe muscular contraction and movement of the umbilicus toward the stimulus.
- Repeat this procedure in the other three quadrants of the abdomen.

▶ Obesity and upper and lower motor neuron pathology can decrease or diminish the response.

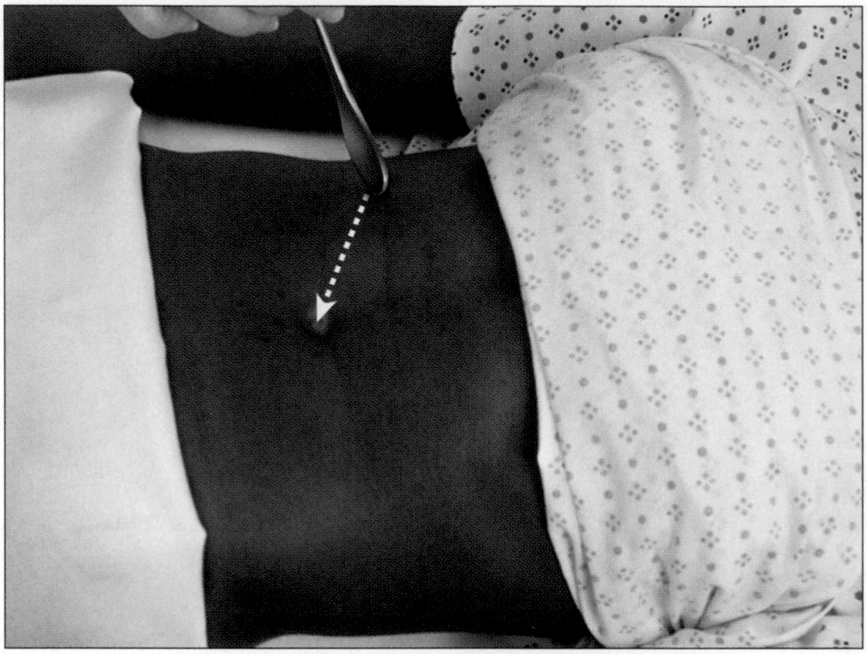

Figure 24.43 ● Abdominal reflex testing pattern.

ADDITIONAL ASSESSMENT TECHNIQUES

CAROTID AUSCULTATION

Auscultation of the carotid arteries may be performed with the assessment of the head and neck or as part of the peripheral vascular assessment. You may need to review your assessment notes for findings of carotid artery auscultation. (Refer to Chapter 17 on page 461 for a detailed discussion of this content ⬭.)

▶ A bruit may be indicative of an obstructive disease process such as atherosclerosis. The amount of blood flow to the brain may be diminished. This decrease in oxygen could be responsible for subtle changes in client responses.

MENINGEAL ASSESSMENT

Ask the client to flex the neck by bringing the chin down to touch the chest. Observe the degree of range of motion and the absence or presence of pain. The client should be able to flex the neck about 45 degrees without pain.

▶ When the meningeal membranes are irritated or inflamed, as in meningitis, the client will experience **nuchal rigidity** or stiffness of the neck.

TECHNIQUES AND NORMAL FINDINGS	ABNORMAL FINDINGS SPECIAL CONSIDERATIONS

When the client complains of pain and has a decrease in the flexion motion, you will observe for *Brudzinski's sign*. With the client in a supine position, assist the client with neck flexion. Observe the legs. Brudzinski's sign is positive when neck flexion causes flexion of the legs and thighs.

USE OF THE GLASGOW COMA SCALE

The *Glasgow Coma Scale* assesses the level of consciousness of the individual on a continuum from alertness to coma (see Figure 24.44 ●). The scale tests three body functions: verbal response, motor response, and eye response. A maximum total score of 15 indicates the person is alert, responsive, and oriented. A total score of 3, the lowest achievable score, indicates a nonresponsive comatose individual.

GLASGOW COMA SCALE
BEST EYE-OPENING RESPONSE
4 = Spontaneously
3 = To speech
2 = To pain
1 = No response
(Record "C" if eyes closed by swelling)
BEST MOTOR RESPONSE to painful stimuli
6 = Obeys verbal command
5 = Localizes pain
4 = Flexion—withdrawal
3 = Flexion—abnormal
2 = Extension—abnormal
1 = No response
(Record best upper limb response)
BEST VERBAL RESPONSE
5 = Oriented × 3
4 = Conversation—confused
3 = Speech—inappropriate
2 = Sounds—incomprehensible
1 = No response
(Record "E" if endotracheal tube in place, "T" if tracheostomy tube in place)

Figure 24.44 ●
Glasgow Coma Scale.

▶ **Syncope** is a brief loss of consciousness and is usually sudden. **Coma** is a more prolonged state with pronounced and persistent changes.
▶ A client experiencing any loss of consciousness needs immediate medical interventions.
▶ The Glasgow Coma Scale has limitations. For example, a client with an endotracheal tube or tracheostomy cannot communicate. As a result, the score is carried out according to each individual component of the scale. The verbal response score would then indicate intubation or tracheostomy. In addition, the motor response scale is invalid in a client with a spinal cord injury, and eye opening may be impossible to assess in those individuals with severe orbital injury.

Refer to the Companion Website at **www.prenhall.com/damico** and click on the **Documentation** module for documentation samples and documentation practice exercises.

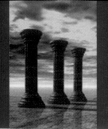

Abnormal Findings

Problems commonly associated with the neurologic system include changes in motor function, including gait and movement, seizures, spinal cord injury, infections, degenerative disorders, and cranial nerve dysfunction. These conditions are described below and in Tables 24.3 and 24.4.

Table 24.3 Problems with Motor Function

GAIT	MOVEMENT
Ataxic Gait A walk characterized by a wide base, uneven steps, feet slapping, and a tendency to sway. This type of walk is associated with posterior column disease or decreased proprioception regarding extremities. Seen in multiple sclerosis and drug or alcohol intoxication.	**Fasciculation** Commonly called a twitch, this is an involuntary, local, visible muscular contraction. It is not significant when it occurs in tired muscles. It can be associated with motor neuron disease.
Scissors Gait A walk characterized by spastic lower limbs and movement in a stiff, jerky manner. The knees come together; the legs cross in front of one another; and the legs are abducted as the individual takes short, progressive, slow steps. This is seen in individuals with multiple sclerosis.	**Tic** Commonly called a *habit,* a tic is usually psychogenic in nature. The involuntary spasmodic movement of the muscle is seen in a muscle under voluntary control, usually in the face, neck, or shoulders.
Steppage Gait Sometimes called the "foot drop" walk. The individual flexes and raises the knee to a higher-than-usual level yielding a flopping of the foot when walking. This usually is indicative of lower motor neuron disease. Seen in individuals with alcoholic neuritis and progressive muscular atrophy.	**Tremor** A rhythmic or alternating involuntary movement from the contraction of opposing muscle groups. Tremors vary in degree and are seen in Parkinson's disease, multiple sclerosis, uremia (a form of kidney failure), and alcohol intoxication.
Festination Gait Referred to as the "Parkinson's walk." The individual has stooped posture, takes short steps, and turns stiffly. There is a slow start to the walk and frequent, accelerated steps. This gait is associated with basal ganglia disease.	**Athetoid Movement** A continuous, involuntary, repetitive, slow, "wormlike," arrhythmic muscular movement. The muscles are in a state of hypotoxicity, producing a distortion to the limb. This movement is seen in cerebral palsy.
	Dystonia Similar to athetoid movements, dystonia involves larger muscle groups. The twisting movements yield a grotesque change to the individual's posture. Torticollis, or wryneck, is an example of dystonia.
	Myoclonus A continual, rapid, short spasm involving a muscle, part of a muscle, or even a group of muscles. Frequently occurs in an extremity as the individual is falling asleep. Myoclonus is also seen in seizure disorders.

Table 24.4 Problems Associated with Dysfunction of Cranial Nerves

CRANIAL NERVE		DYSFUNCTION
I	Olfactory	Unilateral or bilateral anosmia.
II	Optic	Optic atrophy, papilledema, amblyopia, field defects.
III	Oculomotor	Diplopia, ptosis of lid, dilated pupil, inability to focus on close objects.
IV	Trochlear	Convergent strabismus, diplopia.
V	Trigeminal	Tic douloureux, loss of facial sensation, decreased ability to chew, loss of corneal reflex, decreased blinking.
VI	Abducens	Diplopia, strabismus.
VII	Facial	Bell's palsy, decreased ability to distinguish tastes.
VIII	Vestibulocochlear	Tinnitus, vertigo, deafness.
IX	Glossopharyngeal	Loss of "gag" reflex, loss of taste, difficulty swallowing.
X	Vagus	Loss of voice, impaired voice, difficulty swallowing.
XI	Accessory	Difficulty with shrugging of shoulders, inability to turn head to left and right.
XII	Hypoglossal	Difficulty with speech and swallowing, inability to protrude tongue.

SEIZURES

Seizures are sudden, rapid, and excessive discharges of electrical energy in the brain. They are usually centered in the cerebral cortex. Some seizure disorders stem from neurologic problems that occur before or during birth, or they can develop secondary to childhood fevers. In children and adults, seizures can result from a variety of factors including trauma, infections, cerebrovascular disease, environmental toxins, drug overdose, and withdrawal from alcohol, sedatives, or antidepressants. *Epilepsy* is a chronic seizure disorder.

SPINAL CORD INJURIES

The spinal cord extends from the medulla oblongata of the brain stem. As it continues down the back, the cervical, thoracic, and lumbar vertebrae protect it. Spinal cord injuries result from trauma to the vertebrae, which causes dislocation fractures that in turn compress or transect the spinal cord. The most common causes of this type of trauma are automobile and motorcycle accidents, sports accidents such as football and diving accidents, and penetrating injuries such as stab wounds and gunshots. Generally speaking, the higher the level of the injury, the greater the loss of neurologic function. Injuries to the cervical region are the most common and the most devastating.

INFECTIONS OF THE NEUROLOGIC SYSTEM

Infections of the neurologic system include meningitis, myelitis, brain abscess, and Lyme disease. Each of these will be described in the following sections.

Meningitis

Meningitis is caused by a virus or bacteria that infects the coverings, or meninges, of the brain or spinal cord. Meningitis may result from a penetrating wound, fractured skull, or upper respiratory infection, or it may occur secondary to facial or cranial surgery.

In some cases, meningitis may spread to the underlying brain tissues, causing encephalitis. *Encephalitis* is defined as an inflammation of the tissue of the brain. It usually results from a virus, which may be transmitted by ticks or mosquitoes, or it may result from a childhood illness such as chickenpox or the measles.

Myelitis

Myelitis is an inflammation of the spinal cord. Poliomyelitis and herpes zoster infection are two common causes. It may develop after an infection such as measles or gonorrhea, or it may follow vaccination for rabies.

Brain Abscess

A *brain abscess* is usually the result of a systemic infection. It is marked by an accumulation of pus in the brain cells. Most brain abscesses develop secondary to a primary infection. Others result from skull fractures or penetrating injuries, such as a gunshot wound.

Lyme Disease

Lyme disease is an infection caused by a spirochete transmitted by a bite from an infected tick that lives on deer. Its major symptoms are arthritis, a flulike syndrome, and a rash. If untreated, Lyme disease may cause severe neurologic disorders.

DEGENERATIVE NEUROLOGIC DISORDERS

Degenerative neurologic disorders include Alzheimer's disease, amyotrophic lateral sclerosis, Huntington's disease, multiple sclerosis, myasthenia gravis, and Parkinson's disease. These will be discussed in the following paragraphs.

Alzheimer's Disease

Alzheimer's disease is a progressive degenerative disease of the brain that leads to dementia. Although it is more common in people over age 65, its onset may occur as early as middle adulthood. Symptoms include a loss of memory, particularly of recent events, shortened attention span, confusion, and disorientation. Eventually, the client with Alzheimer's disease may experience paranoid fantasies and hallucinations.

Amyotrophic Lateral Sclerosis

Amyotrophic lateral sclerosis, commonly known as Lou Gehrig's disease, is a chronic degenerative disease involving the cerebral cortex and the motor neurons in the spinal cord. The result is a progressive wasting of skeletal muscles that eventually leads to death. Although the cause is unknown, research has implicated viral infection.

Huntington's Disease

Huntington's disease is an inherited disorder characterized by uncontrollable jerking movements, called *chorea,* which literally means dance. It typically progresses to mental deterioration and ultimately death. Symptoms usually first appear in early middle age; thus, those with Huntington's disease often have had children before they know they have the disorder.

Multiple Sclerosis

Multiple sclerosis is the deterioration of the protective sheaths, composed of myelin, of the nerve tracts in the brain and spinal cord. The first attack usually occurs between the ages of 20 and 40. Early symptoms include temporary tingling, numbness, or weakness that may affect only one limb or one side of the body. Other symptoms include unsteadiness, blurred vision, slurred speech, and difficulty in urinating. Some individuals experience repeated attacks that progress in severity. In these individuals, permanent disability with progressive neuromuscular deficits develops.

Myasthenia Gravis

Myasthenia gravis is a chronic neuromuscular disorder involving increasing weakness of voluntary muscles with activity, and some abatement of symptoms with rest. Onset is gradual and usually occurs in adolescence or young adulthood. The precise etiology is unknown, but it is believed that myasthenia gravis is an *autoimmune* disorder, that is, the individual's immune system attacks the individual's own normal cells rather than foreign pathogens. Some of the most common symptoms include ptosis (drooping eyelids), diplopia (double vision), a flat affect, and a weak, monotone voice.

Parkinson's Disease

Parkinson's disease is a degeneration of the basal nuclei of the brain, which are collections of nerve cell bodies deep within the white matter of the cerebrum. These nuclei are responsible for initiating and stopping voluntary movement. Parkinson's disease is characterized by slow movements, continuous "pill-rolling" tremor of the forefinger and thumb, rhythmic shaking of the hands, bobbing of the head, and difficulty in initiating movement. The individual may have a masklike facial expression, difficulty in speaking clearly, and difficulty maintaining balance while walking. Although the precise etiology is unknown, research indicates that environmental toxins, such as carbon monoxide or certain metals, may cause some cases of Parkinson's disease. It may also result from previous encephalitis.

Health Promotion

HEALTHY PEOPLE 2010

FOCUS AREA	PREVALENCE	OBJECTIVES	ACTIONS
Alzheimer's Disease	• Alzheimer's disease occurs in 8 to 15% of adults over 65 years of age. • Alzheimer's disease affects men and women equally; however, the longer life span of women produces more cases of Alzheimer's in women at any specific point in time.	• Increase the number of persons seen in primary healthcare who receive mental health assessment. • Increase the numbers of adults with mental disorders who receive treatment.	• Educational programs for healthcare providers and the public about mental health assessment. • Screening and treatment programs.

CLIENT EDUCATION

The following are physiological, behavioral, and cultural factors that influence neurologic health across the life span. Several factors are cited as trends in *Healthy People 2010*. The nurse provides advice and education to reduce risks associated with the factors mentioned to promote and maintain neurologic health.

LIFE SPAN CONSIDERATIONS

RISK FACTORS

- Low birth weight infants are at risk for neurologic problems including intraventricular hemorrhage. African Americans have a higher incidence of low birth weight infants.
- Head injuries are common causes of neurologic problems in children.
- The incidence of epilepsy is highest in children under 10 years of age but occurs and can be chronic across the age span.

- Reye's syndrome is an illness associated with recovery from viral illness such as influenza, cold, or chickenpox. The development of Reye's syndrome has been linked with the use of aspirin to treat the symptoms of viral illnesses in children. Reye's syndrome results in damage to the brain and generally occurs in children between the ages of 4 and 12.
- Meningitis and encephalitis result from viral and bacterial infection and occur mainly in children and those in crowded living conditions.
- Older adults have decreased reaction time resulting in accident and injury.

CLIENT EDUCATION

- Advise pregnant females, especially African Americans, to seek and participate in prenatal care to prevent low birth weight.

- Educate and inform parents of safety measures for children to prevent head injuries.
- Explain to individuals, parents, and children the types of seizures they experience and the medications required for controls and safety measures to prevent accident or injury.
- Educate parents to read medication labels and avoid aspirin and products with aspirin to decrease the risk of developing Reye's syndrome.

- Advise clients to follow recommendations for *H. influenzae* and pneumococcal vaccinations to reduce risks for meningitis.

- Instruct all clients regarding safety. Include use of seat belts while traveling in a car or driving and the use of safety devices in the home and at work.

CULTURAL CONSIDERATIONS

RISK FACTORS

- Hypertension increases the risk for cerebrovascular problems, including stroke. African Americans have a greater incidence of hypertension.
- Low birth weight infants are at risk for neurologic problems including intraventricular hemorrhage. African Americans have a higher incidence of low birth weight infants.

CLIENT EDUCATION

- Educate clients about screening for hypertension and about the importance of diet and exercise to prevent hypertension.

- Advise pregnant females, especially African Americans, to seek and participate in prenatal care to prevent low birth weight.

ENVIRONMENTAL CONSIDERATIONS

RISK FACTORS

- Stress can increase blood pressure resulting in risk for brain attack (stroke, cerebral vascular accident).
- Medications and remedies, alone or in combinations, may cause neurologic problems or symptoms.
- Stroke (brain attack) occurs with greater frequency in individuals with heart disease, hypertension, and diabetes. Stroke can result in death or functional limitations.

CLIENT EDUCATION

- Instruct clients in stress reduction techniques.
- Educate clients about prescription and over-the-counter medication use, herbs, home remedies, and cultural therapies and the interactions that may lead to neurologic problems.
- Teach clients to recognize and seek help for symptoms of brain attack (stroke).

BEHAVIORAL CONSIDERATIONS

RISK FACTORS

- Accidents at home, at work, or in social situations can result in neurologic problems.
- Alcohol or drug use increases risks for accidents and injury and neurologic disorders.

CLIENT EDUCATION

- Instruct all clients regarding safety. Include use of seat belts while traveling in a car or driving and safety devices in the home and at work.
- Discuss limiting or avoiding the use of alcohol and drugs to reduce the risk of accidents and neurologic problems.

Application Through Critical Thinking

CASE STUDY

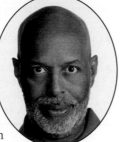

Mr. John Phelps, age 65, is an African American male who comes to the community health clinic. He and his wife Helen recently celebrated their 40th wedding anniversary. He has a 35-year-old daughter, a 32-year-old son, and three grandchildren. Mr. Phelps retired 4 months ago from a busy accounting firm where he worked as a CPA for 25 years. He and his wife have been planning their retirement and are looking forward to traveling across the country to visit family.

Mr. Phelps's chief complaint is tremors that seem to be getting worse over the past few months. He noticed the tremors about 6 months ago and thought they were related to fatigue, since the office was very busy and he was working late hours. He anticipated that the tremors would stop after he retired and became rested. Mrs. Phelps indicates her husband's handwriting has become small and almost illegible and that she had to write several checks for him last week. She also comments that her husband seems depressed about his recent retirement, since he has a "blank look" on his face and his speech is slow. Mari Chung, RN, conducts a focused interview and then proceeds with the physical assessment. She gathers the following objective and subjective data:

- Mood swings
- Tremors, movement of thumb and index finger in a circular fashion
- Shuffling gait, falls easily
- Constipation
- Fatigue
- Loss of 10 lb
- Drooling
- Speaks in a monotone; voice slow, weak, and soft
- Rigidity during passive ROM
- Jerky movements
- Muscle pain and soreness
- Decrease in corneal response
- Posture not erect, forward flexion
- Unable to perform finger-to-nose test and rapid alternating movement
- Difficulty standing from sitting position without assistance

Ms. Chung consults with the clinic physician. After further evaluation, Mr. Phelps is admitted to the neurologic unit of the community hospital with a diagnosis of Parkinson's disease.

► **Complete Documentation**

The following is sample documentation from health assessment of John Phelps.

SUBJECTIVE DATA: Complains of tremors, getting worse over 6 months. He has had some change in his moods, has lost some weight, and is constipated frequently. He has occasional drooling. Experiences muscle pain and soreness. Requires assistance to get up from a chair and falls easily. Wife states writing increasingly illegible. She reports he has become depressed, has a "blank" look, and has slow speech.

OBJECTIVE DATA: Posture not erect—favored flexion, shuffling gait, jerky movements. Voice monotone, slow, weak, soft. Decreased corneal response. Rigidity during passive range of motion (ROM). Unable to perform finger-to-nose and rapid alternating movement tests. Drooling. Weight loss 10 lb since last exam.

► **Critical Thinking Questions**

1. What data was considered in the medical diagnosis of Parkinson's disease?
2. What additional data would be required to confirm a diagnosis of Parkinson's disease?
3. What are the nursing considerations for Mr. Phelps?

► **Applying Nursing Diagnoses**

1. Use the NANDA taxonomy (see Appendix A ∞) to develop two nursing diagnoses from the data provided.

2. *Falls, risk for* and *self-esteem, risk for situational loss* are included as nursing diagnoses in the NANDA taxonomy. Do the data in the case study support these nursing diagnoses? Explain your answer.

► **Prepare Teaching Plan**

LEARNING NEED: The data in the case study revealed that Mr. Phelps has signs and symptoms of Parkinson's disease. His symptoms include tremors, weight loss, fatigue, constipation, falling, and others. He was admitted to the hospital and will begin treatment for his problem. He and his wife will require education about the disease and his care upon discharge.

The case study provides data that is representative of risks, symptoms, and behaviors of many individuals. Therefore, the following teaching plan is based on the need to provide information to members of any community about Parkinson's disease.

GOAL: The participants in this learning program will have increased knowledge about Parkinson's disease and its management.

OBJECTIVES: At the completion of this learning session, the participants will be able to:

1. Describe Parkinson's disease.
2. Identify risk factors associated with Parkinson's disease.
3. List the symptoms of Parkinson's disease.
4. Discuss strategies in management of Parkinson's disease.

ASSESSMENT FORM

		No	Yes	Describe
History:				
	Tremors		X	*6 mos. worsening*
	Mood change		X	*"Depression"*
	Pain		X	*Muscle pain*
	Stiffness		X	*Extremities*
	Speech (change)		X	*Slow, weak*
Describe:	Facial Expression	*"Blank"*		
	ADL	*"Needs assistance to get up from chair"*		
Other:	Constipation			
	Weight loss			
	Falls easily			
Physical Findings:		**Yes**	**No**	**Describe**
	Posture (erect)		X	*Forward flexion*
	Gait (smooth)		X	*Shuffling*
	Movement (smooth/coordinated)		X	*Jerky—finger-nose, rapid alt. movement*
	CN (intact)		X	*Decreased corneal reflex*

APPLICATION OF OBJECTIVE 4: Discuss strategies in management of Parkinson's disease

Content	Teaching Strategy	Evaluation
• Medication is used to manage problems with tremor and movement.	• Lecture	• Written examination.
• Surgery may improve movement.	• Discussion	May use short answer, fill-in, or multiple-choice items or a combination of items.
• Deep brain stimulation refers to implantation of a device to reduce trembling.	• Audiovisual materials • Printed materials	If these are short and easy to evaluate, the learner receives immediate feedback.
• Self-care includes a healthy diet. Fiber reduces problems with constipation. Including folate in the diet or as a supplement may protect against Parkinson's disease. Eating and swallowing carefully reduces risk of choking.	Lecture is appropriate when disseminating information to large groups. Discussion allows participants to bring up concerns and to raise questions.	
• Regular exercise improves mobility, balance, range of motion, and emotional well-being.	Audiovisual materials such as illustrations reinforce verbal presentation.	
• Reduce the risk of injury from falls by making the home environment safe (no throw rugs, install handrails, and grab bars).	Printed materials, especially to be taken away with learners, allow review, reinforcement, and reading at the learner's pace.	
• Seek assistance from physical and occupational therapists for guidelines to improve ease of ambulation and carrying out daily tasks.		
• Communication requires speaking louder than believed necessary. Practice reading aloud. Seek assistance from a speech pathologist.		
• The Patient Education Institute offers an online tutorial regarding Parkinson's disease. Link to their Website through the Companion Website.		

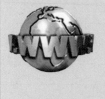

Please refer to the Companion Website at www.prenhall.com/damico and click on Chapter 24, the Application Through Critical Thinking module, to complete the following activities related to this case study:
- ▶ **Critical Thinking questions**
- ▶ **Extended Nursing Diagnosis challenge**
- ▶ **Documentation activity**
- ▶ **Teaching Plan for Objectives 1, 2, and 3**

EXPLORE MediaLink

Additional resources for this chapter are found on the Student CD-ROM accompanying this textbook and on the Companion Website.

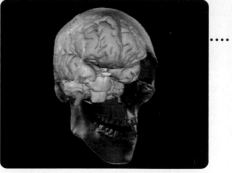

CD-ROM CONTENT

Content for this chapter includes:
Objectives
Key Concepts
NCLEX-RN® Review Questions
Model Documentation Forms
Audio Glossary
Animations
  Brain
  Central Nerves
  Upper Extremity Nerves
  Lower Extremity Nerves
  Neuro Synapse
Games and Challenges
Clinical Spotlight Videos
  Extrapyramidal Signs
  Tremor
  Tardive Dyskinesia
Head-to-Toe Physical Examination Video

COMPANION WEBSITE CONTENT

www.prenhall.com/damico

Content for this chapter includes:
Objectives
NCLEX-RN® Review Questions
Client Interaction Case Study Challenge
Application Through Critical Thinking
  Case Study Teaching Plan Challenge
MediaLinks
MediaLink Application
Tool Box
  Cranial Nerves
  Problems with Motor Function
  Problems Associated with Dysfunction of Cranial Nerves
  Chapter Documentation Form Example
  Health Promotion
    Healthy People 2010
    Client Education
New York Times

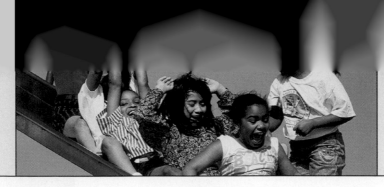

25
Assessment of Infants, Children, and Adolescents

MEDIALINK

www.prenhall.com/damico

The CD-ROM in the back of this textbook and the Media-Link website contain NCLEX-RN® review questions, interactive exercises, case study challenges, animations, videos, documentation and checklist forms, and review materials. For a complete listing of the media content specific to Chapter 25, see the Explore MediaLink at the end of the chapter.

The previous chapters in this book include techniques used to elicit health histories and perform physical assessment of adult clients. Much of the information from previous chapters is appropriate for pediatric clients. However, children are not "little adults," and significant differences exist between infants, children, adolescents, and adults. These differences include variations in physiology, development, and cognition that must be incorporated into the nursing assessment. This chapter uses the word *parent* to represent parents, caregivers, or guardians.

The head-to-toe approach to physical assessment is useful in many situations and with different types of clients, but it may not work with young children. Adults and adolescents will usually sit on an examination table, wear a paper gown, and follow the nurse's instructions. However, infants and toddlers often refuse to sit still or cooperate.

Young children do not have the cognitive or verbal ability to describe symptoms or comply with complex instructions. Nurses must possess strong assessment skills in order to overcome the communication and situational challenges involved in pediatric physical assessment. This chapter focuses on the health history questions, physical assessment and examination techniques, and developmental information necessary to obtain an accurate and comprehensive health status assessment of infants, children, and adolescents. Reducing the number of deaths during childhood and adolescence is included in the goals of the *Healthy People 2010* initiatives. Actions and interventions to achieve these goals are addressed in the *Healthy People 2010* feature on page 816.

CHILDHOOD DEVELOPMENTAL STAGES

Babies are not born with the ability to walk, talk, and independently care for themselves. Just as the brain is not fully mature at birth, all of the major organ systems are immature and develop throughout childhood. The most dramatic development changes occur primarily in infancy and adolescence, although each stage of childhood is marked by unique changes. Knowledge of the normal physical, psychological, and cognitive development of children is essential. It may be helpful to review the material in Chapter 3. ∞

Newborns are children between birth and 1 month of age. **Infants** are children between 1 and 12 months of age. Infancy is characterized by dramatic changes in height and weight, and the development of gross physical and social skills. Young children have **cephalocaudal** physical growth. That is, their development progresses in a head-to-toe fashion. Development and growth begin proximally before developing distally. For example, fine motor skills follow gross motor skills, and the ability to grasp precedes the ability to stand or walk. **Toddlers** are children who are at least 1 year old but who have not yet reached 3 years of age. Toddlerhood is marked by slower, steadier growth, fine motor skill improvement, and language development. **Preschoolers** are children between 3 and 5 years of age. The preschool years are characterized by motor and language skill refinement and beginning social skill development. **School-age** children are between 6 and 10 years old. The major developmental tasks of school-age children involve cognitive and social growth. **Adolescence** is characterized by periods of rapid growth, sexual maturation, and cognitive refinement. Adolescence is the period between 11 and 21 years of age.

NUTRITIONAL ASSESSMENT

It is not set in stone that a nutrition assessment must proceed in a set order. When assessing children, it may be helpful to conduct the nutrition history portion before the physical assessment in order to establish rapport and make the child more comfortable with the process. Rapport is essential, especially when assessing an adolescent. Infants and younger children need a caretaker present to assist with the assessment and to answer questions. Adolescents may be more comfortable having privacy during the assessment. It is best to discuss the assessment arrangement with the adolescent and caregiver separately to allow the adolescent to give an unpressured answer. A caregiver can be interviewed separately if appropriate. When there are known existing nutritional issues, such as disordered eating or obesity, the nurse should be sensitive to the needs of the child and caregiver. Both must feel their respective needs to provide information are met.

NUTRITIONAL HISTORY

A diet recall, food frequency, and food diary can all remain appropriate tools when assessing dietary intake in children. School-age children and children in day care should be assessed for food habits on at-home days as well as days away from home. Differences in intake may also exist for weekend days in the child who is not in school or day care full-time. Children who participate in many outside activities may have varying nutritional habits throughout the week with missed meals, meals on the run, or frequent take-out meals contrasting with more regular eating patterns on other days. The nurse should inquire about the child's schedule and activities in order to determine the extent of variation and need for additional data. Table 25.1 outlines specific data to gather for infants, children, and adolescents during the nutritional history and focused interview.

PHYSICAL ASSESSMENT

The parameters of the physical assessment in children primarily are the same anthropometric measurements and clinical observations as in the adult with references and standards that are unique to age. Growth rate during the first year of life is most rapid compared to later childhood and adolescence. Developmental milestones have important nutrition implications throughout childhood and should become part of a complete assessment.

Anthropometric Measurements

Anthropometric measurements in children should be obtained using equipment appropriate for the pediatric population. Recumbent length and weight measurements are needed in the infant and young child. Weight should be measured without a diaper. Older children can have standing height and weight measured as described. Children with musculoskeletal disorders and contractures can have knee height measured. Skinfold measurements should be done using calipers calibrated to 0.2 mm since small changes in measurement can cause changes in assessment classification. The World Health Organization

---

Table 25.1	Nutritional History Data for Assessment of Infants, Children, and Adolescents

Breast-fed baby:
- Number and lengths of feedings
- Number of wet diapers
- Iron source by 4–6 months
- Vitamin C source concomitant to iron for improved absorption
- Vegan mother—assess for her vitamin B_{12} source

Bottle-fed baby:
- Type and amount of formula
- Iron source by 4–6 months (formula or fortified cereal)
- Vitamin C source concomitant to iron for improved absorption

Assess for intake of solids at age 4–6 months and thereafter. Note type, amount, intolerances, or allergies.

Assess for effect of any medical condition on diet: feeding difficulties, therapeutic diet, food/nutrient as medication interactions, altered nutrient needs.

Assess nutrition knowledge and beliefs of caregiver, including religious and cultural influences.

Assess whether feeding skills are appropriate to developmental stage. Note delays. Note whether food texture is appropriate for development (chewing and swallowing abilities, self-feeding, sitting upright).

Assess for inappropriate feeding practices:
- Sleeping with bottle (assess for baby-bottle tooth decay)
- Solids before age 4–6 months or not after 7–9 months
- Solids added to formula in bottle
- Cow's milk before age 12 months
- Honey before age 1 (botulism risk)
- Fat restriction
- Inappropriately textured foods for developmental stage
- Foods likely to cause choking: hot dogs, grapes, nuts, whole raw vegetables (e.g., carrots), gum, hard candy, chunks of unpeeled fruit
- Supplements not prescribed by healthcare provider
- Use of food for punishment or reward
- All meals and snacks: portion, preparation method

- Meal and snack pattern: frequency, number, missed meals
- Liquid intake: volume, type, presence of caffeine or alcohol intake, sugary drinks

> **ALERT!**
> *It is recommended that children limit juice intake to 12 oz per day. Excess intake of juice is associated with obesity.*

- Food intolerances/allergies
- Therapeutic diet
- Use of supplements: type, dose, frequency
- Self-prescribed diet or restrictive eating habits (especially in adolescents)

> **ALERT!**
> *Adolescents may choose to follow a vegetarian diet for a number of reasons. Ask about this. While religious, ethical, and health beliefs are often cited, many adolescents choose a vegetarian diet to mask attempts at weight loss or disordered eating.*

- Family, child, and caregiver beliefs and knowledge about food, including cultural or religious influences.
- Body satisfaction (older children and adolescents). Ask: "What do you think about your body/body weight? Have you ever tried to gain or lose weight? Tell me what you tried."
- Activity level. Note amount and type. Assess adequacy of intake for active children. Include assessment of daily "screen time" (time spent watching television, playing computer games, playing on the computer).

> **ALERT!**
> *Increased screen time is associated with incidence of overweight and obesity in children.*

(WHO) recommends weight for height as the standard in measuring children since skinfold and circumference measurements are prone to errors that could result in misclassification of nutritional health.

Head circumference is a measurement unique to assessing growth in children at or under 3 years of age. Beyond age 3, head circumference is not a valid tool to assess growth and nutritional status.

Anthropometric measurements have age-specific references established by the CDC and WHO. In children under 20 years of age, references are described using charts with age-specific **percentiles** for height, weight, BMI, and, for children under 36 months, head circumference. Percentiles are used to assess growth rate and health of weight for height. Percentile charts are derived from the distribution of data from population studies and are age- and gender-specific descriptions of anthropometric measurements. Newer infant growth charts are more representative of the population-matched prevalence of breast-fed infants compared to charts published before 2000. Breast-fed infants normally grow at a slightly slower rate than formula-fed babies do. Infants, children, and adolescents can be compared to their age-matched peers to determine their individual percentile within the population. A best use of percentile charts is in monitoring individual growth over time. Normally, children will remain within a narrow percentile range for each measurement over the course of childhood. For example, a child assessed sequentially in the 25th percentile for height (length) for age may have a small frame and parents with small stature and may not be at risk for poor nutritional health. A child sequentially in the 50th percentile for height for age who drops to the 25th percentile may be at risk for undernutrition. A significant drop or increase in percentile category is cause for further investigation to assess for undernutrition or overnutrition. Overweight and obesity in children is defined as BMI for age greater than the 85th percentile and the 95th percentile, respectively. Undernutrition is defined as BMI for age less than the 5th percentile. Separate growth references exist for children with some chronic diseases and for knee-height estimates of stature.

Clinical Examination

Clinical signs of possible poor nutritional health include those in Table 9.5 on pages 146–149 as well as some unique findings. ⚭ Certain diseases and conditions, such as HIV infection, congenital heart disease, or premature birth, can predispose children to nutritional risk. During the clinical exam, the nurse should be mindful of the potential negative influences of existing medical issues on nutritional health. Undernutrition can occur due to insufficient intake, increased nutrient losses, or increased nutritional needs that are not met. Insufficient intake can occur for a variety of reasons. Feeding difficulties, as with cleft palate, food intolerances, and food insecurity, are among the many contributors to poor intake. Nutrient losses can occur with malabsorptive conditions as well as drug-nutrient interactions. Unmatched increased nutritional needs, such as with chronic fever, fracture, or wound healing, will lead to undernutrition.

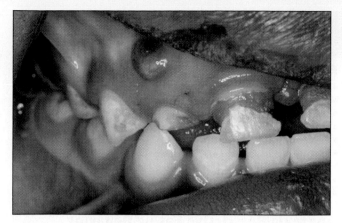

Figure 25.1 ● Baby-bottle tooth decay.

Bottle-fed children should be assessed for signs of baby-bottle tooth decay (see Figure 25.1 ●). Caries can result from the inappropriate practice of putting children to sleep with a bottle containing more than water.

Insufficient vitamin D status from lack of intake or little exposure to sunlight can lead to changes in bone formation that affect a growing child. Rickets, rachitic rosary, pigeon-breast formation of the rib cage, and widened bone epiphyses can occur. Signs and symptoms consistent with disordered eating should also be included in the assessment of older children and adolescents. Box 25.1 outlines clinical findings of disordered eating.

An assessment of development in younger children and pubertal status in older children can be included in a nutritional assessment. Poor nutritional health can negatively affect sexual maturation, growth, and muscle development in the adolescent. A determination of sexual maturity can be included in the assessment as discussed on page 808.

Feeding skills coincide with developmental skills and determine the type of foods a young child can handle. Foods included in the diet should be developmentally appropriate. Introduction of solid foods into the diet should not occur until age 4 to 6 months when an infant can sit with support and transfer food to the rear of the mouth for swallowing. As the ability to chew improves around age 9 to 12 months, more texture-appropriate foods can be introduced. Solids introduced too soon can result in aspiration. Delays in development may impact nutritional health if diet is not carefully monitored. Developmental milestones that impact nutritional health are discussed on page 795.

LABORATORY MEASUREMENTS

The nutritional components of a laboratory assessment in children are the same as described for the general population. Iron deficiency anemia is found in up to 9% of young children. Decreased intake of iron-rich foods and increased needs during growth contribute to the prevalence of anemia. Adolescent males require additional iron as muscle mass and blood volume increase. Adolescent females require additional iron to compensate for menstrual losses. Screening for iron deficiency is done at age 9 to 12 months and again 6 months later. Children

Box 25.1	Clinical Findings Consistent with Eating Disorders

Bulimia/Binge Purge Behavior

- Bloodshot eyes
- Broken blood vessels on the face
- Swollen parotid glands or "chipmunk cheeks"
- Dental erosion
- Hoarse voice
- Scarring on the dorsal surface of the hand from teeth during purge attempts
- Poor or lacking gag reflex
- Weight fluctuations

Anorexia/Restrictive Eating Behavior

- Cold intolerance
- Lanugo, soft white hair growth on body
- Pedal edema
- Dry skin
- Alopecia
- Bradycardia
- Hypotension
- Amenorrhea in nonpregnant postmenarcheal females
- Loss of strength and muscle tone

General Eating Disorder Findings

- Body dissatisfaction. Ask: "How do you feel about your weight?" followed by "Have you ever tried to gain or lose weight? Tell me what you did."
- Constipation
- Bloating
- Fatigue

born prematurely or with special healthcare needs, those not fed an iron-fortified formula or fortified cereal, or those being fed cow's milk before 12 months of age should be screened. Children suspected of being at risk for lead poisoning should have both lead and iron status checked because of the association between the two.

PHYSICAL VARIANTS IN CHILDHOOD

Children are physically different from adults. The following sections include discussion of common physical variants in childhood.

INTEGUMENT

The skin is one of the last systems to develop in utero. Infants have less developed corneum stratum and a thinner epidermis than older children and adults. As a result, infants and newborns are more prone to heat and water loss from skin evaporation, and cold stress from radiant heat loss. The thinner epidermis allows for increased transdermal absorption of substances and medications placed on the skin. It is essential to use special caution with topical medications and preparations in infants under 6 months of age because of the potential for systemic absorption. The sebaceous glands do not begin to function until around the first birthday, causing infants to be at

greater risk for heat intolerance. The apocrine sweat glands and sebaceous glands do not fully function until puberty.

Milia are tiny (less than 0.5 mm), smooth, white cysts of the hair follicle as depicted in Figure 11.3 on page 186. ◯◯ They are often present at birth and are common on the forehead and nose. Milia on the gums are called Epstein's pearls or "witches teeth." Milia are normal infant variations. **Lanugo** is a covering of fine hair in newborns that is most prominent on the upper chest, shoulders, and back. Lanugo disappears within the first few weeks of life. Premature infants generally have more lanugo than full-term infants. **Salmon patches,** also known as stork bites, are small macules and patches caused by visible intradermal capillaries. This normal variant occurs in 30 to 50% of newborns. The most common locations for salmon patches are the forehead, the eyelids, the upper lip, the nasal bridge, and the nape of the neck. Anything that causes the skin to flush, such as fever or crying, will cause these lesions to be more noticeable. Salmon patches spontaneously resolve during infancy in all but a few children. **Mongolian spots** are areas of dark bluish pigmentation that are common in African American, Asian, and Hispanic children (refer to Figure 11.4 on page 186 ◯◯). These benign patches are caused by increased concentrations of melanocytes and can be found anywhere on the body, but are most common at the base of the spine. Mongolian spots are darkest in the newborn period, and they fade during the first 2 years of life. **Acrocyanosis** is a commonly seen, normal finding in newborns and infants. During times of stress, especially exposure to cold environments, the hands and feet appear cyanotic and are often accompanied by increased mottling of the distal arms and legs. Nurses must distinguish this benign condition from true cyanosis that is accompanied by a bluing of the tongue and oral mucous membranes. **Vernix caseosa** is a cheesy-white substance that coats the skin surfaces at birth. Vernix consists of a combination of epithelium cells and sebum. It is generally more pronounced in term and postterm infants.

The integumentary assessment of older children and adolescents is similar to that of adults. **Morbilliform,** or "measles-like," rashes consist of erythematous, confluent macules and papules. Morbilliform rashes are caused by viruses and occur most often in toddlers and preschoolers. **Atopic dermatitis,** also know as **eczema,** is a chronic skin disorder characterized by intense itching, patches, erythema, and papules that typically begins in the first year of life as depicted in Figure 25.2 ●. Infantile eczema is common on the face, the neck, the popliteal space, and the antecubital space. By the school-age years, eczema presents with the same distribution noted in adults.

HEAD, EYES, EARS, NOSE, AND THROAT

The bones of the cranium are not fused at birth. The infant's skull has openings, called fontanelles and sutures, which protect the brain during birth and allow for skull and brain growth during infancy. The **posterior fontanelle** is located in the superior occiput and may not be palpable at birth. It is usually 1 to 2 cm in diameter and closes by 2 months of age. The **anterior fontanelle** is a 2- to 4-cm diamond-shaped opening, also known as a "soft spot," located at the top of the skull.

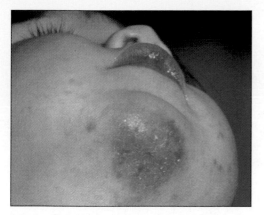

Figure 25.2 ● Chronic eczema.

The skin covering the anterior fontanelle should be even with the skull surface. The anterior fontanelle normally closes between 9 and 18 months of age. Children with premature or delayed fontanelle closure require further evaluation and assessment.

The **cranial sutures** are palpable gaps between the bones of the skull. The **metopic sutures** separate the frontal and temporal bones. The **lambdoidal sutures** separate the temporal and occipital bones. The **sagittal suture** lies in the middle of the skull and crosses the anterior and posterior fontanelles as illustrated in Figure 25.3 ●. **Craniosynostosis** is a condition that results in cranial deformity due to premature fusion of the cranial bones. In craniosynostosis, the skull appears flattened as a body ridge develops along the suture lines (see Figure 12.17 on page 254 ⚭). If untreated, this disorder results in impaired brain growth and dignitive impairment. The nurse should promptly refer any child with suspected craniosynostosis for further evaluation and treatment.

Newborns who are large for gestational age, those born vaginally, and those with birth histories of cephalopelvic disproportion or prolonged or difficult labors often have misshaped skulls from trauma or compression during labor and delivery. **Caput succedaneum** is characterized by edema that results from a collection of fluid in the tissue at the top of the skull. The swelling associated with caput succedaneum crosses the cranial suture lines. **Cephalohematomas** are blood collections inside of the skull's periosteum and do not cross suture lines. Children with cephalohematomas are at increased risk of developing jaundice during the first week of life.

The head is the largest body surface area in infants. Heat loss and cold stress can result from leaving a newborn's head uncovered in cool environments. The head remains disproportionately large in comparison to the body until approximately 5 years of age. As a result, young children are top heavy and prone to minor head injury from falls.

The lymph nodes are present at birth, but differentiation and growth of lymphatic tissue occurs primarily between ages 4 and 8 years. As such, preschoolers and school-age children often have "shotty" lymph nodes. Shotty nodes are noninfected, nontender, slightly enlarged lymph nodes that move when palpated and feel firmer than normal. Most children under 6 to 7 years have palpable, shotty femoral or cervical lymph nodes. Newborns and infants with a history of internal fetal monitoring during labor often have palpable occipital lymph nodes. Enlarged, noninfected tonsils are common in children ages 4 to 8.

The maxillary and ethmoid sinuses are present at birth, but they are proportionately smaller than in adults. The sphenoid sinuses develop before age 5 and the frontal sinuses by age 10. Children rarely have infections of the ethmoid sinuses. The frontal sinuses cause infection only in older school-age and adolescent children. Children under the age of 5 years often have

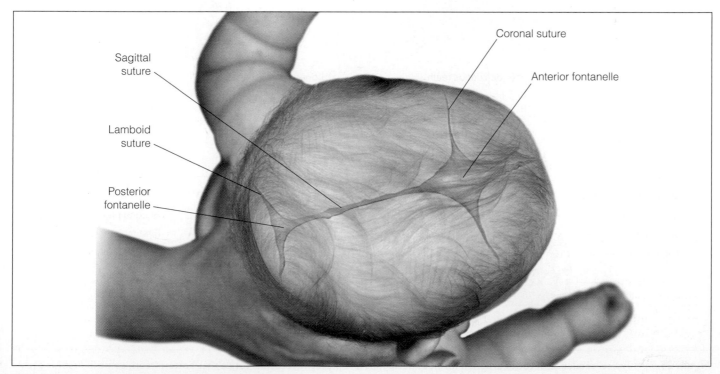

Sagittal suture

Coronal suture

Anterior fontanelle

Lamboid suture

Posterior fontanelle

Figure 25.3 ● Sutures and fontanelles of the skull.

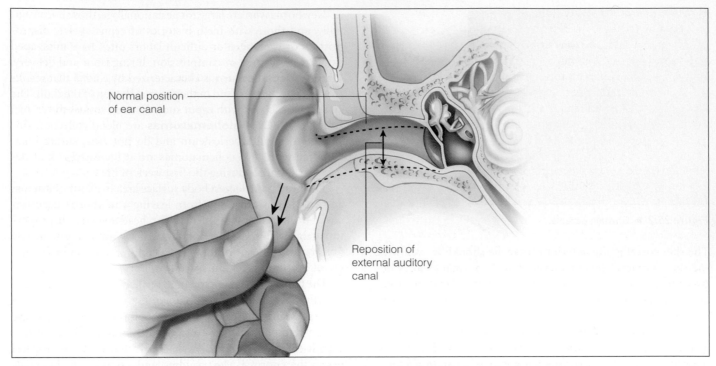

Figure 25.4 ● Positioning of external auditory canal for tympanic membrane visualization.

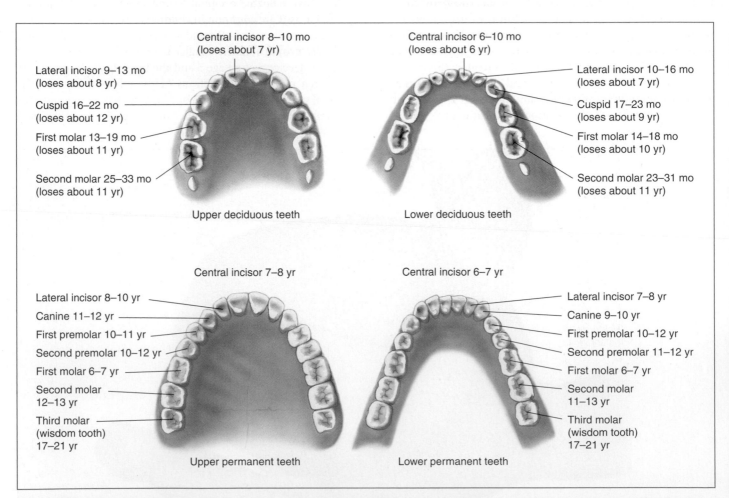

Figure 25.5 ● Typical sequence of tooth eruption for both deciduous and permanent teeth. Notice that bottom teeth come in first for each kind of tooth, incisors, cuspids, and molars.

yellow-green nasal discharge during upper respiratory infections because they cannot efficiently clear their nasal passages.

The external auditory canals of children are smaller and less straight than adults. The nurse should pull the earlobe down and back when examining the tympanic membrane with the otoscope of children under the age of 4 years as illustrated in Figure 25.4 ●. The eustachian tubes of infants, toddlers, and preschoolers are shorter, straighter, and more level than those in older children and adults. This normal variant, in combination with increased frequency of colds and respiratory infections, results in an increased incidence of **otitis media,** or middle ear infections, in children under the age of 4. The occurrence of otitis media peaks between 6 and 18 months of age. Children with middle ear infections typically present with fever, decreased appetite, irritability, and the inability to sleep lying down. The tympanic membrane appears opaque, bulging, and yellow-orange or red colored during otitis media episodes (see Figure 14.31 on page 334 ◯◯). The tympanic membrane is a vascular tissue that appears red with infection, fever, or any condition that results in skin flushing. Children with red tympanic membranes and no purulent discharge in the middle ear space do not have bacterial otitis media.

Teeth first erupt between 4 and 6 months of age. Normally, children lose their primary teeth, also known as baby teeth, in the order they erupt. There is no medical significance associated with the order of tooth eruption. As long as a child cuts the first tooth by 15 months of age, no further evaluation is necessary. Most children lose their first primary tooth by 7 years of age. Figure 25.5 ● shows a typical sequence of tooth eruption for both deciduous and permanent teeth.

Infants have shorter necks than older children and adults. The thyroid gland cannot be palpated until adolescence. Infants do not develop good head control until approximately 4 months of age. Most cases of meningitis occur in children under 3 years of age, but it is difficult to elicit Brudzinski's sign in young children because of their shorter necks (see Figure 25.6 ●). The nurse should promptly refer any child under the age of 2 years with high fever and altered neurologic signs for additional evaluation.

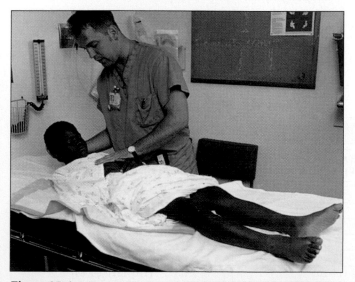

Figure 25.6 ● To test Brudzinski's sign, the nurse flexes the neck of the adolescent while in a supine position.

Babies can see at birth, but the visual acuity of newborns is not as sharp as adults. Children typically have 20/20 vision by the age of 7 years. Uncoordinated eye gaze is normal until 4 months of age. An infant who cannot focus on objects at birth needs further evaluation. A whitened red reflex occurs with congenital cataracts. Infants and preschool children with the cancer retinoblastoma often present a history of a diminished red reflex or a "white glow" in the pupil.

VITAL SIGNS

Accurate heart rates and respiratory rates must be taken for 1 minute. The nurse takes an apical pulse for children under 1 year of age. Infants have irregular breathing patterns characterized by frequent, brief rate accelerations or decelerations. This is a normal variant that disappears during the first few months of life. Blood pressure accuracy depends on the selection of an appropriate sized cuff. Blood pressure cuffs must be wide enough to cover at least 80 to 100% of the upper arm (from the acromion process to the olecranon process). The length of the blood pressure cuff should be large enough so that half of the circumference of the arm does not exceed 40% of the cuff's length, as shown in Figure 25.7 ●. If the cuff is too narrow, the reading will be falsely high. If the cuff is too wide, it will be falsely low. Blood pressure readings should be done with the child's arm supported at the heart level. The diastolic pressure is recorded as the point when the Korotkoff sounds disappear. See Table 25.2 for a listing of the normal childhood vital signs.

RESPIRATORY SYSTEM

Lung development is complete in healthy full-term newborns; however, there are significant differences between child and adult respiratory tracts. Infants have thinner, less muscular chest walls with a more noticeable xiphoid process. Breath sounds are louder and harsher. Referred sounds from the upper airways are common. The anterior-posterior chest diameter is approximately equal in infants, and the ribs appear more horizontal. Infants are obligate nose breathers until 6 months of age; they cannot breathe through their mouths. The nurse should carefully assess children under the age of 6 months with nasal congestion for signs of respiratory distress. Abdominal breathing is common until age 6 years. Thoracic breathing begins in the school-age years.

Children have smaller, more pliant airways until early adolescence. Until that time, children are more prone to airway collapse and blockage. Oxygen needs are higher in small children because their increased metabolic rates result in higher oxygen consumption. It is important to carefully assess and manage children who show signs of dyspnea and respiratory distress. The risk of respiratory failure is greatest in infants, toddlers, and preschoolers, but children of all ages experience respiratory failure much more quickly than adults.

ALERT!

Children are much more likely to die from respiratory failure than cardiovascular collapse. Any child with altered sensorium should be immediately evaluated for respiratory compromise.

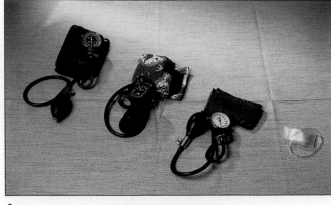

A

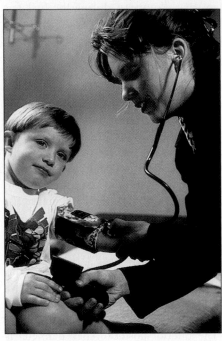

B

Figure 25.7 ● A. Blood pressure cuffs are available in various types and sizes for infants and children. B. Measuring blood pressure with an aneroid manometer.

Choanal atresia is a congenital defect that results in a thin membrane that obstructs the nasal passages. If undetected or untreated, severe respiratory distress results. All newborns must be carefully assessed for nasal patency. **Laryngomalacia** or **tracheomalacia** are congenital defects of the cartilage in the larynx and trachea, respectively. Infants with laryngo- or tracheomalacia have airways that easily collapse. Parents frequently describe children with laryngo/tracheomalacia as "noisy breathers." Continuous inspiratory and expiratory stridor that improves during the first year of life characterizes these abnormalities.

CARDIOVASCULAR SYSTEM

Prenatally, the blood shunts away from the heart and liver through the **ductus venosus,** the **ductus arteriosus,** and the **foramen ovale.** When newborns take their first breath, increased thoracic pressure closes these shunts, although the ductus venosus may remain open for 12 to 72 hours after birth. **Sinus arrhythmia,** also known as heart period variability, presents with heart rate increases during inspiration and decreases during expiration. This normal variant is common until early adulthood and results from parasympathetic enervation of the heart. Cardiac output is more dependent on heart rate than stroke volume in children. Therefore, bradycardia results in rapid decompensation and should be considered life threatening. Children in shock experience hypotension later than adults because the elasticity of a child's blood vessels is greater.

The thinner chest wall of children causes heart sounds to seem louder. Infants have a point of maximal impulse (PMI) that is difficult to assess and is located approximately one intercostal space higher than in adults. An S_2 split with inspiration may be detected in children under the age of 6. The physiological S_2 split disappears with expiration. Any S_2 split that persists throughout the cardiac cycle merits further evaluation. Preadolescents may have a physiological S_3 gallop that results from vibrations during rapid ventricular filling.

Seventy percent of children will have a detectable innocent, or functional, murmur sometime during childhood. Any condition that increases metabolism, like fever or anemia, will make innocent murmurs more pronounced. By definition, **innocent murmurs** arise from increased blood flow across normal heart structures. All innocent murmurs have the following characteristics: they are grade I–II/VI in intensity, are systolic (with the exception of the venous hum), and are not associated with thrills or other cardiac symptoms. See Table 25.3 for a description of the most common innocent murmurs.

A number of congenital cardiac defects occur in the newborn period. **Coarctation of the aorta** results in the narrowing of the aorta with decreased femoral pulses and bounding upper extremity pulses. Also noticeable are discrepancies in blood pressure and oxygen saturation between the up-

Table 25.2	Normal Childhood Vital Signs		
AGE	**HEART RATE (BEATS PER MIN)**	**RESPIRATORY RATE (BREATHS PER MIN)**	**BLOOD PRESSURE RANGE (95th PERCENTILE)**
Newborn	90–160	30–50	(60–90)/(40–60)
1–11 months	85–170	24–45	(94–104)/(50–60)
1–2 years	70–150	22–38	(98–109)/(56–63)
3–5 years	72–140	21–30	(100–115)/(59–71)
6–10 years	68–130	18–24	(105–123)/(67–80)
11–14 years	65–120	14–20	(110–131)/(64–84)
≥15 years	55–100	14–20	(113–130)/(50–84)

NAME	LOCATION	TIMING	CHARACTERISTICS
Venous hum	Upper left or right sternal borders near the clavicles	Continuous	Loudest in sitting position—disappears when child is supine. May also disappear with light pressure on jugular vein or when child turns his or her head to the side.
Still's murmur	Apex or left lower sternal border	Systolic ejection	Most common innocent murmur. May change with position changes.
Pulmonary flow	Pulmonic area or upper left sternal border	Systolic	Usually heard in newborns. Disappears with Valsalva's maneuver.

Table 25.3   Common Innocent Heart Murmurs

per and lower extremities. The nurse should carefully assess all infants and newborns for cardiac murmurs, altered pulse intensity, and cyanosis. It is important to promptly refer any child with suspected congenital heart disease.

ALERT!

Congestive heart failure (CHF) in infants may be the first sign of an acyanotic congenital heart defect. Common symptoms of CHF include sweating and fatigue while feeding, and frequent respiratory tract congestion.

BREASTS

Inverted nipples are evident at birth and common until adolescence. Because of circulating maternal estrogen and prolactin, male and female infants may have enlarged nipples and/or a milky white discharge from their nipples that is commonly called "witches' milk." This condition will resolve within 1 to 2 weeks after birth when maternal hormone levels decrease.

Thelarche, or breast budding, is often the first pubertal sign in females. Breast development follows a clear pattern described by the Tanner stages as illustrated in Figure 25.8 ●. **Gynecomastia** is the benign development of breast tissue in males and results in a tender, mobile knot under the areola in

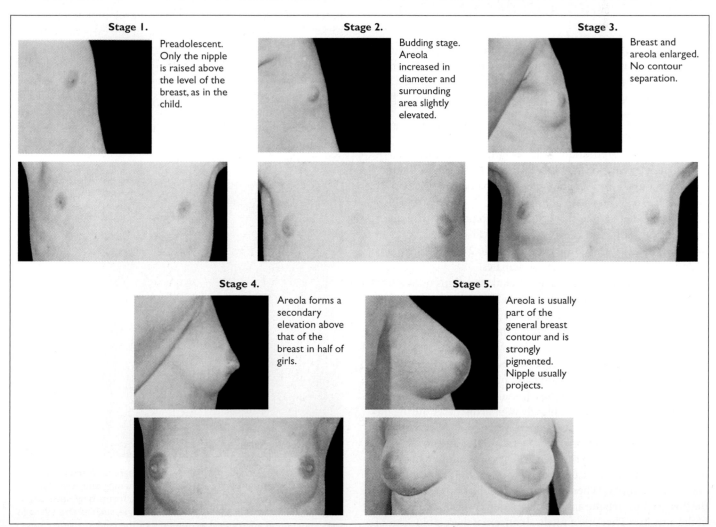

Stage 1.
Preadolescent. Only the nipple is raised above the level of the breast, as in the child.

Stage 2.
Budding stage. Areola increased in diameter and surrounding area slightly elevated.

Stage 3.
Breast and areola enlarged. No contour separation.

Stage 4.
Areola forms a secondary elevation above that of the breast in half of girls.

Stage 5.
Areola is usually part of the general breast contour and is strongly pigmented. Nipple usually projects.

Figure 25.8 ● Tanner stages of breast development.

as many as one third of adolescent males (see Figure 16.27 on page 419 ⚭). This condition is more common in overweight males and in teens who use performance-enhancing steroids.

ABDOMEN

Typically, the umbilical cord will dry and fall off within 3 weeks of birth. The liver edge may be palpable at the right lower costal margin because the thoracic cage of young children is smaller. Any liver edge palpable more than 2 cm below the costal margin indicates hepatomegaly and should be evaluated. **Umbilical hernias** cause a protrusion at the umbilicus and are visible at birth (see Figure 19.30 on page 547 ⚭). Umbilical hernias are common in children with African and Mediterranean heritage. More than 95% resolve spontaneously before 6 years of age. Umbilical hernias require no medical intervention since they do not incarcerate. Toddlers and infants have prominent abdomens that result in a potbelly appearance (see Figure 19.7 on page 518 ⚭). This variance diminishes by age 5 years. Infectious mononucleosis is most common in school-age children. Splenomegaly results in up to 25% of acute mononucleosis cases. Enlarged spleens are vulnerable to trauma because they no longer fit completely behind the thoracic cage. Careful abdominal assessment is indicated in any child with suspected mononucleosis.

GENITOURINARY AND REPRODUCTIVE SYSTEMS

Children do not have adult bladder capacities (approximately 700 ml) until adolescence. A quick way to estimate a child's bladder capacity is to use the following formula: the child's age (in years) plus or minus 2 oz. For example, a 4-year-old child has a bladder capacity of 2 to 6 oz:

$$\text{Age in years} \pm 2 \text{ oz} = 4 \pm 2 = 2 \text{ to } 6 \text{ oz}$$

On average, children attain bladder sphincter control at approximately 3 years for females and age 3 1/2 for males. Bladder training requires bladder sphincter control. Normal urine output for children is at least 2 ml/kg/hr.

Minimal genital growth occurs prior to puberty. The onset of genital development is expected by age 11 in females and 13 in males. Refer to the Tanner stages, Table 21.2, page 588, for males and Table 22.1, page 629 for females.

Uncircumcised males have unretractile foreskins until 2 to 3 years of age. **Cryptorchidism** is the failure of one or both testicles to descend through the inguinal canal during the final stages of fetal development. This condition is more common in premature infants and is detectable at birth. Males with undescended testicles should be referred for surgical evaluation by 6 months of age because there is an increased risk of testicular cancer in retained testicles, and spontaneous descent is rare after this age.

Infant females may have a bloody vaginal discharge during the first 2 weeks of life. This "false menses" is the result of exposure to maternal estrogen and progesterone. **Labial adhesions** occur when the labia minora fuse together. They are common in preadolescent females because decreased estrogen levels result in labial and genital atrophy. When present, labial adhesions extend from the posterior fourchette and look like a skin covering of all or part of the introitus. They are of medical concern if there is blockage of urinary flow or if they result in recurrent urinary tract infections.

MUSCULOSKELETAL SYSTEM

The human skeleton does not fully ossify until 18 years of age. As a result, most children's skeletons are more cartilaginous and structurally weaker than adults' skeletons. During trauma, preadolescent children are more likely to fracture a bone than injure a ligament, muscle, or tendon. Bone growth occurs at the **epiphyseal plates** located in the ends of the bones. Fractures of the epiphyseal plates can result in bone growth failure and limb length discrepancy. Muscular development increases with age and completes after puberty.

Genu varum, or bowlegs, is common until 1 or 2 years of age. Preschoolers and school-age children under 7 years of age are often knock-kneed, also known as **genu valgum** Both genu varum and genu valgum are normal findings in children from the age groups previously listed. Because of well-developed fat pads, children under the age of 2 years appear flatfooted.

Scoliosis is a lateral curvature of the lumbar or thoracic spine that is more common in children with neuromuscular deficits. Screening for scoliosis should begin by age 5 years and continue annually until after puberty because increases in height may worsen the spinal curvature. Figure 25.9 ● depicts a teenage girl with mild scoliosis.

Developmental dysplasia of the hip is a congenital disorder that results from inadequate development of the hip socket. This disorder often manifests in the early newborn period, but it may be noted anytime under 2 years of age.

Muscular dystrophy is an X-linked genetic disorder that results in progressive loss of muscle function. Males are affected four times more likely than females. Both smooth and skeletal muscles are affected. The first signs of muscular dystrophy are often noted around age 3 when a child shows muscle weakness and impaired gait.

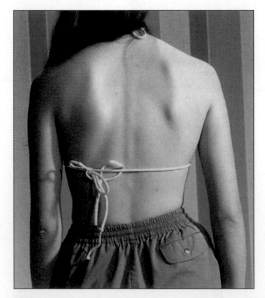

Figure 25.9 ● A child may have varying degrees of scoliosis. For mild forms, treatment will focus on strengthening and stretching. Moderate forms will require bracing. Severe forms may necessitate surgery and fusion. Clothes that fit at an angle, such as this teenage girl's shorts, and anatomical asymmetry of the back provide clues for early detection.

NEUROLOGIC SYSTEM

Myelin is a fatty substance that covers the neurons of the brain and spinal cord. Myelin speeds nerve impulse conduction. The myelin sheath grows until 2 to 3 years of age. Infants have a number of primitive reflexes that gradually disappear as the brain matures (see Table 25.4). Developmental milestones are

Table 25.4	Primitive Reflexes of Early Childhood		
REFLEX	**HOW TO ELICIT**	**AGE WHEN DISAPPEARS**	**EXAMPLE**
Tonic Neck	Turn the infant's head to one side while the infant is supine. The infant will extend the arms and legs on the side the head is turned to while flexing the opposite arm and leg.	2 to 6 months	Tonic neck
Palmar Grasp	Infant will grasp fingers or objects placed in the palm of the hand.	3 to 4 months	Palmar grasp
Plantar Grasp	Infant will curl toes when the base of the toes is touched.	6 to 8 months	Plantar grasp

(continued)

Table 25.4	Primitive Reflexes of Early Childhood *(continued)*		
REFLEX	**HOW TO ELICIT**	**AGE WHEN DISAPPEARS**	**EXAMPLE**
Moro (startle)	Infant will extend the arms with the fingers spread and flex the legs with loud sounds or if the infant's body drops suddenly.	4 to 6 months	Moro
Rooting	Lightly stroke the infant's cheek. Infant will turn the head with the mouth open toward the stroked side.	3 to 4 months	
Stepping	Infant will flex the leg and take steps if the the infant is upright with the feet touching a surface.	4 to 5 months	Stepping
Babinski	Gently stroke the plantar surface of the foot from heel to toe. Infants will extend and fan the toes and flex the foot.	18 to 24 months	Babinski

Table 25.5	Major Developmental Milestones of Childhood
MILESTONE	**AGE ATTAINED**
Visually tracks objects	Birth to 2 months
Smiles socially	2 months
Places objects in mouth	3 to 4 months
Babbles and coos	4 months
Extends forearms to support upper body when prone	4 to 5 months
Rolls from front to back	4 to 5 months
Rolls from back to front	5 to 6 months
Sits with support	6 to 7 months
Transfers objects from one hand to another	6 to 7 months
Sits without support	7 to 8 months
Supports weight when stands	7 to 8 months
Pulls self to standing position	8 months
Creeps or crawls	8 to 9 months
Attains pincer grasp	9 months
Cruises (walks holding on to furniture/objects)	9 to 10 months
Plays "peekaboo" and "pat-a-cake"	10 months
Says one word	11 months
Walks independently	12 to 15 months
Runs/climbs	14 to 18 months
Goes up and down stairs two feet per step	2 years
Goes up and down stairs alternating feet	3 years
Pedals tricycle	3 years
Copies circle	3 years
Prints name	5 years

Table 25.6	Sleep Requirements for Children and Adolescents	
AGE	**AVERAGE HOURS OF SLEEP PER 24 HOURS**	
Newborn	16	
3 months	15	
12 months	13.5	
2 years	11.5	
6 years	9.5	
12 years	11.5	

related to brain development. As a general rule, children acquire and refine gross motor skills before fine motor skills. Table 25.5 lists the major developmental milestones of childhood. Children require more sleep than adults. Table 25.6 lists the normal sleep requirements for infants and children.

SPECIAL CONSIDERATIONS

The nurse must consider the psychosocial and cultural factors that impact the health of infants, children, and adolescents. These are described in the following sections.

PSYCHOSOCIAL CONSIDERATIONS

Children and adults have different understandings of health and illness. It is common for children to believe they are ill because of bad thoughts or behaviors. The belief that illness is a punishment for wrongdoing is common. Young children cannot identify or modify health risks. Children do not have the cognitive ability to understand cause and effect relationships until late school age or early adolescent. Parents and guardians function as proxies for their children in most healthcare decisions.

Nurses should use a caring, supportive, yet firm approach with children. Whenever possible, play should be incorporated into nursing procedures. It is helpful to allow children to touch and manipulate equipment. Adhesive bandages or empty syringes can be provided for playacting with dolls. The nurse should encourage children to talk about their fears and concerns. Painful procedures should not be performed while a child is seated on a parent's lap. Children need to know they are safe from painful experiences when they are with their parents.

When a child is ill, parents suffer from increased stress that results from interrupted sleep, concern for the child's well-being, and frustration at the inability to understand what is hurting or bothering their child. Each of these factors may impact a parent's ability to recall information or to follow complex instructions. Nurses should consider parental stress levels when developing care plans.

CULTURAL CONSIDERATIONS

Most of the world's cultures value children. However, there is significant variation between cultures with respect to what constitutes acceptable child behavior and expectations for health or caregiving. Nurses must be aware of the cultural influences on children and families. For example, European cultures encourage independence at an early age whereas other groups, such as Asians, Hispanics, and Arab Americans, stress a strong commitment to family. Commonly, children from these cultural groups are taught to respect elder family members and to place the needs of the family before their personal needs. Hispanics and Native Americans tend to be very permissive with their children, especially with male children.

All of the dominant American cultures view mothers as the primary child caregivers. Overall, females are viewed as nurturers who are responsible for guiding and caring for children. It is common for mothers to make the decisions regarding home care of child illness and complaints. However, many groups, including Arab Americans, have patriarchal hierarchies where the father must be consulted prior to any professional healthcare decisions.

Many cultures have taboos against physical assessment of postpubertal children by healthcare providers of different genders. The nurse must identify and respect privacy, modesty, and cultural issues of the individual.

Cultural Considerations

African American

- Newborns may have pustular melanosis, characterized by pustules that rupture to leave 2- to 3-mm brown macules. These brown marks will disappear spontaneously within 3 to 4 months.
- Hair texture will become coarser with tighter curls over the first 6 months of life.
- Mongolian spots are commonly located over the lower back and buttocks; they will begin to fade by age 2 or 3.
- Infants should be tested for sickle cell anemia at birth.
- Most are born with dark gray-brown eyes that will not change much as the baby gets older.
- Hypertension and insulin-resistant diabetes are more common in African American youth.

Asian

- As a sign of respect, many Asian parents may be reluctant to disagree with or displease a healthcare provider.
- Direct eye contact may be viewed as impolite.
- Mongolian spots are common.
- Most infants have dark gray eye color at birth.
- Vietnamese families believe the head is sacred. The nurse should avoid touching the head of the mother and baby without first asking permission.
- Chinese practice cupping, where a heated cup is placed over the skin to draw out illness. Vietnamese use coin rubbing, where a coin is rubbed on the trunk. Neither practice should be considered abuse.
- Many Asian families use the concept of hot and cold illnesses. Certain illnesses are considered to be hot or cold, and treatments should counter the effect of the illness. Therefore, hot illnesses should be treated with cold medicines and foods, whereas cold illnesses should be treated with hot medicines and foods.

Hispanic

- Most infants have dark gray-brown eye color at birth.
- Mongolian spots are common.
- Infants should be tested for sickle cell anemia at birth.
- Many Mexican Americans consider it bad luck for a person to touch a child's head.

- Many Hispanic families use the concept of hot and cold illnesses. Certain illnesses are considered to be hot or cold, and treatments should counter the effect of the illness. Therefore, hot illnesses should be treated with cold medicines and foods, whereas cold illnesses should be treated with hot medicines and foods.
- Modesty may be important and should be respected.
- Some groups believe that complimenting a child without touching him or her can cause the "evil eye."
- Many consider fat to be healthy, especially in women and young children.

Native American

- Many Native Americans have strong beliefs that children should be allowed to develop at their own rate. Parents may be reluctant to force a child to stop bottle or pacifier use or to start toilet training.
- Mongolian spots are common.
- Hypothyroidism is more common in Native Americans (1 in 700). Newborn testing and vigilance for symptoms of hypothyroidism are recommended.
- It is taboo to purchase any clothing or items for the newborn prior to birth. This varies from the Western culture.
- Hypertension and insulin-resistant diabetes are more common in Native American youth.
- Direct eye contact may be avoided as a sign of respect.

Middle Eastern

- Direct eye contact may be viewed as impolite or improper, especially with members of the opposite sex.
- Physical examination by individuals of different gender is taboo after adolescence.
- Thalassemias are more common in children of Middle Eastern heritage than in children of European descent.
- Modesty may be important and should be respected.
- Females may defer to the male head of the family for healthcare decisions.

All Races and Cultures

- Babies within all races and cultures are born with lighter, pinker skin. The true color of the baby will develop over the first year.
- All cultures and ethnic groups have folk beliefs that center around childbirth and child rearing. The nurse should assess for positive folk practices and incorporate them into nursing care.

Gathering the Data

The basic components of a health history are the same whether the nurse works with children or adults. However, a number of variations must be incorporated into the pediatric health history. This section focuses on the unique issues involved in taking the history of a child.

It is essential that the nurse determine the relationship between the child who seeks healthcare and the adult who presents with the child. One must never assume legal or family ties between children and adults who accompany them. Nannies, babysitters, friends, siblings, and stepparents often transport children to healthcare appointments. State law determines which individuals can legally consent to medical treatment of a minor child. Federal privacy laws limit access to protected health information. Direct questions of relationships is the easiest way to ensure compliance with the legal and ethical concerns regarding the medical treatment of children.

FOCUSED INTERVIEW

Many children are nonverbal or possess limited language ability; therefore, nurses depend on parents and guardians for health history information. This can limit the specificity of the history information. However, it is important to ask preschoolers and older children about their chief complaint and symptoms even though the information they provide may not be as detailed as the information provided by their parents or guardians. This chapter uses the word *parent* to represent parents, caregivers, or guardians.

The nurse should determine if the parent is stressed or distracted prior to the health interview. Many parents of ill children are sleep deprived because of their child's altered sleep patterns. Sleep deprivation can result in altered recall, limited ability to follow complex questions, and diminished ability to remember verbal instructions. The presence of other children can be distracting, especially if the children are loud, active, or irritable. Nurses can distract energetic or fussy children with books, crayons, or toys.

The nurse should listen carefully to the parent and use openended questions to elicit health information. Parents know their children better than anyone else. They are able to detect subtle differences in their child's behavior. It is essential to pay special attention to the chief complaints that parents provide. A thorough physical assessment is based on the issues and concerns raised in the health history.

The nurse should call the child by his or her name and use words that the child understands. For example, most preadolescents are not familiar with the word *abdomen*, but most children use the word *tummy* or *belly* from infancy. Instead of asking "Does your head hurt?" the nurse should ask the child to touch the head where it hurts. It is necessary to be patient. Children often pause between words or repeat phrases when they are excited or nervous.

Children who are at least 10 years old should be given the option of being examined without their parents present. The client is the child, not the parent. The nurse's legal and ethical responsibility is to the child first. The nurse must respect the confidentiality of the information provided by older children and be aware of state and federal laws regarding parental notification. The parent and the child should be told what the nurse can and cannot keep confidential. For example, statements like "What you and I talk about will be between the two of us, unless you tell me that you are thinking about harming yourself or someone else, or if you tell me that someone is hurting you" help establish rapport and boundaries to the nurse-child and nurse-parent relationship. If a nurse is required to report health interview information to others (e.g., public health departments or child protective service agents), the nurse should always inform the child of the need to share the information with others prior to actually doing so. Failure to do so can jeopardize the rapport between nurse and child.

FOCUSED INTERVIEW QUESTIONS	RATIONALES

The following section provides sample questions and bulleted follow-up questions. A rationale for each question is provided. The list of questions is not all-inclusive, but rather represents the types of questions required in a comprehensive focused interview related to the neurologic system. As these questions are asked, the subjective data obtained helps to identify client strengths or risks associated with the neurologic system described in Healthy People 2010.

QUESTIONS ABOUT THE BIRTH HISTORY

All children under 6 years of age, children with congenital defects, and children who have developmental or neurologic delays require a documented birth history. The birth history includes the following questions:

1. *For the mother of the child:*
   - Did you have prenatal care?
   - How much weight did you gain during the pregnancy?
   - Were there any complications during the pregnancy?
   - Were you ill during the pregnancy?
   - Did you use any medications, alcohol, drugs, or herbal/complementary medicines during pregnancy?

▶ Poor or absent prenatal care is associated with an increased risk of developmental delay and neurologic conditions. Exposure to **teratogens** (substances known to cause birth defects) is associated with genetic defects, congenital abnormalities, and physical and mental syndromes, especially when the exposure occurs during the first trimester of pregnancy. Most of the organ systems develop during the third to eighth week of pregnancy. Exposure to teratogens is especially worrisome when it occurs during this gestational period. Maternal illness can impact embryonic/fetal development during any gestational age. The nurse should note infectious diseases and illnesses that cause high fevers or alter placental blood flow.

FOCUSED INTERVIEW QUESTIONS	RATIONALES
2. How was your labor and delivery? What was your child's due date?	▶ Premature and postmature infants have an increased risk of hypoglycemia. Pregnancies that last at least 37 weeks are considered full term. The nurse should determine the child's birth weight and Apgar scores. Very low birth weight is correlated with negative health outcomes of prematurity such as significant respiratory complications and neurologic deficits. It is important to note the type of delivery (vaginal versus cesarean section). If the child was born by cesarean section, the nurse should ask why the cesarean was performed. The nurse should also ask if the child was admitted to the regular nursery, the special care nursery, or the intensive care unit. Cerebral palsy and other developmental disorders occur more often in children with traumatic birth histories.
3. How did your child do after the birth? • How are you doing with the changes since the baby was born? • How did your husband or partner, parents, siblings, and family members adapt to the new baby?	▶ The nurse should determine if the child needed medical care to assist with feeding, breathing, and so on. The nurse also asks about hearing and vision problems. Did the child receive medications associated with ototoxicity (like vancomycin or gentamicin): Untreated or complicated neonatal jaundice can result in neurologic damage. Separation, illness (maternal or infant), or stress often impact early parental-child attachment. Pediatric nurses and physicians often notice postpartum depression.
4. Is there anything else about the pregnancy, labor, or delivery that you think I should know about?	▶ This question allows parents to add information they feel is pertinent but that they perceived was not covered by the preceding questions.

QUESTIONS RELATED TO ILLNESS OR INFECTION

1. What brings you here today? • How long has the child been ill? • What symptoms does the child have and how have they changed since the beginning of the illness? • Follow-up questions should include timing of the symptoms (day vs. night, at rest vs. when playing), activity levels, effect on the child's appetite and temperament, and whether symptoms disrupt the child's sleep. The nurse should ask verbal children why they are there. • Do the child's symptoms happen during the day, at night, or both? • What is the child's activity level like? • How is the child eating? • How is the child drinking? • Does the child seem crabbier than usual? • Is the child having a hard time sleeping because of the symptoms?	▶ These questions establish the chief complaint and the history of the present illness. ▶ Commonly, small children will complain of a "tummy ache" or "my throat hurts" while parents may be concerned about fussiness or altered sleep patterns. Postnasal drip causes cough that worsens with activity, when arising from bed, or when supine. Preadolescent children will complain of stomach pain when they are gassy, if they are nauseated, or if they actually feel abdominal pain. Children with sore throats often present with a history of normal fluid intake but decreased solid food intake. Anxious or frightened preschool and school-age children may complain of headache or stomachache.
2. Has the child been exposed to other people with the same symptoms?	▶ The nurse should determine if the child attends day care or group babysitting and the number of hours per week. *This helps to identify the origin of infectious diseases.*

FOCUSED INTERVIEW QUESTIONS

RATIONALES

3. **Have you given your child any medicines?**
   - If so, what medicines, what doses, and what frequency?
   - Do you use herbal or complementary medicine?

► Many parents do not think it is important to inform nurses about over-the-counter and herbal preparations since they are readily available. There is limited data on the safety of herbal and complementary medicine in children.

QUESTIONS RELATED TO WELL CHILDREN AND HEALTH PROMOTION

1. **How is the child doing?**
   - Do you have concerns about the child's hearing, vision, physical development, or speech?

► These questions help to identify parental concerns and expectations. Parents often compare their child's abilities to those of other children. They may have unrealistic expectations related to inappropriate age comparisons or incorrect understanding of normal child development. Parents may notice subtle, developmental differences that are difficult to assess in clinical settings.

2. **How does the child do in school?**
   - Does the child seem to make friends and get along with other children?

► This is an easy way to get an overall sense of social and cognitive functioning in an older child.

3. **Does the child play sports?**
   - What types of activities does the child like to do? Does the child like to eat foods from all of the food groups (dairy, fruits, vegetables, meats, and grains)?
   - How much milk, soda, and tea does the child drink?
   - How often does the child eat fast food?
   - What types of beverages does the child drink?
   - How much juice, milk, tea, or soda does the child drink every day?

► These items help identify children at risk for nutritional deficiencies and health problems related to inactivity.

4. **For adolescent children, the nurse should ask about sexual activity (including age of first activity and risky sexual behavior), and tobacco, drug, and alcohol use.**

► Adolescence is a time of experimentation and limit testing. Initial drug, alcohol, and substance use often occurs before age 21. Many adolescents are sexually active, have multiple sexual partners, or do not consistently use birth control or protection against sexually transmitted disease. Most adolescents will not disclose information regarding these topics unless they are specifically questioned about these behaviors.

CLIENT INTERACTION

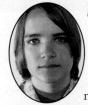

INTERVIEW

Jay Cole is a 15-year-old male who presents to the clinic with a complaint of a breast mass. He has a family history of breast cancer in his 63-year-old maternal grandmother, and his mother is anxious about his recent breast development. Jay's weight is 220 lb and he is 5'11" tall. Jay is quiet and appears withdrawn. When the nurse places him in the examination room, his mother comes along and starts to describe Jay's complaints.

Nurse: Hi. My name is Ms. Wallace and I am your nurse today. How are you today, Jay?

Jay's mother: Hi! We are so concerned about Jay!

Nurse: Jay, I need you to take your shirt off so that I can examine your chest. I have a gown that you can put on.

Jay: Does my mom have to stay in here? I am kind of embarrassed to have her here.

Jay's mother: Why would you be embarrassed? It isn't like I haven't seen your chest before, But, I will wait outside. We are very worried about him. His breasts started growing about 2 months ago and the problem keeps getting worse. Jay, I will be right outside if you change your mind.

Nurse: Jay, do you want to get into the gown now or after we talk? I'll leave the room then and you can get ready in private.

Jay: Thanks.

Jay changes into the gown and the nurse reenters the room.

Nurse: So Jay, I see it says here that you have a breast lump. Tell me about that.

Jay (avoiding eye contact): My chest is growing and it almost looks as bad as a girl's. And my mom is totally freaked about it because my grandmother died of breast cancer and she thinks this is cancer too.

Nurse: When did you first notice this?

Jay: About 2 months ago after I started at the gym.

Nurse: Do you think you have breast cancer?

Jay: No, I don't. But I am worried that I am going to stay like this. And, it hurts some when I touch my breasts.

Nurse: Does it only hurt when you touch them?

Jay: Yes, it only hurts when I touch them.

Nurse: Are there any other symptoms or problems?

Jay: No.

Nurse: Are you taking any medicines right now?

Jay: Um . . . well nothing regular. Are you going to tell my mom what we talk about?

Nurse: Jay, you need to be honest with me so we can help you. Unless you tell me you are thinking about hurting yourself or someone else, or if someone is hurting you, our conversation is between you and me.

Jay: Well this guy at the gym gave me some medicine that he said would help me get more muscles and lose weight faster. He said it isn't bad because it is a prescription medicine. He was just saving me the trouble of getting it from here.

Nurse: What is the name of the medicine?

Jay: I don't know. It's a shot I use once a week.

Nurse: So you inject this medicine?

Jay: Yes, but I use clean needles and I don't share with anyone. I don't want to get sick, just get a better body.

Nurse: Thanks for being honest with me. I won't ask anything else unless you have something else to add.

Jay: Nope.

ANALYSIS

The start of the clinical interaction went well when the nurse introduced herself to Jay. However, she did not introduce herself to the mother. Also, the mother did not allow Jay to answer the questions the nurse asked. Once the mother left the room, Jay was more open to communication. The nurse used appropriate strategies to elicit health information, including use of open-ended statements and respect for client confidentiality and privacy.

Please refer to the Companion Website at **www.prenhall.com/damico** and click on Chapter 25, the **Client Interaction** module, to answer questions about this case. In addition, see other resources for this chapter including NCLEX review questions and other interactive exercises and materials.

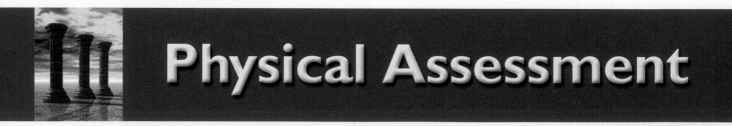

Physical Assessment

The skills and equipment needed to assess a child are the same as those needed for adult physical assessment. This section focuses on physical assessment techniques that are unique to pediatric clients. Refer to the previous text chapters for greater system-specific details.

ASSESSMENT TECHNIQUES AND FINDINGS

There are many ways to make the examination fun. Children should be allowed to touch equipment. For example, the nurse can ask a young child to put the otoscope's "hat" (i.e., speculum) on the light. Before examining the tympanic membrane, the nurse can ask toddlers and preschoolers if they have elephants or cartoon characters in their ear. Young children can be encouraged to take deep breaths by having them blow bubbles or blow out the light on the otoscope. Toys can be used to distract children. Examples include finger puppets, small animals placed on the stethoscope, and whistles or small music boxes. It is important to keep toys with small pieces out of the reach of infants, toddlers, and preschoolers.

HELPFUL HINTS

- Children have the same needs as adults to protect their modesty and privacy.
- Explain procedures and techniques in words that are understandable for children.
- Young children are more comfortable and compliant when they sit on their parents' laps.
- Establish rapport with the parent and child before initiating any physical examination.
- A flexible approach to assessment is essential. Begin with the least threatening examinations.
- Keep painful or invasive procedures at the end of the assessment.
- Auscultate the thorax of the sleeping child.
- Allow children to touch equipment. Use games for examinations, such as asking children if they have elephants in their ears before examining the tympanic membrane.
- Use toys, for example, finger puppets, as distractions.
- Use Standard Precautions.

TECHNIQUES AND NORMAL FINDINGS	ABNORMAL FINDINGS SPECIAL CONSIDERATIONS

GENERAL SURVEY

Observe the child's interaction with the adults present. How does the child react to them? If the child is ill, is he or she consolable? How comfortably do the adults interact with the child? Does the child's development match the chronological age? Assess the child's vital signs.

▶ Poor eye contact between child and adult may indicate impaired attachment. Seriously ill and septic children are often irritable and inconsolable.

GROWTH AND DEVELOPMENT

1. **Obtain accurate height and weight.**

    - Measure the recumbent length of children under 2 years old. Have the child lie supine on the examination table. Hold the child's leg straight with the hips and knees extended. Mark and measure the distance between the heel and the top of the head as shown in Figure 25.10 ●. Make sure the child is flat during the measurement. Plot recumbent length on the growth charts for children between birth and 36 months of age.

▶ Assess for height and weight discrepancies. Height and weight should be within one standard deviation of each other. For example, a child whose height is at the 50th percentile should weigh between the 25th and 75th percentile. Reduced height velocity may indicate endocrine deficiencies or chronic renal disease. Poor weight gain may indicate nutritional deficiency, impaired parental-infant interaction, or chronic congestive heart disease. Overweight and obese children have increased risk of developing type 2 diabetes and acquired cardiovascular disease.

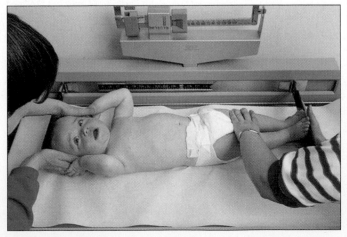

Figure 25.10 ●
Nurse taking a recumbent height of a toddler.

TECHNIQUES AND NORMAL FINDINGS

- Obtain a standing height for children older than 2 years. (*Note:* Some children between 24 and 36 months of age will not be able to stand still long enough to get an accurate reading. Recumbent height is better in this situation.) Make sure the child's heels are flat against the wall. Use a stadiometer for the highest accuracy. Plot standing heights on growth charts for children between 2 and 18 years of age.

- Use an infant scale to weigh children under 2 years. Infants and toddlers should be naked except for a clean, dry diaper. Use a robe for preschoolers, school-age children, and adolescents. *Note:* A single height or weight measurement cannot be used to determine insufficient growth patterns. Children with a body mass index (BMI) less than the 5th percentile for age are underweight. Children with a BMI greater than the 95th percentile for their age are overweight.

2. **Measure head circumference for children under 2 years old.**

   - Hold the measuring tape taut against the child's skull from the forehead (just above the eyebrows) across the parietal region, and over the occipital prominence. Plot the measurement on the growth chart as shown in Figure 25.11 ●.

▶ Any child whose head circumference is below the 5th percentile has **microcephaly**. Microcephaly may be caused by genetic disorders or intrauterine exposure to cocaine or alcohol. Any child whose head circumference is above the 95th percentile has **macrocephaly**. Macrocephaly is associated with hydrocephalus, brain tumor, and increased intracranial pressure. Any child with microcephaly, with macrocephaly, or who has greater than 1 standard deviation change in head circumference percentile should be referred for medical evaluation.

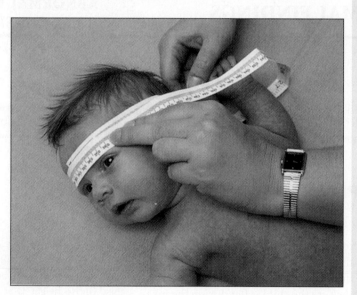

Figure 25.11 ●
Head circumference landmarks.

TECHNIQUES AND NORMAL FINDINGS	ABNORMAL FINDINGS SPECIAL CONSIDERATIONS

SKIN, HAIR, AND NAILS

1. **Inspect the skin for color and the presence of lesions, birthmarks, or discolorations.**
   - Use a measuring tape to determine the exact size of lesions and birthmarks. Carefully document the appearance, distribution, and characteristics of all skin lesions. Cyanosis is best detected by inspecting the mucous membranes. Detect jaundice by inspecting the sclera or by noting a yellow undertone after skin blanching.

▶ Contact diaper rashes occur on the skin surfaces that touch the diaper and typically do not involve the skin folds. Diaper rashes caused by *Candida albicans* are characterized by beefy erythema that concentrates in the intertriginous folds and have small red satellite lesions along the rash margins.

▶ Strawberry hemangiomas initially present during the first few weeks after birth as red macules that blanch with pressure and grow into spongy, vascular nodules. Strawberry hemangiomas grow until approximately 1 year of age and spontaneously resolve by age 9.

▶ Mongolian spots are blue-black patches that are most common at the base of the spine in African American, Hispanic, and Asian infants (refer to Figure 11.4 on page 186 ⬭).

▶ Acne vulgaris appears on the face, neck, upper back, upper chest, and upper arms of preadolescents and adolescents.

▶ Newborn jaundice that appears within 24 hours of birth, in children with maternal ABO/Rh incompatibility, or that persists more than 2 to 3 weeks after birth must be carefully evaluated because of the increased risk of significant complications and underlying disease.

▶ The presence of more than five café au lait lesions may indicate neurofibromatosis. Viral exanthems are morbilliform rashes common in preschool children.

▶ The classic viral exanthem is a nonpruritic, erythematous, macular rash that worsens with skin flushing, coalesces to give a lacy appearance, begins on the trunk and spreads to the extremities, and blanches with light pressure.

2. **Inspect the hair and nails for texture, distribution, and moisture.**
   - Infants who cannot sit upright independently may have areas of friction alopecia on the occiput caused by rubbing and friction. Newborns have thin, brittle nails.

▶ Nail clubbing indicates chronic hypoxemia. Growth of pubic hair, facial hair, and axillary hair in a prepubescent child indicates endocrinologic disease. Areas of alopecia with hair follicle breakage at the skin level characterize tinea capitis, also known as scalp ringworm.

HEAD AND NECK

1. **Inspect and palpate the skull for the presence of deformity.**
   - The scalp should be smooth, intact, round, smooth, and free of lesions. Fontanelles and sutures, if present, should be smooth and flat.

▶ Premature closure of the cranial sutures causes craniosynostosis, a condition characterized by abnormal skull flattening and altered brain growth (see Figure 12.17 on page 254 ⬭). Birth trauma may result in cephalohematoma or caput succedaneum.

TECHNIQUES AND NORMAL FINDINGS	ABNORMAL FINDINGS SPECIAL CONSIDERATIONS

2. Palpate the lymph nodes of the head and neck.

- Assess the lymph nodes of the head and neck in the same order as the adult. Before the exam, ask young children if they have "tickles" in their neck. Shotty lymph nodes are a normal variant in preschoolers and school-age children. Shotty nodes are noninfected, nontender, slightly enlarged lymph nodes that move when palpated and feel firmer than normal. Most children under 6 to 7 years old have palpable, shotty femoral or cervical lymph nodes. Enlarged, non-infected tonsils are common in 4- to 8-year-old children.

▶ Anterior cervical and tonsillar lymphadenopathies are common in children with upper respiratory tract infection. Newborns and infants with a history of internal fetal monitoring during labor often have palpable occipital lymph nodes. Mononucleosis causes lymphadenitis of the anterior and posterior cervical chains.

EYES AND VISION

1. Inspect the eyes for symmetry, position, and movement.

- Note the position of the eyes in relation to the upper margin of the external ear. Normally, the outer canthus of the eye will be even with or slightly higher than the upper margin of the ear. Both eyes should be approximately the same size and shape. Note the presence of discharge, lesions, or edema.

- Nonconvergent strabismus is normal in children under 2 months of age. Assess for esotropia (inward gaze) and exotropia (outward gaze) with the corneal light reflection test and the cover-uncover test. Figure 25.12 ● illustrates normal and abnormal corneal light refraction. Elicit the corneal light reflection by standing about 2 ft in front of the child; ask the child to look at you while you shine the light from the otoscope in his or her eye. The light reflection should be in the same position, slightly medial to the center of the pupil, in both eyes. Asymmetry of the light reflexes indicates eye deviation. To perform the cover-uncover test, have the child stare at an object approximately 3 ft in from of him or her. Cover one eye with your hand for at least 10 seconds. Remove your hand and determine the presence of eye movement.

▶ Low-set ears are associated with various genetic disorders including Down syndrome. *Dacryostenosis* is the congenital blockage of the tear ducts and is a normal variant until 9 months of age. Children older than 9 months who have symptoms of dacryostenosis should be referred to ophthalmology for evaluation. It presents with unilateral increased tearing and nonpurulent crusting. Refer children older than 3 months with strabismus for ophthalmologic evaluation. Esotropia causes the covered eye to move inward (medially), and exotropia causes the covered eye to move outward (laterally) during the cover-uncover test. Periorbital cellulitis is a fast-progressing, serious bacterial infection of the periorbital tissues. Carefully assess all children with edema and erythema of the eye for fever, altered ocular movement, and lymphadenitis.

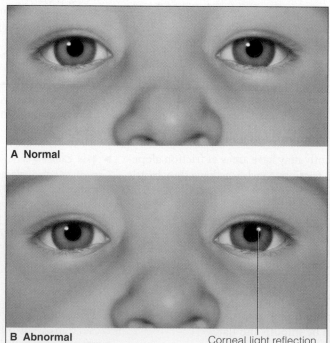

Figure 25.12 ● Normal and abnormal corneal light reflection test.

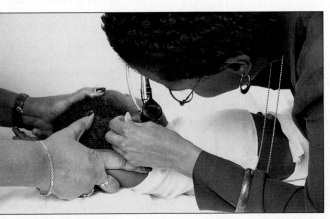

TECHNIQUES AND NORMAL FINDINGS

**ABNORMAL FINDINGS
SPECIAL CONSIDERATIONS**

2. **Assess the inner eye structures.**
   - Assess the red reflex. Inspect the cornea for translucency. The pupils should be equally round and reactive to light accommodation.

   ▶ An absent or "white glow" red reflex may indicate the presence of a retinoblastoma. Congenital cataracts cause the cornea to appear hazy.

3. **Assess vision.**
   - Use modified Snellen charts to assess the vision of children older than 3 to 4 years. Assess the ability to track objects with a blinking light made by rapidly moving your finger in front of the otoscope light. Normal newborns visually track moving objects. Chapter 13 of this text provides a thorough discussion of the eye. ⚭

EARS AND HEARING

1. **Assess the outer ear.**
   - Inspect and palpate the auricle. Note the presence of lesions and nodules. Assess ear position. Determine patency of the external auditory canal.

   ▶ Small, abnormally shaped and low-set ears occur with many genetic syndromes and renal malformations. *Mastoiditis,* and acute infection of the mastoid bone, causes the external ear to protrude forward. Preschoolers frequently insert foreign objects, like beads or rocks, in the external auditory canal.

2. **Inspect the auditory and canal and tympanic membrane.**
   - Restrain young or uncooperative children (see Figure 25.13 ●). Young children have more narrow auditory canals that angle downward. To assess the tympanic membrane of children under the age of 4 years, pull the tragus of the external ear down and back. Carefully insert the speculum of the otoscope into the ear following the curve of the auditory canal. Assess the tympanic membrane for the following: color, opacity, mobility, position, and the presence of fluid or other abnormal findings. Use a speculum that fits tightly into the ear canal and gently press the bulb insufflator to assess tympanic membrane mobility. Look for dimpling, or inward movement, of the tympanic membrane lateral to the umbo. Normal tympanic membranes are pearly-gray, transparent, mobile, and neutrally positioned. The tympanic membrane is a vascular organ; it will redden with conditions that cause flushing (fever, crying, etc.).

   ▶ Reddening of the tympanic membrane, in the absence of purulent discharge, does not indicate the presence of middle ear infection. Otitis media causes full, orange-yellow colored tympanic membranes with decreased motility. Otitis media with effusion, or serous otitis media, is the presence of nonpurulent fluid in the middle ear space caused by edema of the eustachian tubes. Otitis media with effusion results in tympanic membranes that are amber-colored, immobile, and in neutral to full positions. Figure 14.31 on page 334 depicts otitis media. ⚭ Otitis externa, or "swimmer's ear," results in pain with pinna manipulation and erythematous, edematous ear canals with or without purulent discharge. Figure 14.30 on page 333 shows otitis externa. ⚭

Figure 25.13 ●
Parent restraint of a young child during examination of the ear.

3. **Assess hearing.**
   - Use standardized hearing tests for children older than 4 years. Assess infants for the startle reflex or blinking with loud noises. To assess hearing in preschoolers, stand approximately 4 ft behind the child and whisper simple commands or ask simple questions.

   ▶ Refer any abnormalities or parental concerns about hearing for further evaluation.

TECHNIQUES AND NORMAL FINDINGS	ABNORMAL FINDINGS SPECIAL CONSIDERATIONS

NOSE AND SINUSES

1. Assess the nose for nasal patency and septal deviation.

- Children under 6 months of age are obligate nose breathers. They will develop respiratory distress with blocked nasal passages. Determine and document the presence, color, and consistency of any nasal discharge.

▶ Unilateral nasal discharge may indicate septal deviation, foreign body, or nasal polyps, Pale, boggy nasal turbinates occur with nasal allergies. Infection typically results in erythematous, edematous nasal turbinates, and mucosa. Purulent nasal discharge commonly occurs at the end of viral upper respiratory infection and is caused by effective clearing of the nasal passages.

2. Assess the sinuses.

- The maxillary and ethmoid sinuses are present at birth, but they are proportionately smaller than in adults. The sphenoid sinuses develop before age 5 and the frontal sinuses by age 10. Children rarely have infections of the ethmoid sinuses. The frontal sinuses cause infection only in older school-age and adolescent children. Transillumination of the sinuses is not recommended because of poor sensitivity and specificity.

▶ Sinus pressure and tenderness of greater than 10 days' duration indicates sinusitis.

MOUTH AND THROAT

1. Assess the mouth and teeth.

- Inspect and palpate the palate of newborns. Determine the location and order of the teeth. Document the presence of lesions and discharge. Movement of the uvula, tongue, and lips should be symmetrical.

▶*Macroglossia* occurs with congenital hypothyroidism and Down syndrome. White plaques on the gums and buccal mucosa characterize oral thrush, caused by *Candida albicans* infection.

2. Assess the pharynx and tonsils.

- Ask the child to open the mouth, and demonstrate what you want the child to do. Orient young children to the oropharyngeal exam by examining the mouth of a parent or a doll. Preschool and younger children are frightened by the oral exam; therefore, always assess the oropharynx last. Determine the presence and characteristics of postnasal drainage on the posterior pharynx. Children between 3 and 8 years of age often have enlarged, noninfected tonsils.

▶ Strep throat infection, caused by group A beta-hemolytic *Streptococcus pyogenes*, may cause yellow tonsillar exudates, erythematous and edematous pharynx, red tongue with prominent taste buds (strawberry tongue), and petechial hemorrhages on the soft palate near the uvula. *Epiglottitis* is an acute life-threatening infection caused by infection with *Haemophilus influenzae* type B that results in infection and edema of the epiglottis. Symptoms include high fever, marked stridor, and respiratory distress.

ALERT!

Never assess the oropharynx of a preschool child with suspected epiglottis because coughing, crying, or gagging precedes acute respiratory failure.

CHEST AND LUNGS

1. Inspect the chest.

- Young children under the age of 6 years have round chests with prominent xiphoid processes. Abdominal breathing is common until age 6. Thoracic breathing begins in the school-age years. Infants have irregular breathing patterns that increase and decrease often. Pay special attention to respiratory effort and the presence of accessory muscle use. Note the presence of supernumerary nipples (if more than two).

▶*Apnea* is the cessation of breathing for greater than 20 seconds. Funnel chest (pectus excavatum) causes a depression of the lower part of the sternum. Pigeon chest (pectus carinatum) causes bowing of the sternum. Illustrations of pigeon chest and funnel chest can be found in Box 15.3 on pages 386–387. ∞ Wide spacing of the nipples occurs with genetic syndromes such as Turner's syndrome.

TECHNIQUES AND NORMAL FINDINGS	ABNORMAL FINDINGS SPECIAL CONSIDERATIONS

2. Auscultate the chest.

- Lung sounds are louder in children because of their thinned chest wall. Listen carefully in all lung fields, including the apex of the lungs. Children can be encouraged to take deep breaths by blowing bubbles or blowing out the otoscope light.

▶ Referred sounds from upper airway congestion are common and are often described as "chest rattling." To distinguish upper airway congestion from lower airway congestion, listen at the trachea and near the mouth. Lung sounds are always loudest at the point of origin.

CARDIOVASCULAR

1. Assess the child for cyanosis and chest pulsations, and determine the PMI.

- Central cyanosis is more pronounced in the mucous membranes. Apical pulsation is normal in young children. The PMI of children under 4 years of age is difficult to assess and is located approximately one intercostal space higher than in adults.

▶ Pericardial heaves are always abnormal findings. Children with heaves should be referred to cardiology for evaluation.

2. Palpate pulses for symmetry, rate, and rhythm.

- Evaluate the symmetry and amplitude of the femoral pulses in newborns, infants, and toddlers.

▶ Coarctation of the aorta causes a narrowing of the descending aorta and results in diminished femoral pulses and bounding radial pulses.

3. Auscultate heart sounds.

- Sinus arrhythmia presents with heart rate increases during inspiration and decreases during expiration. An S_2 split with inspiration may be detected in children under the age of 6. The physiological S_2 split disappears with expiration. Any S_2 split that persists throughout the cardiac cycle merits further evaluation. Preadolescents may have a physiological S_3 gallop that results from vibrations during rapid ventricular filling. Refer to Table 25.3 for the common innocent heart murmurs.

▶ See Table 25.7 for common pathologic heart murmurs.

Table 25.7	Common Pathologic Heart Murmurs	
NAME	**LOCATION**	**TIMING/ASSOCIATED CHARACTERISTICS**
Pulmonary valve stenosis	Upper left sternal border	Ejection click in early systole.
Aortic valve stenosis	Midsternum and upper right sternal border	Early systolic ejection click. Growth failure with congestive heart failure.
Tetralogy of Fallot	Mid- to upper left sternal border	Continuous murmur. Cyanosis and poor weight gain.
Ventricular septal defect	Lower left sternal border	Pansystolic murmur. Signs of congestive heart failure and poor growth if large.
Artial septal defect	Upper left sternal border	Systolic ejection murmur.
Patent ductus arteriosus	Upper left sternal border	Continuous murmur. Bounding pulses.

ABDOMEN

1. Inspect abdominal contour and movement.

- Infants and toddlers have prominent abdomens that result in a potbelly appearance. Umbilical hernias cause a protrusion at the umbilicus and are visible at birth.

▶ Umbilical hernias are common in children of African and Mediterranean descent.

2. Ausculate the abdomen.

- Use deeper pressure for children with ticklish abdomens. Bowel sounds are present in all quadrants.

▶ Absence of bowel sounds require further evaluation.

TECHNIQUES AND NORMAL FINDINGS	ABNORMAL FINDINGS SPECIAL CONSIDERATIONS

3. Palpate the abdomen.

- The lower liver edge is palpable 1 to 2 cm below the costal margin in most infants. Detect the presence of tenderness or masses.

▶ Constipation may result in a palpable cigar-shaped mass in the left lower quadrant. *Wilms' tumor* is a malignancy of the kidney commonly diagnosed in infants and toddlers. The most common presentation of Wilms' tumor is parental history of an abdominal mass felt during bathing or diaper changes. Refer children with suspected Wilms' tumor for immediate evaluation.

GENITALIA

1. Inspect the external genitalia.

- Genital maturation follows distinct patterns described by the Tanner stages as illustrated in Table 21.2 on page 588 and Table 22.1 on page 629. ∞ Examination of the female internal genitalia is rare in children who are not sexually active. Refer to Chapter 22 for detailed information about the female pelvic examination. ∞ Examine the genitalia with the child in the supine position.

- *Males:* Determine the location of the urethral meatus. The normal urethra is centered at the tip of the glans penis. The scrotum should be symmetrical and should have a uniform color.

▶ *Males:* Chordee is a fixed downward curving of the penile shaft. Hypospadias presents with an abnormal positioning of the urethral opening along the ventral glans or shaft of the penis as illustrated in Figure 25.14 ●. Scrotal swelling may be caused by hydrocele or inguinal hernia.

> **ALERT!**
>
> *The foreskin of uncircumcised males will not retract until the child is between 2 and 4 years old. Do not forcefully retract the foreskin of infants and toddlers. In older children with retractile foreskins, always return the foreskin to the natural position after urethral or glans examination.*

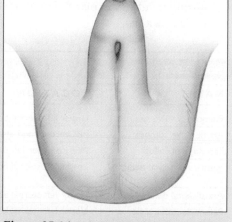

Figure 25.14 ● In hypospadias, the urethral canal is open on the ventral surface of the penis.

- *Females:* Facilitate inspection of the perineal area by placing the child supine with knees and hips flexed and externally rotated. This position is also referred to as the frog-leg position. To visualize the perivaginal area, grasp the labia majora between your thumb and forefinger and gently pull the labia majora up and out. Inspect the vaginal opening and the urethral meatus. Determine hymen patency. Newborns may present with a clear mucoid or blood-tinged vaginal discharge. Exposure to maternal hormones in utero causes "false menses."

▶ *Females:* Foreign bodies commonly cause malodorous, blood-tinged vaginal discharge. Vaginal foreign bodies, with the exception of those caused by retained toilet paper, are suspicious for sexual abuse. Box 25.2 lists signs of sexual abuse in children.

TECHNIQUES AND NORMAL FINDINGS

ABNORMAL FINDINGS
SPECIAL CONSIDERATIONS

2. **Palpate the external genitalia.**
   - *Males:* Verify testicular positioning in the scrotum (see Figure 25.15 ●). Foreskin retraction is impossible at birth. Normal foreskin retraction occurs between 2 and 3 years of age.

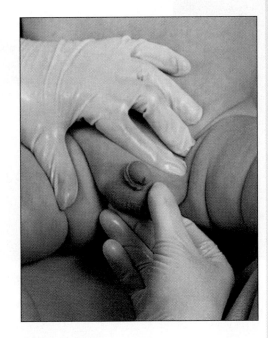

Figure 25.15 ● Palpating the scrotum for descended testicles and spermatic cords.

   - *Females:* Inguinal hernias cause a painful swelling of the labia majora in females.

▶ *Males:* Hydrocele causes a painless, nonreducible, serous fluid accumulation in the scrotum. No treatment is necessary unless the hydrocele persists after the child's first birthday. Inguinal hernias cause a mass at the external inguinal ring. Incarcerated, or nonreducible, inguinal hernias are surgical emergencies that merit immediate surgical evaluation. Refer children with reducible inguinal hernias for surgical evaluation within 1 to 2 weeks. Cryptorchidism, or undescended testicle, is more common in preterm infants. Refer children with undescended testicles between 6 and 12 months of age for medical evaluation.

▶ *Females:* Decreased estrogen production and genital atrophy cause labial adhesions. Labial adhesions present as a fused labia majora that obscures all or most of the perivaginal area. Refer any child with labial adhesions that impair urinary outflow for further evaluation and treatment.

TECHNIQUES AND NORMAL FINDINGS	ABNORMAL FINDINGS SPECIAL CONSIDERATIONS

MUSCULOSKELETAL

1. **Observe the child's gait and movements.**

   • Movements should be coordinated and equal. Ask preschoolers and older children to duck walk. The duck walk involves squatting and moving forward while flapping the upper arms. Any child who can duck walk has normal range of motion of the major joints, and normal muscle strength and coordination.

2. **Assess the upper extremities and neck.**

   • Notice symmetry and coordination of hand grip. Assess range of motion. Bilaterally inspect muscle symmetry and note the presence of weakness, masses, and swelling. Determine shoulder strength by having the child push, pull, and shrug the shoulders against resistance.

▶ *Polydactyly* is the presence of extra finger or toe (see Figure 25.16 ●). *Syndactyly* is webbed fingers or toes (see Figure 25.17 ●). Birth trauma may result in a brachial plexus injury. One type of brachial plexus injury is *Erb's palsy*, a transient condition that results in paralysis of the shoulder and upper arm. Infants with Erb's palsy present with an intact palmar grasp and the inability to move the upper arm. Entire brachial plexus palsy results in no movement of the shoulder, arm, and hand. Unfortunately, this type of brachial plexus injury has a poor prognosis.

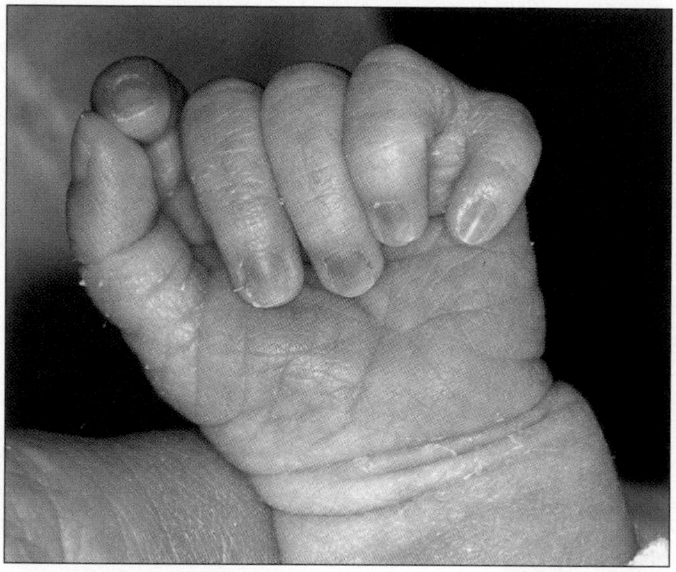

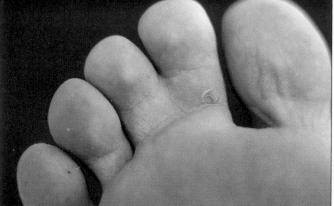

Figure 25.16 ● Polydactyly.

Figure 25.17 ● Syndactyly.

3. **Assess the lower extremities.**

   • Assess range of motion. Bilaterally inspect muscle symmetry and note the presence of weakness, masses, and swelling. Determine hip strength by having the child push and pull against resistance with the knees and hips flexed. Check for pelvic girdle weakness by assessing for Gower's sign. *Gower's sign* is the inability to get up from a seated or squatting position without pushing up with the arms (see Figure 25.18 ●). Children under 2 years of age appear flatfooted. Genu varum, or bowlegs, is common until 1 to 2 years of age. Preschoolers and school-age children under 7 years old are often knock-kneed, also known as genu valgum.

▶ Metatarsus adductus results in a C-shaped appearance of the foot that is caused by adduction of the forefoot. *Osgood-Schlatter* is a disorder of older children and adolescents caused by repetitive strain at the insertion of the quadriceps ligament at the tibial tubercle. It is more common in active children, especially those who participate in activities that require running, jumping, and squatting. Children with Osgood-Schlatter present with knee pain and tenderness over the tibial tubercle.

TECHNIQUES AND NORMAL FINDINGS	**ABNORMAL FINDINGS SPECIAL CONSIDERATIONS**

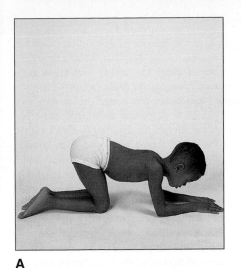

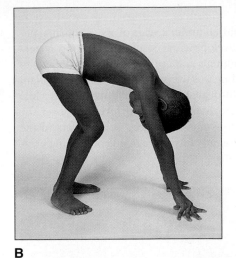

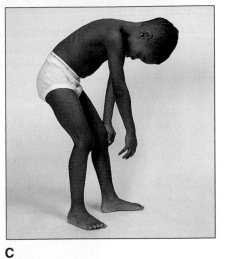

A   B   C

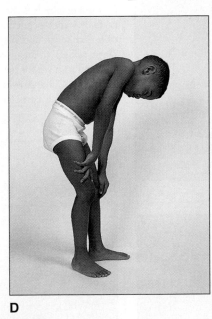

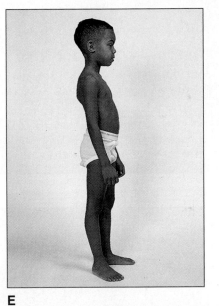

D   E

Figure 25.18 ● Gower's maneuver. Since the leg muscles of children with muscular dystrophy are weak, these children must perform the Gower's maneuver to raise themselves to a standing position. A and B. The child first maneuvers to a position supported by arms and legs. C. The child next pushes off the floor and rests one hand on the knee. D and E. The child then pushes himself upright.

TECHNIQUES AND NORMAL FINDINGS

ABNORMAL FINDINGS
SPECIAL CONSIDERATIONS

4. Assess the hips.

- Careful hip assessment is critical in children under 2 years of age. Abnormal development of the acetabulum causes developmental dysplasia of the hip. Determine symmetry of the fat folds of the gluteus and upper thighs. Place infants in a supine position with their legs extending toward you. To perform the Ortolani maneuver, flex the hips and knees at a 90-degree angle and abduct the hips while placing your thumb over the greater trochanter and your forefinger over the lesser trochanter. To perform the Barlow maneuver, keep your fingers in the same position and adduct the hip while gently lifting the thigh and placing pressure on the trochanter (see Figure 25.19 ●).

▶ None of the following signs indicate definitive diagnosis of hip dysplasia. Refer any child with these findings for further evaluation and treatment. Unequal fat folds occur with improper acetabular placement as shown in Figure 25.20 ●. A manual or audible clunk is positive for Ortolani's sign and Barlow's sign. Place the infant supine and bend both knees with the feet together. Positive Galeazzi and Allis' signs present with unequal knee heights. *Legg-Calvé-Perthes disease* results from an avascular necrosis of the femoral head in children between 7 and 12 years of age. This disorder presents with refusal to bear weight on the affected side, altered gait, and pain with internal rotation and flexion of the hip. Slipped capital femoral epiphysis is the most common hip disorder of adolescents. It is more common in obese children and results in a limp or complete refusal to bear weight on the affected side and pain with internal rotation and flexion of the hip. Children with these disorders often present with a complaint of anterior thigh or knee pain.

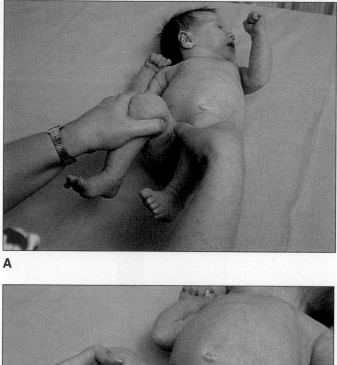

A

B

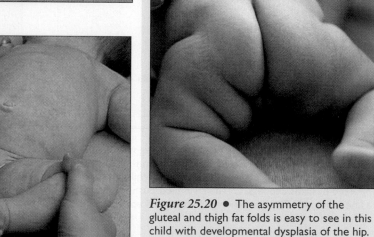

Figure 25.20 ● The asymmetry of the gluteal and thigh fat folds is easy to see in this child with developmental dysplasia of the hip.

Figure 25.19 ● Ortolani-Barlow maneuver. A. Place the infant on his or her back and flex the hips and knees at a 90-degree angle. Place a hand over each knee with the thumb over the inner thigh, and the first two fingers over the upper margin of the femur. Move the infant's knees together until they touch, and then put downward pressure on one femur at a time to see if the hips easily slip out of their joints or dislocate. B. Slowly abduct the hips, moving each knee toward the examining table. Any resistance to abduction or a clunk felt on palpation can be an indication of a congenital hip dislocation.

| **TECHNIQUES AND NORMAL FINDINGS** | **ABNORMAL FINDINGS SPECIAL CONSIDERATIONS** |

ALERT!

Assess the hip of any child with a complaint of anterior thigh or knee pain.

---

5. **Assess the spine.**
   - Have the child stand with feet together and assess for symmetry of the trunk, spine, hips, and scapula. Stand in front of the child and ask him or her to bend forward with the arms extended until the fingers touch the floor. Carefully inspect the back, hips, and scapula for asymmetry.

▶ Scoliosis is a lateral curvature of the spine that usually presents during adolescence. Children with scoliosis present with uneven shoulders, hips, or scapula.

NEUROLOGIC

1. **Assess the child's mental status.**
   - Determine the orientation of younger children by asking, "Is it time for breakfast, lunch, or dinner?" or "Who is your friend?" Note the child's energy level and ability to follow instructions. Normal preschoolers are active and alert and able to follow simple commands.

2. **Assess the child's development and determine the presence of infant reflexes.**
   - Table 25.4 on page 793 depicts and describes primitive reflexes in early childhood.

3. **Assess cranial nerve functioning and deep tendon reflexes.**
   - Examine the cranial nerves and deep tendon reflexes with the same techniques discussed in Chapter 24 of this text. ⚲ Deep tendon reflexes are difficult to assess in young children because of their tendency to tense their muscles during the procedure. Tell preschoolers that you can make their legs "dance" before assessing the patellar reflex.

4. **Assess for coordination, sensation, and movement.**
   - Ask if the child feels "tickles" during light stimulation. Ask children older than 3 years to draw a circle.

   Many of the techniques provided in previous chapters are used during the pediatric health assessment. Remain flexible and take opportunities to assess specific systems when they present. Make the physical examination fun. Children will be less anxious and more cooperative if they view the nurse in a positive light.

▶ Any change in the mental status, reflexes, cranial nerve function, and sensation and movement require further evaluation.

Refer to the Companion Website at **www.prenhall.com/damico** and click on the **Documentation** module for documentation samples and documentation practice exercises.

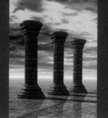

Abnormal Findings

$\mathscr{A}$ number of abnormalities occur commonly during childhood. The following discussion includes descriptions of the typical assessment findings of some of the more common childhood abnormalities. Refer to pediatric nursing textbooks for more detailed and comprehensive information.

Otitis Media

Otitis media, or middle ear infections, results from bacterial or viral infection and is the leading cause of community-based nursing visits (see Figure 14.31 on page 334 ⊙). Acute otitis media (AOM) is a frequent complication of allergic rhinitis and upper respiratory infection whose peak incidence occurs between 6 and 18 months of age. The eustachian tubes connect the middle ear to the posterior pharynx, and are shorter, straighter, and more level in young children than those in older children and adults. AOM results from the accumulation of middle ear fluid that contains viruses or bacteria. Children with middle ear infections typically present with pain, fever, decreased appetite, irritability, and altered sleep patterns. The tympanic membrane appears opaque, bulging, and yellow-orange or red colored during otitis media episodes. The tympanic membrane is a vascular tissue that appears red with infection, fever, or any condition that results in skin flushing. Children with red tympanic membranes and no purulent discharge in the middle ear space do not have bacterial otitis media. Risk factors for AOM include the following: bottle or pacifier use after 6 months of age, day care attendance, exposure to cigarette smoke, personal history of Down syndrome, cleft lip, or cleft palate. Most cases of AOM result in antibiotic therapy although recent clinical guidelines allow for watchful waiting for low-risk children.

Allergic Rhinitis

Allergic rhinitis is an immune hypersensitivity disorder that results from exposure to an allergen. Immune complex response results in the release of histamine, which causes increased mucous production, nasal congestion, lacrimation, and sneezing. Allergic rhinitis occurs in children from infancy through adolescence. Common clinical findings include darkening of the periorbital tissue under the eyes (also known as "allergic shiners"), periorbital edema, erythematous conjunctiva, clear nasal discharge, edematous and pale often blue-tinged nasal turbinates, and a cobblestone appearance of the posterior pharynx. Important findings include child or family history of atopic disease (asthma, allergy, eczema, hives) and history of recent exposure to pollen, animal dander, insect bites, or new goods. Parents of children with allergies often report sneezing "fits" where the child sneezes multiple times in succession, mouth breathing, and halitosis. The cornerstone therapy for allergic rhinitis is removal of the offending substances. Toddlers and older children may be treated with antihistamines, nasal corticosteroids, and leukotriene modifiers.

Asthma

Asthma is one of the most common chronic illnesses in childhood. Asthma is characterized by airway hypersensitivity, bronchospasm, and airway inflammation (see Figure 15.25 on page 388 ⊙). Initial asthma episodes may present from infancy through adolescence. Common asthma triggers include allergens (foods, pollens, danders, mold, grasses, weeds, and cockroaches), smoke, and viruses. Children with acute asthma episodes present with expiratory wheezes, dyspnea (retractions, nasal flaring, and grunting), tachypnea, and prolonged expiratory phases. Risk factors for asthma include infection with respiratory syncytial virus (RSV) and personal or family history of atopy. Asthma therapy is tailored to the severity and frequency of symptoms and includes inhaled bronchodilators, inhaled corticosteroids, leukotriene modifiers, and trigger avoidance.

Acne Vulgaris

Bacterial infections with *Propionibacterium acnes* and sebaceous gland occlusion cause acne vulgaris. Acne typically occurs on the face, upper chest, upper back, neck, and upper
arms of adolescents. Acne is common during adolescence because of the influence of androgens on sebaceous gland secretion. Acne lesions may be open comedones (blackheads),
closed comedones (whiteheads), and cysts (see Figure 25.21 ●).
Common acne treatments include cleansing with mild soap,
keratolytics like benzoyl peroxide, and topical antibiotic
therapy.

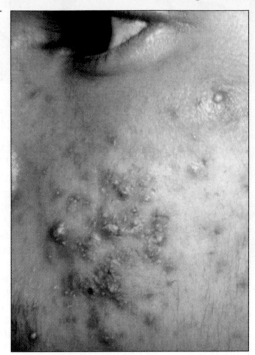

Figure 25.21 ● Open and closed comedones of acne.

Scalp Ringworm (Tinea Capitis)

Tinea capitis is a superficial fungal infection of the scalp hair
follicles that results in areas of alopecia characterized by hair
follicle breakage at the skin surface (see Figure 11.77 on
page 225 ⬭). The peak incidence occurs during school age.

Epidermal scaling may occur inside the bald spots. Treatment
of this disorder includes oral antifungals such as griseofulvin
and selenium sulfide shampoo.

Acute Gastroenteritis

Acute gastroenteritis (AGE) is an acute, common diarrhea disease that may or may not be accompanied by vomiting. Nine
percent of hospital admissions during childhood result from
episodes of AGE. Additional symptoms include abdominal
pain, cramping, and fever. Pertinent history findings include
frequency and amount of diarrhea, vomiting, magnitude and
duration of fever, and presence and location of abdominal
pain. Exposure to infectious substances (*Salmonella, Shigella,*
etc.) and people with similar symptoms, as well as questions
regarding hydration status, are important parts of the history.
Abdominal examination may reveal hyperactive bowel
sounds. Assessment of hydration status is essential and should
include documentation of level of consciousness, presence of
thirst, time and amount of last urination, vital signs (heart

rate and blood pressure), skin turgor, and capillary perfusion
of less than 2 seconds.

ALERT!

*Level of consciousness is the most accurate indicator of dehydra-
tion. Vital signs, skin turgor, and capillary perfusion will be present only with moderate to severe dehydration and indicate risk of
cardiovascular collapse.*

Nursing management of gastroenteritis focuses on the
correction of electrolyte imbalances with oral rehydration
therapy intravenous fluid resuscitation, and administration of
an age-appropriate diet in a nondehydrated child.

Health Promotion

HEALTHY PEOPLE 2010

FOCUS AREA	PREVALENCE	OBJECTIVES	ACTIONS
Fetal and Infant Deaths	• In 1997, there was a rate of 7.2 infant deaths per 1,000 live births. • In 1997, two thirds of all infant deaths took place during the first 28 days of life. • There are four causes for more than half of all infant deaths: birth defects, short gestation/low birth weight, SIDS, and respiratory distress syndrome. • After the age of 1 month, the leading cause of death is SIDS. • In 1997, infant mortality rate among African Americans was 2.3 times that of white infants.	• Reduce the number of fetal and infant deaths to include all deaths, neonatal deaths, postneonatal deaths, deaths related to birth defects, deaths related to congenital heart defects, and deaths due to SIDS.	• Educate to stop smoking and avoid alcohol while pregnant. • Recognize at-risk populations, and risk screening and intervention to focus on this group. • Educate to focus on those at risk for SIDS.
Child Deaths	• In 1997, children between the ages of 1 and 14 had a death rate of 25.1 per 100,000 children. • The leading cause of death in this population was injury. • The leading fatal injuries are motor vehicle accidents, firearms, drownings, fires, and burns. • Other leading causes of death include birth defects, malignant neoplasms, and heart disease.	• Reduce the number of deaths in children between the ages of 1 and 9.	• Educate to include accident prevention, correct use of child car safety seats, prevention of drowning, and prevention of fires and burns. • Educate to prevent firearm storage within reach of children. • Educate parents to use active supervision as a mechanism to decrease injury risk.
Adolescent Deaths	• In 1998, there were 22.1 deaths per 100,000 adolescents between the ages of 10 and 14. • The leading cause of death was motor vehicle accidents. • Other causes were falls, drownings, poisonings, homicides, suicides, AIDS, malignant neoplasms, heart disease, and combination illnesses.	• Reduce the number of preventable deaths in adolescents ages 10 through 19.	• Educate teens and parents about automobile safety. • Encourage automobile safety belt use. • Counsel about high-risk behaviors for falls, drownings, poisonings, AIDS, and homicides. • Recognize teens in need of psychological counseling and suicide prevention. • Counsel adolescents about sexuality, substance use, risk-taking behavior, and STD prevention.

816

FOCUS AREA	PREVALENCE	OBJECTIVES	ACTIONS
Adolescent Deaths (*continued*)	• In 1998, there were 70.6 deaths per 100,000 adolescents between the ages of 15 and 19. • The leading cause of death for this age group was motor vehicle accidents. • Other causes were the same as those identified for the group between the ages of 10 and 14 years.		• Educate to decrease teen violence.

CLIENT EDUCATION

A number of risk factors impact children's health. Most of the *Healthy People 2010* leading health indicators have implications for infants, children, and adolescents. Targeted and individualized nursing interventions can effectively decrease the impact of these risk factors.

BEHAVIORAL CONSIDERATIONS

RISK FACTORS

- Use of these substances is linked with sexually transmitted diseases.
- Very low birth weight is associated with the use of illicit drugs during pregnancy.
- Preterm birth is associated with alcohol and drug use.

- Heavy alcohol use is associated with fetal alcohol syndrome, one of the leading preventable causes of mental retardation in children.
- Alcohol/illicit drug use by pregnant females is associated with child irritability, poor coordination, hypotonia, and neurological disorders.

CLIENT EDUCATION

- Counsel female clients of childbearing age to avoid the use of alcohol and illicit drugs prior to and during pregnancy.

- Review with the mother the potential outcomes of alcohol/illicit drug use on the baby and birth process.
- Encourage counseling or referral to a rehabilitation center to help with illicit drug cessation.

- Assess for substance use (including but no limited to alcohol, steroids, and street drugs) and encourage abstinence from substance use and risk-taking behavior in school-age and adolescent children.

ENVIRONMENTAL CONSIDERATIONS

RISK FACTORS

- Cigarette smoking is the single most preventable cause of disease and death in the United States.
- Environmental smoke contributes to the development of asthma, middle ear infections, and bronchitis in children.
- Smoking during pregnancy can result in miscarriages, premature birth, and SIDS.

CLIENT EDUCATION

- Review the impact of smoking on the developing fetus, the infant, and the adolescent or adult.
- Encourage the use of smoking cessation techniques for parents and children.
- Recommend counseling to aid with smoking cessation, if applicable.

LIFE SPAN CONSIDERATIONS

RISK FACTORS

- Regular physical activity is a proven method to decrease the risk of cardiovascular disease and diabetes.

- In the last decades, the percentage of time American children spend engaging in physical activity during and outside school has decreased.

CLIENT EDUCATION

- Assess and document frequency and type of physical activity.
- Encourage activities that can be done with family members (e.g., evening walks, family games).
- Help children and parents identify activities that can be done for 30 minutes at a time 3 to 5 times a week.

Application Through Critical Thinking

CASE STUDY

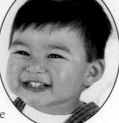

*L*eon is a healthy 18-month-old who presents to the outpatient clinic for his well-child examination. His mother reports that Leon was born at 40 weeks' gestation after an uncomplicated pregnancy and vaginal delivery. Leon has met each developmental milestone at the normal age. Leon's mother tells the nurse that Leon is "a bundle of energy." He sleeps approximately 10 hours each night and takes a 2- to 3-hour nap in the afternoon. He began walking at 13 months of age, and he now runs and climbs. His mother reports that Leon is "very picky" and will not eat "anything that is good for him." She reports that "Leon is healthy as a horse" and that he has never been ill "except for two ear infections last winter and colds every 2 months or so." Leon lives at home with his mother, his father (his parents are not married), and his older sister Martha (4 years old). The mother denies family problems.

▶ Complete Documentation

The following is a sample of the documentation from Leon's visit.
SUBJECTIVE DATA: Child presents for 18-month well-child examination. Birth history and past medical history negative for significant findings. 24-hour diet recall is as follows: breakfast—1 blueberry waffle, 1/2 banana, 8 oz whole milk; morning snack—6 oz "fish" crackers and water; lunch—1 serving macaroni and cheese, 1/2 cup fruit cocktail (in fruit juice, not heavy syrup), and 8 oz whole milk; afternoon snack—1 apple and 6 oz apple juice; dinner—1/2 boneless, skinless chicken breast, 1 serving green beans, tossed salad, 1 dinner roll, 8 oz whole milk. He uses a sippy cup and a pacifier. Sleeps 12 to 13 hours per 24 hours. Mother denies concerns with Leon's health or development, but is concerned about the adequacy of his dietary intake. Has soft, formed bowel movements daily. Wets at least 8 diapers every 24 hours.
OBJECTIVE DATA: Weight 28 lb (70th percentile), height 33.5 in. (80th percentile).

▶ Critical Thinking Questions

1. Is Leon's growth and development normal?
2. Describe the nursing actions needed for Leon's heart murmur. Include discussion of management and evaluation parameters.
3. Document the above information using the SOAP format.

ASSESSMENT FORM

Vital Signs: *P 92—RR 24.*

Head: *Anterior fontanelle nonpalpable.*

Eyes: *Bilateral red reflux extra ocular movement intact (EOMI).*

Nose: *Patent. No discharge noted.*

Mouth: *16 teeth, large second molar bulges. Tonsils 2+, pharynx pink and moist.*

Ears: *TMs pearly gray in a neutral position with normal movement. No fluid noted.*

Lymphatic: *Shotty anterior cervical nodes.*

Lungs: *Breath sounds clear.*

Heart: *Regular rate and rhythm. Clear S1, S2. II/VI systolic ejection murmur heard along left lower sternal border when child supine. Murmur disappears when upright. Femoral pulses equal bilaterally, 2+ intensity.*

Abdomen: *Soft, nondistended with potbelly appearance. No palpable tenderness or masses.*

Spine: *Negative for asymmetry, tenderness, or masses.*

Genitalia: *Tanner 1 male with descended testes bilaterally.*

Musculoskeletal: *Full range of motion in all extremities. Normal muscle mass. Coordinated gait. Genu varum present.*

Neurologic: *Speech 70% understandable. Uses one- to two-word sentences. Runs and climbs. Follows one-step commands. 2+ patellar, bicep, tricep DTRs. Cranial nerves I–XII intact.*

▶ Applying Nursing Diagnoses

1. Use the NANDA taxonomy (see Appendix A ∞) to identify one wellness diagnosis and one problem-oriented nursing diagnosis from the data provided in this case study.
2. From the date provided in this case, is the nursing diagnosis *alteration in cardiovascular function* (as stated in the NANDA taxonomy) a legitimate diagnosis? Explain your answer.
3. Through a subjective interaction with the mother, the nurse learns that the child has never been sick except for two ear infections in the last 2 months and "he seems to constantly have a runny nose." From this information, use the NANDA taxonomy to formulate at least two nursing diagnosis that would be appropriate for this child's illness episodes.

► *Prepare Teaching Plan*

LEARNING NEED: From the information obtained from the health history, the child has had two episodes of ear infections in 2 months and "seems to constantly have a runny nose."

GOAL: The child will experience a decrease in the number of ear infections and colds.

OBJECTIVES: At the completion of the session, the mother of the child will:

1. Identify risk factors for upper respiratory and ear infection.
2. Identify ways to reduce the spread of infection between family members.

APPLICATION OF OBJECTIVE 1: Identify risk factors for upper respiratory and ear infection

Content	Teaching Strategy and Rationale	Evaluation
• Children under the age of 2 years have smaller eustachian tubes and more frequent upper respiratory infections because of their immature immune system. Review the causes of upper respiratory infections in children. Review how a child of 9 months is not able to expectorate and effectively clear the nasal passages.	• One-on-one discussion with the mother. • Provide printed material. • Provide pamphlets about proper hand washing.	• The mother states she will return home and disinfect or clean Leon's toys. • The mother states she will keep track of the number of colds and ear infections that both of her children have. • The mother identifies Leon's risk factors for upper respiratory infection and ear infection. • The mother identifies strategies that she can use to modify these risk factors.
• Children of this age group frequently place objects in the mouth, thus making them more susceptible to viral illness transmission. Bottle and pacifier use after the age of 6 months increases the risk of ear infection. Other risk factors include day care attendance, exposure to cigarette smoke, allergies, and cleft lip/cleft palate.		
• Children often spread infection to other children. Leon has a sister who is 4 years old. Review the mechanism of transmission of microorganisms between individuals.		
• There are a few simple things that can be done to help reduce the number of colds and ear infections that Leon is having. Everyone should use good hand-washing techniques after using the bathroom, after blowing the nose, after coughing, and anytime the hands are obviously soiled.		
• If the daughter has a cold, it is best to keep her away from Leon and his toys. This might be difficult, but it will help Leon.		
• Leon needs plenty of fluids to keep his secretions thin. This will help clear them out of his nose and sinuses and could reduce the buildup that is leading to ear infections.		
• Noncompliance with therapy for otitis media increases the risk of subsequent resistant infection. Teach parents to give prescribed medicines as ordered and to follow up with the provider as recommended.		

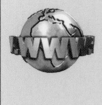

Please refer to the Companion Website at www.prenhall.com/damico and click on Chapter 25, the Application Through Critical Thinking module, to complete the following activities related to this case study:
► Critical Thinking questions
► Extended Nursing Diagnosis challenge
► Documentation activity
► Teaching Plan for Objective 2

EXPLORE MediaLink

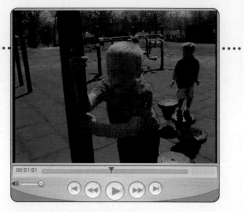

Additional resources for this chapter are found on the Student CD-ROM accompanying this textbook and on the Companion Website.

CD-ROM CONTENT

Content for this chapter includes:
Objectives
Key Concepts
NCLEX-RN® Review Questions
Model Documentation Forms
Audio Glossary
Animations
   Ear and Otoscope
   Child Ear Anatomy
Games and Challenges
Clinical Spotlight Videos
   Growth and Development
   Using the Snellen E Chart
   Nutritional Status of Children
   Health Promotion and Health Maintenance
Head-to-Toe Physical Examination Video

Client Interaction Case Study Challenge
Application Through Critical Thinking
   Case Study Teaching Plan Challenge
MediaLinks
MediaLink Application
Tool Box
   Chapter Documentation Form Example
   Health Promotion
      Healthy People 2010
      Client Education
New York Times

COMPANION WEBSITE CONTENT

www.prenhall.com/damico

Content for this chapter includes:
Objectives
NCLEX-RN® Review Questions

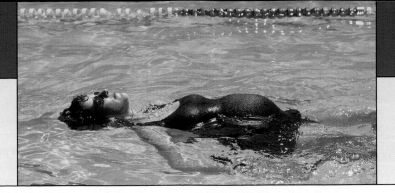

26

The Pregnant Female

MEDIALINK

www.prenhall.com/damico

The CD-ROM in the back of this textbook and the Media-Link website contain NCLEX-RN® review questions, interactive exercises, case study challenges, animations, videos, documentation and checklist forms, and review materials. For a complete listing of the media content specific to Chapter 26, see the Explore MediaLink at the end of the chapter.

*P*regnancy and the postpartum period offer a unique opportunity for health promotion, disease prevention, and changes in lifestyle behaviors through the actions of the nurse. For the vast majority of childbearing females, pregnancy and postpartum are normal processes that can be enhanced through education, healthcare, and supportive intervention. Changes in personal lifestyle behaviors and healthcare can influence not only the course of the pregnancy and the health of mother and child, but also the health behaviors of the entire family in the future. Knowledge of variations in body systems during the three trimesters of pregnancy and postpartum periods will enable the nurse to differentiate normal from abnormal changes. The risk for and development of many pathologic conditions in pregnancy and postpartum can be ascertained and prevented by a careful, thorough interview. Past medical, obstetric, gynecologic, family, genetic, and social history will influence the focus of the physical assessment examination and teaching. Knowledge of lifestyle and health practices, nutrition and exercise history, environmental exposures, and current symptoms will also guide assessment and teaching.

The physical assessment also provides an opportunity for client education and clarification of misperceptions. Cultural, familial, and personal beliefs can be discussed as appropriate during the history and examination. Whether the nurse is perceived as kind and personal, or cold and bureaucratic, knowledgeable and helpful, or ill informed and ineffective will influence the client's willingness and ability to implement health recommendations. This life transition is also an opportunity for sharing much joy and excitement with childbearing families. The nurse can influence a whole generation through caring, accurate, and appropriate assessment and intervention (see Figure 26.1 ●).

Healthy People 2010 goals in maternal and infant health focus on the areas of fetal and infant deaths, maternal deaths and illnesses, prenatal care, obstetric care, and breastfeeding. The prevalence of certain problems, the target objectives, and some actions to achieve the goals are summarized in the *Healthy People 2010* feature on page 868.

NUTRITIONAL ASSESSMENT

A comprehensive nutritional history is important when assessing the nutritional health of a pregnant female. Diet recall and food frequency questionnaires remain important tools to use to assess intake. Assessment of preconception diet should also be obtained in general detail as it provides the foundation for nutritional health in early pregnancy and beyond. Table 26.1 outlines specific data to be assessed when conducting a nutritional history of a pregnant female. Lactation needs are also addressed.

PHYSICAL ASSESSMENT

The clinical examination of a pregnant female should include parameters to assess the nutritional health of the client and weight gain patterns necessary to support a healthy pregnancy.

Anthropometric Measurements

Weight, weight history, and gestational weight gain pattern and amount are important considerations during pregnancy. Preconception weight, height, and BMI are necessary to determine gestational weight gain goals. In pregnant adolescents, **gynecologic age** should be determined to assess whether linear growth may still be occurring. Gynecologic age is the difference between current age and age at menarche. Young women with a gynecologic age of 3 years or less are considered to still be completing linear growth and will have competing nutritional needs between their own growth and that of the fetus. Weight gain guidelines are outlined in Table 26.2. Adolescents and African American females are encouraged to strive for the upper limits of weight gain for their BMI due to the incidence

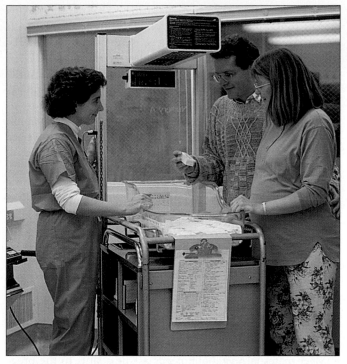

Figure 26.1 • Nurse with pregnant client and family.

Table 26.1 Nutritional History Data for Gestation and Lactation

Assess for Specific Foods and Nutrients

- Folic acid—fortified flour and cereals, orange juice, green leafy vegetables, legumes
- Calcium and vitamin D—dairy, fortified juices, fortified soy products
- Iron—meats, poultry, shellfish, fortified cereals and grains, legumes, dried fruit
- Vitamin B_{12} if vegan—must be synthetic, plant sources not bioavailable
- Fluids, include alcohol
- Caffeine—coffee, tea, cola and other soda, cocoa, chocolate, OTC medications
- Mercury—recommendation is to limit large cold/fresh water fish to 12 oz/week

Assess for Eating Patterns and Behaviors

- Weight gain with any prior pregnancies
- Restrictive eating, missed meals, dieting attempts
- Cultural beliefs related to food and pregnancy
- Food aversions
- Pica
- Gastrointestinal complaints and any resultant alterations in diet

Assess for Supplement Use

- Prenatal vitamin compliance
- Iron supplement compliance
- Other vitamins—high intake of vitamin A is teratogenic
- Herbs—most untested in pregnant or lactating females
- Remedies for any pregnancy symptoms

of low birth weight babies in those populations. Adolescents should gain weight early and continuously. Shorter women (62 inches or less) are encouraged to gain weight at the lower end of their BMI range. Weight gain guidelines for other racial and ethnic groups have had insufficient research focus to establish a consensus. For each client, the nurse should develop individual weight gain guidelines.

During the physical assessment the nurse can screen for factors for low weight gain patterns. Smoking, alcohol consumption, drug use, lack of social support, and depression have all been associated with low weight gain. An adolescent trying to hide a pregnancy may be at risk for low weight gain.

The nurse can also ask questions about the presence of physical symptoms that may be affecting nutritional status. Gastrointestinal discomfort, nausea and vomiting, constipation, and heartburn occur during pregnancy and can alter dietary intake and food tolerance. Follow-up questions should seek information on remedies used to relieve symptoms. A

pregnant female with a history of an eating disorder and hyperemesis gravidarum should be screened for current signs of an eating disorder. Box 26.1 outlines physical findings with an eating disorder.

LABORATORY MEASUREMENTS

Laboratory assessment of the pregnant female should routinely include screening for iron deficiency anemia. The increased iron needs during pregnancy put many females at risk for iron deficiency. Hemoglobin and hematocrit decrease until the end of the second trimester due to expansion of blood volume and

Table 26.2 Gestational Weight Gain Recommendations

BMI	WEIGHT GAIN PATTERN (LB) FIRST TRIMESTER/SECOND WEIGHT GAIN AMOUNT (LB)	AND THIRD TRIMESTER
<19.8	28–40	5/slightly >1
19.8–26	25–35	3.5/1
26–29	15–25	2/0.66
>29	At least 15, not >25	Determine individually
Twins	35–45	At least 1/week throughout
Triplets	50	At least 1/week throughout

Adapted from National Academy of Science 1990, Luke B & Leurgans S 1996, American Dietetic Association 2002, Branco AT et al 1998, Edwards LE et al 1996, Schieve CA et al 2000.

Box 26.1	Clinical Findings Consistent with Eating Disorders

Bulimia/Binge-Purge Behavior

- Bloodshot eyes
- Broken blood vessels on the face
- Swollen parotid glands of "chipmunk cheeks"
- Dental erosion
- Hoarse voice
- Scarring on the dorsal surface of the hand from teeth during purge attempts
- Poor or lacking gag reflex
- Weight fluctuations

Anorexia/Restrictive Eating Behavior

- Cold intolerance
- Lanugo, soft white hair growth on body
- Pedal edema
- Dry skin
- Alopecia
- Bradycardia
- Hypotension
- Amenorrhea in nonpregnant postmenarcheal females
- Loss of strength and muscle tone

General Eating Disorder Findings

- Body dissatisfaction. Ask: "How do you feel about your weight?" followed by "Have you ever tried to gain or lose weight? Tell me what you did."
- Constipation
- Bloating
- Fatigue

red cell mass during pregnancy. Pregnancy-specific standards for normal hemoglobin and hematocrit values should be used (see Table 26.3).

Fasting plasma glucose and, if found to be above 105 mg/dl, subsequent glucose tolerance is performed between weeks 24 and 26 of the pregnancy to assess for gestational diabetes. Both the nutritional health of the mother and the outcome of the pregnancy can be negatively affected if diet changes are not instituted in females found to have gestational diabetes.

Plasma lipid levels increase during pregnancy as normal physiology and may be unrelated to nutrition, requiring no intervention.

Special consideration should be given to screen for plasma lead in females who report **pica,** the eating of nonfood items or

Table 26.3	Gestational Hemoglobin and Hematocrit References for Anemia	
	FIRST AND THIRD TRIMESTERS	**SECOND TRIMESTER**
Hemoglobin (g/dl)	<11	<10.5
Hematocrit (%)	<33	<32

Reference CDC/MMWR 1998

ice, as consumption of earth or clay can be a source of environmental contamination. Females following a **vegan** diet, with no consumption of animal products, are at risk for vitamin B_{12} deficiency unless the diet is fortified or supplemented. Plant sources of vitamin B_{12} are not considered biologically available. Women without added synthetic vitamin B_{12} should be assessed for vitamin B_{12} status. Pregnant females with a history of phenylketonuria should have a plasma assay for phenylalanine to screen for elevated levels. Elevated phenylalanine levels are harmful to fetal brain development.

ANATOMY AND PHYSIOLOGY REVIEW

In order to implement programs of maternal-infant care to promote health, the nurse must understand the adaptations that occur in the female body during pregnancy and postpartum. The anatomical and physiological changes during the 40 weeks of pregnancy serve three important functions:

- Maintain normal maternal physiological function
- Meet maternal metabolic needs as she adapts to the pregnancy
- Meet the growth and development needs of the fetus

An examination of the changes in each body system during pregnancy and postpartum will enable the nurse to interpret findings in the interview and assessment.

THE PLACENTA

The physiological and anatomical changes in pregnancy are due to the hormones secreted by the fetus and placenta and the mechanical effects of the growing fetus. The human placenta is a unique organ that promotes and provides for fetal growth and development. Its functions include metabolism, transport of gases and nutrients, and secretion of hormones. It develops from the fertilized ovum, but generally also includes the maternal uterine lining at the site of implantation. The **placenta** is an ovoid organ that weighs approximately one sixth of the fetus and covers one third of the inner surface area of the uterus at term. Implantation of the fertilized egg, called a *blastocyst,* in the endometrium or lining of the uterus begins 6 days after fertilization. The umbilical blood vessels and placenta develop. Two arteries and a vein exit the fetus at the umbilicus, forming the umbilical cord, and insert in the center of the placenta (see Figure 26.2 ●). The fetal vessels branch out into treelike chorionic villi where the fetal capillaries are the sites of exchange between the maternal and fetal circulations. The fetal and maternal circulations are kept essentially separate by the placental membrane covering the villi. The exchange of nutrients from the maternal to the fetal circulation takes place here, as well as passage of waste products such as carbon dioxide and uric acid from the fetal to maternal circulation. The placenta, in conjunction with the fetus and maternal uterine lining, also produces hormones such as human chorionic gonadotropin (hCG), estrogen, progesterone, relaxin, prolactin, and other hormones.

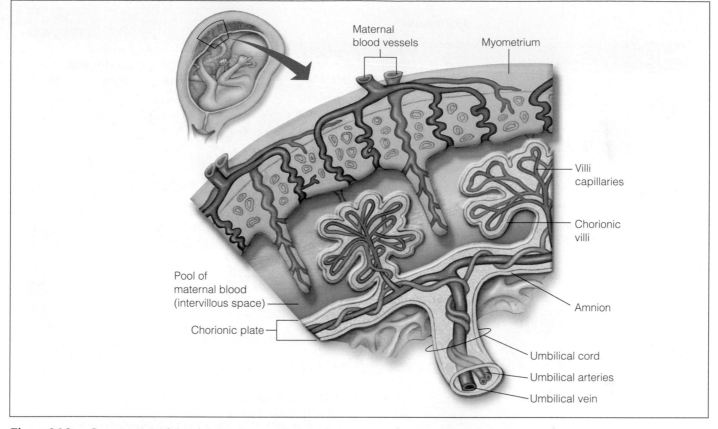

Figure 26.2 ● Cross section of the placenta.

FETAL DEVELOPMENT

Pregnancy is divided into three trimesters, each lasting approximately 13 weeks (3 months in lay terms). The age of the fetus can be referred to in weeks beyond fertilization, used in discussion of fetal development, or **gestational age,** the age in weeks from the last normal menstrual period, more commonly used in prenatal care.

The first 2 weeks after fertilization are the early embryo stage, and disruptions in development, such as from environmental agents, usually cause death, or miscarriage. From 2 to 8 weeks after fertilization the **embryo** is in the stage of *organogenesis*. During this period a **teratogen,** an agent such as a virus, a drug, a chemical, or radiation that causes malformation of an embryo or fetus, may induce major congenital anomalies. The fetal stage is from 8 weeks until birth (see Figure 26.3 ●).

By the end of the first trimester, all major systems have formed. **Viability,** the point at which the fetus can survive outside the uterus, may occur as early as 22 weeks or at the weight of 500 g. During the fetal period the body grows, and differentiation of tissues, organs, and systems occurs.

Although fetal movement can be detected as early as 7 weeks through diagnostic techniques, **quickening,** the fluttery initial sensations of fetal movement perceived by the mother, usually occurs at approximately 18 weeks, possibly earlier in females who have given birth before.

The fetal heart begins beating at 22 days. During assessment, the fetal heartbeat can be heard via Doppler starting between 7 and 12 weeks of pregnancy, and with a **fetoscope,** a specialized stethoscope for listening to fetal heart sounds, beginning at approximately 18 weeks of gestation. The *uterine souffle,* the sound of the uterine arteries, which is synchronous with the maternal pulse, may be heard, as well as the funic souffle, the sound of the umbilical vessels that is synchronous with the fetal heartbeat.

Fetal circulation prior to birth has three shunts that enable the fetus to maximize oxygenation from the maternal circulation since lungs are not yet functional for oxygen exchange. Oxygenated blood from the placenta is carried via the umbilical vein to the fetus, entering at the umbilicus. The fetal liver is partially bypassed by the **ductus venosus,** so that highly oxygenated blood continues on to the heart. More highly oxygenated blood flows into the second shunt, the **foramen ovale,** which connects the fetal right atrium to the fetal left atrium. The other half of the blood continues to the right ventricle. The more highly oxygenated blood from the umbilical vein continues to the left ventricle and is shunted across the **ductus arteriosus** into the descending aorta. In this way, only a small part of the blood flow enters the pulmonary bed. The oxygenated blood then perfuses the rest of the fetal body, and returns to the placenta via the umbilical arteries (see Figure 26.4 ●).

REPRODUCTIVE SYSTEM CHANGES

In addition to the fetus and placenta, extensive changes occur in the reproductive organs. The uterus, cervix, fallopian tubes, and vagina undergo massive changes in size and function.

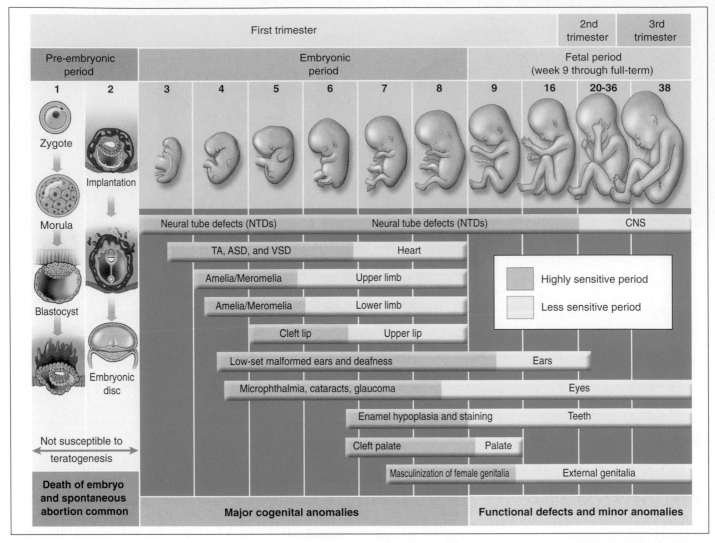

Figure 26.3 ● Fetal development.

Uterus

The uterus is profoundly transformed in pregnancy. The criss-cross muscle fibers of the body of the uterus increase in size and number due to the effects of progesterone and estrogen. The uterus increases in size from 70 grams (2.5 oz) to 1,000 grams (2.2 lb), and from 7.5 cm (3 in.) long, 5 cm (2 in.) wide, and 2.5 cm (1 in.) deep to 25 cm (10 in.) long, 20 cm (8 in.) wide, and 22.5 cm (9 in.) deep, and its capacity increases from 10 ml to 5,000 ml. During the second and third trimesters the growing fetus also mechanically expands the uterus.

Early in pregnancy the uterus retains its nonpregnant pear shape, but becomes more globular by 12 weeks. Bimanual palpation is used to assess the size of the uterus during the early weeks. The early sizes can be compared to fruits: 6 weeks, lemon; 8 weeks, small orange; 10 weeks, large orange; 12 weeks, grapefruit. The growing uterus can be palpated abdominally by about 10 to 12 weeks, at which time the top of the uterus or **fundus** is slightly above the symphysis pubis. The female begins to "show" externally at approximately 14 to 16 weeks, later for a **primigravida,** a female pregnant for the first time, and earlier for a **multigravida,** a female who has been pregnant two or more times. At 16 weeks, the fundus is halfway between the symphysis

and umbilicus. Between 20 and 22 weeks, the fundus reaches the umbilicus. Fundal height increases until 38 weeks. The distance from the symphysis pubis to the fundus is measured with a measuring tape to assess fetal growth and dating in pregnancy. **McDonald's rule** for estimating fetal growth states that after 20 weeks in pregnancy, the weeks of gestation approximately equal the **fundal height** in centimeters (see Figure 26.5 ●). Between 38 and 40 weeks, **lightening,** or the descent of the fetal head into the pelvis, occurs, and the fundal height drops slightly.

Throughout pregnancy the uterus softens, as does the region that connects the body of the uterus and cervix, referred to as **Hegar's sign. Piskacek's sign** is the irregular shape of the uterus due to the implantation of the ovum. The decidua or lining of the uterus becomes four times thicker during pregnancy. Amenorrhea, or the absence of menstruation, one of the first signs of pregnancy, occurs. The contractility of the uterus increases due to the action of estrogen. **Braxton Hicks contractions,** painless and unpredictable contractions of the uterus that do not dilate the cervix, start in the first trimester, are palpable to the nurse by the second trimester, and are felt by the mother usually starting in the third trimester. **Ballottement,** a technique of palpation, where the examiner's hand is used to push against the

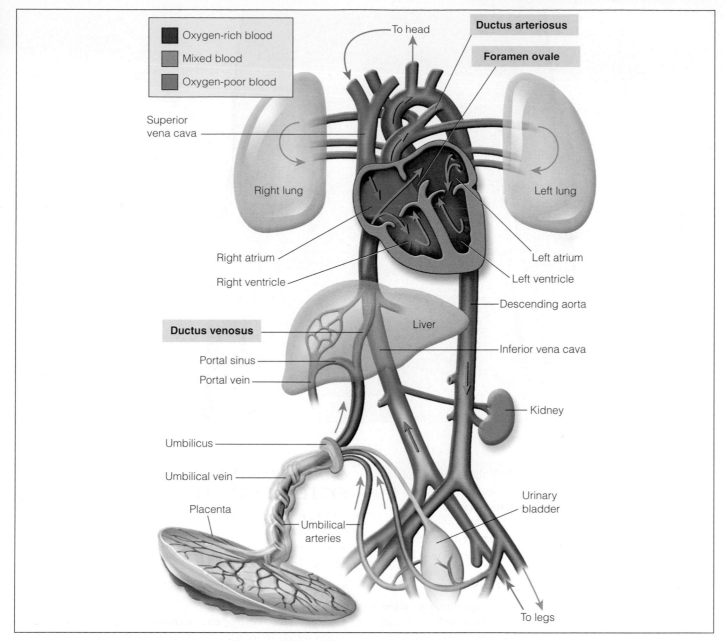

Oxygen-rich blood
Mixed blood
Oxygen-poor blood

To head
Ductus arteriosus
Foramen ovale
Superior vena cava
Right lung
Left lung
Right atrium
Left atrium
Right ventricle
Left ventricle
Descending aorta
Ductus venosus
Liver
Portal sinus
Inferior vena cava
Portal vein
Kidney
Umbilicus
Umbilical vein
Urinary bladder
Placenta
Umbilical arteries
To legs

Figure 26.4 ● Fetal circulation.

uterus and detect the presence or position of a fetus by its return impact, can be elicited after about 20 weeks, because the **amniotic fluid,** a clear, slightly yellowish liquid that surrounds the fetus, is greater in comparison to the still small fetus.

Cervix and Vagina

The cervix, or opening of the uterus, develops a protective **mucous plug** during pregnancy, due to the action of progesterone, which also causes **leukorrhea,** a profuse, nonodorous, nonpainful vaginal discharge that protects against infection. Increased glycogen in vaginal cells predisposes the mother to yeast infections in pregnancy. **Goodell's sign** is the softening of the cervix starting at about 6 weeks. At the same time, increased vascularity causes the cervix and vagina to appear bluish (**Chadwick's sign**). Due to these changes the cervix is more friable and may bleed slightly with sexual intercourse or vaginal

examination. Near the end of pregnancy, cervical **ripening,** or softening, and **effacement,** or thinning, occurs in preparation for labor. Progressive **dilation,** or opening of the cervix, does not usually occur until the onset of active labor. Externally, the labia majora, labia minora, clitoris, and vaginal introitus enlarge because of hypertrophy and increased vascularity.

CHANGES IN BREASTS

One of the first symptoms in pregnancy is breast tenderness, enlargement, and tingling, which is noticeable at 4 to 6 weeks' gestation. These changes are caused by the growth of the alveoli and ductal system and the deposition of fat in the breasts under the influence of estrogen and progesterone. The nipple and the **areola,** the pink circle around the nipple, darken in color in pregnancy, and the sebaceous glands on the areola, **Montgomery's tubercles,** enlarge and produce a secretion that

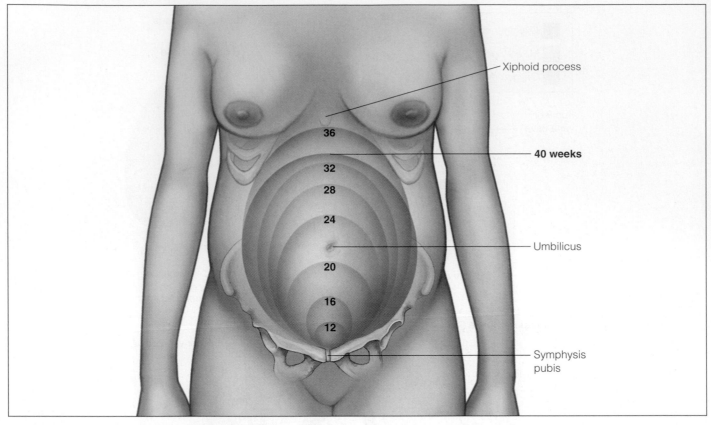

Figure 26.5 ● Fundal height in pregnancy.

protects and lubricates the nipples. With the doubling of the blood flow to the breasts, the vascular network above the breasts enlarges and becomes more visible. **Colostrum,** a yellowish specialized form of early breast milk, is produced starting in the second trimester, and is replaced by mature milk during the early days of lactation after the delivery of the baby (see Figure 26.6 ●).

RESPIRATORY SYSTEM CHANGES

Mechanical and biochemical changes during pregnancy allow the respiratory needs of both mother and fetus to be met. The enlarging uterus lifts the diaphragm up 4 cm, the transverse diameter of the chest increases, the ribs flare, and the subcostal angle increases. The increasing hormonal levels of progesterone and relaxin allow these changes in the thorax.

The respiratory-stimulating properties of progesterone contribute to the following:

- A slight increase in respiratory rate of about 2 breaths per minute
- A lowered threshold for carbon dioxide contributing to a sense of dyspnea by the pregnant female
- Decreased airway resistance
- Increased tidal volume and inspiratory capacity
- Decreased expiratory volume

The vital capacity is unchanged, but oxygen consumption is increased 20 to 60%. The pregnant female may report great fatigue, particularly in the first trimester, due to these changes. Hyperventilation may occur, and rales in the base of the lung may be heard as a result of compression by the growing uterus.

CARDIOVASCULAR AND HEMATOLOGIC SYSTEM CHANGES

The most significant hematologic change is an increase in blood and plasma volume of 30 to 50% beginning at 6 to 8 weeks and is greater in multiple pregnancies. This change is facilitated by three factors:

- The increased progesterone leads to decreased venous tone.
- The increased progesterone combined with increased estrogen results in increased sodium retention and an increase in total body water.
- The shunt of blood to uteroplacental circulation provides physical space for increased plasma volume.

Other hematologic changes include the following:

- A 25 to 33% increase in red blood cells (RBCs)
- Decrease in hemoglobin and hematocrit or **physiologic anemia** caused by plasma volume increase outpacing the increase in RBCs
- Gradual increase in reticulocytes
- Increased white blood cells (WBCs)
- Hypercoagulable state caused by increased activity of most coagulation factors and decreased activities of factors that inhibit coagulation

Physical changes in the cardiac system include cardiac enlargement caused by the increased blood volume and accompanying increase in cardiac output. The upward displacement of the di-

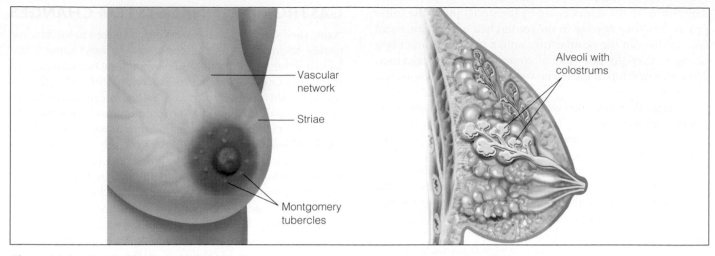

Figure 26.6 ● Breast changes in pregnancy.

aphragm by the growing uterus shifts the heart upward and to the left. Most pregnant females will have an S_1 sound that is louder. Systolic murmurs are usually heard. A murmur over the mammary vessels, the **mammary souffle,** due to increased blood flow, is occasionally heard. The heart rate gradually increases by 10 to 20 beats per minute (bpm) over the course of the pregnancy.

Blood pressure remains the same at the beginning of pregnancy. The decrease in vascular resistance leads to a decrease in diastolic blood pressure that reaches its nadir, or lowest point, during the second trimester and gradually returns to baseline by the time of delivery.

The changes in hemodynamics can cause orthostatic stress when the female changes position from sitting to standing or lying to sitting. **Supine hypotension syndrome,** also known as the vena cava syndrome, occurs when pressure from the pregnant uterus compresses the aorta and the inferior vena cava when the female is in the supine position (see Figure 26.7 ●). She may experience dizziness, syncope, and a significant drop in heart rate and blood pressure.

Decreased peripheral resistance leads to increased filling in the legs, but the pressure of the growing uterus on the femoral veins restricts venous return, leading to increased dependent edema, and varicosities in the legs, vulva, and rectum (hemorrhoids).

INTEGUMENTARY SYSTEM CHANGES

Hormonal and mechanical factors cause the integumentary changes seen with pregnancy. Categories of change include alterations in pigmentation, connective tissue, vascular system, secretory glands, skin, hair, and pruritus. The changes are not usually pathologic, but are a source of concern to expectant mothers.

Alterations in pigmentation, the most common integumentary changes in pregnancy, are caused by the increase in estrogen and progesterone early in pregnancy, and by the increase in placental hormones and melanocyte-stimulating hormone, as well as others, later in pregnancy. Any areas of pigmentation in the body will usually become darker for females of all skin colors, including the areolae, axillae, perineum, and inner thighs. The *linea alba,* a tendinous line that extends midline from the symphysis pubis to the xiphoid, darkens with the progression of the fundus up through the abdomen, and becomes the **linea nigra.** *Melasma,* also called chloasma or the "mask of pregnancy," occurs in a butterfly pattern over the forehead, nose, and cheeks. There is a strong genetic predisposition, and it is also seen with the use of combined oral contraceptive pills. Freckles, nevi, and scars may also darken in pregnancy.

A change in connective tissue is **striae gravidarum,** also known as stretch marks, pinkish-purplish streaks that are

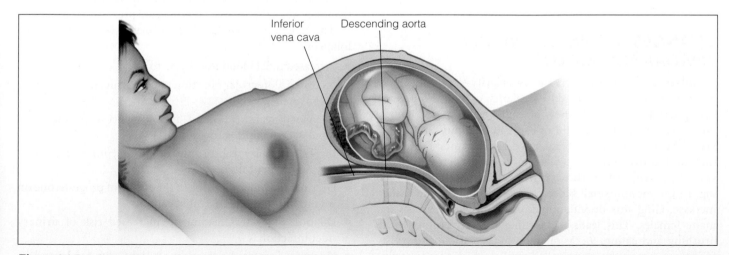

Figure 26.7 ● Supine hypotension in pregnancy. The weight of the uterus compresses the vena cava, trapping blood in the lower extremities.

depressions in the skin. Caused by the stretching of the collagen in skin, they develop in the second half of pregnancy and fade to silver in the postpartum; unlike most integumentary changes, they do not resolve completely after pregnancy. They may develop in the lower abdomen, breasts, thighs, and buttocks.

Vascular alterations that affect the integumentary system are spider angiomas or nevi, and palmar erythema. Spider angiomas or nevi are arterioles dilated at the center, with branches radiating outward, appearing on the face, neck, and arms. They fade after pregnancy, but do not usually disappear. They often occur with palmar erythema, a reddening or mottling of the palms or fleshy side of the fingers, which occurs after the first trimester, has a genetic predisposition, and regresses by the first week after birth.

Alterations in secretory glands in pregnancy include a decrease in apocrine sweat gland activity in the axillae, abdomen, and genitalia. The eccrine sweat glands in the palms, soles, and forehead increase in activity due to increases in thyroid and metabolic activity, allowing for dissipation of increased heat. Some females experience a "glow" in their skin during pregnancy, while some experience an increase in acne due to increased sebaceous gland activity.

A skin change that sometimes occurs in the second half of pregnancy is the development of soft, pedunculated, flesh-colored or pigmented skin tags. They occur on the sides of the face and neck, on the upper axillae, between and under the breasts, and in the groin.

Due to the hormonal influence of estrogen in pregnancy, more hairs enter the growth phase. Some females experience mild hirsutism and report thicker hair. Consequently, more than the usual number of hairs reach maturity and fall out in the postpartum period during months 1 to 5. Usually all hair regrows by 6 to 15 months postpartum. Occasionally nails become soft or more brittle.

Pruritus, itching, is common in the abdomen in the third trimester, and if severe must be distinguished from rare dermatologic disorders in pregnancy such as cholestasis of pregnancy, pruritic urticarial papules and plaques of pregnancy (PUPPP), herpes gestationis, and prurigo of pregnancy. Figure 26.8 ● depicts integumentary changes in pregnancy.

CHANGES IN THE EAR, NOSE, THROAT, AND MOUTH

An increase in estrogen increases vascularity throughout the body in pregnancy. Increased vascularity of the middle ear may cause a feeling of fullness or earaches. Increased blood flow (hyperemia) to the sinuses can cause rhinitis and epistaxis. The sense of smell is heightened in pregnancy. Edema of the vocal cords may cause hoarseness or deepening of the voice. Hyperemia of the throat can lead to an increase in snoring. In the mouth, small blood vessels and connective tissue increase. Gingivitis or inflammation of the gums occurs in many females. This leads to bleeding and discomfort with brushing and eating. Occasionally a hyperplasic overgrowth forms a mass on the gums called epulis, which bleeds easily and recedes after birth.

GASTROINTESTINAL SYSTEM CHANGES

Nausea and vomiting are common beginning at 4 to 6 weeks, and usually resolve by 12 weeks' gestation. The exact cause is unknown, although hormonal and psychological factors have been implicated. Other gastrointestinal changes occur during the second and third trimesters. *Ptyalism,* an increase in saliva production, may occasionally occur with nausea and vomiting. The pregnant female may also report pica, an abnormal craving for and ingestion of nonnutritive substances such as starch, dirt, or ice. Mechanical pressure from the growing uterus contributes to displacement of the small intestine and reduces motility. The increased secretion of progesterone further reduces motility because of decreased gastric tone and increased smooth muscle relaxation; thus, the emptying time of the stomach and bowel is prolonged, and constipation is common. Progesterone's relaxing effect on smooth muscle also accounts for the prolonged emptying time of the gallbladder, and gallstone formation may result. *Pyrosis,* or heartburn, the regurgitation of the acidic contents of the stomach into the esophagus, is related to the enlarging uterus displacing the stomach upward and to the relaxation of the esophageal sphincter. Hemorrhoids are another common finding in the third trimester, resulting from the increasing size of the uterus creating pressure on the pelvic veins. If the mother is constipated, the pressure on the venous structures from straining to move the bowels can also lead to hemorrhoids.

Nutritional demands of the pregnancy and fetus increase the maternal requirements. Each day, the mother requires an increased intake of 300 calories, and 15 g or more of protein. Most nutrient requirements increase from 20 to 100%. The recommended weight gain for females of average weight is 25 to 35 lb, 28 to 40 lb if underweight, and 15 to 25 lb if overweight.

URINARY SYSTEM CHANGES

The growing uterus causes displacement of the ureters and kidneys, especially on the right side. A slower flow of urine through the ureters causes physiological hydronephrosis and hydroureter. Estrogen causes increased bladder vascularity, predisposing the mucosa to bleed more easily. Urinary frequency occurs in the first trimester as the uterus grows and puts pressure on the bladder. Relief from frequency occurs after the uterus moves out of the pelvis, only to return in the third trimester when the enlarged uterus again presses on the bladder.

The functional changes in the urinary system include the following:

- Increased renal blood flow by 35 to 60%
- Increased glomerular filtration rate by as much as 50% above prepregnancy levels
- Decreased reabsorption of filtered glucose in the renal tubules, contributing to glycosuria
- Increased tubular reabsorption of sodium, promoting necessary retention of fluid
- Decreased bladder tone due to the effects of progesterone on smooth muscle, and increased capacity
- Dilation of ureters leading to increased risk of urinary tract infection
- Nocturia, increased urination at night, due to dependent edema resolving while recumbent

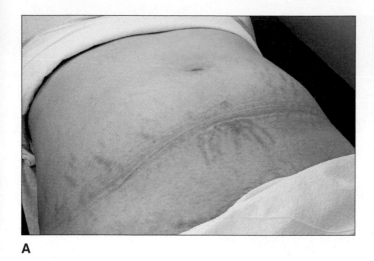

A

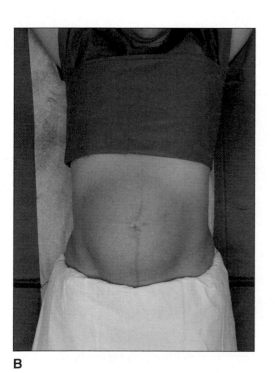

B

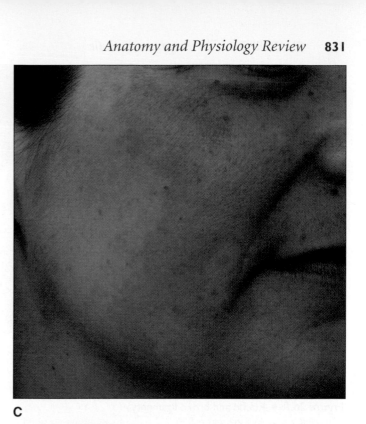

C

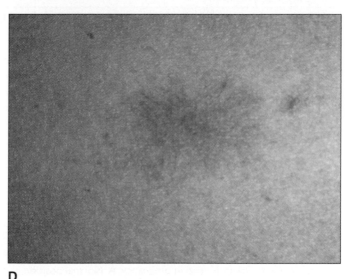

D

Figure 26.8 ● Integumentary changes in pregnancy. A. Striae. B. Linea nigra. C. Melasma. D. Spider angioma.

MUSCULOSKELETAL CHANGES

Anatomical changes in the musculoskeletal system result from the influence of hormones, growth of the fetus, and maternal weight gain. Round ligaments, which attach to the uterus just under the fallopian tubes and insert in the groin, may cause sharp, shooting lower abdominal and groin pain in early pregnancy as the uterus enlarges. As pregnancy advances, the growing uterus tilts the pelvis forward, increasing the lumbosacral curve and creating a gradual lordosis, and the stretching of the broad ligament attaching the uterus to the sacrum may cause back pain (see Figure 26.9 ●). The enlarging breasts pull the shoulders forward, and the client may assume a stoop-shouldered stance. The pelvic joints and ligaments are relaxed by progesterone and relaxin. The rectus abdominis muscles that run vertically down the midline of the abdomen may separate during the third trimester. This is called **diastasis recti ab-**

dominis and may allow the abdominal contents to protrude (see Figure 26.10 ●). The weight of the uterus and breasts, along with the relaxation of the pelvic joints, changes the client's center of gravity, stance, and gait. Muscle cramps and ligament injury are more frequent in pregnancy. Shoe size, especially width, may increase permanently.

NEUROLOGIC SYSTEM CHANGES

Neurologic changes frequently associated with pregnancy include the following:

- Increase in frequency of vascular headaches
- Entrapment neuropathies due to mechanical pressures in the peripheral nervous system
  - Sciatica, pain, numbness, or tingling feeling in the thigh, caused by pressure of the growing uterus on the sciatic nerve

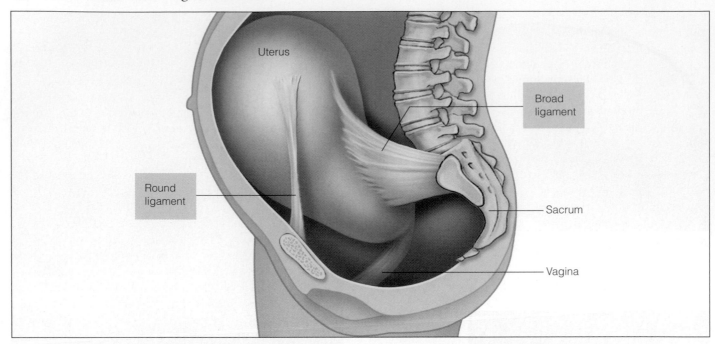

Figure 26.9 ● Round and broad ligaments.

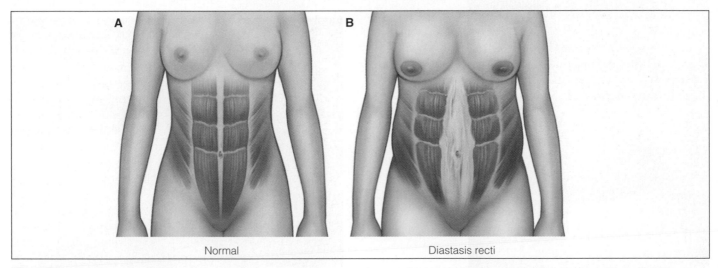

Figure 26.10 ● Diastasis recti in pregnancy. A. Normal position in nonpregnant female. B. Diastasis recti abdominis in pregnant female.

• Carpal tunnel syndrome, pressure on the median nerve beneath the carpal ligament of the wrist, causing burning, tingling, and pain in the hand

● Change in corneal curvature, increased corneal thickness/edema, or change in the tear production, causing changes in optical prescription

● Increased total sleep time and insomnia in first and third trimesters

● Leg cramps, which may be caused by inadequate intake of calcium

● Dizziness and light-headedness, which may be associated with supine hypotension syndrome and vasomotor instability

ENDOCRINE SYSTEM CHANGES

Changes in the endocrine system facilitate the metabolic functions that maintain maternal and fetal health throughout the pregnancy. Human chorionic gonadotropin (hCG), the hormone that is detected by pregnancy tests, is secreted by tissue surrounding the embryo soon after implantation. It serves as a messenger to the corpus luteum to maintain progesterone and estrogen production until the placenta starts to produce these hormones at approximately 5 weeks. It also may be involved in the suppression of maternal immunologic rejection of the fetal tissue.

The fetus and placenta become additional sites for synthesis and metabolism of hormones. The pituitary, thyroid, parathyroid, and adrenal glands enlarge because of estrogen stimulation and increased vascularity. Increases in the production of thyroid hormones, particularly T_3 and T_4, increase the basal metabolic rate (BMR), cardiac output, vasodilation, heart rate, and heat intolerance. The BMR may increase by eightfold.

Changes also occur in the metabolism of protein, glucose, and fats due to the increasing production of human placental lactogen (hPL) by the placenta. Throughout pregnancy, protein is metabolized more efficiently to meet fetal needs. In the second trimester, insulin production increases in response to the rising glucose levels, and falls to nonpregnant levels at the end of pregnancy. In addition, the mother's body tissues develop a decreased sensitivity to insulin, sometimes referred to as the diabetogenic state of pregnancy. This ensures an adequate supply of glucose, which the fetus requires in large amounts. A disruption in this delicate homeostatic balance results in gestational diabetes mellitus. A form of glucose-sparing called accelerated starvation causes the metabolism of fats stored in pregnancy, which makes more glucose available to the fetus, but puts the pregnant female at greater risk of ketosis; ketones are harmful to the fetal brain. Pregnant females are at increased risk of lipolysis during pregnancy secondary to hypoglycemia or prolonged fasting.

After birth, *oxytocin,* secreted by the posterior pituitary, stimulates uterine contractions and causes milk ejection in the mammary glands. Prolactin, secreted by the anterior pituitary, increases production of breast milk after delivery.

CULTURAL VARIATIONS

At the time of pregnancy and birth, females in all stages of acculturation to the mainstream culture will hear the call of their roots. Culturally competent nurses will know specifics about individual cultural groups, not to stereotype clients but to gain a perspective on what issues might pertain to the individual. Table 26.4 summarizes beliefs about pregnancy, childbirth, the postpartum period, and the newborn for cultural, racial, and ethnic groups with over 1 million members according to the 2000 U.S. Census. Sources of diversity within groups include timing of immigration, urban or rural origin, socioeconomic status, educational level, religion, strength of ethnic identity, family style, and personal characteristics.

LABORATORY TESTS IN PREGNANCY

Several types of laboratory tests can be performed during pregnancy. Table 26.5 provides information about these various tests, when they should be performed during pregnancy, the normal and abnormal values, and any client education that is needed as follow-up.

THE POSTPARTUM FEMALE

The critical role of the nurse in assisting clients through the maternity cycle continues after the birth with postpartum assessment.

ANATOMY AND PHYSIOLOGY REVIEW

During the postpartum period, the reproductive organs return to the nonpregnant state through the process of involution. Immediately after the birth of the placenta, the uterine fundus is located midway between the symphysis pubis and the umbilicus. The fundus rises to the umbilicus by 12 hours later, and decreases approximately 1 cm or fingerbreadth per day until it is nonpalpable externally by 10 days. The contracted uterus is firm, preventing postpartum hemorrhage through ligation of the uterine arteries by the contraction. The uterus is longer and wider in mothers who have a cesarean section and shorter in mothers who breast-feed.

The uterine lining or endometrium returns to the nonpregnant state through the process of a postpartum vaginal discharge called lochia. The initial *lochia rubra* contains blood from the placental site, amniotic membrane, cells from the decidua basalis, vernix and lanugo from the infant's skin, and meconium. It is dark red and has a fleshy odor, and lasts anywhere from 2 days to 18 days. Next the discharge becomes pinkish and is called *lochia serosa.* It is composed of blood, placental site exudates, erythrocytes, leukocytes, cervical mucus, microorganisms, and decidua, and lasts approximately a week. Finally, the discharge becomes whitish-yellow, *lochia alba,* and is composed of leukocytes, mucus, bacteria, epithelial cells, and decidua. Most females will have vaginal discharge from 10 days to 5 or 6 weeks.

The cervix closes over the next 2 weeks, and the vagina regains the folds or rugae. Decreased lubrication and lacerations or surgical incisions to the perineum cause discomfort. Hemorrhoids caused by pelvic pressure during pregnancy or pushing during childbirth may occur. Gastric motility slows during labor and resumes afterward. Bowel movements usually restart after 2 to 3 days postpartum. The urethra may be bruised, swollen, or damaged by childbirth or episiotomy.

After birth, the breasts become engorged or full due to swelling of the lymphatic tissue and initial milk production. At days 2 to 4 the mature milk starts to be produced by the alveoli, with a lower protein and immunoglobulin content and higher fat content than the initial colostrum, and engorgement occurs.

The hormones estrogen and progesterone, secreted by the placenta, decrease rapidly after birth. Prolactin, which controls milk production, increases after birth. Oxytocin acts on the smooth muscle of the uterus and muscle cells surrounding the breast alveoli. In nonbreastfeeding mothers menses return at 6 to 10 weeks postpartum. In lactating mothers, menses usually does not return for 12 or more weeks; with exclusive breast-feeding and introduction of solid foods after 6 months, amenorrhea may last a year or more. Eighty percent of first menses in lactating mothers are preceded by anovulatory cycles due to the action of prolactin. These hormonal swings, combined with role changes and exhaustion, contribute to emotional fragility, expressed as "baby blues."

In the circulatory system, it may take up to 6 weeks for slowed blood velocity and relaxed veins to return to the nonpregnant state, so a risk of thromboembolism remains during the postpartum period. In the renal system, diuresis occurs days 2 to 5, and decreased bladder tone and urinary retention can be worsened by birth trauma.

THE BUBBLESHE HEAD-TO-TOE POSTPARTUM ASSESSMENT

With all the physiological changes occurring in the postpartum period, a thorough postpartum assessment plays an important role in healthcare. The mnemonic BUBBLESHE can be used to remember the steps in assessing a postpartum client.

Table 26.4 Cultural Beliefs and Childbearing

CULTURE (U.S. POPULATION 2000)	PREGNANCY	BIRTH	POSTPARTUM/ NEWBORN
African Americans (34.7 million)	Pregnancy is respected and highly valued; pica occasionally occurs; late entry to care seen in teen and low socioeconomic groups.	Usually in the hospital; typically presents late in labor with father of baby (FOB) and female relatives; FOB usually unlikely to provide labor support spontaneously.	Rest encouraged; female relative, especially maternal grandmother, will stay with new mother; herbal teas used; avoidance of drafts practiced; breast-feeding uncommon; mothers are typically caregivers.
Native Americans (2.5 million)	High birth rate; pregnancy is sacred period with traditional rituals and taboos such as avoiding negative thoughts, dead animals, inactivity; pregnancy seen as normal process that does not require medical intervention; also entry to care problems related to transportation and health problems; smoking, fetal alcohol syndrome, and diabetes significant problems.	Usually in hospital, occasionally birth center; medicine person may be called upon to assist; certified nurse-midwives attend many deliveries with emphasis on active participation; placenta and umbilical cord may be saved for burial.	Lying-in period observed in some lying-itribes; acculturation decreasing use of such traditional practices as mothering helper after birth; infants wrapped tightly in blankets or cradleboards; amulets or juniper bracelets to provide protection to infant may be used.
Arab Americans (1.2 million)	Chastity until marriage highly valued and enforced; pregnancy brings increased social status; strenuous activity is avoided; strong emotions believed to hurt pregnancy; cravings are satisfied; care sought for confirmation of pregnancy and problems but not preventive care.	Husband does not participate in labor support but is close by; female relatives provide labor support; a rug to bite on may be used for pain, and herbal drinks offered; vocalization and prayers allowed; placenta considered part of human remains and burial preferred.	A 40-day lying-in period observed; postpartal females considered impure and no sexual intercourse while bleeding; strenuous activity and drafts avoided; breast-feeding for 2 years common; special foods encouraged including fresh goat's milk, candied sesame seed butter, and chicken soup; infant wrapped with cotton umbilical band and massaged with olive oil; amulet pouches pinned to clothing.
Central Americans (1.7 million)	Pregnant females given attention; avoidance of cool air, "hot" foods, strong emotions, and moonlight recommended in some Latin cultures.	Loud vocalization of pain common; pregnant woman's mother and female relatives often present for birth; fathers usually passive.	*La cuarenta,* 40-day lying-in period, may be observed; "cold" foods, drafts, strong emotional states avoided; foods offered may include chicken soup, bananas, and meat; herbal teas and baths may be used for mother and child; public breast-feeding accepted.
Chinese (2.4 million)	Good nutrition, activity restriction, and positive thought during pregnancy recommended; iron supplements believed to harden bones and complicate delivery; may use ginseng in third trimester; prenatal care expected and practiced.	Father and family members may wait outside delivery room; placenta has no significance; mothers may be reluctant to vocalize pain or ask for pain medication.	One-month postpartum period observed; goal of decreasing yin or cold air through consumption of "hot" foods such as ginger, chicken soup, eggs, fish, pork recommended; rice wine avoided for 2 weeks; no going outdoors and windows are kept closed; grandmothers provide support and advice.
Colombians (470,684; largest group of South Americans, 1.3 million)	Usual activities and diet maintained until term; some believe fright should be avoided and cravings satisfied.	Females may eat and drink little during labor due to fear of vomiting; family members not expected to be present at delivery; analgesia welcome but not expected by low-income women.	*Quarentena* for 40 days observed; if women go outside, may cover ears with cotton; breast-feeding common, but not usually over a year; amulets against evil eye such as bead bracelet may be used.
Cubans (1.2 million)	Avoidance of loud noises, strenuous activities, and people with deformities recommended; fresh fruit and low-salt foods recommended.	Pregnant woman's mother present; acculturated fathers may participate; prefer physician provider; pain expressed loudly.	Mother and infant housebound for 41 days; pregnant woman's mother and sisters provide care; new mother protected from stress.
Filipinos (1.9 million)	Pampering pregnant females is a social value; prolonged sitting or sleeping discouraged; sexual intercourse taboo during last 2 months of pregnancy; in late pregnancy, "slippery" foods such as fresh eggs encouraged for easier birth.	Traditionally, fathers not present; pregnant women encouraged to be assertive and vocal during labor; traditional placental burial not usually practiced in U.S. hospitals.	Bathing and activity are restricted in the postpartum period of 10 days; breast-feeding, sometimes to toddlerhood, is common; pelvic binder may be used for 6 weeks; cold drinks and cold drafts avoided; *hilot* may provide massage and perineal hygiene; religious medals or tiger tooth pendant may be pinned to infant's clothing.

Table 26.4	Cultural Beliefs and Childbearing *(continued)*		
CULTURE (U.S. POPULATION 2000)	**PREGNANCY**	**BIRTH**	**POSTPARTUM/ NEWBORN**
Koreans (1.1 million)	Seaweed soup is popular pregnancy food, but many foods are forbidden, including duck, eggs, crab, and rabbit; rest promoted.	Traditionally stoic, Koreans in North America are more vocal in modern times; fathers traditionally not present; only warm food and water consumed.	Exposure to cold and water avoided in postpartum period of 3 to 8 weeks; perineal ice packs may be refused; strong preference for sons; infant's whole body covered to prevent exposure to cold air.
Mexicans (20.6 million)	Moderate activity is encouraged; medications including iron and vitamins may be avoided; excellent self-care promoted, including exercise, rest, good nutrition, avoidance of smoking, drugs, and alcohol; grandmothers and female relatives provide domestic support in late pregnancy.	Loud verbal repetition of "aye, yie, yie" used for pain relief; ambulation recommended; fathers present at birth but do not provide labor support.	A 40-day lying-in period, *la cuarentena*, observed; new mothers discouraged from getting out of bed for several hours after birth; showers discouraged for several days; breast-feeding common; chiles and beans avoided; herbal teas offered to infant; admiring infant without touching puts infant at risk of evil eye.
Puerto Ricans (3.4 million)	Pregnant females indulged; cravings and morning sickness common; some females refrain from sexual activity in the second and third trimesters; extended family may be involved in prenatal care.	Hygiene and modesty valued in labor; extended family present in labor.	During the *cuarentena*, family assists mother; hair not washed during this period; chicken broths and other soups offered to mother; bottle-feeding more common; beans, eggs, and starches avoided during breast-feeding; amulet neck chain may be worn by infant.
South Asian Indians (1.7 million)	Pregnancy is healthy state; heavy lifting and shock proscribed; grandmothers important source of advice; Ayurvedic practitioners consume "cold" foods such as milk products, fruits, and vegetables; pregnant woman may return to her mother's home at end of pregnancy; medicinal oils and massage may be given to pregnant women; Hindus have a special ritual for pregnant women in third trimester.	Light eating advised during labor; traditionally fathers not involved in birthing process; sex of child not told to mother until after placenta delivers; ambulation encouraged in early labor; afterbirth burial traditions not usually observed in North America; Muslim male relatives recite words in right and left ear of newborn to confirm child is Muslim.	A lying-in period of 40 to 56 days is observed; special cooling dishes provided to new mother using ingredients such as herbs and clarified butter; birth celebration party may be held; infant charms may be worn to ward off evil eye; massage for mother and child may be provided; breast-feeding for 6 months to 2 years encouraged.
Vietnamese (1.1 million)	A regimen of "cold" and "hot," and "tonic" and "wind" foods is recommended during pregnancy; sexual intercourse taboo; male personnel may intimidate females in prenatal care.	Father not traditionally present at birth; female relatives provide support; laboring females stoic; natural childbirth preferred, but anesthesia accepted.	Recuperation period is 3 months; mothers do not take full shower for 1 to 3 months; hot, salty towels may be applied to vaginal area; breast-feeding common for up to 1 year, with "cold" or "windy" foods avoided; the newborn should not be given compliments due to fear of evil spirits; the head of the newborn should not be touched.

Source: Adapted from St. Hill, P., Lipson, J. G., & Meleis, A. I. (2003). *Caring for women cross-culturally.* Philadelphia: F. A. Davis; and Lipson, J. G., Dibble, S. L., & Minarik, P. A. (1996). *Culture & nursing care.* San Francisco: UCSF Nursing Press. Population figures from U.S. Census Bureau.

B Breast

U Uterus

B Bowel

B Bladder

L Lochia

E Episiotomy/ perineum

S Support system

H Homans' sign and extremities

E Emotional state

In preparation for the postpartum assessment, the nurse gathers the following supplies: lab coat, stethoscope, black ink pen, and penlight. Prior to entering the room, it is important to review the data needed to fill out the assessment flow sheet (data on pain, UTI symptoms, voiding, stooling, flatus, bleeding, support system, bonding, etc.) as well as the physical assessment. Establishing a good rapport with the client is important, along with the physical exam. The nurse should project caring and confidence, and use eye contact.

Throughout all aspects of the assessment the nurse must be sure to maintain the client's privacy and dignity.

Assess the vital signs, and auscultate the lungs, the heart, and the abdomen. Inspect the IV/saline lock site. Examine the client's breast, palpate for costovertebral angle tenderness, and palpate the fundus.

Inspect the lower extremities for vascular changes, perform the Homans' test and assess for edema. Place the client in a lateral praction to inspect the perineum and rectum.

Table 26.5 Tests in Pregnancy

NAME OF TEST	TIMING OF TEST IN PREGNANCY	NORMAL VALUE	ABNORMAL VALUES	SPECIAL TEACHING
Blood Type, Rh Factor, and Antibody Screen	Initial OB visit and 28 weeks for Rh-negative females	A, B, AB, O, Rh+ or −; no irregular antibodies	Irregular antibodies found	If not her first pregnancy, inquire about previous Rh immune globulin (RhoGAM) administration if Rh−.
Hematocrit	Initial OB visit and 36 weeks	33 to 44%	Outside range	Eat iron-rich foods. Report any bleeding.
Hemoglobin	Initial OB visit and 36 weeks	11 to 14 g/dl	Outside range	Effects of pregnancy on iron needs.
RBC	Initial OB visit	100 to 400 ng/ml cells	Outside range	Red cell indices will also be examined to R/O hemoglobinopathies.
WBC	Initial OB visit	6 to 16×10^3/mm^3	Outside range	Report signs of infection.
Platelets	Initial OB visit	130,000 to 300,000/ml	Outside range	Report abnormal bleeding from gums, bruising.
HIV	Offered at initial OB visit and prn	Negative	Positive Confirmed by further testing: Western blot	Specific informed consent obtained prior to testing. Advise of dramatic decrease in vertical (mother to child) transmission with medication.
Hepatitis B	Initial OB visit	Negative	Positive	Inform client of sexual transmissibility. Explain importance of prophylaxis for infant.
Gonorrhea	Initial OB visit; third trimester if high risk	Negative	Positive	Educate client about infection. Empathetic listening if +. Stress importance of compliance and partner treatment.
Chlamydia	Initial OB visit; third trimester if high risk	Negative	Positive	Address STD prevention.
Rubella Titer	Initial OB visit	Immune	Nonimmune	Recommend maternal immunization after birth. Stress the avoidance of pregnancy for 3 months after immunization. Avoid first-trimester exposure to infection due to risk of congenital rubella syndrome.
Tuberculin Skin Testing	Initial OB visit if high risk	Negative	Positive induration > 10 mm in nonimmunocompromised client	Educate mother about infection. Teach respiratory precautions. Encourage smoking cessation.
Urinalysis	Initial OB visit	Negative	Presence of protein, glucose, ketones, RBCs, WBCs	
Urine Culture	Initial OB visit	Negative	Positive bacteria > 100,000 col	Wipe from front to back during toileting. Report urgency, flank pain, frequency, burning upon urination.
Papanicolaou Smear	Initial OB visit	Negative	Epithelial cell abnormalities or neoplasms present	Refrain from intercourse or douching 2 to 3 days prior to test (for accuracy). Discuss individualized schedule of testing.
RPR/VDRL FTA-ABS (Syphilis)	Initial OB visit; third trimester	Nonreactive	Reactive FTA-ABS reports a ratio	Educate about infection stages and treatment; advise compliance and abstinence during treatment; reinforce importance of follow-up.

Table 26.5	Tests in Pregnancy *(continued)*			
NAME OF TEST	**TIMING OF TEST IN PREGNANCY**	**NORMAL VALUE**	**ABNORMAL VALUES**	**SPECIAL TEACHING**
Multiple Marker Genetic Screen	15 to 20 weeks' gestation; first trimester for PAPP-A and Free Beta	No increased risk	Elevated risk	Discuss conditions screened for and limitations of test. Emphasize need for diagnostic testing if screen is positive.
50-g Glucose Challenge Test	24 to 28 weeks; may be done at initial prenatal visit for clients with increased risk of GDM	≤140 (some are using 135 mm/dl)	>140	Not fasting; blood drawn exactly 1 hour after glucose is drunk.
3-Hour GTT	Follow-up to elevated 1-hour screen	Fasting <95 mg/dl 1-hr <180 mg/dl 2-hr <155 mg/dl 3-hr <140 mg/dl	Two or more values met or exceeded	Three days of unrestricted carbohydrates and physical activity; fasting prior to test; no smoking or caffeine before and during test; inform re: schedule of blood draws.
Group B Streptococcus	Third trimester/35 to 37 weeks	Positive	Negative	IV antibiotics will be given in active labor to decrease risk of transmission to infant.
Ultrasound	Optional, frequently at 15 to 20 weeks, dependent on rationale	Normal	Abnormal	Client can decide whether gender of child should be revealed; some ultrasound studies require vaginal probe; nuchal translucency test at 11 weeks is to screen for chromosomal abnormalities.

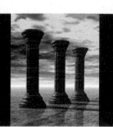

Gathering the Data

The role of the nurse in assessment of the pregnant female includes collecting subjective data from the focused interview. Objective data is obtained from the physical assessment. Objective data is also obtained from secondary sources such as health records, the results of laboratory tests, and radiologic and ultrasound studies. Preparation includes gathering equipment, positioning, and informing the client about the physical examination.

FOCUSED INTERVIEW

At the first prenatal visit, a very thorough interview is conducted. Important information that may dramatically affect the health of the fetus and mother can be obtained; the quality of the relationship with the client for the entire pregnancy is begun. The environment for the interview should be comfortable, quiet, private, and relaxing.

FOCUSED INTERVIEW QUESTIONS

The following sections provide sample questions for each of the categories identified above. A rationale for each of the questions is provided. The list of questions is not comprehensive but represents the type of questions required in a comprehensive prenatal focused interview.

RATIONALES

FOCUSED INTERVIEW QUESTIONS	RATIONALES

CONFIRMATION OF PREGNANCY

Prior to the provision of a prenatal interview and physical assessment, it must be ensured that the client is indeed pregnant. Pregnancy can be determined through urine and serum pregnancy tests, as well as signs and symptoms of pregnancy.

Urine pregnancy tests test for the beta subunit of hCG, and can be accurate 7 days after implantation, or can indicate pregnancy before the missed menstrual period. These tests produce results in 1 to 5 minutes and are 99% accurate. Serum pregnancy tests may indicate pregnancy as soon as 7 to 9 days after ovulation, or just after implantation. This test can be qualitative, with a value of positive or negative, or quantitative, with a level of hCG reported. Serum progesterone can also be obtained if necessary; nonviable pregnancies have lower levels than normal pregnancies.

Presumptive signs of pregnancy are symptoms the client reports that may have multiple causes other than pregnancy. These presumptive signs include amenorrhea, breast tenderness, nausea and vomiting, frequent urination, quickening, or the client's perception of fetal movement, skin changes, and fatigue. Probable signs are elicited by the nurse and have few causes other than pregnancy. Probable signs include positive pregnancy test, abdominal enlargement, Piskacek's sign, Hegar's sign, Goodell's sign, Chadwick's sign, and Braxton Hicks contractions. Positive signs of pregnancy have no possible explanation other than pregnancy. These include hearing the fetal heart with Doppler, fetoscope, or ultrasound, fetal movements verified by the examiner, and visualization of the fetus via ultrasound or radiology.

DEMOGRAPHICS

For the purposes of identification, statistics, billing, and record keeping, the following information must be collected for each pregnant client.

1. **What is your complete name and nickname?**

   ▶ Knowing the client's nickname is important during stressful situations such as labor.

2. **What is your address?**

3. **What is your date of birth?**

   ▶ This also screens for age-related complications.

4. **What is your race or ethnicity?**

   ▶ See Chapter 4 for more detail regarding questions about race and ethnic identity. ⌾ This question also screens for race/ethnicity-related genetic disorders.

5. **Do you work outside the home? How many hours per week do you work? Describe your activities at work.**

   ▶ This also screens for occupational hazards to the mother and fetus.

6. **Are you married, single, divorced, or widowed, or do you have a partner?**

   ▶ Questions 6 to 10 provide information about the client's support system.

7. **What is your baby's father's name?**

8. **What is your partner's name, if that is a different person?**

9. **Who is your emergency contact, and what is their phone number?**

10. **Who lives at home with you?**

11. **What is your religion?**

    ▶ This provides information that may relate to maternity care, such as attitudes toward blood products.

12. **How many years of school have you completed?**

    ▶ This information will assist in the development of the teaching plan.

FOCUSED INTERVIEW QUESTIONS

RATIONALES

MENSTRUAL HISTORY

1. When was the date of your last menstrual period?

▶ The estimated date of birth (EDB), also known as the estimated date of delivery (EDD), estimated date of confinement (EDC), or due date, is usually calculated by using the first day of the last menstrual period (LMP), which may also be useful in estimating gestational age.

2. Do you know the date you ovulated?

▶ This can help determine due date.

3. Do you know the date you conceived?

▶ This also can assist in dating the pregnancy.

4. Were you using any methods of contraception at the time you conceived?

▶ Although oral contraceptive pills have not shown any adverse effects on pregnancy, their use does affect the timing of ovulation. An IUD in place at the time of conception can cause complications in the pregnancy.

5. Describe your usual menstrual cycle.

▶ The typical menstrual cycle is 28 days in length. Prolonged, shortened, or irregular menstrual cycles affect the EDB. If the LMP was not normal for the client, it may have been implantation bleeding or a menstrual dysfunction. Some prenatal charts ask for last NORMAL menstrual period (LNMP) to assist in dating the pregnancy.

6. Have you had any cramping, bleeding, or spotting since your LMP?

▶ Cramping, bleeding, or spotting may indicate a problem with hormonal support of the endometrium and may lead to a spontaneous abortion.

7. How old were you when you got your first menstrual period?

▶ The number of years since **menarche,** or age of first menstrual period, helps determine physical maturity of the client.

CALCULATING ESTIMATED DATE OF BIRTH AND GESTATIONAL WEEKS

A pregnancy lasts approximately 266 days from conception, or 280 days from the LMP, based on a 28-day cycle. **Nägele's rule** can be used to compute the EDB based on the LMP (see Box 26.2). To use this approximate guide to determine the due date, 7 days are added to the day of the month of the first day of the LMP, 3 is subtracted

Box 26.2	**Using Nägele's Rule to Compute an Estimated Date of Birth (EDB)**

EXAMPLE: LMP = January 29, 2005

Rule = first day of LMP + 7, number of month − 3 (year of LMP + 1 if January 1 is passed during pregnancy)

Jan 29
    30   Day 1   Month Dec = 12th month
    31   2   Jan = 13 (if LMP is in January, February, or March,
Feb 1   3   Feb = 14 add 12 to month to prevent negative
     2   4   number) 14 − 3 = 11 = November
     3   5
     4   6
     5   7

Due date = November 5, 2005

FOCUSED INTERVIEW QUESTIONS	RATIONALES

from the number of the month (12 is added to the month number if the LMP occurs in January, February, or March), and the year of the due date is the year of the LMP, plus one year if January 1 is passed during the pregnancy.

A gestational wheel is a two-layer, round, computational device, usually made of laminated paper, which can also be used to compute the EDB and weeks of gestation. Each day of the month in the year has a line on the outer wheel, and each day of the week of the pregnancy has a line on the inner wheel. Zero weeks and days indicates the LMP, and exactly 40 weeks indicates the EDB on the inner wheel. If the zero or LMP line on the inner wheel is aligned with the date of the LMP on the outer wheel, the EDB can be found by determining which date lines up with exactly 40 weeks. If the LMP or EDB is correctly lined up with its date on the outer wheel, the current date on the outer wheel will line up with the gestational age (e.g., 36 weeks and 4 days, often recorded as 36.4 or 36 4/7, based on a 7-day week).

The third way that the EDB can be determined is through the use of ultrasound ("sonograms") in the first half of pregnancy. The EDB should be shared as soon as it is determined with the client, along with its degree of certainty. The fact that a due date actually is the middle day of a month straddling the due date by 2 weeks on each side should be emphasized.

OBSTETRICAL AND GYNECOLOGICAL HISTORY

1. Have you experienced any discomfort or unusual occurrences since your LMP?

▶ The client's response allows the nurse to evaluate whether the symptoms reported are expected or if they suggest development of a complication. The client will most likely report subjective signs of pregnancy, such as absence of menstrual periods, nausea, vomiting, breast tenderness, fatigue, abdominal enlargement, or urinary frequency. Client teaching and other nursing interventions can also be identified.

REACTION TO PREGNANCY

1. Was this pregnancy planned?

▶ Confirmation of pregnancy usually causes ambivalent feelings whether or not the pregnancy was planned. If the pregnancy was unplanned, the nurse needs to assess the mother's desire to maintain the pregnancy and explain available options.

2. How do you feel about this pregnancy? How does your family and partner [if applicable] feel about the pregnancy?

▶ This discussion can strengthen the relationship between the nurse and the client, and provide important cues to the home environment of the client.

PAST OBSTETRICAL HISTORY

1. Have you been pregnant before? If so, how many times?

▶ Multiparity, especially if there have been more than four previous pregnancies, increases the maternal risks of antepartal and postpartal hemorrhage and fetal/neonatal anemia. Teaching needs are also affected by the client's previous experiences.

FOCUSED INTERVIEW QUESTIONS	**RATIONALES**

2. Have you had any spontaneous or induced abortions?
   - If so, how far along in weeks were you?
   - Did you have any follow-up such as a D&C (dilation and curettage procedure)?

▶ Previous history of persistent spontaneous abortion (miscarriage or stillbirth) places the client at higher risk for subsequent spontaneous abortions. Induced abortions may cause trauma to the cervix and may interfere with cervical dilation and effacement during labor.

3. Describe any previous pregnancies, including the length of the pregnancy, the length of labor, problems during pregnancy, medications taken during pregnancy, prenatal care received, type of birth, and your perception of the experience.

▶ Discussion of the client's previous pregnancies helps the nurse anticipate needs and complications of the current pregnancy.

4. Describe your birth experience, including labor or delivery complications, the infant's condition at birth, the infant's weight, and whether the infant required additional treatment or special care after birth.

▶ Reviewing the client's previous birth experience(s) helps to anticipate needs and complications of the current pregnancy and to assess the client's current knowledge base and the success with which the client integrated the previous birth experience into her life experiences. An example of a previous complication that would impact the current pregnancy is group B streptococcus (GBS) colonization. If a client has a history of GBS colonization of the vagina in a previous pregnancy, her baby has a risk for early-onset infection that has serious morbidity and mortality, so she will need to be treated in labor with antibiotics.

5. Do you attend or plan to attend prenatal education classes?

▶ Assessment of prenatal education provides information on the client's current knowledge base and attitude toward education for self-care.

6. What are your expectations for this pregnancy?

▶ Identification of the client's desires helps the nurse provide guidance in formulating the birth plan in the present pregnancy.

PAST GYNECOLOGICAL HISTORY

1. When was your most recent Pap smear and what was the result?

▶ Abnormal Pap smears must be followed up during pregnancy as at any time.

2. At what age did you become sexually active?

▶ This influences risk for certain conditions.

3. What is your current number of sexual partners?

▶ This addresses risk for sexually transmitted infections.

4. How would you describe your sexual orientation: heterosexual, bisexual, or lesbian?

▶ This affects the types of risks incurred and helps determine what kind of education is offered.

5. What types of safer sex methods do you use and how often do you use them?

▶ This determines how much teaching in this area is required.

6. What methods of birth control have you used in the past? How satisfied were you with each method?

▶ This will influence teaching on this topic later in the pregnancy.

7. Have you ever had a sexually transmitted disease?
   - What was the treatment?
   - Were your partners treated and notified?

▶ Untreated STDs can cause complications in pregnancy.

8. Were you exposed to diethylstibestrol (DES) while your mother was pregnant with you?

▶ Females with exposure to diethylstilbestrol (DES), given from the 1940s to 1970s to prevent miscarriage, may have uterine anomalies.

9. Have you had any problems with or surgeries on your breasts, vagina, fallopian tubes, ovaries, or urinary tract?

▶ Problems in the genitourinary system may impact pregnancy. Fibroids will affect the measurement of fundal height during pregnancy. Some types of vaginitis can cause preterm labor.

FOCUSED INTERVIEW QUESTIONS	RATIONALES

10. Have you ever been raped? Did you receive any care afterward?

► A history of sexual abuse is linked to complications in pregnancy and may influence a client's psychological adaptation to pregnancy.

11. Do you have a history of infertility?

► Many causes of previous infertility can impact the current pregnancy. For example, pelvic inflammatory disease increases a client's risk of an ectopic pregnancy.

PAST MEDICAL HISTORY AND FAMILY HISTORY

1. Have you or any members of your family or your partner's family had any of the following conditions:
   - hypertension
   - heart disease
   - asthma
   - kidney or gallbladder problems
   - diabetes mellitus
   - blood or bleeding disorders
   - hepatitis
   - cancer
   - infectious diseases such as HIV
   - tuberculosis
   - chickenpox
   - allergies?

► The nurse needs to assess the family medical history to identify and investigate risk factors thoroughly. Preexisting maternal conditions may increase maternal and fetal risk.

► **Hypertension:** Mild to moderate hypertension poses the risk of intrauterine growth restriction (IUGR) and fetal death. When combined with smoking, there is an increased risk of placental abruption, when the placenta shears off the uterus, which is highly dangerous to mother and child.

► **Heart Disease:** Mitral valve prolapse complicated by regurgitation requires antibiotic prophylaxis to prevent bacteremia (bacterial infection of the blood).

► **Asthma:** The nurse should ask if asthma is well controlled and how stable medication levels have been, and note which medications are currently being used. Asthma can cause fetal growth restriction and may necessitate serial ultrasounds to follow growth in the intrapartum period. Meperdine and morphine for pain relief, and prostaglandin $F_{2\alpha}$ to control postpartum hemorrhage, are not recommended for use by clients with asthma.

► **Kidney and Gallbladder Disease:** Previous occurrences of urinary tract infection may increase risk for asymptomatic bacteriuria, the presence of bacteria in the urine without the usual symptoms of cystitis of urinary frequency, burning upon urination, and flank pain. Asymptomatic bacteriuria may lead to pyelonephritis (kidney infection). Urinary tract infections in pregnancy are associated with preterm labor and birth, low birth weight, anemia, amnionitis (infection of the membrane inside the uterus), hypertension, and preeclampsia. Gallbladder problems may be exacerbated in pregnancy.

► **Diabetes:** Pregestational diabetes (diabetes that was present before the pregnancy) is associated with fetal anomalies and pregnancy loss.

► **Blood and Bleeding Disorders:** Blood disorders such as anemia are associated with urinary tract infections, preterm delivery, low birth weight, preeclampsia, and perinatal mortality, if the anemia occurs before the third trimester. Females with sickle cell anemia and thalassemia have an increase in maternal and perinatal mortality and morbidity. If the client has sickle cell trait, she may have an increase in UTIs and iron and folate deficiency anemia. Female clients with thalassemia minor should be monitored for anemia.

► **Hepatitis:** If a pregnant client has a past history of hepatitis B and is part of the 6 to 10% that go on to become carriers, there is a risk of transmission to the newborn, as well as to her sexual partners. The infant should receive hepatitis B immunoglobulin as well as the HBV vaccine.

FOCUSED INTERVIEW QUESTIONS

2. What medications have you taken since your last menstrual period?

3. Have you ever had a blood transfusion?

RATIONALES

▶ **Cancer:** If cancer of the cervix was treated with cone biopsy, the client is at risk for preterm labor. *Infections:* HIV transmission to the newborn can be dramatically reduced by treatment in pregnancy. Tuberculosis treatment in pregnancy decreases neonatal mortality and morbidity. If the client does not report a history of varicella (chickenpox) and is not immune by blood test, she is susceptible to infection during pregnancy, which can be very harmful to the fetus or newborn. Varicella-zoster immune globulin can be given to exposed mothers and infants.

▶ **Allergies:** Allergies are identified in the prenatal period in the case that medications are recommended during the perinatal period. The nurse should note the type of reaction.

▶ This will help identify any teratogenic exposures as well as medications for illnesses and symptoms. Drugs in pregnancy are rated in risk categories A, B, C, D, and X (see Box 26.3).

Box 26.3	Drugs in Pregnancy: Risk Categories

A: Adequate and well-controlled studies in pregnant women have not shown an increased risk of fetal abnormalities.

B: Animal studies have revealed no evidence of harm to the fetus; however, there are no adequate and well-controlled studies in pregnant women, or animal studies have shown an adverse effect, but adequate and well-controlled studies in pregnant women have failed to demonstrate a risk to the fetus.

C: Animal studies have shown an adverse effect and there are no adequate and well-controlled studies in pregnant women, or no animal studies have been conducted and there are no adequate and well-controlled studies in pregnant women.

D: Adequate well-controlled or observational studies in pregnant women have demonstrated a risk to the fetus. However, the benefits of therapy may outweigh the potential risk.

X: Adequate well-controlled or observational studies in animals or pregnant women have demonstrated positive evidence of fetal abnormalities. The use of the product is contraindicated in women who are or who may become pregnant.

▶ This will help identify increased risk for abnormal antibody reactions, or bloodborne pathogens.

FOCUSED INTERVIEW QUESTIONS	RATIONALES

4. **What infections and immunizations have you had?**
   - Did you have chickenpox as a child?

▶ Some infections such as rubella can cause birth defects. If the client has hepatitis B, her newborn may need hepatitis B immunoglobulin and vaccine after birth. Prior immunizations and exposures affect the client's risk for contracting certain infections during pregnancy. Chickenpox, or varicella, can cause abnormalities in the fetus if contracted between 8 and 20 weeks in pregnancy.

5. **Review of systems questions: For each body system the nurse should discuss benign as well as worrisome changes in pregnancy. For example: Describe any changes you have experienced regarding your skin, digestion, bowel function, muscles and joints or vision.**

▶ This discussion will ensure that the pregnant client recalls each system and provides an important teaching opportunity.

GENETIC INFORMATION

In order to obtain information to determine genetic risk factors, the nurse will ask the client about three generations of her family. This is called a medical family tree or genetic pedigree. These questions refer to her brothers and sisters, her mother and father, her aunts and uncles on both sides, her grandparents and their siblings, all of her children, and all of her cousins on both sides. This information is also needed for the baby's father's family.

1. **Please tell me the date of birth and, if applicable, death, as well as any health problems or diseases for each of these individuals. For those who have died, tell me what the cause was, and date of death.**

▶ Three generations of medical history are needed to determine recessive as well as dominant genetic diseases.

2. **Do you or the baby's father, or anybody in your families, have any of the following conditions:**
   - sickle cell anemia or trait
   - thalassemia
   - Down syndrome
   - cystic fibrosis
   - Huntington's disease
   - muscular dystrophy
   - Tay-Sachs
   - hemophilia
   - any other blood or genetic disorders?

▶ Sometimes charting the medical family tree will not jog the memory of the client, but a specific mention of the condition will.

3. **What is your ethnic background?**

▶ Tay-Sachs occurs more frequently in Ashkenazi Jews, cystic fibrosis trait occurs in 1 in 29 northern European Caucasians, and the sickle cell trait occurs in 1 in 8 African Americans (see Table 26.6).

FOCUSED INTERVIEW QUESTIONS

RATIONALES

Table 26.6	Genetic Disorders and Traits with Increased Frequency by Ethnicity	

ETHNIC GROUP/ GEOGRAPHIC LOCATION	GENETIC DISORDERS AND TRAITS WITH INCREASED FREQUENCY
Africans and Descendants	Sickle cell anemia Alpha- and beta-thalassemia G6PD Fy (Duffy) antigen Rh positive Arcus cornea Café au lait spots Clubbing of digits Polydactyly Vitiligo Abnormal separation of sutures Earlobe absent Keloid Hereditary hypertrophic osteoarthropathy Scaphocephaly Alpha-antitrypsin deficiency
Europeans and Descendants	Cystic fibrosis Neural tube defects Congenital spherocytic anemia PTC taster Red-green color vision defect Alpha$_1$-antitrypsin deficiency Baldness Cleft lip and palate Hemophilia A Congenital dislocation of the hip Hereditary spherocytosis Phenylketonuria XYY syndrome
Ashkenazi Jews	Tay-Sachs disease Niemann-Pick disease Gaucher's disease Canavan's disease Torsion dystonia Familial dysautonomia Nonclassical 21-hydroxylase deficiency Bloom syndrome Hereditary breast cancer
Sephardic and Oriental Jews	G6PD Familial Mediterranean fever Gaucher's disease Beta-thalassemia Laron-type dwarfism
Puerto Rican	Sickle cell anemia
Mediterranean	Sickle cell anemia Alpha-thalassemia
Southeast Asian	Alpha-thalassemia Beta-thalassemia
Italian	Beta-thalassemia
Greek	Beta-thalassemia
Middle Eastern	Sickle cell anemia
French Canadian	Tay-Sachs disease Familial hypercholesterolemia
Lebanese	Familial hypercholesterolemia
Denmark	Alpha$_1$- antitrypsin deficiency
Hispanic	Sickle cell anemia
Scotland	Phenylketonuria
Finland	Phenylketonuria Gyrate atrophy
Japan	Phenylketonuria

Source: Mahowald, M. B., McKusick, V. A., Scheuerle, A. S., & Aspinwall, T. J. (2001). *Genetics in the clinic: Clinical, ethical, and social implications for primary care.* St. Louis, MO: Mosby; Lea, D. H., Jenkins, J. F., & Francomano, C. A. (1998). *Genetics in clinical practice: New directions for nursing and health care.* Boston: Jones & Bartlett; Nussbaum, R. L., McInnes, R. R., & Willard, H. F. (2001). *Thompson & Thompson genetics in medicine.* Philadelphia: W. B. Saunders.

FOCUSED INTERVIEW QUESTIONS	RATIONALES

LIFESTYLE AND SOCIAL HEALTH PRACTICES

1. **How much do you smoke per day? Does anyone in your household smoke?**

   ▶ Smoking doubles the risk of a low birth weight baby and increases the risk of ectopic pregnancy or placental complications. It also increases the infant's risk of SIDS, asthma, and autism after birth. Secondhand smoke exposure also may contribute to low birth weight.

2. **Since the start of pregnancy, how many alcoholic drinks have you consumed each day?**

   ▶ Any amount of alcohol consumption during pregnancy can cause fetal alcohol syndrome and related disorders, composed of physical, neurologic, and behavioral defects in the infant.

3. **What recreational drugs have you used since your last menstrual period? This includes marijuana, cocaine, heroin, prescription painkillers, methadone, and so on.**

   ▶ Cocaine and other drugs have been shown to cause miscarriage and multiple fetal defects.

4. **Have you ever been emotionally or physically abused by your partner or someone important to you?**
   - Within the last year, have you been pushed, shoved, slapped, hit, kicked, or otherwise physically hurt by someone?
   - If yes, by whom?
   - Within the last year, have you been forced to have sex?
   - If yes, by whom?
   - Are you afraid of your partner or anyone else?

   ▶ All female clients should be screened during each trimester for abuse. At least 4 to 8% of females report abuse during pregnancy, which makes abuse more common than most complications screened for in pregnancy such as diabetes and hypertension. Abuse can cause miscarriage, fetal trauma, maternal stress, smoking, and drug abuse. Risk factors for abuse in pregnancy include unintended pregnancy, unhappiness with pregnancy, young maternal age, single maternal status, higher parity, late or absent entry to care, and substance abuse. The nurse should notify the physician or midwife of any positive findings, and work together to develop a plan of care.

NUTRITION AND EXERCISE HISTORY

1. **What kind of exercise do you currently engage in? How many days per week for how many minutes do you do it?**

   ▶ Current recommendations state all pregnant clients should be screened for risk factors such as heart disease, lung disease, cervix that dilates prematurely, preterm labor, multiple births, frequent vaginal bleeding, placenta previa, or hypertension. If no high-risk conditions exist, all normal pregnant clients should be counseled to engage in an accumulated 30 minutes of moderate exercise on most if not all days each week. Exercise in pregnancy can prevent complications such as gestational diabetes, and build stamina for labor. Sports that are not safe in pregnancy include soccer, vigorous racquet sports, gymnastics, basketball, ice hockey, horseback riding, kickboxing, downhill skiing, and scuba diving. Females should not perform any exercises that require lying on the back after the first trimester.

ALERT!

If a pregnant female experiences any of the following conditions during exercise, she should stop exercising and call her healthcare provider:

- *bleeding from the vagina*
- *difficulty or labored breathing BEFORE she exercises*
- *dizziness, headache, or chest pain*
- *muscle weakness, calf pain, or swelling*
- *preterm labor symptoms*
- *decreased movement of the fetus*
- *leakage of fluid from the vagina*

FOCUSED INTERVIEW QUESTIONS	RATIONALES

2. **Describe everything you have consumed for the past 24 hours. Include water, vitamins, and supplements.**

| Table 26.7 | Recommended Daily Allowances (RDAs) of Major Nutrients by Women's Age Groups and in Pregnancy |

FEMALE RDA (BY AGE)	15–18	19–24	25–50	51+	PREGNANT
Calories	2200	2200	2200	1900	+300
Protein	44	46	50	50	60
Vitamin E	8	8	8	8	10
Vitamin K	55	60	65	65	65
Vitamin C	60	60	60	60	70
Thiamin	1.1	1.1	1.1	1.0	1.5
Riboflavin	1.3	1.3	1.3	1.2	1.6
Niacin	15	15	15	13	17
Vitamin B_6	1.5	1.6	1.6	1.6	2.2
Folate	180	180	180	180	400
Vitamin B_{12}	2.0	2.0	2.0	2.0	2.2
Iron	15	15	15	10	30
Zinc	12	12	12	12	15
Selenium	50	55	55	55	65

Source: Office on Women's Health in the Department of Health and Human Services *www.4women.gov*

ALERT!

Great nutrition is vital to the health of every mother and fetus during pregnancy. The nurse should give the client a "gold spoon" (plastic, of course) to remind her how valuable every bite is during pregnancy.

▶ During pregnancy, females should include the following in their diet: four or more servings of fruits and vegetables for vitamins and minerals; four or more servings of whole-grain or enriched bread and cereal for energy; four or more servings of milk and milk products for calcium; three or more servings of meat, poultry, fish, eggs, nuts, dried beans, and peas for protein (see Table 26.7 for RDAs in pregnancy). Clients often need education on portion size: one serving equals one slice of bread, a potato the size of a computer mouse, ¾ cup of juice, 1 cup milk, 2 to 3 oz of meat or poultry, ½ cup beans, or ½ cup vegetables, for example.

Caffeine is a stimulant found in coffee, tea, chocolate, and many medications. In large quantities it may cause miscarriage or low birth weight babies and dehydration for the mother, and should be avoided. Calcium needs increase 40% in pregnancy. Dairy foods are an excellent source of calcium; other excellent sources include collard greens, sesame seed meal, black-strap molasses, bok choy and other greens, soybeans, and tortillas. It is important that females consume eight glasses of water each day. Sodium is a required nutrient in pregnancy, 2,000 to 8,000 mg; pregnant females should salt foods to taste and not consume overly processed highly salted foods.

Females should avoid consuming nonfood items such as clay, cornstarch, laundry starch, dry milk of magnesia, paraffin, coffee grounds, or ice. Pregnant females should also avoid these foods: swordfish, shark, king mackerel, and tilefish due to potentially risky levels of mercury; more than 6 oz of albacore ("white") tuna per week; game fish unless first checking its safety with the local health department; raw fish, especially shellfish (oysters, clams); undercooked meat, poultry, or seafood; hot dogs and deli meats (such as ham, salami, and bologna); soft-scrambled eggs and all foods made with raw or lightly cooked eggs; soft cheeses such as Brie, feta, Camembert, Roquefort, and Mexican-style, unless they are labeled as made with pasteurized milk; unpasteurized milk and any foods made from it; unpasteurized juices; and raw sprouts, especially alfalfa sprouts, if there is a danger of salmonellosis and *E. coli* infections. Everyone, but especially pregnant females, should practice safe food handling, including hand washing, keeping refrigerator temperature below 40°F, cleaning the refrigerator regularly, refrigerating and freezing food promptly, and avoiding cross-contamination between cooked and uncooked foods, to avoid listeriosis and other foodborne infections.

FOCUSED INTERVIEW QUESTIONS

RATIONALES

Some herbal supplements and vitamin supplements can be a problem during pregnancy. As research in herbs in pregnancy is continuing, it is recommended that females check with their healthcare provider prior to consuming herbal teas and supplements. A partial list of common herbs known to be harmful in pregnancy includes aloe vera, black cohosh, blue cohosh, comfrey, dong quai, goldenseal, mugwort, pennyroyal, and wild yam. Although most healthcare providers recommend that pregnant clients consume a prenatal vitamin during pregnancy, some vitamin supplements (such as vitamin A) can cause harm if consumed beyond the recommended daily allowance.

ENVIRONMENTAL EXPOSURE

1. **What kind of chemicals are you exposed to in your home and workplace?**

▶ To prevent birth defects and miscarriage, pregnant females should avoid cigarette smoke, lead (in water and paint), carbon monoxide, mercury, pesticides, insect repellents, some oven cleaners, solvents such as alcohol and degreasers, paint, paint thinners, benzene, and formaldehyde. If the pregnant female must be around these substances, she should minimize her exposure by ensuring good ventilation, wearing protective gear such as face mask and gloves, and checking with the water or health department about the quality of the drinking water. For x-rays, 5 rads is the level of exposure believed to be necessary to cause birth defects; dental, chest, or mammogram x-rays are less than 0.02 rads of exposure. Federal guidelines prohibit exposure in the workplace to more than 0.5 rads accumulated during pregnancy, if the pregnant female has notified her employer of her pregnancy (see Figure 26.11 ●).

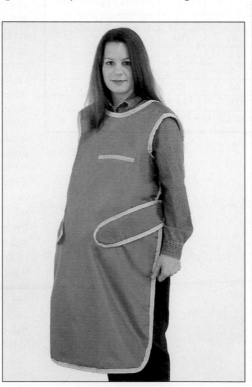

Figure 26.11 ● Pregnant woman wearing a lead apron.

CLIENT INTERACTION

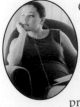

Olu Adams, age 16, presents for a return prenatal visit at 20 weeks' gestation. The prenatal record indicates that this is her first pregnancy, she lives with her parents in a nearby apartment building, and she is in 10th grade. Besides her unplanned adolescent pregnancy, the problems identified so far in this pregnancy include a urinary tract infection that was treated with antibiotics, and a total weight gain of 10 lb; she is 5'7" tall and weighed 120 lb at the beginning of the pregnancy.

INTERVIEW

Nurse: Hi, Ms. Adams. Have a seat and tell me how you have been doing since your last visit.

The nurse leads the client to a chair in the examination room, and pulls up a stool to sit beside the client. The teenager stares down at her lap.

Ms. Adams: Fine.

Nurse: Have you had any vaginal bleeding, contractions, or pelvic pressure?

The client shrugs.

Nurse: Any more problems with peeing, like burning, or peeing more frequently than usual?

The client shakes her head.

Nurse: Is your mom or the baby's father in the waiting room?

Ms. Adams: Nah.

Nurse: Ms. Adams? *Nurse waits for Olu to look up.* Have you felt the baby move yet? It would feel like a little tickle on the middle of your belly.

Ms. Adams: (face lights up, her voice is louder) Yes, I am feeling that! Is it the baby?

Nurse: Yes, it probably is. Tell me about it.

Ms. Adams: In the mornings for about the last week I feel something brushing my insides. And I don't feel so sick anymore.

Nurse: Well, that is certainly good news. Why don't you sit on the exam table and we will listen to the baby's heartbeat and see how much your baby has grown since the last visit.

Ms. Adams: I hope you can tell me how big the baby is now.

ALERT!

Research indicates that clients are often not clear on the signs of preterm labor.

The nurse should discuss the signs of preterm labor with all clients at every prenatal visit after 20 weeks.

- *More than six contractions per hour. This may feel like "the baby balling up," menstrual cramps, backache, or diarrhea.*
- *Leaking fluid, vaginal bleeding, or increased vaginal discharge.*
- *Pelvic pressure, heaviness, or suprapubic pain.*

ANALYSIS

The nurse was appropriate in sitting beside the client and providing a time away from the examination table for questions. Her initial question about preterm contractions was probably not well understood by a client of this age and education level. The nurse's question about urinary symptoms was at a more appropriate level, but yes/no questions to teenagers or any uncommunicative client are not the best choice. The nurse tried to elicit information about the client's family, but again with a closed question. When the client became more animated about quickening, the nurse wisely provided an open-ended question that led to a more productive interchange with the client. The nurse can now go on to find out what the client knows about topics that are relevant at this point in pregnancy: symptoms of preterm labor, continuing importance of good nutrition, results of laboratory tests from last visit, and fetal development, among other possible topics. During pregnancy, a great deal of teaching is done with the pregnant client and her family. In order to ensure that all topics are covered, many obstetric practices use a teaching checklist (see Box 26.4).

Box 26.4	**Pregnancy Teaching Checklist**
GESTATIONAL AGE/ TIMING OF VISIT	**TEACHING TOPICS**
Initial prenatal visit	Welcome
	Types of providers and scope of practice
	Hours of office/clinic
	Phone number, after-hours contact number
	Warning signs in first trimester
	Schedule of prenatal care and laboratory studies
	Safe medications in pregnancy
	Resources: Pregnancy and childbirth classes
	Nutritional requirements in pregnancy; request 3-day food diary
	Exercise in pregnancy
	Discomforts in pregnancy and relief measures
	Dental care
	Abuse screen
	Benefits of breast-feeding
	Bathing and clothing
Second prenatal visit	Explanation of test results
	Discuss 3-day food diary
	Psychological adaptation to pregnancy
	Body mechanics
Throughout pregnancy	Fetal growth and development
	Sexuality/partner relationship
	Traveling while pregnant
15 to 20 weeks	Second trimester laboratory testing
	Genetic tests
	Ultrasound
	Warning signs in second trimester
	Abuse screen
21 to 34 weeks	Preterm labor signs
	Preparation for birth
	Car seats
	Breast-feeding instructions if appropriate
	Home preparation for newborn
	28 week and 36 week testing
35 to 42 weeks	Signs of labor
	Sibling preparation for birth
	Abuse screen
	Breast preparation

Please refer to the Companion Website at **www.prenhall.com/damico** and click on Chapter 26, the **Client Interaction** module, to answer questions about this case. In addition, see other resources for this chapter including NCLEX review questions and other interactive exercises and materials.

The room should be warm and private. For prenatal blood tests, a variety of collection tubes and collection equipment will be required, and differs for each site.

The nurse should ask the client to empty her bladder and explain how to collect a clean-catch urine specimen. If this is the client's first gynecologic exam, the nurse should explain the components and general purposes of the physical exam to the client, using pictures and the equipment as necessary, and ask the client if she has any special needs or questions about the exam. It is important to provide privacy while the client puts on the gown with the opening in back and lays a drape across her lap.

For the initial parts of the physical exam the client can be sitting (see Figure 26.12 ●) and later be assisted to a semi-Fowler's position on the examination table. During the pelvic part of the exam, the client should be assisted to the lithotomy position. Some clients may need to have this exam in the side-lying position with top knee bent. The nurse assists the client in placing her feet in the stirrups, which should be padded if possible. The legs should be symmetrically and comfortably positioned. The client can then be instructed to move her buttocks down to the end of the table until about 0.5 inch is hanging over the edge. For the initial part of the pelvic exam, it is helpful to tell the client what she will feel before the nurse touches her ("You will feel me touching your leg, you will feel me touching your labia," etc.). Some clients will be more relaxed if they assist in the insertion of the speculum (see Figure 26.13 ●).

Remember to use Standard Precautions throughout the assessment.

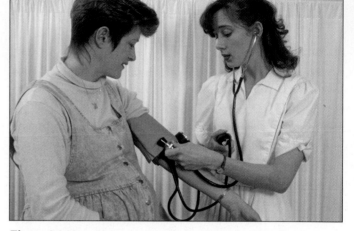

Figure 26.12 ● Blood pressure measurement in pregnancy.

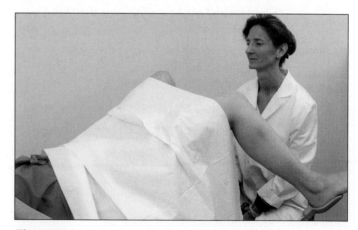

Figure 26.13 ● Pregnant female in lithotomy position.

EQUIPMENT

examination gown and drape
sphygmomanometer
adjustable light source
high-performance stethoscope
centimeter tape measure
reflex hammer
fetoscope or fetal Doppler and ultrasonic gel
urine collection containers
urine testing strips
perineal cleansing wipes
otoscope and specula
tongue depressor

For the pelvic exam, the nurse will need the following materials:

clean, nonsterile examination gloves
labeled slides and fixative or labeled containers for cytology
slide for vaginitis check
potassium hydroxide solution
saline drops
plastic or metal speculum
spatula
cytology brush or cervical broom
tissues
hand mirror (optional per client preference)
water-soluble lubricant
cervical culture swabs

HELPFUL HINTS

- Ask the client to empty her bladder before the examination.
- Explain the purposes and processes of each part of the examination. Use pictures or diagrams as needed.
- Assist the client to the sitting, lying, and lithotomy positions.
- Explain what the client will feel before touching her.
- The nurse must be sure to maintain the client's dignity throughout the examination.
- The side-lying position may be used to examine the perineum and rectum of the postpartum client.

TECHNIQUES AND NORMAL FINDINGS	**ABNORMAL FINDINGS SPECIAL CONSIDERATIONS**

GENERAL SURVEY

1. **Measure the client's height and weight.**
   - At the initial exam, take these measurements to establish a baseline. In the first trimester, the client should gain 4 to 6 lb. The client should gain 1 lb per month in both the second and the third trimesters, for a total weight gain of about 25 to 35 lb, if she is normal weight at conception.

   ▶ A gain of 6.6 lb or more per month may be associated with a large for gestational age baby or developing preeclampsia. A gain of less than 2.2 lb per month may cause preterm birth, small for gestational age infant, or IUGR.

2. **Assess the client's general appearance and mental status.**
   - Tiredness and ambivalence are normal in early pregnancy. Most females express well-being and energy during the second trimester. During the third trimester, most report increased fatigue and concern regarding upcoming birth.

   ▶ It is important to watch for signs of depression such as decreased appetite, persistent feelings of sadness, guilt or worry, and suicidal thoughts.

3. **Take the client's vital signs.**
   - The respiratory rate may increase slightly during pregnancy, the heart rate increases, and the blood pressure may drop to below prepregnancy baseline during the second trimester.

   ▶ Blood pressure should not be greater than 140/90. This could be a sign of gestational hypertension or, if accompanied by significant proteinuria, preeclampsia.

ALERT!

As preeclampsia worsens, multiple systems of the body are affected, producing symptoms such as (from head to toe) the following:

- *headache unrelieved by acetaminophen*
- *blurred vision, dizziness, or vision changes*
- *dyspnea, or difficulty breathing*
- *epigastric (upper abdominal) pain*
- *nausea, vomiting, or malaise ("I don't feel right")*
- *sudden weight gain or sudden, severe edema of face, hands, and legs*

Signs noted by healthcare providers include hypertension greater than 140/90, proteinuria ≥ +1, oliguria (decreased urine output), hyperreflexia, and abnormal laboratory values such as elevated liver enzymes and uric acid.

---

4. **Test the client's urine for glucose and protein.**
   - Occasional mild glycosuria or trace protein can be normal findings in pregnancy.

   ▶ Persistent glycosuria may indicate gestational diabetes and necessitates follow-up. Greater than trace protein may indicate preeclampsia. If the client has lost weight, it is important to check the urine for ketones, indicating ketoacidosis, which is harmful to the fetus.

5. **Observe the client's posture.**
   - Increasing lordosis is a normal adaptation to pregnancy.

6. **Assist the client to a sitting position.**

SKIN, HAIR, AND NAILS

1. **Observe the skin, hair, and nails for changes associated with pregnancy.**
   - These include linea nigra, striae, melasma, spider nevi, palmar erythema, and darkened areola and perineum. Softening and thinning of nails is common. Hair may become thicker in pregnancy.

   ▶ Bruises may indicate physical abuse. Lesions may indicate infection. Scars along veins may indicate intravenous drug abuse.

TECHNIQUES AND NORMAL FINDINGS	ABNORMAL FINDINGS SPECIAL CONSIDERATIONS

HEAD AND NECK

1. **Inspect and palpate the neck.**
   - Slight thyroid gland enlargement is normal in pregnancy.

▶ Enlarged or tender lymph nodes may indicate infection or cancer. Marked thyroid gland enlargement may indicate hyperthyroidism.

EYES, EARS, NOSE, MOUTH, AND THROAT

1. **Inspect the eyes and ears.**
   - There are no visible changes associated with pregnancy.

▶ Redness or discharge may indicate infection.

2. **Inspect the nose.**
   - Increased swelling of nasal mucosa and redness may accompany the increased estrogen of pregnancy.

▶ Epistaxis may occur if the vascular increase is extreme.

3. **Inspect the mouth.**
   - Hypertrophy of gum tissue is normal.

▶ Epulis nodules or poor condition of teeth warrant referral to a dentist. Pale gums may indicate anemia. Redness or exudates may indicate infection.

4. **Inspect the throat.**
   - The throat should appear pink and smooth.

THORAX AND LUNGS

1. **Inspect, palpate, percuss, and auscultate the chest.**
   - Note diaphragmatic expansion and character of respirations. Later in pregnancy, pressure from the growing uterus produces a change from abdominal to thoracic breathing.
   - Observe for symmetrical expansion with no retraction or bulging of the intercostal spaces. Confirm that the lungs are clear in all fields.

▶ Unequal expansion or intercostal retractions are signs of respiratory distress. Rales, rhonchi, wheezes, rubs, and absent or unequal sounds may indicate pulmonary disease.

THE HEART

1. **Auscultate the heart.**
   - Confirm that the rhythm is regular and that the rate is from 70 to 90 bpm. The heart rate in pregnancy increases 10 to 20 bpm above the baseline. Short systolic murmurs are due to increased blood volume and displacement of the heart.

▶ Irregular rhythm, dyspnea, or markedly decreased activity tolerance may indicate cardiac disease.

2. **Position the client.**
   - Assist the client into a semi-Fowler's position, and pull out the bottom of the table extension so the client may lie backwards on the slightly elevated head rest.

TECHNIQUES AND NORMAL FINDINGS	**ABNORMAL FINDINGS SPECIAL CONSIDERATIONS**

BREASTS AND AXILLAE

1. **Inspect the breasts.**
   - Normal changes include enlargement, increased venous pattern, enlarged Montgomery tubercles, presence of colostrum after 12 weeks, striae, and darkening of nipple and areola (see Figure 26.6).

   ▶ Flat or inverted nipples can be treated with breast shells in the last month of pregnancy.

   ▶ Bloody discharge or fixed, unchanging masses or skin retraction could indicate breast cancer.

2. **Palpate the breasts and axillae.**
   - Breasts are more tender to touch and more nodular during pregnancy.

EXTREMITIES

1. **Inspect and palpate the extremities.**
   - Varicose veins in the lower extremities are normal with pregnancy. Mild dependent edema of the hands and ankles is common in pregnancy. Inspect and palpate the extremities for raised or tender veins. Palpate for ankle or lower leg edema.

   ▶ Raised, hard, tender, warm, painful, or reddened veins may indicate thrombophlebitis. Marked edema may indicate preeclampsia.

NEUROLOGIC SYSTEM

1. **Percuss the deep tendon reflexes.**
   - Reflexes should be +1/+2 and bilaterally equal.
   - Refer to Chapter 24 for more detail. ∞

   ▶ Hyperreflexia and clonus are signs of preeclampsia.

ABDOMEN AND FETAL ASSESSMENT

1. **Inspect and palpate the abdomen.**
   - The uterus becomes an abdominal organ after 12 weeks in pregnancy. Uterine contractions are palpable after the first trimester. Palpate uterine contractions by laying both hands on the abdomen. The *frequency* of contractions is determined by measuring the interval from the beginning of one contraction to the beginning of the next contraction. Indent the uterus with a finger to measure *intensity* or strength of contractions. The strength can be classified as mild, moderate, or strong. These distinctions can be described by comparing the rigidity of the uterus to the firmness of certain other body features. Mild contractions are comparable to the firmness of the nose, moderate contractions feel like the chin, and strong contractions are as hard and unyielding as the forehead. The *duration* of contractions is measured from the beginning to the end of the contraction.

   ▶ Liver enlargement is abnormal.

   ▶ More than five contractions per hour may indicate preterm labor.

2. **Assess fetal growth through fundal height assessment.**
   - Prior to 20 weeks, fundal height is measured by indicating the number of fingerbreadths or centimeters above the symphysis pubis or below the umbilicus. Once the uterus rises above the umbilicus, a tape measure is used.
   - The 0 line of the measuring tape is placed at the superior edge of the symphysis pubis.
   - The other hand is placed at the xiphoid with the ulnar surface against the abdomen. When the superior edge of the uterus is encountered by the descending hand, the top of the uterus has been located.

TECHNIQUES AND NORMAL FINDINGS

- The measuring tape is stretched from the top of the symphysis pubis to the fundus. The superior aspect of the tape is held between the middle fingers of the hand that is resting perpendicular to the fundus. The fundal height in centimeters is noted and compared to the weeks of pregnancy. Uterine size in centimeters is approximately equal to the weeks of pregnancy. The uterus should measure within 2 units of the weeks of pregnancy (see Figure 26.14 ●).

▶ If the uterus is more than 2 cm larger or smaller than the weeks of pregnancy, a growth disorder such as IUGR or macrosomia, multiple gestation, amniotic fluid disorders, incorrect dating, fetal malpresentation, or anomalies may be occurring.

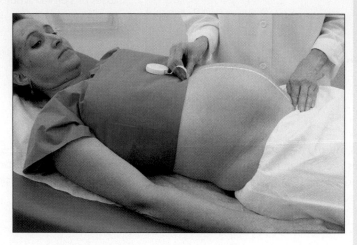

Figure 26.14 ●
Fundal height
measurement.

3. **Assess fetal activity.**
   - After 24 weeks, fetal movement is palpable by the examiner. Maternal perception of movement occurs between 16 and 18 weeks in pregnancy.

▶ The *fetal alarm signal* occurs when there is no fetal movement for 8 hours, fewer than 10 movements in 12 hours, a change in the usual pattern of movements, or a sudden increase in violent fetal movements followed by a complete cessation of movement. Immediate evaluation of the fetus should take place.

4. **Assess fetal lie, presentation, and position.**
   - **Leopold's maneuvers** utilize a specialized palpation of the abdomen sequence to answer a series of questions to determine the position of the fetus in the abdomen and pelvis after 28 weeks' gestation.
     - *First Leopold's maneuver: What is in the fundus?* With the client in a supine position, stand facing her head. Place the ulnar surface of both hands on the fundus, with the fingertips pointing toward the midline. Palpate the shape and firmness of the contents of the upper uterus. A longitudinal lie will find the head or breech in the fundus. A round, firm mass is the fetal head. A soft, irregular mass is the fetal breech. Nothing in the fundus indicates a transverse lie. The fetus can also be oblique, at an oblique angle to the midline (see Figure 26.15 ●).

TECHNIQUES AND NORMAL FINDINGS	ABNORMAL FINDINGS SPECIAL CONSIDERATIONS

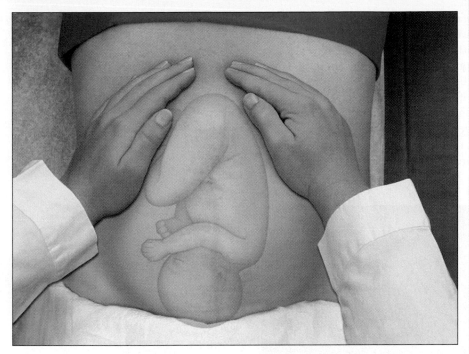

Figure 26.15 ● First Leopold's maneuver.

• *Second Leopold's maneuver: Where is the fetal back?* Move the hands down the sides of the abdomen along the uterine contour. A smooth, long, firm, continuous outline is found on the side with the fetal back. Irregular, lumpy, moving parts are found on the side with the fetal small parts, or feet and hands. Note whether the back is found on the client's left or right side; if an indentation about the size of a dinner plate is seen at the midline and movements are at the center of the abdomen, the fetal back may be against the mother's spine (posterior position) (see Figure 26.16 ●).

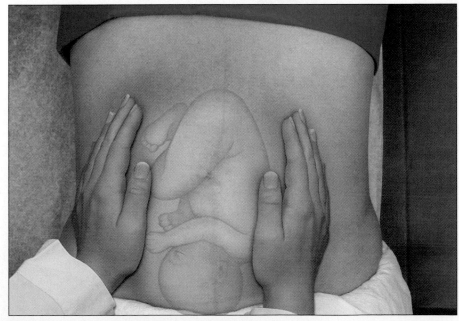

Figure 26.16 ● Second Leopold's maneuver.

TECHNIQUES AND NORMAL FINDINGS	ABNORMAL FINDINGS SPECIAL CONSIDERATIONS

- *Third Leopold's maneuver: What part of the fetus is presenting at the pelvis?* Next, slide your hands down to the area above the symphysis pubis to determine the "presenting" part of the fetus, the part of the fetus entering the pelvic inlet. Palpate the shape and firmness of the presenting part. Use the thumb and third finger of one hand to grasp the presenting part. This may require pressing into the area above the symphysis pubis with some pressure. Try to move the presenting part with one hand and see if the part of the fetus in the fundus moves with it using the other hand. If the breech is presenting, the whole mass of the fetus will move when the presenting part is moved, and it will feel irregular and soft above the symphysis pubis. If a hard, round, independently movable mass is palpated in the pelvis, it is the head (see Figure 26.17 ●).

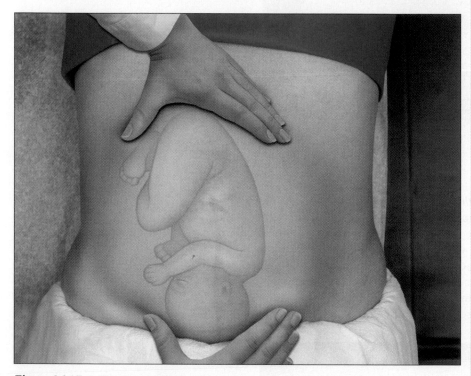

Figure 26.17 ● Third Leopold's maneuver.

- *Fourth Leopold's maneuver: How deep in the pelvis is the presenting part?* Now, face the client's feet. Place the ulnar surface of your two hands on each side of the client's abdomen. Follow the uterine/fetal contour to the pelvic brim. If the fingers come together above the superior edge of the symphysis pubis, the presenting part is floating above the pelvic inlet. If the fingers snap over the brim of the pelvis before coming together, the presenting part has descended into the pelvis. A prominent part on one side is the *cephalic prominence* if the presenting part is the fetal head; this indicates a face presentation if felt on the same side as the back. If a prominence is felt on both sides, the forehead is presenting. If no prominence is felt or the prominence is felt on the same side as the small parts, the fetus is well flexed, with the chin on the chest (flexion) (see Figure 26.18 ●).

| **TECHNIQUES AND NORMAL FINDINGS** | **ABNORMAL FINDINGS SPECIAL CONSIDERATIONS** |

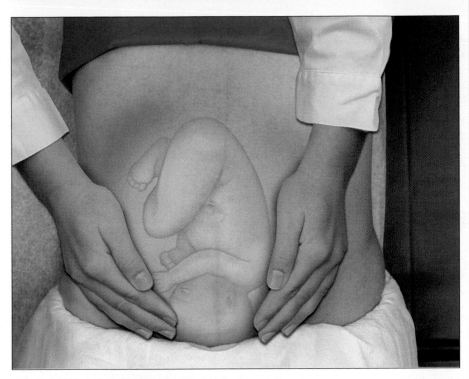

Figure 26.18 ● Fourth Leopold's maneuver.

- *Fetal position.* The position of the fetus is the relationship of the presenting part to the four quadrants of the maternal pelvis. The fetus can be in the left or right half of the maternal pelvis, and in the anterior, posterior, or transverse portion of the pelvis. Three notations are used to designate the fetal position. The first notation is L or R for left or right, indicating in which half of the maternal pelvis the presenting part is found. The second notation is a letter abbreviating the part of the fetus that is presenting at the top of the pelvis. The most common notations for presenting part are O, indicating occiput, or the back of the head in a flexed position; S, indicating sacrum for a breech presentation; Sc, indicating scapula in a transverse lie; and M, indicating mentum or face presentation. The third notation indicates if the presenting part is in the anterior, posterior, or transverse portion of the pelvis. For example, a position of LOA indicates that the presenting part is the occiput, and it is in the left half of the anterior part of the pelvis.

5. Estimate fetal weight.

- Estimating fetal weight by abdominal palpation is only an approximation. It is done in conjunction with fundal height measurement and ultrasound to detect growth abnormalities.

- Use Leopold's maneuvers to assess fetal size. Experience can be gained by palpating undressed term and preterm infants in the nursery. Compare your estimates with the known weights of the infants. One research study showed that in term clients, intrapartum sonographic prediction of birth weight offered no advantage over estimated fetal weight obtained by abdominal palpation.

▶ Large for gestational age (LGA) or small for gestational age (SGA) infants must be further evaluated.

6. Auscultate fetal heart rate.

- Once the position of the fetus has been determined, the fetal heart tones (FHTs) can be located. They are usually heard loudest over the left scapula of the fetus, so this is the area that should be auscultated (see Figure 26.19 ●).

TECHNIQUES AND NORMAL FINDINGS	**ABNORMAL FINDINGS SPECIAL CONSIDERATIONS**

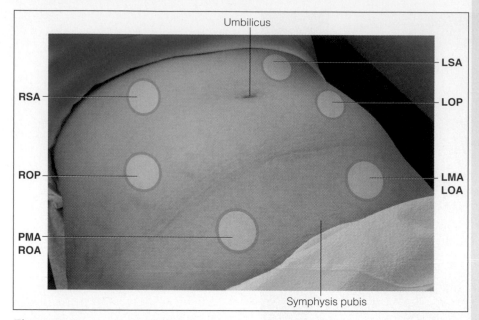

Figure 26.19 ● Location of fetal heart tones for various fetal positions.

- Place the fetoscope or fetal Doppler in the location where the FHTs are most likely to be heard given the findings of Leopold's maneuvers. Place ultrasonic gel, warmed if possible, on the Doppler prior to placement on the abdomen.

▶ If the fetal heartbeat is not found by 12 weeks with a fetal Doppler, or 20 weeks with a fetoscope, ultrasound evaluation of the fetal viability may be indicated. Other causes could be incorrect dating of pregnancy, or retroverted uterus.

- Auscultate the FHT for one minute.

▶ Irregular heartbeats, tachycardia (heart rate above 160 bpm), bradycardia (heart rate below 120 bpm, or 110 bpm in postterm fetuses), or decelerations in fetal heart rate below the baseline should be followed up with electronic fetal monitoring.

7. **Assist the client into the lithotomy position for the next portion of the assessment.**

EXTERNAL GENITALIA

1. **Inspect the external genitalia.**
   - Normal findings include enlargement of the clitoris and labia, gaping vaginal introitus for multiparas (clients who have given birth before), scars on perineum from previous births, small hemorrhoids, and darkened pigmentation. (see Figure 26.20 ●).

   ▶ Varicosities can occur in the labia and upper thighs. Lesions may indicate sexually transmitted infection. Redness may indicate vaginitis.

   - Ask the client to bear down, and note any bulges of the vaginal walls or cervix outside the vagina.

   ▶ The cervix or vaginal walls may protrude from the vagina in cases of uterine, bladder (cystocele), or rectal (rectocele) prolapse. If the cervix is at the introitus, it is graded as a first-degree uterine prolapse. In a second-degree prolapse, the uterus descends through the introitus. In a third-degree prolapse, the entire uterus is outside the vagina.

TECHNIQUES AND NORMAL FINDINGS

ABNORMAL FINDINGS SPECIAL CONSIDERATIONS

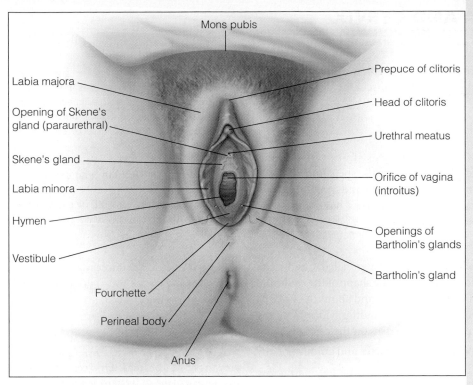

Figure 26.20 • External female genitalia.

2. Palpate Bartholin's gland, urethra, and Skene's glands.

- Insert a gloved index finger into the vagina. Press thumb and index finger together at the 5-o'clock and 7-o'clock positions at the vaginal introitus. Note any masses or discharge (see Figure 26.21 •).
- Insert the index finger into the vagina and press upward toward the urethra. Milk the urethra and Skene's glands for discharge or swelling.

► Note any masses or discharge that may indicate infection.

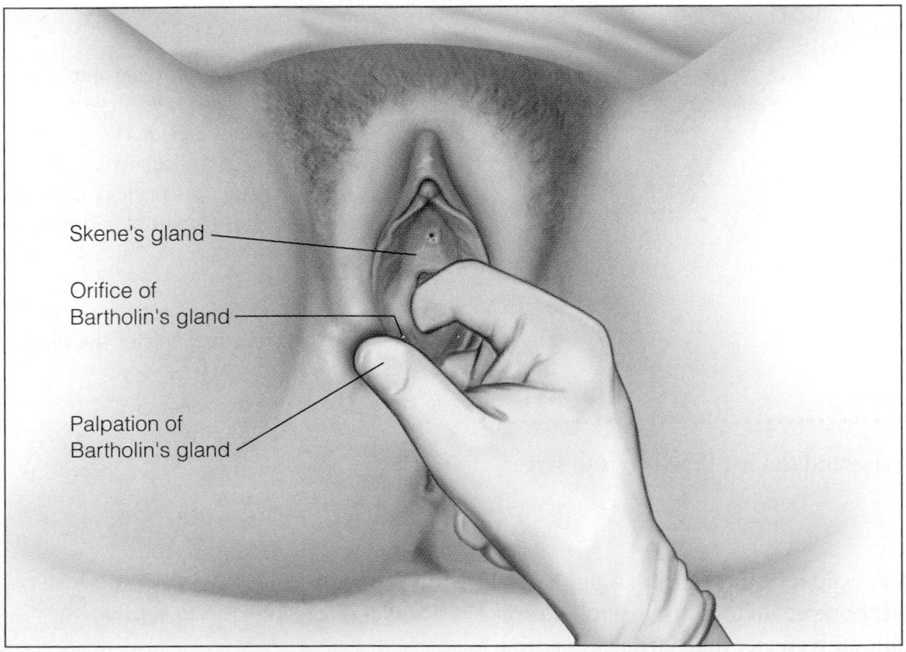

Figure 26.21 • Palpation of Bartholin's gland, urethra, and Skene's glands.

TECHNIQUES AND NORMAL FINDINGS	ABNORMAL FINDINGS SPECIAL CONSIDERATIONS

INSPECTION OF VAGINA AND CERVIX

1. Observe the vagina.

- The vagina may also be bluish in pregnancy. Note the color, consistency, odor, and amount of discharge. Increased whitish, odorless discharge (leukorrhea) is normal in pregnancy.

▶ White, clumping discharge or gray, green, bubbly, fishy-smelling discharge is indication of vaginitis or sexually transmitted infections. The client may complain of itching, burning, dyspareunia or pain on intercourse, or pelvic pain.

2. Visualize the cervix.

- Select the appropriate speculum for the client. Lubricate the speculum with water only. (See Chapter 22 for more instructions on inserting the speculum. ⊙⊙) The speculum can be warmed by warm water, the nurse's hands, the light source, or a heating pad kept in the speculum drawer.

▶ Lubricating gels interfere with some cytologic tests.
▶ A speculum that is too cold or too warm is detrimental to the client's comfort.

3. Inspect the cervix.

- Expected changes in pregnancy include a bluish coloring called Chadwick's sign, or a slitlike cervical opening (os) for multiparas. The shape of the os should match the obstetric history. The os will usually be round and about the size of a pencil tip for a primigravida. The os is usually slitlike in multigravidas. Note any lacerations, ulcerations, erosions, polyps, or other masses on the cervix.

▶ Note any dilation of the cervix.
▶ Polyps may rupture and cause vaginal bleeding during pregnancy.

- Note the color and texture of the cervix, and note character and amount of any discharge from the os.

▶ A rough, reddened texture may represent the growth of cells from the internal cervical canal to the outside of the os (ectopy). It is seen in multiparas, and females who use oral contraceptives. If the speculum is pushed too deeply into the fornices or corners of the vagina, the internal canal may also appear; this eversion should be eliminated by pulling the speculum back slightly.

- If the cervix is covered with secretions, and you will be obtaining a Papanicolaou (Pap) smear, use a gauze pad on a sponge stick or a large swab to blot the cervix.

- Note the size, position, shape, and any friability (bleeding) of the cervix. The cervix should be 2 to 3 cm in diameter.

▶ Increased friability is common in pregnancy.

4. Obtain the Pap smear and cervical cultures.

- See Chapter 22 for guidelines.

▶ Due to the risks of sexually transmitted infections to the fetus during pregnancy, cervical cultures are frequently obtained. The cervical brush is the best method for collection of endocervical cells during pregnancy. Cotton swabs interfere with the growth of chlamydia.

5. Proceed to pelvic assessment.

- Unlock and remove speculum.

▶ If the speculum is not closed prior to removal, there is uncomfortable stretching for the client.

PALPATION OF PELVIS

Some nurses with advanced training assess the size and shape of the pelvis to screen for problems during birth.

1. Assess the angle of the pubic arch.

- Place the thumbs at the midline of the lower border of the symphysis pubis (see Figure 26.22 ●). Follow the edge of the pubic bone down to the ischial tuberosity. Estimate the angle of the pubic arch. A pubic arch greater than 90 degrees is best for vaginal birth.

▶ An angle less than 90 degrees may be more difficult for a fetus to navigate in labor.

| **TECHNIQUES AND NORMAL FINDINGS** | **ABNORMAL FINDINGS SPECIAL CONSIDERATIONS** |

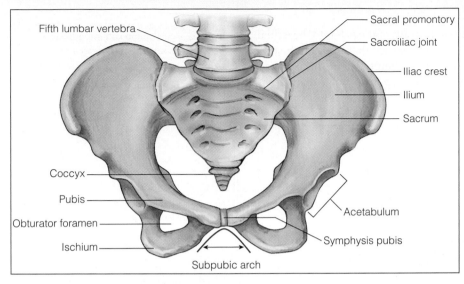

Figure 26.22 • Internal structures of the female pelvis for landmarks.

2. **Lubricate the gloved fingers.**
   • Apply a teaspoon or more of lubricating jelly to the index and middle fingers.

3. **Estimate the angle of the subpubic arch.**
   • Insert the index and middle fingers slightly into the vagina, palmar side up. Keep the fingers separated slightly to prevent pressure on the urethra. Palpate the inner surface of the symphysis pubis. Using both thumbs, externally trace the descending sides of the pubis down to the tuberosities. The symphysis pubis should be at least two fingerbreadths wide, and parallel to the sacrum, without any abnormal thickening (see Figure 26.23 •).

▶ An anterior or posterior tilting, or width less than two fingerbreadths, is abnormal.

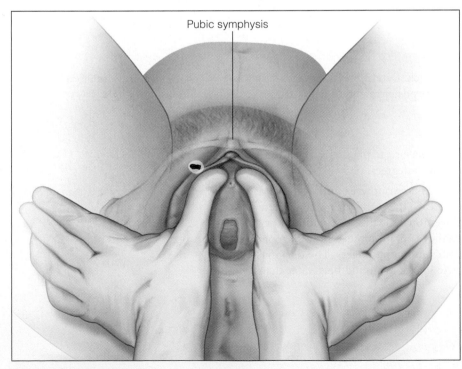

Figure 26.23 • Estimation of angle of subpubic arch.

TECHNIQUES AND NORMAL FINDINGS

4. **Assess the interspinous diameter.**

   - Turn the fingers to the side and follow the lateral walls of the pelvis to the ischial spine. (As the fingers go deeper into the vagina, ensure that the thumb stays away from the perineum.) Determine if the spine is blunt, flat, or sharp. Sweep your fingers across the pelvis to the opposite ischial spine. Average diameter is approximately 10.5 cm (see Figure 26.24 ●).

▶ A pointy ischial spine can impede labor.
▶ A smaller diameter may mean a contracted pelvis.

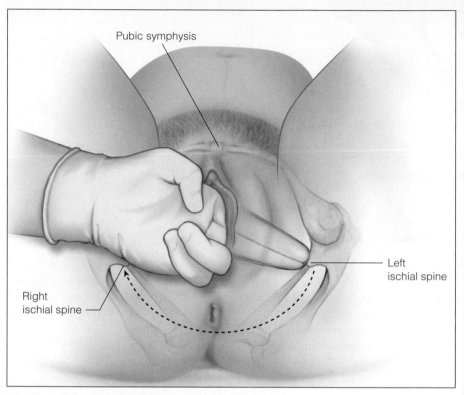

Pubic symphysis

Left ischial spine

Right ischial spine

Figure 26.24 ● Assessing the interspinous diameter.

5. **Assess the curvature of the sacrum.**

   - Sweep your fingers upward as far as you can reach. Determine if the sacrum is concave, flat, or convex. Note if the coccyx at the posterior end of the sacrum is movable or fixed by pressing down on it.

▶ A hollow sacrum provides more room for the fetus moving through the pelvis.

6. **Measure the diagonal conjugate.**

   - Next, position the fingers in the back of the vagina next to the cervix. Drop your wrist so your fingers are at an upward angle of 45 degrees.

   - Reach as far toward the sacrum as you can, and raise your wrist until your hand touches the symphysis pubis. If your fingers reach the sacral promontory, note the distance from the tip of your middle finger touching the sacral promontory to the symphysis pubis. If you cannot reach the sacral promontory, the diagonal conjugate is greater than the length of your examining fingers. The diagonal conjugate is an approximation of the pelvic inlet and should be greater than 11.5 cm (see Figure 26.25 ●).

▶ A diagonal conjugate of less than 11.5 cm may prevent a vaginal birth.

TECHNIQUES AND NORMAL FINDINGS	ABNORMAL FINDINGS SPECIAL CONSIDERATIONS

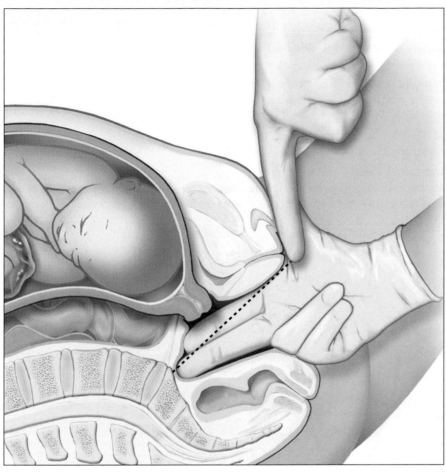

Figure 26.25 • Measuring the diagonal conjugate.

PALPATION OF CERVIX, UTERUS, ADNEXA, AND VAGINA

1. **Assess the cervix.**

   • Run your fingers around the cervix, and feel the length, width, consistency, and opening. The cervix is usually 1.5 to 2 cm long and 2 to 3 cm wide. In multiparas, the outside of the os may be open up to 2 to 3 cm.

   • Assess the texture and position of the cervix. It should be smooth.

   • Move the cervix from side to side with your fingers.

▶ The cervix is softer during pregnancy (Goodell's sign). It becomes even softer and jellylike as the client approaches labor. The outer opening of the cervix may be open but the internal os should be closed prior to term, 37 weeks of pregnancy or more. A shortened cervix is also a symptom or predictor of possible preterm labor.

▶ Note the roughness of ectopy or any nodules or masses. Nabothian cysts may become infected or be a sign of cervicitis. Normal variations include a retroverted uterus, which will have an anterior cervix, and an anteverted uterus, which will have a posterior cervix.

▶ Cervical motion tenderness (CMT) is a sign of pelvic inflammatory disease and other abnormalities.

TECHNIQUES AND NORMAL FINDINGS

2. **Perform bimanual palpation of the uterus.**

- Place the non-dominate hand on the abdomen halfway between the umbilicus and the symphysis pubis. Press the palmar surface of the fingers toward the fingers in the vagina.

- Insert the fingers of the dominate hand into the vagina. Move the fingers to the sides of the cervix, palmar surfaces upward, and press upward toward the abdomen.

- Estimate the size, consistency, and shape of the uterus captured between your hands. The uterus softens in pregnancy, and the isthmus, the area between the cervix and the upper body of the uterus, is compressible (Hegar's sign).

- The uterus will feel about the size of an orange at 10 weeks' gestation, and a grapefruit at 12 weeks' gestation. If the gestation is beyond the first trimester, abdominal fundal height measurement is used (see Figure 26.26 ●).

▶ If the uterine size is not consistent with what is expected for the gestation, then incorrect dating, multiple gestation, or fibroids are suspected.

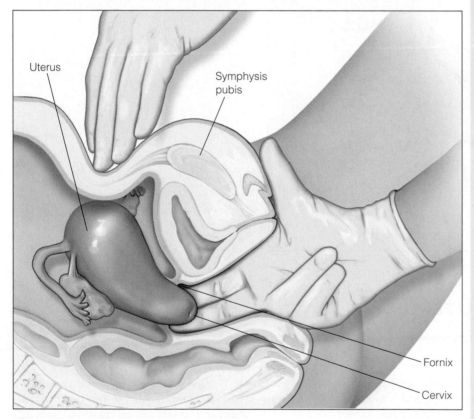

Uterus

Symphysis pubis

Fornix

Cervix

Figure 26.26 ● Bimanual palpation of the uterus.

3. **Palpate the adnexa.**

- The fallopian tubes and ovaries, or adnexa, sometimes cannot be palpated, especially after the uterus enters the abdominal cavity as pregnancy progresses.

▶ Any adnexal masses are abnormal and require referral. Bilateral pain is a symptom of pelvic inflammatory disease. During pregnancy an enlarged fallopian tube could indicate ectopic or tubal pregnancy and must be referred to a physician.

4. **Assess vaginal tone.**

- Withdraw your fingers to just below the cervix, and ask the client to squeeze her muscles around your fingers as hard and long as she can. Normal strength is demonstrated by a snug squeeze lasting a few seconds and with upward movement. This provides an opportunity to teach the client about pelvic floor strengthening exercises.

| **TECHNIQUES AND NORMAL FINDINGS** | **ABNORMAL FINDINGS SPECIAL CONSIDERATIONS** |

ANUS AND RECTUM

1. **Perform the rectovaginal exam.**
   - The exam is sometimes deferred, but it enables the nurse to evaluate internal structures more deeply, and is especially important if any fistulas are noted in the vagina, or if an early pregnancy is in a retroflexed or retroverted uterus.

2. **Measure the intertuberous diameter of the pelvic outlet.**
   - This part of the pelvic assessment is done at the end of the internal exam. As you gently withdraw your hand, make a fist with your thumb on the downward side, and press it in between the ischial tuberosities. A diameter of 11 cm is average, and 8.5 cm or greater usually is adequate. You must know the diameter of your fist to make this determination (see Figure 26.27 ●).

   ▶ A diameter smaller than 8.5 cm may inhibit fetal descent during expulsion.

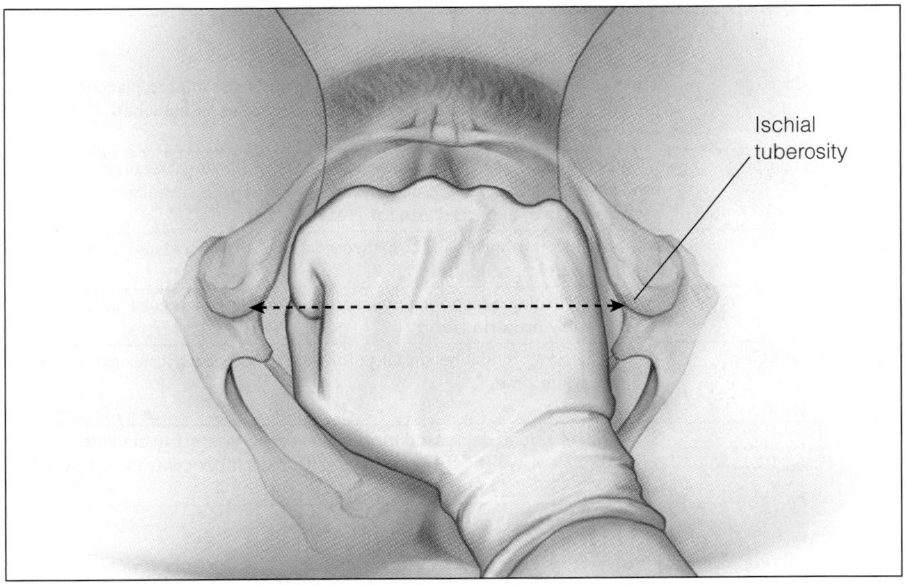

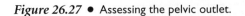

Ischial tuberosity

Figure 26.27 ● Assessing the pelvic outlet.

3. **Inspect the rectum.**
   - Hemorrhoids are common in pregnancy.

   ▶ Thrombosed hemorrhoids are tender, swollen, and bluish in color.
   Candida (yeast), moving trichomonads, or epithelial cells covered with black bacterial spots are abnormal findings.
   KOH will destroy cell membranes and other structures, but not the hyphae of *Candida* infections.

4. **Conclude the exam.**
   - Dispose of speculum, swabs, and gloves in a biohazard container. Use the tissue to wipe the client's perineum, or offer tissues to her to do so. Offer your hand to assist her to the sitting position, and leave the room so she can dress in privacy. Share your findings with her.

Refer to the Companion Website at **www.prenhall.com/damico** and click on the **Documentation** module for documentation samples and documentation practice exercises.

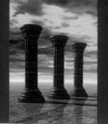

Abnormal Findings

$\mathcal{D}$isease processes can result in abnormal assessment findings, or abnormal laboratory results. Cultural variations may lead to unexpected psychosocial adaptation and behaviors if the nurse is not familiar with cultural groups and sources of variation.

Common Complications in Pregnancy

During pregnancy the role of the nurse is to educate the client to prevent complications of pregnancy and to assist in the screening process to detect complications, identify risk factors, and effectively implement treatment if complications develop. Table 26.8 describes the common complications of pregnancy.

Table 26.8	Common Complications in Pregnancy	
COMPLICATION	**DESCRIPTION**	**ASSESSMENT FINDINGS**
First Trimester		
Spontaneous Abortion	Loss of pregnancy; lay term is miscarriage.	Vaginal bleeding accompanied by cramping and loss of fetus, placenta, and membranes through dilated cervix. No heart tones heard when expected. Fundal height less than expected.
Ectopic Pregnancy	Implantation of fertilized ovum in fallopian tube or other abnormal location.	Client complains of pelvic pain, vaginal bleeding; bimanual exam reveals tenderness in adnexa; mass palpated near uterus; may reveal gestational sac smaller than expected size for gestational age.
Anemia	Deficiency in iron, folate, or B_{12}.	Abnormal iron values in CBC; tachycardia; client reports fatigue, light-headedness, pica, cold intolerance.
Substance Abuse	Use of illicit drugs, alcohol.	Positive screening questionnaire; inappropriate affect; irregular prenatal care; possibly preterm labor.
Molar Pregnancy/ Gestational Trophoblastic Disease	Abnormal growth of placental trophoblast.	Vaginal bleeding; fundal height large for dates; fetal heart tones not heard at appropriate time.
Mood Disorders	Depression	Symptoms present: depressed mood, diminished interest in activities, sleep disorders, weight changes, fatigue, decreased concentration, suicidal ideation.
Second and Third Trimester		
Premature Dilation of the Cervix	Passive, painless dilation of cervix during second trimester.	History of second-trimester loss; short cervix; abnormal cervical ultrasound findings.
Preeclampsia	Multisystem reaction to vasospasm.	Elevated blood pressure above 14/90 after 20 weeks; proteinuria >1 dipstick; pathologic edema of face, hands, and abdomen unresponsive to bed rest.
Gestational Diabetes	Glucose intolerance during pregnancy.	Abnormal screen; positive history; glycosuria.
Preterm Labor	Uterine contractions at 20 to 37 weeks that cause cervical change.	Uterine contractions more frequent than every 10 minutes; change in cervical/vaginal discharge; progressive cervical change: effacement > 80%, dilation > 2 cm; short cervix; positive fetal fibronectin or salivary estriol test.
Intrauterine Growth Restriction	Fetal growth below norms.	Fundal height less than expected; weight gain less than recommended.
Placental Abnormalities	Abnormal placental implantation including placenta previa, when placenta is implanted over cervix, and abruptio placenta, when placenta detaches from uterus	Vaginal bleeding; abdominal pain; non-reassuring fetal heart rate pattern; abnormal ultrasound.

Common Complications in the Postpartum Period

Several, common complications are found during the postpartum period. These complications are discussed in Table 26.9.

Table 26.9	Common Complications in the Postpartum Period
COMPLICATION	**ASSESSMENT FINDINGS**
Postpartum Hemorrhage	Estimated blood loss (EBL) reported to be greater than 500 cc at birth for vaginal delivery or greater than 1,000 cc after cesarean birth; a 10% decrease in hematocrit between admission and postpartum; vaginal bleeding that saturates more than one menstrual pad per hour is considered excessive bleeding; uterine fundus may be relaxed or "boggy," even after circular massage if caused by uterine atony; if caused by lacerations of genital tract, fundus may be firm but bleeding continues.
Preeclampsia	Elevated blood pressure; excessive edema in hands or face; proteinuria greater than +1; headaches, blurred vision, abdominal pain, dyspnea.
Subinvolution of the Uterus	Uterine fundus is above expected level; at 6 weeks postpartum, uterus has not returned to nonpregnant size.
Disseminated Intravascular Coagulation (DIC)	Bleeding from IV site, gums, or nose; petechiae; tachycardia, diaphoresis; decreased platelets and abnormal clotting factor values.
Endometriosis	Fever, tachycardia, chills; extreme pelvic pain when fundus assessed; increased or foul-smelling lochia.
Deep Vein Thrombophlebitis	Unilateral pain in lower extremity; warmth, redness, swelling over vein; vein feels cordlike; Homans' sign may be positive (see Figure 26.28 ●).

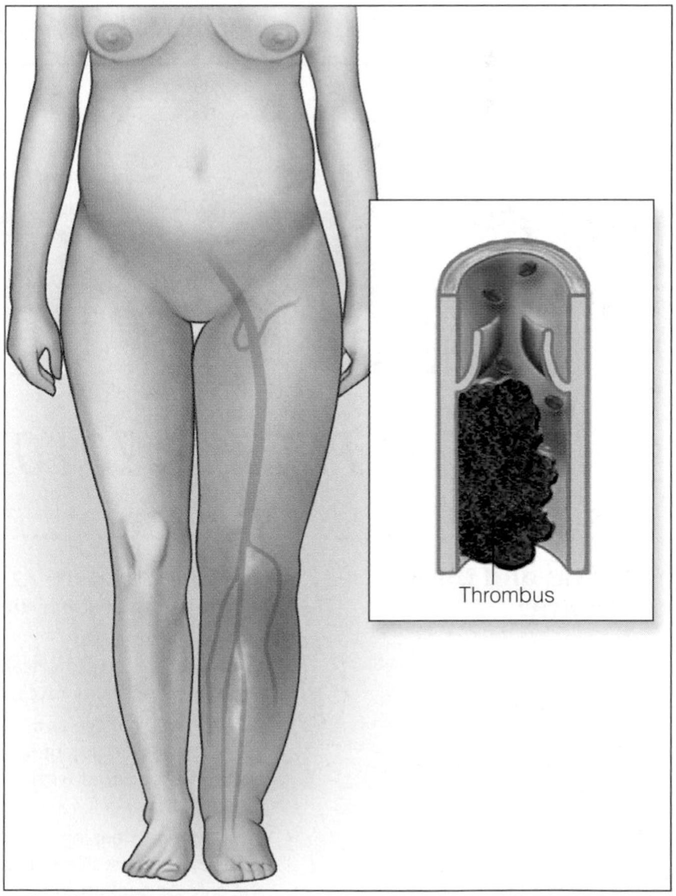

Thrombus

Figure 26.28 ● Deep vein thrombophlebitis.

(continued)

Table 26.9	Common Complications in the Postpartum Period *(continued)*
COMPLICATION	**ASSESSMENT FINDINGS**
Hematoma	Bulging, bluish, painful area in perineum.
Mastitis	Unilateral red streaks on breast; flulike symptoms, fever; mastalgia (breast pain) (see Figure 26.29 ●).

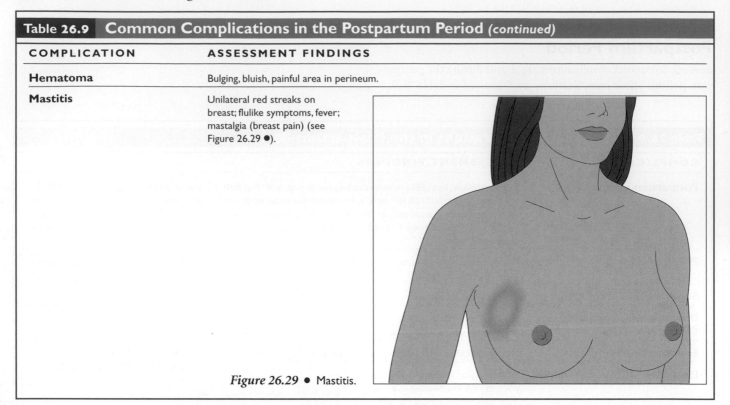

Figure 26.29 ● Mastitis.

Health Promotion

HEALTHY PEOPLE 2010

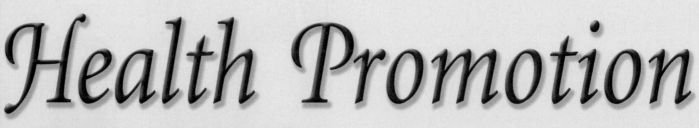

FOCUS AREA	PREVALENCE	OBJECTIVES	ACTIONS
Fetal and Infant Deaths	• Infant mortality rate is 7.2 deaths per 1,000 live births. • There is a large gap between African American and white mortality rates. • Young maternal age and low educational attainment are also associated with increased mortality. • A nonprone sleeping position (that is, sleeping on the side or back rather than the stomach) greatly decreases the risk of SIDS.	• Reduce infant mortality to 4.5 per 1,000 live births. • Reduce racial disparities in mortality rates.	• Preconception counseling regarding folic acid and alcohol consumption. • Identify risk factors in prenatal care. • Prevent and treat substance abuse. • Promote folic acid intake. • Advise adequate and appropriate weight gain in pregnancy. • Screen for vaginal infections and domestic violence. • Offer smoking cessation programs. • Advise parents to avoid prone sleeping position for infants. • Ensure administration of prenatal corticosteroids to women with anticipated preterm birth.

Maternal Deaths and Illnesses	• Maternal mortality rate is 7.1 per 100,000 live births. • The maternal complications rate is 31.2 per 100 deliveries. • The maternal mortality rate among African Americans is 3.6 times that of whites.	• Reduce maternal mortality rate to 3.3 deaths per 100,000. • Reduce rate of complications per 100 deliveries to 24.	• Prevent ectopic pregnancy through better treatment of STDs. • Prevent and treat postpartum depression. • Increase access to care to reduce disparities.
Prenatal Care	• The percentage of pregnant women that receive prenatal care in the first trimester is 83%.	• Increase initiation of prenatal care in the first trimester to 90%.	• Educate young women about the need to begin prenatal care early. • Educate adolescents about unwanted pregnancy prevention. • Offer childbirth education classes.
Obstetric Care	• Approximately 18% of women giving birth for the first time and 72% of the women with previous cesareans delivered via cesarean.	• Reduce risk of cesarean birth to low-risk women to 15% of first-time mothers and 65% of women with previous cesareans.	• Monitor cesarean rates and outcomes of cesarean births. • Advocate use of doulas in maternity care.
Breast-feeding	• Approximately 64% of mothers breast-feed in the early postpartum period, 29% at 6 months, and 16% at 1 year. • The highest rates are found among mothers with high educational achievement, and the lowest among mothers younger than 21 and with low educational achievement.	• Approximately 75% will be breast-feeding at discharge, 50% at 6 months, and 25% at 1 year.	• Educate pregnant clients and the community about breast-feeding. • Provide ongoing education and support to new mothers about breast-feeding, including consequences of artificial nipples and formula. • Provide information about lactation resources, including lactation consultants and community support groups. For more information, link to these resources through the Companion Website. • Implement breast-feeding-friendly maternity ward policies. • Advocate support from employers and community. • Promote media portrayal of breast-feeding as the norm, such as the National Breastfeeding Campaign. For more information, link through the Companion Website.

CLIENT EDUCATION

During pregnancy, the advice and education provided by the nurse regarding physiological, cultural, behavioral, and environmental risk factors is especially vital. Risk factors and *Healthy People 2010* goals can be used to formulate nursing actions for health promotion and client education.

LIFE SPAN CONSIDERATIONS: PREGNANCY

RISK FACTOR

- Pregnancy discomforts include vomiting, breast tenderness, leukorrhea, changes in nasal mucosa, excessive salivation, edema, varicosities, hemrorrhoids, constipation, backache, leg cramps, dizziness, and dyspnea.

CLIENT EDUCATION

- Provide information about specific remedies for each experience.
- Counsel clients to seek healthcare intervention for prolonged or unusual symptoms.
- Instruct clients regarding hygiene, body mechanics, and other measures to reduce the risk of injury and discomfort during pregnancy.
- Counsel clients to include fiber and fluids in daily intake to reduce risks for GI and GU problems.
- Recommend supportive undergarments and devices to reduce breast-related problems.

CULTURAL CONSIDERATIONS

RISK FACTORS

- African American mothers experience much higher rates of infant mortality, compared to non-Hispanic, white mothers.
- Asian American and Pacific Islander women experience language barriers in most prenatal care settings.
- Hispanic women have an increased risk of developing gestational diabetes.

CLIENT EDUCATION

- Encourage early and regular prenatal care.

- Implement culturally competent care models.
- Provide translation services.
- Encourage early screening.
- Provide education about diet and exercise.

BEHAVIORAL CONSIDERATIONS

RISK FACTORS

- Decreased rest contributes to anxiety and health problems.

- Restrictive clothing may lead to problems with circulation or falls.

- Food selection and the amount of intake have consequences for the health of the fetus and mother.

- Lack of exercise increases the risk of obesity, gestational diabetes, and pregnancy discomfort.
- Lack of information for travel can lead to fetal or maternal injury.

- Substance abuse is harmful to fetus and mother.

- Questions about sexual activity during pregnancy can increase anxiety.
- Pregnant couples may have little experience with safe and effective parenting skills.

CLIENT EDUCATION

- Advise clients of the need for 8 to 10 hours of sleep.
- Recommend a side-lying position during pregnancy.
- Advise the client to select and wear loose fitting, cotton clothing.
- Explain the importance of low-heeled, supportive footwear in preventing slips, falls, and injury.
- Provide recommended dietary guidelines for pregnant and postpartal clients.
- Advise pregnant clients to take folic acid to promote fetal growth and prevent maternal anemia.
- Provide guidelines for safe and effective exercise in pregnancy.
- Provide a list of prohibited athletic activities in pregnancy.
- Advise clients to avoid air travel in the final weeks of pregnancy.
- Counsel clients to use safety equipment as recommended for pregnancy.
- Provide information about the hazards of substance abuse.
- Counsel or provide recommendations for smoking cessation and addiction services.
- Advise clients to consult with healthcare providers before using OTC medications and products.
- Educate clients about symptoms that may indicate problems
- Provide information about sexual activity during pregnancy.

- Recommend attendance at childbirth education and parenting classes throughout the pregnancy.

ENVIRONMENTAL CONSIDERATIONS

RISK FACTORS

- Substances such as cancer treatment drugs, lead, ethylene glycol ethers, and ionizing radiation can affect the health of the mother and fetus.
- Some foods, such as seafood, raw fish, and cheese, may affect the health of the mother and fetus during pregnancy.
- Infectious diseases during pregnancy can harm the fetus.

CLIENT EDUCATION

- Teach clients how to recognize and avoid hazardous substances.
- Provide details about foods to avoid during pregnancy.
- Counsel clients to avoid exposure to infectious diseases, such as measles, chickenpox, hepatitis.
- Educate clients regarding handwashing, food preparation, and other hygiene measures.

Application Through Critical Thinking

CASE STUDY

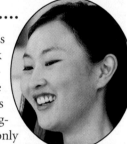

Susan Li, gravida 1, para 1, age 22, is married to a 23-year-old sales clerk who is required to work as much as possible due to family financial problems. She has 2 years of college education and was working as a waitress prior to this pregnancy. She speaks very good English. Her only local family member is her sister who also works full time. The rest of her family is in China. She gave birth to a 7 lb 4 oz female infant 24 hours ago. Her blood loss at birth was 400 cc, and her placenta delivered intact. A first-degree laceration occurred during birth and was repaired, and a small cluster hemorrhoid developed during the pushing stage of labor. She had an unmedicated birth, and breast-fed her baby girl in the delivery room, and two times since for approximately 5 minutes each time. No family members have been to see her since the birth.

▶ Complete Documentation

The case study information is documented on page 872.

▶ Critical Thinking Questions

1. What should the nurse's priority assessments for Susan be during this postpartum assessment exam at 24 hours after birth?
2. Susan complains that her stitches and hemorrhoids are painful at the level of 7 on a 10-point pain scale. Describe the recommended nursing assessment and relief measures.
3. At 5 weeks postpartum, her sister brings Susan to the clinic nurse. Susan tells the nurse she feels hopeless and overwhelmed and has been irritable and anxious for the past 3 weeks. What should the nurse's action be?

▶ Applying Nursing Diagnoses

1. *Ineffective breastfeeding* is a NANDA nursing diagnosis that applies to this client. Provide the related factors and defining characteristics for this diagnosis statement.

2. List one additional physical and one psychosocial diagnosis for this client based on the case study.
3. Rank these three nursing diagnoses in order of importance:
   a. Pain, Acute related to Episiotomy, and Hemorrhoids
   b. Ineffective Breast-feeding
   c. Interrupted Family Processes

▶ Prepare Teaching Plan

LEARNING NEED: Ms. Li has just delivered her first child. She is physically stable but is experiencing severe perineal pain. She has a small hemorrhoid that may be contributing to her pain. She has begun breast-feeding but has not established it yet. She is receiving no support from her family at this time. Like most new mothers, she has pain, self-care, knowledge deficit, social support, and breast-feeding needs that must be addressed by the nurse. The following teaching plan is focused on individual care and education for Ms. Li.

GOAL: The new mother will demonstrate safe care of herself and her newborn, and the family will experience a successful transition to new parenthood.

OBJECTIVES: Upon completion of this educational session, the participant will be able to:

1. Identify two pharmacologic and two nonpharmacologic measures for perineal pain relief.
2. Describe the components of good latch in breast-feeding, the recommended feeding frequency during the first week of life, and indicators of adequate breast-feeding.
3. List three ways in which family members, friends, and community nurses can provide social support to the new mother and family.
4. Demonstrate the use of a sitz bath and other measures for hemorrhoidal pain relief.
5. Explain the difference between baby blues, postpartum depression, and postpartum psychosis, and list two resources for additional help.

Postpartum Flow Sheet	Client Label *Li, Susan*		

Maternal Data		Allergy___ *PCN*_____	
Age __ *22* ___	G_*1*T_*0* P _*0*_ A _*I*_ L *0*	Problems Identified:	
Del _*8*/_*15*/_*04*_ Time _*08*:_*14*__ SVD CSEC		1. __ ✓*Social Support*_____	
Incision Type Abd Intact①2③4 Provider *Jones*		2._____	
Blood Type A⑧O − + Rub Imm⑧on		3._____	
Newborn M ⑧⑧SY NICU BR ⑧OR MD: __ *Night* ___		4._____	
		5._____	

Year 2005	Date/Time	8/15 8 am		
Vital Signs	Temp/Pulse/Resp	98.2/76/16		
	Blood pressure	98/62		
Pain Assessment	1-10 scale	6/10		
	Location	perineal		
	Management 1=Pharm 2=Heat/Cold 3=Touch/Massage 4=Position/Movement	1, 2		
Activity	1=Complete bedrest 2=Partial bedrest 3=Out of bed	3		
	ADL 1=Self 2=Assist	2		
Gastrointestinal	Nutrition	Reg		
	Fluid intake	750 ml		
Breasts	Milk tension	Filling		
	Nipple condition	Intact		
Reproductive	Fundus (consistency, height, position)	FF@U-1		
	Lochia (type, amount)	Rubra small		
	Incision Redness Ecchymosis Edema Discharge Approximation Dressing	NA − + − − + NA		
Elimination	UTI Sx	None		
	Voiding	200cc		
	Bowel: (sounds, flatus, stool)	+ + −		
	Hemorrhoids	small		
Extremities	Edema	slight pedal		
	Homans'	−		
Psychosocial	Rest/sleep	Adequate		
	Bonding	+		
	Adaptation Taking in, Taking hold	Taking In		
	Social work consult Y/N	Y		
Signature		E. Crownheart		

APPLICATION OF OBJECTIVE 1: Identify two pharmacologic and two nonpharmacologic measures for perineal pain relief

Content	Teaching Strategy and Rationale	Evaluation
• Sutures are reabsorbed by the body and do not need to be removed.	• Discussion	• Client verbalizes understanding. For example, client states, "I should call the midwife if my stitches start hurting more."
• Ibuprofen or acetaminophen may be used safely by breast-feeding mothers for perineal pain relief. Witch hazel pads assist with drying, and anesthetic sprays may provide topical relief.	• Audiovisual materials	
	• Printed materials	• Client provides counterdemonstration. For example, client sets up sitz bath unassisted in nurse's presence.
	• Group instruction	
	• Individual discussion allows the client to verbalize specific concerns as well as fears.	• Nurse observes client. For example, nurse observes client put infant to breast and obtain good latch, unassisted.
• Cold packs, a peribottle filled with warm water and squirted on the perineum, and sitz baths are also used to decrease perineal pain.	• Videos on the postpartum unit can allow clients to schedule the timing of the teaching, and provide visual instructions for those with limited English.	
• Do not sit cross-legged (tailor-sit) or place undue stretching on stitches until they have healed.		
• Pain should stay the same or get better each day.	• Printed materials can reinforce teaching performed by the nurse and provide a reference for the client later.	
• Increased perineal pain should be reported to the healthcare provider.	• Small teaching groups provide support and can be more time efficient to ensure that all the basic components of postpartum care are taught to all clients. Large lecture classes are not appropriate for new mother-infant dyads.	
• Good hand-washing technique and frequency should be maintained.		

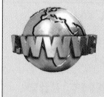

Please refer to the Companion Website at www.prenhall.com/damico and click on Chapter 26, the Application Through Critical Thinking module, to complete the following activities related to this case study:
► Critical Thinking questions
► Extended Nursing Diagnosis challenge
► Documentation activity
► Teaching Plan for Objectives 2, 3, 4, and 5

EXPLORE MediaLink

Additional resources for this chapter are found on the Student CD-ROM accompanying this textbook and on the Companion Website.

CD-ROM CONTENT

Content for this chapter includes:
Objectives
Key Concepts
NCLEX-RN® Review Questions
Model Documentation Forms
Audio Glossary
Clinical Spotlight Videos
  Fetal Life
  Fetal Monitoring
  Preeclampsia
Head-to-Toe Physical Examination Video

COMPANION WEBSITE CONTENT

www.prenhall.com/damico

Content for this chapter includes:
Objectives
NCLEX-RN® Review Questions
Client Interaction Case Study Challenge

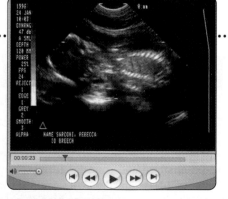

Application Through Critical Thinking
  Case Study Teaching Plan Challenge
MediaLinks
MediaLink Application
Tool Box
  Chapter Documentation Form Example
  Gestational Weight Gain Recommendations
  Recommended Daily Allowances of Major Nutrients by
    Women's Age Groups
  Pregnancy Teaching Checklists
  Health Promotion
    Healthy People 2010
    Client Education
New York Times

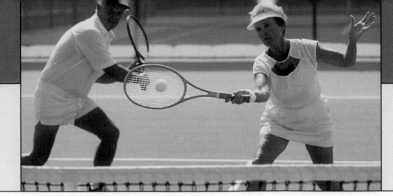

27

Assessing the Older Adult

MEDIALINK

www.prenhall.com/damico

The CD-ROM in the back of this textbook and the Media-Link website contain NCLEX-RN® review questions, interactive exercises, case study challenges, animations, videos, documentation and checklist forms, and review materials. For a complete listing of the media content specific to Chapter 27, see the Explore MediaLink at the end of the chapter.

*I*n the year 2000, 35 million people in the United States, or 12.4% of the population, were 65 years of age or older. Of these, 4.2 million were 85 years or older. This represented an increase of 15 million people in the older generation from 1970. However, the huge growth in the aging population is just beginning. It is estimated that there will be 40 million people 65 years of age or older in 2010, around 55 million in 2020, and between 70 million and 75 million, or 20% of the total population, in the year 2030. In that year, up to 10 million of the older people will be 85 years or older. After that the numbers will continue to climb but at a slower rate (Federal Interagency Forum on Aging-Related Statistics, 2004).

As the population shifts to include this increasing proportion of older adults, the process of aging is no longer viewed as a chronic and terminal disease. It is a normal growth and developmental stage, one that is often filled with happiness and fulfillment (see Figure 27.1 ●). Some of the conditions once tolerated as expected age changes are now being aggressively treated as diseases. Conditions such as incontinence, tooth loss, and some mental confusion can be treated and cured.

The first overarching goal of *Healthy People 2010* is "to increase quality and years of healthy life." However, the report points out that differences in life expectancy between populations of other countries and the United States suggest a substantial need and opportunity for improvement. At least 18 countries with populations of 1 million or more have life expectancies greater than the United States for both men and women (*Healthy People 2010*).

Healthy People 2010 seeks to promote health and reduce chronic disease. Goals will be accomplished through more effective screening programs, education, and treatment management. Several of the goals and focus areas of the plan are pertinent for older people. The *Healthy People 2010* feature on page 901 highlights the focus areas that are particularly applicable to older adults.

THEORIES OF AGING

Theories of aging include those related to environmental influences as well as to cellular changes due to wear and tear, chemical alteration, and genetic influences. In the wear-and-tear theory the body is likened to a machine (Miller, 2004). Over time, cells wear out and cannot be replaced. This eventually leads to death of the entire organism. Within this theory, healthy behaviors have a positive effect because they protect cell wear and tear and may allow cells to repair themselves. When the wear and tear of aging affects the immune system, some believe a greater incidence of cancer, infections, and autoimmune diseases occurs.

In some newer theories, the wear and tear on the cells is expressed by a buildup of detritus, or abnormal collection of malformed or inappropriate molecules within the cells. In the cross-linkage theory, strands of DNA that should remain separate are linked together damaging the DNA and leading to decreased cell function and cell death. In the free radical theory, highly reactive molecules that can be created by irradiation, pollutants, or normal metabolism interact with and damage cellular components. Although these free radicals can be removed by antioxidants including beta-carotene and vitamins C and E, over time the damage that is caused interrupts cellular function enough so that death occurs.

The genetic theories of aging focus on chromosomal differences between persons and chromosomal effects on cellular makeup, function, and longevity. One estimate is that genes have up to 33% influence on longevity and healthy aging, with the remaining influence being composed of environment and other health-related factors (Perls, Kunkel, & Puca, 2002). Genetic theories serve to explain why some families produce people with longer life spans than others.

The apoptosis theory seeks to explain why the process of apoptosis, or the regulation of cells through growth restriction, appears to get out of control in aging. This theory is thought by some to possibly explain the increased incidence of cancer, autoimmune disease, cardiovascular disease, and neurodegenerative diseases seen in aging people (Joaquin & Gollapudi, 2001).

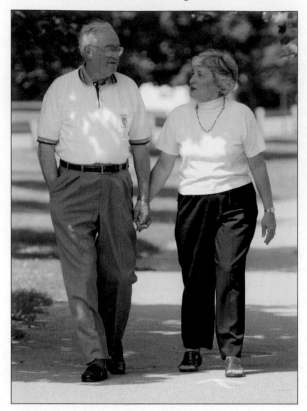

Figure 27.1 ● Older adults.

Miller (2004) concluded the following about biological aging: (1) It affects all living organisms. (2) It is natural, inevitable, irreversible, and progressive with time. (3) The course of aging varies from individual to individual. (4) The rate of aging for different organs and tissues varies within individuals. (5) Biological aging is influenced by nonbiological factors. (6) The processes are different from pathologic processes. (7) Biological aging increases one's vulnerability to disease (p. 49). For these reasons, health assessment of the older adult can be among the most complex and the most fulfilling of nursing care.

ANATOMY AND PHYSIOLOGY REVIEW WITH CHANGES OF AGING

Aging has an impact on all the organs and systems of the body. The following sections describe age-related changes in each of the body systems.

INTEGUMENTARY SYSTEM

Skin-related changes are affected by lifestyle and environmental changes, as well as by normal aging. Exposure to the sun and other radiation, to chemicals, and to the effects of nicotine and alcohol on circulatory function all serve to speed aging skin effects. Over time, corneocytes, which make up 85% of the epidermal cells, become larger and more variable. This alters skin appearance, making it coarser and less smooth. Melanocytes, which protect the skin from radiation and are located in the

basal layer of epidermal tissue, progressively decline in number, thus increasing the risk of radiation changes. The melanocytes tend to clump irregularly leading to patchy pale spots of pigment loss or to denser spots of color, commonly called liver spots, also known as **lentigo senilis.** These skin discolorations due to melanocyte clumping are relatively small in size. The white "freckles" should not be confused with vitiligo, which may affect large areas of the skin (see Figure 11.16 on page 202 ⬤⬤). The rate of epidermal turnover decreases, and the skin becomes thinner and drier.

Wrinkles appear on the face, especially at the corners of the eyes and mouth. This is due to loss of skin elasticity, as well as to loss of underlying subcutaneous tissue. These signs of aging are disliked by many, but some persons see them as marks of experience and wisdom. The face may have bony prominences along the cheeks and jaws, and the eyes may appear sunken due to loss of fat pads around these structures. Eyelids may droop due to loss of skin elasticity or may bulge along the lower lids due to herniation of fat tissue. The nose droops lower. Ears may appear larger than they did when the person was younger. This is due to loss of facial fat deposits, balding, and stretched, pendulous earlobes.

Partial or complete baldness is common, especially in men, and often to a partial extent in women with male pattern baldness genes. Men's beards may remain full, and women may experience increased coarse facial hair growth, especially on the chin. The hair loses its color due to a decrease in melanin production and becomes white or gray. Hair thins all over the body.

The number and functional ability of sweat glands also decrease with aging. This causes less ability of the older person for thermoregulation. Sebaceous glands that help to oil the skin and to prevent loss of water and retard the entry of microorganisms begin to decrease their sebum production. This contributes to the dryness of older skin as well as to opening portals for infection because increasing skin dryness and scaliness can cause pruritus and scratching.

MOUTH, NOSE, AND THROAT

The senses of smell and taste diminish with age because of a decrease in olfactory fibers, taste buds, and saliva production. In some older persons, however, saliva increases, causing the **cheilitis** (angular stomatitis) at the corners of the mouth. Partial or complete loss of teeth may also be found, especially in the oldest adults who lived half of their lives before the use of prophylactic fluoride and other modern dental care. Poor dental health is decreasing, however, now that dental care is improving for people of all ages, and the current generation of older adults has lived most of their lives drinking fluoridated water and observing modern dental hygiene.

Edentulism can give the mouth a pursed or sunken look. Persons both with and without teeth should be examined for gingivitis and signs of periodontal disease. This pathology must be differentiated from normal gums that may recede to an extent, making teeth appear longer.

EYES

Several alterations are associated with normal aging and are not related to vision or eye problems. **Xanthelasma** are soft, yellow plaques on the lids at the inner canthus. These plaques are sometimes associated with high cholesterolemia but usually have no pathologic significance as they appear on persons with normal cholesterol counts. **Pingueculae** are yellowish nodules that are thickened areas of the bulbar conjunctiva caused by prolonged exposure to sun, wind, and dust. They may be on either side of the pupil and cause no problems. However, they must be differentiated from **pterygium,** an opacity of the bulbar conjunctiva that can grow over the cornea and block vision. **Arcus senilis** is a light gray or white ring surrounding the iris at the corneal margin due to the deposition of lipids. This is a common finding that does not affect vision.

A **cataract** is clouding of the lens, which can significantly alter vision in terms of both light perception and clarity of sight. This condition is now easily correctable by outpatient surgery that replaces the lens in a 20- to 30-minute procedure. The lens also loses the ability to accommodate, and many older people cannot focus well on near objects, such as print. **Presbyopia** is the name for this nearsighted vision, and it is treated with reading glasses or bifocals.

EARS

The tympanic membrane may appear more opaque than in a younger person. The client may have difficulty hearing whispered words. This is due to **presbycusis,** the hearing loss that occurs over time and that causes high-frequency sounds not to be heard. Older clients may complain that they do not hear consonants well when listening to normal conversation. This is due to the loss of hair cells in the organ of Corti in the inner ear. However, conductive sound loss can often occur due to an accumulation of earwax that is drier and becomes more impacted than in a younger person. Any older persons complaining of difficulty hearing should be checked for outer ear canal blockage and have their ears cleaned before any further testing is performed.

RESPIRATORY SYSTEM

The stiffening and inelasticity that occurs with aging in all of the soft tissue also affects the lungs. The chest wall does not expand as well, and breaths are therefore shallower. Sagging of nasal and upper airway structures further impedes airflow. Mucus lining the respiratory passages becomes drier. The older person uses more accessory muscles, and therefore must work harder and use more energy to take in air.

The number of capillaries in the pulmonary tissue decreases, and there is less blood flow available for gas exchange. Normal alveoli enlarge and their walls become thinner. Since they are less elastic, it becomes more difficult to maintain positive pressure and keep the small airways open. Gas exchange becomes compromised, especially in the bases of the lungs. The older adult cannot respond well to stress. Anxiety and physical exertion can cause significant demands on the respiratory system, and infection can have devastating effects.

It is important for the older adult to obtain vaccinations against influenza and pneumonia. These two diseases together constitute the fourth leading cause of death in people older than 65 years. The influenza vaccine is formulated every year according to the best prediction of that year's dominant flu strains. Protection is effective for only about 6 months and must be renewed each fall before the start of each flu season. The immunization is effective for most older people but only for those organisms covered in that vaccine. The older person is therefore not protected against other respiratory infections.

The pneumococcal vaccine is recommended for all persons 65 years of age and older. It protects against 23 types of infections that cause 85 to 90% of all cases of pneumonia in the United States and is effective in 75% of older adults (Gross, 2001). Although it was originally considered that the vaccine would give once-a-lifetime immunization, the Centers for Disease Control and Prevention (CDC) now recommends that boosters be given to those people who received their initial immunization more than 5 years ago.

CARDIOVASCULAR SYSTEM

With aging, the heart must pump against a stiffening aorta. There is a gradual rise in blood pressure and a widening of pulse pressure throughout adulthood with mean systolic values for healthy persons peaking between ages 70 and 75 years to a high of 158, followed by a slow decline to within the 140s by age 100. Diastolic pressure stays relatively constant at a little above 80, declining slightly in the advanced elderly. Hypertension is usually defined as blood pressure consistently above 140/90. The incidence of hypertension in older adults is high, and diagnosing it in older persons who may have an increasing high systolic pressure can be important. It is a major risk factor in coronary artery disease, congestive heart failure, renal disease, retinopathy, ruptured aortic aneurysm, and stroke. This should be considered in the diagnosis or treatment of the disease in the client. It has been estimated that middle-aged Americans face a 90% chance of developing hypertension at some point in their lives (Vasan et al., 2002). Almost 13 million or 50% of the people who have the disease are unaware that they have it. Another 7 million are aware but untreated. Of those treated, 58% are not adequately controlled (University of Texas at Austin, 2002).

GASTROINTESTINAL SYSTEM

The intensity of the propulsive esophageal wave decreases in aging. However, it is thought that this does not seriously affect swallowing and digestion. A pathologic cause should be sought if an older person is experiencing esophageal dysfunction.

Gastric emptying times are significantly slowed with aging, however. This can cause feelings of premature fullness and contribute to gastritis and peptic ulcers due to *Helicobacter pylori* infections. Although it was formerly thought that diminished secretion of gastric acid occurred in older people, thereby decreasing the rate of digestion, recent studies indicate that this is not a normal aging finding and that a pathologic cause for the condition should be determined if it occurs (Jensen, McGee, & Brinkley, 2001).

Once food leaving the stomach reaches the small intestine, absorption of some nutrients is slowed in the older person due to atrophy of muscle fibers and mucosal surfaces. Lymphatic and vascular circulation in the villi is reduced, and the villi become flatter and less effective.

In the large intestine, water and electrolytes are absorbed. The walls of the colon become weaker and more flaccid with age. There is less mucous production, and older persons may experience more constipation, especially if they have had a lifetime of poor bowel habits, insufficient fiber intake, and overdependence on laxative use. Continuous overdistention of the bowel and straining to pass stools may result in diverticula formation and hemorrhoids, or even rectal prolapse.

Nutrition

Many older adults are just as interested in the latest nutritional information as are many younger adults. They may be very knowledgeable about reading food labels and as informed about nutritional recommendations for healthy lifestyles as many younger people (see Figure 27.2 ●). But as with younger adults, they may not always follow the recommendations, and fad diets may have more serious side effects on less robust older adults or those with chronic diseases. One way that *Healthy People 2010* hopes to promote health and reduce chronic disease is through nutrition and weight objectives. The first objective is to increase the proportion of adults who are at a healthy weight from the current 42 to 60%. The next objective is to reduce the proportion of adults who are obese from 23 to 15%. Further goals are to increase the amount of fruit, vegetables, whole grains, and calcium in average diets, and to decrease intakes of total fat, saturated fat, and sodium. Another objective

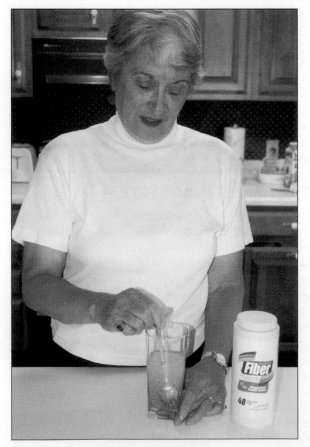

Figure 27.2 ● Adding fiber to the diet.

is to increase food security among U.S. households and to reduce hunger.

Nutritional Assessment

A diet recall, food frequency questionnaire, or more in-depth focused interview can provide complementary information to the laboratory assessment and physical assessment. A careful diet history can uncover risk factors for poor nutritional health. Sensitivity is essential when gathering nutritional history data, as an older adult may be reluctant or embarrassed to divulge personal information. Insufficient funds for food, decline in functional status leading to food preparation challenges, or sadness and depression have all been reported as contributors to malnutrition in older adults, but they may not volunteer whether they are affected by these factors. Table 27.1 outlines important nutritional history data to obtain when assessing the older adult.

Other older clients may have underlying or serious nutritional deficiencies due to lack of knowledge; disease processes that affect digestion and absorption of nutrients; lack of ability to obtain food due to economic, psychological, or mobility problems; edentulism or the pain of periodontal and tooth disease; or alcoholism. The short form of the Geriatric Mini Nutrition Assessment viewed on the Companion Website is a quick way to assess for undernutrition. ◎

The nutritional assessment starts with calculation of body mass index (BMI). This requires measurement of height and weight. This is usually done during the assessment or during the registration process at the beginning of the assessment time. The weight in kilograms divided by the height in meters squared equals the BMI. An older person may be considered underweight if he or she has a BMI less than 23. A client is considered to be obese if he or she has a BMI of 30 or more. Over 22% of adults 60 years of age and older were considered obese in data collected in the first three quarters of 2003. The incidence is highest among non-Hispanic, African American females (Ni et al., 2004). Persons with BMIs over 28 are at significantly higher risk for morbidity and mortality. Because body shape has also been correlated with certain diseases, attention should be given to that if the BMI is elevated. A waist-hip ratio greater than 0.95 puts older adults at high risk for health problems, especially coronary disease (Grodner, Long, & DeYoung, 2004).

Special consideration should be taken when assessing the BMI of an older person who has experienced an **a**mputation. Rubenstein, Harker, Salva, Guigoz, and Vellas (2001) have suggested the following alterations when estimating amputee BMI. The client should be weighed on a scale, and then the following amounts should be used to increase the weight before calculating BMI so that comparisons can be made with existing BMI data. For a client with a single below-the-knee amputation, multiply by 6.0%; single at-the-knee amputation, multiply by 9.0%; single above-the-knee amputation, use 15%; single below-the-elbow amputation, use 3.6%; and single arm amputation, use 6.5%.

Although body weight increases with aging up to the sixth decade of life, it usually decreases in the seventh decade and above. Lean body mass lessens as muscles atrophy, and bone density decreases. Height shrinks due to thinning of the vertebrae and vertebral disks, and due to increasing curvatures of the

Table 27.1	Nutritional Risk Factors on Physical Assessment and Nutritional History in Older Adults (Indicators of poor hydration status are italicized.)		
Face	Sunken eyes	**Sensory**	Impaired vision
	Temporal wasting		Loss of hearing
	Note any changes from Table 9.5		Impaired taste and smell
Mouth	Changes in taste perception (and smell)		**ALERT!**
	Lack of saliva production (xerostomia)		*Taste and smell losses are often related to medications and not aging.*
	Note any mouth changes from Table 9.5		
	Long tongue furrows	**Nervous System**	Note any changes that impair food shopping, preparation, or self-feeding:
Teeth	Caries		• Tremors
	Missing or loose teeth		• Altered gait
	Poorly fitting dentures		• Neuropathy
Chewing and Swallowing Mechanics	Drooling		• Impaired cognition
	Pocketing of food		Confusion, headache, lethargy
	Hoarseness	**Functional Capacity (ADLs, I-ADLs)**	Note any changes that impair food shopping, preparation, or self-feeding:
	Coughing with swallow		• Altered mobility or flexibility
	Complaint of lump in throat		• Pain
Gastrointestinal	Anorexia		• Vision
	Nausea		• Strength
	Vomiting		• Energy level/fatigue
	Diarrhea	**Psychosocial**	Depressive symptoms
	Constipation		Bereavement
	Heartburn		Social isolation
Genitourinary	*Darkened urine*		Dependency
	Low volume urine		Food insecurity
Skin	Decubitus ulcer	**Medical Condition**	Acute or chronic disease
	Poorly healing wounds		Multiple medications
	Note any rashes listed in Table 9.5	**Diet**	Restrictive therapeutic diet
	Dry mucous membranes		**ALERT!**
	Dry axillae		*Most older adults do not need to be on strict therapeutic diets. Each person should be individually evaluated for appropriateness of restrictions, and diet should be liberalized unless contraindicated.*
	ALERT! *Tenting is not an accurate assessment of dehydration in older adults due to altered skin elasticity.*		
Skeleton/trunk	Loss of subcutaneous fat		Missed meals—assess reason
	Muscle wasting		Alcohol
	Note any skeletal changes from Table 9.5		Lack of access to culturally familiar foods

spine. The distribution of fat also changes, with more deposited on the hips and abdomen and less on the face and periphery.

Skinfold thickness and limb measurements are used with mixed results in assessing older adults. Changes in skin integrity and connective tissue as well as loss of muscle tone and fat redistribution can make accurate measurements a challenge. Reference values are available from national survey data and include age, gender, and racial subgroup information. As with younger populations, skinfold and limb measurements are best used to monitor progress or changes in an individual.

LABORATORY MEASUREMENTS. Laboratory measurements for plasma proteins, anemia screening, or nitrogen balance may be included when assessing the elderly population. In particular, any macrocytosis should be evaluated for folic acid and vitamin B_{12} status. Absorption of vitamin B_{12} diminishes with age due to a decreased acid environment in the stomach and decreased production of the intrinsic factor needed for

absorption. Iron absorption also requires an acid medium in the stomach. Medications may further alter gastric acid by buffering the contents or decreasing production.

Fluid Intake

Fluid intake should be assessed along with nutritional intake. Older people may consciously or unconsciously decrease fluid intake because they do not feel thirsty when it is appropriate to drink, because they fear incontinence or nocturia, or because they lack the mobility to have easy access to beverages. Dehydration may lead to confusion, digestion problems, constipation, and bladder infections.

GENITOURINARY SYSTEM

By age 75 to 80, a 50% loss of nephrons has occurred; thus, glomerular filtering is decreased. This has major implications for drug toxicity in older adults. Atherosclerosis of renal arteries can decrease renal blood flow and may lead to atrophy of the kidneys. Tubular function also diminishes, and urine is not as effectively concentrated as at a younger age; maximum specific gravity may be only 1.024.

Urinary incontinence can cause embarrassment and lead to social isolation, infection, and skin breakdown. It is the leading cause of institutionalization into long-term care facilities. It is related to diminished bladder elasticity, bladder capacity, and sphincter control, as well as to cognitive impairment. Stretching of perineal muscles due to childbirth and obesity further contributes to stress incontinence in females. Prostatic enlargement, which occurs in 95% of all males by age 85, results in problems of urinary retention with frequent overflow voiding, especially during the night.

Endocrine changes, described in the following section, affect size, lubrication, and function of genital structures in both men and women. Decreased hormone production affects both libido and performance.

ENDOCRINE SYSTEM

Areas of concern regarding function of the endocrine system in the older adult include sleep, fatigue, and sexual function.

Sleep

One of the myths of aging is that older people need less sleep than younger ones. This is not true, although the pattern and quality of sleep does change. Often older adults will either have trouble getting to sleep or wake up in the middle of the night and not be able to get back to sleep. Many older people take one or more naps. This frequently makes their total sleep time equal that of a younger person. However, if they are not able to nap during the day due to scheduling of jobs and activities, and if they continue to have trouble with sleep patterns at night, they may become sleep deprived. Clients should be questioned about their sleep patterns and whether they feel they are getting enough satisfying sleep. Hypnotic medication may be useful for short-term treatment. However, lifestyle changes may be necessary, such as change of bedtimes, change of environment, and inclusion of some sort of formal exercise. Naps of 1 hour or less should be used judiciously. Nutritional intake should be examined, and large, heavy meals omitted near bedtime. A small protein and carbohydrate snack, to increase serotonin levels, can be helpful before going to sleep.

Normal age changes cause a decreased amount of growth hormone to be produced during sleep. Further endocrine changes cause a decrease in dopamine, an increased release of somatostatin, a lessening of the feedback inhibition of adrenocorticotropic hormone (ACTH) by glucocorticoids, a decrease in estrogen production, a diminished availability of testosterone, a decrease in sperm production, and an increase in follicle-stimulating hormone (FSH) (Terry & Halter, 1994). Women become menopausal, with greater vaginal dryness and more rapid loss of vaginal vasoconstriction. Men usually have decreased sperm production, decreased volume of seminal fluid, less testosterone production, and increased blood levels of FSH. Changes in collagen and the vascular endothelium may impair erection stiffness or frequency. Both men and women may experience body image changes secondary to illness, surgery, or psychosocial factors.

Fatigue

Whenever an older person complains of feeling tired, weak, or unwell, the thyroid should also be screened for malfunction. Some symptoms that many people expect with aging, such as weight loss, slowed mental functioning, slowed physical movement, and feeling unwell, may be signs of thyroid malfunction. Although it was once thought to affect mainly younger adults, the rate of hyperthyroidism is actually higher in older people than in younger ones (Burke & Walsh, 1997).

Sexual Function

All of these changes may decrease sexual function. However, one study showed that at least half of married couples over the age of 60 have sexual relations at least monthly, and 53% of unmarried men and 41% of unmarried women have relations at least weekly (Janus & Janus, 1993). Once the assessment interview has become comfortable for both the client and the interviewer, the older persons should be asked about their sexual health. The interviewer should consider the culture of the client and try to determine the level of interest that the client has in sexual activities. Some clients may not wish to pursue such activities due to the loss of a longtime partner. Others may be very interested, but too shy to bring the subject up. Much too often, this area of health is omitted from assessment. Sometimes this is due to embarrassment, not only on the part of the client, but largely on the part of the person doing the health assessment, who may feel that this is not a proper topic to discuss with an older person.

Some causes of sexual dysfunction, such as medication use, can be easily changed. More is known about the effect of medications on male sexual dysfunction than on female dysfunction. It is thought that medications may diminish female lubrication, decrease libido, or interfere with achieving orgasm (Miller, 2004). Medications that may cause erectile dysfunction include antidepressants such as serotonin reuptake inhibitors, monoamine oxidase inhibitors, and tricyclic antidepressants; tranquilizers; anticholinergics; phenothiazines; and antihypertensives such as beta-adrenergic blockers. Cimetidine may cause erectile dysfunction as well as gynecomastia. Imipramine may reduce libido; methyldopa may inhibit erection by reducing pelvic blood flow (Doerfler, 1999).

MUSCULOSKELETAL SYSTEM

By the age of 80, about 30% of muscle mass is lost. Coupled with structural loss is loss of neurons that control muscle function. Thus, there is a decline in both strength and agility.

Bone loss also increases due to increased resorption, diminished calcium absorption, impaired osteoblast activity, and decreased bone marrow cells. Decreased estrogen production in women and decreased testosterone production in men speed this bone loss. Bone fractures can occur with minimal force. The vertebrae and intervertebral disks dry and flatten, providing less support and resulting in a shortening of several inches of height after age 65.

Weight-bearing joints suffer from the wear and tear of repeated use, especially if subjected to heavy weights. There is decreased viscosity of synovial fluid, and degeneration of supporting collagen and elastin cells. All of this contributes to inflexibility and the aches and pains of osteoarthritis. Gait can become unsteady, and falls become a safety issue.

NEUROLOGIC SYSTEM

The conduction of neurologic impulses slows with aging. This decreases reaction time, slows learning, and may decrease short-term memory. However, the idea that all older persons lose mental capacity is wrong and causes much harm. Any decrease in mental acuity should be investigated to determine its pathologic cause. Too often older people and their families suffer needlessly with conditions that can be treated and relieved. Often the fear of mental incapacity alone decreases quality of life for the older person. Many older persons contribute significantly to their own happiness and to that of their families and society by continuing to provide the intelligence and experience that they have gained over their lifetimes, even if they provide it at a somewhat slower rate.

Aging does bring a series of losses, however, and that can lead to depression. These losses can include loss of spouse and friends through death or illness, loss of occupation or living arrangement due to functional disability, loss of body image, loss of favored recreation, and loss of independence. Of all persons 65 years of age or older, 2.5% report having experienced serious **psychological distress** within the last 30 days, with women more likely affected than men (Ni et al., 2004). Clients should be asked whether they have had such distress and whether they have been medically treated for it.

The interview should give the nurse opportunity to form some opinion of the mental processes of the client. The client's mood and affect should be assessed, along with the ability to concentrate on the questions being asked, to reason competently, and to recall both recent and remote memories.

Recalls about sleep patterns, daily activities, diet intake, medications, and bowel patterns all give some measure of clients' memory and reasoning powers. Clients in early stages of memory loss and even dementia, however, may be able to convey adequate mental ability, especially to persons doing the assessment who may not have known them over time. Changes in mental status may be missed unless a formal instrument is used to compare against norms and to use as a baseline measure for future trend comparisons. This type of testing should not be done at the very outset of the interview, even though it is described at this point in this chapter. Likewise, mental screening should not be done at the very end of the assessment when the client may be tired. The screening should be done toward the end of the verbal part of the interview, when the client has learned to feel comfortable with the interviewer and a rapport has developed. Many older clients, whether experiencing signs of mental decline or not, are very fearful of such a condition. If they believe that they actually have symptoms, they may be even more reticent to participate in formal testing.

The **Mini–Mental State Examination (MMSE)** (Folstein et al., 1975) is one screening instrument of cognitive reasoning that has been used extensively for 30 years. It is familiar to most practitioners and rates well as a reliable and valid tool for detecting dementia and delirium relating to organic disease. It is easy to use. It takes less than 10 minutes to administer and requires no special testing materials other than paper and pencil.

One problem with the MMSE is that it is so widely used that clients may become irritated when they find themselves taking the test over and over. It also becomes easy for anyone, young or old, with dementia or not, to become confused between the answers on one test and the next when they are given too close together. Were the words to be remembered *ball*, *bat*, and *chair*, or was that from the test given yesterday?

Older clients who take the test on a periodic basis begin to learn the scoring system and keep track of their scores. They may become fearful of this progression of numbers and resist giving an opportunity for comparison if they feel it will show decline.

Gathering the Data

*C*omprehensive health assessment of the older adult includes the interview and physical assessment. Subjective data is gathered during the focused interview, in which the client's own words and perceptions are recorded. Objective data is collected during physical assessment, from client records, results from laboratory, and other diagnostic studies.

GUIDELINES FOR INTERVIEWING OLDER ADULTS

It is important to respect the older client's worth and individuality (see Figure 27.3 ●). He or she should initially be interviewed alone and considered to be mentally competent unless mental status is previously known. If caregivers or

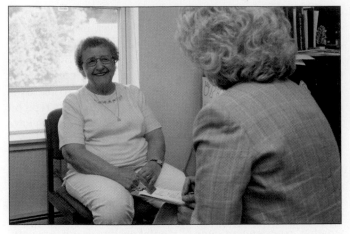

Figure 27.3 • Establishing rapport with the older adult.

family members remain in the room for the interview, the client may not feel comfortable telling the "whole truth." When the client is very frail, the nurse may tend to address the spouse or adult child of the client rather than the client. This may happen unconsciously when the client is slow to answer or does not interact as quickly as the nurse would wish. Frailness does not necessarily mean an inability to respond appropriately, however, ignoring the client at the beginning of the interview is not a way to gain trust and gather information. If it is established in the initial, private interview that the client is unable to communicate sufficiently to supply the nurse with all of the needed information, then it is appropriate to meet later with family or other caregivers. The nurse should consider cultural differences when asking about state of health and functional abilities, and save sensitive subjects, like sexual and cognitive function, until rapport has been established.

The temperature of the room should be in a comfortable range, with the client dressed appropriately for that temperature. A robe, blanket, or slippers may be necessary if the patient is not wearing street clothes. Thin paper or cotton examining gowns often make the older client feel uncomfortably chilly and less able to attend to the health history questions.

In order to facilitate clients' abilities to see and hear clearly, the nurse should make sure they are wearing their glasses or hearing aids that are turned on, minimize background noise, turn off background music, and shut the door or screen the area. Once both participants are seated, the client should have his or her back to the window or strong light source. Thus, glare is reduced, and the light falls upon the face of the examiner. If the older person is known to have a vision impairment, additional lighting may be needed. Eye contact should be maintained at eye level. The interviewer should sit if the client is sitting or lying, and be sure that the client has a back support.

The nurse should address the client by his or her last name. It is also appropriate for the nurse doing the assessment to introduce him- or herself by using a last name. It makes the older person more at ease and trusting to know that the person doing the assessment is approaching it in a professional manner. Other titles, such as Col. or Dr., should also be retained. As rapport is established, a more informal approach can develop.

Once the comforts of seating, lighting, and environmental distractions are cared for, it is important to know whether the client is in pain and whether pharmaceutical or alternative pain therapies should be considered before conducting the interview. It is also important to consider sleepiness and the effects of any recent medication.

The interview precedes the physical assessment; this allows the client and nurse time to become comfortable with each other. After the initial questions and fact-finding are done, and rapport is established, the physical assessment may be started. It often prompts information if questions about function are asked while that body system is being physically assessed.

Asking clients how they assess their own health may yield insight into functionality problems or lack thereof. Often older people are more satisfied with their health than might be apparent. In 2003 almost 40% of all adults 65 years or older in the United States rated their own health as excellent or very good. The number is significantly higher for Caucasian persons than for those who are African American or Hispanic (Ni et al., 2004).

FOCUSED INTERVIEW

Subjective data is collected during the focused interview. The nurse organizes the questions for the client, family members, and caregivers. Following is a sample of questions to be used during the focused interview.

FOCUSED INTERVIEW QUESTIONS	RATIONALES
QUESTIONS FOR THE CLIENT	
1. What is the main reason you have come to see me today?	▶ This question will elicit information in an open-ended manner, although it is important to remember that fear or embarrassment may cause clients' deep concerns to be withheld until trust and comfort increase. Starting with only one concern allows time to establish rapport before going on to further issues.

FOCUSED INTERVIEW QUESTIONS	**RATIONALES**
2. **Can you tell me more about that? Why are you concerned about that?**	▶ The nurse should ask follow-up questions to each point that the client raises. Not only is data lost without these, but a lack of real concern is conveyed to the client if the interviewer does not follow up, and information sharing begins to lessen.
3. **Tell me about what you do during a typical day.** • When do you wake up? • When do you get up? • When do you dress? • When and what do you eat? • When do you start daily activities? Tell me what they are.	▶ These questions need to be broken into specific sections to find out information not only about physical health habits, such as sleep, diet, mobility, and other basic activities of daily living, but also about psychological health, energy, and interaction and socialization with other people.
4. **How long do you usually sleep?** • Do you feel satisfied with your night's sleep? • How often and how long do you nap in the daytime?	▶ Many older people awaken early, but may get up for a cup of coffee and read the newspaper and then return to bed and sleep, not really starting their day until several hours later. So only asking what time they wake up in the morning might elicit an answer of 5 a.m. but not give an accurate picture of their sleep-wake cycle.
5. **How much exercise, planned or informal, do you do during the day?**	▶ Over 28% of adults 65 to 74 years of age reported that they engaged in some form of regular leisure-time physical activity in the year 2000. Almost 18% of those 75 years and over participated, with almost twice as many men exercising than women (Ni et al., 2004).
6. **Do you experience any pain, dizziness, or difficulties when you try to exercise?** • Do you have any of these symptoms when you are at rest? • Do you feel energetic or tired most of the time? • If you are tired, can you relate it to any specific cause?	▶ The answers to these questions can lead to the need for further laboratory or other diagnostic testing to determine physical cause, but may also relate to psychological and social interaction difficulties that must be addressed.
7. **Where do you live? With whom do you live? What is your place in the household?**	▶ The nurse should follow up any responses that might hint at elder or spousal abuse and also follow up any responses that indicate housing is a problem.
8. **Are you responsible for your own care needs and personal business, or do you depend on someone else?**	▶ In the United States, in the first three quarters of 2003, persons who reported needing some help with personal care were as follows: 3.3% of those 65 to 74 years of age, 6.4% of those 75 to 84 years of age, and 22.9% of those 85 years and older.
9. **Do you have a job, either within or outside the home?** • Are you happy doing it? Do you receive compensation for the job? • Does the workplace environment and work situation seem safe?	▶ These questions provide information about activity and socioeconomic status, as well as safety. They also give insight into personal satisfaction and sense of worth.
10. **Do you smoke, drink alcohol, or use recreational drugs?** • If so, how much and for how long? • Have you ever done any of these things in the past? • If so, when did you stop?	▶ During the period from January to September 2003, 10.5% of men 65 years and older, and 8.5% of women that age reported that they smoked. During that same period, 6.5% of men and 1.3% of women reported that they had five or more drinks in one day at least once during the previous year. Recreational drug use also cannot be overlooked whether the use is current or in the past. Ten and one half percent of adults 65 years and older have been tested for HIV in the United States (Ni et al., 2004) actually has the virus.

FOCUSED INTERVIEW QUESTIONS	RATIONALES
11. **What prescribed and over-the-counter medications do you take routinely or occasionally?**	▶ When discussing prescribed medications, the nurse must determine whether the client actually takes them as ordered. Inconvenient scheduling, confusion, ignorance, or thrift are all reasons why older adults may not be taking prescribed medications. Such medications can be extremely expensive, and the prescriptions may never have been filled, or the client may cut pills in half or take them on a delayed schedule. If possible, the client should bring all of his or her pill bottles to the interview. Not only will the names and amounts of the prescribed medications be more accurately known, but also attention can be paid to the dates on which the prescriptions were filled and whether the amount of medication in the bottle matches what should be there at the time of the interview. The nurse should make sure the client understands what each medication is for and assess whether any special instructions for taking them are being followed.
12. **Do you have any problem holding your urine? How many times at night do you get up to urinate?**	▶ This is often a concern that causes embarrassment. The question should be asked late in the interview once rapport has been established. Urinary incontinence may have significant impact on quality of life and functional ability. Negative answers to earlier functionality questions may give hints of this problem that should be followed up.
13. **Do you have any problems with constipation or moving your bowels? What is your normal bowel pattern?**	▶ Asking whether the client feels he or she has constipation problems yields information about elimination expectations as well as actual problems. Here is an opportunity to teach about the variations of normality and ways that regular elimination can be established. Answers to these questions may also hint at laxative abuse.
14. **Do you experience any pain or discomfort in any particular part of your body?** ● How often do you feel this? ● What initiates it? ● How long does it last? ● What do you do to help it feel better? ● How would you rate the quantity of pain on a scale of 0 to 10, with 0 being no pain and 10 being the worst imaginable pain? ● How would you describe the quality of the pain? ● What adjectives would you use?	▶ Suggestions might be *sharp*, *stabbing*, *burning*, *aching*, *throbbing*, *radiating*, *cramping*, and so on. It is especially important to consider cultural differences when clients are talking about their pain and to determine exactly where the pain is and when it occurs.
15. **Do you have times that you feel especially sad or lonely? (Depending on the answer to this question, the nurse should follow up with questions about what clients do to relieve the feeling. Do they have social support? Do they ever consider the end of their lives?)**	▶ Following up may lead to the opportunity to ask whether the client has ever thought of taking his or her own life. Depression and suicide are major concerns with elderly people, especially those who have debilitating illnesses or those who have lost a significant person. The nurse can use the Yesavage/Brink Geriatric Depression Scale to assess further if this seems warranted (see Figure 27.4 ●).

FOCUSED INTERVIEW QUESTIONS

RATIONALES

1. Are you basically satisfied with your life? (no)
2. Have you dropped many of your activities and interests? (yes)
3. Do you feel that your life is empty? (yes)
4. Do you often get bored? (yes)
5. Are you hopeful about the future? (no)
6. Are you bothered by thoughts that you just cannot get out of your head? (yes)
7. Are you in good spirits most of the time? (no)
8. Are you afraid that something bad is going to happen to you? (yes)
9. Do you feel happy most of the time? (no)
10. Do you often feel helpless? (yes)
11. Do you often get restless and fidgety? (yes)
12. Do you prefer to stay home at night, rather than go out and do new things? (yes)
13. Do you frequently worry about the future? (yes)
14. Do you feel that you have more problems with memory than most? (yes)
15. Do you think it is wonderful to be alive now? (no)
16. Do you often feel downhearted and blue? (yes)
17. Do you feel pretty worthless the way you are now? (yes)
18. Do you worry a lot about the past? (yes)
19. Do you find life very exciting? (no)
20. Is it hard for you to get started on new projects? (yes)
21. Do you feel full of energy? (no)
22. Do you feel that your situation is hopeless? (yes)
23. Do you think that most persons are better off than you are? (yes)
24. Do you frequently get upset over little things? (yes)
25. Do you frequently feel like crying? (yes)
26. Do you have trouble concentrating? (yes)
27. Do you enjoy getting up in the morning? (no)
28. Do you prefer to avoid social gatherings? (yes)
29. Is it easy for you to make decisions? (no)
30. Is your mind as clear as it used to be? (no)

Figure 27.4 ● Geriatric depression scale.

Source: Adapted with permission from Yesavage, J. A., & Brink, T. L. (1983). Development and validation of a geriatric depression screening scale: A preliminary report. *Journal of Psychiatric Research, 17*:41. Copyright © 1983, Pergamon Journals Ltd.

16. Do you have any concerns about your memory or thinking powers?

▶ This is a very sensitive question for many older people. Almost all will answer that they have such concerns. The interview up to this point will yield information from which the person doing the assessment can make conclusions about this topic. If the client does voice concerns, it is important to ask for specific examples to determine whether the client suffers from actual mental impairment or simply self-ageism and fear of possible mental decline. The MMSE can be used as a quick screening tool.

QUESTIONS FOR FAMILY MEMBERS OR CAREGIVERS

These questions will need to be tailored as appropriate according to the competence and functionality exhibited by the client in the client interview. Independent older people who are cognitively intact can be expected to give their own accurate interview answers. However, questions that go unsatisfied during the interview, or that seem to elicit confused or inaccurate answers, need to be followed up. This follow-up should be done privately with the family caregivers while the older person waits in another room. Examples of additional questions to caregivers are:

FOCUSED INTERVIEW QUESTIONS	RATIONALES
1. **Have you noticed any forgetfulness or changes in the way (the client) normally does things?** • Has (the client) stopped doing any of his or her normal activities? • Have you noticed any unusual behaviors?	▶ Responses can help the nurse identify changes in mental status or deterioration of function, which might put the client at risk for injury.
2. **Do you have any concerns about (the client) that you wish to tell me but do not want to discuss in front of him or her?**	▶ This gives family members permission to share fears or to ask questions that they are reluctant to mention for fear of worrying the older person.

CLIENT INTERACTION

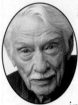

John Powell, age 77, comes to the clinic with a chief complaint of "having no pep and feeling blue." The intake sheet shows that Mr. Powell is a retired metal worker whose wife died last year. He had a negative physical examination last month. He is dressed for this appointment in a paper gown that was given to him when he registered. The nurse has not previously met him. Following is an excerpt of the focused interview.

INTERVIEW

Nurse: Good afternoon, John. It's nice to meet you. Sit up here on the examining table and let's find out why you're feeling depressed.

Mr. Powell looks at the nurse and then away. He appears uncomfortable, but does not speak. He climbs up slowly onto the examining table while holding the gown closed behind him.

Nurse: According to your record, you were doing fine last month. Has anything happened to change that?

Mr. Powell: Well, no. Things are about the same. (Keeps his eyes looking downward.)

Nurse: Let's check to see how your thinking processes are doing today. (*Performs the MMSE and Mr. Powell scores a 29.*)

Nurse: Well, your cognition seems fine. Next we'll check your depression scale.

Mr. Powell: (*looking away and mumbling*): Well, I'm not much for all these tests. There's really nothing the matter with me. I guess I'm just old.

ANALYSIS

The nurse in this situation is apparently trying to get quickly to the core of Mr. Powell's problem. However, she has not allowed time for a positive rapport to develop. She began the interview by calling the client whom she was just meeting for the first time by his first name, without asking his preference or introducing herself. She positioned the client without a back support on the examining table while he was wearing only a thin, paper, backless gown. Although Mr. Powell indicated by his quietness and body language that he was uncomfortable, the nurse immediately proceeded with testing his cognition. This is often a sensitive evaluation and needs to be performed only after a comfortable relationship between the client and the nurse has been established. This was not done in this encounter, but Mr. Powell did well in the MMSE. The nurse then immediately plunged into another screening tool for depression. What was needed, in fact, was the establishment of respectful communication. Mr. Powell needed to feel that the nurse was sincerely interested in his problems, so that he would feel comfortable giving her cues to his problems.

Please refer to the Companion Website at **www.prenhall.com/damico** and click on Chapter 27, the **Client Interaction** module, to answer questions about this case. In addition, see other resources for this chapter including NCLEX review questions and other interactive exercises and materials.

ASSESSMENT TECHNIQUES AND FINDINGS

Before beginning the physical assessment, the nurse should wash his or her hands in warm water, warm the stethoscope, ask whether the client needs to void before the examination, and ask whether the client is warm enough and comfortable.

EQUIPMENT

examination gown	sphygmomanometer
drape	centimeter measuring device
examination gloves	tongue blade
examination light	cotton
penlight	vision screener
stethoscope	tuning fork
ophthalmoscope	reflex hammer
otoscope	sharp and dull objects
substances to taste and smell	

HELPFUL HINTS

- To prevent discomfort due to temperature sensitivity, the nurse should provide gowns and wraps of sufficient warmth. Older adults may remain clothed and remove only what is necessary for a particular examination.
- Lying or sitting on a hard examining table is difficult for many older adults. A bed that can be elevated or a table with a padded mattress can be used.
- The client's energy should be conserved by organizing the assessment so activities are grouped for a minimum of position changes.
- Many older adults are uncomfortable with a much younger examiner, especially if the examiner is of the opposite sex. The nurse should maintain a mature and professional attitude while demonstrating care and concern.
- A great deal of information about the client's functional abilities can be obtained by observation of movements, the ability to carry out requests, and communication and interaction with the examiner. This also provides information about the ability to hear and understand requests.
- Explain each step of the procedure and ask questions about the findings. Older adults are often more at ease when asked to explain a scar or physical alteration.
- Consider the client's need or desire to have a family member present for the assessment.
- Use Standard Precautions.

TECHNIQUES AND NORMAL FINDINGS	ABNORMAL FINDINGS SPECIAL CONSIDERATIONS

GENERAL SURVEY

1. **Position the client.**
   - The client should be in a comfortable sitting position with some back support. Lighting must be adequate to detect skin color changes, discharge, and lesions.

2. **Observe the client.**
   - Note signs of distress, quality of dress and hygiene, and posture or any physical abnormalities.
   - Note any breath or body odor.
   - Note the client's interactions with family members or caregivers.

▶ Facial grimacing, rocking, rigid posture, pallor, or perspiration could indicate pain. Inappropriate dress, body odor, and inadequate hygiene may indicate cognitive or functional problems. Obvious poor care and poor interaction may indicate elder abuse issues, although this should not be assumed. Culture must also be considered. Physical abnormalities may indicate pathologic conditions. Breath and body odors may also gives clues to illness such as infection or diabetes mellitus, or to excess alcohol intake.

TECHNIQUES AND NORMAL FINDINGS	**ABNORMAL FINDINGS SPECIAL CONSIDERATIONS**

3. **Evaluate the client's nutritional status.**
   - Observe for a wasted or apathetic appearance.

   ► Muscle and fat are normally lost with aging, and facial features may sag, but extreme loss may indicate decreased nutrition or be a symptom of disease such as cancer.

   - Measure height and weight and ask about usual values and whether there has been any recent change.
   - Calculate BMI.

   ► Determine classification of BMI. Underweight, overweight, and obesity all indicate risk conditions.

   - Measure waist at the smallest circumference and hips at the largest circumference and calculate waist-hip ratio.

   ► Increased waist-hip ratio has been found to correlate with cardiovascular risk.

   - Assess hydration by looking at skin for dryness, flakiness, or scaling as well as tenting when skin is pinched up. Check oral mucous membranes for dryness.

   ► Dehydration is a common problem in older adults who may not experience thirst appropriately or who may withhold fluids due to nocturia or urinary incontinence. It may also be a sign of problems with caregiving. Dehydration can lead to cognitive problems. Alcohol intake may decrease other food and fluid intake as well as lead to dehydration due to diuresis.

4. **Measure vital signs.**
   - Take the blood pressure in both arms with the client reclining, sitting, and standing. Allow a minute or two between each measurement.

   ► Orthostatic hypotension (a drop of 20 mm Hg or more when standing) may occur in older adults as a result of medications or vascular impairment.

   ALERT!

   It is important to assist the client to a sitting or standing position before retaking the blood pressure and to be cautious that the client does not fall.

   - Use an appropriately sized cuff. A child cuff may be used for very thin persons; a thigh cuff can be used for extremely fatty upper arms.
   - Take the pulse both apically and radially and compare, checking for pulse deficit. Note regularity and strength of beats at both sites.

   ► Weak beats and arrythmias may not be conducted to the radial pulse. Consider the effect that any of the client's medications may have on pulse rate. For example, beta-blockers or digoxin may slow the pulse, whereas adrenergics may increase the rate.

   - Take oral temperature, being sure that the client's mouth is closed around the device.

   ► In the absence of illness, body temperature in older adults is lower than at a younger age. The mean is 36.2°C (97.2°F). Because temperature regulation is not as effective in older adults, however, attention should be paid to whether the client has just come in from the cold or is overly bundled on a warm day.

   - Count respirations for a full minute at a time other than when the thermometer is in the client's mouth. It is best to count the respirations after listening to the last beat of the apical pulse.

   ► It may be difficult for the client to hold an electronic thermometer or even keep his or her mouth closed tightly around a lighter one and still breathe normally. Be sure that clients do not think you want them to take deep breaths when you are listening to their apical pulse.

TECHNIQUES AND NORMAL FINDINGS	ABNORMAL FINDINGS SPECIAL CONSIDERATIONS

- Ask the client to rate his or her current pain on a scale of 0 to 10, with 0 being no pain at all and 10 being the most pain imaginable.

▶ Pain is an important vital sign to measure with all clients. It is especially important in older persons who may experience acute as well as chronic conditions and who may not report the pain because they believe it is a normal part of aging.

INTEGUMENTARY SYSTEM

1. **Inspect the skin for color.**
   - Note any overall redness, cyanosis, jaundice, pallor, or transparency.
   - Check for erythema on bony prominences and in moist areas such as the groin and under the breasts.

▶ Skin in older adults is normally paler and more transparent, but pallor can indicate anemia, malnutrition, or edema. Redness can indicate an inflammation, skin infection, or beginning decubitus ulcer. Differentiate visible veins, especially on lower extremities, from cyanosis or ecchymosis.

ALERT!

Although it is insulting to wear gloves for casual, upper body inspection, gloves should be worn when examining areas that cannot be easily visualized and that might contain open wounds or body fluids, such as scalp, under the breasts, and between the toes.

2. **Palpate the skin.**
   - Note moisture or dryness, scaliness, texture, and thinness.

▶ Skin dryness and scaliness may indicate dehydration, malnutrition, or conditions such as eczema or psoriasis.

   - Note overall temperature as well as individual areas, especially on the periphery. Compare bilaterally.

▶ Overall skin temperature is usually cooler than in younger adults. However, cold spots, especially on the periphery, may indicate circulatory disease.

ALERT!

Skin can be extremely thin and fragile, especially in very old people. This is especially true in persons taking long-term corticosteroids. Care must be taken to avoid tearing and bruising.

3. **Measure and describe all skin lesions.**
   - Look for lesions that are common and nonsignificant in aging skin: cherry angiomas, senile lentigines, seborrheic keratoses, and acrochordons. (See Chapter 11. ⌦) Describe and measure these so that new lesions or changes can be identified later. Inspect precancerous actinic keratoses for cancerous lesions such as melanoma or basal or squamous cell carcinomas. Identify any areas of trauma, decubitus, or vascular ulcers.

▶ Herpes zoster is more common in older adults. Look for painful, red vesicular or pustular lesions that may be in a line or in patches on the thorax, front or back. Ecchymoses, petechiae, or purpura may indicate a bleeding disorder. Excessive bruising or burns may be signs of abuse, falling, or cognitive problems.

TECHNIQUES AND NORMAL FINDINGS

ABNORMAL FINDINGS SPECIAL CONSIDERATIONS

4. **Inspect the hair.**
   - Observe the amount, distribution, and color of hair.
   - Note excessive or total loss of hair; abnormal location of hair, especially gender related; and dry, brittle, or coarse hair.

▶ Hair usually becomes gray or white due to loss of melanocytes. Be sure to check the color at the roots if it is dyed. Balding of hair in men and thinning of head hair in women is common. However, hairiness increases in the nose and ears. Women may experience an increase of facial hair, especially on the chin. Excessive hair changes may indicate hormonal disorders, use of gonadotropic hormones for cancer chemotherapy, or excessive use of corticosteroids. Dry, brittle hair may indicate malnutrition. Dull, coarse hair could indicate hypothyroidism. Disheveled hair may indicate lack of care or mental impairment.

5. **Inspect the nails and nail beds.**
   - Note the condition, hygiene, nail-bed angle, and blanching.

▶ Nails become thicker and may be more brittle. However, extreme brittleness and tearing may indicate a protein deficiency. Very thick nails are seen in vascular insufficiency and diabetes. Long, dirty nails are signs of caregiver or self-care neglect. Increased nail-bed angle (clubbing) is related to chronic lung or cardiac diseases.

HEAD AND NECK

1. **Observe the face.**
   - Aging changes result in more wrinkles and a softer, more jowly appearance.

▶ Excessive sagging and drooping, especially when it is unilateral, may indicate a stroke or other neurologic damage.

2. **Inspect the nose and nares.**
   - Note color, size, and any excessive dryness.

▶ Dryness is a sign of senile rhinitis, and redness in the nares may indicate chronic allergy. The nose tends to get larger with age, but a swollen papular, red nose indicates rhinophyma, a severe rosacea of the lower half of the nose. Usually seen in males, rhinophyma is characterized by lobulated overgrowth of sebaceous glands and epithelial connective tissue.

3. **Evaluate the client's sense of smell.**
   - Use identifiable substances such as coffee, mint, or lemon.

▶ Smell and taste diminish with age, but perceiving unusual odors may be a sign of temporal lobe epilepsy. An inability to distinguish pungent, common odors could be related to neurologic dysfunction such as stroke.

TECHNIQUES AND NORMAL FINDINGS	ABNORMAL FINDINGS SPECIAL CONSIDERATIONS

4. Inspect the oral mucous membranes, gums, throat, and tongue.

- Note color, exudate, swelling, and lesions.
- Have the client say "ah" as you depress the tongue with a tongue blade. Check for symmetrical elevation of the soft palate.

▶ Pale mucous membranes can indicate malnutrition or anemia; white patches could be precancerous leukoplakia. If the client's own teeth are present, redness and spongy swelling with recession of the gum from the neck of the tooth indicate periodontal disease. If the client is wearing dentures, redness and leukoplakia are signs of poorly fitting, irritating dentures. A bright red tongue could indicate thiamine (B_1) or vitamin C deficiency; a dark red, swollen tongue with white or yellow adherent patches is a sign of fungal infection, which older people taking antibiotics commonly experience. A dry and red tongue with longitudinal furrows indicates dehydration, especially in people taking diuretics or having elevated blood sugar levels. Unequal elevation or loss of elevation of the soft palate occurs with impairment of cranial nerves IX and X, seen with cerebral vascular accident. In this case, the person is at risk for choking and aspiration.

5. Palpate and auscultate the carotid arteries.

- Proceed gently, palpating one artery at a time.
- Auscultate with the bell of the stethoscope.
- Note any bruits.

▶ Bruits are signs of carotid stenosis and impending cerebral vascular accident. If you hear bruits, check the aortic and pulmonic valve areas of the chest for murmurs, which may be radiating into the neck.

6. Inspect and palpate the neck veins.

- Assess the veins first with the client lying flat and then with the client elevated above a 45-degree angle.
- Note any firmness and distention.

▶ All vessels enlarge with age and are more visible because of decreased subcutaneous tissue, but they are normally soft and compressible. If the veins are flat when the client is supine, suspect dehydration. If the neck veins are visible, firm to the touch, or tortuous when the client is elevated 45 degrees, suspect increased venous pressure and right-sided heart failure.

7. Evaluate the range of motion of the neck.

- Do not overextend the neck.

▶ Limited range of motion in the neck is often related to cervical arthritis, degenerative disk disease, or muscle spasm. Overextension may be painful. It may also decrease blood flow to basal arteries if any are stenosed. If kyphosis is present, hyperextension of the neck is difficult. Dizziness may also occur with motion if there are any preexisting inner ear pathologies.

TECHNIQUES AND NORMAL FINDINGS	ABNORMAL FINDINGS SPECIAL CONSIDERATIONS

EYE

1. **Inspect the eyelids, cornea, and iris.**
   - Note the position of the lid on the iris, identifying any tumors or cloudiness of the cornea, rings over the limbus, irregularities of the iris, and inturning or drooping of lids.

▶ The eyelids cover more of the iris in the aging eye because of decreased muscle tone, but frank ptosis in which the upper lid covers a considerable portion of the pupil, especially if unilateral, is a sign of dysfunction of cranial nerves III and IV, possibly due to cerebral vascular accident (brain attack). Bilateral ptosis may be due to ocular myasthenia gravis. Pterygium is not significant, nor is arcus senilis. Cloudiness over the pupil could be due to beginning cataracts. Irregularities of the iris may be genetic in origin but more likely due to previous surgery for glaucoma. Entropion and ectropion are the result of loss of muscle tone.

2. **Check the pupils for size, equality, and reactivity.**
   - Note both consensual and direct response to light. Ensure that the room is dimly lighted and that the client is facing away from sources of outside light.

▶ Pupils decrease in size with age, and because of their smallness it may be difficult to elicit pupillary constriction. Lack of consensual response or inequality of size may indicate damage to cranial nerve III. Unusually small pupils (smaller than 2 mm) may be due to ophthalmic miotic medications for glaucoma.

3. **Measure visual acuity.**
   - Be sure that the light is now comfortably bright.
   - Use a handheld Rosenbaum or Jaeger card, testing each eye separately while the client has glasses on. Then test both eyes together.
   - Note if the client holds the screening card more than the recommended 14 inches in order to read.

▶ Loss of accommodation and power (holding the screener more than 14 inches away from eyes and requiring bright light to read by), called presbyopia, is a normal finding. However, the client should be asked when last he or she had a full vision screening and reading glasses prescription update. Loss of central vision indicates macular degeneration. Blurring or cloudiness could be related to glaucoma, diabetic retinopathy, or cataracts.

4. **Check peripheral fields of vision.**
   - Especially note any losses of either left or right fields of vision.

▶ A right or left hemispheric stroke can result in a loss in the contralateral visual field. Bilateral loss of peripheral vision may indicate cataracts or glaucoma.

5. **Inspect the fundus of the eye with an ophthalmoscope.**
   - Note any dark areas in the red reflex, changes in the optic disc, and appearance of the blood vessels.

▶ Tiny pupils make funduscopic inspection difficult. Changes of aging include narrower and straighter vessels. Black spots in the red reflex are signs of opacities as may be seen in cataracts. "Cupping" of the disc is a sign of glaucoma, and a "fuzzy disc" indicates cerebral edema. Narrowing and tapering of the arterioles are seen in hypertensive disease, and small red spots or creamy round lesions are punctate hemorrhages and exudate seen in diabetic retinopathy.

TECHNIQUES AND NORMAL FINDINGS	ABNORMAL FINDINGS SPECIAL CONSIDERATIONS

6. Gently palpate the eyeball.

- Ask the client to close his or her eyes. Note tension or firmness.

▶ Very soft or boggy eyeballs indicate dehydration, whereas rock-hard orbits could mean glaucoma.

EAR

1. Inspect the outer ear, ear canal, and tympanic membrane.

- Use an otoscope to inspect the ear canal and tympanic membrane.
- Note any excessive cerumen or changes in the tympanic membrane.

▶ Excessive cerumen may cause a conductive hearing loss. Cerumen tends to be drier in older adults and may not be easy to remove. Improper ear-cleaning habits (e.g., use of cotton swabs) can pack cerumen tightly in the canal, interfering with hearing and obscuring visualization of the tympanic membrane. Scarring and sclerosis of the tympanic membrane from repeated inflammation or infection give a darkened appearance or dark lines.

2. Evaluate the client's hearing.

- Use the whisper, Rinne, and Weber tests. Use a 512 or 1024 tuning fork.

▶ Hearing loss with aging begins with diminished perception of high-frequency sounds. Subtle changes are found when using higher-frequency tuning forks. Sensorineural losses are more common than conductive losses in older adults because of loss of hair cells in the organ of Corti. This loss is called presbycusis. In sensorineural hearing loss, the Rinne test is normal (AC>BC), but the Weber test shows the sound lateralizing to the good ear or equal in both if hearing is diminished bilaterally.

RESPIRATORY SYSTEM

1. Inspect the shape of the thorax.

- Look for increased anterior to posterior diameter and spinal curvature abnormalities that may affect respiration.

▶ Loss of bone density and weakened thoracic musculature result in an increased anteroposterior diameter. Severe barrel chest is a sign of chronic obstructive pulmonary disease. Also, kyphosis and scoliosis may decrease lung expansion. (See Chapter 15. ⚭)

2. Assess the chest wall and ribs.

- Assess pain or tenderness to touch, crepitus, or bruising.
- Palpate for tactile fremitus.

▶ Pain upon palpation of the ribs is a sign of pathologic fractures of the ribs, which can occur without any major trauma in the client with osteoporosis. Also look for bruising in conjunction with rib pain, which could be due to falls or physical abuse.

Increased fremitus, especially in the periphery, indicates fluid accumulation or tissue consolidation.

TECHNIQUES AND NORMAL FINDINGS	ABNORMAL FINDINGS SPECIAL CONSIDERATIONS

3. **Percuss the lung fields.**

- Check for hyperresonance or dullness.

▶ Anticipate hyperresonance in the older adult with chronic obstructive pulmonary disease. Dullness indicates fluid accumulation from pulmonary edema or retained secretions. Dullness could also indicate tissue consolidation from a tumor or mass.

4. **Auscultate the lung fields.**

- Auscultate all lung fields and note characteristics of sounds.

▶ Scattered rales in the bases are quite common in healthy older adults. Rales that extend upward and do not temporarily clear with cough suggest pulmonary edema. Scattered or discrete rales can be due to alveolar or small airway exudate. Coarse, loud rales may be signs of pulmonary fibrosis seen in people with long-standing lung disease. Because lung expansion decreases with age, breath sounds are not heard as far down as in younger adults. If the person has increased trapped air from emphysema, which is present to some degree in the very old as a normal finding, breath sounds and vocal resonance will be diminished. Difficulty hearing any breath sounds, harsh rhonchi, or bronchovesicular breath sounds in the periphery are indicative of advanced chronic lung disease.

When listening to breath sounds, care should be taken to allow the older adult to intersperse the necessary deep breaths with shallower ones so that the client does not hyperventilate and become dizzy. Care should also be taken to keep the client warm and not overly exposed.

BREASTS

1. **Assess the female and male breasts.**

- Note changes in symmetry, lumps or thickening of tissue, lesions or sores, inflammation, changes in the nipples, or drainage from open lesions or from the nipples. (See Chapter 16. ∞)

▶ Hormonal changes can increase breast tissue in males and put them at risk for breast cancer; however, the incidence is still very low for males. Females on postmenopausal hormone therapy are also at increased risk for breast cancer, especially if female relatives have had it. Decreased fat in the female breast may make masses easier to feel. Risk for all cancers increases with age, and early identification of tumors is vital.

| **TECHNIQUES AND NORMAL FINDINGS** | **ABNORMAL FINDINGS SPECIAL CONSIDERATIONS** |

CARDIOVASCULAR SYSTEM

1. **Auscultate the precordium.**
   - Auscultate at five points on the precordium. Listen for S_1 and S_2.
   - Check for murmurs, clicks, and S_3 or S_4 gallops.
   - Using the bell of the stethoscope, listen for low-pitched murmurs during S_3 and S_4.
   - Using the diaphragm, listen for high-pitched murmurs, clicks, and snaps.
   - If you hear a murmur, inch the stethoscope away from the site in several directions to check for radiation. Describe murmurs using specified criteria. (See Chapter 17. ⬯)

   ▶ Murmurs, usually holosystolic and grade 3 without radiation, and S_3 are common in older people because of decreased cardiac muscle tone. Loud murmurs grade 4 or greater and with thrills or radiation suggest a failing heart, valvular stenosis, or incompetency. Murmurs that radiate from the apex to the anterior axillary area are usually of mitral origin. Murmurs that radiate from the base near the sternal border, right or left, up into the neck are usually related to aortic or pulmonic valve disease. Clicks and snaps are opening sounds and point to aortic or mitral calcifications. A fixed splitting of the second heart sound (not heard just on inspiration, but throughout the respiratory cycle) is noted in pulmonary hypertension or chronic obstructive pulmonary disease.

2. **Take the apical pulse.**
   - Note rate and rhythm.

   ▶ Arrythmias are quite common in healthy elders. Abnormally slow rates could indicate heart block or sinus arrest, especially if accompanied by syncope. Fast or grossly irregular rhythms point to potentially serious tachyarrythmias, especially if accompanied by chest pain or dizziness. After periods of immobilization, increased heart rate can indicate decompensation.

ABDOMEN

1. **Inspect the abdomen.**
   - Observe for shape, symmetry, and pulsations.

   ▶ Flaccid or "potbelly" abdomen is common because of loss of collagen and muscle, and deposition of fat. A scaphoid and flaccid abdomen is seen in the very old with additional fat loss but may also be a sign of rapid weight loss accompanying malnutrition or cancer. A distended abdomen is seen with fluid in the peritoneal cavity (ascites) or excessive gas. Asymmetry may indicate tumors, hernia, constipation, or bowel obstruction. Although the slight up-and-down pulsation from a normal aorta is more readily seen in clients with thin abdominal walls, lateral pulsations or soft, pulsatile masses indicate an aortic aneurysm. Visible tortuous veins on the abdominal wall near the umbilicus, in conjunction with a firm and distended abdomen, indicate portal hypertension with ascites.

TECHNIQUES AND NORMAL FINDINGS	ABNORMAL FINDINGS SPECIAL CONSIDERATIONS
2. Auscultate the abdomen. • Note the number and quality of bowel sounds. • Check for vascular bruits over the aorta, in flank areas for renal arteries and over the groin for femoral and iliac arteries.	▶ Bowel sounds may be hypoactive. Borborygmi may be due to bleeding or inflammatory bowel disease. High-pitched hyperactive bowel sounds accompanied by colicky pain and distention are signs of small bowel obstruction, which occurs most often in older males. Bruits heard over any of the arteries are signs of stenosis or aneurysms.
3. Percuss the abdomen. • Percuss the four quadrants of the abdomen and note tympany and dullness over most of the abdomen.	▶ Because of the normally thinner abdominal wall, tympany may be more noticeable but should still be within normal ranges. Areas of dullness in the lower left quadrant and sigmoid area are probably related to stool, but it is essential to rule out tumors. Shifting dullness, especially when accompanied by firm dullness, suggests ascites. Dullness above the symphysis pubis could indicate a full bladder.
4. Palpate the abdomen. • Use light then deep palpation and note tenderness, firmness, rigidity, and masses. • Palpate the costal margin at the right midclavicular line and midsternal line for liver enlargement.	▶ Tenderness with moderate distention could be due to flatus but could also indicate irritation of the stomach or bowel. The thinner abdominal wall of the older adult makes it easier to feel the underlying bowel. A soft mass or small firm masses felt in the left lower quadrant may be stool, especially because constipation is common. Firmness is associated with fluid or excessive gas, but rigidity is a sign of peritoneal inflammation. Distention just above the symphysis pubis may be caused by bladder distention due to prostatic hypertrophy or incomplete emptying. If the liver can be palpated below the costal margins, the liver is probably enlarged. Enlargement may reflect passive congestion due to congestive heart failure or liver disease, especially if the liver feels nodular.

GENITOURINARY SYSTEM

FEMALE

1. Check the underclothing for staining. • If present, note color, amount, and odor.	▶ Staining indicates urinary or bowel incontinence or vaginal discharge.
2. Inspect the external genitals. • Note changes in color, appearance, and odor in the external genitalia. Atrophy of the labia is usual.	▶ Redness, swelling, or odor can indicate incontinence, yeast infections, inadequate self-care, or caretaker neglect. Fecal-like odor could signal a urinary fistula.

TECHNIQUES AND NORMAL FINDINGS	ABNORMAL FINDINGS SPECIAL CONSIDERATIONS

3. Perform a pelvic examination.

- Assist the client into the left lateral position.

▶ Bulging of tissue or muscle into the vagina or rectum indicates cystocele, rectocele, or uterine prolapse. Vaginal atrophy and dryness may make examination painful. Malodorous vaginal discharge could be a sign of cancer or infection.

4. Examine the rectum.

- Note sphincter control.
- Check for hemorrhoids.
- Take a stool sample and check for occult blood.

▶ Sphincter control decreases with age, resulting in incontinence. Rectal cancer is more common in older adults; occult blood in the stool is an early sign of cancer.

MALE

1. Check the underclothing for staining.

- Note color and odor of stains.

▶ Staining indicates incontinence. Small amounts of dried blood could indicate intermittently bleeding hemorrhoids.

2. Examine the external genitals.

- Observe for swelling, redness, or odor.

▶ Testicular and penile atrophy is normal, but swelling could be a sign of infection or prostatic hypertrophy. Swelling, redness, and odor can be a sign of infection, incontinence, poor self-care, or caretaker neglect.

3. Perform a rectal examination.

- Note sphincter control.
- Check for prostate enlargement and any rectal abnormalities such as hemorrhoids.
- Take a stool sample and check for occult blood.

▶ Prostatic hypertrophy can be benign or malignant; encourage the client to have a prostate-specific antigen (PSA) test. Elevated levels usually indicate carcinoma of the prostate. The occult blood test can detect colon cancer, which increases in incidence in men over age 40. Hemorrhoids can cause bright red bleeding as well as a red stain on the stool. A mass in the rectum could be rectal cancer.

MUSCULOSKELETAL SYSTEM

1. Position the client.

- Help the client to a comfortable sitting position while maintaining safety.

2. Assess the spinal column.

- Note abnormal curvatures, deformities, pain or tenderness with palpation of vertebrae, and bruising or other signs of trauma.

▶ Shortening of the spine due to flattening of the disks is very common. Loss of bone matrix and decreased muscle mass and tone can result in increased curvatures such as kyphosis, lordosis, or scoliosis. Arthritis and degenerative disk disease can cause spinal deformities. Pain upon palpation of the vertebrae and generalized back pain indicate pathologic fractures due to osteoporosis. Bruising or unusual lesions on the back could indicate falls or physical abuse.

TECHNIQUES AND NORMAL FINDINGS	ABNORMAL FINDINGS SPECIAL CONSIDERATIONS

3. Assess all joints.

- Assess for pain, heat, redness, swelling, deformity, and range of motion.

▶ Heat, redness, swelling, and pain on movement of joints indicate bursitis or gouty or septic arthritis. Rheumatoid arthritis also produces these symptoms but is more likely to be seen in younger adults. Osteoarthritis causes swelling and joint deformity with early morning stiffness and pain. Hands and weight-bearing joints, such as hips and knees, are most often affected.

4. Assess the muscles.

- Inspect the muscles for size, comparing one side with the other.
- Palpate muscles for tone.

▶ Loss of innervation to specific muscle groups or paralysis from cerebral vascular accident or other neurologic diseases results in atrophy and loss of or increased tone.

5. Assess the feet.

- Note color, skin integrity, any deformities, and signs of inflammation, infection, or ulcerations.
- Palpate pedal pulses.

▶ Bunions and corns are common. If home remedies have been used to treat corns, inflammation and ulceration may result. Pedal pulses may diminish with aging, but the inability to palpate pulses, especially if the feet are red or dusky in color, indicates arterial insufficiency. Pitting edema of feet and legs due to venous incompetency or right-sided heart failure may be present.

NEUROLOGIC SYSTEM

1. Evaluate mental status.

- Do this at the end of the examination when rapport has been well established with the client, as long as the client is not overly tired. If at any point the client seems to be tiring, dividing the examination into two sessions should be considered, and the mental status assessment should be done when the client is rested.
- Use a tool designed for older people such as the MMSE.
- Screen for depression, if indicated.

▶ These tools can identify subtle changes in memory and mental functioning that the client could disguise in ordinary conversation by confabulation. They are especially valuable when compared over successive evaluations. However, clients can get very apprehensive over the possibility of poor performance, and the tools must be used with empathy and understanding.

2. Assess cranial nerves.

- Assess cranial nerves as described in Chapter 24. ⚭ Tests are performed using the same techniques. Findings may include slowed or diminished responses.

3. Evaluate balance and coordination.

- Assess the client's ability to walk heel to toe forward and backward.
- Ask the client to perform the Romberg test first with eyes opened, then with eyes closed.
- Look for swaying and loss of balance.
- Stand close to the client with arms outspread, ready to prevent fall or injury.

▶ The heel-to-toe walk is often impaired and is not indicative of any specific disease, but it can place the person at risk for falls. Older people have a tendency to fall sideways. Falling forward and a propulsive gait are indicative of Parkinson's disease. If the person can correct balance with the eyes open, the defect is probably proprioceptive rather than of basal ganglion or cerebellar origin.

ALERT!

Any time that clients are asked to close their eyes, special care should be taken to protect them from falling.

TECHNIQUES AND NORMAL FINDINGS	ABNORMAL FINDINGS SPECIAL CONSIDERATIONS

4. Inspect for tremors of the head, face, and extremities.

- Note the kind of tremor and whether it is present at rest or primarily with movement.

▶ Gross tremor of the head (head bobbing), jaw, and tongue is called a senile tremor and is not treatable. A resting tremor, which diminishes with willed movement, and a pill-rolling tremor of the hands is seen in Parkinson's disease. People taking bronchodilator drugs have a fine tremor that increases with activity.

5. Evaluate motor strength.

- Assess the client's arm drift. Have the client stand with his or her feet comfortably apart and the arms held straight out at shoulder level. Check arm drift first with the client's eyes closed, then with them open.
- Assess the client's grip and extremity strength against resistance.

▶ Subtle hemiparesis is indicated by slow downward drift and pronation of hand on affected side when the eyes are closed; if the client is able to correct drift when the eyes are opened, suspect proprioceptive dysfunction (sensory-position sense). Unilateral diminished grip and loss of strength against resistance can indicate a stroke.

6. Evaluate sensation.

- Assist the client to a sitting position.
- Ask the client to close his or her eyes for all sensory evaluation.
- Check various sites for sensitivity to touch (use sharp and dull objects) and vibration (use a tuning fork on joints). Ask the client to identify where sensation is felt by pointing or verbally identifying the location.
- Assess stereognosis by asking the client to close the eyes and identify a key or other familiar object placed in the client's hand.
- Assess graphesthesia by asking the client to identify numbers you write with your finger on each of the client's hands.
- Evaluate proprioception by having the client identify the position to which you move a toe or finger.

▶ Sensation and discrimination normally decrease in elderly people, as does vibratory sense in the toes. Suspect neurologic disease such as cerebrovascular accident if sensation is absent in any area, especially unilaterally. Diminished or absent sensation symmetrically in lower extremities is a sign of diabetic peripheral neuropathy.

7. Evaluate reflexes with a reflex hammer.

- Note diminished or increased reflexes.

▶ Reflexes normally diminish with aging. If they are absent, suspect upper motor neuron disease; if they are hyperactive, especially with clonus, suspect lower motor neuron disease.

8. Evaluate sleep sufficiency.

- Does the client nap? When? How long? How many hours are spent asleep at night? Does the client rate his or her sleep as sufficient in terms of both quality and quantity?

▶ Poor sleep quality can be rated on a scale of 0 to 10, similar to pain rating. Zero represents totally adequate sleep with no sleep quality problems. Ten represents totally inadequate sleep quality, usually related to severe insomnia.

▶ It is important to ask when the client rises and starts the day's activities, not just when he or she awakens. Many older people wake up early, but fall back to sleep before rising.

Refer to the Companion Website at **www.prenhall.com/damico** and click on the **Documentation** module for documentation samples and documentation practice exercises.

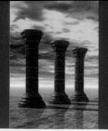

Abnormal Findings

*A*bnormal findings common in older adults include skin lesions, insulin resistance syndrome, diabetes mellitus, and drug and alcohol abuse.

SKIN LESIONS

The aging skin is subject to a variety of lesions. (See Chapter 11.) The cause is unknown but may be related to altered DNA causing a change in cell types. Xanthelasma is a tiny, tumorlike fatty deposit on the eyelid that may be related to hyperlipidemia. **Acrochordons,** or skin tags, are pedunculated, flesh-colored lesions of collagen and subcutaneous tissue that occur on the neck, back, axillary area, and eyelids. **Actinic keratoses** are normal aging growths, especially in fair skins, but are considered precancerous. They appear as calluslike red, yellow, or flesh-colored plaques on exposed areas such as ears, cheeks, lips, nose, upper extremities, or balding scalp. **Seborrheic keratoses** are benign, greasy, wartlike lesions that are yellow-brown in color. They can appear anywhere on the body, but are seen more frequently on the neck, chest, and back. Vascular lesions can include **cherry angiomas,** which are nonsignificant tiny red spots, either macules or papules, rarely larger than 3 to 4 mm, seen usually on the trunk. Another more serious vascular lesion is **senile purpura,** which can occur spontaneously or in response to minimal trauma in the very old client with fragile blood vessels. It is a coalescence of petechiae that begins as tiny individual red-to-purple spots caused by rupture of small capillaries. The petechiae converge from large purple to brown patches.

Cheilitis (angular stomatitis) is seen in persons who have poorly fitting dentures or who are not swallowing saliva well due to stroke or muscular weakness. This is marked by sore, reddened, cracked skin at either end of the mouth, and is due to excess salivation and *Candida* infection.

INSULIN RESISTANCE SYNDROME

Insulin resistance syndrome is a disorder in which there is a whole complex of symptoms that relate together, including obesity, heart disease, hypertension, gout, polycystic ovaries, and type 2 diabetes. Insulin resistance syndrome is difficult to understand and to treat. It involves more than just transient hyperglycemia. The hyperinsulinemia resulting from the increased blood sugar levels causes hypoglycemia if meals are delayed. This may cause excess production of adrenal hormones (Lerman-Garber et al., 2000), which increases the heart rate and causes physical tremors.

The enzyme lipoprotein lipase, which helps break down triglycerides, is also altered in the presence of hyperinsulinemia. Thus, elevated triglyceride levels are found in persons experiencing the condition, especially in those who have central obesity. Such persons also show higher than usual incidence of atherosclerosis and gout. Each of these conditions is associated with increased risk for heart disease. In the first case, this is due to stenosis caused by plaque buildup. In the second, it is due to the role of uric acid in thrombotic tendency (Longo-Mbenza, Luila, Mbete, & Vita, 1999).

Polycystic ovary syndrome is also related to hyperinsulinemia. In the presence of excess insulin levels, androgens are formed leading to male pattern hair loss, excessive body hair, and ovarian cysts. There is an increased potential for endometrial hyperplasia and malignancy. Even though the older woman may have undergone menopause, taking a good menstrual history, with attention to irregular menstrual cycles and infertility, may identify possible polycystic ovary syndrome in an older, obese, hypertensive, hyperinsulinemic woman who may be experiencing insulin resistance syndrome.

Diabetes Mellitus

The chance of becoming diabetic doubles with every decade of life. A very small percentage of older clients have type 1 diabetes, but 16.7% of all persons 65 years and older in the United States have type 2 diabetes. The incidence is higher in men than in women, in most populations, and non-Caucasians are about 20% more likely to develop the disease (Ni et al., 2004). American and Canadian Indians have the highest incidence of type 2 diabetes. Estimates of incidence in this population vary greatly. It has been estimated that 24.6% of American Indian women 65 years and older have the disease, as compared to 19.8% of the elderly American Indian men. In Pima Indians, the most widely studied American Indian group, the prevalence of type 2 diabetes is thought to be about 50% in adults between the ages of 30 and 64 years (National Diabetes Information Clearinghouse, 2004), and rates increase with aging.

Although there is a genetic link with this type of diabetes, with over 90% of clients with type 2 diabetes having a family history of the disease, nutritional factors over time greatly contribute to incidence. These factors include overeating, intake of a high-fat diet, and physical inactivity.

Diabetes is diagnosed when random blood sugars are above 200 mg/dl and are not accounted for by intake. An older adult usually demonstrates a higher glucose tolerance curve than do younger persons. Urine tests are not reliable because the renal threshold also rises in aging, so the absence of sugar in urine does not clear the person of having diabetes. Examination of glycohemoglobin A values shows the amount of

blood glucose that is stored in hemoglobin and indicates the average blood glucose level for the previous 120-day period. It is useful not only when diagnosing but also when treating the client and checking for effectiveness of health maintenance activities.

Drug and Alcohol Abuse

Of adults 65 years and older, 6.5% of men and 1.3% of women report having had more than five drinks of alcohol in one day at least once in the last year (Ni et al., 2004). This must be considered when performing a nutritional assessment. The client should be asked the amount and type of alcoholic beverages he or she may drink. Although intake of one glass of wine or beer is associated with increased well-being, excessive alcohol intake will lead to undernutrition and to serious complications, such as pancreatitis or liver disease. If the client reports a high daily

alcohol intake, the **CAGE** questionnaire (Ewing, 1984), which has been extensively validated against psychiatric criteria for alcoholism and alcohol abuse, may be used. The designer of the questionnaire recommends that even one "yes" identifies the need for further workup: (**C**) Have you ever had to **Cut Back** on your drinking? (**A**) Have people **Annoyed You** with criticism about your drinking? (**G**) Have you ever felt **Guilty** about your drinking? (**E**) Have you ever needed to start the day with a drink (an **Eye-Opener**)?

Health Promotion

HEALTHY PEOPLE 2010

FOCUS AREA	PREVALENCE	OBJECTIVES	ACTIONS
Diabetes	• Diabetes is most common in those over the age of 60. • An increase in the number of individuals with diabetes is expected as the population of the United States ages. • Type 2 diabetes is associated with increases in obesity and inactivity in older populations.	• Increase the number of individuals with diabetes who receive education. • Decrease the number of cases of newly diagnosed diabetes. • Reduce the number of diabetes-related deaths. • Increase the number of individuals who have eye, dental, and foot examinations.	• Formal education for those with diabetes and community-based education regarding diabetes. • Education about nutrition, weight management, and exercise to decrease the risk for type 2 diabetes. • Education about comorbidities (heart disease, kidney disease) as well as diabetic management. • Regular eye, dental, and foot examinations.
Injury and Violence Prevention	• Falls are the most common form of injury and hospital admissions for older adults. • Falling has been the leading cause of injury deaths in those 65 years of age and older. • Hip fracture is the most common injury from falls in the older adult population. • Almost half of older adults hospitalized for hip fracture do not return home or live independently following the fracture.	• Reduce deaths from falls. Reduce hip fractures among older adults. • Reduce disability from unintentional injury.	• Promotion of safety in the home and environment through education during individual healthcare visits and community programs. Education of older adults about risks for falls, including visual changes, medication effects, and changes in neuromuscular function.

| **Mental Health and Mental Disorders** | • Depression rates are higher among older adults who experience other health problems, such as hip fracture or heart disease.

• Dementias, such as Alzheimer's, and other severe forms of loss of mental ability occur among persons 65 and older and increase with aging. | • Increase the number of persons seen in primary healthcare who receive mental health screening and assessment. | • Education about the need for mental health screening. Education about the types of mental health screening. Community programs for older adults and caregivers about the risks for mental disorders and availability of assessment and treatment. |
| **Immunization** | • Although infectious diseases are no longer the most common causes of death, pneumonia and influenza remain among the top 10 causes of death for older adults. In 2000, pneumonia and influenza were responsible for 3.3% or 58,557 deaths among people 65 years of age and older. | • Increase the number of older adults who receive vaccination for influenza and pneumonia. | • Education about the risks for influenza and pneumonia in the older adult population. Individual and community programs to promote the need for vaccination. Provision of vaccines through low-cost community programs. |

CLIENT EDUCATION

The following physiological, behavioral, and cultural factors affect geriatric health. Several of these factors are cited as trends in *Healthy People 2010*. The nurse provides advice and education to reduce risks associated with the factors and to promote and maintain cardiovascular health.

LIFE SPAN CONSIDERATIONS

RISK FACTORS

- The incidence of chronic diseases such as arthritis, diabetes, and hypertension increases with aging.

- The incidence of cardiovascular disease increases with aging. Almost 80% of clients with coronary artery disease are 65 years of age or older.
- Changes in the neuromuscular system including changes in strength, reaction time, gait, vision, and hearing increase the risks for accident and injury.

CLIENT EDUCATION

- Support and provide education for older adults and families about screening, assessment, and management of chronic diseases.
- Encourage older adults to participate in regular screening for risks associated with cardiovascular disease. Explain the association of age-related changes with cardiovascular health.
- Provide information about the physical changes that accompany aging and advise older adults to participate in regular health screenings, including vision and hearing. Educate older adults and their families about ways to increase safety in the home and environment.

CULTURAL CONSIDERATIONS

RISK FACTORS

- Hypertension is a risk factor for coronary artery disease. Hypertension occurs more frequently in African Americans and Hispanics than in other groups.

- Obesity is increasing in older adults in the United States and occurs most frequently in African American women. The incidence of diabetes is highest in Native Americans, Hispanics, and African Americans.

CLIENT EDUCATION

- Tell clients that hypertension is often referred to as the "silent killer" because it is asymptomatic in most individuals. Clients need to participate in blood pressure screening, especially African Americans and Hispanics, who are at greater risk.
- Advise clients with a diagnosis of hypertension to be monitored regularly and to take medication as prescribed to decrease risks associated with hypertension.
- Provide information about nutrition to maintain healthy body weight and body fat percentage to clients of all ages. Recommendations for weight reduction and exercise programs should be provided to obese clients.
- Provide education about diet and exercise to assist clients with diabetes to decrease the risks and promote diagnosis and management of diabetes.

ENVIRONMENTAL CONSIDERATIONS

RISK FACTORS

- Older adults, especially those with chronic diseases, take many prescribed and over-the-counter medications.
  Medication interactions and adverse effects can result in complications, injury, and death.
- As a result of sensory changes, such as decreased vision, altered touch perception, and adaptability to light and dark, older adults are at risk for falls and injury.

CLIENT EDUCATION

- Educate older adults about each medication. Encourage older adults to discuss all medications with all healthcare providers. Advise older adults to keep a list of all medications at hand for health visits.
- Promote safety in the home. Educate older adults about expected changes in sensory abilities. Discuss changes that may affect the ability to be independent in activities of daily living, such as driving.

BEHAVIORAL CONSIDERATIONS

RISK FACTORS

- Smoking is a risk factor in development of cardiovascular disease. Smokers have double the mortality rate from myocardial infarction than nonsmokers.
- Lack of physical activity increases the risk for developing diseases that predispose one to cardiovascular disease, such as diabetes, obesity, and hypertension, and alone can increase the risk for heart disease.
- Changes in diet, especially the exclusion of fruits, vegetables, and roughage, can occur as older adults have dental changes that affect chewing. Decreased fluid intake may accompany the desire to control incontinence or urinary dribbling that may occur with prostate changes in older males or decreased muscular control in older females. Decreased food and fluid intake increases the risk for constipation, electrolyte imbalances, anemia, skin disorders, and other problems associated with nutrition.

CLIENT EDUCATION

- Participate in education to prevent smoking and assist clients who are looking for ways to stop smoking.
- Encourage regular exercise in clients of all ages. Exercise reduces the risks for cardiovascular disease by promoting healthy weight, maintains healthy blood pressure, and reduces the risk for development of diabetes.
- Inform older adults about nutritional needs. Encourage fluid intake of at least four glasses of water daily. Provide information about bladder control. Advise older adults to have regular screenings for problems related to nutrition, such as dental examination, testing for anemia, and screening for electrolyte imbalances.

Application Through Critical Thinking

CASE STUDY

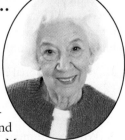

$\mathcal{M}$ary Sutton is an 83-year-old grandmother of five who lives alone in a senior high-rise apartment in downtown Philadelphia. Her husband died 15 years ago. She has two daughters who live in Washington, DC, and Baltimore. They visit her every month or so, and she talks to them on the phone weekly. Mrs. Sutton has always been proud of her independence and has stated firmly that, although she loves her family, she would never want to move in with either of her daughters and lose this independence.

She retired from her position as an executive secretary to a bank president when she was 67 years old, and has been busy up until recently volunteering in several community projects, as well as visiting friends and caring for her own daily needs. She has come to the clinic for a routine physical examination. Everyone in the clinic looks forward to her visits, because she frequently brings homemade cookies and is always smiling and friendly.

Mrs. Sutton's health has been fairly good up until now, although she has experienced angina and arthritis pain in the past. She is being treated for hypertension with atenolol 25 mg (beta-blocker) and nifedipine 10 mg (calcium channel blocker) each day, as well as furosemide 40 mg (loop diuretic). Her blood pressure is usually 140/80. She takes allopurinol 200 mg (antihyperuricemic) to control symptoms of gout, and simvastatin 40 mg for hyperlipidemia. She also takes a daily low-dose enteric-coated aspirin, has nitroglycerin tablets, and takes ibuprofen as needed for pain. She is on a low-fat, low-salt diet

Today Mrs. Sutton seems quieter and smiles less than normal. She apologizes when she comes in that she was unable to bring any homemade goodies as she did not have a chance to go out to buy more sugar and eggs. When asked how she has been feeling, she answers "okay." But when asked about some of her volunteer activities, she states that she has not been able to get involved as much as before. She is dressed nicely, although in quiet colors, and does not appear ill. Her hair is combed neatly, although she apologizes that she did not get a chance to get her monthly permanent wave at the beauty parlor. She has no specific complaints.

When Mrs. Sutton weighs in, the nurse finds that she has lost 10 lb since her last visit 3 months ago. Her vital signs are as follows: BP 152/85—P 74—RR 18—T 99.8—Pain 4. All of these values are elevated since her last visit. Her muscle strength is somewhat diminished but adequate. Her gait is slow, steady, and balanced.

Examination of her head, neck, and throat reveals no abnormalities or signs of inflammation or illness, although her skin is dry and she appears to have more wrinkles than the nurse remembers her having. Her hearing is unchanged, as is her vision. She is wearing bifocals that were updated 6 months ago. Her teeth appear to be in good condition and she does not exhibit any bad mouth odor. However, her mucous membranes are somewhat pale and dry. Her lung fields are clear and her respirations are not labored. Her breasts are soft and without palpable masses. When listening to her heart, the nurse hears the systolic murmur that has been present for some time. It does not seem to have changed from the previous visit. Her abdomen is soft and not distended. No bruits or abnormal sounds are auscultated, although bowel sounds are somewhat hypoactive. No tenderness, firmness, rigidity, or masses are palpated.

Although Mrs. Sutton was asked to remove her clothing and put on an examination gown before the physical assessment, she chose to keep on her underpants. When asked to slide these down so that her genitourinary system could be assessed, she became somewhat flustered and anxious, but did so. The nurse sees that she has a wad of damp tissue inside her pants. There is no obvious stain on the pad, but there is a strong odor of urine. The skin of her perineum and thighs is inflamed with a red, papular rash. When asked how long she has had the rash, she states that it has been getting worse for the last 2 months and that nothing she has tried has helped it. When asked what she has tried she answers, "cornstarch or talcum powder, witch hazel, and soap."

The nurse asks why she is using the tissues. Mrs. Sutton answers that it is just a way to stay clean. The nurse then asks if she has any trouble holding her urine, and Mrs. Sutton says, "Of course. I'm 83, aren't I?" The nurse asks whether there is anything else that she does to help this, and she says that she puts pads on all the chairs she sits on and on her bed at night. She also says that she does not allow herself to drink water after 3 p.m. Upon further questioning she starts to wipe tears from her eyes and says that she cannot go out anymore and visit her friends because she is afraid of ruining their furniture. She admits that this is why she has given up her volunteer activities and why she does not get out to the store or the hairdresser anymore. She does not have her friends come to her apartment because she is embarrassed to have them see the pads on the furniture, and sometimes she is afraid that there is a bad odor. She ends by saying, "It's not fun to be old and have to be like this."

As the nurse questions Mrs. Sutton about the specifics of her urinary incontinence, it is learned that this problem has been increasing since shortly after the last clinic visit. Mrs. Sutton states she loses urine every time that she laughs, sneezes, coughs, carries heavy bundles, or even stands up quickly. This happens more when she is tired and when her bladder is full. Some days she skips taking her furosemide pill because it makes the problem worse. The rash is very annoying; it itches and stings at times. Lately her urine has started to burn her when she voids. Because of these symptoms, Mrs. Sutton has curtailed all social activity.

The rest of the physical assessment is normal. Her cognitive ability has not changed and she does not score highly on the depression screening scale. However, her affect is sad, and her enthusiasm for life is missing.

▶ Complete Documentation

The following is sample documentation for Mary Sutton.

SUBJECTIVE DATA: 83-year-old female with no complaints; seen for routine physical assessment. States urinary incontinence and rash for 3 months that is unrelieved by talcum powder, witch hazel, or soap. States incontinence episodes occur with laughing, sneezing, coughing, carrying heavy bundles, or standing up quickly. Reports that she restricts fluid intake after 3 p.m., sometimes withholds furosemide, and has withdrawn from community involvement and confined herself to her home for fear of embarrassment from wetness and odor. Sees the reason for this as "old age." Also states she has recently felt pain on voiding.

OBJECTIVE DATA: Vital signs slightly elevated since last visit 3 months ago. Mucous membranes are pale and dry. All other systems are within normal limits for client except for a red, papular rash on perineum and upper, inner thighs, and strong urine odor on wadded tissues in underpants. Client's cognition is good, and her depression screening is normal. Her affect is sad and her personality more listless than normal for her. Her hair is not "permed" as usual, and her clothes are less colorful than is normal for her. A urinalysis yielded the following abnormal information: hazy, amber urine with a specific gravity of 1.035 that tested positive for bacteria. Other urine values were normal.

▶ Critical Thinking Questions

Clustering the objective and subjective data obtained from the interview will lead to several nursing diagnoses. However, Mrs. Sutton has also given some hints that may require follow-up to obtain additional information.

1. What additional information would help the nurse to plan care for this client?
2. How should information be clustered to guide decision making?
3. What recommendations would you provide for this client?

▶ Applying Nursing Diagnoses

1. *Stress urinary incontinence* is a nursing diagnosis in the NANDA taxonomy. Do the data for Mary Sutton support this diagnosis? If so, identify the data.
2. Another NANDA diagnosis is *impaired social interaction*. Do the data for Mrs. Sutton support this diagnosis? If so, identify the data.

3. Another NANDA diagnosis is *impaired skin integrity*. Do the data for Mrs. Sutton support this diagnosis? If so, identify the data.
4. Use the NANDA taxonomy in Appendix A to develop additional diagnoses for Mrs. Sutton. ∞
5. Identify the data required for the PES (problem, etiology, signs or symptoms) statement.

▶ *Prepare Teaching Plan*

LEARNING NEED: Mary Sutton came to the clinic for a routine physical assessment. She was experiencing stress incontinence, which had caused her embarrassment, fear, sorrow, inflammation, dehydration, possible infection, and social isolation. Mrs. Sutton saw this incontinence as a normal part of aging, causing her to adopt a hopeless attitude and not to seek treatment. Although she initially denied any health problems, her significant problems were found upon genitourinary examination and follow-up questioning. In addition to the incontinence and rash, the issue of Mary's self-ageism must be addressed so that she can learn how to control her stress incontinence, clear up her rash, and once again enjoy her vibrant, outgoing lifestyle.

The case study presents a problem that is all too common among both older women and older men. It is frequently underreported and undertreated due to ageism on the part of both the client and the provider. The following teaching plan on managing stress incontinence can be used for all clients experiencing this problem, but it is directed toward an older woman.

GOAL: The participant will be able to control her incontinence.

OBJECTIVES: Upon completion of this educational session, the participant will be able to:

1. State normal voiding patterns for older adults.
2. Identify causes of stress incontinence.
3. Describe measures to manage stress incontinence.
4. Describe measures to protect skin from incontinence episodes.

APPLICATION OF OBJECTIVE 1: State normal voiding patterns for older adults

Content	Teaching Strategy and Rationale	Evaluation
• Incontinence is not "normal" in older people. • The amount of urine that an older person can store comfortably in his or her bladder is between 200 and 300 ml. • This is less than the 350 to 450 ml held comfortably by younger adults due to thickening of the bladder wall with age, which makes distention more difficult. • The presence of urine in the bladder triggers the neurologic control to void. • Given normal kidney function, the amount of urine produced each hour depends on the amount of fluid taken in. This alters the times between voidings. • Some fluid is lost through sweat, respiration, and bowel movements, so the intake does not exactly match the output. • Medications, such as diuretics, increase the amount of urine produced. • Drinks that contain caffeine or alcohol also increase urine production.	• Lecture • Discussion • Audiovisual materials • Printed materials • Samples of equipment Lecture is appropriate when disseminating information to large groups. Discussion allows participants to bring up concerns and to raise questions. Audiovisual materials, such as illustrations of the structures of the urinary system, reinforce verbal presentation. Printed material, especially to be taken away with learners, allows review, reinforcement, and reading at the learner's own pace.	• Having learners state orally the various points that they have learned is the best way to test their knowledge. This eliminates any problems with reading, writing, or the anxiety caused by a formal test situation. • Some learners in the early stages may not feel comfortable using the vocabulary or discussing out loud a topic area that they still find embarrassing or shameful. For them, written questions may be best.

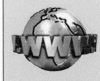

Please refer to the Companion Website at www.prenhall.com/damico and click on **Chapter 27**, the **Application Through Critical Thinking** module, to complete the following activities related to this case study:
▶ **Critical Thinking questions**
▶ **Extended Nursing Diagnosis challenge**
▶ **Documentation activity**
▶ **Teaching Plan for Objectives 2, 3, and 4**

EXPLORE MediaLink

Additional resources for this chapter are found on the Student CD-ROM accompanying this textbook and on the Companion Website.

CD-ROM CONTENT

Content for this chapter includes:
Objectives
Key Concepts
NCLEX-RN® Review Questions
Model Documentation Forms
Audio Glossary
Clinical Spotlight Videos
 Parkinson's Disease
 Alzheimer's Disease
Head-to-Toe Physical Examination Video

COMPANION WEBSITE CONTENT

www.prenhall.com/damico

Content for this chapter includes:
Objectives
NCLEX-RN® Review Questions

Client Interaction Case Study Challenge
Application Through Critical Thinking
 Case Study Teaching Plan Challenge
MediaLinks
MediaLink Application
Tool Box
 Chapter Documentation Form Example
 Health Promotion
  Healthy People 2010
  Client Education
New York Times

2005–2006 NANDA-APPROVED NURSING DIAGNOSES

Activity Intolerance
Activity Intolerance, Risk for
Adaptive Capacity: Intracranial, Decreased
Adjustment, Impaired
Airway Clearance, Ineffective
Anxiety
Anxiety, Death
Aspiration, Risk for
Attachment, Parent/Infant/Child, Risk for Impaired
Body Image, Disturbed
Body Temperature: Imbalanced, Risk for
Bowel Incontinence
Breastfeeding, Effective
Breastfeeding, Ineffective
Breastfeeding, Interrupted
Breathing Pattern, Ineffective
Cardiac Output, Decreased
Caregiver Role Strain
Caregiver Role Strain, Risk for
Communication, Readiness for Enhanced
Communication: Verbal, Impaired
Confusion, Acute
Confusion, Chronic
Constipation
Constipation, Perceived
Constipation, Risk for
Coping: Community, Ineffective
Coping: Community, Readiness for Enhanced
Coping, Defensive
Coping: Family, Compromised
Coping: Family, Disabled
Coping: Family, Readiness for Enhanced
Coping (Individual), Readiness for Enhanced
Coping, Ineffective
Decisional Conflict (Specify)
Denial, Ineffective
Dentition, Impaired
Development: Delayed, Risk for
Diarrhea
Disuse Syndrome, Risk for
Diversional Activity, Deficient
Dysreflexia, Autonomic
Dysreflexia, Autonomic, Risk for
Energy Field Disturbance
Environmental Interpretation Syndrome, Impaired
Failure to Thrive, Adult
Falls, Risk for
Family Processes, Dysfunctional: Alcoholism
Family Processes, Interrupted

Family Processes, Readiness for Enhanced
Fatigue
Fear
Fluid Balance, Readiness for Enhanced
Fluid Volume, Deficient
Fluid Volume, Deficient, Risk for
Fluid Volume, Excess
Fluid Volume, Imbalanced, Risk for
Gas Exchange, Impaired
Grieving, Anticipatory
Grieving, Dysfunctional
Grieving, Risk for Dysfunctional
Growth, Disproportionate, Risk for
Growth and Development, Delayed
Health Maintenance, Ineffective
Health Seeking Behaviors (Specify)
Home Maintenance, Impaired
Hopelessness
Hyperthermia
Hypothermia
Identity: Personal, Disturbed
Infant Behavior, Disorganized
Infant Behavior: Disorganized, Risk for
Infant Behavior: Organized, Readiness for Enhanced
Infant Feeding Pattern, Ineffective
Infection, Risk for
Injury, Risk for
Knowledge, Deficient (Specify)
Knowledge (Specify), Readiness for Enhanced
Latex Allergy Response
Latex Allergy Response, Risk for
Lifestyle, Sedentary
Loneliness, Risk for
Memory, Impaired
Mobility: Bed, Impaired
Mobility: Physical, Impaired
Mobility: Wheelchair, Impaired
Nausea
Neurovascular Dysfunction: Peripheral, Risk for
Noncompliance (Specify)
Nutrition, Imbalanced: Less than Body Requirements
Nutrition, Imbalanced: More than Body Requirements
Nutrition, Imbalanced: More than Body Requirements, Risk for
Nutrition, Readiness for Enhanced
Oral Mucous Membrane, Impaired
Pain, Acute
Pain, Chronic
Parenting, Impaired
Parenting, Readiness for Enhanced
Parenting, Risk for Impaired
Perioperative Positioning Injury, Risk for
Poisoning, Risk for

Post-Trauma Syndrome
Post-Trauma Syndrome, Risk for
Powerlessness
Powerlessness, Risk for
Protection, Ineffective
Rape-Trauma Syndrome
Rape-Trauma Syndrome: Compound Reaction
Rape-Trauma Syndrome: Silent Reaction
Religiosity, Impaired
Religiosity, Readiness for Enhanced
Religiosity, Risk for Impaired
Relocation Stress Syndrome
Relocation Stress Syndrome, Risk for
Role Conflict, Parental
Role Performance, Ineffective
Self-Care Deficit: Bathing/Hygiene
Self-Care Deficit: Dressing/Grooming
Self-Care Deficit: Feeding
Self-Care Deficit: Toileting
Self-Concept, Readiness for Enhanced
Self-Esteem, Chronic Low
Self-Esteem, Risk for Situational Low
Self-Esteem, Situational Low
Self-Mutilation
Self-Mutilation, Risk for
Sensory Perception, Disturbed (Specify: Visual, Auditory,
    Kinesthetic, Gustatory, Tactile, Olfactory)
Sexual Dysfunction
Sexuality Patterns, Ineffective
Skin Integrity, Impaired
Skin Integrity, Risk for Impaired
Sleep Deprivation
Sleep Pattern Disturbed
Sleep, Readiness for Enhanced
Social Interaction, Impaired
Social Isolation
Sorrow, Chronic
Spiritual Distress

Spiritual Distress, Risk for
Spiritual Well-Being, Readiness for Enhanced
Spontaneous Ventilation, Impaired
Sudden Infant Death Syndrome, Risk for
Suffocation, Risk for
Suicide, Risk for
Surgical Recovery, Delayed
Swallowing, Impaired
Therapeutic Regimen Management: Community, Ineffective
Therapeutic Regimen Management, Effective
Therapeutic Regimen Management: Family, Ineffective
Therapeutic Regimen Management, Ineffective
Therapeutic Regimen Management, Readiness for Enhanced
Thermoregulation, Ineffective
Thought Processes, Disturbed
Tissue Integrity, Impaired
Tissue Perfusion, Ineffective (Peripheral)
Tissue Perfusion, Ineffective (Specify: Renal, Cerebral,
    Cardiopulmonary, Gastrointestinal, Peripheral)
Transfer Ability, Impaired
Trauma, Risk for
Unilateral Neglect
Urinary Elimination, Impaired
Urinary Elimination, Readiness for Enhanced
Urinary Incontinence, Functional
Urinary Incontinence, Reflex
Urinary Incontinence, Risk for Urge
Urinary Incontinence, Stress
Urinary Incontinence, Total
Urinary Incontinence, Urge
Urinary Retention
Ventilation, Impaired Spontaneous
Ventilatory Weaning Response, Dysfunctional
Violence: Other-Directed, Risk for
Violence: Self-Directed, Risk for
Walking, Impaired
Wandering

Source: NANDA Nursing Diagnoses: Definitions and Classification, 2005–2006. Philadelphia: North American Nursing Diagnosis Association. Used with permission.

BACKGROUND

Standard Precautions synthesize the major features of UP (Blood and Body Fluid Precautions) (designed to reduce the risk of transmission of bloodborne pathogens) and BSI (designed to reduce the risk of transmission of pathogens from moist body substances) and applies them to all patients receiving care in hospitals, regardless of their diagnosis or presumed infection status. Standard Precautions apply to (1) blood; (2) all body fluids, secretions, and excretions except sweat, regardless of whether or not they contain visible blood; (3) nonintact skin; and (4) mucous membranes. Standard Precautions are designed to reduce the risk of transmission of microorganisms from both recognized and unrecognized sources of infection in hospitals.

STANDARD PRECAUTIONS

Use Standard Precautions, or the equivalent, for the care of all patients.

A. HANDWASHING

1. Wash hands after touching blood, body fluids, secretions, excretions, and contaminated items, whether or not gloves are worn. Wash hands immediately after gloves are removed, between patient contacts, and when otherwise indicated to avoid transfer of microorganisms to other patients or environments. It may be necessary to wash hands between tasks and procedures on the same patient to prevent cross-contamination of different body sites.

2. Use a plain (nonantimicrobial) soap for routine handwashing.

3. Use an antimicrobial agent or a waterless antiseptic agent for specific circumstances (e.g., control of outbreaks or hyperendemic infections), as defined by the infection control program.

B. GLOVES

Wear gloves (clean, nonsterile gloves are adequate) when touching blood, body fluids, secretions, excretions, and contaminated items. Put on clean gloves just before touching mucous membranes and nonintact skin. Change gloves between tasks and procedures on the same patient after contact with material that may contain a high concentration of microorganisms. Remove gloves promptly after use, before touching noncontaminated items and environmental surfaces, and before going to another patient, and wash hands immediately to avoid transfer of microorganisms to other patients or environments.

C. MASK, EYE PROTECTION, FACE SHIELD

Wear a mask and eye protection or a face shield to protect mucous membranes of the eyes, nose, and mouth during procedures and patient-care activities that are likely to generate splashes or sprays of blood, body fluids, secretions, and excretions.

D. GOWN

Wear a gown (a clean, nonsterile gown is adequate) to protect skin and to prevent soiling of clothing during procedures and patient-care activities that are likely to generate splashes or sprays of blood, body fluids, secretions, or excretions. Select a gown that is appropriate for the activity and amount of fluid likely to be encountered. Remove a soiled gown as promptly as possible, and wash hands to avoid transfer of microorganisms to other patients or environments.

E. PATIENT-CARE EQUIPMENT

Handle used patient-care equipment soiled with blood, body fluids, secretions, and excretions in a manner that prevents skin and mucous membrane exposures, contamination of clothing, and transfer of microorganisms to other patients and environments. Ensure that reusable equipment is not used for the care of another patient until it has been cleaned and reprocessed appropriately. Ensure that single-use items are discarded properly.

F. ENVIRONMENTAL CONTROL

Ensure that the hospital has adequate procedures for the routine care, cleaning, and disinfection of environmental surfaces, beds, bedrails, bedside equipment, and other frequently touched surfaces, and ensure that these procedures are being followed.

Category IB

G. LINEN

Handle, transport, and process used linen soiled with blood, body fluids, secretions, and excretions in a manner that prevents skin and mucous membrane exposures and contamination of clothing, and that avoids transfer of microorganisms to other patients and environments.

Category IB

H. OCCUPATIONAL HEALTH AND BLOODBORNE PATHOGENS

1. Take care to prevent injuries when using needles, scalpels, and other sharp instruments or devices; when handling sharp instruments after procedures; when cleaning used instruments; and when disposing of used needles. Never recap

used needles, or otherwise manipulate them using both hands, or use any other technique that involves directing the point of a needle toward any part of the body; rather, use either a one-handed "scoop" technique or a mechanical device designed for holding the needle sheath. Do not remove used needles from disposable syringes by hand, and do not bend, break, or otherwise manipulate used needles by hand. Place used disposable syringes and needles, scalpel blades, and other sharp items in appropriate puncture-resistant containers, which are located as close as practical to the area in which the items were used, and place reusable syringes and needles in a puncture-resistant container for transport to the reprocessing area.

2. Use mouthpieces, resuscitation bags, or other ventilation devices as an alternative to mouth-to-mouth resuscitation methods in areas where the need for resuscitation is predictable.

I. PATIENT PLACEMENT

Place a patient who contaminates the environment or who does not (or cannot be expected to) assist in maintaining appropriate hygiene or environmental control in a private room. If a private room is not available, consult with infection control professionals regarding patient placement or other alternatives.

Source: Excerpted from Guidelines for Isolation Precautions in Hospitals, January 1996. Centers for Disease and Precaution
http://www.cdc.gov/ncidod/hip/ISOLAT/std_prec_ excerpt.htm

STANDARD PRECAUTIONS†,‡

Use Standard Precautions for the care of all patients

AIRBORNE PRECAUTIONS

In addition to Standard Precautions, use Airborne Precautions for patients known or suspected to have serious illnesses transmitted by airborne droplet nuclei. Examples of such illnesses include:

- Measles
- Varicella (including disseminated zoster)†
- Tuberculosis‡

DROPLET PRECAUTIONS

In addition to Standard Precautions, use Droplet Precautions for patients known or suspected to have serious illnesses transmitted by large particle droplets. Examples of such illnesses include:

- Invasive *Haemophilus influenzae* type b disease, including meningitis, pneumonia, epiglottitis, and sepsis
- Invasive *Neisseria meningitidis* disease, including meningitis, pneumonia, and sepsis

Other serious bacterial respiratory infections spread by droplet transmission, including:

- Diphtheria (pharyngeal)
- Mycoplasma pneumonia
- Pertussis
- Pneumonic plague
- Streptococcal (group A) pharyngitis, pneumonia, or scarlet fever in infants and young children

Serious viral infections spread by droplet transmission, including:

- Adenovirus†
- Influenza
- Mumps
- Parvovirus B19
- Rubella

CONTACT PRECAUTIONS

In addition to Standard Precautions, use Contact Precautions for patients known or suspected to have serious illnesses easily transmitted by direct patient contact or by contact with items in the patient's environment. Examples of such illnesses include:

Gastrointestinal, respiratory, skin, or wound infections or colonization with multidrug-resistant bacteria judged by the infection control program, based on current state, regional, or national recommendations, to be of special clinical and epidemiologic significance

Enteric infections with a low infectious dose or prolonged environmental survival, including:

- *Clostridium difficile*
- For diapered or incontinent patients: enterohemorrhagic *Escherichia coli* O157:H7, *Shigella*, hepatitis A, or rotavirus

Respiratory syncytial virus, parainfluenza virus, or enteroviral infections in infants and young children

Skin infections that are highly contagious or that may occur on dry skin, including:

- Diphtheria (cutaneous)
- Herpes simplex virus (neonatal or mucocutaneous)
- Impetigo
- Major (noncontained) abscesses, cellulitis, or decubiti
- Pediculosis
- Scabies
- Staphylococcal furunculosis in infants and young children
- Zoster (disseminated or in the immunocompromised host)†

Viral/hemorrhagic conjunctivitis

- Viral hemorrhagic infections (Ebola, Lassa, or Marburg)

Source: Centers for Disease Control and Prevention Fundamentals of Isolation Precautions, http://www.cdc.gov/ncidod/hip/ISOLAT/ isopart2.htm
† Certain infections require more than one type of precaution.
‡ See CDC *"Guidelines for Preventing the Transmission of Tuberculosis in Health-Care Facilities."* (23)
Contents *These precautions last reviewed and updated by CDC, April 1, 2005.*

Table D.1   **Blood Pressure Levels for Girls by Age and Height Percentile. Use the child's height percentile for the age and sex from a standard growth chart. A blood pressure value at 50th percentile for the child's age, sex, and height percentile is considered the midpoint of the normal range. A reading above the 95th percentile indicates hypertension.**

AGE (YEAR)	BP PERCENTILE	Systolic BP (mmHg) Percentile of Height							Diastolic BP (mmHg) Percentile of Height						
		5TH	10TH	25TH	50TH	75TH	90TH	95TH	5TH	10TH	25TH	50TH	75TH	90TH	95TH
1	90th	97	97	98	100	101	102	103	52	53	53	54	55	55	56
	95th	100	101	102	104	105	106	107	56	57	57	58	59	59	60
2	90th	98	99	100	101	103	104	105	57	58	58	59	60	61	61
	95th	102	103	104	105	107	108	109	61	62	62	63	64	65	65
3	90th	100	100	102	103	104	106	106	61	62	62	63	64	64	65
	95th	104	104	105	107	108	109	110	65	66	66	67	68	68	69
4	90th	101	102	103	104	106	107	108	64	64	65	66	67	67	68
	95th	105	106	107	108	110	111	112	68	68	69	70	71	71	72
5	90th	103	103	105	106	107	109	109	66	67	67	68	69	69	70
	95th	107	107	108	110	111	112	113	70	71	71	72	73	73	74
6	90th	104	105	106	108	109	110	111	68	68	69	70	70	71	72
	95th	108	109	110	111	113	114	115	72	72	73	74	74	75	76
7	90th	106	107	108	109	111	112	113	69	70	70	71	72	72	73
	95th	110	111	112	113	115	116	116	73	74	74	75	76	76	77
8	90th	108	109	110	111	113	114	114	71	71	71	72	73	74	74
	95th	112	112	114	115	116	118	118	75	75	75	76	77	78	78
9	90th	110	110	112	113	114	116	116	72	72	72	73	74	75	75
	95th	114	114	115	117	118	119	120	76	76	76	77	78	79	79
10	90th	112	112	114	115	116	118	118	73	73	73	74	75	76	76
	95th	116	116	117	119	120	121	122	77	77	77	78	79	80	80
11	90th	114	114	116	117	118	119	120	74	74	74	75	76	77	77
	95th	118	118	119	121	122	123	124	78	78	78	79	80	81	81
12	90th	116	116	117	119	120	121	122	75	75	75	76	77	78	78
	95th	119	120	121	123	124	125	126	79	79	79	80	81	82	82
13	90th	117	118	119	121	122	123	124	76	76	76	77	78	79	79
	95th	121	122	123	124	126	127	128	80	80	80	81	82	83	83
14	90th	119	120	121	122	124	125	125	77	77	77	78	79	80	80
	95th	123	123	125	126	127	129	129	81	81	81	82	83	84	84
15	90th	120	121	122	123	125	126	127	78	78	78	79	80	81	81
	95th	124	125	126	127	129	130	131	82	82	82	83	84	85	85
16	90th	121	122	123	124	126	127	128	78	78	79	80	81	81	82
	95th	125	126	127	128	130	131	132	82	82	83	84	85	85	86
17	90th	122	122	123	125	126	127	128	78	79	79	80	81	81	82
	95th	125	126	127	129	130	131	132	82	83	83	84	85	85	86

BP, blood pressure

*The 90th percentile is 1.28 SD, 95th percentile is 1.645 SD, and the 99th percentile is 2.326 SD over the mean.

National Heart, Lung, and Blood Institute. (2004). Blood pressure tables for children and adolescents from the fourth report on the diagnosis, evaluation, and treatment of high blood pressure in children and adolescents. www.nhlbi.nih.gov/guidelines/hypertension/child_tbl.htm, accessed 6/11/2004.

Table E.1 Blood Pressure Levels for Boys by Age and Height Percentile. Use the child's height percentile for the age and sex from a standard growth chart. A blood pressure value at 50th percentile for the child's age, sex, and height percentile is considered the midpoint of the normal range. A reading above the 95th percentile indicates hypertension.

AGE (YEAR)	BP PERCENTILE	Systolic BP (mmHg) Percentile of Height							Diastolic BP (mmHg) Percentile of Height						
		5TH	10TH	25TH	50TH	75TH	90TH	95TH	5TH	10TH	25TH	50TH	75TH	90TH	95TH
1	90th	94	95	97	99	100	102	103	49	50	51	52	53	53	54
	95th	98	99	101	103	104	106	106	54	54	55	56	57	58	58
2	90th	97	99	100	102	104	105	106	54	55	56	57	58	58	59
	95th	101	102	104	106	108	109	110	59	59	60	61	62	63	63
3	90th	100	101	103	105	107	108	109	59	59	60	61	62	63	63
	95th	104	105	107	109	110	112	113	63	63	64	65	66	67	67
4	90th	102	103	105	107	109	110	111	62	63	64	65	66	66	67
	95th	106	107	109	111	112	114	115	66	67	68	69	70	71	71
5	90th	104	105	106	108	110	111	112	65	66	67	68	69	69	70
	95th	108	109	110	112	114	115	116	69	70	71	72	73	74	74
6	90th	105	106	108	110	111	113	113	68	68	69	70	71	72	72
	95th	109	110	112	114	115	117	117	72	72	73	74	75	76	76
7	90th	106	107	109	111	113	114	115	70	70	71	72	73	74	74
	95th	110	111	113	115	117	118	119	74	74	75	76	77	78	78
8	90th	107	109	110	112	114	115	116	71	72	72	73	74	75	76
	95th	111	112	114	116	118	119	120	75	76	77	78	79	79	80
9	90th	109	110	112	114	115	117	118	72	73	74	75	76	76	77
	95th	113	114	116	118	119	121	121	76	77	78	79	80	81	81
10	90th	111	112	114	115	117	119	119	73	73	74	75	76	77	78
	95th	115	116	117	119	121	122	123	77	78	79	80	81	81	82
11	90th	113	114	115	117	119	120	121	74	74	75	76	77	78	78
	95th	117	118	119	121	123	124	125	78	78	79	80	81	82	82
12	90th	115	116	118	120	121	123	123	74	75	75	76	77	78	79
	95th	119	120	122	123	125	127	127	78	79	80	81	82	82	83
13	90th	117	118	120	122	124	125	126	75	75	76	77	78	79	79
	95th	121	122	124	126	128	129	130	79	79	80	81	82	83	83
14	90th	120	121	123	125	126	128	128	75	76	77	78	79	79	80
	95th	124	125	127	128	130	132	132	80	80	81	82	83	84	84
15	90th	122	124	125	127	129	130	131	76	77	78	79	80	80	81
	95th	126	127	129	131	133	134	135	81	81	82	83	84	85	85
16	90th	125	126	128	130	131	133	134	78	78	79	80	81	82	82
	95th	129	130	132	134	135	137	137	82	83	83	84	85	86	87
17	90th	127	128	130	132	134	135	136	80	80	81	82	83	84	84
	95th	131	132	134	136	138	139	140	84	85	86	87	87	88	89

BP, blood pressure

*The 90th percentile is 1.28 SD, 95th percentile is 1.645 SD, and the 99th percentile is 2.326 SD over the mean.

National Heart, Lung, and Blood Institute. (2004). Blood pressure tables for children and adolescents from the fourth report on the diagnosis, evaluation, and treatment of high blood pressure in children and adolescents. www.nhlbi.nih.gov/guidelines/hypertension/child_tbl.htm, accessed 6/11/2004.

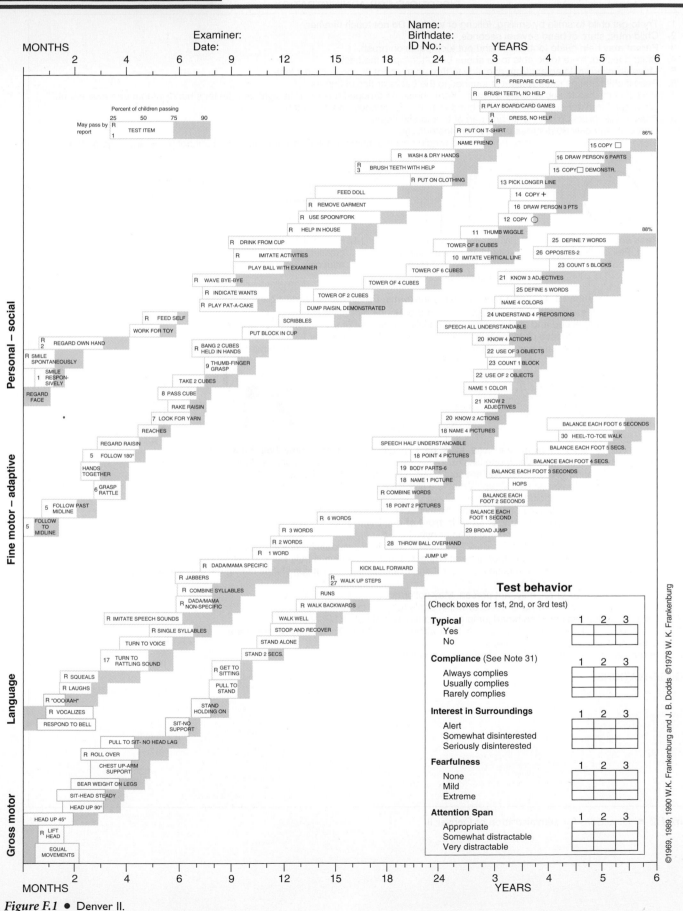

Figure F.1 ● Denver II.

DIRECTIONS FOR ADMINISTRATION

1. Try to get child to smile by smiling, talking or waving. Do not touch him/her.
2. Child must stare at hand several seconds.
3. Parent may help guide toothbrush and put toothpaste on brush.
4. Child does not have to be able to tie shoes or button/zip in the back.
5. Move yarn slowly in an arc from one side to the other, about 8" above child's face.
6. Pass if child grasps rattle when it is touched to the backs or tips of fingers.
7. Pass if child tries to see where yarn went. Yarn should be dropped quickly from sight from tester's hand without arm movement.
8. Child must transfer cube from hand to hand without help of body, mouth, or table.
9. Pass if child picks up raisin with any part of thumb and finger.
10. Line can vary only 30 degrees or less from tester's line.
11. Make a fist with thumb pointing upward and wiggle only the thumb. Pass if child imitates and does not move any fingers other than the thumb.

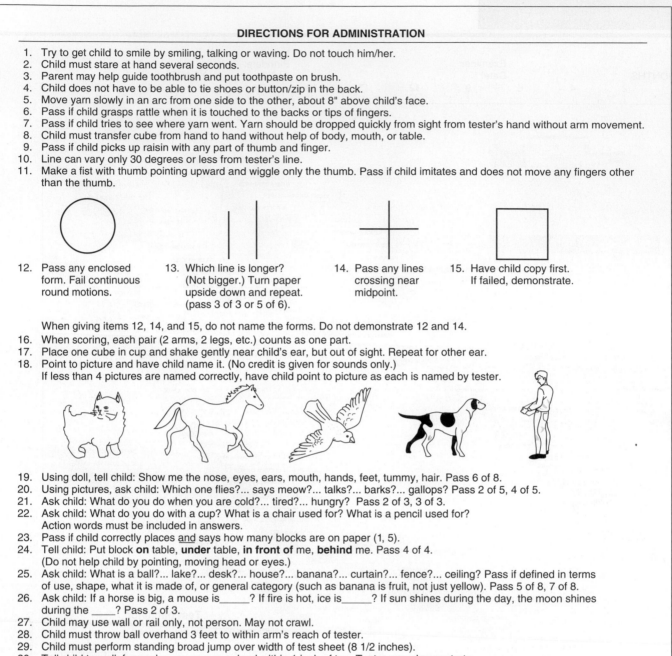

12. Pass any enclosed form. Fail continuous round motions.
13. Which line is longer? (Not bigger.) Turn paper upside down and repeat. (pass 3 of 3 or 5 of 6).
14. Pass any lines crossing near midpoint.
15. Have child copy first. If failed, demonstrate.

When giving items 12, 14, and 15, do not name the forms. Do not demonstrate 12 and 14.

16. When scoring, each pair (2 arms, 2 legs, etc.) counts as one part.
17. Place one cube in cup and shake gently near child's ear, but out of sight. Repeat for other ear.
18. Point to picture and have child name it. (No credit is given for sounds only.)
    If less than 4 pictures are named correctly, have child point to picture as each is named by tester.

19. Using doll, tell child: Show me the nose, eyes, ears, mouth, hands, feet, tummy, hair. Pass 6 of 8.
20. Using pictures, ask child: Which one flies?... says meow?... talks?... barks?... gallops? Pass 2 of 5, 4 of 5.
21. Ask child: What do you do when you are cold?... tired?... hungry? Pass 2 of 3, 3 of 3.
22. Ask child: What do you do with a cup? What is a chair used for? What is a pencil used for?
    Action words must be included in answers.
23. Pass if child correctly places <u>and</u> says how many blocks are on paper (1, 5).
24. Tell child: Put block **on** table, **under** table, **in front of** me, **behind** me. Pass 4 of 4.
    (Do not help child by pointing, moving head or eyes.)
25. Ask child: What is a ball?... lake?... desk?... house?... banana?... curtain?... fence?... ceiling? Pass if defined in terms of use, shape, what it is made of, or general category (such as banana is fruit, not just yellow). Pass 5 of 8, 7 of 8.
26. Ask child: If a horse is big, a mouse is_____? If fire is hot, ice is_____? If sun shines during the day, the moon shines during the _____? Pass 2 of 3.
27. Child may use wall or rail only, not person. May not crawl.
28. Child must throw ball overhand 3 feet to within arm's reach of tester.
29. Child must perform standing broad jump over width of test sheet (8 1/2 inches).
30. Tell child to walk forward, ⬭⬭⬭⬭ → heel within 1 inch of toe. Tester may demonstrate.
    Child must walk 4 consecutive steps.
31. In the second year, half of normal children are non-compliant.

OBSERVATIONS:

Figure F.2 ● Directions for administration of Denver II.

NESTLÉ NUTRITION SERVICES

Nestlé

Mini Nutritional Assessment
MNA®

Last name: _____ First name: _____ Sex: _____ Date: _____

Age: _____ Weight, kg: _____ Height, cm: _____ I.D. Number: _____

Complete the screen by filling in the boxes with the appropriate numbers.
Add the numbers for the screen. If score is 11 or less, continue with the assessment to gain a Malnutrition Indicator Score.

Screening

A Has food intake declined over the past 3 months due to loss of appetite, digestive problems, chewing or swallowing difficulties?
0 = severe loss of appetite
1 = moderate loss of appetite
2 = no loss of appetite ☐

B Weight loss during the last 3 months
0 = weight loss greater than 3 kg (6.6 lbs)
1 = does not know
2 = weight loss between 1 and 3 kg (2.2 and 6.6 lbs)
3 = no weight loss ☐

C Mobility
0 = bed or chair bound
1 = able to get out of bed/chair but does not go out
2 = goes out ☐

D Has suffered psychological stress or acute disease in the past 3 months
0 = yes   2 = no ☐

E Neuropsychological problems
0 = severe dementia or depression
1 = mild dementia
2 = no psychological problems ☐

F Body Mass Index (BMI) (weight in kg) / (height in m)^2
0 = BMI less than 19
1 = BMI 19 to less than 21
2 = BMI 21 to less than 23
3 = BMI 23 or greater ☐

Screening score (subtotal max. 14 points) ☐ ☐
12 points or greater   Normal – not at risk – no need to complete assessment
11 points or below   Possible malnutrition – continue assessment

Assessment

G Lives independently (not in a nursing home or hospital)
0 = no   1 = yes ☐

H Takes more than 3 prescription drugs per day
0 = yes   1 = no ☐

I Pressure sores or skin ulcers
0 = yes   1 = no ☐

J How many full meals does the patient eat daily?
0 = 1 meal
1 = 2 meals
2 = 3 meals ☐

K Selected consumption markers for protein intake
• At least one serving of dairy products (milk, cheese, yogurt) per day?   yes ☐   no ☐
• Two or more servings of legumes or eggs per week?   yes ☐   no ☐
• Meat, fish or poultry every day   yes ☐   no ☐
0.0 = if 0 or 1 yes
0.5 = if 2 yes
1.0 = if 3 yes ☐ . ☐

L Consumes two or more servings of fruits or vegetables per day?
0 = no   1 = yes ☐

M How much fluid (water, juice, coffee, tea, milk...) is consumed per day?
0.0 = less than 3 cups
0.5 = 3 to 5 cups
1.0 = more than 5 cups ☐ . ☐

N Mode of feeding
0 = unable to eat without assistance
1 = self-fed with some difficulty
2 = self-fed without any problem ☐

O Self view of nutritional status
0 = views self as being malnourished
1 = is uncertain of nutritional state
2 = views self as having no nutritional problem ☐

P In comparison with other people of the same age, how does the patient consider his/her health status?
0.0 = not as good
0.5 = does not know
1.0 = as good
2.0 = better ☐ . ☐

Q Mid-arm circumference (MAC) in cm
0.0 = MAC less than 21
0.5 = MAC 21 to 22
1.0 = MAC 22 or greater ☐ . ☐

R Calf circumference (CC) in cm
0 = CC less than 31   1 = CC 31 or greater ☐

Assessment (max. 16 points) ☐ ☐ . ☐

Screening score ☐ ☐

Total Assessment (max. 30 points) ☐ ☐ . ☐

Malnutrition Indicator Score
17 to 23.5 points   at risk of malnutrition ☐
Less than 17 points   malnourished ☐

Ref.: Guigoz Y, Vellas B and Garry PJ. 1994. Mini Nutritional Assessment: A practical assessment tool for grading the nutritional state of elderly patients. *Facts and Research in Gerontology.* Supplement #2:15-59.
Rubenstein LZ, Harker J, Guigoz Y and Vellas B. Comprehensive Geriatric Assessment (CGA) and the MNA: An Overview of CGA, Nutritional Assessment, and Development of a Shortened Version of the MNA. In: "Mini Nutritional Assessment (MNA): Research and Practice in the Elderly". Vellas B, Garry PJ and Guigoz Y, editors. Nestlé Nutrition Workshop Series. Clinical & Performance Programme, vol. 1. Karger, Bâle, in press.

© Sociéte des Produits Nestlé S.A., Vevey, Switzerland, Trademark Owners

Interpreting the MNA® score

The MNA was specifically designed to identify elderly people at risk of malnutrition and guide nutritional intervention in order to improve nutritional status.

MNA score > 23.5	MNA score 17-23.5	MNA score < 17
Satisfactory nutritional status. (see 1)	Malnutrition risk with good prognosis given early intervention. (see 2)	Protein energy malnutrition. (see 3)

1

Repeat MNA every 3 months. Provide guidelines for a balanced diet.

back to top

2

Analyse the MNA results to identify the reasons for the low score.

Perform a detailed diet history / interview.

▲ Does their medication interfere with their food intake?
▲ Do they have difficulty preparing or obtaining their meals?
▲ Does their mental status interfere with their oral intake?
▲ Is their diet unbalanced?
▲ Do they have shin lesions?
▲ Discuss these issues with their physician and / or provide the patient with the appropriate resources or educational information.
▲ Follow up with a repeat MNA in 3 months.

back to top

3

Analyse the score as described above. Perform a dietary interview. Investigate for other causes of malnutrition, e.g. disease states, increased metabolic needs, nutritional intervention must be initiated immediately. Consider use of nutritional supplements to enhance oral diet and or initiation of enteral tube feeding.

back to top

MNA Home Page
▶ Introduction

▼ Clinical practice
User Guide
MNA Forms
MNA Score
Feedback

▲ Research & validation
▲ News
▲ References
▲ Links

Nestlé
NUTRITION

Glossary

abdomen The largest cavity of the body that contains organs and structures belonging to various systems of the body

abduction A movement of a limb away from the midline or median plane of the body, along the frontal plane

accessory digestive organs The structures connected to the alimentary canal by ducts—the liver, gallbladder, and pancreas—that contribute to the digestive process of foods

accommodation The ability of the eye to automatically adjust clear vision from far to near or a variety of distances

acetabulum A rounded cavity on the right and left lateral sides of the pelvic bone

acini cells Glandular tissue in each breast that produce milk

acrochordons (Skin tags) Pedunculated, flesh-colored lesions of collagen and subcutaneous tissue that occur on the neck, back, axillary area, and eyelids

acrocyanosis A normal finding in newborns and infants in which during times of stress, especially exposure to cold environments, the hands and feet appear cyanotic and are often accompanied by increased mottling of the distal arms and legs

acromegaly A disorder caused by overproduction of growth hormone by the pituitary gland. The result may be enlargement of the skull and cranial bones, enlargement of the lower jaw, and enlargement of the lips, tongue, hands, and feet

actinic keratoses Normal aging growths, especially in fair skins, that are considered precancerous;. they appear as calluslike red, yellow, or flesh-colored plaques on exposed areas such as ears, cheeks, lips, nose, upper extremities, or balding scalp

acute pain Pain that lasts only through the expected recovery period from illness, injury, or surgery, whether it has a sudden or slow onset and regardless of the intensity

adduction The movement of a limb toward the body midline

adolescence The period between 11 and 21 years of age

adolescent The transition period from childhood to adulthood, 12 to 19 or 20 years of age

adventitious sounds Added sounds heard during auscultation of the chest. These sounds are superimposed on normal breath sounds and may indicate an underlying airway problems or diseases

aerobic exercise Activity in which oxygen is metabolized to produce energy

air conduction The transmission of sound through the tympanic membrane to the cochlea and auditory nerve

alimentary canal A continuous, hollow, muscular tube, that begins at the mouth and terminates at the anus

Allen's test Test used to determine patency of the radial and ulnar arteries

alopecia areata Sudden patchy or complete loss of body hair for unknown cause. Occurs most often on scalp although it may occur over the entire body

amniotic fluid A clear, slightly yellowish liquid that surrounds the fetus during pregnancy

anabolism A condition that occurs when the intake of protein and calories exceeds the nitrogen loss

anaerobic exercise Activity in which the energy required is provided without using inspired oxygen

analgesia The absence of pain sensation

anesthesia The inability to perceive the sense of touch

angle of Louis Also called the sternal angle. A horizontal ridge formed at the point where the manubrium joins the body of the sternum

angular stomatitis A clinical finding of poor nutrition; cracks at the corner of the mouth

anorexia nervosa A complex psychosocial and physiological problem characterized by a severely restricted intake of nutrients and a low body weight

anosmia The absence of the sense of smell, which may be due to cranial nerve dysfunction, colds, rhinitis, or zinc deficiency, or it may be genetic

anteflexion Abnormal variations of uterine position in which the uterus folded forward at about a 90-degree angle, and the cervix is tilted downward

anterior fontanelle A small diamond-shaped area, also known as a "soft spot," located at the top of the skull where the bones of the skull have not as yet closed. This area protects the brain during birth and allows for skull and brain growth during infancy

anterior triangle A landmark area of the anterior neck bordered by the mandible, the midlline of the neck, and the anterior aspect of the sternocleidomastoid muscles

anteversion Normal uterine position where the uterus is tilted forward, cervix tilted downward

anthropometrics Any scientific measurement of the body

anus The terminal end of the large intestine exiting the body

apocrine glands Glands in the axillary and anogenital regions that are dormant until the onset of puberty, and produce a secretion made up of water, salts, fatty acids, and proteins, which is released into hair follicles

aqueous humor A clear, fluidlike substance found in the anterior segment of the eye that helps maintain ocular pressure

arcus senilis A light gray ring around the outer pupil due to the deposition of lipids

areola A circular pigmented field of wrinkled skin containing the nipple

arterial aneurysm A bulging or dilation caused by a weakness in the wall of an artery

arterial insufficiency Inadequate arterial circulation, usually due to the buildup of fatty plaque or calcification of the arterial wall

arteries Tubular elastic-walled vessels that carry oxygenated blood throughout the body

ascites An abnormal collection of fluid in the peritoneal cavity

assessment The first step of the nursing process. This includes the collection, organization, and validation of subjective and objective data

assimilation The adoption and incorporation of characteristics, customs, and values of the dominant culture by those new to that culture

astigmatism A condition in which the refraction of light is spread over a wide area rather than on a distinct point on the retina

atlas The first cervical vertebra which carries the skull

atopic dermatitis (Eczema) A chronic skin disorder characterized by intense itching, patches, erythema, and papules that typically begins in the first year of life

atrioventricular (AV) node Node, located in the wall of the right atrium, capable of initiating electrical impulses in the event of SA node failure; intricately connected to the bundle of His

atrioventricular valves Valves that separate the atria from the ventricles within the heart

atrophic papillae A clinical finding of poor nutritional health

attending Giving full-time attention to verbal and nonverbal messages

auricle The external portion of the ear

auscultation Using a stethoscope to listen to the sounds produced by the body

axillary tail (Tail of Spence) Breast tissue which extends superiolaterally into the axilla

axis The second cervical vertebra (C_2) which supports the movement of the head

Babinski response The fanning of the toes with the great toe pointing toward the dorsum of the foot; considered an abnormal response in the adult that may indicate upper motor neuron disease

ballottement A palpation technique used to detect fluid or examine floating body structures by using the hand to push against the body

Bartholin's glands (Greater vestibular glands) Glands located posteriorly at the base of the vestibule that produce mucus, which is released into the vestibule and actively promotes sperm motility and viability

Bell's palsy A temporary disorder affecting cranial nerve VII and producing a unilateral facial paralysis

biology Genetic background, gender, race and ethnicity, family history, and problems occurring throughout life

blepharitis The inflammation of the eyelids

blood pressure Pressure caused by waves of blood as it ebbs and flows within the systemic arteries

Blumberg's sign The experience of sharp stabbing pain as the compressed area returns to a noncompressed state

bone conduction The transmission of sound through the bones of the skull to the cochlea and auditory nerve

brain stem Located between the cerebrum and spinal cord, contains the midbrain, pons, and medulla oblongata and connects pathways between the higher and lower structures

Braxton Hicks contractions Painless and unpredictable contractions of the uterus that do not dilate the cervix

bronchial sounds Loud, high-pitched sounds heard in the upper airways and region of the trachea. Expiration is longer in duration than inspiration

bronchophony Auscultation of voice sounds, patient says "ninety-nine" and normal lung sound will be muffled

bronchovesicular sounds Sounds that are medium in loudness and pitch, heard as ausculation moves from the large central airways toward the periphery of the lungs. Inspiration and expiration are equal in duration

bruit A group of heart sounds that elicit a loud blowing sound. This is an abnormal finding, most often associated with a narrowing or stricture of the carotid artery usually associated with atherosclerotic plaque

bulbourethral glands (Cowper's glands) Small, round glands located below the prostate within the urethral sphincter, just before ejaculation, they secrete a clear mucus into the urethra that lubricates the urethra and increases its alkaline environment

bundle branches Expressways of conducting fibers that spread the electrical current through the ventricular myocardial tissue

bundle of His atrioventricular node Nodes that are intricately connected and function to receive the current that has finished spreading throughout the atria

bursae Small, synovial-fluid-filled sacs that protect ligaments from friction

calcaneus A tarsal bone of the foot, also known as the heel bone

calculi Stones that block the urinary tract, usually composed of calcium, struvite, or a combination of magnesium, ammonium, phosphate, and uric acid content in water

capillaries The smallest vessels of the circulatory system that exchange gases and nutrients between the arterial and venous systems

caput succedaneum A condition that is characterized by edema that results from a collection of fluid in the tissue at the top of the skull

cardiac conduction system The heart's conduction system which can initiate an electrical charge and transmit that charge via cardiac muscle fibers throughout the myocardial tissue

cardiac cycle The events of one complete heartbeat, the contraction and relaxation of the atria and ventricles

cardiac output The amount of blood ejected from the left ventricle over 1 minute

cartilaginous joint Bones joined by cartilage

catabolism A condition that occurs when there is a negative nitrogen balance

cataract A condition in which the lens continues to thicken and yellow, forming a dense area that reduces lens clarity resulting in a loss of central vision

central nervous system Nervous system of the body that consists of the brain and the spinal cord

cephalocaudal Head to toe, direction

cephalohematomas Blood collections inside of the skull's periosteum that do not cross suture lines

cerebellum Located below the cerebrum and behind the brainstem, it coordinates stimuli from the cerebral cortex to provide precise timing for skeletal muscle coordination and smooth movements; also assists with maintaining equilibrium and muscle tone

cerebrum The largest portion of the brain, responsible for all conscious behavior

cerumen Yellow-brown wax secreted by glands in the external auditory canal

cervical os The inferior opening; the vaginal end of the canal

cervix Round part of the uterus that projects 2.5 cm into the vagina

Chadwick's sign Vascular congestion that creates a blue-purple blemish or change in cervical coloration

cheilitis Angular stomatitis; inflammation of the lip

cheilosis An abnormal condition of the lips characterized by scaling of the surface and by the formation of fissures in the corners of the mouth

cherry angiomas Vascular lesions, nonsignificant tiny red spots, either macules or papules, rarely larger than 3 to 4 mm, seen usually on the trunk

chloasma A skin condition that develops during pregnancy resulting in hyperpigmented patches on the face. Also referred to as melasma, gravidum, or "the mask of pregnancy"

choanal atresia A congenital defect that results in a thin membrane that obstructs the nasal passages

choroid The middle layer, the vascular-pigmented layer of the eye

chronic pain Pain that is prolonged, usually recurring or persisting over 6 months or longer, and interferes with functioning

circumduction The movement in which the limb describes a cone in space: while the distal end of the limb moves in a circle, the joint itself moves only slightly in the joint cavity

client record A legal document used to plan care, to communicate information between and among healthcare providers, and to monitor quality of care

clitoris The primary organ of sexual stimulation, it is a small, elongated mound of erectile tissue located at the anterior of the vestibule

clonus Rhythmically alternating flexion and extension; confirms upper motor neuron disease

clubbing Flattening of the angle of the nail and enlargement of the tips of the fingers is a sign of oxygen deprivation in the extremities

coarctation of the aorta A congenital cardiac defect in the newborn that results in the narrowing of the aorta with decreased femoral pulses and bounding upper extremity pulses, and causes discrepancies in blood pressure and oxygen saturation between the upper and lower extremities

cochlea A spiraling chamber in the inner ear that contains the receptors for hearing

cognitive theory How people learn to think, reason, and use language

cold sores Vesucykar that occurs on the lip or corner of the mouth. Caused by a herpes simplex virus

colostrum Thick, yellow discharge that may leak from breasts in the month prior to birth in preparation for lactation

coma A prolonged state of unconciousness, with pronounced and persistent changes

communication Exchange of information, feelings, thoughts, and ideas

concreteness Speaking to the client in specific terms rather than in vague generalities

confidentiality Protecting information, sharing only to those directly involved in client care

consensual constriction The simultaneous response of one pupil to the stimuli applied to the other

convergence Movement of the two eyes so that the coordination of an image falls at corresponding points of the two retinas

cornea The clear, transparent part of the sclera that forms the anterior part of the eye, considered to be the window of the eye

cortex The outer portion of each kidney composed of over 1 million nephrons, which form urine

costovertebral angle (CVA) The area on the lower back formed by the vertebral column and the downward curve of the last posterior rib

cranial sutures Palpable gaps between the bones of the skull

craniosynostosis A condition that results in cranial deformity due to premature fusion of the cranial bones

cremasteric reflex A reflexive action that may cause the testicles to migrate upward temporarily; cold hands, a cold room, or the stimulus of touch could cause this response

critical thinking A process of purposeful and creative thinking about resolutions of problems or the development of ways to manage situations.

cryptorchidism The failure of one or both testicles to descend through the inguinal canal during the final stages of fetal development

cues Bits of information that hint at the possibility of a health problem

cultural competence The capacity of nurses or health service delivery systems to effectively understand and plan for the needs of a culturally diverse client or group

culture The nonphysical traits, such as values, beliefs, attitudes, and customs, that are shared by a group of people and passed from one generation to the next

Cushing's syndrome Abnormality where increased adrenal hormone production leads to a rounded "moon" face, ruddy cheeks, prominent jowls, and excess facial hair

cutaneous pain Pain that originates in the skin or subcutaneous tissue

cuticle A fold of epidermal skin along the base of the nail that protects the root and sides of each nail

cystocele A hernia that is formed when the urinary bladder is pushed into the anterior vaginal wall

dandruff White or gray dead scaly skin flakes of epidermal cells

database An electronic storage unit that contains subjective and objective data gathered about a client's medical history and physical examination findings

deep somatic pain Pain that is diffuse and arises from ligaments, tendons, bones, blood vessels, and nerves, which tends to last longer than cutaneous pain

depression For the musculoskeletal system, this is the movement in which the elevated part is moved downward to its original position

dermatome An area of skin innervated by the cutaneous branch of one spinal nerve

dermis A layer of connective tissue that lies just below the epidermis

development An orderly, progressive increase in the complexity of the total person. It involves the continuous, irreversible, complex evolution of intelligence, personality, creativity, sociability, and morality

developmental dysplasia of the hip A congenital disorder that results from inadequate development of the hip socket

diaphoresis Profuse perspiration or sweating that may occur during exertion, fever, pain, and emotional stress and in the presence of some metabolic disorders such as hyperthyroidism

diastasis recti abdominus The rectus abdominis muscles that run vertically down the midline of the abdomen may separate during the third trimester and may allow the abdominal contents to protrude

diastole The phase of ventricular relaxation in which the ventricles relax and are filled as the atria contract. This is also associated with the bottom number of a blood pressure reading

diastolic pressure The lowest arterial blood pressure of the cardiac cycle occuring when the heart is at rest

diet recall A remembrance of all food, beverages, and nutritional supplements or products consumed in a set period of time such as a 24-hour period

dilation Progressive opening of the cervix

diplopia Double vision

dislocation A displacement of the bone from its usual anatomical location in the joint

diversity The state of being different

diverticula A condition caused by continuous overdistention of the bowel and straining to pass stools

documentation The recording of information about a client. This is a legal document used to plan care, to communicate information between and among healthcare providers, and to monitor quality of care.

dorsiflexion Flexion of the ankle so that the superior aspect of the foot moves in an upward direction

Down syndrome A chromosomal defect that causes varying degrees of mental retardation; its prominent facial features include slanted eyes, a flat nasal bridge, a flat nose, a protruding tongue, and a short neck

ductus arteriosus The third shunt in fetal circulation that shunts blood into the descending aorta

ductus venosus A shunt in fetal circulation that enables the fetus to maximize oxygenation from the maternal circulation

dullness A flat percussion tone that is soft and of short duration

dysphagia Difficulty swallowing

dyspnea Shortness of breath or difficulty getting one's breath

dysreflexia An alteration in urinary elimination that affects clients with spinal cord injuries at level T_7 or higher

ecchymosis Bruising resulting from the escape of blood from a ruptured blood vessel into the tissues

eccrine glands Glands which produce a clear perspiration mostly made up of water and salts, which they release into funnel-shaped pores at the skin surface

ectropion The eversion of the lower eyelid caused by muscle weakness

eczema (Atopic dermatitis) A chronic skin disorder characterized by intense itching, patches, erythema, and papules that typically begins in the first year of life

edema An increased accumulation of fluid in a dependent part that is caused by an accumulation of fluid in the intercellular spaces

effacement Thinning of the cervix occuring near the end of pregnancy in preparation for labor

egophony Ausculation of voice sounds; when client says "E," normal lungs sound like "eeeeee"

electrocardiogram (ECG) Electrical representations of the cardiac cycle are documented by deflections on recording paper

elevation Lifting or moving superiorly along a frontal plane

embryo Child during any development stage of pregnancy prior to birth

emmetropia The normal refractive condition of the eye

empathy Understanding, being aware, being sensitive to the feelings, thoughts, and/or experiences of another

encoding The process of formulating a message for transmission to another person

endocardium The innermost layer of the heart, a smooth layer that provides an inner lining for the chambers of the heart

entropion The inversion of the lid and lashes caused by muscle spasm of the eyelid

enuresis Involuntary urination, such as bed-wetting, that occurs after 4 years of age

epicardium   The outer layer of the heart wall that is also called the visceral pericardium

epidermis   The outer layer of skin on the body

epididymis   A comma- or crescent-shaped system of ductules emerging posteriorly from the testis which holds the sperm during maturation.

epididymitis   A common infection in males characterized by a dull, aching pain

epiphyseal plates   Plates located in the ends of the bones

epispadias   A condition in which the urethral meatus is located on the superior aspect of the glans

epitrochlear node   Node located on the medial surface of the arm above the elbow that drains the ulnar surface of the forearm and the third, fourth, and fifth digits

esophagitis   Inflammatory process of the esophagus, caused by a variety of irritants

esophoria   Inward turning of the eye toward the nose

ethnicity   The awareness of belonging to a group in which certain characteristics or aspects such as culture and biology differentiate the members of one group from another

ethnocentrism   The tendency to believe one's way of life, values, beliefs, and customs are superior to those of others

eupnea   The regular, even-depth, rhythmic pattern of inspiration and expiration; normal breathing

eustachian tube   The bony and cartilaginous auditory tube that connects the middle ear with the nasopharynx. This helps to equalize the air pressure on both sides of the tympanic membrane

eversion   A movement in which the sole of the foot is turned laterally

exophoria   Outward turning of the eye

extension   A bending movement around a joint that increases the angle between the bone of the limb at the joint

false reassurance   The client is assured of a positive outcome with no basis for believing in it

fetoscope   A specialized stethoscope for listening to fetal heart sounds, beginning at approximately 18 weeks of gestation

fever blisters   Lesions or blisters on the lips may be caused by the herpes simplex virus

fibrous joint   Bones joined by fibrous tissue

fifth vital sign   The assessment of pain with other vital sign evaluations

flag sign   Dyspigmentation of the mouth or a part of the mouth

flatness   A dull percussion tone that is soft and has a short duration

flexion   A bending movement that decreases the angle of the joint and brings the articulating bones closer together

focused interview   An interview that enables the nurse to clarify points, to obtain missing information, and to follow up on verbal and nonverbal cues identified in the health history

food frequency questionnaire   A questionnaire that assesses intake of a variety of food groups on a daily, weekly, or longer basis

food security   A parameter used in nutritional assessment, free access to adequate and safe food

foramen ovale   The second shunt in fetal circulation prior to birth which connects the fetal right atrium to the fetal left atrium

formal teaching   Organized information sharing that occurs in response to an identified learning need of an individual, group, or community

fracture   A partial or complete break in the continuity of the bone from trauma

fremitus   The palpable vibration on the chest wall when the client speaks

friction rub   A rough, grating sound caused by the rubbing together of organs or an organ rubbing on the peritoneum

functional assessment   An observation to gather data while the client is performing common or routine activities

fundal height   Size of the fundus; after 20 weeks' pregnancy, the weeks of gestation equal the fundal height in centimeters

fundus   The inner back surface of the internal eye

galactorrhea   Lactation not associated with childbearing or breast feeding

general survey   Impressions based on what is seen, heard, or smelled during the initial phase of assessment

genital warts   Raised, moist, cauliflower-shaped papules

genogram   A pictorial representation of family relationships and medical history

genu valgum   Knock knees, a condition of the musculoskeletal system where the knees touch each other but the ankles do not

genu varum   Bowlegs, a condition of the musculoskeletal system where the ankles touch each other but the knees do not

genuineness   The ability to present oneself honestly and spontaneously

gestational age   The age of the fetus, which can be referred to in weeks from the last normal menstrual period

gliding   The simplest type of joint movements. One flat bone surface glides or slips over another similar surface. The bones are merely displaced in relation to one another

glomeruli   Tufts of capillaries in the kidneys

glomerulus   Tufts of capillaries of the kidneys that filter more than one liter (1 L) of fluid each minute

glossitis   Inflammation or redness of the tongue. Often seen in malnutrition

goiter   Enlargement of the thyroid gland that is commonly visible as swelling of the anterior neck. The cause is often lack of iodine intake

Goodell's sign   An increase in cervical vascularity that contributes to the softening of the cervix during pregnancy

growth   Measurable physical change and increase in size; indicators of growth include height, weight, bone size, and dentition

gynecologic age   The difference between one's current age and age at menarche

gynecomastia   Benign temporary breast enlargement in one or both breasts in males

hair   A thin, flexible, elongated fiber composed of dead, keratinized cells that grow out in a columnar fashion

hallux valgus   The great toe is abnormally adducted at the metatarsophalangeal joint

health   A state of complete physical, mental, and social well-being

health assessment   A systematic method of collecting data about a client for the purpose of determining the client's current and ongoing health status, predicting risks to health, and identifying health-promoting activities

health history   Information about the client's health in his or her own words and based on the client's own perceptions. Includes biographical data, perceptions about health, past and present history of illness and injury, family history, a review of systems, and health

health pattern   A set of related traits, habits, or acts that affect a client's health

health promotion   Behavior motivated by the desire to increase well-being and actualize human potential

Healthy People 2010   A report and program sponsored by the United States Department of Health and Human Services, focusing on health promotion of individuals, families, and communities

heart   An intricately designed pump composed of a meticulous network of synchronized structures. The heart is responsible for receiving unoxygenated blood from the body and returning oxygenated blood to the body

heart murmurs   Atypical sounds of the heart often indicating a functional or structural abnormality

Hegar's sign   The softening of the uterus and the region that connects the body of the uterus and cervix that occurs throughout pregnancy

helix   The external large rim of the auricle of the ear

hematuria   Blood in the urine

hemorrhoids   A mass of dilated veins in swollen tissue caused by continuous overdistention of the bowel and straining to pass stools

hepatitis   An inflammatory process of the liver caused by viruses, bacteria, chemicals, or drugs

hernia   A protrusion of an organ or structure through an abnormal opening or weakened area in a body wall

holism   Considering more than the physiological health status of a client, including all factors that impact the client's physical and emotional well-being

Homans' sign   Diagnostic maneuver in which pain may increase with sharp dorsiflexion of the foot

hydrocephalus   The enlargement of the head caused by inadequate drainage of cerebrospinal fluid, resulting in abnormal growth of the skull

hymen   A thin layer of skin within the vagina

hyoid   A bone that is suspended in the neck approximately 2 cm (1 in.) above the larynx

hypalgesia   Decreased pain sensation

hyperalgesia   Excessive sensitivity to pain

hyperesthesia   An increased sensation

hyperextension   A bending of a joint beyond 180 degrees

hyperopia   A condition in which the light rays focus behind the retina. Also called farsightedness

hyperresonance   Abnormally loud auscultatory tone that is low and of long duration

hyperthermia   Body temperature that is greater than expected. Also called a fever, it may be caused by an infection, trauma, surgery, or a malignancy

hyperthyroidism   The excessive production of thyroid hormones, resulting in enlargement of the gland, exophthalmos (bulging eyes), fine hair, weight loss, diarrhea, and other alterations

hypodermis   A cellular layer of subcutaneous tissue consisting of loose connective tissue. Stores approximately half of the body's fat cells, cushions the body against trauma, insulates the body from heat loss, and stores fat for energy

hypospadias   A condition in which the urethral meatus is located on the underside of the glans

hypothermia   Body temperature that is less than expected. This is usually a response to prolonged exposure to cold

hypothyroidism   Metabolic disorder causing enlarged thyroid due to iodine deficiency

immunocompetence   A biochemical assessment laboratory measurement used in nutritional assessment

incontinence   The inability to retain urine; may be classified as functional, reflex, stress, urge, or total

infant   A child from 1 month of age through 11 months of age

infective endocarditis   A condition caused by bacterial infiltration of the lining of the heart's chambers

informal teaching   Occurs as a natural part of a client encounter, may provide instructions, explain a question or procedure, or reduce anxiety

inguinal hernia   When a separation of the abdominal muscle exists, the weak points of these canals afford an area for the protrusion of the intestine into the groin region

innocent murmurs   Heart sounds that arise from increased blood flow across normal heart structures, they are grade I–II/VI in intensity, are systolic (with the exception of the venous hum), and are not associated with thrills or other cardiac symptoms

inspection   The skill of observing the client in a deliberate, systematic manner

interactional skills   Actions that are used during the encoding/decoding process to obtain and disseminate information, develop relationships, and promote understanding of self and others

interdependent relationship   Relationships in which the individual establishes bonds with others based on some single factor such as trust or a common goal

interpretation of findings   Making determinations about all of the data collected in the health assessment process

interview   Subjective data gathering, including the health history and focused interview, including primary and secondary sources

intractable pain   Pain that is highly resistant to relief

introitus   Vaginal opening

inversion   A movement in which the sole of the foot is turned medially or inward

iris   The circular, colored muscular aspect of the eye's middle layer located in the anterior portion of the eye

iritis   The circular, colored muscular aspect of the middle layer of the eye that is located in the anterior portion of the eye

joint   (Articulation) The point where two or more bones in the body meet

keratin   A fibrous protein which gives the epidermis its tough, protective qualities

kidneys   Bean-shaped organs located in the retroperitoneal space on either side of the vertebral column

koilonychia   A clinical finding of poor nutrition; spoon-shaped ridges in the cardia

kyphosis   An exaggerated thoracic dorsal curve that causes asymmetry between the sides of the posterior thorax

labia   A dual set of liplike structures lying on either side of the vagina

labial adhesion   A condition common in preadolescent females which occurs when the labia minora fuse together

lambdoidal sutures   Palpable gaps between the bones of the skull that separate the temporal and occipital bones

landmarks   Thoracic reference points and specific anatomical structures used to help provide an exact location for the assessment findings and an accurate orientation for documentation of findings

lanugo   A fine, downy fine hair in newborns that is most prominent on the upper chest, shoulders, and back

laryngomalacia   Congenital defect of the cartilage in the larynx

leading health indicators   Factors that impact individual and community health and wellness

left atrium   The left atrium of the heart is the chamber that receives oxygnated blood from the pulmonary system.

left ventricle   The left ventricle, the most powerful of all heart chambers, pumps the oxygenated blood outward through the aorta to the periphery of the body

lens   A biconvex (convex on both surfaces), situated directly behind the pupil, is a transparent and flexible structure that separates the anterior and posterior segments of the eye

lentigo senilis   (Liver spots) Patchy pale spots of pigment loss or denser spots of colorlentigo senilis. These skin discolorations due to melanocyte clumping are relatively small in size

Leopold's maneuvers   A special palpation sequence of the abdomen used to determine the position of the fetus after 28 weeks' gestation

leukorrhea   A profuse, nonodorous, nonpainful vaginal discharge that protects against infection

lightening   The descent of the fetal head into the pelvis

linea nigra   A dark line running from the umbilicus to the pubic area; increased pigmentation of the areolae and nipples

listening   Paying undivided attention to what the client says and does

lobule   A small flap of flesh at the inferior end of the auricle of the ear

lordosis   An exaggerated lumbar curve of the spine that compensates for pregnancy, obesity, or other skeletal changes

lunula   A moon-shaped crescent which appears on the nail body over the thickened nail matrix

lymph   Clear fluid that passes from the intercelluar spaces of the body tissue into the lymphatic system

lymph nodes   Rounded lymphoid tissues that are surrounded by connective tissue. Lymph nodes are located along the lymphatic vessels in the body

lymphadenopathy   The enlargement of lymph nodes which is often caused by infection, allergies, or a tumor

lymphatic vessels Vessels that extend from the capillaries. Their purpose is to collect lymph in organs and tissues

macrocephaly Any child whose head circumference is above the 95th percentile; the condition is associated with hydrocephalus, brain tumor, and increased intracranial pressure

macula Appears as a hyperpigmented spot on the temporal aspect of the retina and is responsible for central vision

malnutrition An imbalance, whether a deficit or excess, of the required nutrients of a balanced diet

mammary ridge "Milk line," which extends from each axilla to the groin

mammary soufflé A murmur over the mammary vessel due to increased blood flow, occasionally heard during pregnancy

manual compression test A maneuver to determine the length of varicose veins

manubrium The superior or upper portion of the sternum

mapping The process of dividing the abdomen into quadrants or regions for the purpose of examination

Marfan's syndrome A degenerative disease of the connective tissue, which over time may cause the ascending aorta to either dilate or dissect, leading to abrupt death

mastoiditis Inflammation of the mastoid that may occur secondary to a middle ear or a throat infection

McDonald's rule A method for estimating fetal growth that states that after 20 weeks in pregnancy, the weeks of gestation approximately equal the fundal height in centimeters

mediastinal space The area where the heart sits obliquely within the thoracic cavity between the lungs and above the diaphragm

mediastinum Part of the thorax, or thoracic cavity, that contains the heart, trachea, esophagus, and major blood vessels of the body

medulla The inner portion of the kidney, composed of structures called pyramids and calyces

melanin Skin pigment produced in the melanocytes in the stratum basale

menarche Age of first menstrual period

meninges Three connective tissue membranes that cover, protect, and nourish the central nervous system

metopic sutures Palpable gaps between the bones of the skull that separate the frontal and temporal bones

microcephaly Any child whose head circumference is below the 5th percentile, may be caused by genetic disorders or intrauterine exposure to cocaine or alcohol

middle adulthood The period of a person's life when 40 to 65 years of age

midposition Uterine position which lies parallel to the tailbone, with the cervix pointed straight

milia Harmless skin markings on newborns; areas of tiny white facial papules due to sebum that collects in the openings of hair follicles

Mini-Mental State Examination (MMSE) A screening instrument of cognitive reasoning for detecting dementia and delirium relating to organic disease

miosis Excessive or prolonged constriction of the pupil of the eye

mongolian spots Gray, blue, or purple spots in the sacral and buttocks areas of newborns which fade during the first year of life

Montgomery's glands (tubercles) The sebaceous glands on the areola, which enlarge and produce a secretion that protects and lubricates the nipples

morbilliform "Measleslike" rashes

multigravida A female who has been pregnant two or more times

mucous plug A protective covering of the cervix that develops during pregnancy due to progesterone

muscular dystrophy An X-linked genetic disorder that results in progressive loss of muscle function

mydriasis Excessive or prolonged dilation of the pupil of the eye

myocardium The second, thick, muscular layer of the heart, made up of bundles of cardiac muscle fibers reinforced by a branching network of connective tissue fibers called the fibrous skeleton of the heart

myopia (Nearsightedness) A condition in which the light rays focus in front of the retina

Nägele's rule A formula that can be used to compute the fetus' expected date of birth (EDB) based on the mother's last menstrual period (LMP)

nails Thin plates of keratinized epidermal cells that shield the distal ends of the fingers and toes

nasal polyps Smooth, pale, benign growths found along the turbinates of the nose

neuropathic pain Pain resulting from current or past damage to the peripheral or central nervous system rather than a particular stimulus

newborns Children between birth and 1 month of age

nociception The physiological processes related to pain perception

nociceptors The receptors that transmit pain sensation

nocturia Nighttime urination

nonverbal communication Nonspoken language used to share information and ideas. This may include gestures, facial expressions, and mannerisms that inform others of emotions, feelings, and responses

nuchal rigidity Stiffness of the neck as experienced when the meningeal membranes are irritated or inflamed

nursing diagnosis The second step of the nursing process, whereby the nurse uses critical thinking and applies knowledge from the sciences and other disciplines to analyze and synthesize the data

nursing process A systematic, rational, dynamic, and cyclic process used by the nurse for planning and providing care for the client

nutritional health Using vitamins, foods, nutrients, or herbs to achieve or maintain good health

nystagmus Rapid fluttering or constant involuntary movement of the eyeball

obesity Weight of 20% or more above recommended body weight

objective data Data observed or measured by the professional nurse, also known as overt data or a sign since it is detected by the nurse. This data can be seen, felt, heard, or measured

older adulthood The period of a person's life when over 65 years of age

oliguria Diminished volume of urine

opposition The movement of touching the thumb to the tips of the other fingers of the same hand

optic atrophy Degeneration of the optic nerve resulting in a change in the color of the optic disc and decreased visual acuity

optic disc The creamy yellow area on the retina of the eye where the optic nerve leaves the eye

orchitis Inflammation of the testicles

ossicles Bones of the middle ear: the malleus, the incus, and the stapes

otitis externa Swimmer's ear, infection of the outer ear or ear canal

otitis media Middle ear infections

ovaries Almond-shaped glandular structures that produce ova, as well as estrogen and progesterone

overnutrition Excessive intake or storage of essential nutrients

overweight A weight of 10% to 20% in excess of recommended body weight

oxygen saturation The percentage of oxygen in the blood

pain A highly unpleasant sensation that affects a person's physical health, emotional health, and well-being

pain rating scale Assessment of the intensity of pain using a standardized measurement tool. The tools, which may be numbers, words, or pictures, provide the client the opportunity to describe the degree of discomfort

pain reaction Responses to pain, including the autonomic nervous system and behavioral responses to pain

pain sensation The acknowledgement of pain, often known as pain threshold

pain threshold The point at which the sensation of pain is perceived

pain tolerance The maximum amount and duration of pain that an individual is able to endure without relief

palate The anterior portion of the roof of the mouth formed by bones

palpation The skill of assessing the client through the sense of touch to determine specific characteristics of the body

palpebrae The eyelid

palpebral fissure The opening between the upper and lower eyelids

papilledema Swelling and protrusion of the blind spot of the eye caused by edema

paranasal sinuses Mucous-lined, air-filled cavities that surround the nasal cavity and perform the same air-processing functions of filtration, moistening, and warming

paraphrasing Restating the client's basic message to test whether it was understood

paraurethral glands (Skene's glands) Glands located just posterior to the urethra that open into the urethra and secrete a fluid that lubricates the vaginal vestibule during sexual intercourse

paronychia An inflammation of the cuticle, sometimes caused by infection

peau d'orange "Orange peel" appearance caused by edema from blocked lymphatic drainage in advanced cancer

pediculosis capitis Small parasitic insects that live on the scalp and neck, often called head lice

penis The male organ used for both elimination of urine and ejaculation of sperm during reproduction

percentiles Comparisons of various measurement values used to assess growth rate and healthy weights versus height

percussion "Striking through" a body part with an object, fingers, or reflex hammer, ultimately producing a measurable sound

pericardium A thin sac composed of a fibroserous material that surrounds the heart

perineum The space between the vaginal opening and anal area or between the scrotum and anus

periorbital edema Swelling of the soft tissue in the periorbital area. Often, the swelling is found in the dependent tissue space

peripheral nervous system System of the body that consists of the cranial nerves and spinal nerves

peripheral vascular system Blood vessels of the body that together with the heart and the lymphatic vessels make up the body's circulatory system

peritoneum A thin, double layer of serous membrane in the abdominal cavity

peritonitis A local or generalized inflammatory process of the peritoneal membrane of the abdomen

Peyronie's disease Disease which causes the shaft of the penis to be crooked during an erection

phantom pain Painful sensation experienced in a missing body part (amputation) or paralyzed area

phimosis Condition in which the foreskin of a penis cannot be fully retracted

physical assessment Hands-on examination of the client; components are the survey and examination of systems

physical environment Consists of all the things that are experienced through the individual's senses and some harmful elements such as radiation, ozone, and radon

physiologic anemia Decrease in hemoglobin and hematocrit caused by plasma volume increase outpacing the increase in red blood cells (RBCs)

pica Abnormal craving for or eating of nonfood items such as chalk or dirt

pingueculae Yellowish nodules that are thickened areas of the bulbar conjunctiva caused by prolonged exposure to sun, wind, and dust. They may be on either side of the pupil and cause no problems

pinna The external portion of the ear

Piscacek's sign The irregular shape of the uterus due to the implantation of the ovum

placenta A vascular organ that connects the fetus to the mother prior to birth. Also mediates the exchange nutrients between the mother and fetus one third of the inner surface area of the uterus at term and mediates metabolic exchanges between the fetus and uterus

plantar flexion Extension of the ankle (pointing the toes) away from the body

pleximeter The device that accepts the tap or blow from a hammer

plexor A hammer or tapping finger used to strike an object

positive regard The ability to appreciate and respect another person's worth and dignity with a nonjudgmental attitude

posterior fontanelle A small diamond-shaped "soft spot" on the infant's skull located in the superior occiput which protects the brain during birth and allows for skull and brain growth during infancy

posterior triangle A landmark area of the posterior neck bordered by the trapezius muscle, the sternocleidomastoid muscle, and the clavicle

preinteraction The period before first meeting with the client in which the nurse reviews information and prepares for the initial interview

presbycusis High frequency hearing loss that occurs over time. Often associated with aging

presbyopia Decreased ability of the eye lens to change shape to accommodate for near vision

preschooler A child between 3 and 5 years of age

primary lesions The initial lesion of a disease

primary prevention Interventions that occur to promote health and well-being before a problem occurs

primary source The client is the best source because he can describe personal symptoms, experiences, and factors leading to the current concerns

primigravida A female pregnant for the first time

prolapsed uterus Condition in which the uterus may protrude right at the vaginal wall with straining, or it may hang outside of the vaginal wall without any straining

pronation Movement of the forearm so that the palm faces down, posteriorly or inferiorly

prostate gland Organ that borders the urethra near the lower part of the bladder it lies just anterior to the rectum and is composed of glandular structures that continuously secrete a milky, alkaline solution

protein-calorie malnutrition A nutrient deficiency resulting from undernutrition

protraction A nonangular anterior movement in a transverse plane

pruritis Itching, usually due to dry skin, that may increase with age

psychoanalytic theory Defines the structure of personality as consisting of three parts: the id, the ego, and the superego

psychological distress A mental condition that can be brought about by many factors including loss of spouse and friends through death or illness, loss of occupation or living arrangement due to functional disability, loss of body image, loss of favored recreation, or loss of any other item of significance

psychosocial functioning The way a person thinks, feels, acts, and relates to self and others. It is the ability to cope and tolerate stress, and the capacity for developing a value and belief system

psychosocial health Being mentally, emotionally, socially, and spiritually well

psychosocial theory States that culture and society influence development across the entire life span

pterygium An opacity of the bulbar conjunctiva that can grow over the cornea and block vision

ptosis One eyelid drooping

pulse Wave of pressure felt at various points in the body due to the force of the blood against the walls of the arteries

Purkinje fibers Fibers that fan out and penetrate into the myocardial tissue to spread the current into the tissues themselves

quickening The fluttery initial sensations of fetal movement perceived by the mother

race The identification of an individual or group by shared genetic heritage and biological or physical characteristics

radiating pain Pain perceived at one location that then extends to nearby tissues

rales/crackles Discontinuous sounds which are intermittent, non-musical, and brief

Raynaud's disease A condition in which the arterioles in the fingers develop spasms, causing intermittent skin pallor or cyanosis and then rubor (red color)

rectal prolapse A condition caused by continuous overdistention of the bowel and straining to pass stools, whereby the lower rectal tissue may be forced out of the body through the anus

rectocele A hernia that is formed when the rectum pushes into the posterior vaginal wall

referred pain Pain felt in a part of the body that is considerably removed or distant from the area actually causing the pain

reflecting A communication technique used in letting the client know that the nurse empathizes with the thoughts, feelings, or experiences expressed

reflexes An automatic stimulus-response that involves a nerve impulse passing from a peripheral nerve receptor to the spinal cord and then outward to an effector muscle without passing through the brain. The muscle typically contracts following stimulation of the nerve receptor

resonance A long, low-pitched hollow sound elicited with percussion over the lungs

respiratory cycle Consists of an inspiratory and expiratory phase of breathing

respiratory rate The number of times the individual inhales and exhales during a one-minute period of time

retina The third and innermost membrane, the sensory portion of the eye, a direct extension of the optic nerve

retraction A nonangular posterior movement in a transverse plane

retrobulbar neuritis An inflammatory process of the optic nerve behind the eyeball

retroflexion Abnormal variation of uterine position in which the uterus is folded backward at about a 90-degree angle, cervix tilted upward

retroversion Normal variation of uterine position in which the uterus is tilted backward, cervix tilted upward

rhonchi A range of whistling or snoring sounds heard during auscultation when there is some type of airway obstruction. Types of rhonchi include sibilant wheezes, sonorous rhonchi, and stridor

rickets A clinical finding associated with poor nutritional health resulting in bowed legs

right atrium A thin-walled chamber located above and slightly to the right of the right ventricle that forms the right border of the heart. The right atrium receives unoxygenated blood from the periphery of the body

right ventricle Part of the heart formed triangularly that comprises much of the anterior or sternocostal surface of the heart. The right ventricle pushes unoxygenated blood out to the pulmonary vessels. This is where oxygenation occurs

ripening Softening of the cervix near the end of pregnancy in anticipation of birth

role development The individual's capacity to identify and fulfill the social expectations related to the variety of roles assumed in a lifetime

Romberg's test A test that assesses coordination and equilibrium

rotation The turning movement of a bone around its own long axis

S₁ The first heart sound (lub) is heard when the AV valves close. Closure of these valves occurs when the ventricles have been filled

S₂ The second heart sound (dub) occurs when the aortic and pulmonic valves close, they close when the ventricles have emptied their blood into the aorta and pulmonary arteries

sagittal suture Palpable gap between the bones of the skull that lies in the middle of the skull and crosses the anterior and posterior fontanelles

salmon patches (Stork bites) Small macules and patches caused by visible intradermal capillaries

school age A child between 6 and 10 years old

sclera The outermost layer of the eye, an extremely dense, hard, fibrous membrane that helps to maintain the shape of the eye

scoliosis A lateral curvature of the lumbar or thoracic spine that is more common in children with neuromuscular deficits

scrotum A loosely hanging, pliable, pear-shaped pouch of darkly pigmented skin located behind the penis that houses the testes, which produce sperm

sebaceous glands Oil glands that secrete sebum, an oily secretion, which generally is released into hair follicles

seborrheic keratoses Benign, greasy, wartlike lesions that are yellow-brown in color; they can appear anywhere on the body, but are seen more frequently on the neck, chest, and back

secondary lesions Skin condition or changes to the skin that occurs following a primary lesion

secondary prevention Focus on early diagnosis of health problems, and prompt treatment with the restoration of health

secondary sources A person or record beyond the client that provides additional information about the client

seizures Sudden and rapid physical manifestations (as convulsions or loss of consciousness), resulting from excessive discharges of electrical energy in the brain

self-concept The beliefs and feelings one holds about oneself

semilunar valves Valves that separate the ventricles from the vascular system

seminal vesicles A pair of saclike glands, located between the bladder and rectum, that are the source of 60% of the semen produced

senile purpura A more serious vascular lesion which can occur spontaneously or in response to minimal trauma in the very old client with fragile blood vessels

sinoatrial (SA) node The node located at the junction of the superior vena cava and right atrium that initiates the electrical impulse

sinus arrhythmia (Heart period variability) Presents with heart rate increases during inspiration and decreases during expiration

smegma A white, cheesy sebaceous matter that collects between the glans of the penis and the foreskin

social environment Interactions between individuals and others as well as the institutions in an individual's community, including churches, schools, transportation systems, and protective services

somatic protein Another term for muscle mass or skeletal muscle

spermatic cord A cord composed of fibrous connective tissue; its purpose is to form a protective sheath around the nerves, blood vessels, lymphatic structures, and muscle fibers associated with the scrotum

spermatocele A cyst located in the epididymis

sphygmomanometer An instrument used to measure arterial blood pressure

spinal cord A continuation of the medulla oblongata that has the ability to transmit impulses to and from the brain via the ascending and descending pathways

sprain A stretching or tearing of the capsule or ligament of a joint due to forced movement beyond the joint's normal range

sternum The flat, narrow center bone of the upper anterior chest

strabismus A condition in which the axes of the eyes cannot be directed at the same object

strain A partial muscle tear resulting from overstretching or overuse of the muscle

striae gravidarium   Also known as stretch marks, these pinkish-purplish skin depressions in connective tissue develop in the second half of pregnancy

stress   Perceived or physical response to environmental factors. It is the body's response to thoughts and feelings that may result in a behavioral or physiological response

striae   (stretch marks) A change in connective tissue resulting in silvery, shiny, irregular markings on the skin. Often seen in obesity, pregnancy, and ascites

stroke volume   The amount of blood that is ejected with every heartbeat

subculture   Groups that exist within larger culture. Subcultures are composed of individuals who have a distinct identity based on some characteristic such as occupation, a medical problem, or a specific ethnic heritage

subjective data   Information that the client experiences and communicates to the nurse, known as covert data or symptoms

subluxation   A partial dislocation of the bones in a joint such as the head of the radius which may occur when a child is dangled by his or her hands

summarizing   Tying together the various messages that the client has communicated throughout the interview

supination   Movement of the forearm so that the palm faces up, anteriorly or superiorly

supine hypotension syndrome   (vena cava syndrome) Occurs when pressure from the pregnant uterus compresses the aorta and the inferior vena cava when the female is in the supine position

suspensory ligament   (Cooper's ligaments) Ligaments that extend from the connective tissue layer, through the breast, and attach to the fascia underlying the breast

sutures   Nonmovable joints that connect two bones

syncope   Brief loss of consciousness, usually sudden

synovial joint   Bones separated by a fluid-filled joint cavity

systole   The phase of ventricular contraction in which the ventricles have been filled, then contract to expel blood into the aorta and pulmonary arteries. This is also associated with the top number of a blood pressure reading

systolic pressure   The highest arterial blood pressure during the height of a ventricular contraction; the first number in a blood pressure reading

temperature   The degree of hotness or coldness within the body as measured by a thermometer.

tendon   Tough fibrous bands that attach muscle to bone, or muscle to muscle

teratogen   An agent that causes birth defects, such as a virus, a drug, a chemical, or radiation

terminal hair   Dark, coarse, long hair that appears on eyebrows, the scalp, and the pubic region

tertiary prevention   Activity aimed at restoring the individual to the highest possible level of health and functioning

testes   Two firm, rubbery, olive-shaped structures that manufacture sperm and are thus the primary male sex organs

thalamus   The largest subdivision of the diencephalon, which is the gateway to the cerebral cortex. The location where all input channeled to the cerebral cortex is processed

thelarche   Breast budding, often the first pubertal sign in females

thrill   Soft vibratory sensations assessed by palpation with either the fingertips or palm flattened to the chest

thyroid gland   The largest gland of the endocrine system which is butterfly shaped and is located in the anterior portion of the neck

toddler   Child who is at least 1 year old but who has not yet reached 3 years of age

tophi   Gout-related hard nodules that may appear over the joint

torticollis   A spasm of the sternocleidomastoid muscle on one side of the body, which often results from birth trauma

tracheal sounds   Harsh, high-pitched sounds heard over the trachea when the client inhales and exhales

tracheomalacia   Congenital defect of the cartilage in the trachea

tragus   A small projection on the external ear that is positioned in front of the external audiotory canal

tympanic membrane   Also called the eardrum, this membrane separates the external ear and middle ear

tympany   A loud, high-pitched, drumlike tone of medium duration characteristic of an organ that is filled with air

umbilical hernia   A protrusion at the umbilicus, visible at birth

undernutrition   Insufficient intake or storage of essential nutrients. Also referred to as malnutrition.

ureters   Mucous-lined narrow tubes approximately 25 to 30 cm (10 to 12 in.) in length and 6 to 12 mm (0.25 to 0.5 in.) in diameter whose major function is transporting urine from the kidney to the urinary bladder

urethra   A mucous-lined tube that transports urine from the urinary bladder to the exterior

urethral stricture   Condition indicated by pinpoint appearance of the urinary meatus

urinary retention   A chronic state in which the client cannot empty his or her bladder

uterine tubes   Ducts on either side of the uterus' fundus; also known as fallopian tubes

uterus   A pear-shaped, hollow, muscular organ that is located centrally in the pelvis between the neck of the bladder and the rectal wall

uvula   A fleshy pendulum that hangs from the edge of the soft palate in the back of the mouth. The uvula moves with swallowing, breathing, and phonation

vagina   A long, tubular, muscular canal that extends from the vestibule to the cervix at the inferior end of the uterus, its major function is serving as the female organ of copulation, the birth canal, and the channel for the exit of menstrual flow

varicocele   A varicose enlargement of the veins of the spermatic cord causing a soft compressible mass in the scrotum. This may lead to male infertility

varicosities   Distended and dilated veins that have a diminished blood flow and an increased intravenous pressure

vegan   Dietary choice in which no animal products are consumed

veins   Tubular walled vessels that carry deoxygenated blood from the body periphery back to the heart

vellus hair   Pale, fine, short hair that appears over the entire body except for the lips, nipples, palms of hands, soles of feet, and parts of external genitals

venous insufficiency   Inadequate circulation in the venous system usually due to incompetent valves in deep veins or a blood clot in the veins

verbal communication   Spoken language to share information and ideas

vernix caseosa   A cheesy-white substance that coats the skin surfaces at birth

vesicular sounds   Soft and low-pitched breath sounds heard over the periphery, inspiration is longer than expiration

viability   The point at which the fetus can survive outside the uterus

visceral layer   The inner layer, which lines the surface of the heart

visceral pain   Pain that results from stimulation of pain receptors deep within the body such as the abdominal cavity, cranium, or the thorax

visual field   Refers to the total area of vision in which objects can be seen while the eye remains focused on a central point

vital signs   The systematic measurement of temperature, pulse, respirations, blood pressure, and pain status

vitiligo   A skin condition identified by patchy depigmented skin over various areas of the body

vitreous humor   A refractory medium, a clear gel within the eye that helps maintain the intraocular pressure and the shape of the eye, and transmits light rays through the eye

wellness   A state of life that is balanced, personally satisfying, and characterized by the ability to adapt and to participate in activities that enhance quality of life

wheezes   High-pitched squeaky or sibilant breath sounds, heard on expiration

whispered pectoriloquy   Auscultation of voice sounds, patient whispers "one, two, three," normal lung sounds will be faint, almost indistinguishable

xanthelasma   Soft, yellow plaques on the lids at the inner canthus, which are sometimes associated with high cholesterolemia

xerophthalmia   A clinical finding of poor nutrition, dry mucosa

young adult   The period of a person's life between 20 and 40 years of age

Chapter 1

Alfaro-LeFevre, R. (2003). *Critical thinking and clinical judgment: A practical approach.* Philadelphia: Saunders.

American Nurses Association (ANA). (2004). *Nursing's agenda for health care reform.* Retrieved May 20, 2004, from nursingworld. org/readroom/rnagenda.htm.

Andrews, J. D. (1995-2000). *Cultural, ethnic, and religious reference manual for health care providers. Sample chapter. Jamarda resources.* Retrieved August 2, 2004, from www.jamard-aresources.com/basic.htm.

Bandman, E., & Bandman, B. (1995). *Critical thinking in nursing* (2nd ed.). Norwalk, CT: Appleton & Lange.

Clark, M. J. (2003). *Community health nursing: Caring for populations* (4th ed.). Upper Saddle River, NJ: Prentice Hall.

Common teaching methods. From McCarthy, P. (1992). *Getting the most out of your HIV/AIDS trainings.* East Bay Aids Education Training Center. Retrieved August 2, 2004, from www.hcc.hawaii.edu/intranet/committees/FacDevCom/guidebk/teachtip/comteach.htm.

Coty, E., Davis, J. L., & Angell, L. (2000). *Documentation: The language of nursing.* Upper Saddle River, NJ: Prentice Hall.

Daniels, G. A. (1997). *Nursing process: Nursing diagnosis.* Retrieved April 24, 2004, from www.rsu.edu/faculty/LAndrews/ndx.ppt.

Duke University School of Nursing. NANDA data retrieved April 24, 2004, from www.duke.edu/~goodw010/vocab/NANDA.html.

Harkreader, H., & Hogan, M. (2003). *Fundamentals of nursing: Caring and clinical judgment* (2nd ed.). Philadelphia: Saunders.

Kozier, B., Erb, G., Berman, A., & Snyder, S. (2004). *Fundamentals of nursing: Concepts, process and practice* (7th ed.). Upper Saddle River, NJ: Prentice Hall.

Leavell, H. R., & Clark, E. G. (1965). *Preventive medicine for the doctor in the community.* New York: McGraw-Hill.

Lehne, R. (2004). *Pharmacology for nursing care* (5th ed.). Philadelphia: Saunders.

Leininger, M. M. (Ed.). (1991). *Culture care diversity and universality: A theory of nursing.* New York: National League for Nursing Press.

Lewis, S., Heitkemper, M., & Dirksen, S. (2004). *Medical-surgical nursing: Assessment and management of clinical problems* (6th ed.). St. Louis, MO: Mosby.

Nightingale, F. (1969). *Notes on nursing: What it is and what it is not.* New York: Dover Books. (Original work published 1860.)

Orem, D. E. (1971). *Nursing: Concepts of practice.* Hightstown, NJ: McGraw-Hill.

Pender, N. J., Murdaugh, C. L., & Parsons, M J. (2002). *Health promotion in nursing practice* (4th ed.). Upper Saddle River, NJ: Prentice Hall.

Potter, L., & Martin, C. (2003). *Health literacy fact sheets.* Center for Health Care Strategies. Retrieved August 2, 2004, from www.healthliteracy.com/hlmonth/fact.html.

Potter, P., & Perry, A. (2002). *Basic nursing: Essentials for practice* (5th ed.). St. Louis, MO: Mosby.

Roy, C., & Andrews, H. (1999). *The Roy adaptation model* (2nd ed.). Stamford, CT: Appleton & Lange.

United States Department of Health and Human Services (USDHHS). (2000). *Healthy People 2010: Understanding and improving health.* Retrieved May 2004 from www.health.gov/healthypeople.

United States Preventive Services Task Force. (1996). *Guide to preventive services* (2nd ed.). Introduction. Patient education and counseling for prevention. Washington, DC: U.S. Department of Health and Human Services. Office of Disease Prevention and Health Promotion. Retrieved April 24, 2004, from www.vnh.org/GCP52/toc.htm.

University of New Orleans, Social studies web site. (2004). *150 teaching methods.* Retrieved June 15, 2004, from www.uno.edu/SS/homePages/MethodsIndex. html.

Valanis, B. (1999). *Epidemiology in health care* (3rd ed.). Stamford, CT: Appleton & Lange.

Vanetzian, E. (2001). *Critical thinking: An interactive tool for learning medical-surgical nursing.* Philadelphia: F.A. Davis.

Winninghan, M., & Preusser, B. (2001). *Critical thinking in medical-surgical settings* (2nd ed.). St. Louis, MO: Mosby.

World Health Organization (WHO). (1947). *Constitution of the World Health Organization.* Geneva, Switzerland: Author.

Chapter 2

Ainsworth, B. E., Hasbue, W. L., Teor, A. S., et al. (1993). Compendium of physical activities: Clarification of energy costs of human physical activities. *Medicine and Science in Sports and Exercise, 25*(1), 71–80.

Ainsworth, B. E., Haskell, W. L., Leon, A. S., Jacobs, D. R., Montoye, H. J., Sallis, J. F., & Paffenbarger, R. S. J. (1993). Compendium of physical activities: Classification of energy costs of human physical activities. *Medicine and Science in Sports and Exercise, 25,* 71–80.

Becker, M. H. (Ed.). (1974). *Historical origins of the health belief model. The health belief model and personal health behavior.* Thorofare, NJ: Charles B. Slack.

Bell, A. J., Talbot-Stern, J. K., & Hennessey, A. (2000). Characteristics and outcomes of older patients presenting to the emergency department after a fall: A retrospective analysis. *Medical Journal of Australia, 173*(4), 176–177.

Borg, G. (1998). *Perceived exertion and pain scales.* Champaign, IL: Human Kinetics. Retrieved January 2004 from www.cdc.gov/nccdphp/dnpa/physical/measuring/perceived_exertion.htm.

Center for Disease Control and Prevention. (2005). *Physical activity for everyone: Recommendations.* Retrieved July 15, 2005, from www. cdc.gov.nccdphp/dnpa/physical/recommendation.

Chan, A. W. K., Pristack, E. A., & Welt, J. (1994). Detection by the CAGE of alcoholism or heavy drinking in primary care outpatients and the general population. *Journal of Substance Abuse, 6*(12), 123–135.

Companion web site: Bowles Center for Alcoholic Studies http://www.med.unc.edu/alcohol.

Dunn, H. (1973). *High level wellness.* Arlington, VA: R. W. Beatty, Ltd.

Edelman, C., & Mandel, C. (1998). *Health promotion throughout the life span* (4th ed.). St. Louis, MO: Mosby.

Ewing, J. A. (1984). Detecting alcoholism: The CAGE questionnaire. *JAMA, 252,* 1905–1907.

Fiore, M. (2000). *Treating tobacco dependency. A public service clinical practice guideline.* USDHHS. Retrieved August 2, 2004, from www.surgeongeneral. gov/tobacco/.

Health promotion models [Special issue]. (2000). *International Electronic Journal of Health Education, 3,* 180–193.

Hyner, G. C., Peterson, K. W., Travis, J. W., Dewey, J. E., Foerster, J. J., & Framer, E. M. (Eds.). (1999). *SPM handbook of health assessment tools.* Pittsburgh, PA: The Society of Prospective Medicine & The Institute for Health and Productivity Management.

Kozier, B., Erb, G., Berman, A., & Burke, K. (2004). *Fundamentals of nursing: Concepts, process and practice* (7th ed.). Upper Saddle River, NJ: Prentice Hall.

Leavell, H. C., & Clark, E. G. (1965). *Preventive medicine for the doctor in the community* (3rd ed.). New York: McGraw-Hill.

Mersy, D. J. (2003). Recognition of alcohol and substance abuse. American Family Physician, April 1:67 (&) 1529–32.

Murray, R. B., & Zentner, J. P. (2001). *Health assessment and promotion strategies through the life span.* Upper Saddle River, NJ: Prentice Hall.

National Center for Injury Prevention and Control. (2000). *Falls and hip fractures among older adults.* Retrieved August 2, 2004, from www.cdc.gov/ncipc/factsheets/falls.htm.

National Institute on Drug Abuse. (2002). *Research Report Series—Prescription Drugs: Abuse and Addiction. Trends in prescription drug abuse.* USDHHS. Retrieved August 2, 2004, from www.nida.nih.gov/ResearchReports/Prescription/prescription5.html#Trends.

Pender, N. J., Murdaugh, C. L., & Parsons, M. A. (2002). *Health promotion in nursing practice.* Upper Saddle River, NJ: Prentice Hall.

Rosenstock, I. M. (1974). Historical origins of the health belief model. In M. H. Becker (Ed.), *The health belief model and personal health behavior.* Thorofare, NJ: Charles B. Slack.

Sharp, L. K., & Lipsky, M. S. (2002). Screening for depression across the lifespan: A review of measures for use in primary care settings. *American Family Physician, 66*(2), 1001–1008.

Travis, J., & Ryan, S. (1988). *The wellness workbook* (2nd ed.). Berkeley, CA: Ten Speed Press.

United States Department of Health and Human Services (USDHHS). (2004). *Healthy People 2010: Understanding and improving health.* Retrieved May 2004 from www.health. gov/healthypeople.

Chapter 3

BMI. Retrieved June 2004 from www.nblbi. nih.gov/guidelines/obesity/bmi_tbl.htm.

Bretherton, I. (1992). The origins of attachment theory. *Developmental Psychology, 28,* 759–775.

Clinical growth charts. (2000). Retrieved June 2004 from www.cdc.gov/growthcharts.

Family practice notebook. Retrieved June 2004 from www.fpnotebook.com/PED88.htm.

Kozier, B., Erb, G., Berman, A. J., & Burke, K. (2004). *Fundamentals of nursing: Concepts, process and practice* (7th ed.). Upper Saddle River, NJ: Prentice Hall.

Lutz, C., & Prztulski, K. (2001). *Nutrition and diet therapy* (3rd ed.). Philadelphia: F. A. Davis.

Murray, R. B., & Zentner, J. P. (2000). *Health assessment and promotion strategies, through the life span.* Upper Saddle River, NJ: Prentice Hall.

O'Sullivan, A. L., & Krisman-Scott, M. A. (2001). *Adolescent health.* Retrieved June 2004 from www.nursingworld.org/mods/mod500/ceadabs. htm.

Purnell, L. D., & Paulanka, B. J. (1998). *Transcultural health care: A culturally competent approach.* Philadelphia: F. A. Davis.

Soren, K. (2001). The adolescent years. In *Columbia University College of Physicians and Surgeons home medical guide.* Retrieved June 2004 from www.healthsciences.columbia.edu/texts/guide/toc/toc08.html.

Valdivia, R. (1999). *The implications of culture on developmental delay.* The ERIC Clearinghouse on Disabilities and Gifted Children. Retrieved June 2004 from www.eric.org.

Chapter 4

American Nurses Association. (2003). *Cultural diversity in nursing practice.* Retrieved September 20, 2003, from www.nursingworld. org/readroom/position/ethics/etcldv.htm.

Campina-Bacotte, J. (2003). Many faces: Addressing diversity in health care. *Online Journal of Nursing Issues, 8*(1). Retrieved January 2, 2004, from www.nursingworld.org/ojin/topic20/tpc20_2.htm.

Catalano, J. T. (2000). *Nursing now: Today's issues, tomorrow's trends* (2nd ed.). Philadelphia: F. A. Davis.

Cook, C. (2003). The many faces of diversity: Overview and summary. *Online Journal of Issues in Nursing, 8*(1). Retrieved January 2, 2004 from www.nursingworld.org/ojin/topic20/tpc20ntr.htm.

Diversity Rx. (2003). *Overview of models and strategies for overcoming linguistic and cultural barriers to health care.* Retrieved October 10, 2003, from www.diversity.org.

Kozier, B., Erb, G., Berman, A. J., & Burke, K. (2004). *Fundamentals of nursing. Concepts, process and practice* (7th ed.). Upper Saddle River, NJ: Prentice Hall.

Leininger, M., & McFarland, M. (2002). *Transcultural nursing: Concepts, theories, research and practice* (3rd ed.). New York: McGraw-Hill.

Murray, R. B., & Zentner, J. P. (2001). *Health assessment and promotion strategies through the lifespan.* Upper Saddle River, NJ: Prentice Hall.

Office of Minority Health, CDC, DHHS. (2003a). *About minority health.* Retrieved September 20, 2003, from www.cdc.gov/omh/AMH/AMH.htm

Office of Minority Health, CDC, DHHS. (2003b). *Cultural competence.* Retrieved October 10, 2003, from www.omhrc.gov/cultural/index. htm.

Office of Minority Health, CDC, DHHS. (2003c). *Definitions of racial and ethnic populations.* Retrieved www.cdc.gov/omh/Populations/definitions.htm.

Purnell, L. D., & Paulanka, B. J. (1998). *Transcultural health care: A culturally competent approach.* Philadelphia: F. A. Davis.

Spector, R. E. (2004). *Cultural diversity in health and illness* (6th ed.). Upper Saddle River, NJ: Prentice Hall.

U.S. Census Bureau. (2000). U.S. Census Report. Retrieved August 2, 2004, from www.census.gov/.

U.S. Department of Health and Human Services, OPHS, Office of Minority Health. (2001). *National standards for culturally and linguistically appropriate services in health care. Final report.* Retrieved Sept. 2003 from www.omhrc.gov/cultural/cultural4.htm.

Chapter 5

American Academy of Family Physicians. (2004). *Mind/body connection: How your emotions affect your health.* Retrieved April 1, 2004, from http://Familydoctor.org/Familydoctor.org/782.xml.

Anadarajah, G., & Hight, E. (2000). *Spirituality and medical practice: Using the HOPE questions as a practical tool for spiritual assessment.* Retrieved www.aafp.org/.

Clark, M. (2003). *Community health nursing: Caring for populations* (4th ed.). Upper Saddle River, NJ: Prentice Hall.

Donatelle, R. J. (2006). *Health: The basics* (6th ed.). San Francisco, CA: Benjamin/Cummings.

Ellison, C. W., & Paloutzian, R. F. (1982). *The spiritual well being scale.* Life Advance, Inc. Retrieved August 2, 2004, from www.lifeadvance.com/applications.htm.

Hodge, D. R. (2001). Spiritual assessment: A review of major qualitative methods and a new framework for assessing spirituality. *Social Work, 46*(3), 8037–8046.

International Council of Nurses. (2005). Fact sheet genetics and nursing. Retrieved July 17, 2005, from www.icn.ch/matters_genetics. htm.

Joint Commission on Accreditation of Healthcare Organizations. (2004). *Spiritual assessment.* Retrieved August 2, 2004, from www. jcaho.org/accredited+organizations/hospitals/standards/hospital+faqs/provision+of+care/assessment/spiritual+assessment.htm.

Kozier, B., Erb, G., Berman, A., & Burke, K. (2004). *Fundamentals of nursing: Concepts, process and practice* (7th ed.). Upper Saddle River, NJ: Prentice Hall.

Life Advance. (1982). *The spiritual well-being scale.* Retrieved December 22, 2003, from www. lifeadvance.com/applications.htm.

QOLID Quality of Life Instruments Database. (2004). *List of generic instruments.* Retrieved February 13, 2005, from www.qolid. org/general/htm.

McDowell, I., & Newell, C. (1996). *Measuring health: A guide to rating scales and questionnaires* (2nd ed.). New York: Oxford University Press.

McSherry, W., & Ross, L. (2001). Dilemmas of spiritual assessment: Considerations for nursing practice. *Journal of Advanced Nursing, 38*(5), 479–488.

Murray, R. B., & Zentner, J. P. (2000). *Health assessment and promotion strategies through the life span* (7th ed.). Upper Saddle River, NJ: Prentice Hall.

President's Council on Physical Fitness and Sports. (2003). *Fitness Fundamentals: Guidelines for Personal Exercise Programs.* Washington DC.

Roy, C., & Andrews, H. (1999). *The Roy adaptation model* (2nd ed.). Stamford, CT: Appleton & Lange.

Stoll, R. I. (1979). Guidelines for spiritual assessment. *American Journal of Nursing, 79*(9), 1574–1577.

Taylor, E. J. (2002). *Spiritual care: Nursing theory, research, and practice.* Upper Saddle River, NJ: Prentice Hall.

United States Department of Health and Human Services. *CDC Core Healthy Day Measures.* Centers for Disease Control and Prevention. National Center for Chronic Diseases Prevention and Health Promotion. Retrieved October 6, 2005, from www.cdc.gov/hrqo/hrqo/14_measures.htm.

Chapter 6

Barbarito, C., & D'Amico, D. (2000). *Comprehensive health assessment: A student workbook.* Dubuque, IA: Kendall/Hunt Publishing.

Kozier, B., Erb, G., Berman, A. J., & Burke, K. (2004). *Fundamentals of nursing: Concepts, process and practice* (7th ed.). Upper Saddle River, NJ: Prentice Hall.

Lewis, S., Heitkemper, M., & Dirksen, S. (2004). *Medical-surgical nursing: Assessment and management of clinical problems* (6th ed.). St. Louis, MO: Mosby.

National Institute for Occupational Safety and Health (NIOSH). (1998). *Preventing allergic reactions to natural rubber latex in the workplace.* Retrieved April 20, 2004, from www.cdc.gov/niosh/latexalt.html.

United States Department of Health and Human Services (USDHHS). (1999). *Latex allergy: A prevention guide.* Retrieved April 20, 2004, from www.cdc. gov/niosh/98-113.html.

Wilson, S., & Giddens, J. (2001). *Health assessment for nursing practice* (2nd ed.). St. Louis, MO: Mosby.

Winninghan, M., & Preusser, B. (2001). *Critical thinking in medical-surgical settings* (2nd ed.). St. Louis, MO: Mosby.

Chapter 7

Craven, R., & Hirnle, C. (2002). *Fundamentals of nursing: Human health and function* (4th ed.). Philadelphia: Lippincott, Williams & Wilkins.

Environmental Protection Agency. (2004). *Frequently asked questions about mercury fever thermometers.* Retrieved February 21, 2004, from www.epa.gov/glnpo/bnsdocs/hg/thermfaq. html.

Harkreader, H., & Hogan, M. (2003). *Fundamentals of nursing: Caring and clinical judgment* (2nd ed.). Philadelphia: W. B. Saunders.

Kozier, B., Erb, G., Berman, A. J., & Burke, K. (2004). *Fundamentals of nursing: Concepts, process, and practice* (7th ed.). Upper Saddle River, NJ: Prentice Hall.

Lewis, S., Heitkemper, M., & Dirksen, S. (2004). *Medical-surgical nursing: Assessment and management of clinical problems* (6th ed.). St. Louis, MO: Mosby.

Medical Indicators, Inc. (2004). *How to use NexTemp single-use, disposable thermometers.* Retrieved February 2, 2004, from www.medicalindicators. com/html/NTHowto.html.

MedWay Interactive Educational Services. SSB Healthcare Division. (2004). *Pulse oximetry and the oxyhemoglobin dissociation curve.* Retrieved April 10, 2004, from www.continuingeducation.com/nursing/pulseox/pulseox. pdf.

Murray, R. B., & Zentner, J. P. (2000). *Health assessment and promotion strategies, through the life span.* Upper Saddle River, NJ: Prentice Hall.

Potter, P., & Perry, A. (2001). *Fundamentals of nursing* (5th ed.). St. Louis, MO: Mosby.

Smith, S. F., & Duell, D. (2004). *Clinical nursing skills* (6th ed.). Upper Saddle River, NJ: Prentice Hall.

Chapter 8

Acello, B. (2000). Meeting JCAHO standards for pain control. *Nursing, 30*(3), 52–54.

American Academy of Pediatrics and the Canadian Paediatric Society. (2000). Prevention and management of pain and stress in the neonate. *Pediatrics, 105*(2), 454–461.

American Pain Society. (1999). *Principles of analgesic use in the treatment of acute pain and cancer pain* (4th ed.). Glenview, IL: Author.

Andrews, M. M., & Boyle, J. S. (2003). *Transcultural concepts in nursing care* (4th ed.). Philadelphia: Lippincott Williams & Wilkins.

Ball, J. W., & Bindler, R. C. (2003). *Pediatric nursing: Caring for children* (3rd ed.). Upper Saddle River, NJ: Prentice Hall.

Bergh, I., & Sjostrom, B. (1999). A comparative study of nurses' and elderly patients' ratings of pain and pain tolerance. *Journal of Gerontological Nursing, 25*(5), 30–36.

Bieri, D., Reeve, R., Champion, G., Addicoat, L., & Ziegler, J. B. (1990). The Faces Pain Scale for the assessment of the severity of pain experienced by children: Development, initial validation, and preliminary investigation for ratio scale properties. *Pain, 41*, 139–150.

Cox, F. (2001). Clinical care of patients with epidural infusions. *Professional Nurse, 16*, 1429–1432.

Eliopoulos, C. (2005). *Gerontological nursing* (6th ed.). Philadelphia: Lippincott.

Hawthorn, J., & Redmond, K. (1998). *Pain causes and management.* Oxford, England: Blackwell Science.

Herr, K. (2002). Chronic pain in the older patient: Management strategies. *Journal of Gerontological Nursing, 28*(2), 28–34.

Hockenberry-Eaton, M., Barrere, P., Brown, M., Bottomly, S. J., & O'Neill, J. B. (1999). *Cancer pain management in children.* Houston, TX: Baylor College of Medicine. Retrieved July 30, 2004, from www.childcancerpain.org/content.cfm?content=assess01.

Johnson, M., Maas, M., & Moorhead, S. (Eds.). (2000). *Nursing outcomes classification* (2nd ed.). St. Louis, MO: Mosby.

LaDuke, S. (2002). Undertreated pain: Could it land you in court? *Nursing, 32*(9), 18.

Life's End Institute: Missoula Demonstration Project. (1998–2003). *Pain assessment scale.* Missoula, MT: Life's End Institute. Retrieved July 30, 2004, from www.lifes-end.org/pain_scale.phtml.

McCaffery, M., Ferrell, B. R., & Pasero, C. (2000). Nurses' personal opinions about patients' pain and their effect on recorded assessments and titration of opioid doses. *Pain Management Nursing, 1*(3), 79–87.

McCaffery, M., & Pasero, C. (1999). *Pain: Clinical manual* (2nd ed.). St. Louis, MO: Mosby.

McCloskey, J. C., & Bulechek, G. M. (Eds.). (2000). *Nursing interventions classification* (3rd ed.). St. Louis, MO: Mosby.

Melzack, R., & Wall, P. D. (1965). Pain mechanisms: A new theory. *Science, 150*, 971–979.

North American Nursing Diagnosis Association (NANDA) International. (2003). *NANDA nursing diagnoses: Definitions and classification 2003–2004.* Philadelphia: Author.

Paice, J. A. (2002). Controlling pain. Understanding nociceptive pain. *Nursing, 32*(3), 74–75.

Partners Against Pain. (2004). *Eighteen multilanguage pain scales.* Stanford, CT: Purdue Pharma L. P. Retrieved July 30, 2004, from www.partnersagainstpain.com/index-pc.aspx?sid=12&aid=7692.

Pasero, C. (2000). Continuous local anesthetics. *American Journal of Nursing, 100*(8), 22–23.

Pasero, C., & McCaffery, M. (2002). Pain control: Monitoring sedation. *American Journal of Nursing, 102*(2), 67–68.

Puntillo, K. A., White, C., Morris, A. B., Perdue, S. T., Stanik-Hutt, J., Thompson, C. L., et al. (2001). Patients' perceptions and responses to procedural pain: Results from Thunder Project II. *American Journal of Critical Care, 10*, 238–251.

Rhiner, M., & Kedziera, P. (1999). Managing breakthrough pain: A new approach. *American Journal of Nursing, 99*(3), Supplement 3–12.

Taylor, L. J., & Herr, K. (2002). Evaluation of the Faces Pain Scale with minority older adults. *Journal of Gerontological Nursing, 27*(4), 15–23.

Tucker, K. L. (2001). Deceptive placebo administration. *American Journal of Nursing, 101*(8), 55–56.

U.S. Department of Health and Human Services. (1992). *Clinical practice guidelines: Acute pain management in adults: Operative procedures: Quick reference guide for clinicians* (Publication No. 92–0019). Rockville, MD: Public Health Service Agency for Health Care Policy and Research.

Wong, D. L., Hockenberry-Eaton, M., Wilson, D., Winkelstein, M. L., & Schwartz, P. (2001). *Essentials of pediatric nursing* (6th ed.). St. Louis, MO: Mosby.

Chapter 9

American Diabetes Association. (2002). Position statement: Gestational diabetes mellitus. *Diabetes Care, 24*, S77-S79.

American Medical Directors Association (AMDA). (2001). *Altered nutritional status: Clinical practice guideline.* Author.

Beck, F. K., & Rosenthal, T. C. (2002). Prealbumin: A marker for nutritional evaluation. *American Family Physician, 65*, 1575-1578.

Bianco, A. T., Smilen, S. W., Davis, Y., Lopez, S., Lapinski, R., & Lockwood, C. J. (1998). Pregnancy outcome and weight gain recommendations for the morbidly obese woman. *Obstetrics and Gynecology, 91*, 97-102.

Bracken, M. B., Triche, E. W., Belanger, K., Hellenbrand, K., & Leaderer, B. P. (2003). Association of maternal caffeine consumption with decrements in fetal growth. *American Journal of Epidemiology, 157*, 456-466.

Brenner, N. D., McManus, T., Galuska, D. A., Lowry, R., & Wechsler, H. (2003). Reliability and validity of self-reported height and weight among high school students. *Journal of Adolescent Health, 32*, 281-287.

Brown, J. K., Feng, J., & Knapp, T. R. (2002). Is self-reported height or arm span a more accurate alternative measure of height? *Clinical Nursing Research, 11,* 417-432.

Calle, E. E., Thun, M. J., Petrelli, J. M., Rodriguez, C., & Heath, C. W. (1999). Body-mass index and mortality in a prospective cohort of U.S. adults. *New England Journal of Medicine, 341,* 1097-1105.

Census Bureau Reports. (2003). *Poverty, income see slight changes, child poverty rate unchanged.* Retrieved October 14, 2003, from www.census.gov/Press-Release/www/2003/cb03-153.html.

Centers for Disease Control (CDC). (1998). Recommendations to prevent and control iron deficiency in the United States. *Morbidity and Mortality Weekly Review, 47,* RR-3.

Centers for Disease Control, National Center for Health Statistics. (2000). *Anthropometry procedures manual.* Retrieved October 30, 2003, from www.cdc.gov/nchs/data/nhanes/bm.pdf.

Centers for Disease Control, National Center for Health Statistics. *Health, United States, 2003.* Retrieved November 4, 2003, from www.cdc.gov/nchs/hus.htm.

Centers for Medicare and Medicaid Services (CMS). (2000). *Minimum data set manual* (version 2.0). Retrieved October 16, 2003, from www.cms.hhs.gov/medicaid/mds20/mds0900b.pdf.

Chumlea, W. C., Roche, A. F., & Mukherjee, D. (1984). *Nutritional assessment of the elderly through anthropometry.* Columbus, OH: Ross Laboratories.

Council on Practice Quality Management/American Dietetic Association. (1994). ADA's definitions for nutrition screening and nutrition assessment. *Journal of the American Dietetic Association, 94,* 838-839.

Covinsky, K. E. (2002). Malnutrition and bad outcomes. *Journal of General Internal Medicine, 17,* 956-957.

Covinsky, K. E., Covinsky, M. H., Palmer, R. M., & Sehgal, A. R. (2002). Serum albumin concentration and clinical assessments of nutritional status in hospitalized older people: Different sides of different coins? *Journal of the American Geriatric Society, 50,* 631-637.

Crogan, N. L., Corbett, C. F., & Short, R. A. (2002). The minimum data set: Predicting malnutrition in newly admitted nursing home residents. *Clinical Nursing Research, 11,* 341-353.

Dennison, B. A., Rockwell, H. L., & Baker, S. L. (1997). Excess fruit juice consumption by preschool-aged children is associated with short stature and obesity. *Pediatrics, 99,* 15-22.

DeOnis, M. (2000). Measuring nutrition status in relation to mortality. *Bulletin of the World Health Organization, 78,* 1271-1275.

Deurenberg, P., Deurenberg-Yap, M., & Guricci, S. (2002). Asians are different from Caucasians and from each other in their body mass index/body fat percent relationship. *Obesity Reviews, 3,* 141-146.

Dietz, W. H., & Bellizzi, M. C. (1999). Introduction: The use of body mass index to assess obesity in children. *American Journal of Clinical Nutrition, 70* (S), 123S-125S.

Edwards, L. E., Hellerstedt, W. L., Alton, I. R., Story, M., & Himes, J. H. (1996). Pregnancy complications and birth outcomes in obese and normal-weight women: Effects of gestational weight change. *Obstetrics and Gynecology, 87,* 389-394.

Franko, D. L., & Spurrell, E. B. (2000). Detection and management of eating disorders during pregnancy. *Obstetrics and Gynecology, 95,* 942-946.

Fryzek, J. P., Lipworth, L., Signorello, L. B., & McLaughlin, J. K. (2002). The reliability of dietary data for self- and next-of-kin respondents. *Annals of Epidemiology, 12,* 278-283.

Gallagher, D., Heymsfield, S. B., Heo, M., Jebb, S. A., Murgatroyd, P., & Sakamoto, Y. (2000). Healthy percentage body fat ranges: An approach for developing guidelines based on body mass index. *American Journal of Clinical Nutrition, 72,* 694-701.

Gans, K. M., Ross, E., Barner, C. W., Wylie-Rosett, J., McMurray, J., & Eaton, C. (2003). REAP and WAVE: New tools to rapidly assess/discuss nutrition with clients. *Journal of Nutrition, 133,* 556S-562S.

Gilbody, S. M., Kirk, S. F. L., & Hill, A. J. (1999). Vegetarianism in young women: Another means of weight control? *International Journal of Eating Disorders, 26,* 87-90.

Grindel, C. G., & Costello, M. C. (1996). Nutrition screening: An essential assessment parameter. *Medsurg Nursing, 5,* 145-156.

Hu, P., Seeman, T., Harris, T. B., & Reuben, D. B. (2003). Does inflammation or undernutrition explain the low cholesterol-mortality association in high-functioning older persons? MacArthur studies of successful aging. *Journal of the American Geriatric Society, 51,* 80-84.

Huffman, G. B. (2002). Evaluating and treating unintentional weight loss in the elderly. *American Family Physician, 65,* 640-650.

Institute of Medicine. (1990). *Nutrition during pregnancy: Part I: weight gain.* Washington, DC: National Academy Press.

Jeejeebhoy, K. N. (2000). Nutritional assessment. *Nutrition, 16,* 585-590.

Kristal, A. R., Andrilla, H. A., Koepsell, T. D., Diehr, P. H., & Cheadle, A. (1998). Dietary assessment instruments are susceptible to intervention-associated response set bias. *Journal of the American Dietetic Association, 98,* 40-43.

Kubena, K. S. (2000). Accuracy in dietary assessment: On the road to good science. *Journal of the American Dietetic Association, 100,* 775-776.

Kuczmarski, M. F., Kuczmarski, R. J., & Najjar, M. (2001). Effects of age on validity of self-reported height, weight, and body mass index: Findings from the third National Health and Nutrition Examination Survey 1988-1994. *Journal of the American Dietetic Association, 101,* 28-34.

Lean, M. J., & Han, T. S. (2002). Waist worries. *American Journal of Clinical Nutrition, 76,* 699-700.

Luke, B., & Leurgans, S. (1996). Maternal weight gains in ideal twin outcomes. *Journal of the American Dietetic Association, 96,* 178-181.

Lyne, P. A., & Prowse, M. A. (1999). Methodological issues in the development and use of instruments to assess client nutritional status or the level of risk of nutritional compromise. *Journal of Advanced Nursing, 30,* 835-842.

McGee, S., Abernethy, W. B., & Simel, D. L. (1999). Is this client hypovolemic? *Journal of the American Medical Association, 281,* 1022-1029.

Mini Nutrition Assessment. *Tool and information on usage.* Retrieved June 26, 2005, from www.mna-elderly.com.

Must, A., Spadano, J., Coakley, E. H., Field, A. E., Colditz, G., & Dietz, W. H. (1999). The disease burden associated with overweight and obesity. *Journal of the American Medical Association, 282,* 1523-1529.

Nawaz, H., Chan, W., Abdulrahman, M., Larson, D., & Katz, D. L. (2001). Self-reported weight and height: Implications for obesity research. *American Journal of Preventative Medicine, 20,* 294-298.

NHLBI Obesity Education Initiative Expert Panel. *Clinical guidelines on the identification, evaluation, and treatment of overweight and obesity in adults—the evidence report.* Retrieved November 4, 2003, from www.nhlbi.nih.gov/guidelines/obesity/ob_home.htm.

Novotny, J. A., Rumpler, W. V., Riddick, H., Hebert, H., Rhodes, D., Judd, J. T., et al. (2003). Personality characteristics as predictors of underreporting of energy intake on a 24-hour dietary recall interview. *Journal of the American Dietetic Association, 102,* 1146-1151.

Nutrition Screening Initiative. *Tool and information on usage.* Retrieved October 13, 2003, from www.aafp.org/nsi.xml.

Omran, M. L., & Morley, J. E. (2000). Assessment of protein-energy malnutrition in older persons, Part II: Laboratory evaluation. *Nutrition, 16,* 131-140.

Osterkamp, L. K. (1995). Current perspective on assessment of human body proportions of relevance to amputees. *Journal of the American Dietetic Association, 95,* 215-218.

Persson, M. D., Brismar, K. E., Katzarski, K. S., Nordenstrom, J., & Cederholm, T. E. (2002). Nutritional status using mini nutritional assessment and subjective global assessment predict mortality in geriatric clients. *Journal of the American Geriatric Society, 50,* 1996-2002.

Position of the American Dietetic Association and Dietitians of Canada: Vegetarian diets. (2003). *Journal of the American Dietetic Association, 103,* 748-765.

Position of the American Dietetic Association: Liberalized diets for older adults in long-term care. (2002). *Journal of the American Dietetic Association, 102,* 201-204.

Position of the American Dietetic Association: Nutrition and lifestyle for a healthy pregnancy outcome. (2002). *Journal of the American Dietetic Association, 102,* 1479-1490.

Prentice, A. M., & Jebb, S. A. (2001). Beyond body mass index. *Obesity Reviews, 2,* 141-147.

Russell, R. M., Rasmussen, H., & Lichtenstein, A. H. (1999). Modified food guide pyramid for people over 70 years of age. *Journal of Nutrition, 129,* 751-753.

Sahyoun, N., Lin, C., & Krall, E. (2003). Nutritional status of the older adult is associated with dentition status. *Journal of the American Dietetic Association, 103,* 61-66.

Sahyoun, N. R., Jacques, P. F., Dallal, G. E., & Russell, R. M. (1997). Nutrition screening initiative checklist may be a better awareness/educational tool than a screening one. *Journal of the American Dietetic Association, 97,* 760-764.

Satia-About, J., Patterson, R. E., Neuhouser, M. L., & Elder, J. (2002). Dietary acculturation: Applications to nutrition research and dietetics. *Journal of the American Dietetic Association, 102,* 1105-1118.

Schieve, L. A., Cogswell, M. E., Scanlon, K. S., Perry, G., Ferre, C., Blackmore-Prince, C., et al. (2000). Prepregnancy body mass index and pregnancy weight gain: Associations with preterm delivery. *Obstetrics and Gynecology, 96,* 194-200.

Shenkin, A., Cederblad, G., Elia, M., & Isaksson, B. (1996). Laboratory assessment of protein energy status. *Clinica Chimica Acta, 253,* S5-S59.

Spear, B. A. (2002). Adolescent growth and development. *Journal of the American Dietetic Association, 102*(S), S23-S29.

Stang, J. (2002). Assessment of nutritional status and motivation to make behavior changes among adolescents. *Journal of the American Dietetic Association, 102*(S), S13-S22.

Stevens, J., Cai, J., Pamuk, E. R., Williamson, D. F., Thun, M. J., & Wood, J. L. (1998). The effect of age on the association between body-mass index and mortality. *New England Journal of Medicine, 338,* 1-7.

Sullivan, D. H., Bopp, M. M., & Roberson, P. K. (2002). Protein-energy undernutrition and life-threatening complications among the hospitalized elderly. *Journal of General Internal Medicine, 17,* 923-932.

Sullivan, D. H., Sun, S., & Walls, R. C. (1999). Protein-energy undernutrition among elderly hospitalized clients. *Journal of the American Medical Association, 281,* 2013-2019.

Taylor Baer, M., & Bradford Harris, A. (1997). Pediatric nutrition assessment: Identifying children at risk. *Journal of the American Dietetic Association, 97*(S2), S107-S115.

Thomas, D. R., Zdrowski, C. D., Wilson, M. M., Conright, K. C., Lewis, C., Tariq, S., & Morley, J. E. (2002). Malnutrition in subacute care. *American Journal of Clinical Nutrition, 75,* 308-313.

Tomkins, A. (2003). Assessing micronutrient status in the presence of inflammation. *Journal of Nutrition, 133,* 1649S-1655S.

United States Department of Health and Human Services (USDHHS). (2000). *Healthy People 2010.* Retrieved November 4, 2003, from www.healthypeople. gov/Document/tableofcontents.htm#volume1.

U.S. Department of Agriculture and Department of Health and Human Resources. *Dietary Guidelines for Americans 2005.* Washington, DC. Retrieved June 26, 2005, from http://health.gov/dietaryguidelines/dga2005/.

U.S. Department of Health & Human Services. U.S. Department of Agriculture. *Dietary Guidelines for Americans, 2005.* Retrieved June 26, 2005, from www.healthiers. gov/dietaryguidelines.

Vellas, B., Guigoz, Y., Garry, P. J., Nourhashemi, F., Bennahum, D., Lauque, S., & Albarede, J. L. (1999). The Mini Nutrition Assessment and its use in grading the nutritional state of elderly clients. *Nutrition, 15,* 116-122.

Volpato, S., Leveille, S. G., Corti, M., Harris, T. B., & Guralnik, J. M. (2001). The value of serum albumin and high-density lipoprotein cholesterol in defining mortality risk in older persons with low serum cholesterol. *Journal of the American Geriatric Society, 49,* 1142-1147.

Wagner, D. R., & Heyward, V. H. (1999). Measures of body composition in blacks and whites: A comparative review. *American Journal of Clinical Nutrition, 71,* 1392-1402.

Wagner, D. R., & Heyward, V. H. (2000). Techniques of body composition assessment: A review of laboratory and field methods. *Research Quarterly for Exercise and Sport, 70,* 1-17.

Whitaker, R. C., Wright, J. A., Pepe, M. S., Seidel, K. D., & Dietz, W. H. (1997). Predicting obesity in young adulthood from childhood and parental obesity. *New England Journal of Medicine, 337,* 869-873.

Willett, W. C., Dietz, W. H., & Colditz, G. A. (1999). Guidelines for healthy weight. *New England Journal of Medicine, 341,* 427-434.

World Health Organization (WHO). (1999). *Management of malnutrition: A manual for physicians and other senior health workers.* Retrieved November 4, 2003, from www.who. int/ nut/documents/manage_severe_malnutrition_ eng.pdf.

Zhu, S., Wang, Z., Heshka, S., Moonseong, H., Faith, M. S., & Heymsfield, S. B. (2002). Waist circumference and obesity-associated risk factors among whites in the third National Health and Nutrition Examination Survey: Clinical action thresholds. *American Journal of Clinical Nutrition, 76,* 743-749.

Zlotkin, S. (2003). Clinical nutrition 8: The role of nutrition in the prevention of iron deficiency anemia in infants, children and adolescents. *Canadian Medical Association Journal, 168,* 59-63.

Chapter 10

Barkauskas, V., Baumann, L., & Darling-Fischer, C. (2002). *Health and physical assessment* (3rd ed.). Philadelphia: Mosby.

Bikley, L. S. (2004). *Bates guide to physical examination and history taking* (8th ed.). Philadelphia: Lippincott.

Brammer, L. M., Abrego, P., & Shostrum, E. (1993). *Therapeutic counseling and psychotherapy* (6th ed.). Upper Saddle River, NJ: Prentice Hall.

Carkhuff, R. R. (2000). *The art of helping in the 21st century.* Amherst, MA: Human Resources Development Press.

Cormier, L. S., Cormier, W. H., & Weiser, R. J. (1984). *Interviewing and helping, skills for health professionals.* Belmont, CA: Wadsworth.

Doenges, M. A., & Moorhouse, M. F. (1990). *Nursing diagnosis with interventions* (3rd ed.). Philadelphia: F.A. Davis.

Duke University. (2000). GIFT, Genetics Interdisciplinary Faculty Training. Retrieved April 20, 2004, from http://gift.duke.edu.

Gordon, M. (1990). Toward theory based diagnostic categories. *Nursing Diagnosis, 1*(1), 5–11.

Gotler, R. S., Medalie, J. H., Zyzarnski, S. J., Kikano, G., Acheson, L. S., & Stange, K. C. (2001). Focus on the family, Part I: What is your family focus style? *Family Practice Management, 8*(3), 49–51.

Leasia, M. S., & Monahan, F. D. (2002). *A practical guide to health assessment* (2nd ed.). Philadelphia: W.B. Saunders.

Lutz, C., & Przytulski, K. (2001). *Nutrition and diet therapy* (3rd ed.). Philadelphia: F.A. Davis.

Murray, R. B., & Zentner, J. P. (2001). *Health promotion strategies throughout the life span* (7th ed.). Upper Saddle River, NJ: Prentice Hall.

Naryan, M. C. (2003). Cultural assessment and care planning. *Home Healthcare Nurse, 21*(9), 611–620.

Orem, D. E. (1991). *Nursing concepts and practice* (4th ed.). St. Louis, MO: Mosby.

Ramor, M., & Brown, C. M. (2003). Physical examination for the occupational health nurse: Skills update. *American Association of Occupational Health Nurses Journal, 5*(9), 390–403.

Rogers, C. R. (1951). *Client-centered therapy.* Boston: Houghton Mifflin.

Rogers, C. R. (1957). The necessary and sufficient conditions of therapeutic personality change. *Journal of Consulting Clinical Psychology, 21,* 95–103.

Chapter 11

Aging changes in hair and nails. Retrieved November 14, 2003, from www.nln.nih.gov/ medlineplus/ency/article/004005.htm.

Barkauskas, V., Baumann, L., & Darling-Fischer, C. (2002). *Health and physical assessment* (3rd ed.). Philadelphia: Mosby.

Bickley, L. S. (2003). *Bates guide to physical examination and history taking* (8th ed.). Philadelphia: Lippincott.

Kaplan, D. L. (2003). Dermclinic: A photo quiz to hone dermatologic skills. *Consultant, 43*(8), 969–977.

Kozier, B., Erb, G., Berman, A., & Snyder, S. (2004). *Fundamentals of nursing: Concepts, process, and practice* (7th ed.). Upper Saddle River, NJ: Prentice Hall.

Marieb, E. (2004). *Human anatomy and physiology* (4th ed.). Redwood City, CA: Benjamin/Cummings Publishing Company.

Proper skin care. Retrieved December 2, 2003, from www.MayoClinic.com.

Purnell, L. D., & Paulanka, B. J. (1998). *Transcultural health care: A culturally competent approach.* Philadelphia: F. A. Davis.

Schafer, R. C. (2000). *Skin and nail trauma and related disorders.* Retrieved December 10, 2003, from www.chiro.org.

Seidel, H., Ball, J. W., Dains, J. E., Benedict, W. G., et al. (2003). *Mosby's guide to physical examination* (5th ed.). St. Louis, MO: Mosby.

Skin care for African Americans. Retrieved December 2, 2003, from www.aad.org.

Skin, hair and nail insights. Retrieved December 2, 2003, from www.aad.org.

Tortora, G. J., Grabowski, S. R., & Prezbindowski, K. S. (2002). *Principles of anatomy and physiology* (10th ed.). New York: John Wiley & Sons.

Turnbull, R. (2000). Skin assessment in children: A methodical approach. *Nursing Times, 96*(41), 33–34.

Chapter 12

Bikley, L. S. (2004). *Bates guide to physical examination and history taking* (8th ed.). Philadelphia: Lippincott.

Gray, H. (2000). *Gray's anatomy.* New York: Barnes & Noble Books.

Johns Hopkins Medicine. *Cleft lip and palate.* Retrieved September 22, 2003, from www.hopkinsmedicine.org.

Kozier, B., Erb, G., Berman, A. J., & Burke, K. (2004). *Fundamentals of nursing: Concepts, process and practice* (7th ed.). Upper Saddle River, NJ: Prentice Hall.

Marieb, E. (2000). *Human anatomy and physiology* (5th ed.). Redwood City: Benjamin/Cummings Publishing Company.

Thyroid disease. Retrieved February 22, 2004, from www.clevelandclinic.org/health/health-info/docs.

Thyroid problems and pregnancy. Endocrine disease and endocrine surgery. Retrieved February 22, 2004, from www.endocrineweb.com.

United States Department of Health and Human Services (USDHHS). *Healthy People 2010: Understanding and improving health.* Retrieved May 2002 from www.health.gov/healthypeople.

Chapter 13

American Academy of Ophthalmology. (2002). *Health tips on how often to have an eye exam.* Retrieved November 9, 2002, from www.medem.com.

American Academy of Pediatrics. (2002). *Vision: Aged 4 to 7 months.* Retrieved November 29, 2002, from www.medem.com; www.preventblindness.org www.childrensvision.com.

Bikley, L. S. (2004). *Bates guide to physical examination and history taking* (8th ed.). Philadelphia: Lippincott.

Eye conditions. (2002). Retrieved November 29, 2002, from www.eyemdlink.com.

Marieb, E. N. (2004). *Human anatomy and physiology.* Redwood City, CA: Benjamin/Cummings.

Murray, R. B., & Zentner, J. P. (2000). *Health assessment and promotion strategies through the life span.* Upper Saddle River, NJ: Prentice Hall.

National Eye Institute. *Strategic plan on reducing health disparities FY 2000–2004.* Retrieved (date) from www.nei.nih.gov/resources/strategicplans/disparities.htm

Purnell, L. D., & Paulanka, B. J. (1998). *Transcultural health care: A culturally competent approach.* Philadelphia: F. A. Davis.

Tortora, G. J., Grabowski, S. R., & Prezbindowski, K. S. (2002). *Principles of anatomy and physiology* (10th ed.). New York: John Wiley & Sons.

United States Department of Health and Human Services (USDHHS). (2000). *Healthy People 2010: Understanding and improving health.* Retrieved May 2002 from www.health.gov/healthypeople.

Chapter 14

Bikley, L. S. (2004). *Bates guide to physical examination and history taking* (8th ed.). Philadelphia: Lippincott.

Gray, H. (2000). *Gray's anatomy.* New York: Barnes & Noble Books.

Kozier, B., Erb, G., Berman, A. J., & Burke, K. (2004). *Fundamentals of nursing: Concepts, process and practice* (7th ed.). Upper Saddle River, NJ: Prentice Hall.

Lewis, S., Heitkemper, M., & Dirksen, S. (2004). *Medical surgical nursing* (6th ed.). St. Louis, MO: Mosby.

Marieb, E. (2003). *Human anatomy and physiology* (6th ed.). Redwood City, CA: Benjamin/Cummings Publishing Company.

Tortora, G. J., Grabowski, S. R., & Prezbindowski, K. S. (2002). *Principles of anatomy and physiology* (10th ed.). New York: John Wiley & Sons.

United States Department of Health and Human Services (USDHHS). (2000). *Healthy People 2010: Understanding and improving health.* Retrieved May 2002 from www.health.gov/healthypeople.

Vargas, C. M., Kramarow, E. A., & Yellowitz, J. A. (2001). The oral health of older Americans. *Aging Trends* (no. 3). Hyattsville, MD: National Center for Health Statistics.

Chapter 15

American Lung Association. (2000b). *Fact sheet: American Indians/Alaskan Natives and lung disease.* Retrieved from www.lungusa.org/diseases/nativelung/factsheet/html.

American Lung Association. (2000a). *Fact sheet: African Americans and lung disease.* Retrieved from www.lungusa.org/diseases/africanlung/factsheet/html.

Bickley, L. S. (1999). *Bates guide to physical examination and history taking* (7th ed.). Philadelphia: Lippincott.

CDC's Core Curriculum on Tuberculosis. (2000). In *Guidelines from the Centers for Disease Control core curriculum on tuberculosis* (4th ed.). Retrieved from http://ethnomed.org/ethomed/clin.topics/th/cdc.tst.html.

Gibbons, M. (2001). Racial disparities in health care a vexing problem. *Advance for Respiratory Care Practitioners.* Retrieved from www.advanceforrep.com/pastarticles/dec17.01cover.html.

Gray, H. (1995). *Anatomy descriptive and surgical* (15th ed.). New York: Barnes & Noble Books.

Jackson, C. (1996). *Linguistic and cultural management aspects of tuberculosis screening and management for refugees and immigrants.* Presented at International Union Against Tuberculosis and Lung Disease Conference. Retrieved from http://ethnomed.org/ethnomed/clin.topics/th/th/html.

Lewis, S., Heitkemper, M., & Dirksen, S. (2005). *Medical surgical nursing, assessment and management of clinical problems* (6th ed.). St. Louis, MO: Mosby.

Marieb, E. (2000). *Human anatomy and physiology* (5th ed.). Redwood City, CA: Benjamin/Cummings Publishing.

Meyers, R. (2000). *Master guide for passing the respiratory care credentialing exam* (4th ed.). Upper Saddle River, NJ: Prentice Hall.

Potter, P., & Perry, A. (2001). *Fundamentals of nursing* (5th ed.). St. Louis, MO: Mosby.

Respiratory diseases in *Healthy People 2010.* Centers for Disease Control. Retrieved from www.health.gov/healthypeople/document/HTML/Volume2/24Respiratory.htm.

Seidel, H., et al. (1995). *Mosby's guide to physical examination* (3rd ed.). St. Louis, MO: Mosby.

Tortoro, G. J., Grabowski, S. R., & Prezbindowski, K. S. (2002). *Principles of anatomy and physiology* (10th ed.). New York: John Wiley & Sons.

Chapter 16

American Cancer Society. (2001). *Breast cancer facts and figures 2001–2002.*

American Cancer Society. (2003). *Guidelines for the early detection of cancer.* Retrieved October 3, 2003, from www.cancer.org/docroot/NWS/content/NWS. 2.1x.american.

American Cancer Society. (2004). *Breast self-exam is too valuable to discard, experts say.* Retrieved May 2, 2004, from www.cancer.org/docroot/NWS/content/update/NWS.1.

Bikley, L. S. (2004). *Bates guide to physical examination and history taking* (8th ed.). Philadelphia: Lippincott.

Breast cancer and mammography information. Retrieved October 3, 2003, from www.cdc.gov.cancer/nbvvedn/info-bc.htm.

Freund, K. M. (2004). *Clinical breast exam/BSE.* Retrieved July 13, 2004, from www.annieappleseedproject.org/rattecofelin.html.

Growth and development: Breast conditions. Retrieved October 2003 from www.lpch.org/diseasehealthinfo/healthlibrary/growth/brcond.html.

Kozier, B., Erb, G., Berman, A. J., & Burke, K. (2004). *Fundamentals of nursing: Concepts, process and practice* (7th ed.). Upper Saddle River, NJ: Prentice Hall.

Male breast cancer. (2003). Retrieved July 13, 2004, from www.cancer.gov/cancertopics/pdq/treatment/malebreast/healthprofessional.

Mammograms and other breast imaging procedures. (2003). Retrieved October 2003 from www. cancer.org/docroot/CRI.

National Cancer Institute. (2004). *Breast cancer risk assessment tool.* Retrieved July 13, 2004, from http://bcra.nci.nih.gov/brc/.

Purnell, L. D., & Paulanka, B. J. (1998). *Transcultural health care: A culturally competent approach.* Philadelphia: F. A. Davis.

Seidel, H., et al. (2002). *Mosby's guide to physical examination* (3rd ed.). St. Louis, MD: Mosby.

United States Preventive Services Task Force (USPSTF). (2002). *Breast cancer screening.* Retrieved July 13, 2004, from www.ahrq.gov/clinic/uspstf/uspsbrca.htm.

Chapter 17

Beery, T. A. (2000). The evolving role of genetics in the diagnosis and management of heart disease. *Nursing Clinics of North America, 35*(4), 963–973.

Bikley, L. S. (2004). *Bates guide to physical examination and history taking* (8th ed.). Philadelphia: Lippincott.

Carey, B. E. (2002). Incidence and epidemiology of congenital cardiovascular malformation in the newborn and infant. *Newborn Infant Nursing Reviews, 2*(2), 54–59.

Gray, H. (2000). *Gray's anatomy.* New York: Barnes & Noble Books.

Heredity as a risk factor. Retrieved July 13, 2004, from www.Americanheart.org.

Kozier, B., Erb, G., Berman, A. J., & Burke, K. (2000). *Fundamentals of nursing: Concepts, process, and practice* (7th ed.). Upper Saddle River, NJ: Prentice Hall.

Kuznar, K. A. (2004). Peripheral arterial disease. *Advance for Nurses, 4*(13), 17–22.

Lewis, S., Heitkemper, M., & Dirksen, S. (2000). *Medical surgical nursing.* St. Louis, MO: Mosby.

Marieb, E. (2003). *Human anatomy and physiology* (6th ed.). Redwood City, CA: Benjamin/Cummings Publishing Company.

Seidel, H., Ball, J., Dains, J., Benedict, W. (2002). *Mosby's guide to physical examination* (5th ed.). St. Louis, MO: Mosby.

Chapter 18

Bikley, L. S. (2002). *Bates guide to physical examination and history taking* (8th ed.). Philadelphia: Lippincott.

Futterman, L. G., & Lemberg, L. (2002). Peripheral arterial disease is only the tip of the atherosclerotic "iceberg." *American Journal of Critical Care, 11*(4), 390–394.

Gray, H. (2000). *Gray's anatomy.* New York: Barnes & Noble Books.

Kozier, B., Erb, G., Berman, A. J., & Burke, K. (2004). *Fundamentals of nursing: Concepts, process and practice* (7th ed.). Upper Saddle River, NJ: Prentice Hall.

Lewis, S., Heitkemper, M., & Dirksen, S. (2000). *Medical surgical nursing: Assessment and management of clinical problems* (6th ed.). St. Louis, MO: Mosby.

Marieb, E. (2003). *Human anatomy and physiology* (6th ed.). Redwood City, CA: Benjamin/Cummings Publishing Company.

Seidel, H., et al. (2002). *Mosby's guide to physical examination* (3rd ed.). St. Louis, MO: Mosby.

Seventh report of the Joint National Committee on Prevention, Detection, Evaluation, and Treatment of High Blood Pressure (JNC 7) Express. Retrieved July 14, 2004, from www.nhlbi.nih.gov/guidelines/hypertension/jncintro.htm; www.agingwell.state. ny.us/prevention/hypertension.htm.

United States Department of Health and Human Services (USDHHS). *Healthy People 2010: Understanding and improving health.* Retrieved July 14, 2004, from www.healthypeople.gov.

Chapter 19

Food safety. Retrieved July 14, 2004, from www.healthypeople.gov/Document/HTML/Volume1/10Food.htm.

Gastrointestinal diseases in minority patients. Retrieved July 14, 2004, from http://home.fuse.net/bell0039/advisor19.html.

H pylori and peptic ulcer. Retrieved July 14, 2004, from www.digestive.niddk.nih.gov/ddiseases/pubs/hpylori/.

Kozier, B., Erb, G., Berman, A., & Snyder, S. J. (2004). *Fundamentals of nursing: Concepts, processes, and practice* (7th ed.). Upper Saddle River, NJ: Prentice Hall.

Lewis, S. M., Heitkemper, M. M., & Dirksen, S. R. (2004). *Medical-surgical nursing: Assessment and management of clinical problems* (6th ed.). St. Louis, MO: Mosby.

Marieb, E. N. (2000). *Human anatomy and physiology* (5th ed.). Redwood City, CA: Benjamin/Cummings.

Murray, R. B., & Zentner, J. P. (2000). *Health assessment and promotion strategies, through the life span.* Upper Saddle River, NJ: Prentice Hall.

NIH guide: Liver and biliary disease among women and minorities. Retrieved July 14, 2004, from www.grants.nih.gov/grants/guide/pa-files/PA-98-086.html.

Chapter 20

Bianchi, D. W., Crombleholme, T. M., & D'Alton, M. E. (2000). *Fetology: Diagnosis and management of the fetal patient* (pp. 641–647). New York: McGraw-Hill.

Gray, H. (2000). *Gray's anatomy.* New York: Barnes & Noble Books.

Kozier, B., Erb, G., Berman, A. J., & Burke, K. (2004). *Fundamentals of nursing: Concepts, process and practice* (7th ed.). Upper Saddle River, NJ: Prentice Hall.

Lewis, S. M., Heitkemper, M. M., & Dirksen, S. R. (2004). *Medical-surgical nursing: Assessment and management of clinical problems* (6th ed.). St. Louis, MO: Mosby.

Marieb, E. (2000). *Human anatomy and physiology* (5th ed.). Redwood City, CA: Benjamin/Cummings Publishing Company.

National Kidney and Urological Disease Information Clearinghouse. Urinary Tract Infections in Adults. Retrieved July 2004 from http://kidney.niddk.nih.gov/kudisease/pubs/utiadult/index.htm.

Seidel, H., Ball, J., Dains, J., Benedict, W., et al. (2002). *Mosby's guide to physical examination* (5th ed.). St. Louis, MO: Mosby.

United States Department of Health and Human Services (USDHHS). (2000). *Healthy People 2010: Understanding and improving health.* Retrieved July 16, 2004, from www.health.gov/healthypeople.

Chapter 21

Bikley, L. S. (2004). *Bates guide to physical examination and history taking* (8th ed.). Philadelphia: Lippincott.

Cancer reference information. Retrieved July 15, 2004, from www.cancer.org/docroot/home/index.asp.

Gray, H. (2004). *Gray's anatomy.* New York: Barnes & Noble Books.

Kozier, B., Erb, G., Berman, A., & Snyder, S. J. (2004). *Fundamentals of nursing: Concepts, processes, and practice* (7th ed.). Upper Saddle River, NJ: Prentice Hall.

Lewis, S. M., Heitkemper, M. M., & Dirksen, S. R. (2004). *Medical-surgical nursing: Assessment and management of clinical problems* (6th ed.). St. Louis, MO: Mosby.

Marieb, E. (2000). *Human anatomy and physiology* (6th ed.). Redwood City, CA: Benjamin/Cummings Publishing Company.

Murray, R. B., & Zentner, J. P. (2000). *Health assessment and promotion strategies, through the life span.* Upper Saddle River, NJ: Prentice Hall.

Purnell, L. D., & Paulanka, B. J. (1998). *Transcultural health care: A culturally competent approach.* Philadelphia: F. A. Davis.

Tortora, G. J., Grabowski, S. R., & Prezbindowski, K. S. (2002). *Principles of anatomy and physiology* (10th ed.). New York: John Wiley & Sons.

Chapter 22

Bikley, L. S. (2004). *Bates guide to physical examination and history taking* (8th ed.). Philadelphia: Lippincott.

Female genital mutilation. Retrieved from www.who.int/inf-fs/en/fact241.html.

Gray, H. (2004). *Gray's anatomy.* New York: Barnes & Noble Books.

Ignatavicus, D., & Workman, M. L. (2006). *Medical-surgical nursing: Critical thinking for collaborative care* (5th ed.). St. Louis, MO, Elsevier/Saunders.

Kozier, B., Erb, G., Berman, A., & Snyder, S. J. (2004). *Fundamentals of nursing: Concepts, processes, and practice* (7th ed.). Upper Saddle River, NJ: Prentice Hall.

Lewis, S. M., Heitkemper, M. M., & Dirksen, S. R. (2004). *Medical-surgical nursing: Assessment and management of clinical problems* (6th ed.). St. Louis, MO: Mosby.

Marieb, E. (2000). *Human anatomy and physiology* (5th ed.). Redwood City, CA: Benjamin/Cummings Publishing Company.

National Institutes of Health (NIH). (2000). *What you need to know about ovarian cancer.* NIH Publication No. 00–1561, pp. 4–14. Bethesda, MD.

Purnell, L. D., & Paulanka, B. J. (1998). *Transcultural health care: A culturally competent approach.* Philadelphia: F. A. Davis.

www.cancer.org.

www.cdc.gov/od/oc/media/pressrel/fs020509.htm.

www.niaid.nih.gov/factsheets/stdpid.htm.

Chapter 23

Bikley, L. S. (2004). *Bates guide to physical examination and history taking* (8th ed.). Philadelphia: Lippincott.

Evaluating limping in children. www.dynomed.com/encyclopedia/pediatric.orthopedics; www.orthoinfo.aaos.org.

Marieb, E. (2003). *Human anatomy and physiology* (6th ed.). Redwood City, CA: Benjamin/Cummings Publishing Company.

The National Women's Health Information Center. Washington, DC: U.S. Public Health Service's Office on Women's Health, 1998. *Women of Color Health Data Book.* Retrieved January 20, 2003, from www.4woman.gov.owh/pub/woc/elderly.htm.

Potter, P., & Perry, A. (2001). *Fundamentals of nursing* (5th ed.). St. Louis, MO: Mosby.

Potter, P., & Perry, A. (2002). *Basic nursing: Essentials for practice* (5th ed.). St. Louis, MO: Mosby.

Purnell, L. D., & Paulanka, B. J. (1998). *Transcultural health care: A culturally competent approach.* Philadelphia: F. A. Davis.

Questions and answers about arthritis and rheumatic diseases. (2002). www.niams.nih.gov/hi/topics/arthritis/artrheu.htm.

Seidel, H., et al. (2002). *Mosby's guide to physical examination* (3rd ed.). St. Louis, MO: Mosby.

Tortora, G. J., Grabowski, S. R., & Prezbindowski, K. S. (2002). *Principles of anatomy and physiology* (10th ed.). New York: John Wiley & Sons.

United States Department of Health and Human Services (USDHHS). (2000). *Healthy People 2010: Understanding and improving health.* Retrieved July 16, 2004, from www.health.gov/healthypeople.

United States Department of Health and Human Services. National Institutes of Health. National Heart, Lung and Blood Institute. Diseases and Conditions Index. (2003). Sickle Cell Anemia. Retrieved February 16, 2004, from www.nhlbi.nih.gov/health/dci/Diseases/Sca/SCA_WhatIs.html.

Chapter 24

Bikley, L. S. (2004). *Bates guide to physical examination and history taking* (8th ed.). Philadelphia: Lippincott.

Brain attack. Retrieved July 20, 2004, from www.ninds.nih.gov/health_and_medical/pubs/stroke_bookmark.htm.

Geriatric assessment tools. Retrieved July 20, 2004, from www.medicine. uiowa.edu.

Gray, H. (2004). *Gray's anatomy.* New York: Barnes & Noble Books.

Kozier, B., Erb, G., Berman, A. J., & Burke, K. (2004). *Fundamentals of nursing: Concepts, process and practice* (7th ed.). Upper Saddle River, NJ: Prentice Hall.

Lucile Packord Children's Hospital (2001-2005). Neurological disorders, seizures, and epilepsy. Retrieved February 5, 2003, from www.lpch.org/diseasehealthinf/healthlibrary/neuro/seizep.htm.

Marieb, E. (2000). *Human anatomy and physiology* (5th ed.). Redwood City, CA: Benjamin/Cummings Publishing Company.

Merck manual of geriatrics. (2001-2005). Chapter 38. Mental status examination. Retrieved March 26, 2003 from www.Merck.com.

Neurologic disorders. Retrieved February 15, 2003, from www.pch.org/diseases healthinfo/healthlibrary/neuro.html.

Tortora, G. J., Grabowski, S. R., & Prezbindowski, K. S. (2002). *Principles of anatomy and physiology* (10th ed.). New York: John Wiley & Sons.

Wong, D. (1995). *Whaley & Wong's nursing care of infants and children* (5th ed.). St. Louis, MO: Mosby.

Chapter 25

American Academy of Pediatrics, Council on Child and Adolescent Health. (1988). Age limit of pediatrics. *Pediatrics, 81*(5), 736.

Bickley, L. S., & Szilagyi, P. G. (Eds.). (2003). *Bates' guide to physical examination and history taking* (8th ed.). Philadelphia: Lippincott, Williams & Wilkins.

Blake, J. (1992). Gynecologic examination of the teenager and young child. *Obstetrics and Gynecologic Clinics of North America, 19,* 27.

Burns, C. E., Brady, M. A., Dunn, A. M., & Starr, N. B. (2000). *Pediatric primary care: A handbook for nurse practitioners* (2nd ed.). Philadelphia: W.B. Saunders.

Coylar, M. R. (2003). *Well-child assessment for primary care providers.* Philadelphia: F.A. Davis.

Flynn, J. T. (2003). Recognizing and managing the hypertensive child. *Contemporary Pediatrics, 20*(8), 38–60.

Green, M., & Palfrey, J. S. (Eds.). (2002). *Bright futures: Guidelines for health supervision of infants, children and adolescents* (2nd ed.). Arlington, VA: National Center for Education in Maternal Child Health.

Harris, J. P. (1994). Consultation with the specialist: Evaluation of heart murmurs. *Pediatrics in Review, 15*(12), 490–494.

Kurdahi Zahr, L., & Hattar-Pollara, M. (1998). Nursing care of Arab children: Consideration of cultural factors. *Journal of Pediatric Nursing, 13*(6), 349–355.

National High Blood Pressure Education Program. (1996). *Update on the task force report (1987) on high blood pressure in children and adolescents: A working group report from the national high blood pressure education program.* NIH Publication: No. 96-3790. Bethesda, MD; National Institutes of Health National Heart, Lung, and Blood Institute.

Pizzutillo, P. D. (1997). *Practical orthopedics in primary practice.* New York: McGraw-Hill.

Reece, R. M., & Ludwig, S. (2001). *Child abuse: Medical diagnosis and management* (2nd ed.). Philadelphia: Lippincott, Williams & Wilkins.

Chapter 26

American Pregnancy Association. *Natural herbs and vitamins during pregnancy.* Retrieved April 18, 2004, from www.americanpregnancy.org/pregnancyhealth/naturalherbsvitamins.html.

Barnhard, Y., Bar-Hava, I., & Divon, M. Y. (1996). Accuracy of intrapartum estimates of fetal weight effect of oligohydramnios. *Journal of Reproductive Medicine, 41,* 907–910.

Blackburn, S. (2003). *Maternal, fetal, and neonatal physiology* (2nd ed.). St. Louis, MO: Saunders.

Centers for Disease Control and Prevention. (2002). *Intimate partner violence during pregnancy.* Retrieved July 20, 2004, from www.cdc.gov/reproductivehealth/violence/ipvdp.htm.

Centers for Disease Control and Prevention. (2003). *Folic acid: Topic home.* Retrieved March 25, 2004, from www.cdc.gov/node.do/id/0900f3ec80010af9.

Creasy, R. K., & Resnik, R. (Eds.). *Maternal-fetal medicine* (4th ed.). Philadelphia: W. B. Saunders.

Cunningham, F. G., Gant, N. F., Leveno, K. J., Gilstrap, L. C., Hauth, J. C., & Wentstrom, K. D. (2001). *Williams obstetrics* (21st ed.). New York: McGraw-Hill.

Engstrom, J. L. (1993). Fundal height measurement: Part 1—Techniques for measuring fundal height. *Journal of Nurse-Midwifery, 38*(1), 5–16.

Engstrom, J. L., & McFarlin, B. L. (1993). Fundal height measurement: Part 2—Intra-Interexaminer reliability of three measurement techniques. *Journal of Nurse-Midwifery, 38*(1), 17–22.

Engstrom, J. L., Piscioneri, L., Low, L., McShane, H., & McFarlin, B. (1993). Fundal height measurement: Part 3—The effect of maternal position on fundal height measurements. *Journal of Nurse-Midwifery, 38*(1), 25–27.

Freda, M., Andersen, F., Damus, K., & Merkatz, I. R. (1993). Are there differences in information given to private and public prenatal clients? *American Journal of Obstetrics and Gynecology, 169*(1), 155–160.

Godlee, F. (2003). *Clinical evidence concise.* London: BMJ Publishing Group.

Green, C. J., & Wilkinson, J. M. (2004). *Maternal newborn nursing care plans.* St. Louis, MO: Mosby.

Hale, T. W. (2004). *Medications and mother's milk: A manual of lactational pharmacology.* Amarillo, TX: Pharmasoft Medical Publishing.

Knowles, M. S. (1992). Applying principles of adult learning in conference presentations.

Lea, D. H., Jenkins, J. F., & Francomano, C. A. (1998). *Genetics in clinical practice: New directions for nursing and health care.* Boston: Jones & Bartlett.

Leitich, H., Brunbauer, M., Bodner-Adler, B., Kaider, A., Egarter, C., & Husslein, P. (2003). Antibiotic treatment of bacterial vaginosis in pregnancy: A meta-analysis. *American Journal of Obstetrics and Gynecology, 188*(3), 752–758.

Lipson, J. G., Dibble, S. L., & Minarik, P. A. (1996). *Culture & nursing care.* San Francisco: UCSF Nursing Press.

Littleton, L. Y., & Engebretson, J. C. (2002). *Maternal, neonatal, and women's health nursing.* Albany, NY: Delmar.

Lowdermilk, D. L., & Perry, S. E. (2004). *Maternity & women's health care* (8th ed.). St. Louis, MO: Mosby.

Luxner, K. L. (2005). *Delmar's maternal-infant nursing care plans* (2nd ed.). Australia: Thomson Delmar Learning.

Mahowald, M. B., McKusick, V. A., Scheuerle, A. S., & Aspinwall, T. J. (2001). *Genetics in the clinic: Clinical, ethical, and social implications for primary care.* St. Louis, MO: Mosby.

Mamelle, N., Segueilla, M., Munoz, F., & Berland, M. (1997). Prevention of preterm birth in clients with symptoms of preterm labor—The benefits of psychological support. *American Journal of Obstetrics and Gynecology, 177*(4), 947–952.

March of Dimes. *Smoking during pregnancy.* Retrieved January 29, 2004, from www.marchofdimes. com/professionals/681_1171.asp.

Margulies, R., & Miller, L. (2001). Fruit size as a model for teaching first trimester uterine sizing in bimanual examination. *American College of Obstetricians and Gynecologists, 98*(2), 341–344.

Mattson, S., & Smith, J. E. (2000). *Core curriculum for maternal-newborn nursing* (2nd ed.). Philadelphia: W. B. Saunders.

McCance, K. L., & Huether, S. E. (1998). *Pathophysiology* (3rd ed.). St. Louis, MO: Mosby.

McFarlin, B. (1994). Intrauterine growth retardation: Etiology, diagnosis, and management. *Journal of Nurse-Midwifery, 39*(2), 52S.

Miller, D. W., Yeast, J. D., & Evans, R. L. (2003). The unavailability of prenatal records at hospital presentation. *Obstetrics & Gynecology, 101*(4), 87S.

Moore, K. L., & Persaud, T. V. N. (1998). *Before we are born: Essentials of embryology and birth defects* (5th ed.). Philadelphia: W. B. Saunders.

NANDA, International. *NANDA nursing diagnoses: Definitions and classification 2003–2004.* Philadelphia: Author.

Nussbaum, R. L., McInnes, R. R., & Willard, H. F. (2001). *Thompson & Thompson genetics in medicine.* Philadelphia: W. B. Saunders.

Office on Women's Health. *Pregnancy and nutrition.* Retrieved March 24, 2004, from www.4women. gov.

Robertson, L., Flinders, C., & Godfrey, B. (1986). *Laurel's kitchen: A handbook of vegetarian cookery and nutrition.* Petaluma, CA: Nilgiri Press.

Rorie, J. L., Paine, L. L., & Barger, M. K. (1993). Primary care for women: Cultural competence in primary care services. *Journal of Nurse-Midwifery, 41*(2), 92–100.

Sinclair, C. (2004). *A midwife's handbook.* St. Louis, MO: Saunders.

Star, W. L., Shannon, M. T., Lommel, L. L., & Gutierrez, Y. M. (1999). *Ambulatory obstetrics* (3rd ed.). San Francisco: UCSF Nursing Press.

St. Hill, P., Lipson, A., & Meleis, A. I. (2003). *Caring for women cross-culturally.* Philadelphia: F. A. Davis.

Toppenberg, K. S., Hill, D. A., & Miller, D. P. American Academy of Family Physicians. (1999). Retrieved April 18, 2004, from www.aafp.org/ afp/990401ap/1813.html.

U.S. Census Bureau. (2000a). *Profiles of general demographic characteristics.* Retrieved June 12, 2004, from www.census.gov/Press-Release/www/2001/demoprofile.html.

U.S. Census Bureau. (2000b). *Quick table: Ancestry: 2000.* Retrieved June 12, 2004, from http://factfinder.census.gov/servlet/QTTable?_bm=y&-geo_id=01000US&-qr_name=DEC_2000_SF3_U_QTP13&-ds_name=DEC_2000_SF3_U&-_lang=en&-redoLog=false&-_sse=on.

U.S. Census Bureau. (2000c). *Quick table: Hispanic or Latino by type.* Retrieved June 12, 2004, from http://factfinder.census.gov/servlet/QTTable?_bm=y&-geo_id=01000US&-qr_name=DEC_2000_SF1_U_QTP9&-ds_name=DEC_2000_SF1_U&-_lang=en&-redoLog=false&-_sse=on.

U.S. Census Bureau. (2000d) *Quick table: Race alone or in combination.* Retrieved June 12, 2004, from http://factfinder.census.gov/servlet/QTTable?_bm=y&geo_id=01000US&-qr_name=DEC_2000_SF1_U_QTP5&-ds_name=DEC_2000_SF1_U&-_lang=en&-redoLog=false&-_sse=on.

U.S. Department of Agriculture Food Safety and Inspection Service. (2001). *Listeriosis and pregnancy: What is your risk?* Retrieved April 18, 2004, from www.fsis.usda.gov/OA/pubs/lm_tearsheet.htm.

U.S. Nuclear Regulatory Commission. (1999). *Instruction concerning prenatal radiation.* Retrieved April 18, 2004, from www.nrc.gov/reading-rm/doc-collections/reg-guides/occupational-health/active/8-13/08-013.pdf.

U.S. Preventive Services Task Force. *Screening: Bacterial vaginosis in pregnancy.* Retrieved March 25, 2004, from www.ahrq.gov/clinic/uspstf/uspsbvag. htm.

Varney, H., Kriebs, J. M., & Gegor, C. L. (2004). *Varney's midwifery* (4th ed.). Sudbury, MA: Jones & Bartlett.

Walsh, L. (2001). *Midwifery: Community-based care during the childbearing year.* Philadelphia: W. B. Saunders.

Whitley, N. (1985). *A manual of clinical obstetrics.* Philadelphia: Lippincott.

Chapter 27

Burke, M. M., & Walsh, M. B. (1997). *Gerontologic Nursing* (2nd ed.). St. Louis, Mosby Co.

Doerfler, E. (1999). Male erectile dysfunction: A guide for clinician management. *Journal of the American Academy of Nurse Practitioners, 11*(3), 117–123.

Ewing, J. (1984). Detecting alcoholism: The CAGE questionnaire. *Journal of the American Medical Association, 252* (14), 1905–1907.

Federal Interagency Forum on Aging-Related Statistics. (November 2004). *Older Americans 2004: Key Indicators of Well-Being.* Federal Interagency Forum on Aging-Related Statistics, Washington, DC: U.S. Government Printing Office.

Folstein, M., Folstein, S. E., & McHugh, P. R. (1975). Mini-mental state: A practical method for grading the cognitive state of patients for the clinician. *Journal of Psychiatric Research, 12*(3), 189–198.

Grodner, M., Long, S., & DeYoung, S. (2004). *Foundations and clinical applications of nutrition: A nursing approach.* St. Louis, MO: Mosby.

Gross, P. (2001). Vaccines for pneumonia and new antiviral therapies. *Medical Clinics of North America, 86*(6), 1531–1544.

Janus, S., & Janus, C. (1993). *The Janus report on sexual behavior.* New York: Wiley & Sons.

Jensen, G., McGee, M., & Brinkley, J. (2001). Gastrointestinal disorders in the elderly. Nutrition in the elderly. *Gastroenterology Clinics, 30,* 313–334.

Joaquin, A., & Gollapudi, S. (2001). Functional decline in aging and disease: A role for apoptosis. *Journal of the American Geriatrics Society, 49,* 1234–1240.

Lerman-Garber, I., Valivia Lopez, J., Flores Rebollar, A., Gomez Perez, F., Antonio Rull, J., & Hermosillo, A. (2000). Evidence of a linkage between neurocardiogenic dysfunction and reactive hypoglycemia. *La Revistade Investigacion Clinica, 52*(6), 603–610. (English translation)

Longo-Mbenza, B., Luila, E., Mbete, P., & Vita, E. (1999). Is hyperuricemia a risk factor of stroke and coronary heart disease among Africans? *International Journal of Cardiology, 71*(1), 17–22.

Miller, C. A. (2004). *Nursing for wellness in older adults: Theory and practice* (4th ed.). Philadelphia: Lippincott Williams & Wilkins.

National Diabetes Information Clearinghouse. (2004). *Diabetes in American Indians and Alaska Natives.* Retrieved from http://diabetes.niddk.nih.gov/dm/pubs/americanindian/index.htm.

Ni H., Coriaty-Nelson, Z., Shiller, J., Cohen, R., & Barnes, P. (2004). *Early release of select estimates based on data from the January-September 2003 National Health Interview Survey.* National Center for Health Statistics. (March 2004). Retrieved March 2005 from www.cdc.gov/nchs/data/nhis/earlyrelease2004.pdf. Currently published in Schiller, J., Adams, P., & Coriaty-Nelson, Z. (April 2005). Summary health statistics for the U.S. population: National health interview survey 2003. *Vital and Health Statistics,* Series 10, number 24. Retrieved October 15, 2005, from www.cdc.gov/nchs/data/series/sr_10/sr10_224.pdf.

Perls, T., Kunkel, L., & Puca, A. (2002). The genetics of exceptional human longevity. *Journal of the American Geriatrics Society, 50*(2), 359–368.

Rubenstein, L., Harker, J., Salva, A., Guigoz, Y., & Vellas, B. (2001). Screening for undernutrition in geriatric practice: Developing the short-form mini-nutritional assessment (MNA-SF). *Journal of Gerontology: Biological and Medical Sciences, 56*(6), M366.

Terry, L. C. and Halter, J. B. (1994). *Aging of the Endocrine System.* In Hazzard, W. R., Bierman, E. L., Blass, J. P., Ettinger, W. H., and Halter, J. B. (eds.). Principles of Geriatric Medicine and Gerontology, 3rd edition., pages 791–806, New York, McGraw Hill.

University of Texas at Austin, School of Nursing, Nurse Practitioner Program. (2002). *Screening for hypertension in adults.* Retrieved from www. guideline.gov.

Vasan, R., Beiser, A., Seshadri, S., Larson, M., Kannel, W., D'Agostino, R., & Levy, D. (2002). Residual lifetime risk for developing hypertension in middle-aged women and men: The Framingham Heart Study. *Journal of the American Medical Association, 287*(8), 1003–1010.

Frontmatter

iii Andrea Booher / Stone / Getty Images **iv** Vital Pictures / Image Bank / Getty Images **vi** Clarissa Leahy / Stone / Getty Images **viii** Jim Cummins / Taxi / Getty Images **xii** John Kelly / Image Bank / Getty Images **xiii** Mike Powell / Allsport Concepts / Getty Images.

Chapter 1: Health Assessment

CO1 Ryan McVay/Getty Images, Inc. **Critical Thinking:** Lisa Peardon/Getty Images/Digital Vision. **1-13** Getty Images, Inc.

Chapter 2: Wellness and Health Promotion

CO2 C.Garroni Parisi/Das Fotoarchive/Peter Arnold, Inc. **2-3** Reprinted with permission, *Wellness Workbook,* Travis & Ryan, Ten Speed Press, Berkeley, CA © 1981 by John W. Travis, MD (**http://www.thewellspring.com**). **2-4** Hyner, G. C., Peterson, K. W., Travis, J. W., Dewey, J. E., Foerster, J. J., & Framer, E. M. (Eds.). (1999). *SPM Handbook of Health Assessment Tools.* Pittsburgh, PA: The Society of Prospective Medicine & The Institute for Health and Productivity Management. Reprinted with permission from Occupational Health Strategies. **2-6** Pender, Nola J.; Murdaugh, Carolyn L.; Parsons, Mary Ann, *Health Promotion in Nursing Practice*, 4th ed., © 2002. Reprinted by permission of Pearson Education, Inc., Upper Saddle River, NJ. **Critical Thinking:** John Coletti/Getty Images–Photodisc.

Chapter 3: Health Assessment Across the Life Span

CO3 R. W. Jones/Corbis RF. **3-3** © Patrick J. Watson. **3-5** Michael Newman/PhotoEdit. **3-6** Bill Aron/PhotoEdit. **3-7** Tony Freeman/PhotoEdit. **Critical Thinking:** Thomas Barwick/Getty Images–Photodisc.

Chapter 4: Cultural Considerations

CO4 David Young-Wolff/PhotoEdit. **4-1** Bob Daemmrich/Stock Boston. **4-2** Stockbyte. **Critical Thinking:** Caroline Woodham/Getty Images–Photodisc.

Chapter 5: Psychosocial Assessment

CO5 Jim Cummins/Getty Images, Inc.–Taxi. **5-1** from *Health The Basics*, 5th ed. by Rebecca J. Donatelle. © 2003 Pearson Education, Inc. Reprinted by permission. **5-2** from *Health The Basics*, 5th ed. by Rebecca J. Donatelle. © 2003 Pearson Education, Inc. Reprinted by permission. **Critical Thinking:** Comstock/Corbis–Comstock Images Royalty Free.

Chapter 6: Techniques and Equipment

CO6 © Robbie Jack/Corbis/Bettmann. **6-11** Elena Dorfman/Pearson Education. **T6-1E** Photography courtesy of Brinkmann Instruments, Inc. **Critical Thinking:** Getty Images Inc.–Rubberball Royalty Free.

Chapter 7: General Survey

CO7 Sylvain Grandadam/Getty Images Inc.–Stone Allstock. **7-15** From Hockenberry, M. J., Wilson, D., Winkelstein, M. L.:*Wong's Essentials of Pediatric Nursing*, 7th ed., St.Louis, 2005, p.1259. Used with permission. Copyright Mosby. **Critical Thinking:** Ryan McVay/Getty Images–Photodisc.

Chapter 8: Pain Assessment

CO8 Robert E. Daemmrich/Bob Daemmrich Photography, Inc. **Critical Thinking:** Photodisc Blue/Getty Images–Photodisc.

Chapter 9: Nutritional Assessment

CO9 Ralf Schultheiss/Getty Images Inc.–Stone Allstock. **9-4** Reprinted with permission from OMRON Healthcare, Inc. **9-5** BOD POD® Body Composition Tracking System. Reprinted with permission from Life Measurement, Inc. **T9-5A** Centers for Disease Control and Prevention (CDC). **T9-5B** Centers for Disease Control and Prevention (CDC). **T9-5C** Centers for Disease Control and Prevention (CDC). **T9-5D** Centers for Disease Control and Prevention (CDC). **T9-5E** E. H. Gill/Custom Medical Stock Photo, Inc. **T9-5F** Centers for Disease Control and Prevention (CDC). **T9-5H** Custom Medical Stock Photo, Inc. **T9-5I** Dr. M. A. Ansary/Photo Researchers, Inc. **T9-5J** Centers for Disease Control and Prevention (CDC). **T9-5K** O Damika/Medical-On-Line Ltd. **Critical Thinking:** Getty Images/Digital Vision.

Chapter 10: The Health History

CO10 David Woolley/Getty Images Inc.–Stone Allstock. **Critical Thinking:** Kevin Peterson/Getty Images–Photodisc.

Chapter 11: Skin, Hair, and Nails

CO11 Dannielle Hayes/Omni-Photo Communications, Inc. **11-03** © Patrick J. Watson. **11-04** NMSB/Custom Medical Stock Photo, Inc. **11-05** Copyright © 1994, Carroll H. Weiss. All rights reserved. **11-06** © Patrick J. Watson **11-09** Zuber/Custom Medical Stock Photo, Inc. **11-10** Levy/Phototake NYC **11-11** Leonard Lessin/Peter Arnold **11-12** SPL/Photo Researchers, Inc. **11-15** Custom Medical Stock Photo, Inc. **11-26** Logical Images/Custom Medical Stock Photo, Inc. **11-29** H. C. Robinson/Science Photo Library/Photo Researchers, Inc. **11-30** Custom Medical Stock Photo, Inc. **11-31** Logical Images/Custom Medical Stock Photo, Inc. **11-32** Logical Images/Custom Medical Stock Photo, Inc. **11-33** Logical Images/Custom Medical Stock Photo, Inc. **11-34** Logical Images/Custom Medical Stock Photo, Inc. **11-53** Charles Stewart & Associates. **11-54** Charles Stewart & Associates. **11-55** Custom Medical Stock Photo, Inc. **11-56** P. Barber/Custom Medical Stock Photo, Inc. **11-57** Custom Medical Stock Photo, Inc. **11-58** Logical Images/Custom Medical Stock Photo, Inc. **11-59** Custom Medical Stock Photo, Inc. **11-60** Custom Medical Stock Photo, Inc. **11-61** SIU Bio Med/Custom Medical Stock Photo, Inc. **11-62** Logical Images/Custom Medical Stock Photo, Inc. **11-63** NMSB/Custom Medical Stock Photo, Inc. **11-64** NMSB/Custom Medical Stock Photo, Inc. **11-65** © Patrick J. Watson. **11-66** National Archives and Records Administration. **11-67** Edward H. Gill/Custom Medical Stock Photo, Inc. **11-68** NMSB/Custom Medical Stock Photo, Inc. **11-69** Zeva Oelbaum/Peter Arnold, Inc. **11-70** Zeva Oelbaum/Peter Arnold, Inc. **11-71** Kenneth E. Greer/Visuals Unlimited. **11-72** Phototake NYC. **11-73** Visuals Unlimited. **11-74** Courtesy of Elizabeth A. Abel, M.D., from the Leonard C. Winograd Memorial Slide Collection, Stanford University School of Medicine. **11-75** Phototake NYC. **11-76** Greenhill/Mediscan/Medical-On-Line Ltd. **11-77** SPL/ Photo Researchers, Inc. **11-78** NMSB/Custom Medical Stock Photo, Inc. **11-79** Courtesy of Dr. Hikka Helovuo, K. Kakkarainen, and K. Pannio. Oral Microbiol. Immuno. 8:75-79, (1993). **11-80** NMSB/Custom Medical Stock Photo, Inc. **11-81** Dr. P. Marazzi/Photo Researchers, Inc. **11-82** Logical Images/Custom Medical Stock Photo, Inc. **11-83** Logical Images/Custom Medical Stock Photo, Inc. **11-84** Custom Medical Stock Photo, Inc. **11-85** Custom Medical Stock Photo, Inc. **11-86** Logical Images/Custom Medical Stock Photo, Inc. **11-87** Custom Medical Stock Photo, Inc. **Client Interaction:** SW Productions/Getty Images– Photodisc. **Critical Thinking:** Jess Alford/ Getty Images–Photodisc.

Chapter 12: Head, Neck, and Related Lymphatics

CO12 Julie Toy/Getty Images Inc.–Stone Allstock. **12-16** M.A. Ansary/Custom Medical Stock Photo, Inc. **12-18** © Dr. William H. Daughaday, University of California/Irvine. American Journal of Medicine (20) 1956. With permission of Excerpta Medica Inc. **12-19**

Chapter 24: Neurologic System

CO24 Jake Martin/Getty Images, Inc.–Allsport Photography. **Client Interaction:** Marc Romanelli/Getty Images–Photodisc. **Critical Thinking:** Ryan McVay/Getty Images–Photodisc.

Chapter 25: Assessment of Infants, Children, and Adolescents

CO25 Bob Daemmrich/Getty Images Inc.–Stone Allstock. **25-01** Gill/Custom Medical Stock Photo, Inc. **25-02** Dr. H. C. Robinson/Photo Researchers, Inc. **25-08** From Van Wieringen et al.: *Growth Diagrams 1965.* Courtesy of Wolters-Noordhoff, the Netherlands. **25-16** Science Photo Library/Photo Researchers, Inc. **25-17** Custom Medical Stock Photo, Inc. **25-21** Custom Medical Stock Photo, Inc. **Client Interaction:** Tim Jones/Getty Images–Photodisc. **Critical Thinking:** Getty Images/Digital Vision.

Chapter 26: The Pregnant Female

CO26 Leanne Temme/Photolibrary.Com. **26-08D** Logical Images/Custom Medical Stock Photo, Inc. **26-11** Photo courtesy of Techno–Aide. **26-12** Custom Medical Stock Photo, Inc. **Client Interaction:** Geoff Manasse/Getty Images–Photodisc. **Critical Thinking:** Stockdisc/Getty Images, Inc.–Stockdisc.

Chapter 27: Assessing the Older Adult

CO27 Arthur Tilley/Getty Images, Inc.–Taxi. **Client Interaction:** Kevin Peterson/Getty Images–Photodisc. **Critical Thinking:** Elke Van de Velde/Getty Images–Photodisc.

Index

Page numbers followed by italic *f* indicate figures and those followed by italic *t* indicate tables or boxes.

Vitreous humor, 265, 265f
Voice sounds, auscultation, 379
Voiding patterns, 561–62. See also Urinary system
Vomiting, 523, 830
Vulvovaginitis, 635

W

Waist circumference, 142–43, 143f
Warts, genital, 611, 611f
Water-hammer pulse, 501t
WAVE tool, 152
WBC (white blood cell count), in pregnancy, 836t
Weber test, 325, 325f, 893
Wechsler Preschool and Primary Scale of Intelligence–Revised (WPPSI-R), 67t
Weight. See also Anthropometrics
  average acceptable for adults, 112t
  gain
    causes, 564
    gestational, recommendations, 823t, 830
  history, 140
  loss
    causes, 520
    percentage, 140, 140t
  measurement, 111, 112f, 140, 802
  normal growth
    infants, 49
    preschoolers, 54
    school-age children, 57
    toddlers, 52

Wellness. See also Health promotion
  critical thinking application
    case study, 44–45
    questions, 45
  definition, 23
  theories
    Dunn, 23, 23f
    Leavell and Clark, 23–24
    Travis and Ryan, 24, 24f
Wheal, 213, 213f
Wheezes, 378, 378t
Whisper test, 323, 323f
Whispered pectoriloquy, 379
White blood cell count (WBC), in pregnancy, 836t
White matter, 731
WHO. See World Health Organization
Wide split S$_2$, 430t
Wilms' tumor, 808
Witch's milk, 401
Wong/Baker "Faces" pain rating scale, 120f
Wood's lamp, 102f, 207, 207f
World Health Organization (WHO), definition of health, 3
WPPSI-R (Wechsler Preschool and Primary Scale of Intelligence–Revised), 67t
Wrist. See also Hand and fingers
  abnormal findings
    carpal tunnel syndrome. See Carpal tunnel syndrome
    Dupuytren's contracture, 701, 720, 720f
    ganglion, 699
    ulnar deviation, 720, 720f

anatomy and physiology, 670, 677f
physical assessment techniques and normal findings
  inspection, 698
  muscle strength, 702, 702f
  palpation, 698–99, 699f
  Phalen's test, 701, 701f
  range of motion, 700–701, 700f, 701f
  Tinel's sign, 701, 701f

X

Xanthelasma, 146t, 453, 876–77, 900
Xerophthalmia, 146t
Xiphoid process, 437, 438f

Y

Yeast infections, 634
Young adult:
  definition, 61
  development
    cognitive, 61
    physiological, 61
    psychosocial, 61, 61f
    tasks, 61
  health assessment
    periodic health examination, 60t, 62t
    principles, 61

Z

Zosteriform lesions, 220, 220f. See also Lesions, skin

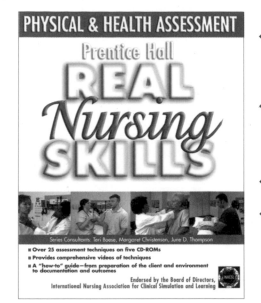
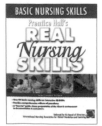 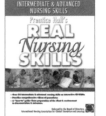 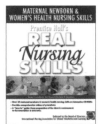 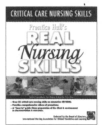 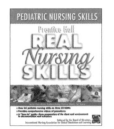